Oxford Textbook of

Correctional Psychiatry

Oxford Textbook of

Correctional Psychiatry

SECOND EDITION

EDITED BY

Reena Kapoor, MD

Professor of Psychiatry
Yale University School of Medicine

Anthony C. Tamburello, MD

Clinical Professor of Psychiatry
Rutgers – Robert Wood Johnson Medical School

James L. Knoll, IV, MD

Clinical Professor of Psychiatry and Behavioral Sciences
SUNY Upstate Medical University

Jeffrey L. Metzner, MD

Clinical Professor Emeritus of Psychiatry
University of Colorado School of Medicine

OXFORD
UNIVERSITY PRESS

OXFORD
UNIVERSITY PRESS

Oxford University Press is a department of the University of Oxford.
It furthers the University's objective of excellence in research, scholarship,
and education by publishing worldwide. Oxford is a registered trade mark of
Oxford University Press in the UK and certain other countries.

Published in the United States of America by Oxford University Press
198 Madison Avenue, New York, NY 10016, United States of America.

CIP data is on file at the Library of Congress

ISBN 978-0-19-777400-7

DOI: 10.1093/med/9780197774007.001.0001

Printed by Integrated Books International, United States of America

MIX
Paper
FSC FSC® C183721

The manufacturer's authorized representative in the EU for product safety is
Oxford University Press España S.A., Parque Empresarial San Fernando de Henares,
Avenida de Castilla, 2 – 28830 Madrid (www.oup.es/en or product.safety@oup.com).
OUP España S.A. also acts as importer into Spain of products made by the manufacturer.

We dedicate this book to all correctional health care staff, medical students, residents, and fellows who share our passion for providing psychiatric care for incarcerated persons, for strengthening the reputation of this field, and for promoting the science of correctional medicine.

Contents

Foreword

I have worked at the intersection of mental health and criminal justice policy for more than 5 decades and have had the opportunity to collaborate with many talented and dedicated forensic psychiatrists and psychologists as they have struggled to overcome impediments to care for an increasing number of defendants and prisoners suffering from distressing disorders. I have watched "correctional psychiatry" move to the center of the profession's challenges and commitments. I was therefore pleased to have the opportunity to write the Foreword to the first edition of this richly informative textbook when it was published a decade ago. In that Foreword, I expressed hope that the nation was poised to invest in a range of community services that might enable the courts to rely less on penal incarceration and more on (a) civil interventions in nonpunitive and less restrictive residential settings and (b) leveraged use of criminal sanctions in outpatient settings. Although promising innovations have taken root in some localities (and are highlighted in this text), courts, jails, hospitals, penal facilities, community programs, and system-involved patients and their families continue to face daunting challenges.

"Mass incarceration" continues to be one of the most disturbing challenges facing our nation. The huge scale of this problem has become increasingly evident, not only to correctional psychiatrists, but also to every informed and ethically engaged citizen. Indeed, our nation's penal population remains the largest in the world despite falling incarceration rates in the past decade (Fair & Walmsley, 2024). Readers may be disheartened to learn that the United States still accounts for approximately 16% of all the world's prisoners, even though we account for only 4% of the world's population (Fair & Walmsley, 2024). This distinct form of "American exceptionalism" does not have its roots in the founding, the Civil War, or the First or Second World Wars. It is distinctly connected to crime policy implemented by our nation during the last third of the 20th century.

Between the 1970s and the late 2000s, the rate of incarceration in this country more than quadrupled. More than 2.3 million people were incarcerated in U.S. jails, state prisons, and federal prisons in 2009, when the incarceration rate peaked (Walmsley, 2013). By 2019, the incarcerated population had decreased to 2.1 million (Fair & Walmsley, 2024), and the COVID-19 pandemic in 2020 created a precipitous population drop—approximately 14%—as jails and prisons released individuals in an effort to prevent and contain infection (Nellis, 2024). Incarceration levels have since rebounded, with approximately 1.9 million people incarcerated in the United States in 2024 (Sawyer & Wagner, 2024). Although startling, these figures don't reveal the full scope of mass incarceration and its impact on the lives of incarcerated individuals, their families, and their communities: In 2022, about 7 million individuals were booked into (and released from) local jails (Zeng, 2023). About 3.7 million persons were on probation or parole (Sawyer & Wagner, 2024). Altogether, 5.7 million individuals are under correctional supervision at any given moment. How did this happen? What can (or should) be done about it?

As indicated earlier, U.S. crime policy took a strongly punitive turn at all levels of criminal justice administration in the late 1970s and thereafter for another 3 decades or so. It has been marked by an increase in arrests, especially for drug crimes; higher rates of incarceration per arrest; and increasing severity of sentences for crimes involving violence and drug trafficking. Mandatory prison terms increased markedly in the 1980s, and during the 1990s, more than half of the states, as well as Congress, enacted "three strikes" laws (or even "two strikes" laws), mandating terms of 25 years or longer for offenders covered by these laws.

Most states also abolished, or significantly limited, opportunity for discretionary release (indeterminate sentences) in favor of so-called "truth in sentencing" laws that required prisoners to serve at least 85% of the actual sentence. Ameliorative principles and procedures, including any overt attempt at rehabilitation, were erased from the prevailing practice of criminal punishment. Perhaps the most misguided component of this "get tough on crime" policy was criminalization of offending by "older" teens (ages 14 to 17). This turn toward mass incarceration by youngsters has had huge costs, of course, and these costs (like the costs of street crime itself) fall unevenly on marginalized individuals from poor communities; unfortunately, the association between mass incarceration and race is inescapable.

According to a survey by researchers from the Bureau of Justice Statistics (BJS), more than half of all incarcerated people in U.S. jails and prisons have a current, treatable "mental health problem" (James & Glaze, 2006). Another study estimates that between one third and one half of state and federal prisoners have a "mental illness," as compared with about 18% of the general population (Kolodziejczak & Sinclair, 2018). Another BJS study found that 41% of all state and federal prisoners had a history of "mental health problems" (43% of state prisoners and 23% of federal prisoners; Maruschak et al., 2016). Other surveys consistently show that at least 15% of incarcerated people have a serious or acute mental illness (Maruschak et al., 2016; Steadman et al., 2009; 12% to 15% of state prisoners had serious psychological distress within the past 30 days).

Although the causal connection between deinstitutionalization of mental health services and the increased prevalence of mental illness in prisons remains in dispute, there is little doubt that a significant proportion of people with mental illness in local jails are being arrested and held in custody due to gaps in mental health services that could have prevented or ameliorated the acute crises that landed these adults in jail. It is also recognized that mental health challenges and repeated criminality are rooted in similar social determinants, including poverty, racism, poor education, and exposure to criminal offending by role models. Moreover, confinement and the stresses of prison life tend to make the individual's clinical situation worse, especially for those with serious mental illness. In short, one of the most pronounced effects of mass incarceration has been a substantial increase in the pressures on prison health systems during incarceration and then on community services of all kinds after prisoners are released. These pressures are especially high for prisoners who need mental health services.

All these factors have placed psychiatrists and their clinical teams on the front lines of our society's effort to cope with the clinical needs and humanitarian challenges associated with mass incarceration. The needs are huge, and the capacity of correctional agencies to respond to them is often severely constrained. Quality of care varies widely across the country, as does the financial capacity of state- and locally funded systems. Although there are several accrediting bodies, a minority of facilities (out of more than 3,000) have been accredited (American Correctional Association, n.d.; Sawyer & Wagner 2024), and serious questions have been raised about the methods and value of the accreditation process (Office of the Inspector General, U.S. Department of Justice, 2023). These challenges are both individual and collective.

At the individual level, correctional psychiatrists must respond daily to the demands of conscience. The larger the population under care, the greater the gaps in service, the greater the patient's suffering, and the greater the psychiatrist's moral distress. Clinical skill is only the minimum prerequisite for the job. Psychiatrists also need the ability to cope with scarcity and to manage resources in an ethically responsible way, and they must learn how to use their voices effectively to advocate for change within the organization responsible for health care delivery, as well as within the correctional agency. They may often encounter an authoritarian culture where caring is not the overriding value. At the collective level, psychiatry and the allied professions must stand up for the needs and rights of the patients and for the psychiatrists and other professionals who bear the responsibility for serving those needs.

There are a few bright spots in this very gloomy picture. One is a significant increase in the dedication and skill of mental health professionals who have devoted their time—and perhaps their careers—to improving correctional psychiatry, thereby helping to lay a foundation for long-term improvement. As mentioned at the outset of this Foreword, there has also been a significant decline in the rate of incarceration over the last 10 to 15 years. Having reached a peak in the late 2000s, the adult incarceration rate in the United States (which includes federal and state prisons, as well as local jails) declined 13% between 2007 and 2015 (Gelb & Stevenson, 2017), indicating a reversal of the growing incarceration rate even before the pandemic-related changes of 2020 and 2021. The nation's imprisonment rate fell 8.2%, while the violent crime and property crime rate fell 14.6%. (Gelb & Stevenson, 2017). These findings may be thin and may not be sustained due to an erosion of access to care or an increase in offending. However, they represent a beacon of hope, especially when greater reliance on treatment is reinforced by advances in therapeutic methods and support from the bench and from prosecutors.

Do correctional psychiatrists (and other correctional health care providers) stand alone in facing these challenges? Fortunately, psychiatrists and their professional comrades do have allies. One source of encouragement is an occasional victory in the state appellate courts or in the federal courts. The threat of a lawsuit aiming to remediate inadequate medical and mental health care can still provide an incentive for negotiation when the conditions fall below minimally acceptable standards. The federal courts remain accessible notwithstanding the limitations imposed by Congress in the Prison Litigation Reform Act (1996). The California litigation leading to and following the Supreme Court's decision in *Brown v. Plata* (2011) demonstrates that, if necessary, the federal courts will order states to reduce the number of prisoners in overcrowded, underserved facilities to ensure adequate health care. Although subsequent litigation efforts related to prisoners' mental health have not always been as successful (e.g., *Johnson v. Prentice*, 2023), litigation remains an important avenue for reform.

A second source of encouragement is the energy and skill of public interest organizations, such as the Vera Institute of Justice, and top-notch litigators, including the American Civil Liberties Union's National Prison Project, the Equal Justice Initiative, and the Special Litigation Section of the U.S. Department of Justice's Civil Rights Division. They represent a revival of spirit, energy, and humanitarian ideals in justice reform litigation. This reawakening is also evident in recent statements and standards issued by, or under the auspices of, professional organizations including the American Correctional Association (2003), the American Bar Association (2010), the National Commission on Correctional Health Care (2016), and the American Psychiatric Association (2016). A particularly potent initiative was undertaken by the American Psychiatric Association in 2023 (APA, 2023).

A third source of influential support has been provided by several major philanthropic foundations that have explored the causes and consequences of the growth of incarceration in the United States and have highlighted the way forward. One important contribution to this discussion is a still-timely report by the National Research Council, *The Growth of Incarceration in the United States* (National Research Council, 2014). More recent examples include reports by the Vera Institute of Justice (2018) and the Liman Center for Public Interest Law and Correctional Leaders Association (2022), as well as web-based resources compiled by the Prison Policy Initiative (http://www.prisonpolicy.org) and The Sentencing Project (http://www.sentencingproject.org).

A fourth potentially beneficial influence is political. There is always the risk that crime rates will rise, especially during a recession. However, a healthy economy typically provides an opportunity for innovation—by calling attention to the high costs of incarceration—in financial as well as human terms. Providing rehabilitative services during confinement and ensuring a seamless transition in health care services (and other rehabilitative services) upon release facilitate successful reentry into the community. Indeed, intensified implementation of the Affordable Care Act could play an important role in facilitating reentry (National Research Council, 2014), as can prisoner reentry programs supported under the Second Chance Act and the Justice Reinvestment Act (Pew Center on the States, 2012; Council of State Governments Justice Center, 2013). Recently, the Center for Medicare and Medicaid Services' "Section 1115 Waiver" program for justice-involved persons has created a pathway for federal reimbursement of health care and transitional case management services provided during an individual's last 90 days of incarceration. California was the first state to apply for this funding, and many others have followed suit (Kaiser Family Foundation, 2024).

These are hopeful signs that the number of incarcerated individuals with serious mental illness will decline in the years ahead. For the foreseeable future, however, publication of the *Oxford Textbook of Correctional Psychiatry* responds to an urgent need for authoritative guidance by psychiatrists and professional staff in facilities and communities across the country. It also facilitates recruitment of new generations of young psychiatrists, psychologists, and other mental health professionals to pursue training experiences in correctional settings, including as part of internships, residencies, and forensic fellowships.

The new edition of the *Oxford Textbook of Correctional Psychiatry* will serve equally well as a reference book and a reader for concentrated study. It is hard to imagine that practitioners will encounter a clinical, ethical, or organizational challenge relating to the patient, the treatment, or the setting that has not been addressed in this volume. New topics have been added. They include telepsychiatry, pandemic management in corrections, staff wellness, posttraumatic stress disorder and trauma-informed care, peer support programs for incarcerated people, immigrants and immigration detention, and jail-based competency restoration. In addition, the book creates a solid foundation in improving practice that goes beyond existing guidelines and resources.

I hope and expect that the psychiatrists, psychologists, and other clinicians who choose to serve patients in correctional settings will become the next generation of advocates for humanitarian values in corrections, leaders of the profession, and allies of proponents of criminal justice reform. If I may shift into "first person," I applaud you and I hope that this volume will serve your needs, inspire you, and help point the way forward for generations to come.

Richard J. Bonnie
Harrison Foundation Professor Emeritus of Law, Medicine, and Public Policy
Director Emeritus, Institute of Law, Psychiatry and Public Policy
University of Virginia School of Law

REFERENCES

American Bar Association. (2010). *Standards for treatment of prisoners.*

American Correctional Association. (n.d.). *The Commission on Accreditation for Corrections.* https://www.aca.org/ACA_Member/ACA/ACA_Member/Standards_and_Accreditation/SAC_Commission.aspx#:~:text=Currently%2C%20ACA%2C%20through%20the%20Commission,and%20sizes%20under%20ACA's%20standards

American Correctional Association. (2003). *Standards for adult correctional institutions.*

American Psychiatric Association. (2016). *Psychiatric services in jails and prisons* (3rd ed.).

American Psychiatric Association. (2023, March). *Position statement on engaging law enforcement personnel and correctional staff to address mental health and racial inequities in jails and prisons.*

Brown v. Plata, 563 U.S. 493 (2011).

Council of State Governments Justice Center. (2013). *Reentry matters: Strategies and successes of Second Chance Act grantees across the United States.*

Fair, H., & Walmsley, R. (2024). *World prison population* (14th ed.). World Prison Brief. https://www.prisonstudies.org/sites/default/files/resources/downloads/world_prison_population_list_14th_edition.pdf

Gelb, A., & Stevenson, P. (2017). *US adult incarceration rate declines 13% in 8 years.* https://www.pewtrusts.org/en/research-and-analysis/articles/2017/01/12/us-adult-incarceration-rate-declines-13-percent-in-8-years

James, D. J., & Glaze, L. E. (2006). *Mental health problems of prison and jail inmates.* U.S. Bureau of Justice Statistics. https://bjs.ojp.gov/content/pub/pdf/mhppji.pdf

Johnson v. Prentice, 601 U.S. _____ (2023).

Kaiser Family Foundation. (2024). *Medicaid waiver tracker: Approved and pending Section 1115 waiver applications by state.* https://www.kff.org/medicaid/issue-brief/medicaid-waiver-tracker-approved-and-pending-section-1115-waivers-by-state/

Kolodziejczak, O., & Sinclair, S. J. (2018). Barriers and facilitators to effective mental health care in correctional settings. *Journal of Correctional Health Care: Official Journal of the National Commission on Correctional Health Care, 24*(3), 253–263.

Liman Center for Public Interest Law and Correctional Leaders Association. (2022). *Time-in-cell: A 2021 snapshot of restrictive housing.* https://law.yale.edu/sites/default/files/area/center/liman/document/time_in_cell_2021.pdf

Maruschak, L. M., Bronson, J., & Alper, M. (2016). *Indicators of mental health problems reported by prisoners.* https://bjs.ojp.gov/sites/g/files/xyckuh236/files/media/document/imhprpspi16st.pdf

National Commission on Correctional Health Care. (2016). *Standards for mental health services in correctional facilities.*

National Research Council. (2014). *The growth of incarceration in the United States.* https://nap.nationalacademies.org/catalog/18613/the-growth-of-incarceration-in-the-united-states-exploring-causes

Nellis, A. (2024). *Mass incarceration trends.* The Sentencing Project. https://www.sentencingproject.org/reports/mass-incarceration-trends/

Office of the Inspector General, U.S. Department of Justice. (2023, November). *Audit of the Federal Bureau of Prisons contract awarded to the American Correctional Association.* https://oig.justice.gov/sites/default/files/reports/24-009.pdf

Pew Center on the States. (2012). *Time served: The high cost and lower return of long prison terms.*

Sawyer, W., & Wagner, P. (2024). *Mass incarceration: The whole pie 2024.* Prison Policy Initiative. https://www.prisonpolicy.org/reports/pie2024.html

Steadman, H. J., Osher, F. C., Robbins, P. C., Case, B., & Samuels, S. (2009). Prevalence of serious mental illness among jail inmates. *Psychiatric Services (Washington, D.C.), 60*(6), 761–765.

Vera Institute of Justice. (2018). *Reimagining prison.* https://www.vera.org/reimagining-prison-web-report

Walmsley, R. (2013). *World prison population list.* International Center for Prison Studies.

Zeng, Z. (2023). *Jail inmates in 2022—Statistical tables.* Bureau of Justice Statistics, Office of Justice Programs, U.S. Department of Justice. https://bjs.ojp.gov/document/ji22st.pdf

Acknowledgments

We thank each of the contributors to this textbook for their strong work to provide the best available resource for our readers. We also thank Peter Stevenson, Adam Breivik, and Katie Lakina from Oxford University Press for their support and guidance through this project. We thank our colleagues and coworkers, including mental health and other medical staff, nurses, administrators, correctional officers, nonuniformed correctional staff, and chaplains who partner with us to care for our patients. Finally, we thank the incarcerated persons who, through our work together, have become our best teachers.

Reena Kapoor would like to thank her beloved family, friends, and colleagues in the Yale Law & Psychiatry Division for their decades of support, guidance, and good humor.

Anthony Tamburello would like to thank his wife, Kelly, for her support and tolerance. He owes a debt of gratitude to a long list of mentors, including but not limited to John K. Frost, David Eskin, William Hobbs, Bruce Cohen, Paul McHugh, Jeffrey Janofsky, Christiane Tellefsen, Annette Hanson, and Rusty Reeves.

James Knoll would like to thank Professor Fred Cohen and Joel Dvoskin for helping to inspire interest in correctional mental health law, practice, and research. He is grateful to all the hard-working, well-intended correctional officers and other correctional staff who are unsung heroes.

Jeffrey Metzner would like to thank his late wife, Linda, and son, Dylan, for their tolerance and support during his many years of monitoring/consulting to correctional systems across the country. Special thanks to his *Coleman* family and numerous friends in the American Academy of Psychiatry and the Law.

We acknowledge Robert Trestman, Kenneth Appelbaum, and Jeffrey Metzner for their work in establishing the first edition of this textbook, which was well received by the correctional mental health clinician community.

Contributors

Joel T. Andrade, PhD
Falcon, Inc.

Elie G. Aoun, MD
Division of Law, Medicine and Psychiatry
Columbia University

CJ Appleton, MS
Assistant Professor
Sanford School of Public Policy
Duke University

Bruce A. Arrigo, PhD
Department of Criminal Justice & Criminology
University of North Carolina at Charlotte

Peter Ash, MD
Department of Psychiatry and Behavioral Sciences
Emory School of Medicine

Dean Aufderheide, PhD, MPA
Florida Department of Corrections

Rebecca A. Ballard, MD, FACCP, CCHP-P
Centurion Health

Virginia Barber Rioja, PhD
Center for Justice Innovation

Sharen Barboza, PhD
Barboza Consulting, LLC

Lisa C. Barry, PhD, MPH
UConn Center on Aging
University of Connecticut

Lama Bazzi, MD, MRO

Adam Bernstein, MD
Department of Psychiatry
SUNY Upstate Medical University

Ingrid A. Binswanger, MD, MPH, MS
Department of Medicine
University of Colorado School of Medicine
Institute for Health Research, Kaiser Permanente Colorado

Jennifer S. Bradford, MD, MPH
Department of Family Medicine and Community Health
UMass Memorial Health

Brittany Brizendine, PsyD, MBA
California Department of Corrections and Rehabilitation

Sarah M. Broom, PhD

Jeremiah W. Burkhart, PsyD
Department of Psychiatry and Behavioral Medicine
Carilion Clinic—Virginia Tech Carilion School of Medicine
U.S. Army Reserve

Paul R. S. Burton, MD
San Quentin, California Department of Corrections and Rehabilitation

Philip J. Candilis, MD, DFAPA
Saint Elizabeths Hospital
Washington DC.
Department of Behavioral Health
George Washington University School of Medicine and Health Sciences

Charles D. Cash, JD, LLM
Professional Risk Management Services

Michael K. Champion, MD
Department of Psychiatry
John A. Burns School of Medicine, University of Hawai'i at Manoa

Reema Dedania, MD, MPH
Department of Psychiatry and Behavioral Sciences
Emory School of Medicine

James F. DeGroot, PhD
Georgia Department of Corrections

Charles Dike, MD, MPH, FRCPsych
Department of Psychiatry
Yale School of Medicine

Henry A. Dlugacz, MSW, JD
Department of Psychiatry and Behavioral Sciences
New York Medical College

Doris A. Dumond, MA
Consultants for Improved Human Services

Robert W. Dumond, MA
Department of Psychology
Southern New Hampshire University

Joel Dvoskin, PhD
Department of Psychiatry
University of Arizona College of Medicine

Bernice S. Elger, MD, Dr. habil, dipl. theol.
Institute of Biomedical Ethics, University of Basel
Center for Legal Medicine, University of Geneva

Stephanie Eng, MD
Department of Psychiatry
Weill Cornell Medical Center

Barbara Fair, MSW, LCSW
Stop Solitary CT

Zoe R. Feingold, PhD
Center for Justice Innovation

Jamie Fellner, JD
United States Program
Human Rights Watch (retired)

Elizabeth B. Ford, MD
Department of Psychiatry
Columbia University Vagelos College of Physicians & Surgeons

Sadé D. Frazier, DO
Department of Psychiatry
Rutgers—Robert Wood Johnson Medical School

Erik J. Garcia, MD
Department of Internal Medicine
UMass Memorial Health

Lindsey Gilling, PhD, MSc
Department of Psychology
Glasgow Caledonian University

Graham D. Glancy, MB, ChB
Department of Psychiatry
University of Toronto, Windsor

Annette L. Hanson, MD
Department of Psychiatry
University of Maryland School of Medicine

Haseeb Haroon, MD
California Department of State Hospitals

Lindsay M. Hayes, MS
Hayes Consulting

George W. Hebert, PhD
Department of Counseling/Department of Physician Assistant Studies
Louisiana State University Health Sciences Center—New Orleans

Nadeen Ibrahim, BA
National Institute on Drug Abuse, Summer Research Internship Program

André Ivanoff, PhD
School of Social Work
Columbia University

Daniel Jackson, MD
Regional Forensic Unit
Rochester Psychiatric Center

Mohamedu F. Jones, LLM
Pannone Lopes Devereaux & West LLC

Jayesh Kamath, MD, PhD
Department of Psychiatry
University of Connecticut Health Center

Reena Kapoor, MD
Department of Psychiatry
Yale School of Medicine

Emily A. Keram, MD
Department of Psychiatry and Biobehavioral Sciences
University of California, Los Angeles

Rose Kleman, PhD, MPA
Kleman Consulting, LLC

James L. Knoll IV, MD
Department of Psychiatry
SUNY Upstate Medical University

Catherine M. Knox, MN, RN

Thomas Kocienda, PsyD
Connecticut Department of Correction

Vikram Kumar, MD
Mid-Hudson Forensic Psychiatric Center
Department of Psychiatry
SUNY Upstate Medical University

William Kuo, LCSW, LICSW
DBT-Linehan Board of Certification, Certified Clinician

Danielle B. Kushner, MD
Department of Psychiatry
NYU Grossman School of Medicine

Rakesh Lamba, MBBS, FRCPC
Division of Forensic Psychiatry
Department of Psychiatry
University of British Columbia

Melissa J. Lavoie, MD
Department of Psychiatry
University of Maryland School of Medicine

Catherine F. Lewis, MD
Department of Psychiatry
University of Connecticut Health Center

Darren L. Lish, MD
Department of Psychiatry
University of Colorado School of Medicine

Ashley J. B. MacLean, MD
Department of Psychiatry
UMass Chan Medical School

Michael P. Maloney, PhD
Department of Psychiatry and the Biobehavioral Sciences
The David Geffen School of Medicine
University of California

Maria Masotta, PsyD
Clinical and Forensic Psychology Private Practice

William R. McBride, DO
Traumatic Brain Injury—Polytrauma Department
Corporal Michael J. Crescenz VA Medical Center

Barbara E. McDermott, PhD
Department of Psychiatry and Behavioral Sciences
University of California

Donald E. McLawhorn Jr., MD, PhD
Department of Psychiatry
University of Rochester Medical Center

Jeffrey L. Metzner, MD
Department of Psychiatry
University of Colorado School of Medicine

Jaimie P. Meyer, MD, MS, FACP
Department of Medicine, Section of Infectious Diseases
Yale School of Medicine and Public Health

Nathaniel P. Morris, MD
Department of Psychiatry and Behavioral Sciences
University of California, San Francisco
San Quentin, California Department of Corrections and Rehabilitation

Nicole Mushero, MD, PhD
Department of Medicine, Section of Geriatrics
Boston University Chobanian & Avedisian School of Medicine

Rosa E. Negrón Muñoz, MD
Department of Child and Adolescent Psychiatry
University of South Florida

Michael A. Norko, MD, MAR
Department of Psychiatry
Yale School of Medicine

Maureen L. O'Keefe, MA
Elevation Research

Daisy Ort, PhD
Department of Psychology
Columbia University

Jason D. Ourada, MD
Nebraska Department of Correctional Services

Ira K. Packer, PhD
Department of Psychiatry
University of Massachusetts Medical School

Marcus R. Patterson, PsyD
Patterson Forensic Psych Consulting

Raymond F. Patterson, MD
St. Elizabeths Hospital
Department of Behavioral Health

Luca Pauselli, MD
Department of Psychiatry
Hackensack Meridian School of Medicine

John Penezic, PsyD

Joseph V. Penn, MD, CCHP-MH
Department of Psychiatry
Correctional Managed Care
University of Texas Medical Branch

Mary Perrien, PhD
Safe Society Solutions

Tasha R. Phillips, PsyD
Department of Psychiatry
University of Massachusetts Medical School

Debra A. Pinals, MD
Department of Psychiatry
University of Michigan Medical School
National Association of State Mental Health Program Directors

Lindsay M. Poplinski, DO
District of Columbia
Department of Behavioral Health

Badr Ratnakaran, MBBS
Department of Psychiatry and Behavioral Medicine
Carilion Clinic—Virginia Tech Carilion School of Medicine

Rusty Reeves, MD
Department of Psychiatry
University Correctional Health Care
Rutgers University—Robert Wood Johnson Medical School

Erik Roskes, MD
Department of Psychiatry
University of Maryland School of Medicine

Merrill Rotter, MD
Department of Psychiatry
Albert Einstein College of Medicine

Fabian M. Saleh, MD
Department of Psychiatry and Behavioral Sciences
The Johns Hopkins University School of Medicine

Henry Schmidt III, PhD
Behavioral Affiliates, Inc.

Charlotte M. Schwarz, MD
Department of Psychiatry
Yale School of Medicine

Charles L. Scott, MD
Department of Psychiatry & Behavioral Sciences
University of California, Davis

Harshit Sharma, MD
Department of Psychiatry
Icahn School of Medicine at Mount Sinai

Savannah Shaw

Sarah Shelton, PsyD, MPH, MSCP
Department of Clinical Psychopharmacology
The Chicago School

Anthony C. Tamburello, MD
Rutgers University—Robert Wood Johnson Medical School
University Correctional Health Care

Faye S. Taxman, PhD
Department of Criminology, Law and Society
Center for Advancing Correctional Excellence
George Mason University

Stuart D. M. Thomas, PhD
School of Global, Urban, and Social Studies
RMIT University

Lindsay D. G. Thomson, MBChB, MPhil, MD, FRCPsych
Division of Psychiatry
The University of Edinburgh
The State Hospitals Board for Scotland and the Forensic Network

Jennifer M. Tippett, PsyD
Graduate School of Professional Psychology
University of Colorado

Todd Tomita, MD, FRCPC
Division of Forensic Psychiatry
Department of Psychiatry
University of British Columbia

Robert L. Trestman, PhD, MD
Department of Psychiatry and Behavioral Medicine
Carilion Clinic—Virginia Tech Carilion School of Medicine

Ruben Valencia, PsyD, MBA
Kaiser Permanente

Cecilia Vigil, MD
Department of Psychiatry
Rutgers—Robert Wood Johnson Medical School

Sarah E. Wakeman, MD
Department of Medicine
Harvard Medical School

Brian Wasicek, MD
University of Connecticut

Nancy Wolff, PhD
EJ Bloustein School of Planning and Public Policy
Rutgers, The State University of New Jersey

S. Ananya Yarrapureddy, MD
Department of Psychiatry
University of Connecticut Health Center

Sohrab Zahedi, MD
Department of Psychiatry
University of Connecticut Health Center

James Q. Zhou, MD
Department of Medicine
Massachusetts General Hospital

Abbreviations

3,4-methylenedioxy-methamphetamine (MDMA)
Accreditation Council for Graduate Medical Education (ACGME)
adjustment disorder (AD)
adverse childhood experiences (ACEs)
alcohol use disorder (AUD)
Alcoholics Anonymous (AA)
American Academy of Psychiatry and the Law (AAPL)
American Correctional Association (ACA)
American Psychiatric Association (APA)
antisocial personality disorder (ASPD)
Association of Directors of Medical Student Education in Psychiatry (ADMSEP)
attention-deficit/hyperactivity disorder (ADHD)
behavioral management plan (BMP)
benzodiazepine (BZD)
bipolar disorders (BDs)
body-worn cameras (BWCs)
borderline personality disorder (BPD)
Brain Injury Screening Questionnaire (BISQ)
Brief Jail Mental Health Screen (BJMHS)
Bureau of Justice Statistics (BJS)
Buss–Perry Aggression Questionnaire (BPAQ)
Centers for Disease Control and Prevention (CDC)
Centers for Medicare and Medicaid Services (CMS)
central nervous system (CNS)
Civil Rights of Institutionalized Persons Act (CRIPA)
Clinical Opiate Withdrawal Scale (COWS)
cognitive-behavioral therapy (CBT)
cognitive-behavioral therapy for insomnia (CBT-I)
cognitive processing therapy (CPT)
Collaborative Assessment and Management of Suicidality (CAMS)
Columbia-Suicide Severity Rating Scale (CSSRS)
competent to stand trial (CST)
continuous quality improvement (CQI)
Convention Against Torture and Other Cruel, Inhuman, or Degrading Treatment or Punishment (CAT)
Convention on the Rights of Persons With Disabilities (CRPD)
correctional mental health research (CMHR)
Correctional Mental Health Screen (CMHS)
Crisis Intervention Team (CIT)
crisis stabilization unit (CSU)
delirium tremens (DTs)
Department of Correction (DOC)
Diagnostic and Statistical Manual of Mental Disorders (DSM)
dialectical behavior therapy (DBT)
dual diagnosis motivational interviewing (DDMI)
extended-release buprenorphine (XR-BUP)
extended-release naltrexone (XR-NTX)
Federal Bureau of Investigation (FBI)
fiscal year (FY)
full-time equivalent (FTE)
generalized anxiety disorder (GAD)
Georgia Department of Corrections (GDC)
Geriatric Depression Scale (GDS)
Government Accountability Office (GAO)
Historical Clinical Risk Management-20, Version 3 (HCR-20)
incarcerated persons (IPs)
incompetent to stand trial (IST)
Institute for Juvenile Research (IJR)
integrated dual disorder treatment (IDDT)
intellectual disability (ID)
intermittent explosive disorder (IED)
International Covenant on Civil and Political Rights (ICCPR)
International Covenant on Economic, Social and Cultural Rights (ICESCR)
jail-based competency restoration (JBCR)
Just Detention International (JDI)
lesbian, gay, bisexual, and transgender (LGBT)
Level of Service Inventory-Revised (LSI-R)
licensed independent practitioner (LIP)
major depressive disorder (MDD)
Massachusetts Youth Screening Instrument—Second Version (MAYSI-2)
medically supervised withdrawal (MSW)
medication for opioid use disorder (MOUD)
mental health (MH)
mental health courts (MHCs)
mental illness (MI)
mild cognitive impairment (MCI)
Miller Forensic Assessment of Symptoms of Test (M-FAST)
Millon Clinical Multiaxial Inventory (MCMI)
Mini-International Neuropsychiatric Interview (MINI)
Minnesota Multiphasic Personality Inventory (MMPI)
Minnesota Multiphasic Personality Inventory-2—Restructured Form (MMPI-2-RF)
Montreal Cognitive Assessment (MoCA)
Moral Reconation Therapy (MRT)
motivational interviewing (MI)
narcissistic personality disorder (NPD)
National Commission on Correctional Health Care (NCCHC)
National Detention Standards (NDSs)
National Incident-Based Reporting System (NIBRS)

National Institute for Clinical Excellence (NICE)
National Institute for Occupational Safety and Health (NIOSH)
National Institute of Corrections (NIC)
National Institutes of Health (NIH)
National Prison Rape Elimination Commission (NPREC)
National Research Council (NRC)
neurocognitive disorders (NDs)
no mental illness (NMI)
Office of Juvenile Justice and Delinquency Prevention (OJJDP)
opioid use disorder (OUD)
paranoid personality disorder (PPD)
Personality Assessment Inventory (PAI)
Performance-Based National Detention Standards (PBNDSs)
personality disorder (PD)
pharmacy and therapeutics committees (P&TCs)
phencyclidine (PCP)
posttraumatic stress disorder (PTSD)
pre-exposure prophylaxis (PrEP)
Prison Litigation Reform Act of 1995 (PLRA)
Prison Rape Elimination Act (PREA)
prison-specific activities of daily living (pADLs)
Professional Risk Management Services (PRMS)
Protection of Religious Exercise in Land Use and by Institutionalized Persons Act (RLUIPA)
Psychopathy Checklist-Revised (PCL-R)
Qualified Mental Health Professional (QMHP)
quality assurance (QA)
quality improvement (QI)
Racketeer Influenced and Corrupt Organizations Act (RICO)
randomized controlled trials (RCTs)
Reasoning and Rehabilitation (R&R)
Repeatable Battery for the Assessment of Neuropsychological Status Update (RBANS)
restrictive housing units (RHUs)
risk–need–responsivity (RNR)
security risk group (SRG)
selective serotonin reuptake inhibitor (SSRI)
self-injurious behavior (SIB)
special needs (SN)
Structured Inventory of Malingered Symptomatology (SIMS)
Structured Inventory of Reported Symptoms (SIRS)
substance use disorder (SUD)
Supports Intensity Scale (SIS)
Test of Malingered Memory (TOMM)
therapeutic communities (TCs)
traumatic brain injury (TBI)
Traumatic Brain Injury Questionnaire (TBIQ)
tricyclic antidepressants (TCAs)
United Nations (UN)
urine drug tests (UDTs)
U.S. Customs and Border Protection (CBP)
U.S. Department of Health and Human Services (DHHS)
U.S. Department of Veterans Affairs (VA)
U.S. Food and Drug Administration (FDA)
U.S. Immigration and Customs Enforcement (ICE)
Validity Indicator Profile (VIP)
Wechsler Abbreviated Scale of Intelligence (WASI)
Wechsler Memory Scale (WMS)
World Health Organization (WHO)
World Medical Association (WMA)

Introduction

Ten years after the *Oxford Textbook of Correctional Psychiatry* was first published, we are pleased to present the second edition. In the intervening decade, correctional facilities have navigated a worldwide pandemic and, in some places, concomitantly engaged in large-scale reform projects in numerous social, clinical, and technological domains. Practicing psychiatry in a jail or prison—which was already challenging—has become more complex than ever. Even as overall incarceration rates have declined (Fair & Walmsley, 2024), correctional facilities remain populated with a great many persons with serious mental illness, substance use disorders, personality disorders, and medical conditions. The need for competent and compassionate psychiatrists to care for incarcerated patients remains profound, and because the vast majority of these patients will return to the community, the value of correctional psychiatrists extends far beyond the walls.

Readers of the first edition will notice that the vocabulary used to describe the practice of psychiatry in jails, prisons, and other detention facilities is in flux, as evidenced by variations in language used by the contributors in the second edition. The National Commission on Correctional Health Care's 2021 position statement on the use of humanizing language calls for avoidance of correctional labels like "inmate," "offender," "prisoner," "felon," "convict," and "criminal" to describe incarcerated people. As editors, we have opted to use the term "incarcerated person" for the textbook's second edition and have encouraged contributors to do the same, though some authors have chosen different terminology based on local custom or law (e.g., U.K. laws referring to "mentally disordered offenders") or to refer to a specific subgroup of incarcerated people (e.g., "prisoner" when differentiating that group from individuals detained in jails). Similarly, the National Commission on Correctional Health Care's position statement favors person-centered language related to the use of substances. Research suggests that terms like "addict" and "[substance] abuse" generally introduce more stigma and can be a barrier to treatment (Ashford et al., 2018, 2019; Kelly & Westerhoff, 2010; Kelly et al., 2010). As such, we have opted for language related to substance use disorders that is person centered, nonpejorative, and consistent with *Diagnostic and Statistical Manual of Mental Disorders*, fifth edition, text revision (DSM-5-TR; American Psychiatric Association, 2022) terminology.

We debated vigorously about the title of this textbook, with some editors feeling that the term "correctional" is becoming antiquated because it (a) implies that incarcerated people need to be "corrected" as individuals, downplaying the numerous structural factors (e.g., racism, poverty, policing practices, sentencing laws) that contribute to incarceration, and (b) implies more of a rehabilitative focus than U.S. jails and prisons currently provide. The term "carceral," while not yet in widespread use, has the potential advantage of being more neutral and descriptive of jails and prisons. On the other hand, decades of hard work under the appellations "correctional psychiatry" and "correctional health care" have gone into professionalizing the field, transforming prisons and jails from the workplace of last resort to a rich clinical setting suitable for trainees and highly skilled, experienced practitioners alike. In fact, when the Accreditation Council on Graduate Medical Education proposed a new fellowship in 2023 focused on health care in jails and prisons, it chose "correctional (carceral) medicine" as the title rather than abandoning the older terminology (Accreditation Council on Graduate Medical Education, 2023).

As editors, we ultimately decided that retiring the term "correctional" is premature. As of this writing and to our knowledge, no stakeholding professional organization has adopted "carceral" rather than "correctional psychiatry," and while there are certainly many areas for improvement in the field, we want to highlight the professional identity that correctional psychiatry has earned through decades of incremental improvement. However, out of respect for extant professional differences on this matter, we have permitted contributors to use either the term "correctional" or "carceral" as they prefer.

The *Oxford Textbook of Correctional Psychiatry* is designed for use either as part of an organized course or for self-directed study. While some content has been reorganized based on developments in the field or editorial preferences, every chapter from the first edition is represented in updated form in this second edition, with seven new chapters addressing important and current topics: telepsychiatry, trauma-informed care, peer support programs, immigrants in detention, staff wellness, pandemic management, and jail-based competency restoration. When possible, we brought the original chapter contributors back for this edition, though we welcomed many new voices as well. We are proud to have assembled a distinguished panel of leaders in the field, including clinicians, administrators, systems monitors, researchers, ethicists, attorneys, and individuals with lived experience. Each chapter contains an up-to-date literature review with supportive references and a critical examination of best practices.

Section I: Section I, *Context and Perspective*, provides relevant background. The first chapter reviews the evolution of the U.S. imprisonment system, especially as it related to correctional psychiatry. It examines the history of American prisons, including their shifting purposes, standards, and practices. The chapter goes on to explain how rehabilitation theory has intersected with the diagnosis and treatment of incarcerated persons with psychiatric disorders, discusses the current status of imprisonment in the United States, and looks at how the historical perspective may influence the future of these systems. The second chapter summarizes the historical context of correctional versus community mental health, factors resulting in the increasing management of people with mental illness in correctional settings, and similarities and differences between mental health care in correctional and community settings. Next, formative case law and litigation are discussed, including the legal and constitutional foundation for correctional mental health care in the United States. The next chapter focuses on human rights, with a review of the challenges and controversies that exist in correctional mental health care in North America and internationally and an overview of the key internationally recognized human rights that should inform the work of correctional mental health professionals. The final chapter in this section shares the insights of incarcerated individuals, with autobiographical interviews presenting a narrative in their own words and reflecting themes of human struggle, coping, failure, regret, and hope. This chapter is coauthored by the mother of an incarcerated person, who shares another important perspective about the impact of incarceration on families.

Section II: Section II, *Organization, Structure, and Function of Correctional Institutions*, starts at the point before an individual becomes incarcerated. The first chapter, on diversion programs and alternatives to incarceration, reviews the major models used to divert those with serious mental illness from incarceration, with overviews of drug and mental health courts, jail diversion programs, and alternatives to incarceration for defendants with mental illness. The next chapter discusses distinctions between prisons (postsentence facilities) and jails (housing detainees awaiting trial) in service delivery and treatment challenges. Managing correctional populations is the topic of the following chapter. Jails and prisons share population management challenges with hotels—like the availability of beds to meet the explicit requirements of the persons residing there. In making skillful placement decisions, large facilities and systems recognize safety risks and clinical needs in real time. The chapter discusses these pragmatic issues, particularly in the context of psychiatric management. As in community settings, a continuum of care exists for incarcerated persons with mental illness, which is addressed in the chapter on levels of care. It describes outpatient care, emergency services, day treatment, supported residential housing, infirmary care, and inpatient psychiatric hospitalization and how to successfully adapt each level to meet the mental health needs of incarcerated persons.

The next chapter covers formal disciplinary processes in jails and prisons to address rule breaking and other misbehavior. Because incarcerated persons with mental illness may be more prone to rule infractions due to their illness, they are more likely to receive discipline and be placed in restrictive housing unless specific processes are in place to limit such sanctions. The chapter reviews common segregation practices, the data on the potential effects of restrictive housing on mental illness, and the role of psychiatry in the disciplinary process. The final chapter in this section deals with the cost and financing of correctional mental health care, which must consider both constitutionally mandated care obligations and resource constraints. This chapter includes a discussion of funding models, liability concerns, performance indicators, and copays for incarcerated persons.

Section III: Section III focuses on *Adapting Psychiatric Practice to Correctional Settings*. Each of these topics should be familiar to psychiatrists working in the community, though they may be less familiar with how these concepts are applied to correctional mental health care. The leadoff chapter deals with the many, often unique, ethical concerns that correctional settings present to the psychiatrist. Obligations to the law, professional standards, the community, and public health require a complex appreciation of competing values. Critical topics including informed consent and coercion, dual agency, appropriate access to care, and managing professional boundaries and standards are addressed. The next chapter is a pragmatic discussion of what it is like for psychiatrists to work inside the walls of a jail or prison. The psychiatrist must come to terms with the realities of the correctional setting to feel secure, satisfied with the work, and clinically effective. As with any health care setting, communication is a critical component of effective care delivery, and the following chapter explicitly discusses the inherent cultural differences among interdisciplinary staff, the special challenges to effective communication faced by correctional psychiatrists, and the importance of that communication given the central role that psychiatrists play in the overall mission of jail and prison health care.

In jails and prisons, the process, structure, content, and timing of screenings and assessments are vital parts of the health care system. This chapter reviews the initial mental health screening of persons entering prisons and jails, with a special emphasis on suicide risk screening and follow-up clinical assessments when intake screening suggests a need for treatment or suicide prevention efforts. Learning to conduct an interview is fundamental to psychiatric diagnosis and treatment. The next chapter addresses the challenges, requirements, importance, and complexity of clinical interviews in jails and prisons, with particular attention given to how the correctional population and setting can influence the interview process. While essential reading for trainees, even seasoned clinicians may benefit from this review and discussion. The diagnostic review and revision chapter reimagines incarceration as an opportunity to reexamine medications and diagnoses of people with mental illness whose care may have been confounded by substance use, treatment nonadherence, and other factors in less controlled community environments. This segues into the chapter on transition of medication treatment in the community to correctional settings.

The next chapters address common clinical concerns in correctional settings that may be vexing for health care professionals. Incarcerated persons often seek health care for sleep problems, and appropriate education regarding insomnia evaluation and management is necessary for jail and prison health care staff. This chapter outlines treatment guidelines that apply in community settings, presents an overview of the clinical and ethical issues of insomnia management in correctional institutions, and provides evidence- and ethics-based recommendations. Recognizing when someone is not being truthful is challenging, but detection of malingering helps ensure judicious use of limited resources and improves diagnostic accuracy. The next chapter details the topic of malingering in corrections and examines important skills related to its assessment and management.

What follows is a new chapter on telepsychiatry. Telemedicine is no longer a new technology, and it has been increasingly incorporated into correctional work. While telepsychiatry may improve access to care, psychiatrists using it should be cognizant of related security, technical, and clinical concerns. The next chapter addresses cultural and structural competence as an essential aspect of providing mental health care in correctional settings. Disparities exist in the rate of incarceration of minorities in the United States, with substantial elevations occurring in Black, Latinx, and Native American populations; the correctional psychiatrist must be familiar with cultural and structural factors contributing to these disparities. The last chapter in this section focuses on community reentry. As most incarcerated persons return to the community, it is in society's interest to be concerned with the readiness of formerly incarcerated people to live a productive life. This chapter presents the current understanding of transition support needs and practices to optimize successful community reentry for those with mental illness.

Section IV: Section IV tackles the *Management of Psychiatric Emergencies*. The first chapter focuses on the pragmatics of crisis assessment and management. Crisis calls occur often in correctional settings, with psychiatrists commonly needed for triage and management. The chapter reviews a range of crisis concerns in correctional settings, as well as related best practices. The use of seclusion, restraints, and emergency medication is the topic of the subsequent chapter, including legal precedents that regulate their use and guidance on minimizing their routine application in jails and prisons. Acute hospitalization is the focus of the final chapter in this section. Systems vary in this regard, with some having access to a dedicated secure hospital and others utilizing outside forensic or community hospitals. This chapter discusses models that link psychiatric care across institutional boundaries.

Section V: Matters generally related to *Psychopharmacology* are contained in Section V. The chapter on formulary management details the processes and procedures used to develop, implement, and monitor systems-based prescribing practices by establishing an effective pharmacy and therapeutics committee to weigh the cost, appropriateness, effectiveness, and safety of medications prescribed to incarcerated patients. The following chapter discusses medication administration and management. There are many steps, people, and processes involved in getting the right medication to the right patient within a correctional facility. This chapter reviews the structural, procedural, and clinical concerns of medication administration and management in jails and prisons.

The use of hypnotic agents and controlled substances is the topic of the next chapter. Sleep medications are among the most frequently written prescriptions in the community, and controlled substances such as benzodiazepines and opioid medications have become a major public health concern through overuse and misuse. The chapter describes best practices related to prescribing opioids, benzodiazepines, and both controlled and noncontrolled medications for sleep. The final chapter in this section considers the misuse of noncontrolled medications in correctional settings. The alteration, diversion, and nonmedical use of medications not ordinarily thought to be at risk for such is commonplace in jails and prisons. This chapter presents data on specific classes of medications at risk for, methods of, and approaches to minimize misuse and diversion.

Section VI: Section VI is a series of chapters on *Disorders and Syndromes*, starting with diagnostic prevalence and comorbidity. This chapter outlines the best available data on the correctional prevalence of common mental disorders and considers the key assumptions and methodological challenges involved in ascertaining these rates. The chapter on psychotic disorders discusses their complex and diverse presentation in jails and prisons, including the need to tease out schizophrenia spectrum disorders from the secondary neurotoxic effects of substances. This chapter covers the evidence basis for psychotherapy and psychopharmacology for psychotic disorders in correctional settings. Mood disorders, which represent a substantial portion of all psychiatric care in both community and correctional settings, are the topic of the following chapter. The review includes core management, best practices, and evidence-based therapeutic approaches to the treatment of major depressive and bipolar disorders in jails and prisons. Given the stressful nature of correctional settings, adjustment disorder is a key diagnostic consideration here and is addressed in detail in the next chapter.

The following two chapters cover anxiety disorders and posttraumatic stress disorder. Unrecognized anxiety disorders can result in disruptive behavior and the overuse of general medical health services. Appropriate, available, consistent, and well-integrated assessment, diagnosis, and treatment can be used to successfully manage anxiety disorders that present in correctional settings. In response to the DSM-5's moving of posttraumatic stress disorder out of the anxiety disorders section (which was introduced while the first edition of the textbook was in development), we dedicated a chapter entirely to this topic in this edition, greatly expanding it to consider the wider concept of trauma-informed care. Persons often arrive to correctional facilities already carrying a trauma burden, and many will encounter new trauma during incarceration. An evidence-based and trauma-informed approach promises benefits to patients with posttraumatic stress disorder, a reduction in traumagenesis, and a better work environment for staff.

Personality disorders, the topic of the following chapter, are highly prevalent and problematic in jails and prisons. The chapter zooms in on four personality disorders of particular clinical relevance to correctional psychiatry—borderline personality disorder, antisocial personality disorder, narcissistic personality disorder, and paranoid personality disorder—including specific management concerns and challenges, data on correctional prevalence, appropriate psychotherapy, and potential psychopharmacological interventions. The next chapter addresses the differential diagnosis and management challenges related to attention deficit disorders in a population with highly prevalent comorbid or confounding factors like personality and substance use disorders, presenting a balanced, evidence-based treatment model.

The final two chapters of this section look at the interface of psychiatry and general medical practice, first with an examination of general medical disorders with psychiatric implications, including delirium, and conditions that can mimic or exacerbate mood or psychotic disorders. Next is a review of the psychiatric aspects of chronic pain management in correctional settings. This chapter discusses from a psychiatric perspective the assessment challenges related to highly comorbid substance use disorders, the elements of a chronic pain interview, developing a multidisciplinary treatment plan, cognitive-behavioral interventions, pharmacological strategies, and the tracking of treatment outcomes.

Section VII: Section VII is about *Psychotherapy and Other Nonpharmacological Treatments* and begins with a chapter on applying the recovery model in prisons and jails. While correctional facilities are built around the general principles of sentencing that include retribution, deterrence, and incapacitation, another key purpose of confinement that cannot be overlooked is rehabilitation. This chapter presents feasible and potentially helpful considerations related to recovery-oriented services and discusses the tensions between the concepts of recovery and responsibility when working with incarcerated persons. The chapter on individual psychotherapy discusses practical and fundamental aspects of this practice in the correctional context, including evidence-based paradigms, therapeutic style, strategies to minimize the risks of therapeutic nihilism, and the limits of confidentiality. The next chapter reviews group psychotherapy, which is a standard practice in prisons and, to a lesser degree, jails. This chapter presents group therapies that have been adapted or created for correctional use and discusses appropriate patient selection, required therapist training, sustainability, and outcomes.

Section VIII: While touched upon in many other areas of this text, Section VIII is dedicated to *Substance Use Disorders*, which are collectively the most common mental health disorders in incarcerated persons. The first chapter reviews screening for and common presentations of intoxication and withdrawal syndromes and distinguishes these from other mental disorders. The substances found in facilities vary geographically, as do medical management approaches. Besides direct assessment and treatment, correctional psychiatrists make important contributions by offering educational, clinical, and policy consultations to other staff. The next chapter dives deeper into detoxification or medically supervised withdrawal in correctional facilities.

The section then shifts toward integrated strategies in the chapter on treatment models for substance use disorders, which describes the evolution of these approaches, drug courts, therapeutic communities, pharmacologically supported therapy, harm reduction, and current evidence-based modalities such as cognitive-behavioral interventions. The next chapter deals with dually diagnosed individuals, as substance use disorders and other mental illnesses frequently co-occur, especially in incarcerated persons.

Few facilities offer U.S. Food and Drug Administration–approved medications for substance use disorders in jails and prisons, though this practice is growing in the United States. The next chapter specifically discusses the evidence base, both in the community and in corrections, for pharmacotherapy for substance use disorders, which is also known as medication-assisted treatment or medication for opioid use disorder. This section concludes with a chapter on successful support of the transition back to the community for incarcerated patients with substance use disorders. Ineffective treatment of substance use disorders during incarceration is associated with relapse after release; this chapter discusses best practices to support community reentry.

Section IX: Section IX centers on *Self-Injury, Aggression, and Misconduct.* The chapter on suicide risk reduction presents prevalence, demographics, trends, screening and assessment, and appropriate suicide risk management. Factors unique to correctional settings, such as restrictive housing, facility transfers, loss of community social supports, and peer conflicts, may increase suicide risk in incarcerated persons. Proactive recognition of key risk factors, morbidity and mortality reviews to promote quality improvement initiatives, staff support after an incident, and a staff culture committed to improvement of knowledge and skills are addressed in this chapter. Closely related, the next chapter covers best practices for assessment and intervention for self-injurious behavior, which is one of the greatest management challenges in correctional settings.

The section then shifts to aggression directed toward others. The chapter on aggression reviews the factors that contribute to assaultive behavior in correctional settings. Opportunities for assessment, diagnosis, and treatment of those behaviors, both impulsive and predatory, are also presented. The final chapter of the section describes the use of behavior management plans to reduce the frequency, intensity, or severity of harmful or disruptive behaviors.

Section X: Section X details information of specific relevance for *Distinct Populations* of incarcerated patients, beginning with chapters for women; lesbian, gay, bisexual, and transgender individuals; persons with developmental disabilities; persons with traumatic brain injury; justice-involved youth; elderly individuals; and veterans. These chapters go into depth about each of these groups, including discussions about legal precedents, clinical concerns, and special assessment and treatment needs, ripped from recent headlines. These chapters are followed by a new chapter on immigrants and refugees, many of whom have suffered trauma in their home country or during their travels and arrest yet are often detained in facilities with limited access to mental health services or their support systems. Treatment standards, both actual and aspirational, and related litigation and monitoring are addressed.

The next chapter provides information on sex offenders, the treatment of whom is arguably one of the most challenging undertakings for psychiatrists. Paraphilias may or may not be present, and the stigmatization of sexual crimes by society may be acted out by incarcerated peers through exclusion, intimidation, or violence, which compounds preexisting or leads to de novo mental disorders in these patients. Gangs are a fact of life in jails and prisons, as reviewed in the final chapter on distinct populations. This essential reading for persons working in correctional settings describes the dynamics of gang leadership, membership, and involvement, as well as best practices for collaborative and productive interventions.

Section XI: Section XI includes a range of *Special Topics* and begins with a new chapter on staff wellness. The structural, operational, clinical, and political environments of jails and prisons may contribute to high rates of injury, illness, and burnout of staff. This chapter reviews these risks, as well as systemic, institutional, and individual approaches to reduce these risks. The chapter on forensic and legal issues addresses the intersection of correctional work with the legal system, including malpractice and civil rights actions, consent decrees, and forensic evaluations such as competency to stand trial and sanity. The next chapter shifts to a discussion of psychological testing, which offers substantial value as a helpful adjunct to standard clinical assessments in corrections. This chapter presents the history of psychological testing and the contexts for when it can and cannot be performed. What follows is another new chapter on pandemic management. The global COVID-19 pandemic caused widespread morbidity, mortality, and other consequences that exposed weaknesses in various systems, including correctional mental health care. This chapter describes the operational and clinical innovations that were helpful during the height of COVID-19, with an eye on systems being ready to respond effectively to the next event.

Hunger strikes, which are often used by incarcerated persons as a means of protest, are fielded in the next special topics chapter. Correctional psychiatrists may find themselves with conflicting duties to the hunger-striking patient, the institution, and other health care providers, creating complex tensions and medical ethics concerns that rarely exist in other practice locations. This chapter provides correctional psychiatrists with the historical, clinical, legal, and ethics background for working with hunger strikers. The following chapter deals with the growing recognition of and commitment to eliminate sexual assaults in jails and prisons. Sexual abuse in detention has a profound impact on survivors and, ultimately, society. This chapter examines current knowledge about sexual victimization in America's jails, prisons, and juvenile facilities; discusses the successes and limitations of the Prison Rape Elimination Act of 2003; and makes recommendations to further alleviate the problem.

Next is a new chapter on jail-based competency restoration. Resource constraints in many jurisdictions make hospital-based competency restoration impractical. When needed, jail-based competency restoration may reduce delays in resolving a defendant's legal matters. This chapter describes the best practices for when jail-based competency restoration is appropriate and how best to implement it. The last chapter in this section discusses international perspectives and practice differences, highlighting the importance of learning from other jurisdictions and systems, whatever our geographic location.

Section XII: The textbook concludes with Section XII, *Education, Research, and Quality Improvement.* This section opens with a chapter on correctional health care standards and accreditation. It presents a brief historical narrative on the development and adoption of national jail, prison, and juvenile correctional health care standards; a cogent review of recent jail and prison standards with relevance to psychiatry and mental health; and a discussion of accreditation programs. The next chapter addresses the monitoring of systems and the significant role for quality assurance and improvement. This chapter summarizes the monitoring process in a class action lawsuit settlement agreement, emphasizing the value of developing a quality improvement process that should ultimately eliminate the need for an external monitor.

Correctional settings present opportunities for psychiatrists to assume roles as leaders and educators, as reviewed in the next chapter. The increase in the number of incarcerated persons who require mental health services, the need for dedicated and qualified leadership of complex systems of care, and the importance of education and training in correctional mental health practices have created many administrative and teaching opportunities for psychiatrists. The following chapter shifts attention to the role of clinical trainees in jails and prisons, which are important and worthy training sites for medical students, general psychiatry residents, child and adolescent psychiatry residents, and forensic psychiatry fellows. Research and program evaluation opportunities are addressed in the following chapter. Robust research on mental health disorders of incarcerated persons essentially stopped in the mid-1970s as federal regulations were developed to protect incarcerated persons as human subjects. The chapter discusses the current impact of regulation and makes recommendations for engaging in ethical and useful research in jails and prisons.

The final chapter closes the circle and updates the editors' vision for the future of correctional psychiatry, starting with the context of where we are now. We discuss how standards of care in jails and prisons may change, the development of practice guidelines, innovative correctional approaches like the Norway model, and the integration of technologies like artificial intelligence and machine learning. The appendix contains other available resources for correctional health care, including updated links to relevant guidelines and practice resources. In closing, we encourage the reader to utilize the index when researching a particular topic. The complexities of correctional work necessitated some overlap in content, and contributors may offer a range of insights based on their individual expertise in the context of a more general subject. It is our hope that this comprehensive text will answer your most pressing questions about psychiatric practice in jails and prisons but also will lead you to consider new avenues of inquiry.

REFERENCES

Accreditation Council for Graduate Medical Education. (2023). *Proposed ACGME requirements for graduate medical education in correctional (carceral) medicine.* https://www.acgme.org/globalassets/pfassets/reviewandcomment/correctionalmedicine_rc-07112023.pdf

American Psychiatric Association. (2022). *Diagnostic and statistical manual of mental disorders* (5th ed, text rev.).

Ashford, R. D., Brown, A. M., & Curtis, B. (2018). Substance use, recovery, and linguistics: The impact of word choice on explicit and implicit bias. *Drug and Alcohol Dependence*, *189*, 131–138.

Ashford, R. D., Brown, A. M., McDaniel, J., & Curtis, B. (2019). Biased labels: An experimental study of language and stigma among individuals in recovery and health professionals. *Substance Use & Misuse*, *54*(8), 1376–1384.

Fair, H., & Walmsley, R. (2024). *World prison population* (14th ed.). World Prison Brief. https://www.prisonstudies.org/sites/default/files/resources/downloads/world_prison_population_list_14th_edition.pdf

Kelly, J. F., Dow, S. J., & Westerhoff, C. (2010). Does our choice of substance-related terms influence perceptions of treatment need? An empirical investigation with two commonly used terms. *Journal of Drug Issues*, *40*(4), 805–818.

Kelly, J. F., & Westerhoff, C. M. (2010). Does it matter how we refer to individuals with substance-related conditions? A randomized study of two commonly used terms. *International Journal on Drug Policy*, *21*(3), 202–207.

National Commission on Correctional Health Care. (2021). *Use of humanizing language in correctional health care.* https://www.ncchc.org/wp-content/uploads/Use-of-Humanizing-Language-in-Correctional-Health-Care-2021-1.pdf

SECTION I

Context and perspective

1

History of imprisonment

Bruce A. Arrigo

Introduction

In the United States, the use of criminal confinement as a form of punishment commenced during the colonial era (Parsons, 2022; Rothman, 2002; Scull, 2006). Since then, imprisonment practices have continued to evolve, with fluctuating commitments to punishment's transitory purpose and the variable penal philosophies that justify it. This chapter focuses on the evolution of the U.S. imprisonment system and examines the system's development in relation to correctional psychiatry, beginning with the history of U.S. prisons, including their shifting purposes, standards, and practices. Rehabilitation theory has intersected with the clinical assessment, diagnosis, and treatment of persons experiencing psychiatric disorders while criminally confined. The swelling number of persons with psychiatric disorders found in correctional settings today has converted U.S. jails and prisons into ill-equipped and underfunded de facto institutions that warehouse individuals, much like the reformist-minded era of the 19th century. Commentary is also provided addressing the precarious human rights status of incarcerated persons (IPs) with mental illness in today's U.S. prisons and jails. The chapter concludes by discussing several developing issues in correctional psychiatry, including forensic neuroscience and its role in maximizing effective psychiatric care and correctional treatment, and the emerging relevance of digital technology in the planning of rehabilitative treatment for recovery and reentry. This discussion offers a glimpse into the historical future of the U.S. imprisonment system and correctional psychiatry's role in it.

History of U.S. prisons and punishment

The prisons of the colonial era were rooted in religion, English tradition, and practical wisdom (Meskell, 1999). With relatively small populations to police, the criminal justice system administered swift and public punishments that were intended to humiliate, enslave, or even torture (Pfohl, 2009). Moreover, given the strong sense of kinship that shaped colonial hamlets, punishment existed to deter transgression and to discipline waywardness (Foucault, 1979). Deterrence philosophy was fueled through Calvinist religious doctrine and dogma (Barnes, 1968). For Calvinists, it was wasteful and futile to rely on and invest in a reformist-based penal system because humans were innately sinful, wicked, and evil. Operating from within this no-nonsense and religiously driven framework, the colonies drew from English criminal codes to define specific capital offenses, ranging from murder to blasphemy (Barnes, 1968). For noncapital offenses, retribution increased in severity as recidivism continued, and punishment could eventually result in banishment (Cullen & Gilbert, 1982). This English-based, Calvinist-inspired system of punishment persisted until the late 1700s, when reform movements emerged as a response to rapid population growth and the call for a more humane "corrections" system (Barnes, 1968; Rothman, 2002). Utilitarians such as Jeremy Bentham and John Stuart Mill began criticizing the English system of punishment and imprisonment. They argued that people were not innately cruel or sinful but rather that they were calculating. This calculation meant that people weighed the costs and benefits of committing a crime and made a choice on how best to behave based on this reasoned calculus (Barnes, 1968).

During the post-Revolutionary era, the Italian criminologist Cesare Beccaria emerged as the most significant theorist to influence the U.S. system of corrections (Hirsch, 1982). He had disdain for the English penal system's practice of meting out severe punishment that exceeded the harshness of the crime (Meskell, 1999). Beccaria posited that the source for crime was the criminal code itself and not the individual (Gillin, 1926). Specifically, he maintained that to overcome the arbitrary and draconian criminal codes found in countries such as England, governments should enact legislation that strictly defined punishments, limited the power of judges appropriately, codified laws clearly and publicly, created punishments that instilled fear in potential offenders and thus deterred them from engaging in criminal behavior, and developed punishments that were the least harsh and the least necessary to achieve the goal of deterrence (Gillin, 1926). By the late 1700s, America's acceptance of Beccaria's recommendations led to the revision of its criminal codes and the introduction of a reformist-based system of punishment (Cullen & Gilbert, 1982).

The early U.S. prisons were harsh, often housing men and women together. They lacked discipline, humane treatment, and sanitary living conditions (Rothman, 2002; Scull, 2006). In 1786, following the acceptance of arguments put forward by the classical school of criminology (i.e., the integration of utilitarianism's reasoned calculus and Beccaria's fear of punishment), Benjamin Rush, along with the Society for Assisting Distressed Prisoners, drafted a new criminal code in the United States (Barnes, 1968). One of the most notable correctional facilities to emerge following this codification was the Walnut Street Jail in Philadelphia (Roth, 2006). The origins of its system of punishment and imprisonment can be traced to a law passed by the Pennsylvania legislature on April 5, 1790, based on a Society for Assisting Distressed Prisoners draft report that called for solitary confinement combined with the administration of hard labor (Barnes, 1968). The law specifically instituted hard labor as punishment, called for the segregation of prisoners by gender and type of crime, and permitted solitary confinement for the most serious of offenses (Barnes, 1968). Prisoners in the Walnut Street Jail were required to read the Bible and participate in religious instructions, and they were not allowed to drink alcohol. This model of criminal confinement encouraged introspection and the elimination of bad habits, and it purged the "moral contamination" of IPs through dependence on isolative practices such as solitary confinement (Roth, 2006).

Eventually, the penal culture changed along with the law undergirding the U.S. system. Jails were no longer run for profit, as they had been under the colonial system; the organization of imprisonment was standardized, and IPs were less vulnerable to extortion by their keepers (McGowen, 1995). While the Walnut Street Jail limited solitary confinement to persons with the most egregious offenses, the facility lacked a full-fledged model of prisoner isolative segregation that did not include hard labor (De Beaumont et al., 1833). In other words, isolated IPs still had to work. Sustained imprisonment under these conditions was both demoralizing and dehumanizing. Moreover, while the Walnut Street Jail experienced some success, it lacked proper prison-based controls, suitable plans for expansion, and sufficient financial support. The facility deteriorated in the 1820s and was officially shut down in 1835 (Lewis, 1965).

A new wave of reformers began to take part in shaping the burgeoning U.S. system of imprisonment and punishment. Theory on the origin of crime shifted sharply to a new view of criminality rooted in the ills of a failed social order (Gillin, 1926). From this perspective, the purpose of prison confinement was to advance the well-being of the person sentenced; that is, the aim of criminal confinement was to ensure the safety and to further the good of society as a whole while at the same time correcting (i.e., normalizing) the transgressor (Foucault, 1979). In 1816, a prison was constructed in Auburn, New York, modeled after this philosophy (De Beaumont et al., 1833).

The attempt at solitary confinement without hard labor was unsuccessful at the Auburn Prison. As a penal practice, some questioned whether isolative segregation ultimately led to insanity (Barnes, 1968; see Chapter 10). Eventually, this criticism led to the elimination of isolative segregation as a broadly applied penal practice. Auburn Prison then implemented the congregate system of correctional management (Meskell, 1999). Under the congregate system, prisoners were allowed to work together during the day. However, at night, they were required to sleep in different cells and were prohibited from speaking, effectively preventing communication with others who were incarcerated (Lewis, 1965). The Auburn system used intense observation of prisoners to monitor their behavior, and it relied on consistent discipline throughout the prison to manage and correct misconduct.

The Eastern State Penitentiary in Pennsylvania was constructed in 1821, and it departed from the example set at the Auburn facility (Barnes, 1968). Eastern State Penitentiary implemented a system of imprisonment that focused on the reform of prisoners as soon as they began serving their sentences. IPs were placed in solitary confinement, not allowed to work, and expected to reflect on their criminal wrongdoings. Eventually, they were given permission to work, had access to the Bible, and were taught to read during their incarceration if they entered the prison illiterate (De Beaumont et al., 1833). These reforms were driven by Quaker religious convictions and based on a philosophy of both moral reform and social rehabilitation (Dumm, 1987). Known as the Philadelphia model, this approach to penal practice required less intense supervision of persons incarcerated than did the Auburn model. Both models of correctional management shaped the U.S. prison system throughout much of the 19th century. However, the approach developed at the Auburn Prison was more widely adopted within the United States and came to dominate 19th-century practices (U.S. Department of Justice, 1939). This was due in large part to the health repercussions of isolative segregation without labor (as experienced at Eastern State Penitentiary) and the financial savings that followed from the imprisonment model at Auburn (i.e., the costs per IP were nearly half those of Eastern State Penitentiary).

In the late 1800s through the mid-1900s, a series of international mobilization events and national reform efforts emerged to improve the treatment of IPs. In 1885, an international prison conference in Rome led to radical changes in penal philosophy and practice. During this period, the focus on scientific approaches to the confinement and rehabilitation of prisoners propelled efforts to reduce reliance on incarceration, to pursue alternative sanctions for less severe crimes, and to introduce new strategies such as probation (Ferracuti, 1989). Two more international conferences were held—one in Amsterdam in 1901, the other in London in 1925. These conferences shifted the focus to the IP's psychopathology (Palermo, 2013). This clinical approach to criminal behavior emphasized the role of psychological testing and the relevance of behavioral assessment as sources of knowledge about proper diagnoses, effective treatment, and palliative care. Moreover, these clinical gains fostered the development of alternative approaches to carceral detention, including a new focus on the social reintegration of prisoners (Ferracuti, 1989).

This rehabilitative turn in correctional philosophy led to improvements in prison conditions. Notwithstanding the mostly nominal gains that followed, many deficiencies remained in U.S. correctional institutions up until the 1960s. Indeed, the penal system had reached a point where persons incarcerated were afforded a decent diet, had access to reading materials, benefited from several forms of recreation, and were able to buy certain personal items. However, they served longer sentences, were under constant surveillance, and still lacked access to much-needed health and mental health services, as well as appropriate planning for successful community reentry and ongoing recovery (Parsons, 2022).

As the 20th century progressed, urban centers became more densely populated, and crime rates and jail populations increased. These realities contributed to overcrowded prisons, substandard living conditions, and a heightened threat of violence (Morris, 1995). Once again, the increased prison population led to strict supervision, reduced access to rehabilitative services, and a decline in humane conditions of confinement. U.S. prisons became undisciplined and dangerous, a breeding ground for the recruitment of gang members, for the sale and purchase of drugs, and for the development of a pariah as well as predatory prison economy (e.g., sexual violence; Pardue et al., 2011; Wortley, 2003). To improve these deteriorating conditions, judicial intervention surged from the 1960s to the 1980s (DiIulio, 1990). A coalesced concern for civil liberties, prisoners' rights, and scholarly research documenting the physical and psychological impact of incarceration in the absence of social and psychological supports led to progressive, constitutionally supported reforms within the U.S. penal system (Appelbaum, 1994; Parsons, 2022).

Beginning in the late 20th century, researchers noted that a significant decline in criminality had occurred across the United States. However, unprecedented prison population growth, coupled with rapid correctional facility expansion, continued unabated (D. Garland, 2002). In 2014, by most accounts, the number of criminally confined individuals in jails or prisons exceeded 2.7 million. This figure did not account for the collateral harm that extended to the family members of those incarcerated (Chesney-Lind & Mauer, 2003; Clear & Frost, 2013). Moreover, by the end of the 20th century, the total number of persons with serious mental illness in prisons and jails was larger than the total number of psychiatric hospital patients (Lamb & Weinberger, 1998), making the delivery of effective correctional psychiatric services and social programming both fiscally unsustainable and clinically untenable. These institutional dynamics persisted into the early 21st century, especially when noting that at least 40% of persons with severe mental illnesses had been, at some point in their lives, housed in jails or prisons (Torrey et al., 2010). The same concern for effective correctional psychiatric services when treating justice-involved patients continues today. For example, in a study of the criminal histories of 240 patients with severe mental illnesses served in the public mental health system, Compton and colleagues (2022) found that over 70% had been arrested, with a lifetime average number of arrests of 8.6. In addition, the conditions of imprisonment in the 21st century remain problematic (e.g., overcrowded and underfunded), with an emphasis on retributive penal practices. Examples include reliance on "supermax" secure housing units to mass incarcerate; dependence on long-term disciplinary and administrative segregation to manage dangerousness; and utilization of surveillance technologies and information systems to measure risk, maintain correctional security, and monitor precrime behavior (Arrigo & Sellers, 2021).

Mental illness and the correctional rehabilitation system

Throughout the 19th and early 20th centuries, the purpose of imprisonment in the United States was to rehabilitate (McGee, 1969). Indeed, the very name *penitentiary*—a popular descriptor used during this period—indicated that prisons were more than just a place to house transgressors (Cullen & Gendreau, 2000). Religious values principally motivated this commitment to the rehabilitative ideal until it was professionalized in the 20th century in the form of individual treatment (Palermo, 2013). The professionalization of correctional rehabilitation changed the way recovery and reentry were defined and the conditions under which both occurred.

Throughout the latter portion of the 20th century, individualized rehabilitation dominated prison psychiatry (Gunn, 2000). An important part of this philosophy was determining which antisocial characteristics an IP possessed and which critical thinking errors the individual exhibited. These so-called criminogenic deficits were understood to induce criminal conduct (Andrews & Bonta, 2017). This assessment and diagnostic approach to rehabilitation became a starting point for predicting and controlling criminal susceptibilities, thoughts, and behaviors. The aim of this approach was to better address the IP's clinical needs and to better protect the community's security interests (Cullen & Gendreau, 2000). Important alternatives to (Ward & Brown, 2004) and criticisms of (Arrigo, 2013) this rehabilitation approach exist. Today, however, these needs and this security are the subject of risk management through algorithmic calculation (Werth, 2019) in the service of a penology whose intention advances the administrative imperatives of actuarial justice (Arrigo & Sellers, 2021; Rothschild-Elyassi et al., 2018). Increasingly, IPs, prison institutions, correctional programming, and community reentry planning are mostly monitored and maintained through cutting-edge algorithmic prediction. What this means is that reliance on digital technology, the information sciences, and the tools of data analytics has become standard best practice. However, concerns for legal privacy, unconscious bias in decision-making, social and emotional well-being, and "surveillance creep" are some of the unintended consequences of this penology (Kilgour, 2021; Ward et al., 2022).

Arguably, clinical risk assessment, diagnosis, and treatment have become more sophisticated in the 21st century, given advances in psychopharmacological medicine, actuarial rigor in social science methodologies, and precision in diagnostic techniques and analytics (Stein et al., 2022). Regrettably, however, the fate of IPs with mental illness has not similarly progressed. Incarceration is difficult on one's well-being because of "overcrowding, violence, lack of privacy, lack of meaningful activities, isolation from family and friends, uncertainty about life after prison, and inadequate health services" (Fellner, 2006, p. 391). Researchers continue to report the alarming percentage of persons who suffer from mental illness within the correctional system (Prison Policy Initiative, 2024a; Torrey et al., 2010; see Chapter 31). Indeed, drawing from the available empirical research, Mulvey and Schubert (2017, p. 232) summarized the "broad and entrenched problem" that correctional health care providers confront:

> If being mentally ill means "experiencing symptoms or receiving mental health treatment," estimates are that about 56 percent of state prison inmates and 64 percent of jail inmates are mentally ill.... If the focus is narrowed to serious mental illnesses, such as psychotic symptoms, mania, and severe depression, between 10 and 20 percent of jail inmates and 25 percent of prison inmates are seriously mentally ill.... The prevalence rate of serious mental disorders among jail inmates is somewhere between three and six times that in the general population; the level of disparity in prevalence rates doubles when considering just female detainees.... If substance use disorders are added to the clinical picture, the rates are higher. Over half of both jail and state prison inmates have a substance use disorder. As many as three-fourths of both jail and state prison inmates with mental health problems have also been diagnosed as having a substance use disorder.

Moreover, the swelling number of persons with psychiatric disorders found in correctional settings today has converted jails and prisons into ill-equipped and underfunded de facto institutions that warehouse individuals, much like in the 19th century (Parsons, 2022). While the U.S. justice system has implemented some novel accommodations for persons with psychiatric disorders (e.g., specialized rehabilitation units, diversion through mental health courts), those who experience severe forms of mental illness are often subjected to the same punitive treatment of isolative confinement that was popular during the 19th century (Fellner, 2006; Metzner & Fellner, 2013). Prison segregation only amplifies the lack of adequate care available for those who need or could benefit from mental health treatment, and it exacerbates the detrimental impact such custodial care has on IPs who live with or are susceptible to psychiatric illness (Brown, 2020; Haney, 2017).

The U.S. prison system has always struggled to determine the treatments that could best aid in the recovery and reentry process for the heterogenous population of persons with mental illness (Lamb & Weinberger, 1998; Mulvey & Schubert, 2017). Current correctional policies that target interventions for IPs coping with psychiatric disorders endeavor to balance the ideals of individual liberty and human dignity against the need for institutional safety and the demand for public protection (Lamb & Weinberger, 2017). Mindful of the inadequate delivery of psychiatric services found in many U.S. prisons, several international covenants informed by human rights legal activism have called for an overhaul of policies that affect persons with mental disabilities (Perlin, 2011). In fact, the United Nations Standard Minimum Rules for the Treatment of Prisoners recognizes that some IPs experiencing serious mental illness should not be subjected to imprisonment at all (Fellner, 2006; Haney, 2017). While much of the focus is on improving conditions within correctional institutions, researchers contend that the "most effective way to ensure that the rights of IPs with mental illness are protected is to try to keep them out of prison in the first place" (Fellner, 2006, p. 411). This would require an increase in community-based programming and court-ordered mental health services, a consideration of the IP's mental status in judicial policies such as mandatory minimum sentencing, and a restructuring of the pretrial process in which defendants with mental illness would be identified (Appelbaum, 1994; Mulvey & Schubert, 2017). Thus, while the clinical risk assessment, diagnosis, and treatment of mental disorders in correctional settings arguably have advanced over time, the human rights of IPs with mental illness within the prison system have not so similarly progressed.

Current and developing concerns

The number of African Americans incarcerated under the guise of the Reagan-era War on Drugs campaign has been alarming. To date, the most telling consequence of the War on Drugs initiative is that more than 31 million people have been arrested and convicted for these criminal offenses, leading to systematic mass incarceration that adversely and unequally affects poor people of color (Alexander, 2020). Presently, 48% of people serving life, life without parole, or "virtual life" (i.e., death will occur while confined) sentences are Black (Prison Policy Initiative, 2024b). Immigration, detention, and the care of persons with severe mental illness present additional treatment and best practice concerns for forensic practitioners working within the U.S. correctional system (Ochoa et al., 2010). Confronted with the reality of racialized justice and an imprisonment culture that struggles to cultivate, much less implement, sorely needed rehabilitative prescriptions, correctional psychiatry now increasingly directs its clinical attention to the challenges of treating the psychopathology of internet harassers, cyber-stalkers, and virtual sexual predators (Gunn, 2000; Ticknor, 2018).

Coupled with these novel and mostly untested directions is the application of cognitive neuroscience to forensic and correctional settings (Banich & Compton, 2018; B. Garland, 2011; Gazzaniga, 2009). For example, restoring the capitally sentenced person's competence for purposes of state-sanctioned execution raises serious questions about the legal limits of individual privacy rights, the "soft" science of functional magnetic resonance imaging technology, and medicine's responsibilities to navigate professionally the clinical ethics of both (e.g., Arrigo, 2007). These ethics concerns involve cultural norms (Aggarwal, 2009) and extend to such increasing correctional responsibilities as the prediction of recidivism using neuroimaging (Kiehl et al., 2018).

In addition, digital science has made the management and control of IPs reentering society mostly a matter of mass surveillance and prediction algorithms (Budd & Mancini, 2021). Questions persist about reliance on this actuarial model of rehabilitation, especially when planning for the institutional release of formerly convicted persons with a sex offense to the community, where electronic monitoring facilitates reintegration goals (Budd & Mancini, 2017) while arguably quelling public fears (Lussier & Mathesius, 2019). These are just some of the urgent and emergent concerns in the correctional psychiatry field.

Summary

Prisons in the United States have shifted in their purposes, standards, and practices over time. What began as harsh environments to punish individuals in colonial times had, by the 19th century, evolved to consider rehabilitation and reform. In more recent years, the challenge of managing large numbers of people with mental illness has plagued correctional systems, most of which remain ill-equipped to provide adequate health care. In addition, prison systems have ventured into controversial areas such as forensic neuroscience and the use of digital technology for reentry planning and monitoring. Thorny directions and complex developments such as these await the attention of correctional psychiatry, with implications for the emotional, relational, and social well-being of the kept and their keepers.

REFERENCES

Aggarwal, N. K. (2009). Neuroimaging, culture, and forensic psychiatry. *Journal of the American Academy of Psychiatry and the Law, 37*(2), 239–244.

Alexander, M. (2020). *The new Jim Crow: Mass incarceration in the age of colorblindness.* New Press.

Andrews, D. A., & Bonta, J. (2017). *The psychology of criminal conduct* (5th ed.). Anderson Publishing.

Appelbaum, P. S. (1994). *Almost a revolution: Mental health law and the limits of change.* Oxford University Press.

Arrigo, B. A. (2007). Punishment, freedom, and the culture of control: The case of brain imaging and the law. *American Journal of Law and Medicine, 33*(3), 457–482.

Arrigo, B. A. (2013). Managing risk and marginalizing identities: On the society-of-captives thesis and the harm of social dis-ease. *International Journal of Offender Therapy and Comparative Criminology, 57*(6), 672–693.

Arrigo, B. A., & Sellers, B. G. (Eds.). (2021). *The pre-crime society: Crime, culture, and control in the ultramodern age.* Bristol University Press.

Banich, M. T., & Compton, R. J. (2018). *Cognitive neuroscience*. Cambridge University Press.

Barnes, H. E. (1968). *The evolution of penology in Pennsylvania: A study in American social history*. Patterson Smith.

Brown, E. (2020). A systematic review of the effects of prison segregation. *Aggression and Violent Behavior, 52*, 101389.

Budd, K. M., & Mancini, C. (2017). Public perceptions of GPS monitoring for convicted sex offenders: Opinions on effectiveness of electronic monitoring to reduce sexual recidivism. *International Journal of Offender Therapy and Comparative Criminology, 61*(12), 1335–1353.

Budd, K. M., & Mancini, C. (2021). Mass monitoring: The role of big data in tracking individuals convicted of sex crimes. In B. A. Arrigo & B. G. Sellers (Eds.), *The pre-crime society* (pp. 315–340). Bristol University Press.

Chesney-Lind, M., & Mauer, M. (Eds.). (2003). *Invisible punishment: The collateral consequences of mass imprisonment*. New Press.

Clear, T. R., & Frost, N. A. (2013). *The punishment imperative: The rise and failure of mass incarceration in America*. New York University Press.

Compton, M. T., Graves, J., Zern, A., et al. (2022). Characterizing arrests and charges among individuals with serious mental illnesses in public-sector treatment settings. *Psychiatric Services, 73*(10), 1102–1108.

Cullen, F. T., & Gendreau, P. (2000). Assessing correctional rehabilitation: Policy, practice and prospects, United States. *Criminal Justice, 3*, 109–175.

Cullen, F. T., & Gilbert, K. E. (1982). *Reaffirming rehabilitation*. Anderson Publishing.

De Beaumont, G. A. D., De Tocqueville, C. A., & Lieber, F. (1833). *On the penitentiary system in the United States and its application in France* (F. Lieber, Trans.). Carey, Lea & Blanchard.

DiIulio, J. J. (1990). *Courts, corrections, and the constitution*. Oxford University Press.

Dumm, T. L. (1987). *Democracy and punishment*. University of Wisconsin Press.

Fellner, J. (2006). A corrections quandary: Mental illness and prison rules. *Harvard Civil Rights-Civil Liberties Law Review, 41*, 391–412.

Ferracuti, F. (1989). *Carcere e trattamento* [Prisons and treatment], *Trattato di Criminologia, Medicina Criminologica e Psichiatria Forense* [Treatise on criminology, criminological medicine and forensic psychiatry] (Vol. 11). Giuffre.

Foucault, M. (1979). *Discipline and punish: The birth of the prison* (A. Sheridan, Trans.). Vintage.

Garland, B. (2011). *Neuroscience and the law: Brain, mind, and the scales of justice*. Dana Press.

Garland, D. (2002). *The culture of control: Crime and social order in contemporary society* (Vol. 77). University of Chicago Press.

Gazzaniga, M. S. (2009). *The ethical brain*. Dana Press.

Gillin, J. L. (1926). *Criminology and penology*. Jonathan Cape.

Gunn, J. (2000). Future directions for treatment in forensic psychiatry. *British Journal of Psychiatry, 176*, 332–338.

Haney, C. (2017). "Madness" and penal confinement: Some observations on mental illness and prison pain. *Punishment & Society, 19*(3), 310–326.

Hirsch, A. J. (1982). *From pillory to penitentiary: The rise of criminal incarceration in early Massachusetts*. Michigan Law Review Association.

Kiehl, K. A., Anderson, N. E., Aharoni, E., et al. (2018). Age of gray matters: Neuroprediction of recidivism. *NeuroImage: Clinical, 19*, 813–823.

Kilgour, L. (2021). *Designed to shame: Electronic ankle monitors and the politics of carceral technology*. https://doi.org/10.7298/rwe9-yy43

Lamb, H. R., & Weinberger, L. E. (1998). Persons with severe mental illness in jails and prisons: A review. *Psychiatric Services, 49*, 483–492.

Lamb, H. R., & Weinberger, L. E. (2017). Understanding and treating offenders with serious mental illness in public sector mental health. *Behavioral Sciences & the Law, 35*(4), 303–318.

Lewis, W. D. (1965). *From Newgate to Dannemora: The rise of the penitentiary in New York, 1796–1848*. Cornell University Press.

Lussier, P., & Mathesius, J. (2019). Trojan horse policies: Sexual predators, SORN laws and the American experience. *Psychology, Crime & Law, 25*(2), 133–156.

McGee, R. A. (1969). What's past is prologue. *Annals of the American Academy of Political and Social Science, 381*, 1–10.

McGowen, R. (1995). Well-ordered prison: England, 1780–1865. In N. Morries & D. Rothman (Eds.), *Oxford history of the prison: The practice of punishment in western society* (pp. 79–109). Oxford University Press.

Meskell, M. W. (1999). An American resolution: The history of prisons in the United States from 1777 to 1877. *Stanford Law Review, 51*, 839–865.

Metzner, J. L., & Fellner, J. (2013). Solitary confinement and mental illness in US prisons: A challenge for medical ethics. *Health and Human Rights in a Changing World, 1*, 316–323.

Morris, N. (1995). The contemporary prison. In D. Morris & D. J. Rothman (Eds.), *Oxford history of the prison: The practice of punishment in western society* (pp. 227–259). Oxford University Press.

Mulvey, E. P., & Schubert, C. A. (2017). Mentally ill individuals in jails and prisons. *Crime and Justice, 46*(1), 231–277.

Ochoa, K. C., Pleasants, G. L., Penn, J. V., & Stone, D. C. (2010). Disparities in justice and care: Persons with severe mental illnesses in the US immigration detention system. *Journal of the American Academy of Psychiatry and the Law, 38*(3), 392–399.

Palermo, G. B. (2013). The evolution of punishment and incarceration. In N. Konrad, B. Völlm, & D. N. Weisstub (Eds.), *Ethical issues in prison psychiatry* (pp. 77–102). Springer.

Pardue, A., Arrigo, B. A., & Murphy, D. S. (2011). Sex and sexuality in women's prisons: A preliminary typological investigation. *Prison Journal, 91*(3), 279–304.

Parsons, A. E. (2022). *From asylum to prison: Deinstitutionalization and the rise of mass incarceration after 1945*. UNC Press Books.

Perlin, M. L. (2011). *International human rights and mental disability law: When the silenced are heard*. Oxford University Press.

Pfohl, S. J. (2009). *Images of deviance and social control: A sociological history*. Waveland Press.

Prison Policy Initiative. (2024a). *Mental health: Policies and practices surrounding mental health*. https://www.prisonpolicy.org/research/mental_health/

Prison Policy Initiative. (2024b). *Race and ethnicity: Key statistics*. https://www.prisonpolicy.org/research/race_and_ethnicity/

Roth, M. P. (2006). *Prisons and prison systems*. Greenwood Press.

Rothman, D. J. (2002). *Conscience and convenience: The asylum and its alternatives in progressive America*. Aldine Transaction.

Rothschild-Elyassi, G., Koehler, J., & Simon, J. (2018). Actuarial justice. In M. Deflem (Ed.), *The handbook of social control* (pp. 194–206). John Wiley & Sons.

Scull, A. (2006). *The insanity of place/the place of insanity: Essays on the history of psychiatry*. Routledge.

Stein, D. J., Shoptaw, S. J., Vigo, D. V., et al. (2022). Psychiatric diagnosis and treatment in the 21st century: Paradigm shifts versus incremental integration. *World Psychiatry, 21*(3), 393–414.

Ticknor, B. (2018). *Virtual reality and the criminal justice system: Exploring the possibilities for correctional rehabilitation*. Lexington Books.

Torrey, E. F., Kennard, A. D., Lamb, H. R., & Pavle, J. (2010). *More mentally ill persons are in jails and prisons than hospitals: A survey of the states*. Treatment Advocacy Center.

U.S. Department of Justice. (1939). *The Attorney General's survey of release procedures: Digest of federal and state laws on release procedures*. U.S. Government Printing Office.

Ward, T., Arrigo, B., Barnao, M., et al. (2022). Urgent issues and prospects in correctional rehabilitation practice and research. *Legal and Criminological Psychology*, *27*(2), 103–128.

Ward, T., & Brown, M. (2004). The good lives model and conceptual issues in offender rehabilitation. *Psychology, Crime & Law*, *10*(3), 243–257.

Werth, R. (2019). Risk and punishment: The recent history and uncertain future of actuarial, algorithmic, and "evidence-based" penal techniques. *Sociology Compass*, *13*(2), e12659.

Wortley, R. (2003). *Situational prison control: Crime prevention in correctional institutions*. Cambridge University Press.

2

Mental illness management: The shift from community to corrections

Charles L. Scott*

Introduction

An increasing number of individuals with mental illness are now treated in correctional environments instead of community settings. In the incarcerated population, prevalence estimates of serious mental illness range from 9% to 20% (Beck & Maruschuk, 2000; Diamond et al., 2001; Regier et al., 1990; Steadman et al., 2009), compared to 6% in the community (Kessler et al., 2005). In their survey of state and federal incarcerated persons (IPs), Maruschak et al. (2021) found that 41% had a history of mental health problems. More astonishingly, in 2005, over three times more persons with serious mental illness in the United States were located in jails and prisons than in hospitals (Torrey et al., 2010). It was not always like this. How did U.S. correctional systems become de facto mental health institutions for so many? Scholars point to a number of reasons for the increasing prevalence of mental illness among incarcerated individuals, including deinstitutionalization and limited community resources, prominent court decisions and legislative rulings, and the "revolving door" phenomenon (Talbott, 2004; Yohanna, 2013). This chapter summarizes the historical context of correctional versus community mental health, factors resulting in the increasing management of people with mental illness in correctional settings, and similarities and differences between the provision of mental health care in correctional versus community settings.

Historical context of correctional versus community mental health care

Mental illness has existed in America since the beginning of this nation (de Young, 2010; Eldridge, 1996). Individuals with mental illness living during colonial times often relied on families or friends to care for them. If their relatives or friends could not or would not care for them, they typically became homeless or incarcerated. Until the mid-18th century, this segment of the "insane," as they were called, ended up in the same institutions as criminals—houses of correction and workhouses—even if they had not committed a crime (de Young, 2010).

The establishment of Philadelphia's Pennsylvania Hospital in 1751 marked the start of a new era, one in which the disposition of these two populations differed. Shortly after this general hospital—the nation's first—opened, it accepted patients with mental illness (de Young, 2010; Graham, 2008), almost assuredly diverting some from correctional settings.

Despite a dedicated environment for the treatment of mental illness in the new hospital, patients initially encountered conditions similar to those previously experienced by people with psychiatric problems in correctional settings. For example, they were locked in the "damp and unwholesome" cellar of the hospital (Graham, 2008) and, not uncommonly, chained (de Young, 2010). However, a noteworthy distinction existed between the purposes of confinement in houses of correction and those of the new hospital: Instead of simply enclosing individuals, the hospital attempted to treat their mental illnesses.

By 1773, Virginia had constructed the "Public Hospital for Persons of Insane and Disordered Minds," the country's first building devoted solely to treating individuals with mental illness. The hospital's first patient was transferred from the local jail (Zwelling, 1985), perhaps a progressive recognition that people with mental illness deserve treatment instead of punishment. By today's standards, the available treatments were undoubtedly inadequate. However, the shift represented, if nothing more, a developing contrast in the physical location between those with mental illness and those convicted of a crime.

In the following years, the number of individuals institutionalized for mental illness grew, and states accordingly built more asylums. Most of these institutions emphasized a more humane psychological approach to the custody and care of individuals with psychiatric disease, in accordance with French physician Philippe Pinel's "moral treatment" (de Young, 2010).

Over time, provision of care diverged from this more humane approach. As the number of patients at facilities swelled, asylum populations outgrew their funding, effectively decreasing staff-to-patient

*. The author acknowledges the contributions of Brian Falls, MD, who contributed as a coauthor to this chapter in the book's first edition.

ratios (de Young, 2010). Understaffed hospital units became progressively less equipped to manage their growing populations, and the quality of care provided deteriorated (Wright, 1997). After World War II (de Young, 2010; Torrey et al., 2010), the general public began to increasingly view psychiatric hospitals as cruel (de Young, 2010; Talbott, 2004), "run-down archaic establishments that simply housed the mentally ill" (Testa & West, 2010, p. 33).

Factors resulting in increased management of persons with mental illness in correctional settings

Deinstitutionalization and limited community resources

Increasing public attention to the inhumane conditions of these facilities, along with several other sociocultural and economic factors, led to a shift in the locus of care from public psychiatric hospitals to the community (Koyanagi, 2007). At its peak in 1955, there were 560,000 individuals living in state hospitals across America (Borus, 1981; Koyanagi, 2007; Talbott, 2004). By 2020, the state psychiatric hospital census had dramatically dropped to 40,000 patients (*Use of State Psychiatric Hospitals*, 2021). This movement of individuals from public hospitals into the community came to be known as "deinstitutionalization" (Borus, 1981; Lamb & Bachrach, 2001; Talbott, 2004).

As stated above, several factors led to this phenomenon. After World War II, the public's attention was increasingly drawn to the poor living conditions in state psychiatric hospitals (Scull, 1981). The late 1940s and early 1950s saw the introduction of far more effective treatments, such as lithium and chlorpromazine, which allowed physicians to release some patients safely to the community (de Young, 2010). In the 1960s, a subset of attorneys advocated for the "liberation" of patients from psychiatric hospitals (Geller, 2000; Scull, 1981).

The 1960s also saw the development of programs (e.g., Supplemental Security Income [SSI], Social Security Disability Insurance, Medicaid, and Medicare) that used federal dollars to provide financial assistance for people with mental illness in the community (Koyanagi, 2007). By and large, state hospital patients were not eligible for SSI or Medicaid (Gronfein, 1985). States discharged these patients, thereby shifting the financial burden from state-funded hospitals to these federally funded programs (Gronfein, 1985; Koyanagi, 2007; Searight & Handal, 1988).

Although the intent was to support independent living in the community, deinstitutionalization, in reality, resulted in homelessness and movement into various de facto psychiatric institutions for many patients (Koyanagi, 2007; Lamb & Weinberger, 1998; Searight & Handal, 1988; Szasz, 2007). Such institutions included correctional settings (Lamb & Weinberger, 2005; Talbott, 2004). Although scholars disagree whether a causal relationship exists (Osher & Han, 2002; Prins, 2011), many believe deinstitutionalization is the primary contributor to the growth of psychiatric disorders in jails and prisons (Lamb & Weinberger, 2005; Talbott, 2004). A retrospective study in the 1980s determined that available and appropriate treatment programs in the community were relevant to the success of deinstitutionalization (Braun et al., 1981). However, as state hospital populations transitioned back into communities, states did not sufficiently provide treatment to the ever-growing nonhospitalized population (Cameron, 1989; Koyanagi, 2007).

The U.S. Community Mental Health Act of 1963 provided federal grants to establish community mental health programs in anticipation of the discharge of state hospital patients (Koyanagi, 2007; Slovenko, 2003). Although it theoretically represented a reasonable idea, the program was underfunded (Koyanagi, 2007). President Reagan's Omnibus Budget Reconciliation Act of 1981 overturned the previous administration's Mental Health Systems Act and discontinued the federal government's direct provision of services to people with mental illness (Bazelon Center for Mental Health Law, 2011; Cameron, 1989). Federal mental health spending declined by nearly a third from 1980 to 1982 (Marmor & Gill, 1989). By 1985, the federal government funded only about 11% of community mental health agency budgets (Eichman et al., 1992). In addition, after the passage of 1973's Health Maintenance Organization Act, the growth of managed care organizations decreased inpatient lengths of stay (Parsons, 2006). Between 2009 and 2012, states cut $4.35 billion in public mental health funding, the largest reduction since deinstitutionalization (Glover et al., 2012). This detrimental tide of budget cuts for community mental health treatment has reversed over the last decade. For example, in 2013, the National Institutes for Health provided $2.1 billion in mental health funding, which grew to $4.4 billion in fiscal year 2024 (Mikulic, 2023).

Prominent court decisions and legislative policy

In the 1960s and 1970s, courts increased the threshold for civil commitment, enhancing the right to autonomy and increasing the difficulty of hospitalizing individuals (Perlin, 2007). As a result, involuntary hospitalizations decreased in frequency and duration (Peters et al., 1987). Some persons with mental illness who no longer met civil commitment criteria remained unaided in the community, some unwilling or unable to pursue outpatient treatment. This lack of access to care in the community increased the likelihood of criminal behavior by untreated persons with mental illness. Unsurprisingly, there was an associated growth in correctional populations. California exemplified this pattern; the number of people with psychiatric illness in one county jail doubled within a year of passing a new civil commitment statute, the eponymous Lanterman-Petris-Short Act (Abramson, 1972).

Meanwhile, legislators passed statutes promoting harsher sentencing. Led by Texas in 1974, most states enacted "three-strikes" laws (Tonry, 2013), while the federal government approved lengthy determinate sentences for drug offenders. Passage of drug-related laws throughout the years has led to inflation in drug-related incarcerations (Austin et al., 2000; Lurigio, 2000; Spencer, 1995). U.S. statutes criminalizing drug use and distribution date back a century, since the 1914 passage of the Harrison Act. The Anti-Drug Abuse Act of 1986 mandated a 5- to 40-year sentence, without parole, for first-time offenders convicted of possession with intent to distribute certain quantities of heroin, cocaine, phencyclidine, lysergic acid diethylamide (LSD), or marijuana (Spencer, 1995). The 1994 Violent Crime Control and Law Enforcement Act expanded the use of mandatory minimums for drug and drug-related offenses (Spencer, 1995). The number and duration of drug-related incarcerations have grown with these laws (Austin et al., 2000; Lurigio, 2000; Spencer, 1995) to the point where more than four out of five IPs have a history of drug use (Karberg & James, 2005; Karberg & Mumola, 2006). As the number of incarcerated drug users has risen, so too has the percentage of IPs with psychiatric and substance use diagnoses (Lurigio, 2000).

"Revolving door" incarcerations

The "revolving door" metaphor was initially used to describe frequent rehospitalizations and decreased durations of hospitalizations of homeless individuals with mental illness (Talbott, 1974). However, it has been readapted to reflect the frequent reincarceration of persons with mental illness (Baillargeon et al., 2009). One Texas study examined nearly 80,000 IPs from 2000 to 2006, finding that those with a serious mental illness (major depression, bipolar disorders, schizophrenia, and other psychotic disorders) were approximately twice as likely to be reincarcerated as their peers without these diagnoses (Baillargeon et al., 2009). These data are even more impressive when one considers that IPs with mental illness have fewer chances to commit new crimes that may result in reincarceration because they typically receive longer sentences and spend more time incarcerated than in the community. For example, IPs with mental illness in prison are incarcerated on average for 12 months longer than other offenders (Ditton, 1999).

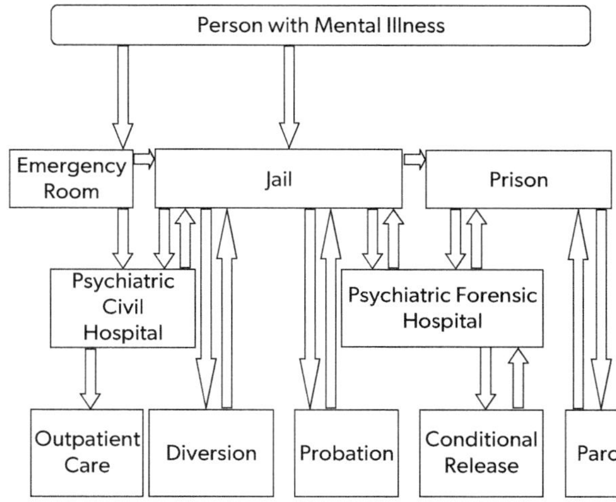

Figure 2.1 Entry and exit points between carceral and community settings.

Correctional and community care linkages

Correctional and community environments have important similarities and distinctions in the provision of mental health care. These two settings, however, are not isolated islands. In fact, persons with mental illness who face possible arrest may travel over interlinking bridges between correctional and community settings. Figure 2.1 outlines some potential entry and exit points between correctional and community care faced by persons with mental illness upon arrest; it is not exhaustive of all potential or likely combinations.

How and why an individual with mental illness enters a correctional setting instead of community treatment depends on factors that include criminal history, mental health history, local jurisdictional attitudes and approaches, police training, and, not infrequently, chance. Consider the following vignette:

> Joe is a 28-year-old man with bipolar disorder and alcohol and methamphetamine use. He lives with his mother and has been treated in the community with a mood stabilizer, which he frequently refuses to take. One evening, after snorting methamphetamine, he became paranoid that his mother was working with the FBI to have him killed. He confronted her; she told him he needed to take his medicine and then tried to call his doctor. He pushed her while grabbing for the phone, and she fell to the floor and bruised her arm. She called 911. When the police arrived, they noticed small bruises and a small cut on her arm. She acknowledged that Joe pushed her, which resulted in the injuries. Joe's mother begged the police to take Joe to the local emergency room because he "needs immediate treatment." She stated that she did not want to press charges, that her injuries were an accident, and that Joe had no intent to harm her.

At this point, the police play a critical role in how Joe's subsequent life will unfold. If they use their discretion and take Joe to the local emergency room instead of jail, Joe may be completely diverted from the criminal justice system. In contrast, if the police decide that Joe should be criminally charged for his actions, they will likely take him to the local jail or detention facility. Depending on Joe's local jurisdiction and available resources, he might be diverted to a mental health court or community treatment (see Chapter 6) or be kept in the jail awaiting charges, where he might not have access to inpatient psychiatric care. Due to Joe's mental illness, his attorney could question Joe's competency to stand trial. If Joe is found incompetent, he may be transferred to a state hospital in some jurisdictions (see Chapter 26), again crossing the threshold between corrections and community. If Joe is found nonrestorable, he might be released to the community for treatment or committed for a longer period, depending on whether he meets statutory criteria for continued commitment. If restored to competency, Joe would reenter the correctional system, where he could accept a plea bargain (if one is offered) or proceed to trial. Because Joe has a major mental illness, his attorney could raise the issue of his mental state and criminal responsibility if allowed by state statute.

If found not criminally responsible for his assault on his mother, Joe will likely return to a state hospital for continued commitment until he is determined safe for release. If found guilty, Joe may serve time in jail or prison. Some states would allow Joe to be involuntarily committed to a state hospital at the end of his prison term as a mentally disordered offender if his mental disorder played a substantial role in his crime and he continued to have symptoms that pose a risk of danger to others. If Joe does not qualify as a mentally disordered offender and is released from prison, he may have strict parole requirements to continue mental health treatment and refrain from using substances. If Joe violates his conditions of parole, he could be returned to prison. In some states, if Joe had committed a qualifying sexual offense, he could be evaluated to determine if he meets criteria for indefinite commitment as a sexually violent predator.

As the above vignette illustrates, incarcerated individuals may shuttle between correctional and community treatment systems, like a vehicle on a complicated highway with numerous on and off ramps and frequent detours. Despite this confusing maze of possibilities, there are several similarities and differences, summarized below, between the provision of correctional and community mental health care.

Similarities and differences between correctional and community mental health care

Standards of care

Both community and correctional mental health providers are expected to follow general standards of care. In addressing whether the standards should differ for incarcerated individuals, the American Psychiatric Association (2016, p. 6) stated:

> The fundamental policy goal for correctional mental health care is to provide the same level of mental health services to each patient in the criminal justice process that should be available in the community. This policy goal is deliberately higher than the "community standard" that is called for in various legal contexts.

Tort law governs the legal resolution of complaints about medical treatment and applies in both correctional and community settings. Negligent torts occur when a clinician's behavior unintentionally causes an unreasonable risk of harm to another. The four elements required to establish medical negligence are commonly known as the "four Ds": Dereliction of Duty that Directly results in Damages.

Correctional mental health care differs in the availability of additional legal mechanisms that IPs may use to address concerns about their care. For example, IPs may sue, claiming that the care provided, or not provided, violates their constitutional rights. In *Estelle v. Gamble* (1976), the U.S. Supreme Court attempted to define the constitutional standard of care for IPs in prison (see Chapter 3). J. W. Gamble was a sentenced prisoner who claimed that his constitutional rights were violated because, in part, an X-ray was not ordered to evaluate his complaint of back pain. The court in *Gamble* noted that, although a failure to conduct an X-ray or use additional diagnostic techniques may represent negligence, the presence of medical malpractice alone does not represent a constitutional violation. The court specifically stated, "Medical malpractice does not become a constitutional violation merely because the victim is a prisoner" (*Estelle v. Gamble*, 1976, p. 429). The court noted that a violation of an IP's constitutional rights was established if prison personnel demonstrated "deliberate indifference" to a prisoner's "serious illness or injury." In the subsequent case of *Farmer v. Brennan* (1994), the U.S. Supreme Court defined deliberate indifference as follows (p. 847):

> A prison official may be held liable under the Eighth Amendment for acting with "deliberate indifference" to inmate health or safety only if he knows that incarcerated persons face a substantial risk of danger of serious harm and disregards that risk by failing to take reasonable measures.

Provision of mental health care

There are many similarities between correctional and community mental health care services. Both systems typically provide appropriate medications, emergency care, hospitalization, medication management, and follow-up care. However, key differences often exist in correctional systems, including restricted formularies due to concerns of medication abuse or cost, alternative involuntary medication procedures, restricted access by visitors, and the inability of mental health providers to control the treatment environment (see Section III). In particular, decisions on the placement of IPs with mental illness may involve important custody considerations such as security level and potential for harm from other IPs (e.g., rival gang members or known enemies). Additional treatment considerations in custodial environments include increased limitations on confidentiality and "dual role" issues when correctional providers need to reveal information for IPs' discipline or placement evaluations (see Chapter 13).

Discharge and follow-up care

Correctional settings are increasingly expected to arrange follow-up care for released IPs. Several cases examining this expectation suggest the following guidelines (*Brad H v. City of New York*, 2000; *Lugo v. Senkowski*, 2000; *Wakefield v. Thompson*, 1999):

1. Provide psychiatric medications sufficient for an inmate to reasonably access a treating provider in the community;
2. Coordinate discharge planning and reentry into the community when feasible; and
3. Consider monitoring and further intervention necessary for treatment that is begun but not completed.

Such increasing expectations for correctional providers pose potential challenges because of key differences when compared to community settings. In particular, IPs' release is generally not under the control of the correctional provider, and in some circumstances, IPs may be released with little or no notice. In addition, depending on the location of the jail or prison, the correctional provider may have a limited, if any, relationship with community treatment providers, particularly when the IP returns to a community far from the correctional institution.

Summary

What began as a good-intentioned separation of criminals and people with mental illness in the late 18th century has ended in mass incarceration of individuals with psychiatric and substance use disorders. The population of incarcerated individuals with psychiatric illness continues to grow in the wake of deinstitutionalization, scant community resources, and a changing legal landscape. Many factors determine how and why individuals with mental illness are treated in correctional settings as opposed to community settings. There are numerous interlinking bridges between these two worlds. Understanding these multiple pathways is crucial for navigating the mental health care delivery systems inside and outside the walls of detention.

REFERENCES

Abramson, M. F. (1972). The criminalization of mentally disordered behavior: Possible side-effect of a new mental health law. *Hospital and Community Psychiatry*, *23*, 101–105.

American Psychiatric Association. (2016). *Psychiatric services in jails and prisons* (3rd ed.).

Austin, J., Clark, J., Hardyman, P., & Henry, D. A. (2000). *Three strikes and you're out: The implementation and impart of strike laws.* https://www.ncjrs.gov/pdffiles1/nij/grants/181297.pdf

Baillargeon, J., Binswanger, I. A., Penn, J. V., Williams, B. A., & Murray, O. J. (2009). Psychiatric disorders and repeat incarcerations: The revolving prison door. *American Journal of Psychiatry*, *166*(1), 103–109.

Bazelon Center for Mental Health Law. (2011). *Funding for mental health services and programs.* http://www.bazelon.org/LinkClick.aspx?fileticket=GzmAbAweikQ%3D&tabid=436

Beck, A. J., & Maruschak, L. M. (2000). *Mental health treatment in state prisons, 2000.* http://www.bjs.gov/content/pub/pdf/mhtsp00.pdf

Borus, J. F. (1981). Sounding Board. Deinstitutionalization of the chronically mentally ill. *New England Journal of Medicine*, *305*, 339–342.

Brad H v. City of New York, 712 N.Y.S.2d 336 (Sup. Ct. 2000); 716 N.Y.S.2d 852 (N.Y. App. Div. 2000).

Braun, P., Kochansky, G., Shapiro, R., Greenberg, S., Gudeman, J. E., Johnson,S.,&Shore,M.F.(1981).Overview:Deinstitutionalization of psychiatric patients, a critical review of outcome studies. *American Journal of Psychiatry*, *138*(6), 736–749.

Cameron, J. M. (1989). A national community mental health program: Policy initiation and progress. In D. Rochefort (Ed.), *Handbook on mental health policy in the United States* (pp. 121–142). Greenwood Press.

de Young, M. (2010). *Madness: An American history of mental illness and its treatment*. McFarland & Company.

Diamond, P. M., Wang, E. W., Holzer, C. E., Thomas, C., & Cruser, D. A. (2001). The prevalence of mental illness in prison. *Administration and Policy in Mental Health and Mental Health Services Research*, *29*(1), 21–40.

Ditton, P. M. (1999). *Mental health and treatment of incarcerated persons and probationers*. Bureau of Justice Statistics. http://www.bjs.gov/content/pub/pdf/mhtip.pdf

Eichman, M. A., Griffin, B. P., Lyons, J. S., Larson, D. B., & Finkel, S. (1992). An estimation of the impact of OBRA-87 on nursing home care in the United States. *Hospital & Community Psychiatry*, *43*(8), 781–789.

Eldridge, L. D. (1996). Crazy brained: Mental illness in colonial America. *Bulletin of the History of Medicine*, *70*(3), 361–386.

Estelle v. Gamble, 429 U.S. 97 (1976).

Farmer v. Brennan, 555 U.S. 825 (1994).

Geller, J. (2000). The last half-century of psychiatric services as reflected in Psychiatric Services. *Psychiatric Services*, *51*(1), 41–67.

Glover, R. W., Miller, J. E., & Sadowski, S. R. (2012). *Proceedings on the state budget crisis and the behavioral health treatment gap: The impact on public substance abuse and mental health treatment systems*. National Association of State Mental Health Program Directors. http://www.nasmhpd.org/docs/Summary-Congressional%20Briefing_March%2022_Website.pdf

Graham, K. A. (2008). *A history of the Pennsylvania Hospital*. History Press.

Gronfein, W. (1985). Psychotropic drugs and the origins of deinstitutionalization. *Social Problems*, *32*(5), 437–454.

Karberg, K. C., & James, D. J. (2005). *Substance dependence, abuse, and treatment of jail incarcerated persons, 2002* (NCJ 209588). Bureau of Justice Statistics. http://www.bjs.gov/content/pub/pdf/sdatji02.pdf

Karberg, K. C., & Mumola, C. J. (2006). *Drug use and dependence, state and federal prisoners, 2004* (NCJ 213530). Bureau of Justice Statistics. http://www.bjs.gov/content/pub/pdf/dudsfp04.pdf

Kessler, R. C., Chiu, W. T., Demler, O., & Walters, E. E. (2005). Prevalence, severity, and comorbidity of twelve-month DSM-IV disorders in the National Comorbidity Survey Replication (NCS-R). *Archives of General Psychiatry*, *62*(6), 617–627.

Koyanagi, C. (2007). *Learning from history: Deinstitutionalization of people with mental illness as precursor to long-term care reform*. Kaiser Commission on Medicaid and the Uninsured. http://www.nami.org/Template.cfm?Section=About_the_Issue&Template=/ContentManagement/ContentDisplay.cfm&ContentID=137545

Lamb, H. R., & Bachrach, L. L. (2001). Some perspectives on deinstitutionalization. *Psychiatric Services*, *52*(8), 1039–1045.

Lamb, H. R., & Weinberger, L. E. (1998). Persons with severe mental illness in jails and prisons: A review. *Psychiatric Services*, *49*, 483–492.

Lamb, H. R., & Weinberger, L. E. (2005). The shift of psychiatric inpatient care from hospitals to jails and prisons. *Journal of the American Academy of Psychiatry and the Law*, *33*(4), 529–534.

Lugo v. Senkowski, 114 F. Supp.2s 111 (N.D. N.Y. September 25, 2001).

Lurigio, A. J. (2000). Drug treatment availability and effectiveness: Studies of the general and criminal justice populations. *Criminal Justice and Behavior*, *27*(4), 495–528.

Marmor, T. R., & Gill, K. C. (1989). The political and economic context of mental health care in the United States. *Journal of Health Politics, Policy and Law*, *14*(3), 459–475.

Maruschak, L. M., Bronson, J., & Alper, A. (2021). *Indicators of mental health problems reported by prisoners; survey of prison inmates, 2016* (NCJ 252643). Bureau of Justice Statistics. https://bjs.ojp.gov/sites/g/files/xyckuh236/files/media/document/imhprpspi16st.pdf

Mikulic, M. (2023). *Total mental health funding by the National Institutes for Health (NIH) from FY 2013 to FY 2024 (2023)*. https://www.statista.com/statistics/716663/mental-health-funding-by-the-national-institutes-for-health/

Osher, F. C., & Han, Y. L. (2002). Jails as housing for persons with serious mental illness. *American Jails Magazine*, *16*(1), 36–41.

Parsons, T. (2006). Length of stay: Managed care agenda or a measure of clinical efficiency? *Psychiatry*, *3*(6), 46–52.

Perlin, M. L. (2007). *Mental disability law: Civil and criminal* (2nd ed.). LexisNexis.

Peters, R., Miller, K. S., Schmidt, W., & Meeter, D. (1987). The effects of statutory change on the civil commitment of the mentally ill. *Journal Law and Human Behavior*, *11*(2), 73–99.

Prins, S. J. (2011). Does transinstitutionalization explain the overrepresentation of people with serious mental illnesses in the criminal justice system? *Community Mental Health Journal*, *47*(6), 716–722.

Regier, D. A., Farmer, M. E., Rae, D. S., Locke, B. Z., Keith, S. J., Judd, L. L., & Goodwin, F. K. (1990). Comorbidity of mental disorders with alcohol and other drug abuse: Results from the Epidemiologic Catchment Area (ECA) study. *Journal of the American Medical Association*, *264*, 2511–2518.

Scull, A. (1981). Deinstitutionalization and the rights of the deviant. *Journal of Social Issues*, *37*(3), 6–20.

Searight, H. R., & Handal, P. J. (1988). The paradox of psychiatric deinstitutionalization: Historical perspective and policy implications. *Journal of Health and Human Resources Administration*, *11*(2), 249–266.

Slovenko, R. (2003). The transinstitutionalization of the mentally ill. *Ohio North University Law Review*, *29*(3), 641–660.

Spencer, M. P. (1995). Sentencing drug offenders: The incarceration addiction. *Villanova Law Review*, *40*(2), 335–381.

Steadman, H. J., Osher, F. C., Robbins, P. C., Case, B., & Samuels, S. (2009). Prevalence of serious mental illness among jail inmates. *Psychiatric Services*, *60*(6), 761–765.

Szasz, T. (2007). *Coercion as cure: A critical history of psychiatry*. Transaction.

Talbott, J. A. (1974). Stopping the revolving door: A study of readmissions to a state hospital. *Psychiatric Quarterly*, *48*, 159–168.

Talbott, J. A. (2004). Deinstitutionalization: Avoiding the disasters of the past (1979 reprint). *Psychiatric Services*, *55*(10), 1112–1115.

Testa, M., & West, S. G. (2010). Civil commitment in the United States. *Psychiatry*, *7*(10), 30–40.

Tonry, M. (2013). *Oxford handbook of crime and criminal justice*. Oxford University Press.

Torrey, E. F., Kennard, A. D., Eslinger, D., Lamb, R., & Pavle, J. (2010, May). *More mentally ill persons are in jails and prisons than hospitals: A survey of the states*. Treatment Advocacy Center and National Sheriffs' Association.

Use of state psychiatric hospitals: NRI's 2020-2021 state profiles. (2021). https://www.nri-inc.org/media/ju5ld0hx/nri_2020_profiles_-_use_of_state_psychiatric_hospitals-_september_2021.pdf
Wakefield v. Thompson, 177 F.3d 1160 (9th Cir. 1999).
Wright, D. (1997). Getting out of the asylum: Understanding the confinement of the insane in the nineteenth century. *Social History of Medicine*, *10*(1), 137–155.
Yohanna, D. (2013). Deinstitutionalization of people with mental illness: Causes and consequences. *American Medical Association Journal of Ethics*, *15*(10), 886–891.
Zwelling, S. S. (1985). *Quest for a cure: The public hospital in Williamsburg, Virginia, 1773–1885*. Colonial Williamsburg Foundation.

3

Formative case law and litigation

Mohamedu F. Jones

Introduction

While it is difficult to measure the accuracy of prevalence rates of incarcerated persons (IPs) with mental illness, according to the Prison Policy Initiative, over 40% of people in prisons and jails have been diagnosed with a mental health disorder (Prison Policy Initiative, 2022). Metzner and Fellner (2010) reported that the presence of comprehensive carceral mental health treatment programs and services is often due to successful class action litigation. This chapter reviews the legal and constitutional background for carceral mental health care in the United States and addresses many of the critical ways these courts affect policy and care delivery on a daily basis.

Background and precedent

Several court decisions have shaped modern carceral mental health care delivery in the United States. Under the Eighth Amendment, officials are obligated to provide convicted prisoners with adequate medical care (*Estelle v. Gamble*, 1976), which extends to mental health treatment (*Bowring v. Godwin*, 1977). Pretrial detainees also have a right to adequate physical and mental health care under the due process clause of the 14th Amendment (*Bell v. Wolfish*, 1979). To prevail on a claim of constitutionally inadequate care, IPs must show that officials acted with deliberate indifference. There are two components to proving deliberate indifference: the objective element (deprivation was sufficiently serious) and the subjective element (officials acted with a sufficiently culpable state of mind; *Farmer v. Brennan*, 1994; *Wilson v. Seiter*, 1991). In practice, given the similar high threshold of proof required to sustain a claim and the goal of adequate health care, the distinction of constitutional basis upon which the right rests between convicted prisoner and pretrial detainee makes little difference.

In 1996, acting under impressions that 42 U.S.C. § 1983 was being abused by frivolous prisoners' lawsuits and clogging up federal courts, and at the urging of several state and local law enforcement and correctional officials, Congress enacted the Prison Litigation Reform Act (PLRA, 1995) to regulate prisoners' litigation that involves federal constitutional rights and outcomes. Boston and Manville (2010, p. 1) described the PLRA as making "litigation by prisoners more difficult, more expensive and less likely to succeed." Provisions of the PLRA that support the authors' conclusion include the requirement for administrative exhaustion prior to filing a complaint and the payment of filing fees.

Limitations were also placed on courts, including restrictions on prospective relief judgments and the use of special masters in the PLRA. In cases where IPs prevail by proving constitutional violations and where a court orders a remedy, the PLRA grants prison officials the right to file a motion to terminate the remedial order at any point after 2 years. Once a motion to terminate is filed, the court has a maximum of 90 days to rule on the motion; otherwise, the remedial order is automatically stayed and is no longer in effect. In ruling on a motion to terminate, a court must find "current and ongoing" constitutional violations to maintain jurisdiction in the matter and enforce its remedial orders. In some instances, this has resulted in an entirely new trial.

The U.S. Supreme Court addressed involuntary transfers of IPs to psychiatric hospitals for acute care in *Vitek v. Jones* (1980). That decision determined that an IP may not be involuntarily transferred to a psychiatric hospital without the following: adequate notice that such a transfer is being considered; a written statement of why the transfer is proposed; and an adversarial hearing before an independent decision-maker, with appointed counsel if the IP cannot afford one. State law and regulations may impose more stringent requirements (see Chapter 26).

In *Washington v. Harper* (1990), the U.S. Supreme Court held that a convicted prisoner may be involuntarily medicated on a nonemergency basis if prison authorities can show that the medication is medically appropriate for treating a serious mental illness that has made the prisoner a danger to self or others. As with transfer to psychiatric hospitals, the standard for the use of involuntary medications is often more stringent based on state law and/or regulations (see Chapter 25).

Evolving legal issues

Since the U.S. Supreme Court proclaimed that IPs have a constitutional right to adequate health care, much has been written about the controlling decisions, their implications and applications by courts, and their implementation in carceral systems. There are, however, discrete issues related to mental health care in carceral settings that patients and providers contend with daily that may not yet be resolved as matters of constitutional law.

Decisions made by courts with limited jurisdiction or limited precedential value include the exclusion of persons with serious mental illness from restrictive housing, an obligation to fulfill discharge services or other forms of discharge planning, and the absence of health care quality improvement as evidence of deliberate indifference. Other areas, such as mental health input in the disciplinary process, clearly influence mental health conditions in institutions but may not necessarily rise to the level of constitutionally required care. In specific instances, notably the nature of structured and unstructured programming in restrictive housing, experienced carceral mental health experts have recommended specified minimum measures necessary for appropriate clinical care. Such measures may not be required by law but support delivery of quality mental health care. A legal overview of these issues is provided in the following sections.

Mental health input in the disciplinary process

The U.S. Supreme Court has held that, following a disciplinary infraction, IPs who violate the rules are not entitled to the full body of constitutional protections in prison disciplinary proceedings available in criminal prosecutions. Minimally, they must be afforded a hearing, timely notice of the offense, and an opportunity to call witnesses and present documentary evidence. Under certain circumstances in the disciplinary proceedings, a counsel substitute or staff assistance may be required to ensure due process protections for IPs.

IPs with mental illness are frequently involved in the disciplinary process because of rule infractions. Mental illness may contribute to the violation; some IPs were psychotic at the time of their rule violation. Legal experts have not identified mental health input in the disciplinary process as a specific requirement of a constitutionally adequate prison mental health care system. No court decision has found IPs with serious mental illness to have a constitutional right to mental health evaluations as part of a prison's disciplinary process. Although it does not appear to be constitutionally required, multiple correctional systems provide for mental health input in their disciplinary process.

Dvoskin and colleagues (1995) have noted, however, that *Powell v. Coughlin* (1991) held that IPs have no right to formal mental health evaluations before undergoing disciplinary hearings. The court in *Matz v. Vandenbook* (2013) questioned whether there was any legal ground that would support a federal court prohibiting prison officials from punishing "prisoners for behavior they cannot control."

Successful lawsuits have resulted in court-ordered or court-approved inclusion of mental health input in the disciplinary process in California, New Jersey, and New York. In *D.M. v. Terhune* (1999), the New Jersey Department of Corrections was required to implement disciplinary regulations to mandate mental health input in the process and to consider whether to refer the IP to a mental health program instead of imposing disciplinary sanctions.

In New York, a court ruling initially required mental health input in the prison disciplinary process. Subsequently, the state amended its regulations to incorporate the court-ordered procedures that require mental health input in the disciplinary process and consideration by the hearing officer of the mental illness of the IP when determining whether to dismiss, find guilty, or reduce the penalty imposed.

The court in *Coleman v. Wilson* (1995) subsequently approved a comprehensive mental health policy and procedure program that included provision of clinical input in the disciplinary process and permitted the hearing officer discretion to consider mental health conditions in mitigation of punishment. The American College of Correctional Physicians (2013) recommends that correctional systems include mental health input in their disciplinary processes.

While it may not be a constitutional right, many carceral mental health experts find mental health input in disciplinary proceedings to be relevant to overall mental health care in institutions and recommend that it form a part of the process. They emphasize, however, that mental health input should not cross a forensic boundary and directly address responsibility for the action. They argue that doing so could create circumstances where the mental health staff become the ultimate decision-makers of culpability. In addition, the National Commission on Correctional Health Care (2016) cautions against health professionals determining an IP's physical or psychological fitness for restrictive housing—a frequent outcome of the disciplinary process.

Obegi (2021, p. 318) has identified what he characterized as "some of the more salient challenges, such as crafting a test of nonresponsibility, identifying which inmates are eligible for assessments of disciplinary responsibility, and addressing professional dilemmas related to the assessment process." Even in the face of these challenges, Tamburello and Haston (2021, p. 323) are unequivocal in their advocacy of mental health input in the disciplinary process: "There should be mental health input into a correctional disciplinary process when an inmate's mental illness may have been a factor."

Mental health care in restrictive housing

In *Palakovic v. Wetzel* (2017), the United States Court of Appeals for the Third Circuit specifically acknowledged the legal and scientific authority recognizing adverse mental health consequences caused by long-term isolation in solitary confinement. There is significant consensus around the risks associated with placing IPs with serious mental illness in segregated housing. A position statement by the American Psychiatric Association (2023) states the following:

> Restrictive housing of incarcerated adults with serious mental illness, with rare exceptions that involve significant danger to others, should be avoided due to the potential for harm to such individuals. If an individual with serious mental illness is placed in restrictive housing, in which one is confined to a cell for 22 or more hours per day, out-of-cell structured therapeutic activities (e.g., mental health/psychiatric treatment) in appropriate programming space and regular unstructured out-of-cell time should be provided to maximize access to clinically indicated programming, treatment, recreation and transfer to a more therapeutic settings [*sic*].

The American College of Correctional Physicians (2013) similarly endorses the exclusion of IPs with serious mental illness from prolonged placement in restrictive housing (i.e., more than 4 weeks).

A substantial body of law continues to evolve on this point. *Braggs v. Dunn* (2019) held that both mental health and carceral professionals have recognized that "long-term isolation resulting from segregation or solitary confinement has crippling consequences for mental health" (p. 1344). The *Braggs* court held that, except in "extenuating circumstances," it was "categorically inappropriate to place prisoners with serious mental illness in segregation" (*Braggs v. Dunn*, 2019, p. 1346). The court in *Madrid v. Gomez* (1995) had earlier held that it is constitutional to place an IP in disciplinary or security segregation for legitimate penological reasons, but it is unlawful to subject IPs in segregation to systematic psychological deprivations, extreme social isolation, and reduced environmental stimulation.

The *Madrid* court excluded IPs from the secured housing units at Pelican Bay State Prison in California who were at a "particularly high risk for suffering very serious or severe injury to their mental health, including overt paranoia, psychotic breaks with reality, or massive exacerbations of existing mental illness" as a result of the conditions in the secured housing unit (*Madrid v. Gomez*, 1995, p. 1266). The *Braggs* court concluded that appropriate mental health staff must be involved in and approve the placement of persons with serious mental illness in restrictive housing and that those IPs "should be moved out of segregation as soon as possible" (*Braggs v. Dunn*, 2019, p. 1347).

Braggs also recognized that appropriate care must be provided when IPs with mental illness are placed in restrictive housing. In *Madrid*, the court found that there was a need for "substantial psychiatric services" in the secured housing unit at Pelican Bay. In a number of systems encountered by the author, policy mandated the minimum clinical and psychiatric contact that had to occur within designated timeframes. In addition, updated treatment plans, including psychotropic medication therapy, had to be completed at specified time intervals.

In assessing whether adequate care is provided in a restrictive housing unit, the court in *Indiana Protection and Advocacy Services Commission v. Commissioner, Indiana Department of Corrections* (2012) pointed out that appropriate mental health treatment in administrative segregation is different from mere mental health monitoring. In the author's experience, ongoing cell-front clinical contacts performed in a perfunctory manner by mental health clinical staff in restrictive housing units, particularly for policy-mandated minimal periodic clinical services, are inadequate irrespective of the reasons. IPs in restrictive housing may sometimes refuse to come out of the cell for reasons directly related to their mental illness, or clinicians may feel compelled to interview patients at the cell front because of high caseloads. IPs may also be seen at the cell front for custody reasons, such as security lockdowns or insufficient escort officers. None of these reasons justify the continued use of the cell front as the default location for clinical interventions by mental health clinicians in a locked unit.

Metzner and Dvoskin (2006) identified screening as a required standard of appropriate care to exclude those suffering from severe mental illness from restrictive housing (where such exclusion is required or permitted) and divert them to special mental health programs, where available. Screenings and timely evaluations are necessary to recognize mental health problems and monitor for any deterioration of mental status because of the conditions. In *Braggs*, the court found that defendants did not have "an effective system for evaluating mental-health risks both when deciding whether to place prisoners in segregation and when determining the length of a segregation placement" (*Braggs v. Dunn*, 2019, p. 1346). IPs in restrictive housing require frequent and ongoing monitoring, which *Morgan v. Rowland* (2006) and *Braggs* recognized must include appropriate rounding on each IP placed there.

Treatment plans must be individualized and preferably developed by a multidisciplinary treatment team. In *Troy v. State of Colorado* (2013), the district court endorsed the need for a multidisciplinary treatment team to include a psychiatrist, while pointing out it could not order it. The author has jointly observed treatment teams with carceral mental health experts in restrictive housing. Observations focused on the composition and involvement of members of the treatment team, including whether or not the assigned primary clinician, psychiatrist, and correctional staff were present and interactive in the multidisciplinary team meeting.

During these observations, we looked for the presence of the patient in the treatment team meeting and whether the patient had an opportunity to participate meaningfully. We noted the availability and use of medical, mental health, and custody records during the meeting. Other areas we measured while observing treatment teams included the presentation by the primary treating clinician; references to and discussions regarding prescribed psychotropic medications, if any; and the individualization and relevance of the treatment plan to diagnosis and treatment goals. We also looked at therapeutic group assignments, if indicated, and their clinical relationships to treatment goals. As observers, we were attentive to whether the treatment team considered a change in the level of care where appropriate, including the need for admission to inpatient care if clinically indicated.

Carceral mental health care experts also emphasize that adequate treatment in restrictive housing units must include sufficient hours of structured out-of-cell therapeutic and unstructured or recreation activities. Metzner and Dvoskin (2006) recommend structured out-of-cell therapeutic activities for at least 10 to 15 hours per week in addition to at least 10 hours of unstructured or recreation activities. The American College of Correctional Physicians (2013) recommends that adequate out-of-cell structured therapeutic activities and adequate time for outdoor exercise in appropriately designed areas should be provided to IPs in restrictive housing.

Other core standards of appropriate care in locked units are suicide prevention protocols such as periodic documented welfare checks that are staggered and not predictable. Welfare checks are observations of affirmative indicators of a "living body." These checks may last for a designated initial period or throughout a stay in restrictive housing.

Discharge planning

Most states provide some form of mental health care discharge planning. In a survey of 43 states, La Vigne and colleagues (2008) found that most states provided discharge medications, with a significantly smaller number of states also making referrals and/or appointments for postrelease health care services. The U.S. Supreme Court, however, has not found a constitutional duty to provide health care after a person is released from incarceration. Specifically, the Supreme Court in *DeShaney v. Winnebago City Department of Social Services* (1989) pointedly declared that any constitutional obligation to provide services to persons in custody is limited to the period during which they are in custody.

The Ninth Circuit Court of Appeals in *Wakefield v. Thompson* (1999) held that carceral officials have an affirmative duty to provide discharge service by providing medications at the time of release for a very limited duration. The court reasoned that the IP's practical ability to secure medication is not immediately restored upon release from prison. Relying on *Wakefield*, the court in *United States v. County of L.A.* (2016) expressly found that there was no reason the same principle laid out in the *Wakefield* case should not apply to mental illness.

The Third Circuit Court of Appeals in *Charles v. Orange County* (2019) vacated the dismissal by a lower court of detainees' claim of deprivation of their constitutional right to a level of continuity of care following their discharge from custody, remanding the matter for further proceedings. The appellate court found the detainees' claim that providing them postrelease services, such as interim medications and referrals, was a required function of constitutionally mandated treatment while in custody to be "plausible." Appelbaum (2020, p. 441) appropriately described *Charles* as the "clearest statement to date of a broader state duty, based on the federal Constitution, to conduct adequate discharge planning before release from a correctional facility." Appelbaum further observed that the *Charles* decision may give rise to "proactive efforts by the states to come into compliance with generally accepted standards so as to avoid having to confront allegations of a failure to … [provide adequate discharge planning] in federal court" (p. 441).

Gilbert v. County of Los Angeles (2022) found that the constitutional obligation of a correctional institution to provide adequate discharge planning is equivalent to its obligation to provide adequate medical and mental health care while an individual is in its custody. In *Brad H v. City of New York* (2000), which remains perhaps the most extensive and far-ranging discharge planning court decision to date, the city consented to providing treatment and supportive services to IPs with mental illness following their release. In addition to psychiatric treatment, which includes outpatient treatment and medications, the city agreed to assist with housing and, in cases of indigence, with the means to obtain services. *Brad H* is distinguishable from non–New York state cases because the principles of institutional mental health care and discharge planning undergirding the settlement agreement in the case were based on New York state statutory and case law.

Despite its limited precedential legal value, *Brad H* may offer a useful blueprint to systems seeking to expand postrelease services to IPs. It may also serve as a valuable aid in negotiations as a framework for effective settlement of postdischarge planning litigation. Carceral officials may also be able to use *Brad H* to formulate policies for the regulation of effective discharge services as clinically indicated for their patients. Mental health staff could potentially use *Brad H* as a practical guide for articulating discharge instructions permissible under institutional policies.

Quality improvement in mental health care

Measuring the quality of care in mental health involves assessments of whether the services provided consistently achieve the desired outcomes in the mental health program (see Chapter 74). Hermann and colleagues (2002) found that fundamental principles of effective quality care models involve monitoring and evaluating processes and outcomes to compare current practice with evidence-based treatment guidelines and outcomes with accepted benchmarks.

From their review of international research on quality indicators and performance measures in the prison setting, Bellas and colleagues (2022) concluded that, as a function of an effective quality improvement system, carceral establishments should develop robust evidence-based indicators that allow for both internal and external comparisons. As performance measurements, these indicators would enable correctional systems to monitor the quality of care they provide and appropriately identify areas for improvement. In addition to the capacity to identify opportunities for improvement, an effective quality improvement system must also have the capacity to develop and implement desired changes.

Several federal district courts have articulated that quality improvement plays an essential role in providing adequate health care in carceral systems. *Grubbs v. Bradley* (1993), *Madrid v. Gomez* (1995), and *Coleman v. Wilson* (1995) identified quality improvement systems as part of the remedy to findings of constitutionally inadequate carceral health care by a court. *Coleman* and *Madrid* held specifically that a correctional system cannot provide adequate mental health care without quality improvement. In *Madrid*, the court found the absence of a functional quality improvement system to be a systemic deficiency and to constitute deliberate indifference. *Grubbs* held that "an appropriate quality assurance plan" was "indispensable" to remedy systemic deficiencies in carceral systems.

In both *Grubbs* and *Coleman*, the court required the development of system-wide quality improvement programs as part of the remedial action plan. In *Plata v. Schwarzenegger* (2008, p. 1092), which involved medical care provided in the California correctional system, the court held that "[a] meaningful peer review procedure is a necessary component of a constitutionally adequate health care system." In *Lewis v. Cain* (2021, p. 51), the court held that the prison's "failure to engage in meaningful quality improvement program and analysis," coupled with other defects, constituted evidence of a constitutional violation.

Laube v. Campbell (2004) emphasized that quality improvement systems implemented in carceral settings must be consistent with nationally accepted standards. *Hadix v. Johnson* (2002) and *Laube* recognized continuous quality improvement (CQI) as an effective model for quality improvement in carceral systems. The *Hadix* court approvingly observed that CQI is widely used in large organizations. Also, the court distinguished CQI from traditional quality assurance, which relies on peer reviews and case audits to evaluate individual performance related to fixed outcome measures to discover and eliminate ineffective individual clinical practices. In contrast, the court characterized CQI as one of the most effective long-term strategies for enhancing quality "by analyzing and adjusting major systems in a never-ending quest for improvement" (*Hadix v. Johnson*, 2002, p. 300). The *Hadix* court specifically recognized that effective CQI is dependent on management information systems that systematically gather and analyze information.

Laube described an appropriate carceral CQI system as one with capacities to quantify performance indicators, analyze them for "opportunities for improvement," and expeditiously implement remedies. The indicators would then be reassessed to measure the results of interventions as part of an ongoing process of assessing corrective action plans, with the objective of preventing future adverse outcomes.

The author has participated in the development of an information management–based CQI system from initial discussions, design, and beta testing through piloting and expected roll-out. The benefits of an effective quality improvement system include assisting in the provision of adequate patient care and supervision, as well as the potential to inoculate a system against litigation.

Summary

Many of the developments in U.S. carceral laws and standards discussed here have been formulated by lower courts and/or advanced by carceral mental health experts. To date, appellate reviews remain sparse, leaving open final resolution of multiple issues. Nevertheless, case law and litigation continue to drive innovations in standards of care and improve the quality of carceral mental health. These reforms have gained wider acceptance as preferred and expected standards of carceral mental health care in jails and prisons and reflect the present-day "evolving standard of decency," in turn becoming touchstones of constitutionally adequate health care across systems.

REFERENCES

American College of Correctional Physicians. (2013). *Position statement regarding restricted housing of mentally ill inmates.* https://accpmed.org/restricted_housing_of_mentally.php

American Psychiatric Association. (2023). *Position statement regarding restrictive housing of incarcerated adults with serious mental illness.* https://www.psychiatry.org/getattachment/de02560f-34fd-420b-b36a 257f1450558a/Position-Restrictive-Housing-of-Adults.pdf

Appelbaum, P. S. (2020). *Discharge planning in correctional facilities: A constitutional right?* https://ps.psychiatryonline.org/doi/10.1176/appi.ps.202000084

Bell v. Wolfish, 441 U.S. 520 (1979).

Bellass, S., Canvin, K., McLintock, K., et al. (2022) Quality indicators and performance measures for prison healthcare: A scoping review. *Health Justice, 10*, 13.

Available at: https://doi.org/10.1186/s40352-022-00175-9

Boston, J., & Manville, D. (2010). *Prisoners' self-help litigation manual.* Oxford University Press.

Bowring v. Godwin, 551 F.2d 44 (4th Cir. 1977).

Brad H v. City of New York, 185 Misc 2d 420 (Sup. Ct. N.Y. County 2000).

Braggs v. Dunn, 367 F. Supp. 3d 1340 (2019).

Charles v. Orange Cnty., 925 F.3d 73 (2d Cir. 2019).

Coleman v. Wilson, 912 F. Supp. 1282, 1308 (E.D. Cal. 1995).

DeShaney v. Winnebago Cty. Dep't of Soc. Servs., 489 U.S. 189 (1989).

D.M. v. Terhune, 67 F. Supp. 2d 401 (D.N.J. 1999).

Dvoskin, J. A., Petrila, J., & Stark-Riemer, S. (1995). Powell v. Coughlin and the application of the professional judgment rule to prison mental health. *Mental and Physical Disability Law Reporter, 19*(1), 108–114.

Estelle v. Gamble, 429 U.S. 97 (1976).

Farmer v. Brennan, 511 U.S. 825 (1994).

Gilbert v. Cntv. of Los Angeles, 2022 U.S. Dist. LEXIS 234978 (2022).

Grubbs v. Bradley, 821 F. Supp 496 (M.D. Tenn. 1993).

Hadix v. Johnson, 2002 LEXIS 21283 213, 300 (S.D. Mich. 2002).

Hermann, R. C., Leff, S. H., & Logodmos, G. (2002). *Selecting process measures for quality improvement in mental healthcare.* Center for Mental Health Services.

Indiana Prot. & Advocacy Servs. Comm'n v. Comm'r, Ind. Dep't of Corr., 2012 U.S. Dist. LEXIS 182974 (S.D. Ind. Dec. 31, 2012).

La Vigne, N., Davies, E., Palmer, T., & Halberstadt, R. (2008). *Release planning for successful reentry: A guide for corrections, service providers, and community groups.* Urban Institute Justice Policy Center. http://www.urban.org/UploadedPDF/411767_successful_reentry.pdf

Laube v. Campbell, 333 F. Supp. 2d 1234, 1263 (M.D. Ala. 2004).

Lewis v. Cain, CIVIL DOCKET NO.: 3:15-CV-318 (M.D. La. Mar. 31, 2021).

Madrid v. Gomez, 889 F. Supp. 1146 (N.D. Cal. 1995); rev'd in part on other grounds 190 F.3d 990 (9th Cir. 1999).

Matz v. Vandenbrook, 2013 U.S. Dist. LEXIS 116930 (W.D. Wis. Aug. 19, 2013).

Metzner, J. L., & Dvoskin, J. (2006). An overview of correctional psychiatry. *Psychiatric Clinics of North America, 29*(3), 761–772.

Metzner, J. L., & Fellner, J. (2010). Solitary confinement and mental illness in U.S. prisons: A challenge for medical ethics. *Journal of the American Academy of Psychiatry and the Law, 38*(1), 104–108.

Morgan v. Rowland, 2006 U.S. Dist. LEXIS 11081 (D. Conn. Mar. 17, 2006).

National Commission on Correctional Health Care. (2016). *Position statement: Solitary confinement (isolation).* https://www.ncchc.org/position-statements/solitary-confinement-isolation-2016/

Obegi, J. H. (2021). Disciplinary responsibility in prison. *Journal of the American Academy of Psychiatry and the Law, 49*(3), 316–322.

Palakovic v. Wetzel. 854 F.3d 209 (3d Cir. 2017).

Plata v. Schwarzenegger, 556 F. Supp. 2d 1087 (N.D. Cal. 2008).

Powell v. Coughlin. 953 F.2d 744 (2d Cir. 1991).

Prison Litigation Reform Act of 1995 (PLRA), 18 U.S.C. § 3626 (1995).

Prison Policy Initiative. (2022). *Chronic punishment: The unmet health needs of people in state prisons.* https://www.prisonpolicy.org/reports/chronicpunishment.html#mentalhealth

Tamburello, A. C., & Haston, L. (2021). Mischief, mayhem and remediation. *Journal of the American Academy of Psychiatry and the Law, 49*, 323–325.

Troy v. State of Colorado, Civil Action No. 10-cv-01005-RBJ-KMT (Col. August 24, 2012), http://solitarywatch.com/wp-content/uploads/2012/08/troy-anderson-v-colorado-doc.pdf

United States v. County of L.A., Case No. CV 15-05903 DDP (JEMx) (2016).

Vitek v. Jones, 445 U.S. 480 (1980).

Wakefield v. Thompson, 177 F.3d 1160 (9th Cir. 1999).

Washington v. Harper, 494 U.S. 210 (1990).

Wilson v. Seiter, 501 U.S. 294 (1991).

4

Human rights

Jamie Fellner and Mohamedu F. Jones

Introduction

The participation of mental health professionals in the interrogation and torture of incarcerated persons (IPs) at Guantanamo led to renewed attention in the United States to their ethical and human rights responsibilities, particularly with regard to the treatment of involuntarily detained persons (Institute on Medicine as a Profession, 2013; Physicians for Human Rights & School of Public Health and Primary Health Care, University of Cape Town Health Sciences Faculty, 2003). Many correctional mental health professionals are unaware of the human rights codified in international treaties—rights that are applicable to correctional policies and practices. This chapter provides an overview of several crucial human rights that should guide their work.

The touchstone of human rights is the dignity of all persons. Human rights treaties to which the United States is a party or a signatory codify the rights that flow from the recognition of human dignity and that public officials must respect in policy and seek to realize in practice. Human rights complement and expand on the ethical principles of beneficence and nonmaleficence.

The human rights framework

In 1948, the international community affirmed the inherent dignity and the equal and inalienable fundamental rights of all persons with the Universal Declaration of Human Rights (United Nations [UN], 1948). Subsequent international and regional treaties codified a range of human rights and established compliance and oversight mechanisms. Treaty bodies, UN-appointed special rapporteurs, and other UN and international entities, academic experts, and nongovernmental organizations have interpreted and applied the treaties in authoritative decisions, statements of principle, rules, guidelines, and reports (Coyle, 2002). They have given special attention to the treatment of people who are involuntarily confined in correctional facilities because of their unique vulnerability to abuse. The single most comprehensive delineation of the human rights standards applicable to carceral systems is the UN Standard Minimum Rules for the Treatment of Prisoners, updated and revised in 2015 and now known as the Nelson Mandela Rules in honor of the late former South African president (UN, 2015; hereafter Mandela Rules).

Several interrelated human rights are particularly relevant to the work of correctional health professionals, including the rights to mental health treatment and rehabilitation; the right to life; the right to freedom from torture or other cruel, inhuman, or degrading treatment or punishment; and the right to be free of discrimination based on disability. These rights are affirmed in the International Covenant on Civil and Political Rights (ICCPR; UN, 1966a); the Convention Against Torture and Other Cruel, Inhuman, or Degrading Treatment or Punishment (CAT; UN, 1984); the International Covenant on Economic, Social and Cultural Rights (ICESCR; UN, 1966b); and the Convention on the Rights of Persons With Disabilities (CRPD; UN, 2006). As a party to the ICCPR and CAT, the United States is bound to comply with them, and as a signatory to the ICESCR and the CRPD, the United States must refrain from action that undermines their purpose. These obligations apply to federal, state, and local agencies.

Dignity

The ICCPR states that persons deprived of their liberty "shall be treated with humanity and with respect for the inherent dignity of the human person" (UN, 1966a). This is not an optional directive, nor is it one that officials can violate on budgetary or staffing grounds (UN Human Rights Committee, 1992). Prisoners retain their dignity and their human rights while incarcerated, with restrictions on those rights permitted only to the extent required by the fact of incarceration itself.

The right to health and rehabilitation

Governments must respect IPs' right to health, which embraces both physical and mental health and well-being. They must protect and promote health needs through policies and practices, including by providing the facilities, staff, and services necessary to meet those needs and by protecting prisoners from unhealthy or dangerous conditions. The health care services should pay particular attention to prisoners with special health care needs that may hamper their rehabilitation (Mandela Rules, R. 25.1). Correctional authorities must provide medical services that "seek to detect and treat physical or mental illnesses or defects from which prisoners may suffer," and "all necessary medical, surgical and psychiatric services including those available in the community shall be provided to the prisoner for that purpose" (Council of Europe Committee of Ministers, 2020, p. 12). The standards of mental health care in a prison should be the same as community standards (UN Committee on Economic, Social and Cultural Rights, 2000; Mandela Rules, R. 24). Mental health staff in prisons should have the same qualifications and credentials as required for mental health care in community settings and should be able to provide treatment with full clinical independence. When the medical condition of an IP deteriorates, prison authorities must act promptly and diligently to identify the illness and initiate appropriate therapy (Abramsky & Fellner, 2003; European Committee for the Prevention of Torture and Inhuman or Degrading Treatment or Punishment, 2011; *Kolesnikovich v. Russia*, 2022). IPs should be transferred to other facilities—carceral or civilian—if the facility in which they are incarcerated does not have the staffing and resources to provide the specialized mental health care appropriate to their needs (Abramsky & Fellner, 2003; *Sy v. Italy*, 2022).

In the carceral context, the right to health is closely linked to the recognition of every IP's potential for change, growth, redemption, and rehabilitation.

> The purposes of a sentence of imprisonment … are primarily to protect society against crime and to reduce recidivism. Those purposes can be achieved only if the period of imprisonment is used to ensure, so far as possible, the reintegration of such persons into society upon release so that they can lead a law-abiding and self-supporting life. (Mandela Rules, R. 4, p. 8)

Mental health professionals should play a crucial role in the rehabilitation of prisoners with, or at risk of developing, mental illnesses and disorders. The right of IPs to adequate mental health treatment is often breached in U.S. correctional facilities.

The right to be free of abuse

Article 7 of the ICCPR prohibits torture and other cruel, inhuman, or degrading treatment or punishment (Fellner, 2015; UN, 1966a). The CAT requires parties to the treaty to

> ensure that education and information regarding the prohibition against torture are fully included in the training of … medical personnel … who may be involved in the custody, interrogation or treatment of any individual subjected to any form of arrest, detention or imprisonment(Article 10.1)

and that "the prohibition be included in the rules or instructions issued in regard to the duties and function of any such person" (UN, 1984, Article 10.2). This prohibition is consistent with the Mandela Rules (R. 32). Health care professionals must document and report cases of torture or cruel, inhuman, or degrading treatment or punishment by any staff to the appropriate medical and administrative authorities (Mandela Rules, R. 34).

The CAT defines torture as

> any act by which severe pain or suffering, whether physical or mental, is intentionally inflicted on a person … by or at the instigation of or with the consent or acquiescence of a public official or other person acting in an official capacity. (UN, 1984, Article 1.1)

The prohibition addresses a continuum of acts inflicting different degrees of pain or suffering, and any ill treatment on that continuum is prohibited (Fellner, 2015). Any act by prison staff that inflicts acute physical or mental suffering beyond that inherent in incarceration may be impermissible.

Authorized prison practices and programs may constitute prohibited abuse. For example, indefinite solitary confinement or the extensive use of pepper spray during a cell extraction constitutes prohibited mistreatment, especially when used against an IP with mental illness (Fellner, 2015). To be consistent with human rights requirements, control and restraint measures should only be used when they are necessary and are the least restrictive option to protect the life or well-being of the IP, other IPs, or staff.

Insufficient, inappropriate, or untimely mental health treatment can also constitute prohibited treatment, whether it is deliberate or the result of negligence, oversight, or ignorance. As the European Committee for the Prevention of Torture and Inhuman or Degrading Treatment or Punishment (2011, p. 38) has noted, inadequate health care can "lead rapidly to situations falling within the scope of the term 'inhuman and degrading treatment.'" The touchstone is the suffering endured by the IP and whether staff's conduct, which includes lack of treatment, caused or aggravated that suffering.

International and national medical organizations have affirmed the ethical obligation of physicians to refrain from countenancing, condoning, participating in, or facilitating torture or other forms of cruel, inhuman, or degrading treatment (American Medical Association, 2022; World Medical Association, 2006; World Psychiatric Association, 1996). Also, in 2022, the National Commission on Correctional Health Care (NCCHC, 2022, p. 1) updated its position statement that correctional health professionals should "not participate in or condone any form of mistreatment of incarcerated people."

When staff know an IP is suffering from a disorder that may make them particularly vulnerable to suicide, staff must do everything that could reasonably be expected to prevent it (*Edwards v. United Kingdom*, 2002; *Renolde v. France*, 2008).

Nondiscrimination based on disability

Many of the provisions of the CRPD are relevant for IPs with mental disabilities (UN, 2006). The CRPD affirms that all persons with any type of disability, including those deprived of their liberty, must enjoy all human rights and fundamental freedoms. Public officials must ensure reasonable accommodation for persons with disabilities, including IPs. The lack of such accommodation in detention facilities is likely to increase the risk of neglect, violence, abuse, torture, and ill treatment (UN General Assembly, 2013). The CRPD also prohibits the abuse and exploitation of persons with disabilities and recognizes the right of every person with disabilities to respect for their physical and mental integrity.

Coping with incarceration can challenge anyone, but IPs with mental disabilities, particularly if they are not receiving appropriate mental health treatment, struggle more than others to adjust to the extraordinary stresses of incarceration, to follow the rules governing every aspect of life, and to respond promptly and fully to staff orders. They may violate carceral rules by refusing to follow orders and by engaging in symptomatic behavior deemed misconduct that warrants punishment, other sanctions, or removal from the general carceral population to a restrictive housing unit (RHU). IPs with mental illness are sanctioned more frequently for disciplinary infractions, subjected to force by carceral staff more frequently than other IPs, and disproportionately isolated in restrictive housing (Fellner, 2015). The mental health care in U.S. carceral systems too often fails to protect the rights of IPs with mental disabilities, which has resulted in relevant successful class action litigation (Metzner, 2002).

Special problem: The use of force against incarcerated persons with mental illness

Carceral staff are authorized to use force to protect the safety and security of the carceral facility. But under international human rights law (as well as the U.S. Constitution), force against any IP should only be used when and to the extent necessary as a last resort and never as punishment. When force is used needlessly, excessively, or punitively, it violates the human right prohibition against torture or other cruel, inhuman, or degrading treatment. It often reflects the failure of carceral authorities to accommodate the needs of IPs with mental disabilities.

Research shows, however, that carceral staff frequently respond with violence when IPs with mental illness engage in minor nonthreatening misconduct, such as urinating on the floor, using profane language, or banging on a cell door. Force has also been used where there is a genuine immediate need to control an IP, but the amount of force was excessive to the need or continued after the IP was brought under control. Such inappropriate use of force has included use of chemical sprays and electric stun guns, prolonged placement in restraint chairs, and physical abuse (Fellner, 2015). For example, in a case involving the repeated use of chemical agents against IPs with mental illness, a court concluded, "If an inmate is gassed when he cannot control his action due to his mental illness, then the force no longer has a necessary penological purpose and becomes brutality" (*Thomas v. Bryant*, 2010, p. 1311). When IPs are unable or unwilling to stop acutely dangerous behavior, carceral policies often permit custody staff to temporarily immobilize them in full body restraints. Such restraints should only be used in extreme and exigent circumstances and as a last resort.

Physical abuse against IPs with mental illness is not inevitable. It is more likely in facilities that lack sufficient mental health services and/or staff to help preclude or mitigate IPs' misconduct. Despite the prevalence of mental illness in carceral populations, custodial staff often do not receive appropriate training regarding the nature of mental illness and how it can affect behavior, and they are infrequently required to use verbal de-escalation techniques or to seek the help of mental health staff when IPs with mental illness engage in misconduct. Custodial staff often respond with force to nondangerous misconduct that is troublesome, bizarre, or disturbing. The conduct may reflect a mental health condition that limits an IP's ability to comply with orders, for example, when IPs do not follow orders because hallucinations and delusions have impaired their connection with reality (Fellner, 2015).

Although it is custodial staff who usually are the ones responsible for using excessive force on IPs, carceral mental health professionals nonetheless have responsibilities to safeguard their patients from abuse. They should not acquiesce to the ill treatment of IPs regardless of who commits it or why. For example, when an IP is not complying with an order because of mental illness and there is no immediate threat of injury to the IP or others, mental health staff who are present should not stand by while custodial staff prepare to use pepper spray. They should intervene to seek the opportunity to talk with the IP in an effort to peacefully secure the end to the misconduct. They should also advocate for rules that require custody staff to give them such an opportunity. Mental health staff should seek to influence carceral policies and practices in other ways as well, for example, to ensure their participation in after-incident reviews to address whether the use of force could have been avoided. Mental health staff should also inform authorities when they believe force has been used excessively or punitively. Carceral authorities should require and encourage such interventions, participation, and reporting by mental health staff, and they should act promptly and decisively to address mental health staff concerns about custodial staff hostility and retaliation when they do speak out.

Restrictive housing

Correctional systems rely on RHUs—also called segregation, isolation, locked-down units, super-maximum security, and solitary confinement, among other terms—to manage or punish IPs who have engaged in conduct the authorities deem threats to carceral safety and security. In the typical RHU, IPs are isolated in small cells for 23 hours a day of unstructured time, idleness, and little or no social contact or stimulation. In recent years, criticism of prolonged and indefinite confinement in RHUs has grown (see Chapter 10). Research suggests RHUs may inflict psychological distress on individuals who have not previously had mental health problems and aggravate the symptoms of those with existing disorders (Fellner, 2015; Kapoor & Trestman, 2016; Metzner & Fellner, 2010). The nature and severity of the harm depend on the characteristics of the individual, the duration of the confinement, and the particular conditions (e.g., size of cell; noise level; access to natural light, books, radio).

Because of their higher rates of rule breaking, IPs with mental disabilities are disproportionally confined in RHUs (Fellner, 2015; Kapoor & Trestman, 2016). Isolation has not been proven to reduce misconduct. Indeed, it can have the paradoxically harmful effect of exacerbating the nature and symptoms of mental illness, yielding further misconduct—which can result in the harmful isolation being continued indefinitely. Many IPs with mental illness held in RHUs will decompensate, requiring crisis care or psychiatric hospitalization—after which they are often returned to an RHU. Not surprisingly, self-injury and suicides occur disproportionately more often in RHUs than elsewhere in prison (Kapoor & Trestman, 2016).

Mental health professionals are frequently unable to mitigate the harm associated with isolation. Although some carceral systems have increased the amount of mental health services available to persons who are separated from the general population, typical mental health services in RHUs are limited to psychotropic medication, a health care clinician periodically stopping at the cell front to ask how the IP is doing (i.e., mental health rounds, often derisively called "walk-bys"), and occasional meetings in private with a clinician. Individual or group therapy and structured educational, recreational, or life skill–enhancing activities are usually not available because of insufficient resources and rules that require IPs to remain in their cells (Kapoor & Trestman, 2016; Metzner & Dvoskin, 2006).

Citing the mental health impacts of isolation, international treaty bodies and human rights experts, including the UN Human Rights Committee (1992, 2006), the UN Committee Against Torture (2006), the UN Special Rapporteur on Torture (UN General Assembly, 2013), and the European Committee for the Prevention of Torture and Inhuman or Degrading Treatment or Punishment (2011), have concluded that solitary confinement (i.e., RHUs) may amount to torture or other cruel, inhuman, or degrading treatment or punishment. Reflecting such views, the Mandela Rules prohibit solitary confinement for 22 hours or more a day without meaningful human contact that is indefinite in duration or that is prolonged, defined as lasting more than 15 days (Mandela Rules, R. 44). The rules further mandate that such confinement should only be used "in exceptional cases as a last resort, for as short a time as possible, and subject to independent review" (Mandela Rules, R. 45.1). Moreover, the "imposition of solitary confinement should be prohibited in the case of prisoners with mental or physical disabilities when their conditions would be exacerbated by such measures" (Mandela Rules, R. 45.2).

Consistent with its recognition of the harm that can come from confinement in restrictive housing, the American Psychiatric Association (2023) recently adopted the following updated position statement:

> Restrictive housing of incarcerated adults with serious mental illness, with rare exceptions that involve significant danger to others, should be avoided due to the potential for harm to such individuals. If an individual with serious mental illness is placed in restrictive housing, in which one is confined to a cell for 22 or more hours per day, out-of-cell structured therapeutic activities (e.g., mental health/psychiatric treatment) in appropriate programming space and regular unstructured out-of-cell time should be provided to maximize access to clinically indicated programming, treatment, recreation and transfer to a more therapeutic setting.

The NCCHC (2016, p. 4) has taken an even stronger position, stating that "prolonged (greater than 15 consecutive days) solitary confinement is cruel, inhumane, and degrading treatment, and harmful to an individual's health." It calls for the elimination of solitary confinement as a means of punishment and states that it should not be used as an administrative security measure when other, less restrictive options are available, and even then, for the shortest time possible, never to exceed 15 days (NCCHC, 2016).

The use of restrictive housing, particularly for persons with mental illness, may pose unique ethical challenges for correctional medical professionals, for example, when they are asked to certify that individual IPs are fit to be placed or kept in RHUs. According to the NCCHC (2016, p. 3):

> The participation of health care staff in actions that may be injurious to an individual's health is in conflict with their role as caregivers. This is especially true when they are called on to determine whether a patient is physically and psychologically well enough to be placed in solitary confinement.

Along with the UN and the World Health Organization, the NCCHC affirms that carceral health care professionals should not participate in any way in practices that constitute torture or other cruel, inhuman, or degrading treatment. Medical staff should never certify IPs as fit for isolation or otherwise participate in segregation decisions or efforts. They should, however, advocate that individuals be removed from restrictive housing if their medical or mental health deteriorates or if necessary services cannot be provided to them as long as they are isolated (NCCHC, 2016; World Health Organization, 2016). To avoid being complicit in conditions of confinement that violate human rights standards, carceral health care professionals should advocate within the carceral system for changed restrictive housing policies, and if that fails, they should undertake public advocacy.

Experience demonstrates that prisons can operate safely and securely without putting IPs with mental illness in typical conditions of segregation. Because of litigation, in some carceral systems, IPs with mental illness who would otherwise be locked in their cell for 23 hours a day are given more time outside their cells, including time in group and other therapeutic interventions. These IPs have improved clinical responses and reduced rates of misconduct (Metzner & Fellner, 2010).

Enforcement of human rights

Unfortunately, there are no direct enforcement mechanisms for internationally recognized human rights in the United States. Lawsuits cannot be predicated on human rights treaties. Treaty bodies and authorities review U.S. treaty compliance (with the help of submissions from nongovernmental organizations) and make recommendations, but they have no power to compel the United States to comply with those recommendations.

Officials nonetheless remain responsible for fulfilling their human rights obligations. Carceral policies should expressly incorporate international human rights standards, and all staff should be trained in them. Effective internal methods of supervision and accountability for compliance with the standards will signal that officials are serious about protecting the rights of IPs. They should also support health professionals to resist pressures to engage in or be complicit with abusive practices and policies. Carceral policies should expressly require the participation of carceral mental health staff in the development of appropriate mental health services but also in the development and application of housing regimes and use of force standards and in reviews of their application. Mental health professionals are not guests in carceral systems. They must be full participants in systemwide efforts to safeguard fully the rights of IPs.

Summary

As the Physicians for Human Rights and School of Public Health and Primary Health Care, University of Cape Town Health Sciences Faculty (2003) have stated, "For health professionals, a human rights framework provides a steady moral compass, a blueprint of a just and humane social order that at its core articulates the principles of the dignity and equality of every human being." Pursuing respect for the rights of IPs with mental illness, carceral mental health professionals can not only improve their treatment and hence their prospects for well-being but also, more generally, help humanize carceral conditions. The more carceral mental health practitioners embrace and advocate for human rights, the greater the likelihood that IPs' rights will be respected and carceral systems will become places where mental health staff can work without compromising their professional standards and ethical responsibilities.

REFERENCES

Abramsky, S., & Fellner, J. (2003). *Ill-equipped: US prisons and offenders with mental illness.* Human Rights Watch.

American Medical Association. (2022). *AMA Code of medical ethics, 9.7.5 torture.* https://code-medical-ethics.ama-assn.org/sites/amacoedb/files/2022-08/9.7.5.pdf

American Psychiatric Association. (2023). *Position statement regarding restrictive housing of incarcerated adults with serious mental illness.* https://www.psychiatry.org/getattachment/de02560f-34fd-420b-b36a 257f1450558a/Position-Restrictive-Housing-of-Adults.pdf

Council of Europe Committee of Ministers. (2020). *European prison rules*. https://rm.coe.int/09000016809ee581

Coyle, A. (2002). *A human rights approach to prison management: Handbook for prison staff.* International Centre for Prison Studies.

European Committee for the Prevention of Torture and Inhuman or Degrading Treatment or Punishment. (2011). *CPT standards*. Council of Europe.

Edwards v. United Kingdom, No. 46477/99, European Court of Human Rights (2002).

Fellner, J. (2015). *Callous and cruel: Use of force against inmates with mental disabilities in US jails and prisons*. Human Rights Watch. https://www.hrw.org/report/2015/05/12/callous-and-cruel/use-force-against-inmates-mental-disabilities-us-jails-and

Institute on Medicine as a Profession. (2013). *Ethics abandoned: Medical professionalism and detainee abuse in the "War on Terror."* Institute on Medicine as a Profession.

Kapoor, R., & Trestman, R. (2016). *Mental health effects of restrictive housing*. Office of Justice Programs, U.S. Department of Justice. https://ojp.gov/ncjrs/virtual-library/abstracts/mental-health-effects-restrictive-housing

Kolesnikovich v. Russia, No. 44694/13, European Court of Human Rights (2022).

Metzner, J. L. (2002). Class action litigation in correctional psychiatry. *Journal of the American Academy of Psychiatry and the Law, 30*, 19–29.

Metzner, J., & Dvoskin, J. (2006). An overview of correctional psychiatry. *Psychiatric Clinics of North America, 29*, 761–772.

Metzner, J. L., & Fellner, J. (2010). Solitary confinement and mental illness in U.S. prisons: A challenge for medical ethics. *Journal of the American Academy of Psychiatry and the Law, 38*(1), 104–108.

National Commission on Correctional Health Care. (2016). *Position statement: solitary confinement (isolation)*. https://www.ncchc.org/position-statements/solitary-confinement-isolation-2016/

National Commission on Correctional Health Care. (2022). *Position statement: Correctional health professionals' response to abuse of incarcerated people*. https://www.ncchc.org/wp-content/uploads/Correctional-Health-Professionals-Response-to-Abuse-of-Incarcerated-People-2022-1.pdf

Physicians for Human Rights and School of Public Health and Primary Health Care, University of Cape Town Health Sciences Faculty. (2003). *Dual loyalty and human rights in health professional practice: Proposed guidelines & institutional mechanisms*. PHR and University of Cape Town. https://s3.amazonaws.com/PHR_Reports/dualloyalties-2002-report.pdf

Renolde v. France, No. 5608/05. European Court of Human Rights (2008).

Sy v. Italy, ECHR 024, European Court of Human Rights (2022).

Thomas v. Bryant, 614 F.3d 1288, 1311 (11th Cir. 2010).

United Nations. (1948). *Universal declaration of human rights*. https://www.un.org/en/about-us/universal-declaration-of-human-rights

United Nations. (1966a). *International covenant on civil and political rights*. https://www.ohchr.org/en/instruments-mechanisms/instruments/international-covenant-civil-and-political-rights

United Nations. (1966b). *International covenant on economic, social and cultural rights*. https://www.ohchr.org/en/instruments-mechanisms/instruments/international-covenant-economic-social-and-cultural-rights

United Nations. (1984). *Convention against torture and other cruel, inhuman or degrading treatment or punishment*. https://digitallibrary.un.org/record/74216?ln=en&v=pdf

United Nations. (2006). *Convention on the rights of persons with disabilities*. https://www.un.org/disabilities/documents/convention/convoptprot-e.pdf

United Nations. (2015). *Standard minimum rules for the treatment of prisoners (the Nelson Mandela Rules)*. https://documents.un.org/doc/undoc/gen/n15/443/41/pdf/n1544341.pdf?token=Y9fziq3dUIQrCWvkNk&fe=true

United Nations Committee Against Torture. (2006). *Consideration of reports submitted by states parties under article 19 of the convention, conclusions and recommendations of the Committee Against Torture, United States of America*. CAT/C/USA/CO/2. https://www.refworld.org/policy/polrec/cat/2006/en/46876

United Nations Committee on Economic, Social and Cultural Rights. (2000). *General comment no. 14: The right to the highest attainable standard of health (art. 12 of the covenant)*. E/C.12/2000/4. https://www.refworld.org/legal/general/cescr/2000/en/36991

United Nations General Assembly. (2013). *Interim report of the special rapporteur of the Human Rights Council on torture and other cruel, inhuman or degrading treatment or punishment*. https://www.unodc.org/documents/justice-and-prison-reform/SPECIAL_RAPPORTEUR_EN.pdf

United Nations Human Rights Committee. (1992). *CCPR general comment no. 20: article 7 (prohibition of torture, or other cruel, inhuman or degrading treatment or punishment)*. https://www.refworld.org/legal/general/hrc/1992/en/11086

United Nations Human Rights Committee. (2006). *Consideration of reports submitted by states parties under article 40 of the covenant, concluding observations of the Human Rights Committee: United States of America*. CCPR/C/USA/CO/3. https://www.refworld.org/policy/polrec/hrc/2006/en/3703

World Health Organization. (2016). *Prisons and health*. https://www.who.int/europe/publications/i/item/9789289050593

World Medical Association. (2006). *WMA Declaration of Tokyo—Guidelines for physicians concerning torture and other cruel, inhuman or degrading treatment or punishment in relation to detention and imprisonment*. https://www.wma.net/policies-post/wma-declaration-of-tokyo-guidelines-for-physicians-concerning-torture-and-other-cruel-inhuman-or-degrading-treatment-or-punishment-in-relation-to-detention-and-imprisonment/

World Psychiatric Association. (1996). *Madrid declaration on ethical standards for psychiatric practice*. https://www.wpanet.org/current-madrid-declaration

5 The lived experience of incarceration

Barbara Fair and Reena Kapoor[*]

Introduction

Incarceration is a stressful and dehumanizing process that affects not only incarcerated individuals but also their families and communities. Even for those who work with incarcerated people regularly, it can be difficult to appreciate the range and intensity of their experiences because staff members typically see only a small part of life in a carceral setting. This chapter gives voice to the experiences of incarcerated persons (IPs) and their families. Currently or formerly incarcerated individuals were interviewed in an open-ended way as part of a project to obtain narrative accounts of how incarceration has affected them. In addition, the mother of a young man with mental illness and repeated incarcerations contributed a written account of her decades-long journey of suffering and recovery. Core elements and themes are presented in the contributors' own words; their names and some details are changed to protect their identities. We hope these stories elucidate the range of adverse experiences that IPs endure, the complexity of healing, and the structural problems that contribute to our current carceral system.

Miles L.—Time

INTERVIEWER: Does time wear on you harder now that you know you're getting on in age?

ML: It does to a point because you're not getting younger and you know it. And time means more now than it did in the past. In the past, I didn't care because I figured I would live forever. And now that I'm gettin' older, I do know that the end is veritably here. So it's harder to do.... One day is like a week, is like a month, is like a year. To where in the past, one day, I really didn't care. I could afford to lose a day, or a week, or a month, or a year.... And there's something about time that you lose, everything that you had when you were younger, your thought pattern changes, the way that you see things change, the way that you deal with things change. As far as when you were young and now that you're old. Whether it has to do with time or just experience, I don't know. I don't know. If it's, you think one way when you're young, and another way when you're older. If it takes growin' up all those years to reach that point, or if it's something that just happens chemically. I don't know.

A long time ago I used to think that [prison] was full of [guards] that were all-knowing. They knew how prison worked. And today I see it for actually what it is, and it's just individuals that have a job to do. And they chose that field, and they've got good days and bad days. And they're not necessarily up on current events, whether they're happening inside or outside. So, they're just as fallible as everybody else.

I think doin' time is, the biggest aspect to that is the time itself, is what you do. Again, you can escape by putting your mind in employment, or education. If you're stuck inside of a room to where you're constantly thinking, and you constantly got 24 hours at a time to do, that's what makes county jail time harder than prison time—is the fact that you're locked up, and you have so much time on your hands.

Pat D.—Access to treatment

PD: I was incarcerated twice. As far as prison goes, I had a short time to do, just a 2-year sentence. No way to get into the mental (health) program, they're all booked up. There's no help there for you.

I look at it this way. I put myself in prison. I was in a treatment program in the community. But in prison, they're not equipped to handle mental health people. They don't carry a lot of my meds. I learned you had to tell them, "I have to have that med. You have to get it for me."

This last time what really hurt me was I had been waiting for this mental health program. I finally got into it. I was so happy. What they concentrated on is what I wanted. I wanted to get something out of prison, other than just working. But

*. The authors acknowledge the contributions of Brad Bogue and Robert Trestman, who interviewed incarcerated persons and wrote this chapter in the textbook's first edition.

they wouldn't switch my work schedule, so there's no way I could do it. They wouldn't switch me because I was good at what I did. I spent 7 months in the kitchen, which was hard, real hard. I didn't get nothing but work.

INTERVIEWER: Did you get to see an individual psychologist or therapist?

PD: There's mental people in there that need help, and they don't get it. They're there a lot longer than I'm going to be there. My heart goes out to them, because it's hard to get help in there. For me, when I have a problem, I need to talk to a therapist now. You know, I could have hurt somebody already. When I hit my peak, I know when it is.

When that one officer that I told, "I need mental health now," he laughed at me. I said, "Man, I'm not joking, I need mental health, I'm going to freaking flip. It's very frustrating. I realize they deal with a lot of people, but when they've been around me 5, 6 months, they know what I am. They know what I'm about.

Regina G.—Loneliness and faith

INTERVIEWER: What was the experience of doing time like?

RG: Discipline. Usual discipline. You're really structured. It's controlled. It was hard. I don't know. It was sad at times. It was happy at times. There are things that you have no control over. You can call family. Something happens. You just have to swallow it, and live through it, get through it the best way you can.

I was put in the safe hole because they had the lesbian act going on there. I disagreed with it, so they PC'd [protective custody] me. I lived in segregation because the girls all turned on me and stuff. I lived in there. I learned to like it there. I felt safe there. I programmed from there. I worked from there. I would just roll out of seg and then go to work and do my programs. I was segregated from the other women. I enjoyed being alone in prison, for the fact that I had time to focus on my behaviors and to focus on what I was going to do, what I had done, and where I was going. I didn't mind being alone. Actually, when they asked me if I wanted to go back into population, I refused. I liked being alone.

I got used to it, and I got strong. I would go to work, and I would tell the Lord, "OK. It's me and you. It's me and you today. You are going to work for me because I'm going to work for you." I would get through it like that, and he would help me through it a lot. But I'm surprised I made it through some of it, some of the things that I did. There's that wood lot, where they would take tree trunks and they'd put them on this big saw, and then they'd cut them in half. Then there was this big table and they'd fall on there, and you'd have to stack them just so. Heavy: I mean heavy. I don't know how I made it through that, but I did.

Actually, when I left there, I missed it, because I got used to it, and I felt good. I felt healthy. I felt strong. I really didn't want to leave. I got attached to a lot of people there.

Prison, to me, it wasn't all a bad experience. To me, it saved my life. It saved my children's future. I'm clean and sober today. I'm good. I'm here. I'm happy.

Rick W.—Penitence and fitting in

RW: There was a time when I went from, for lack of a better term, a straight-laced White guy to being surrounded by mostly murderers and gangbangers. It's just a world I wasn't prepared for, but it was a world that I fit in somehow. I couldn't tell you how, but I was able to take care of myself.

In there, you're in the fishbowl. Everything is ... you don't know who's watching you. You don't know who's observing what.

It's such a small world. If you show any kind of weakness, you're going to get preyed upon, because it's all of society's predators. I was at a maximum-security facility, and that's where all your hard-core predators are.

At the same time, the state takes everything away from you, everything: home, family, material things. They take everything, but what they can't take away from you is your integrity, your character, so if your word's good, your business is good, and you're not about to bullshit, that goes a long way in terms of the respect factor.

You are trying to learn a new world, and it was crippling, but at the same time, you can't show any of that, because as soon as you start showing that, that's when you get preyed upon. All I could do was focus forward. All I wanted to do was wake up the next morning and deal with it then.

You're living with somebody that you don't know, and you don't have any choice but to live with this person. You don't know what they're in for, so you're just trying to get along. Most people that are in prison lack the ability to know how to communicate. You have a whole lot of guys together that absolutely don't know how to communicate with one another. They don't know how to communicate with anybody. Yet, in order to survive, to make this thing work, they have to be able to communicate.

They don't know how to, so it's such chaos.... Then you have staff who haven't got a clue. They don't have ... I don't want to stain all staff, but the majority don't have a clue, not just how to communicate, but they don't have integrity. They don't have professionalism. They don't have the necessary tools just to have the job.

INTERVIEWER: Speak a little about introspection.

RW: When you realize for the first time that you have no character, not bad character, you have no character, and that's like having no credit. It's worse than bad credit. No integrity. No principles. No values. When you find that out for the first time ... I was sick to my stomach. When I looked back on how I treated people, how I treated my wife, how I treated my family ... and I had to go to prison to figure this out. I had to be around the absolute scum of the freaking earth to figure out what kind of a piece of shit I was.

But what it was, was Department of Corrections (DOC) ended up being this big mirror that I had to look at, because all those that were around me, I could find a piece of me in all of them of some sort. It was just so sickening. It was so incredibly ... I just wanted to puke for days, months, years. I couldn't shower that shit off me.

But I wasn't going to allow the judicial system, I wasn't going to allow DOC, I wasn't going to allow convicts, I wasn't going to allow anybody to beat me. The only way that I could throw it all back at them was to be successful. In some form or fashion, I was going to be successful.

Rob B.—A failed system

RB: Every day I fear what life's going to be like when I get out because I worry about other things like I happen to believe ... but I'm cut off from the world still slightly here, that we're losing more and more of our liberties on the outside, that more and more of our freedoms are disappearing, and I look at the price of stuff in stores, and I know that ... what kind of wage am I going to be making? Am I going to be able to afford to pay rent and eat?

Yeah, I live in terror. I don't feel this place is designed to make you a better person or to reintroduce you to society, and somehow I'll just have to deal with it.

INTERVIEWER: You are skeptical about what really is going on?

RB: Yes, but the interesting thing is it makes sense to them. The DOC lobbyists can say, "We need more guards. We need more money." The system is designed for failure.

I'm surrounded by artists in my prison, I mean that. We've got artists picking up garbage on the side of the road. I noticed across the street the VFW has a mural of a battleship. I'm thinking, "Why don't you have a sign-painting crew? Why don't you have a public works crew that does public murals?" There's no imagination in the prison system for the talent they have.

All of this is designed for failure, as far as I'm concerned. It's a rest and recovery center for career criminals, because the people who get along the best here go, "All I do here is smile and lie, and then my 6 months are up, and then I get to go back to crime." All this did was stimulate my mind to where I'm more antisocial, more eccentric, and I notice that that's one thing prison does to people.

INTERVIEWER: Are you saying that prison makes people worse?

RB: Oh yeah. It makes them more creative at defects. This isn't always the case. People who are so self-disciplined, they're never going to commit a crime again. The problem with the system is that you have nonviolent people who are not going to reoffend, and you're trying to drive them insane so that. Yeah. Well, it's like this. I think that it's like the guy who wrote *Empire of the Sun*. He was a psychiatrist. He gets out, he's 15 years old, he's been in captivity for 8 years. He decides he's going to help humanity. He becomes a psychiatrist. He practices psychiatry for a decade and he goes, "What analysis seeks to do to make you normal really doesn't help as much as it would help if people were taught theater, literature, music."

That's how you would teach people to talk to their inner self, to articulate their grievances.

Jason H.—Attitude and endurance

JH: I have done, all told, 7½ years in prison. I got into a gang at 13 and that was my entire life right there. At 13 years old, half my life I'd been in institutions and group homes; my attitude was pretty crappy back then. It was like I found my niche in life and that was my thing.

Looking back on it now, yeah, I wish I could go back in time and slap the old me around a little bit. I guess there's some things that I learned on a positive note from all the gangbanging and all the dumb shit that I did. I've got a different sense of morals than a lot of other people do. A lot of people write off gangsters and gangbangers and people in that life as having no morals. They do, for real. I learned a real high sense of honor from gangbanging.

I remember, I was in prison one day and got called to the front office and told that I was leaving the next day. That I was going to a halfway house. Like a dumb ass, back then, I had rabbit feet real bad. I got to the halfway house, and that night, I took off. I don't even know what I was thinking, but I just took off. I got 2 years for taking off out of the halfway house added to the 18 months.

At 18, I went to prison and still didn't give a damn. I just went in there with an attitude, like, "You know what, man, fuck this shit. Fuck you." I was there 11 months, ended up catching assault on a DOC guard. They didn't take me to court or give me any more time for it, but they sent me into 23-hour-a-day lockdown. For me, it changed how sociable I was. When you're locked down 23 hours a day in a cell by yourself, without even trying to, you become a bit antisocial. Then I ended up doing shit. I did 2½ years in of 3-year term in solitary.

INTERVIEWER: Have you now changed that attitude to not go back?

JH: When you were pointing that out, I feel everything that I'm suffering with right now is an endurance trial. I just feel that I am overcoming my greatest fear, and my greatest fear is for whatever reason going back to who I once was. I'm trying to overcome that by doing positive things instead of negative things. My treasure now is my kids and showing my kids that Dad's different.

Tim S.—The locked door and surviving

TS: When you take that bus in, your autonomy stops. That's when you became a number, and you put on the same clothes as everybody else. You became a wave in a sea of lost souls. You don't know that at the time. You don't realize. It's terrifying. The first time you go in your cell and they close those doors, and you're alone. The brick walls and open bars, and the smells, and the screaming, and the hollering, and it was absolutely just traumatic. You have no identity in prison. You were somebody that just started their prison sentence.

INTERVIEWER: You're like a piece on a board game, and you don't know what the game is.

TS: Absolutely. All you learn is to be hypervigilant towards "respect." You had a whole different set of rules. When you're 18, you're very impressionable. When we went into prison, we were told, this is the way you have to be to be a good, solid convict or you're a piece of shit. You begin to think, "This is what I need to do, and the harder I work towards being a good convict, the faster I become somebody."

You want to survive.

From that first time, I was in and out of community corrections, getting put on probation, or parole, or whatever, violating, and going back to that revolving door system of using drugs, using cocaine, getting a hot UA (i.e., positive urine toxicology), and back to prison.

At 35, I really wanted to make changes. I did a lot of segregation time, a lot of hole time [i.e., restrictive housing], and I still think I've come up pretty well. But you can't be locked in a box and stare at the wall day after day with no human contact, except for when they feed you and when screaming down the tier without it affecting you to some degree.

All those opportunities and all the things that I forfeited, all things to think about those dark nights all night long, they're wasted unless you use it somehow. That's why I'm so set on trying to do something and using my experiences to give back. I haven't wasted that time. I have, still, to a degree, but I'm hoping I can live with it.

When you do time there is a helplessness, a loneliness, a kind of absent feeling, which leaves you feeling empty. It's not really lonely. It's empty. It's kind of an empty kind of void. The only way to fill that empty void is to try to control your inner personal environment, what's going on around you. You can't control any of that stuff.

INTERVIEWER: That makes sense. You make the connections in yourself, that you're not helpless.

TS: You're struggling with all this negativity and humiliation and just trying to search for some sort of value as a human being, some sort of belonging to this world, some sort of attachment to the life or the existence around you. When you give up, when you can't find that way to attach, when you can't find a way to save yourself is when you lose it.

INTERVIEWER: From that experience, just an incredible experience stacking 25 years in prison, what cycles could you think of that are involved in doing time?

TS: I think there are a couple. One is trying to survive each day, trying to get through the day. It's hard. You can't think about tomorrow, but yet you have to hope in tomorrow. You have to put some faith and hope that tomorrow is coming, but you can't really plan for it, because it will drive you crazy because of the amount of time you still have to do. I'll tell you one thing that's been actually a result of doing a lot of prison time. I have a fantastic memory of everything in my life, because I've had a unique opportunity to do nothing but think about things in my life and think about them over and over and over.

The other thing, getting back to the other part of this living, you have to, just do whatever you have to do to get through the day. There's a lot of stuff you turn off until later. I can't do this. I'm just going to turn it off until I get out. You have to do it by day, but at the same time you can't just cancel everything in your life or you succumb to that thing. You have to inspire yourself somehow. You have to hope that tomorrow is going to be better. Otherwise you die. It's such a hard, thin line to ride.

I believe in the whole full circle. That's why I'm so into trying to make change on a larger scale happen. Especially in recovery, we teach best what we most need to learn. By helping others, it keeps you where you need to be. It keeps you grounded in what you need to do for yourself. It's almost selfish helping other people, because you're taking care of yourself.

Regina M.—Emotions, routine, consequences

RM: When I first started, I think it was exciting; it was fun. I was curious what prison would be like, and it was just a real fun experience. Chip on my shoulder, thought I was invincible, 10 feet tall and bulletproof, and I didn't give a shit about anything. I knew I barely had a little tiny 10-year sentence, and I could get through that, no problem. And towards the end, it was more of a nerve-wracking, mind-fucking, lonely, yet crowded place to be.

Towards the end of doing my 10, I was just tired of it. It wasn't fun anymore. It took things that I took for granted and things you missed when you're out there, like stopping and smelling a fucking flower or stopping and getting a burger, just even going for a walk or being able to step outside when you want to.

Those are some of the small things a lot of people on a daily basis take for granted and don't even realize things that you're going to miss when it's all taken away from you.

INTERVIEWER: What do you recall about the experience of doing time? How did you make that work for you?

RM: Routine. I had my day pretty much planned out. I knew what I was going to do. I knew I had to get up for work at 3:00. I'd come back. I had everything planned out. I was so medicated, I was asleep by 5:30, 6:00. I knew I'd be out like that, so my days just flew by. They were just monotone.

INTERVIEWER: Can you recall anything about struggles you might have had with emotions or mind while you were doing time?

RM: Yeah. I lost my children because of doing time, so it was pretty fucking hard for me. Because the days that went by, I realized I would never get back. That I would never know if one of my children fell down and got hurt. You know what I mean? I was pretty mind fucked. Again, that's why I said I was pretty medicated. Numb. All you have time to do is sit and think. Worrying. A lot of it is worrying about what's going on out there, things you have no control over. It's hard to not worry about what's going on out there, that life still goes on.

INTERVIEWER: What do you think people need to hear that would help them?

RM: Just the severity of using drugs. When you're thinking about getting high, you're not thinking about what diseases you could be catching while you're getting high. Or the different risks that you take, or how careless you get with everyday things. How dangerous things really are. You think you want to do what you want to do, but you don't realize how dangerous drugs really are. Or how out of your mind you are: you don't even care about what you're doing. Or the consequences.

Barbara F.—A mother and son's journey

As I write, my son is in the hospital on the psychiatric ward, yet again following an arrest and likely jail outcome. Again, a threatening charge. This is what my life and the lives of his siblings have been for what seems like a lifetime. After spending months in supermax prison, my son was lost to me. He was stolen through state-sanctioned barbarism. I have lived for decades with the broken pieces of him that are still recognizable.

My son's first encounter with prison was at the age of 16 in the 1990s. In those days, jails and prisons were commonly called "the belly of the beast" because once someone entered them, the toxic environment devoured people and operated to kill one's spirit. One's individuality and any sense of humanity were programmatically erased from day 1. Initiation into the DOC reminds me of the institution of slavery. So much of the system embraces remnants of American slavery, with the elimination of one's name, replacing it with a number. Then there are the degrading, dehumanizing, and deeply humiliating cavity searches that send a clear message that one has lost their right to the privacy of their own body. Finally, there is the use of chains, shackles, belly chains, and leg irons—the tools of oppression.

My son's first day of incarceration was the beginning of a journey of chronic stress and coping with being locked away in a cage away from his family. Incarceration exacerbated his mental instability, and the DOC's response was a diagnosis of schizophrenia and a myriad of antipsychotic medications. Much of this journey I suffered alone because I didn't want the rest of the family being aware of his suffering.

At age 17, my son was transferred to a supermax prison after a disciplinary investigation. The supermax was a facility designed to break the spirit of anyone whom officers saw as a threat to the smooth operation of the system. Notorious for its restrictive housing and complete isolation from other human beings, the prison's barbaric practices were hidden from public scrutiny. On any given day, those housed there were primarily African American and Latino men. Self-harm and suicidal attempts were high. I had no prior knowledge of this facility until my son was sent there. Soon after being there, he was writing about the abusive and toxic environment and begging me to get him out because the suffering was becoming too much to bear. I visited him once, and it tore me apart seeing him brought to me surrounded by several officers, chained, and shackled. It took every ounce of strength not to break down in front of him. We got through the visit, and I went outside and screamed into the air, wallowing in pain after seeing how my son was being treated. He was a kid. How can anyone be okay with that type of treatment of another human being?

For weeks, my son wrote home, and suddenly there was nothing. No letters and no calls. I called the DOC commissioner to look into what was going on. I was told he had lost his rights to calls, visits, and letters. This information caused me to almost have a mental breakdown because now I had no way of knowing what was happening to my son.

Families of the incarcerated suffer even though they are not in those cages with their loved one. It was during my son's period of incarceration that I developed panic attacks, sleepless nights, a strong sense of helplessness, as well as crying spells as I tried to cope and get through each day. At night, as I struggled to get to sleep, I felt his spirit crying out for my help. Eventually, with assistance, I was able to get my son out, but not before irrevocable harm was caused.

When my son returned home, he was an emotional and psychiatric mess, a shell of the young talented writer and hip-hop artist who entered that system as a 16-year-old.

As I sit here writing this, I fight back the tears knowing my son is in the grips of the DOC once again. As a licensed clinical social worker, I am quite aware that returning to the spaces that took my son down is deeply traumatic and triggering. But when I bail him out, as I have done so many times in the past, he instinctually returns to that which helps him cope with the harms against him (drugs). So many of these deeply painful experiences have led him down a rathole that he can't seem to pull himself out. The outcome of his lived experiences has led to incarceration, countless psychiatric hospitalizations, and psych meds, which are nothing but band aids for a lost soul. As I watch him struggle to navigate this world in his state of mind, my heart breaks. I dread picking up the phone if I don't recognize the number. Is it someone from the hospital, police department, DOC, or a stranger informing me my son is gone from me forever? Even when it's his number calling, I dread hearing him call to say, "Mom, I just can't do this anymore."

Now in his 40s, my son has been to hell and back several times, and I'm amazed at his resilience. He has been able to bounce back several times to where he is not consumed by addiction. It is that history that keeps me hopeful. I recognize my son will never be who he had the capacity to become before the carceral system swallowed him whole, yet I'm blessed to still have him in my life. I ask myself how many more of our people must experience the evils of America's evil, racist, and harmful carceral system before it is dismantled and someone is held accountable. All I ask is that, as the formerly incarcerated fight for justice, they don't forget about the families who served time on the outside while their loved one was inside. We all are being harmed by this deeply punitive and indifferent carceral system.

Summary

We hope that the stories told in this chapter convey the diversity of experiences of incarceration and the diversity of people who become incarcerated. Ultimately, our aim is to strengthen the relationship between patient and clinician—the therapeutic alliance. Developing appropriate therapeutic alliances with patients has been shown to enhance outcomes in mental health treatment (Baier et al., 2020). The better we understand our patients and can empathize with them, the greater the therapeutic alliance and the greater the likelihood of positive outcomes.

REFERENCE

Baier, A. L., Kline, A. C., & Feeny, N. C. (2020). Therapeutic alliance as a mediator of change: A systematic review and evaluation of research. *Clinical Psychology Review*, *82*, 101921.

SECTION II

Organization, structure, and function of correctional institutions

6

Diversion programs and alternatives to incarceration

Merrill Rotter, Virginia Barber Rioja, and Zoe R. Feingold

Introduction

The reported prevalence of individuals with serious mental illness in jails and prisons ranges from 10% to 25% (Bronson & Berzofsky, 2017; Hirschtritt & Binder, 2017), which is several times higher than in the general population. This overrepresentation of persons with serious mental illness in jails and prisons is often attributed to the downsizing of state hospitals, hospitalization admission criteria that require dangerous behavior, inadequate community treatment resources, and the behaviors associated with comorbid substance use. Over the past 2 decades, however, a body of research has found that the relationship between mental illness and criminal justice contact is more complicated and that criminal justice activity, even among those with serious mental illness, is mostly explained by so-called "criminogenic" (crime-causing) factors similar to individuals without mental illness, including problems with employment, social support, and attitudes or behaviors that predispose to offending behavior (e.g., Peterson & Heinz, 2016).

In addressing the problem proactively, the primary approach has been to divert justice-involved individuals with mental illness into appropriate community care, including both treatment for serious mental illness and interventions for criminogenic factors. This chapter includes a review of the major models used to divert those with serious mental illness from incarceration, paying particular attention to the role of jail-based services in support of these initiatives.

Background

While diversion programming for justice-involved individuals with mental illness began receiving significant attention over the past 2 decades, the establishment of such programs was a recommendation of the National Coalition for Jail Reform as early as the 1970s (Steadman et al., 1999). Early diversion efforts focused on individuals with substance use disorders (SUDs), with the dual goals of improving participants' functioning and protecting public safety. Although many of these early diversion participants with SUDs likely also experienced mental health concerns, programs that explicitly extended alternative-to-incarceration opportunities to individuals with mental illness did not develop until the 1990s.

Whether for individuals with SUDs, mental illness, or co-occurring disorders, diversion programs all require identification of clinical eligibility and referral to clinical services in lieu of incarceration and/or continued criminal justice processing (Steadman et al., 1999). The potential for identification and diversion can occur at several different points in the criminal justice continuum, from initial police contact through incarceration. Jurisdictions across the United States have used the Sequential Intercept Model to determine where there are opportunities to identify individuals with justice involvement who may be eligible for diversion to community treatment. The Sequential Intercept Model is illustrated in *Figure 6.1*.

Recent revisions to the model have added an even further upstream, prepolice contact intercept focused on mobile crisis and other purely clinical interventions aimed at preventing criminal justice contact altogether (Heilbrun et al., 2012). The most relevant intercept for jail-based services is postbooking or court-based diversion, since earlier intercepts, when successful, will preempt admission to the carceral setting. The later intercepts, focused on reentry planning and services, are addressed elsewhere in this text (see Chapters 23 and 50).

Postbooking diversion occurs after an individual is arrested and formal charges are filed (Heilbrun et al., 2012). Because charges have been filed, postbooking diversion programs require a negotiated agreement among the court, the prosecutor's office, and the defense attorney. The offer includes a community treatment alternative to incarceration and a final adjudication of the criminal case. When both the instant offense and the participant's criminal record are less serious, charges may be dropped and a referral to treatment made. More often, the participant must plead guilty, with final sentencing (often to a lesser charge) held in abeyance until completion of mandated treatment. Although alternatives to incarceration can be offered in any court (including non-problem-solving courts), in many jurisdictions similar cases are grouped together and offered diversion through mental health courts (MHCs), which have become the most studied type of court-based diversion program (Steadman et al., 2001). MHCs often use their own staff to divert and monitor clients instead of relying on an external agency.

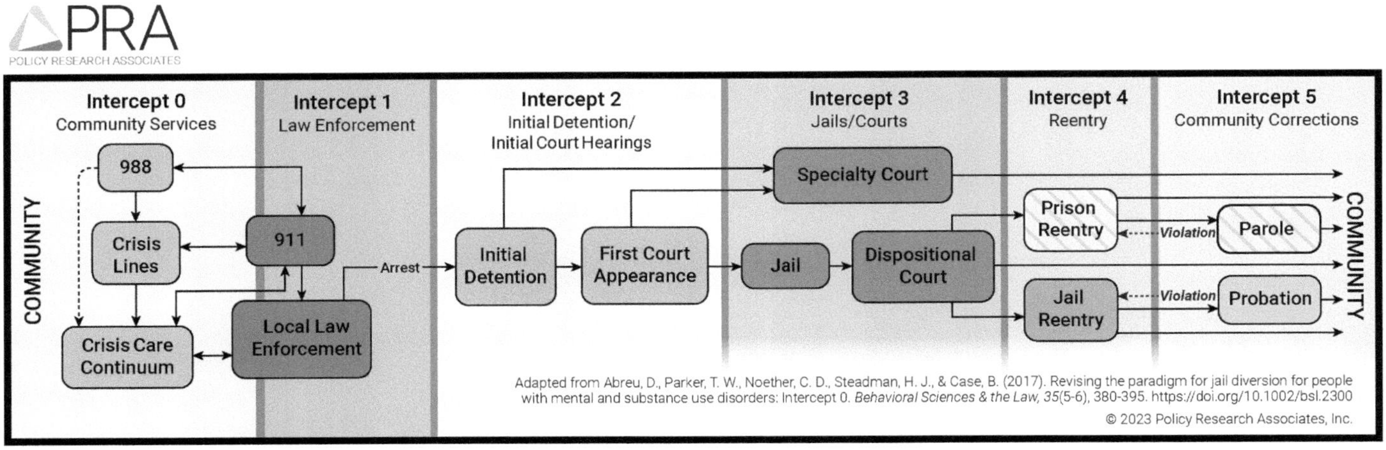

Figure 6.1 Sequential intercept model.

Mental health courts

MHCs are a type of problem-solving court specifically devoted to individuals with mental illness. The premise of problem-solving courts is that public safety goals can be met by directly addressing the problem associated with criminal activity. Examples include courts dedicated to substance use, domestic violence, trafficking (prostitution), and veterans. MHCs were created to address the problem of criminal behavior in persons with untreated or undertreated mental illness. They were established according to the belief that mental illness may mitigate criminal behavior, that jails and prisons are especially noxious environments for individuals with mental illness, and that traditional court sanctions (in particular, remand to jail) are ineffective at best and destructive at worst.

The first MHC in the United States was established in the late 1980s. The Broward County (Florida) Mental Health Court, which opened in 1996, was the first to be studied. Serving defendants charged with misdemeanors, the court improved access to mental health services without defendants feeling coerced into accepting the plea and treatment offered (McGaha et al., 2002).

The popularity of MHCs has grown immensely in the past several decades. While an estimated 200 MHCs were in operation nationwide in 2010, this number increased to 618 at the end of 2022 (National Treatment Court Resource Center, 2023; Redlich, 2013). It is often said, "If you've seen one mental health court, you've seen one mental health court." These courts vary widely based on clinical and legal target populations, length and extent of court mandates, standard plea arrangements, makeup and responsibilities of the court team, venue for identifying participants, assessment and treatment planning, community service availability, and expectations for program completion (Redlich, 2005). The temperament and philosophy of the judge also play an important role in program and client success (Redlich, 2005).

Despite marked variation in their practices, many established MHCs do share several important features. Most MHCs process participants' cases on a single court docket with a specific judge and an assigned prosecutor and defense attorney. MHCs almost always include a clinical team that recommends and makes linkages to treatment, and availability of appropriate clinical placement is ensured before the judge makes a ruling on diversion. Finally, MHCs typically involve specialized court monitoring with possible sanctions for noncompliance (Steadman et al., 2001).

Sanctions and rewards

Sanctions and rewards in a drug court are typically prescribed and straightforward (National Association of Drug Court Professionals, 1997). Sanctions in an MHC are, as a rule, more flexible. The possibility that the violation may be the result of the defendant's underlying mental illness, rather than the flouting of judicial authority, is explicitly taken into account (Barber-Rioja & Rotter, 2014). Minor infractions may lead courts to invoke sanctions that mimic the increased structure and support found in the clinical environment (e.g., increasing the frequency of contact with the case manager or court) or may be more specifically punitive in nature (e.g., completing a writing assignment or lengthening the period of the mandate). Remand to jail is a possible sanction but is usually the last resort, reserved in most courts for situations in which immediate public safety concerns cannot be managed any other way or for more serious breaches of the court order (e.g., absconding or arrest for new charges).

Mental health court research

Several themes emerge from the body of research examining the effectiveness of MHCs. Studies consistently show that MHCs are effective at linking participants to behavioral health services and that MHC participants spend less time incarcerated after diversion when compared to individuals with mental illness who undergo traditional criminal justice processing (Cosden et al., 2003; Frailing, 2010; Lowder et al., 2018). On other metrics, including changes to participants' quality of life (e.g., Matejkowski et al., 2020), reductions in psychiatric symptoms (e.g., Cosden et al., 2003; Steadman & Naples, 2005), and rates of rearrest (Lowder et al., 2018), research shows varied findings. For instance, while some studies show that MHC participants experience improvements in quality of life relative to nondiverted subjects, other studies show no relative improvement in quality-of-life ratings over time (Cosden et al., 2003; Matejkowski et al., 2020). The same mixed results are reported for rearrest rates (e.g., Cosden et al., 2003; Steadman et al., 2011), with several studies showing neutral or nonsignificant outcomes (e.g., lack of significant decrease in rearrest rates relative to nondiverted individuals). While diversion may not always reduce rearrest rates, it does not appear to exacerbate risk relative to traditional criminal justice processing.

The question of *for whom* mental health diversion is most effective emerges often in the MHC literature. Completion of diversion (i.e., graduation) is consistently cited as a key ingredient for MHC success. In fact, many studies indicate that only individuals who fully complete diversion experience postdischarge decreases in recidivism (Burns et al., 2013; Hiday & Ray, 2010). This finding introduces the question of whether individuals who complete diversion have particular characteristics to begin with that decrease their likelihood of rearrest, whether completers' reduced likelihood of recidivism is due to the positive effects of diversion services, or some combination of the two.

There is some evidence to suggest that MHC completers may be different from noncompleters on select characteristics. Across studies, the factors most often associated with greater risk of MHC dropout are the same characteristics that contribute to greater criminogenic risk, such as a more extensive criminal history, younger age, and substance use (Burns et al., 2013; Hiday et al., 2014; Reich et al., 2015). This is perhaps unsurprising, given that the traditional model of MHCs was designed to address primarily the factors associated with mental illness rather than established criminogenic risk factors. Whether a defendant's profile is indicative of program success is, of course, intimately linked to the availability of the necessary services in the community and the defendant's ability to access them. For instance, several studies suggest that housing instability or homelessness at MHC intake increases the likelihood of premature program dropout (e.g., Burns et al., 2013; Reich et al., 2015). Such findings do not necessarily indicate that individuals with unstable housing are less engaged with MHC services or less likely to benefit from diversion but rather that basic social service resources (e.g., stable housing) must be available to retain such individuals in programming. Nevertheless, these findings suggest a need for further study of the exact services and interventions necessary to engage MHC participants adequately in programming and ensure their successful completion of diversion.

Interestingly, one characteristic increasingly thought not to be directly relevant to program success—at least as defined by completion and decreased recidivism—is mental illness. Clinical factors such as primary diagnosis and specific symptoms of serious mental illness show no association with program completion (Comartin et al., 2015; Linhorst et al., 2020; Reich et al., 2013) or recidivism (Comartin et al., 2015; Reich et al., 2013). Additionally, receipt of mental health treatment services does not appear to have a direct influence on likelihood of recidivism following MHC enrollment (Han, 2020; Keator et al., 2013). This, in turn, is in keeping with literature suggesting that symptoms of mental illness are rarely direct drivers of violent or criminal behavior, even among individuals with mental illness already involved in the criminal legal system (e.g., Junginger et al., 2006; Skeem et al., 2013). More often, the direct causal factors implicated in criminal behavior among individuals with mental illness are the same as the factors most often identified in the general offender literature, including social and environmental circumstances (e.g., unemployment and financial instability), the influence of antisocial peers or partners, and substance use problems (e.g., Peterson & Heinz, 2016; Skeem et al., 2013). Indirectly, though, active symptoms of mental illness may increase the likelihood that these direct factors exist and/or may interfere with interventions that address these criminogenic factors.

To this end, many MHCs and diversion programs are including the risk–needs–responsivity paradigm (Andrews & Bonta, 2010) as part of their assessment for program inclusion and treatment planning. This model includes a formal evaluation of recidivism risk to adjust levels of supervision and an explicit review of recidivism-related dynamic factors as targets for intervention. Substance use treatment, vocational and educational support, family involvement, and the availability of prosocial activities and peers have historically been part of many programs. Factors such as antisocial personality disorder and antisocial thinking have received recent attention; governmental grant-making bodies and diversion programs are increasingly including assessment and cognitive-behavioral interventions to address these issues. Cognitive-behavioral change programs such as Interactive Journaling (Proctor et al., 2012), Thinking for a Change (Golden, 2002), Moral Reconation Therapy (Little & Robinson, 1988), and Reasoning and Rehabilitation (Ross et al., 1988) can now be found as part of the treatment expectations for community programs affiliated with diversion projects or delivered by clinicians and case managers within the diversion team.

To date, only one known study exists specifically examining the effects of adherence to risk–needs–responsivity principles on MHC outcomes. Among 196 individuals referred to MHC, Campbell and colleagues (2015) found that MHC participants who received a greater number of services matched to their identified criminogenic needs experienced a lower likelihood of rearrest in the 12 months following MHC enrollment. These findings suggest a promising path forward for MHCs as they continue to expand on the scope of interventions offered and the goals of both addressing clinical need and decreasing criminogenic risk.

As noted previously, one factor that is critical for MHC success is the demeanor of the judge and the atmosphere in the courtroom (Redlich et al., 2005). Rather than acting as a dispassionate arbiter of courtroom rules, the MHC judge presents a more collaborative and even supportive persona to the participant while maintaining ultimate authority over enforcement of the treatment mandate. MHC judges may ask clients about treatment, school, jobs, family, or other areas of importance. It is not unusual for judges to compliment participants on their community-based successes. In such an atmosphere, clients perceive an enhanced sense of voluntariness and fairness.

Whether that positive perception leads to better outcomes is still unclear. The interaction with the judge has been shown to be relevant to success in previous drug court studies, but in MHCs, the research is scarce and results are mixed. Some studies suggest that judges' use of praise and increased eye contact may be related to positive outcomes (Frailing, 2010; Wales & Hiday, 2010), whereas other studies show no differences in participants' perceptions between a judge who made more supportive or praising comments and a judge who did not (Kopelovich et al., 2013).

Jail diversion in general, and MHCs in particular, are not without their detractors. Among the criticisms are that diversion programs engage in "net widening." In this context, individuals who may otherwise have had the opportunity for release (after trial or plea bargain) are offered the opportunity for diversion, find it difficult to refuse, and consequently are kept under judicial supervision with the potential for incarceration for an extended period. Defendants' interests give way to a paternalistic, clinically focused intervention that is inherently coercive. While diversion clients often waive privilege as a prerequisite for program participation, there may still be concerns about sharing confidential clinical information in open court and with the judge and prosecutor. One additional concern is the potential that such information may influence criminal justice decisions if the client ultimately chooses to go to trial or a diversion offer is rescinded.

Recent trends

In recent years, criminal justice practitioners and treatment providers have taken more of a public health approach to the substance use and behavioral problems experienced by MHC clients. These include prebooking diversion, bail reform, and harm reduction.

In 2022, the Conference of Chief Justices and Conference of State Court Administrators passed a resolution calling for members to "support state and community efforts to utilize a public health model rather than a criminal justice approach ... [and] to deflect or divert cases from the court system and into treatment" (National Judicial Task Force to Examine State Courts' Response to Mental Illness, 2022, p. 23). The addition of "deflection" refers to a focus on advocating for systems change—upstream, at intercept 0—that would avoid criminal justice adjudication and detention for individuals with mental illness altogether (e.g., greater access to community-based crisis care, supportive housing, and civil commitment reform). Several states, such as California and New York, have reduced exposure to jail through reducing or eliminating the cash bail system that disproportionately detained people of color and the economically disadvantaged, some of whom also suffer from serious mental illness (Pope, 2023). In some jurisdictions, the needs of individuals with serious mental illness and associated court concerns about adherence to hearing attendance are addressed by pretrial supervised release programs that specifically include mental health supports (Fader-Towe & Osher, 2015). The clinical and criminal justice characteristics of potential diversion candidates who are in jail at the time of diversion consideration are, therefore, evolving.

The increasing focus on harm reduction is another trend that impacts both diversion and related jail-based services (Garcia & Lucas, 2021). Although most MHCs have an expectation of abstinence from drugs and alcohol, which is inconsistent with one of the tenets of harm reduction, MHCs do offer harm reduction by providing an alternative to incarceration, avoidance and/or minimization of jail detention, and minimal use of jail remand as a sanction. Additional harm reduction practices influencing diversion include a willingness to embrace psychopharmacologic interventions for mental illness, medication-assisted treatments (such as suboxone and naltrexone), and dissemination of overdose prevention interventions (i.e., naloxone and fentanyl test strips). This changing landscape of harm reduction expectations and practices has also begun to affect jail-based services that seek to support detainees' successful release to the community (see Chapters 49 and 50).

Mental health diversion and jail-based practices

Jail-based staff can play an important role in supporting mental health diversion, including identification of potential diversion candidates, stabilization and support, and discharge planning coordination. All three activities require active communication with community providers, courts, and court-based teams.

While, as noted above, MHCs differ from one another in structure and integration with jail and the community, some counties have created jail population review teams to increase consistency in practices (e.g., Lucas County, Ohio; Pima County, Arizona). Through a collaborative approach, these teams, which include jail staff and court stakeholders, identify individuals in custody, conduct reviews of all cases, and provide policy or release recommendations (Weill et al., 2022). Furthermore, jail mental health screening and assessment can be helpful in identifying appropriate candidates for diversion. Even though these assessments are conducted primarily for jail treatment purposes, mental health diversion programs often benefit from having access to correctional health care records as part of their review for eligibility and community-based treatment planning determinations. These records provide helpful information about diagnoses, treatment needs, or any social service needs that the jail staff might have already identified and worked on, such as supportive housing applications.

Jail-based clinicians can also support more rapid release through active treatment, about which there is open communication with the court-based team. Clients who are candidates for diversion usually need to be symptomatically stable prior to acceptance by a community-based provider. Treatment adherence, positive response to treatment, and a firm program intake date are often among the criteria for release, so active treatment and symptom reduction early in an individual's incarceration can play a critical role in the diversion decision-making and timing.

Open communication is also important for the sharing of information from the court-based team to the jail-based provider. Clients may present to the court-based team with active symptoms that preclude taking a plea and program placement and/or indicate immediate safety concerns. The team needs to be able to communicate this information easily and effectively to the jail-based provider so that treatment adjustments can be made if indicated. The bidirectional communication and collaboration between the jail-based and court-based teams is also important for clients who were already placed in a diversion program but who may have been remanded to jail during the pendency of their court mandate.

Although jail reentry services are an essential part of jail health care for all detainees, recognized by courts and correctional accreditation agencies (*Brad H. v. City of New York*, 2020; *Charles v. Orange County*, 2019; National Commission on Correctional Health Care, 2018; *Wakefield v. Thompson*, 1999), staffing challenges, rapid turnover, and short or unpredictable lengths of stay make discharge planning difficult (Foellmi & Rotter, 2023). These challenges can be significantly mitigated when individuals are released from incarceration through a mental health diversion program. In these scenarios, the discharge date is known (typically the date of the plea) and the release can be planned. Staffing resource limitations, which are common in jails (Fagan & Ax, 2011; Helms et al., 2016), may be made up for by mental health diversion programs that can provide case management and care coordination services, including linkage to community services and applications for supportive housing or insurance. Jail-based staff can often help with these applications, which may require documentation of the client's current clinical condition and treatment.

Summary

Decreasing the number of individuals with mental illness in the criminal justice system remains a public mental health priority—one that has even reached the U.S. Supreme Court (*Brown v. Plata*, 2011). Diverting individuals with mental illness from jail or prison decreases their exposure to the traumatic carceral environment and addresses security concerns of corrections professionals charged with their care and management. When diversion is coupled with the court-based, problem-solving approach of monitored care and treatment in the community, public safety is improved, and the clinical success of the individual is enhanced. When treatment in the community includes an explicit focus on criminogenic factors, the ability to meet public safety goals is enhanced even further. And when, as recommended, participation in the program and proposed treatment plan is truly voluntary (i.e., clients choose to participate intelligently and competently), these programs are consistent with the mental health recovery approach critical to community stability and long-term success.

Most of the data are clear that diversion can be implemented without exacerbating mental health or public safety concerns and that there are models for client intercept and associated programming. However, given the considerable variability from jurisdiction to jurisdiction in court resources, treatment resources, social supports, political philosophies, and fiscal realities, the types of diversion that will work for one community may not work for another. Jail-based practitioners can support diversion efforts through knowledge of and active participation in the programs in their specific jurisdictions.

REFERENCES

Andrews, D. A., & Bonta, J. (2010). Rehabilitating criminal justice policy and practice. *Psychology, Public Policy, and Law, 16*, 39–55.

Barber-Rioja, V., & Rotter, M. (2014). A therapeutic approach to jurisprudence: A differential thinking model of sanctions and rewards. *International Journal of Forensic Mental Health, 13*(3), 272–278.

Brad H. v. City of New York, 712 N.Y.S. 2d 336 (Sup. Ct. 2000).

Bronson, J., & Berzofsky, M. (2017). *Indicators of mental health problems reported by prisoners and jail inmates, 2011–12*. Bureau of Justice Statistics.

Brown v. Plata, 131 S. Ct. 1910 (2011).

Burns, P. J., Hiday, V. A., & Ray, B. (2013). Effectiveness 2 years postexit of a recently established mental health court. *American Behavioral Scientist, 57*(2), 189–208. https://doi.org/10.1177/0002764212465416

Campbell, M. A., Canales, D. D., Wei, R., Totten, A. E., MacAulay, W. A. C., & Wershler, J. L. (2015). Multidimensional evaluation of a mental health court: Adherence to the risk-need-responsivity model. *Law and Human Behavior, 39*(5), 489–502. https://doi.org/10.1037/lhb0000135

Charles v. Orange County, 925 F.3d 73 (2d Cir. 2019).

Comartin, E. B., Kubiak, S. P., Ray, B., Tillander, E., & Hanna, J. (2015). Short-and long-term outcomes of mental health court participants by psychiatric diagnosis. *Psychiatric Services, 66*(9), 923–929. https://doi.org/10.1176/appi.ps.201400230

Cosden, M., Ellens, J., Schnell, J., Yamini-Diouf, Y., & Wolfe, M. M. (2003). Evaluation of a mental health court with assertive community treatment. *Behavioral Sciences and the Law, 21*, 415–427.

Fader-Towe, H., & Osher, F. (2015). *Improving responses to people with mental illnesses at the pretrial stage*. https://csgjusticecenter.org/publications/improving-responses-to-people-with-mental-illnesses-at-the-pretrial-stage-essential-elements

Fagan, T., & Ax, R. K. (2011). *Correctional mental health handbook*. Sage Publications.

Foellmi, M., & Rotter, M. (2023). Reentry and diversion: From jail to community. In V. Barber-Rioja, A. Garcia-Mansilla, B. Subedi, & A. Batastini (Eds.), *Handbook of mental health assessment and treatment in jails*. Oxford University Press.

Frailing, K. (2010). How mental health courts function: Outcomes and observations. *International Journal of Law and Psychiatry, 33*, 207–213.

Garcia, A., & Lucas, D. (2021). *Bridging the gap: A practitioner's guide to harm reduction in drug courts*. https://www.innovatingjustice.org/publications/harm-reduction-drug-courts

Golden, L. (2002). *Evaluation of the efficacy of a cognitive behavioral program for offenders on probation: Thinking for a Change*. http://www/nicic.org/pubs/2002/018190.pdf

Han, W. (2020). Effect of behavioral health services and neighborhood disadvantages on recidivism: A comparison of mental health court and traditional court participants. *Journal of Experimental Criminology, 16*(1), 119–140. https://doi.org/10.1007/s11292-019-09402-0

Heilbrun, K., Dematteo, D., Yasuhara, K., Brooks-Holliday, S., Shah, S., King, C., Bingham Dicarlo, A., Hamilton, D., & LaDuke, C. (2012). Community-based alternatives for justice-involved individuals with severe mental illness: Review of the relevant research. *Criminal Justice and Behavior, 39*(4), 351–419. https://doi.org/10.1177/0093854811432421

Helms, R., Gutierrez, R. S., & Reeves-Gutierrez, D. (2016). Jail mental health resourcing: A conceptual and empirical study of social determinants. *International Journal of Offender Therapy and Comparative Criminology, 60*(9), 1036–1063.

Hiday, V. A., & Ray, B. (2010). Arrests two years after exiting a well-established mental health court. *Psychiatric Services, 61*(5), 463–468. https://doi.org/10.1176/ps.2010.61.5.463

Hiday, V. A., Ray, B., & Wales, H. W. (2014). Predictors of mental health court graduation. *Psychology, Public Policy, and Law, 20*(2), 191–199. https://doi.org/10.1037/law0000008

Hirschtritt, M. E., & Binder, R. L. (2017). Interrupting the mental illness–incarceration–recidivism cycle. *JAMA, 317*(7), 695–696.

Junginger, J., Claypoole, K., Laygo, R., & Crisanti, A. (2006). Effects of serious mental illness and substance abuse on criminal offenses. *Psychiatric Services, 57*(6), 879–882. https://doi.org/10.1176/ps.2006.57.6.879

Keator, K. J., Callahan, L., Steadman, H. J., & Vesselinov, R. (2013). The impact of treatment on the public safety outcomes of mental health court participants. *American Behavioral Scientist, 57*(2), 231–243. https://doi.org/10.1177/0002764212465617

Kopelovich, S., Yanos, P., Pratt, C., & Hoerner, J. (2013). Procedural justice in mental health courts: Judicial practices, participant perceptions, and outcomes related to mental health recovery. *International Journal of Law and Psychiatry, 36*, 113–120.

Linhorst, D. M., Kondrat, D., Eikenberry, J., & Dirks-Linhorst, P. A. (2020). Associations between legal representation and mental health court outcomes. *American Journal of Criminal Justice, 47*(3), 1–23. https://doi.org/10.1007/s12103-020-09594-6

Little, G. L., & Robinson, K. D. (1988). Moral Reconation Therapy: A systematic step-by-step treatment system for treatment-resistant clients. *Psychological Reports, 62*, 135–161.

Lowder, E. M., Rade, C. B., & Desmarais, S. L. (2018). Effectiveness of mental health courts in reducing recidivism: A meta-analysis.

Psychiatric Services, *69*(1), 15–22. https://doi.org/10.1176/appi.ps.201700107

Matejkowski, J., Han, W., & Conrad, A. (2020). Voluntariness of treatment, mental health service utilization, and quality of life among mental health court participants. *Psychology, Public Policy, and Law*, *26*(2), 185.

McGaha, A., Boothroyd, R. A., Poythress, N. G., Petrila, J., & Ort, T. G. (2002). Lessons from the Broward County Mental Health Court. *Evaluation and Program Planning*, *25*, 125–135.

National Association of Drug Court Professionals. (1997). *Defining drug courts: The key components*. http://www.nadcp.org/sites/default/files/nadcp/KeyComponents.pdf

National Commission on Correctional Health Care. (2018). *Standards for health services in jails: 2018*.

National Judicial Task Force to Examine State Courts' Response to Mental Illness. (2022). *State courts leading change: Report and recommendations*. https://issuu.com/statecourts/docs/mhtf_finalreport

National Treatment Court Resource Center. (2023). *Treatment courts across the United States (2022)*. University of North Carolina Wilmington. https://ntcrc.org/wp-content/uploads/2023/11/2022_NTCRC_TreatmentCourt_Count_Table.pdf

Peterson, J. K., & Heinz, K. (2016). Understanding offenders with serious mental illness in the criminal justice system. *Mitchell Hamline Law Review*, *42*(3), 537–563. http://open.mitchellhamline.edu/mhlr/vol42/iss2/3

Pope, L. G., Pohl, D. J., Ehntholt, A., Boswell, T., Ford, E., Rotter, M., & Compton, M. T. (2023). New York State's Bail Elimination Act of 2019: A retrospective mental health impact assessment. *Impact Assessment and Project Appraisal*, *41*(6), 430–443.

Proctor, L., Hoffmann, N. G., & Allison, S. (2012). The effectiveness of interactive journaling in reducing recidivism among substance-dependent jail inmates. *International Journal of Offender Therapy and Comparative Criminology*, *56*, 317–332.

Redlich, A. D. (2005). Voluntary, but knowing and intelligent. Comprehension in mental health courts. *Psychology, Public Policy and Law*, *11*, 605–619.

Redlich, A. D. (2013). The past, present, and future of mental health courts. In R. L. Wiener & E. M. Brank (Eds.), *Problem solving courts* (pp. 147–161). Springer. https://doi.org/10.1007/978-1-4614-7403-6_9

Redlich, A. D., Steadman, H. J., Monahan, J., Petrila, J., & Griffin, P. A. (2005). The second generation of mental health courts. *Psychology, Public Policy, and Law*, *11*(4), 527–538.

Reich, W. A., Picard-Fritsche, S., Cerniglia, L., & Hahn, J. W. (2013, November). *Predictors of program compliance and re-arrest in mental health courts*. Center for Court Innovation.

Reich, W. A., Picard-Fritsche, S., Lebron, L., & Hahn, J. W. (2015). Predictors of mental health court program compliance and re-arrest in Brooklyn, New York. *Journal of Offender Rehabilitation*, *54*(6), 391–405. https://doi.org/10.1080/10509674.2015.1055035

Ross, R. R., Fabiano, E. A., & Ewles, C. D. (1988). Reasoning and rehabilitation. *International Journal of Offender Therapy and Comparative Criminology*, *32*, 29–35.

Skeem, J. L., Winter, E., Kennealy, P. J., Louden, J. E., & Tatar, J. R. (2013). Offenders with mental illness have criminogenic needs, too: Toward recidivism reduction. *Law and Human Behavior*, *38*(3), 212–224. https://doi.org/10.1037/lhb0000054

Steadman, H. J., Cocozza, J. J., & Veysey, B. M. (1999). Comparing outcomes for diverted and nondiverted jail detainees with mental illness. *Law and Human Behavior*, *23*(6), 615–627.

Steadman, H. J., Davidson, S., & Brown, C. (2001). Mental health courts: Their promise and unanswered questions. *Psychiatric Services*, *52*, 457–458.

Steadman, H. J., & Naples, M. (2005). Assessing the effectiveness of jail diversion programs for persons with serious mental illness and co-occurring substance use disorders. *Behavioral Sciences and the Law*, *23*(2), 163–170. https://doi.org/10.1002/bsl.640

Steadman, H. J., Redlich, A., Callahan, L., Robbins, P., & Vesselinov, R. (2011). Effect of mental health courts on arrest and jail days: A multisite study. *Archives of General Psychiatry*, *68*, 167–172.

Wakefield v. Thompson, 177 F.3d 1160 (9th Cir. 1999).

Wales, H. W., & Hiday, B. R. (2010). Procedural justice and the mental health court judge's role in reducing recidivism. *International Journal of Law and Psychiatry*, *33*, 265–271.

Weill, J., Cissner, A. B., & Naraharisetti, S. (2022). *Population review teams: Evaluating jail reduction and racial disparities across three jurisdictions*. Safety + Justice Challenge and Center for Justice Innovation. https://www.innovatingjustice.org/sites/default/files/media/document/2022/CCI%20PRT%20Report%20Final%204.21.22.pdf

7

Jails and prisons

*Joel A Dvoskin and Sarah M. Broom**

Introduction

Jails and prisons have a constitutional duty to provide necessary mental health services to incarcerated persons (IPs) with serious medical needs, including psychiatric needs, under the 14th and Eighth Amendments to the Constitution, respectively. While the constitutional standard of deliberate indifference is the same in both settings (*Farmer v. Brennan*, 1994), the manner in which jails and prisons carry out their duties may be quite different. This chapter describes the most important differences between jails and prisons and the implications of these differences for providing mental health services to IPs.

Historically, jails have been used to hold defendants for trial and to confine prisoners who have been sentenced for misdemeanors, typically for sentences of less than 1 year. In contrast, prisons are managed by state or federal governments (either directly or by contract) and used for longer term confinement of individuals convicted of a felony offense who are generally serving sentences of 1 year or longer. However, these distinctions are not hard and fast. For example, some prisoners may return to jails intermittently if they still have pending charges or as a transitional period when approaching the end of their sentence. In addition, some states have modified their sentencing guidelines, leading to a significant number of individuals convicted of a felony being housed in county jails. Some state and federal institutions are running combined systems, with pretrial and sentenced individuals housed in the same facilities. As a result, some jails, especially larger ones, have needed to change their mental health service delivery systems to accommodate long-stay prisoners, and some jails have needed to incorporate services that were traditionally thought appropriate for prison mental health services.

The differences between jails and prisons can be examined across several important axes, including the nature of the people who live there, the circumstances of their presence, and the nature of the institution.

Jail versus prison detainees: similar people in different situations

In general, there are few differences between the people who are detained or incarcerated in jails and prisons except for the length of time they have been locked up. After being arrested, people are often delivered to the jail directly by police officers, in some cases after spending a few hours in a police lockup. IPs who are newly admitted to prison in most cases have been in jail for some length of time, where they may have received mental health treatment and are less likely to be under the influence of alcohol or illicit drugs. Due to receiving previous treatment, their symptoms may be better managed with psychotropic medications or behavioral interventions, leading to a less severe presentation and less acute symptoms when they are brought to prison.

Substance abuse poses additional challenges to providers in jail settings. Estimates have found that over 60% of jail detainees are dependent on drugs and alcohol (Toman et al., 2018). As a result of their very recent arrests, it is no surprise that from 62% to 86% of new admissions to jail are under the influence of alcohol, stimulants, or other drugs (Office of National Drug Control Policy, 2013). This creates several challenges for jail mental health providers, some of which are discussed in the chapters on detoxification (Chapter 46) and suicide prevention (Chapter 51). Detainees may be at higher risk of suicide immediately after admission due to the disinhibiting effects of substances. The risk of suicide can also be higher for detainees who are experiencing the painful process of detoxification. An additional challenge is created by the difficulty in diagnosing a person who arrives at the jail under the influence of alcohol, stimulants, or other substances. Even experienced clinicians will have difficulty distinguishing between various forms of preexisting psychotic illness, substance-induced psychosis, and drug-induced disorders, especially in individuals for whom previous records or other sources of collateral information are not immediately available.

*. The authors acknowledge the contributions of Melody C. Brown, who coauthored this chapter in the textbook's first edition.

Steadman and colleagues (2009) found weighted prevalence rates for newly admitted IPs with a serious mental illness of 14.5% for men and 31.0% for women. James and Glaze (2006) stated that 24% of jail inmates reported psychotic symptoms within the 12 months preceding their jail admission; however, it is difficult to know the underlying reason for these reported symptoms (e.g., serious mental illness, drug or alcohol use).

Jails often provide an initial diagnosis, leaving further diagnostic refinement and provision of long-term treatment to the prison setting. However, early detection of mental illness and substance use disorders in jail can lead to better stabilization of symptoms and significantly decreased time spent in initial assessment and treatment planning at prisons. In recent years, one prominent example of this early-detection approach has been the use of medication for opioid use disorder. As discussed in Chapter 49, more individuals are being diagnosed with substance use disorders in the jail setting, and they are being prescribed medication for opioid use disorder (e.g., buprenorphine, methadone, naltrexone) to provide proactive treatment that continues throughout the individual's incarceration and community transition (see Chapter 50). This type of comprehensive treatment, including both medication for opioid use disorder and behavioral therapies, is being encouraged and institutions are implementing it more consistently.

Perhaps the most important difference between jails and prisons, from the perspective of mental health service delivery, is the disparity in turnover, which is much higher in jails than in prisons. The average pretrial jail detainee remains in jail for less than 72 hours (Osher et al., 2002). As a result, although there are similar rates of IPs in jails and prisons, the individuals in jails are constantly rotating. For example, within just the first 6 months of 2023, 30,609 individuals were arrested and booked into the Los Angeles County (California) jails (Los Angeles County Jail System by the Numbers, 2023). This number was much lower than previous years, which researchers attribute to the COVID-19 pandemic. In 2019, upwards of 110,941 individuals were admitted into the Los Angeles County Jail System by the Numbers, 2023, whereas in 2021 California prisons under the jurisdiction of state and federal correctional authorities admitted 25,834 people on new court commitments (Carson, 2023).

Because of the rapid turnover that occurs in jails, mental health professionals spend a far greater percentage of their time doing initial assessments and evaluations, which are much more time-consuming than follow-up visits. Because this work involves complex diagnostic assessment and, in many cases, prescribing psychotropic medications, the American Psychiatric Association (2016) has recommended a significantly larger number of psychiatrists and other prescribers (e.g., advanced practice nurse practitioners and physician's assistants) in jails than prisons. These ratios are described in *Table 7.1*.

Acute versus persistent mental health problems

Because jail detainees are more likely than prison IPs to arrive in an intoxicated or psychotic state and because arrests frequently are the cause and/or effect of extreme emotional distress, mental health professionals in jails are far more likely than their prison counterparts to encounter people suffering from acute psychological distress, including suicidal depression, various forms of psychosis, extreme anxiety, and intoxication. This leads to a significant increase in crisis contacts in jails as compared to prisons. While each of these phenomena can also occur in prisons, prison mental health professionals are more likely to be confronted with serious and persistent mental health problems. It is important to note that acuity does not necessarily refer to severity; here, acuity is used to denote a recent onset or an episode of exacerbated distress. Persistent or chronic disorders such as schizophrenia can be extremely serious, even if the person is not experiencing an acute exacerbation at the moment.

In responding to acute psychological distress, jail mental health professionals have several immediate duties. First, they must assess the person, paying special attention to suicidality or the likelihood of violence toward others. Chapter 15 examines the methods of screening new admissions. As a result of screening, a significant portion of detainees and IPs will be identified as likely needing mental health assessment and treatment. Each of these "positive screens" will, in turn, require assessment by a mental health professional to determine the need for intervention on an emergency or routine basis.

At this stage, diagnosis is much more difficult; even experienced clinicians may have difficulty distinguishing between acute exacerbations of serious mental illness, symptoms brought on by stress or intoxication, and malingering. The clinician's first priority is to keep the patients safe and to stabilize the acute situation, with less emphasis placed on sorting out complex diagnostic challenges.

In contrast, prison mental health professionals are less likely to encounter psychiatric emergencies immediately upon entry to the institution and, in theory, will be able to review mental health treatment records from jail, the community, or previous prison admissions. In both jails and prisons, collateral information from previous treatment records or family is invaluable. Prison mental health providers are now tasked with determining the need for long-term treatment, clarifying diagnoses, optimizing medication regimens, and encouraging treatment adherence. Due to prison IPs having longer sentences, mental health providers are tasked not only with providing routine treatment but also with managing potential crisis contacts that may result from bad news, such as divorce notices, loss of custody or illness in children, or sentences for other crimes. This type of bad news can often increase hopelessness and other risk factors for suicide. In addition to the diagnostic challenges presented by acute distress and intoxication, clinicians are also faced with the difficulty of assessing malingering. Although the reasons

Table 7.1 American Psychiatric Association's recommended psychiatrist-to-patient ratios

Setting	Recommendation for jail	Recommendation for prison
General population	1 FTE psychiatrist for every 75–100 IPs prescribed psychotropic medication	1 FTE psychiatrist for every 150–200 IPs prescribed psychotropic medications
Residential treatment units	1 FTE psychiatrist for every 50 patients	1 FTE psychiatrist for every 50 patients

Note. FTE = full-time equivalent; IP = incarcerated person.

for malingering in jails and prisons are different, the need to make accurate assessments is the same.

Malingering

One of the most vexing and controversial issues in correctional mental health is the assessment of malingering. While discussed in more depth in Chapter 20, it is important to note some differences between jails and prisons in regard to malingering.

Perhaps the best way for clinicians to think about malingering is as a question rather than an answer. In other words, if an IP is purposely and inaccurately presenting as mentally ill, presumably they are doing this to achieve some sort of benefit. For pretrial detainees, it is commonly assumed that they are trying to create the false impression that they are incompetent to stand trial or to support a strategy of pleading not guilty by reason of insanity. In extreme cases, such as first-degree murder, such a strategy might make sense, as commitment to a forensic psychiatric hospital might be preferable to a sentence of life without parole or even death. Other defendants might hope that a finding of incompetence to stand trial would result in a long delay that would hinder prosecution. In some cases, feigning or exaggeration of mental health symptoms would need to be maintained over a long period, given that competency evaluations do not typically occur immediately upon the detainee's arrival at the jail and may take many months to perform because of systemic shortages in the state hospital system (Kois et al., 2023; *Trueblood v. Washington State Department of Social and Health Services*, 2016; see Chapter 71). Competency evaluators use a variety of methods to detect malingered symptoms or disabilities, including psychological testing and reliance upon collateral information; these strategies are discussed in Chapter 20.

In prisons, there is a different set of likely reasons that an IP might feign or exaggerate symptoms or disabilities. The most common of these is a desire to move from one housing location to another that is considered safer or otherwise more desirable. Other reasons include seeking medication for inappropriate purposes (e.g., sale or intoxication) and, in rare cases, efforts to escape (e.g., during transportation to a hospital). Treatment responses in prison might include an assessment of the likely reasons for feigned or exaggerated symptoms and skill-building treatments aimed at improving the IP's manner of preventing or solving problems.

Another common reason IPs might exaggerate symptoms of mental illness is fear. Jails and prisons can be dangerous places, especially for individuals who are unable or unwilling to defend themselves physically. First-time detainees may exaggerate these dangers based on fictional accounts of jails and prisons.

Additionally, many jails and prisons have limited or understaffed mental health services. This may lead a person with a moderate depression or anxiety disorder to exaggerate symptoms in the belief that "gilding the lily" is the only way to get help. When malingering is suspected, it is important to try to understand the reasons the person might feign or exaggerate symptoms or disabilities. Simply put, malingered symptoms and genuine mental disorder can coexist. Even when a person is exaggerating or feigning symptoms, it is dangerous to simply dismiss the possibility that they suffer from a real mental illness.

In both jails and prisons, two very useful strategies can be employed for responding to the possibility of malingering. First and most importantly, all individuals must be kept safe when presenting with symptoms of acute psychological distress, even if there is a strong suspicion that the distress is feigned or exaggerated. If the IP's presentation is based on fear or extreme anxiety, a nonresponsive correctional mental health system might inadvertently communicate to the individual that the only way to end their intolerable psychological distress is through suicide. The assessment of malingering is not an exact science, and the consequences of a false-positive determination of malingering are potentially lethal. The second strategy is to seek collateral information from as many sources as possible. Previous mental health records from jails, prisons, hospitals, and community providers that have treated the person in the past can be useful. In addition, seeking feedback from the custody, program, health care, and support staff who observe the person 24 hours each day can provide valuable insight about the nature and consistency of an IP's reported symptoms.

Special mental health housing

Unlike other aspects of correctional mental health, housing differs less as a function of jail versus prison and more as a function of the size of the institution or system. Jails and prisons require several housing options. As explained in Chapter 51, every jail or prison must provide appropriate housing, often called "suicide watch" cells, for people who are deemed to pose a high or imminent risk of suicide. In large jails and prisons, these cells are often located in a dedicated unit or in part of another type of special housing, such as residential mental health units or medical infirmaries. In smaller jails or for IPs who already reside in specialized mental health housing, suicide watch may be performed within the unit or within general population housing. Wherever they exist, suicide watch cells must be reasonably suicide resistant, with the ability for direct observation by staff or IP companions and for additional precautions such as tear-resistant clothing, paper utensils, and limited access to property. Suicide watch cells must include ease of observation and an absence of places from which an IP can easily suspend a ligature. When a person poses an imminent risk of suicide, there is no substitute for direct observation by staff.

In addition to suicide watch cells, many larger jails and prisons have specialized mental health housing units, often modeled after group homes or residential treatment settings in the community. Specialized mental health housing can serve several purposes. First, separating IPs with mental illnesses can allow for more efficient provision of psychiatric, nursing, and other treatment services. This is especially true for the provision of group therapies aimed at psychosocial rehabilitative and skill-building treatments. Second, it allows for more diligent observation of detainees and IPs who pose a risk of suicide or interpersonal violence. Third, it can prevent detainees and IPs with mental illnesses from being frightened or harmed by predators in the general population.

Equally important, people with serious mental illnesses may be psychologically vulnerable to exacerbations caused by real or perceived dangers posed by IPs in the general population. In large jails and prisons, it is often helpful to create psychologically safer housing alternatives such as residential treatment units. Again, this will vary more as a function of institution size and less as a function of jail versus prison settings.

Treatment: symptom reduction and safety versus skill building and rehabilitation

As discussed in Chapters 42 and 43, correctional mental health services include individual and group therapies, not just psychotropic medication. These therapies have several purposes, including crisis prevention and response, suicide prevention, reduction of idle and unstructured time, and psychosocial skill building.

The relative importance given to each type of therapy depends, in large part, on the setting. Because of the high turnover and higher level of acuity in jails, therapy will largely be aimed at prevention of immediate harm and symptom reduction. While psychotropic medications play an important role in reducing symptoms, it is a mistake to ignore the potential value of individual and group therapies, especially in the treatment of anxiety and depression. Similarly, the management of sleep complaints in jail settings can often benefit from a nonpharmacologic approach initially (see Chapter 19).

In contrast, prison mental health professionals can expect to treat their patients and clients for long periods of time, creating the very real possibility of meaningful skill acquisition in psychologically relevant ways. For example, group therapy implementing cognitive-behavioral approaches, along with other methods, has been found to help IPs to be more effective and to reduce incidences of prison violence (Auty et al., 2017). Individual treatment can be effective in aiding IPs in symptom reduction and maintenance in a challenging environment.

Segregation or restrictive housing

As discussed in Chapter 10, there is some controversy about the extent and nature of psychological harm caused by long-term segregation. However, several professional organizations, including the American Psychiatric Association, have cautioned that such settings pose a risk of exacerbating or causing mental illness or preventing IPs with serious mental illnesses from improving (Bailey et al., 2023). Treatment interventions, both crisis and maintenance, can be more challenging in these settings. Issues of confidentiality, space, and restriction of resources can impede effective interventions in restrictive housing units. Sadly, according to Kaba et al. (2014), a disproportionate number of suicides in jails and prisons occur in restrictive housing, suggesting that people housed in segregated housing require enhanced and periodic observation and interaction.

Despite concerns about the risks associated with restrictive housing, jails and prisons continue to use the strategy to maintain institutional safety. Some IPs even express a preference for restrictive housing, usually due to fears of serious harm if returned to the general population. For various reasons, people with serious mental illnesses are placed in restrictive housing at disproportionally high rates (Gilligan & Lee, 2013; Kapoor & Trestman, 2016).

Because lengths of stay in prison are much longer than in jail, the likelihood of long-term segregation is much higher in prisons. For IPs with serious mental illnesses, court orders and settlement agreements have increasingly required states to create mental health alternatives to traditional segregation (*Disability Advocates, Inc. v. New York State Office of Mental Health, et al.*, 2002; *Disability Law Center, Inc. v. Massachusetts Department of Corrections, et al.*, 2012; *Jones' El v. Berge*, 2002; *Madrid v. Gomez*, 1995).

Jail and prison systems should make plans for mental health alternatives for detainees and IPs with mental illnesses who remain housed in restrictive housing for long periods (New York City Department of Correction, 2013). Many state and federal correctional systems have created alternative programs and housing units for individuals with mental illness, such as step-down programs, which assist with preparing for the general population.

Transition, discharge, and reentry planning

Transition planning, also known as discharge planning or reentry planning (American Association of Community Psychiatrists, 2001), can be a vexing issue for jails and prisons alike, in part because of a community mental health system that is already stressed and inadequately funded to meet existing demand. As a result, people who received regular mental health treatment in prison may have difficulty gaining access to those same services after they are released. Further, many years in prison may have caused preexisting life skills to atrophy to the point that simple tasks such as taking a bus to the clinic become extremely difficult.

Transition planning in jails poses a very different problem. Again, because of the high turnover, there is often very little time in which to plan for the discharge and transition back into the community of a detainee with serious mental illness. The sheer number of discharges is enough to overwhelm the social work staff of most jail mental health services. An additional challenge is the unpredictable timing of release from jail. Cases are routinely dismissed, plea-bargained for time served, or otherwise disposed of, often with little or no warning to jail mental health providers. One good way to address this challenge is to follow the adage "discharge planning begins at admission" and attend to the basic elements of a transition plan during the initial assessment or initial treatment plan for any detainee with serious mental illness (see Chapter 23). The essential elements of such a plan include prescriptions or medications upon release, a safe place to sleep in the community, and assistance with obtaining entitlements such as Social Security Disability Income or Medicaid. The Medicaid Reentry Section 1115 program was created to assist IPs up to 90 days prior to reentry. This program may assist not only with the transition process of reentry but also with aftercare and treatment (Centers for Medicare and Medicaid Services, 2023). One evolving best practice for transition planning includes "community in-reach," whereby case managers or primary clinicians from community mental health providers are able to meet with the detainee in jail prior to release (Dlugacz, 2010; Lennox et al., 2012).

Equally challenging, the lack of adequate social services in most U.S. communities (La Vigne et al., 2008; Steadman & Veysey, 1997) means that there are often inadequate services to which IPs can be referred. Additionally, the U.S. Department of Health and Human Services has noted an increase in inadequate services since the COVID-19 pandemic, which has made an already challenging problem much larger (U.S. Department of Health and Human Services et al., 2022). This also reflects the lack of social and familial support systems for many frequent arrestees with serious mental illness, particularly those who were homeless at the time of their arrest.

Summary

There are many similarities between prisons and jails, especially regarding the constitutional standard for mental health services. However, it is important to recognize the differences to ensure that the unique needs of each kind of institution are met. Predominant among these differences is the very high degree of turnover in jail populations, resulting in dramatic increases in acuity of mental illness and substance misuse, a significantly increased risk of suicide, and increases in workload due to the much higher percentage of initial assessments. As a result, staffing plans for a variety of professions must consider this higher workload if jails are to meet their obligations. In contrast, prison mental health services are more often faced with the realities of serious and persistent mental illnesses and the hopelessness that can come after years of incarceration and in the face of very long sentences. While prison mental health clinicians have more time with which to work than their jail counterparts, they also face significantly greater expectations for treatment that goes beyond crisis response and psychotropic medication.

REFERENCES

American Association of Community Psychiatrists. (2001). *AACP continuity of care guidelines: Best practices for managing transitions between levels of care.*

American Psychiatric Association. (2016). *Psychiatric services in correctional facilities.*

Auty, K. M., Cope, A., & Liebling, A. (2017). Psychoeducational programs for reducing prison violence: A systematic review. *Aggression and Violent Behavior, 33*, 126–143.

Bailey, R. K., Ford, E., Morris, N. P., Metzner, J., & Patterson, R. (2023). *Position statement on restrictive housing of incarcerated adults with serious mental illness.* American Psychiatric Association.

Carson, E. A. (2023). *Prisoners in 2022—Statistical tables.* Department of Justice, Office of Justice Programs, Bureau of Justice and Statistics.

Centers for Medicare and Medicaid Services. (2023). *HHS release new guidance to encourage states to apply for new Medicaid reentry section 1115 demonstration opportunity to increase health care for people leaving carceral facilities.* https://www.cms.gov/newsroom/press-releases/hhs-releases-new-guidance-encourage-states-apply-new-medicaid-reentry-section-1115-demonstration

Disability Advocates, Inc. v. New York State Office of Mental Health, et al., U.S. District Court, Southern District of New York, Case 02 CV 2002 (GEL) (2002).

Disability Law Center, Inc. v. Massachusetts Department of Corrections, et al., U.S. District Court, District of Massachusetts, Case No. 07-10463 (MLW) (2012).

Dlugacz, H. A. (2010). *Reentry planning for offenders with mental disorders.* Civic Research Institute.

Farmer v. Brennan, 511 U.S. 825 (1994).

Gilligan, J., & Lee, B. (2013). *Report to the New York City Board of Correction.* Solitary Watch. https://solitarywatch.org/wp-content/uploads/2013/11/GilliganReport.-Final.pdf

Kaba, F., Lewis, A., Glowa-Kollisch, S., Hadler, J., Lee, D., Alper, H., Selling, D., MacDonald, R., Solimo, A. A., & Venters, H. (2014). Solitary confinement and risk of self-harm among jail inmates. *American Journal of Public Health, 104*, 442–447.

Kapoor, R., & Trestman, R. (2016). *Mental health effects of restrictive housing.* Office of Justice Programs, U.S. Department of Justice. https://ojp.gov/ncjrs/virtual-library/abstracts/mental-health-effects-restrictive-housing

Kois, L. E., Murrie, D. C., Gowensmith, W. N., & Packer, I. K. (2023). A public health perspective to reform the competence to stand trial system. *Psychiatric Services, 74*, 1289–1290.

James, D. J., & Glaze, L. E. (2006). *Mental health problems of prison and jail inmates* (NCJ 213600). Department of Justice, Office of Justice Programs, Bureau of Justice and Statistics.

Jones' El v. Berge, U.S. District Court, Western District of Wisconsin, Case No. 00-C-421-C (2002).

La Vigne, N., Davies, E., Palmer, T., & Halberstadt, R. (2008). *Release planning for successful reentry: A guide for corrections, service providers, and community groups.* Urban Institute Justice Policy Center. http://www.urban.org/UploadedPDF/411767_successful_reentry.pdf

Lennox, C., Senior, J., King, C., et al. (2012). The management of released prisoners with severe and enduring mental illness. *Journal of Forensic Psychiatry and Psychology, 23*(1), 67–75.

Los Angeles County Jail System by the Numbers. (2023). *Los Angeles Almanac.* https://www.laalmanac.com/crime/cr25b.php#:~:text=In%20the%20first%20six%20months,ended%20up%20booked%20into%20jail

Madrid v. Gomez, 889 F. Supp. 1146 (1995).

New York City Department of Correction. (2013, May). *New mental health initiative will intervene and provide treatment for seriously mentally ill among jail population.* http://www.nyc.gov/html/doc/downloads/pdf/NEWS_from_Mental_Health_051313.pdf

Office of National Drug Control Policy. (2013, May). *Arrestee drug abuse monitoring program II: 2012 Annual report.*

Osher, F. C., Steadman, H. J., & Barr, H. (2002). A best practice approach to community reentry from jails for inmates with co-occurring disorders: The APIC Model. *Crime and Delinquency, 48*(3), 379–396. https://doi.org/10.1177/0011128702048003006

Steadman, H. J., Osher, F. C., Robbins, P. C., Case, B., & Samuels, S. (2009). Prevalence of serious mental illness among jail inmates. *Psychiatric Services, 60*, 761–765.

Steadman, H. J., & Veysey, B. M. (1997). *Providing services for jail inmates with mental disorders.* Department of Justice, Office of Justice Programs, Bureau of Justice and Statistics.

Toman, E. L., Cochran, J. C., & Cochran, J. K. (2018). Jailhouse blues? The adverse effects of pretrial detention for prison social order. *Criminal Justice and Behavior, 45*, 316–339. https://doi.org:10.1177/0093854817753018

Trueblood v. Washington State Department of Social and Health Services, 822 F.3d 1037 (2016).

U.S. Department of Health and Human Services, Department of Labor, and Department of Treasury. (2022). *2022 MHPEA report to Congress.* https://www.dol.gov/sites/dolgov/files/EBSA/laws-and-regulations/laws/mental-health-parity/report-to-congress-2022-realizing-parity-reducing-stigma-and-raising-awareness.pdf

8

Population management

Robert L. Trestman[*]

Introduction

Jails and prisons share population management challenges with hotels: What beds are available to meet requirements for which individuals? The management of large facilities and systems must recognize many safety and clinical demands in real time. Levels of security risk; medical, mental health, and addiction treatment needs; and sex offender status, among others, must all be taken into account in placement decisions (Brennan, 2020; Meyers et al., 2023; Shaffer et al., 2019). This chapter discusses such pragmatic issues, particularly in the context of the psychiatric management challenges they present.

Classification of incarcerated persons

A core responsibility of correctional systems is safety and security for incarcerated persons (IPs) and for staff. Several considerations affect placement decisions. Correctional systems increasingly use objective classification systems, with resources developed to help them do this (Bonta & Wormith, 2018). In most facilities and all systems, classification requires computer support. Smaller systems integrate classification with other computerized functions. Some larger systems separate medical and mental health housing management from the security housing system. Whether integrated or separated, from a health systems perspective, the computerized IP management system should interface with the electronic health record (when one exists). The severity and violence of the alleged offense or conviction are primary determinants of classification, but there are other considerations.

SCENARIO: CLASSIFICATION CHALLENGES

BD is a 26-year-old man convicted of aiding in the rape of a 13-year-old girl. BD cooperated with authorities and testified against his codefendant. He has a history of bipolar disorder, cocaine and heroin use disorders, and HIV infection. He has two prior incarcerations for nonviolent crimes but assaulted a cellmate on his previous incarceration. What are the considerations for his housing assignment?

Classification for BD presents several important considerations. His sexual offense involving a 13-year-old girl puts him at risk for assault; other IPs often target child molesters and IPs with mental illness, both of whom tend to fall low on the status hierarchy among IPs. His cooperation with authorities and testimony against his codefendant also put him at risk of retaliation from other IPs. His prior assault on a cellmate, however, complicates the concerns about his safety. He may be a predator as well as a potential victim during his incarceration. The classification decision needs to balance the benefits of removing him from contact with more violent IPs against the risks of housing him with more vulnerable peers. The placement decision must also consider BD's substance use and mental health treatment needs.

Admission and assessment

Much of the work of population management is done at the time of admission into a facility. Court documents are reviewed and prior records retrieved. Custody, medical, and (where indicated) mental health staff interview the IP on intake. Demographics, aliases, and criminal history are detailed. In a jail, the emphasis is on safety and basic medical and mental health needs (see Chapter 7). On intake into a prison, additional concerns include educational activities, programming, and vocational needs (Nur & Nguyen, 2023). Although more sophisticated measures are possible and may be used in selected systems (Pierce, 2016), most correctional facilities and systems use simple 5-point, graded classification scales. There is no uniformity; in some systems, 5 is the most severe, whereas in others the most severe is represented by 1. Typical classification scales include security; educational, vocational, medical, mental health, and addiction needs; and sex offender risk scores. Subscales are also commonly used. The unique requirements of female, transgender, and gender nonconforming IPs are receiving emerging recognition (Routh et al., 2017). All systems keep the genders separate (almost always by sex assigned at birth), but most do not differentiate classification schemes by gender.

*. The author acknowledges the contributions of Kenneth L. Appelbaum, MD, who was a coauthor of this chapter in the first edition of the textbook.

Security

Jails are generally designed as "one size fits all" facilities; housing units range from minimum- through maximum-security levels. Prison systems commonly include a range of facilities, each one designated at a specific security level. In general, IPs accused or convicted of more violent offenses are housed in higher security levels. Higher security comes with greater costs. Minimum-security IPs are usually housed in dormitory settings with lower correctional officer staffing ratios; maximum-security settings are generally double- or single-cell housing with limited movement and more security staff. Security scores typically are composed of several elements, including risk for violence, disciplinary history from previous incarcerations, escape risk, current offense, and gang membership (Tahamont & Frisch, 2019). Inaccurate classification can create significant problems. Underclassification may place other IPs at risk; one unintended consequence of overclassification is the potential for increased risk of rearrest and future incarcerations (Chen & Shapiro, 2007; Gaes & Camp, 2009).

Security risk group

Gang membership typically defines security risk group (SRG) identification, with status or rank in the gang reflecting the level of SRG classification. SRG scoring is often defined as follows: 1, no gang affiliation; 2, prior gang affiliation successfully renounced; 3, active gang member; and 4, gang leader or threat member (Connecticut Department of Correction, 2012). The details of SRG management and concerns are discussed in Chapter 64.

Protective custody and keeping separate

Several groups require protection from other IPs during incarceration. Such groups include law enforcement personnel, IPs with low status among their peers (e.g., sex offenders and those with serious mental illness or cognitive impairment), and informants who testified against gangs, codefendants, or crime organizations. These individuals are often housed in a protective custody unit apart from the general population (Austin, 1998). Protective custody status raises significant concerns. Although it may protect selected individuals, it may be overused. This may occur, for example, when providing appropriate accommodations for an IP in general population proves difficult. Protective custody also typically limits movement and precludes access to programs that would otherwise be available. This is especially problematic for IPs with special needs, such as those with mental impairments. Systems must find ways to ensure their safety without cutting them off from beneficial programming and services.

Distinct from protective custody are individuals who must be kept apart from each other during incarceration. Such "keep-away" concerns may occur for codefendants in a trial, those who physically assaulted each other during incarceration, those known to have preexisting issues from the community (e.g., one IP allegedly killed the sister of another IP), or those affiliated with opposing gangs. Keep-away issues between IPs and staff may occur, for example, when a family member of custody staff becomes incarcerated.

Education

In general, anyone under the age of 18 incarcerated in a U.S. correctional facility without a high school diploma or a General Equivalency Degree (GED) must attend school. Those older than 18 years without a diploma or GED are generally encouraged to go to school. To do so, they must be housed in a facility with educational capacity. The availability of educational programs varies widely among facilities and correctional systems, though many large prison systems now offer educational opportunities beyond high school, often through partnerships with local universities (Gonzalez, 2021; Hackett, 2019). In 2023, the U.S. Department of Education made financial aid in the form of Pell grants available to some incarcerated students, supporting their pursuit of a college education (U.S. Department of Education, 2023).

Treatment needs: mental health, medical, substance use disorder, and sex offender classification

Access to appropriate treatment is always a critical issue; classification helps support such access by creating a designation that allows population management staff to ensure proper IP placement (see Chapter 9). Mental health classification, as with other classifications, should be purely functional and unrelated to diagnosis. On a 5-point scale, the levels, with variability among jurisdictions, may be represented as follows: 1, no past or present treatment needs; 2, no active treatment needs; 3, needs ambulatory level of treatment; 4, requires the equivalent of supported residential housing; and 5, requires infirmary or inpatient level of care. Generally, individuals with a mental health (MH) score of MH-3 or greater will need housing in a facility with dedicated mental health clinicians and nursing staff. Functional levels are dynamic and may change frequently. Someone with bipolar disorder in remission may have MH-3 needs, become acutely manic and be hospitalized for 6 days (during which time the score becomes MH-5), subsequently be discharged to supported housing for 3 weeks (with a score of MH-4), and finally return to the baseline state (MH-3). Some systems also use subcodes that might assist in tracking someone who was on the active caseload of the community mental health authority and will return to the caseload on community release. Another purpose might be to record individuals with a history of suicide attempt to help alert clinical staff upon reincarceration or transfer to a new facility.

Mental health classifications have effects on IPs. In general, IPs get a week of medications for general medical conditions to hold in their cells in a process labeled KOP (keep on person). With few exceptions, nurses administer psychiatric medication individually in directly observed therapy. There are many arguments for and against this approach, but for safety concerns, this has become standard practice. That means that a patient, once prescribed psychiatric medication, must be housed in a facility with nursing support. This may preclude housing in many minimum-security and prerelease facilities. As an unfortunate consequence, some patients choose to stop their medications so they can become eligible for placement in lower security settings. This may lead to decompensation and eventual return to higher security, where they can resume taking their medications.

Exclusion from prerelease settings also deprives IPs on psychotropic medications of the opportunity to develop skills, under supervision, that they will need to self-monitor their medications in the community. These pragmatic concerns reflect the importance of accurate diagnosis, discussion of treatment options, and full and meaningful informed consent with the patient prior to initiating treatment (see Chapters 9 and 16).

The ways in which staff use classification systems, especially for mental health, may raise concerns. For example, consider a patient currently classified as MH-3 who might benefit from a treatment program only available in a residential unit (requiring a MH-4 classification). Yet the patient is not someone who otherwise needs a residential level of care. A clinician may, in an attempt to provide care for that patient, classify the patient as MH-4. While this may sound reasonable, such overclassification may lead to reduced availability of residential beds for those in greater need and unintended effects on parole decisions, leading to longer incarceration. Further, those placed in residential treatment units, similar to those in protective custody, may have restricted access to other programming or vocational opportunities.

Medical classification follows a similar system to mental health. Typical coding reflects the following: 1, no past or current medical treatment needs; 2, no current treatment needs; 3, active treatment well managed with medications with need for predictable access to nursing care 16 hours daily, 7 days per week; 4, chronic illness requiring full-time nursing availability or disability accommodations; and 5, infirmary or inpatient level of care. Subcodes for medical needs may include whether someone is blind or deaf, requires crutches or a sleep apnea machine, and so forth. For example, those with anaphylactic reactions to bee stings might have a subcode or designation as medical-4, with full-time access to nursing care.

Systems must ensure proper use of their clinical beds, including residential beds for mental health needs and infirmary housing, whether for medical or mental health purposes. For example, correctional officers may want to use a designated infirmary bed to house an IP for security purposes or use residential mental health beds for protective custody or to keep IPs apart from potential enemies. Such practices should be avoided, as they reduce the availability of limited infirmary and residential beds and complicate care delivery to patients on those units. Residential programs try to create therapeutic environments where all IPs participate in activities and programming. Boarding nonprogram IPs in these settings can undermine the therapeutic character and mission of the unit.

Treatment of substance use disorders includes consideration of appropriate programming (see Chapter 47). In correctional settings, services range from none through short-term psychoeducation to intensive therapeutic community placement. Given the pandemic nature of substance use treatment needs in corrections, it is a rare system that can provide treatment to all who might benefit from it.

Sex offenders are simply defined as those incarcerated for a sex-related crime (see Chapter 63) and do not necessarily include everyone with inappropriate or violent sexual behaviors. Classification scoring often relates to the criminal charges and history, not to treatment needs. Frequency and level of violence of the behavior are the defining characteristics. Sex offender scoring may be defined as follows: 1, no prior or current sex offense–related charges; 2, noncontact sexual charge (e.g., voyeurism, exhibitionism); 3, one sexual offense with physical contact; 4, a pattern of two or more sexual offenses with physical contact; and 5, a pattern of repeated sexual offenses with gratuitous violence or sadism.

Movement of incarcerated persons

Internal movement

IPs are moved within a facility and between facilities for many reasons. Changes in custody status (i.e., becoming convicted), health status, need for a specific program, or preparation for release each may trigger movement of an IP. For security reasons, most moves are unannounced. Although this decreases the risk of escape planning, it may engender increased anxiety for the affected IP.

Transportation logistics

Movement to and from court, other facilities, and health care facilities for procedures or hospitalizations all require secure transportation. Transportation decisions require judgment: Is an ambulance needed, or can the IP travel to a hospital by correctional vehicle? How many officers are required for transport given the security risk of the individual? Because of security risks, IPs typically do not know the scheduled date or time of nonemergency clinical appointments outside the facility. If psychiatrists, other clinicians, or custody staff divulge this information to an IP, it creates an opportunity for escape planning or other safety breaches and may necessitate rescheduling of the appointment.

Respite care: interstate compacts

For many reasons, IPs in a state prison system may move to another state through an interstate compact agreement. These moves may be requested because of challenging management concerns such as repeated extreme violence or acute protective custody concerns (e.g., a high-profile and unpopular IP) or to access resources more readily available elsewhere. Such transfers often allow for respite of exhausted staff who have managed a difficult IP and may ease conflicts not easily resolved between an IP and a correctional system (e.g., litigated demands or unresolved power struggles).

Community transition: end of sentence, halfway house, parole eligibility, and early release

IPs often get incentives for good behavior as they progress through their incarceration. Avoiding conflict and following institutional rules allow IPs greater eligibility for job and training opportunities. Participation in appropriate programming and therapy is also often reflected in good behavior credits and progress toward rehabilitation. As IPs become eligible for early release or parole, their behavior and program participation are reviewed. If deemed adequate by the review board, the IP may become approved for conditional release to a halfway house or other community-based parole program. Preparation for such transition opportunities may be available only at other facilities, again requiring transfer. Often, as part of this process, the level of community supervision and support needed, on the one hand, and risk of reoffending, on the other, is assessed. This assessment process typically includes formal tools to support such determinations (Goodley et al., 2022; Kroner & Hanson, 2022).

Summary

Population management is a critical component of safety and security in correctional facilities and systems. Multiple factors must be taken into account to address the sometimes conflicting demands of treatment, educational, vocational, and security needs. Systems have been developed to manage these complex concerns with growing efficiency. Increasing integration of evidence-based systems will likely occur in the future.

REFERENCES

Austin, J. (1998). *Objective jail classification systems: A guide for jail administrators*. National Institute of Corrections. https://s3.amazonaws.com/static.nicic.gov/Library/014373.pdf

Bonta, J., & Wormith, J. S. (2018). Adult offender assessment and classification in custodial settings. In J. D. Wooldredge & P. Smith (Eds.), *The Oxford handbook of prisons and imprisonment* (pp. 397–424). Oxford University Press.

Brennan, T. (2020). Review of risk assessment and classification in prisons. In L. A. Gould & J. J. Brent (Eds.), *Routledge handbook on American prisons* (pp. 42–74). Routledge.

Chen, M. K., & Shapiro, J. M. (2007). Do harsher prison conditions reduce recidivism? *American Law and Economics Review*, *9*, 1–29.

Connecticut Department of Correction. (2012). *Objective classification manual, revised*. http://www.ct.gov/doc/lib/doc/PDF/PDFReport/ClassificationManualLibraryCopy.pdf

Gaes, G., & Camp, S. (2009). Unintended consequences: Experimental evidence for the criminogenic effect of prison security level placement on post-release recidivism. *Journal of Experimental Criminology*, *5*, 139–162.

Gonzalez, S. (2021). *Yale prison education program receives $1.5 million Mellon grant*. https://news.yale.edu/2021/04/15/yale-prison-education-program-receives-15-million-mellon-grant

Goodley, G., Pearson, D., & Morris, P. (2022). Predictors of recidivism following release from custody: A meta-analysis. *Psychology, Crime & Law*, *28*(7), 703–729.

Hackett, A. (2019). *Boston College launches prison education program*. https://www.bc.edu/bc-web/bcnews/campus-community/announcements/prison-education-program.html

Kroner, D. G., & Hanson, R. K. (2022). Measuring what matters: Standardised risk levels for criminal recidivism risk. In G. Liell, M. Fisher, & L. Jones (Eds.), *Challenging bias in forensic psychological assessment and testing* (pp. 95–110). Routledge.

Meyers, T. J., Testa, A., & Wright, K. A. (2023). Managing violence: In-prison behavior associated with placement in an alternative disciplinary segregation program. *American Journal of Criminal Justice*, *48*(1), 250–272.

Nur, A. V., & Nguyen, H. (2023). Prison work and vocational programs: A systematic review and analysis of moderators of program success. *Justice Quarterly*, *40*(1), 129–158.

Routh, D., Abess, G., Makin, D., Stohr, M. K., Hemmens, C., & Yoo, J. (2017). Transgender inmates in prisons: A review of applicable statutes and policies. *International journal of offender therapy and comparative criminology*, *61*(6), 645–666.

Shaffer, J. S., Russo, J., Woods, D., & Jackson, B. A. (2019). *Managing the seriously mentally ill in corrections*. RAND Corporation. https://www.rand.org/pubs/research_reports/RR2698.html

Tahamont, S., & Frisch, N. E. (2019). Correctional classification and security. In M. S. Phelps & C. Curry (Eds.), *Oxford research encyclopedia of criminology*. Oxford University Press. https://doi.org/10.1093/acrefore/9780190264079.013.452

U.S. Department of Education (2023). *Confined or incarcerated student fact sheet*. https://fsapartners.ed.gov/sites/default/files/2023-03/ConfinedIncarceratedStudentFactSheet.pdf

9

Levels of care

*Jeffrey L. Metzner**

Introduction

Just as in community settings, correctional systems need a continuum of mental health care. These levels of care generally follow the community mental health center model. The purpose of the Community Mental Health Act of 1963 (CMHA, 1963) was to provide seed funding for community-based mental health care as an alternative to institutionalization. The core set of services included the following:

- Outpatient mental health services, including services for substance use disorders and for specific populations, such as children, elderly individuals, and individuals with chronic mental illness;
- 24-hour-a-day emergency care services;
- Day programs that include partial hospitalization services and other aftercare services following discharge from a higher level of care;
- Access to inpatient psychiatric treatment; and
- Community consultation and education for caretakers.

The CMHA was intended to promote deinstitutionalization of persons with chronic mental illness and establish a model of community-based mental health treatment. It is ironic that the CMHA may have contributed to "transinstitutionalization" into the correctional mental health system due primarily to lack of adequate community-based funding. Many aspects of the community mental health center model, however, can be implemented in correctional settings.

The continuum of care for incarcerated persons (IPs) with mental illness includes outpatient care, emergency services, day treatment, supportive housing, infirmary care, and inpatient psychiatric hospitalization services. This chapter describes each level of care and how it may be adapted to function in correctional settings.

Levels of care: overview

Guidelines developed by the American Psychiatric Association (APA, 2016) define mental health treatment as the use of biological, psychological, and social therapies to treat symptoms of mental illness that cause distress and/or significantly interfere with functioning. Policies and procedures that are consistent with the standards of correctional mental health care provide a structure for offering treatment in a multidisciplinary and eclectic manner (APA, 2016; Metzner, 1998). A comprehensive system of mental health services includes the following (Metzner, 1998):

1. Outpatient treatment service is the least intensive level of care. In some systems, this may include a day treatment program that provides enhanced mental health services similar to a residential program, as described below. In the case of outpatient treatment, participating IPs live in a general population housing unit with other IPs, many of whom are not in need of mental health services.
2. A residential program (i.e., housing unit) within the correctional setting is provided for IPs with chronic mental illness who do not require inpatient treatment but do require enhanced mental health services. Such a designated housing unit can provide a safer and more therapeutic environment for those unable to function adequately within the general incarcerated population.
3. Crisis intervention services include both brief counseling and supervised stabilization. The latter, often provided in an infirmary setting, serves short-term stabilization and/or diagnostic purposes. The length of stay in such settings is generally less than 10 days.
4. A psychiatric inpatient program is the most intensive level of care and is often provided by the state psychiatric hospital system.

The levels of mental health care offered to IPs in jails are often limited by their short stays and the size of the facility. Essential treatment services generally emphasize psychotropic medication management by a psychiatrist and crisis intervention, which may include short-term counseling and transfer to a special needs unit or infirmary. IPs with longer pretrial confinements or sentences might receive more extensive mental health services, including verbal therapies and skill-building activities (APA, 2016; Metzner, 1998). Other essential services include mental health screening and referral assessments (see Chapter 15), a suicide prevention program (see Chapter 51), discharge planning (see Chapter 23), and timely access to a special mental health housing unit or an inpatient psychiatric bed (APA,

*. The author acknowledges the contribution of Kenneth Applebaum, MD, who was the second author of this chapter in the first edition of this textbook.

2016). Jails also need adequate nursing staff for medication administration and often for continuous coverage of special mental health housing units.

Small jails contract with local mental health centers, private practitioners, or for-profit mental health companies to provide services. Unfortunately, especially with private practitioners who often do not understand the needs of a correctional mental health system, the hours contracted are often not enough to provide the necessary services. IPs in need of emergency psychiatric care might be transported to a local emergency department for acute stabilization (e.g., following a suicide attempt), but inpatient psychiatric care in community hospitals is generally unavailable. Inpatient mental health services may be obtained through the forensic division of the public hospital system following negotiations with the state department of mental health or an equivalent governmental agency.

Prison mental health systems provide a more comprehensive system of mental health care than jails due to their different mission, larger incarcerated population, longer duration of incarceration, and greater resources (see Chapter 7). Although prisons require essential mental health services that are similar to those described for jails, they are more likely to provide access to special needs housing, inpatient psychiatric care, and psychosocial rehabilitation treatment for IPs with serious mental illness.

Every IP who receives mental health services needs a written treatment plan. Such a plan is an individualized and often a multidisciplinary statement of short- and long-term goals and the methods to achieve them, including the necessary level of care and discharge planning in residential settings (National Commission on Correctional Health Care [NCCHC], 2015). The comprehensiveness and frequency of treatment plan reviews vary depending on the level of care and the IP's clinical condition. Specific triggers for reviews and revisions include changes in level of mental health care, critical incidents such as suicide attempts, and failure to achieve treatment goals.

Outpatient mental health services

An outpatient clinic provides mental health care to most IPs who receive mental health treatment in a correctional facility. These IPs usually live in the general population and enter outpatient services via the intake mental health screening process, by self-referral, or by staff referral sometime during their incarceration. The latter may occur due to changing environmental stressors, despite a negative intake screening, or following discharge from a higher level of mental health care (e.g., infirmary). Correctional outpatient clinics have a diverse range of treatment programs and philosophies, and they require supervision and a quality improvement process to ensure provision of appropriate services (Smith & Smith, 2006; see Chapter 74).

The development of protocols for psychotropic medications by class (e.g., antidepressants, antipsychotics, mood stabilizers) helps to ensure their appropriate use, especially in the context of monitoring relevant laboratory tests. Due to the high prevalence of substance use among correctional populations, many clinicians discourage use of sedative-hypnotic and antianxiety medications. Other commentators advocate for close monitoring of indications for and response to these medications as part of supervised protocols (Appelbaum, 2009; see also Chapter 29).

Some systems limit individual outpatient psychotherapy to crisis intervention and supportive psychotherapy for IPs with serious mental illnesses because of limited resources. However, regular psychotherapy sessions are often useful for IPs with severe behavioral disorders. Group psychotherapy is a cost-effective form of treatment within a prison setting (Metzner, 1998) and may be beneficial in large jail settings as well.

Staffing for outpatient clinic services should include psychiatrists and other mental health clinicians such as advanced practice registered nurses, psychologists, social workers, and nurses. Clerical staff provide valuable assistance with scheduling and other administrative functions (e.g., obtaining health care records) necessary to operate an effective outpatient clinic. Staffing allocations designed to ensure adequate IP access to needed mental health resources vary based on local differences and needs. Metzner has summarized staffing allocation guidelines developed by the state of New York and by a blue-ribbon consultation panel in Massachusetts (Metzner, 1997). The APA (2016) recommends one full-time psychiatrist for every 75 to 100 IPs in jail with a serious mental illness or 150 to 200 IPs in prison on psychotropic medications (APA, 2016).

An effective approach for approximating discipline-specific staffing needs for a given facility involves determining the type of services provided by that discipline, the time required for each unit of service, and the number of units within a given period. For example, if a facility's social workers typically conduct 90 mental health intake assessments per week and each assessment, on average, takes 20 minutes, then the facility needs 30 hours of social work time per week for this service alone. Similar calculations can be made for other social worker services such as case management encounters and restrictive housing rounds. Dividing the sum of all calculated service hours by the net weekly clinical time provided by a full-time equivalent (FTE) social worker will yield the approximate number of FTEs needed. This determination assumes that an FTE provides, on average, fewer than 40 hours per week of direct service (e.g., 24 hours per week) after accounting for paid time off and time spent on other functions such as meetings and training. The model does not apply to positions that require back-fill post coverage, such as infirmary nurses. A similar approach for determining psychiatric workloads in community mental health settings has been described (Bhaskara, 1999). The above approach is a form of a time and motion study to determine staffing needs (Kalne & Mehendale, 2022).

Sufficient suitable space, supplies, and equipment should be available for outpatient mental health services. This includes program areas that allow for confidential, private assessment and treatment of IPs; group programming; and storage of supplies and equipment (NCCHC, 2015). This principle applies equally to the outpatient programming space for high-security IPs, which generally includes those in locked-down (i.e., segregation or restrictive housing) units (see Chapter 10).

Effective implementation of outpatient mental health services depends on sufficient custody staff for escorting IPs and maintaining safety within the programming areas. These positions should be established by post orders and staffed by regularly assigned officers to foster consistency of practices and compliance with pertinent policies and procedures. Effective collaboration and ongoing communication between health care and custody staff are critical for a safe and secure environment that supports meaningful and efficient treatment.

Timely access to outpatient services is an essential component of an adequate mental health system. This includes a clear, easy-to-use, and readily available referral process, typically beginning with a referral form available on all housing units. The referral form should accurately identify the IP, location of the IP, source of referral, and date of referral, and it should include a brief summary of the reason for the request to be seen (Smith & Smith, 2006). The referral system may be integrated with the health services sick-call request system or may be a separate process through the mental health department. Receipt and triage of oral or written requests for nonemergency mental health services occur within 24 hours. During regular-duty hours, either a qualified mental health professional (i.e., credentialed staff whose scope of practice is consistent with licensure, certification, and/or registration requirements within the relevant jurisdiction) or a qualified health care professional (e.g., physician, physician's assistant, nurse, or nurse practitioner) must perform this function (NCCHC, 2015). On-call coverage during nonduty hours is needed. This is commonly provided on a scheduled rotating basis by the mental health staff, although other options are available depending on the system's size and resources (e.g., via a psychiatric nurse in an inpatient unit if the facility has such a unit).

Many correctional mental health systems triage referrals as emergent, urgent, or routine. Emergent referrals should be seen as soon as possible (generally within 4 hours), urgent referrals within 24 hours, and routine referrals within 7 to 14 business days, based on clinical need. A referral that is noted to require a suicide risk assessment will generally be triaged as emergent if the system does not have the staff resources to place the IP under constant observation until the assessment occurs.

Continuity of care facilitates the establishment of a therapeutic alliance between the IP and clinician, and frequent changes (e.g., more than twice in 12 months) of the IP's psychiatrist and/or primary mental health clinician make this difficult to achieve. Frequent changes occur due to staff recruitment or retention issues and the use of short-term, contract clinicians.

Residential programs for incarcerated persons with serious mental illness

A residential treatment program (often known as a residential treatment unit, intermediate care unit, supportive living unit, special needs unit, psychiatric services unit, or extended outpatient program) is a critical level of care for most prison systems and larger jails. IPs who are appropriate for these units generally have had significant difficulty functioning in a general population environment due to symptoms of serious mental illness (Metzner, 1998).

These programs are designed to provide supportive housing and psychosocial rehabilitation (Cnaan et al., 1988). The admission criteria and goals of these programs often vary. For example, some programs are designed to teach IPs the skills they will need to be mainstreamed back into the general IP population (Lovell et al., 2001). Other programs attempt to mainstream but recognize that a significant percentage (i.e., 40% to 60%) of IPs will need to remain in this level of care throughout their incarceration due to their inability to function in the general population. It has been the experience of this author based on monitoring numerous correctional systems that 10% to 15% of the total mental health caseload will require this level of mental health care on any given day.

Residential treatment programs typically house 30 to 50 IPs, which allows for cost-effective staffing. Essential features include adequate space for staff offices (preferably on or close to the unit), programming, individual and group therapies, indoor and outdoor recreation, a day room, a medication room, other nursing functions such as sick calls, and designated cells near nursing or correctional officers' stations for close observation and/or clinical restraints. These units should be designed so that IPs can be observed from the nurses' office and the correctional officers' station. Important environmental conditions include the ability to maintain reasonable room temperature, adequate ventilation, and proper acoustics to decrease the noise level in treatment and housing areas (Metzner, 1998).

The psychosocial rehabilitation model emphasizes group therapies and activities that promote socialization and productive use of time. Useful treatment modalities include psychoeducation, cognitive-behavioral therapies, socialization skills, art, music, recreation, and substance use and anger management groups. Weekly community meetings help to create a therapeutic milieu. Unstructured out-of-cell time for IPs in these programs should at least equal the amount of recreational time (i.e., outdoor yard) available to general-population IPs at the same security classification and should include an additional 10 hours of out-of-cell structured therapeutic programming per week for each IP. Appropriately credentialed or supervised mental health staff conduct the therapeutic programming. These units also provide individual supportive counseling and access to psychotropic medications that include nonemergency, involuntary medications when appropriate and permitted, especially in high-security settings. A computerized database can help document the number of hours per week that an IP participates in the treatment program. This information will facilitate quality improvement activities and needs assessment processes (see Chapter 74).

Staffing allocations vary based on the size of the unit and the security classification levels of the IPs. The multidisciplinary treatment team typically includes a psychiatrist, nurses, activity therapists, clerks, and other mental health professionals (e.g., psychologists, social workers, occupational therapists, mental health technicians). A taskforce of the APA (2016) recommended that the staffing allocation for a residential treatment unit include 1.0 FTE psychiatrist for every 50 patients. Correctional officers should receive enhanced mental health training for assignment to these programs and be assigned to the unit for at least 6 months for continuity purposes (Appelbaum et al., 2001; Dvoskin & Spiers, 2004). Under these circumstances, it is recommended that custody staff are made full members of the treatment team who attend team meetings, share observations, have access to clinical information, participate in therapeutic activities, and maintain confidentiality and other clinical obligations that do not conflict with security. Appropriate training to support these expectations should be provided. To facilitate a good working relationship between officers and mental health staff, the mental health director of the unit must have meaningful input into selection and retention of these officers.

Providing residential treatment for high-security IPs or those in a locked-down setting such as a supermax facility or a restrictive housing unit is staff intensive and generally requires special physical plant modifications such as the use of "programming modules" (Metzner & Dvoskin, 2006; see Chapter 10). Successful implementation of a residential treatment unit can enhance IPs' participation in work, school, and other programming and can reduce the need for inpatient psychiatric beds, admissions to crisis beds, and the frequency of disciplinary infractions (Condelli et al., 1994; Lovell et al., 2001; Smith et al., 2004).

A few correctional systems have developed residential treatment programs for IPs who have significant behavior problems due to a personality disorder and are generally not appropriate for residential settings that use a psychosocial approach to treat IPs with serious mental illnesses. These programs often use a cognitive-behavioral approach and a phase system that rewards prosocial behaviors with increasing privileges (Andrade, 2009). Depending on the criteria for admission to such programs, the success rate (as measured by less frequent disruptive and/or self-harming behaviors) varies widely. However, since many of these IPs require a disproportionate amount of time from the mental health services, even a low percentage of successful outcomes is often very beneficial to the correctional system and the IP.

Crisis intervention services

Crisis intervention services provide another necessary component of an adequate correctional mental health system. These services must include timely access, when clinically indicated, to housing in a crisis stabilization unit (CSU). Some systems also have an adjacent infirmary-type dormitory that serves as a transition back to general population housing (Smith & Smith, 2006). CSUs generally have single cells and 24/7 coverage by nursing and custody staff, with mental health staff on-site during the usual working hours and on call during off hours. CSUs provide observation (e.g., suicide watch), diagnosis, and treatment functions in a safe and therapeutic environment, as characterized by supportive clinical interventions and a nonpunitive approach. Placing crisis cells in segregation units and routinely using "strip cell" status (e.g., no personal property, use of a suicide smock, no out-of-cell time) are examples of nontherapeutic milieus and should be avoided.

In general, CSUs have a length of stay less than 10 days. In small or resource-poor correctional facilities that have problems with access to psychiatric hospitals, a CSU often also serves as an acute care program, which results in longer lengths of stay. These valuable and scarce mental health care beds should not be used for non–health care purposes (e.g., protective custody, overflow housing) or for prolonged stays following clinical discharge from the crisis unit.

The structure and staffing of CSUs should allow admission of IPs of any classification within the facility or catchment area for regionalized units. Clinical staff should make admission and discharge decisions with input from custody staff, especially regarding discharges. CSUs usually occupy a separate section of general medical infirmaries that house IPs with conditions that require 24/7 nursing care. CSUs, which almost always serve as the primary housing unit for IPs on suicide precautions or watch, need suicide-resistant cells (Metzner & Hayes, 2006) and suicide prevention policies and procedures (see Chapter 51). Because IPs in CSUs have short stays, acute symptoms, a frequent need for clinical stabilization with psychotropic medications, and diagnostic uncertainty, a medical model serves as a useful operating structure. IPs need daily contact with a psychiatrist or other appropriately credentialed mental health clinician, with continuous coverage by a psychiatrist available.

Patterns of admission to a CSU should be reviewed. Some IPs have two or more admissions to a CSU in a 6-month period due to self-injurious behaviors or threats of injuring self or others. Other potentially problematic admissions include IPs who seek new housing for nonclinical reasons such as wanting to escape repayment of a debt. These IPs often precipitate hostility and countertransference from CSU clinical and custody staff that interfere with assessment and treatment. Staff frequently, and sometimes accurately, label these IPs as malingering or having antisocial personality disorders, and they subsequently fail to identify other comorbid symptoms of a significant mental disorder. At times, staff inappropriately impose harsh conditions of confinement (e.g., no mattress or clothing) for such IPs in an attempt to covertly discourage them from remaining in or returning to the CSU. IPs who have CSU stays longer than 10 days or who have multiple admissions within a 6-month period should be considered for a higher level of mental health care and/or a change in their current treatment plan.

CSUs occasionally have problematic custody and clinical practices. Some correctional systems treat all CSU IPs as maximum-security IPs. This practice is based, in part, on the belief that all IPs with mental illness who need CSU care are dangerous and unpredictable. As a result, they lock down these IPs 23 to 24 hours per day, do not provide access to recreational areas, and overly restrict possession of clothing and property unrelated to clinical needs. Mental health staff should educate custody staff regarding these misperceptions and implement policies and procedures that prevent inappropriately restrictive practices. Other common problems include cell-front clinical contacts that lack confidentiality and the absence of clinical interventions other than observation and psychotropic medications (e.g., activity/recreational therapy, individual counseling).

Psychiatric inpatient programs

Inpatient psychiatric hospitalization is the most expensive and intensive level of care, and it is generally the least available to correctional mental health programs due to limited resources. Models used by correctional systems to provide access include the following:

1. An arrangement (e.g., contract or memorandum of agreement, statutory provisions) with the state department of mental health or equivalent agency to provide either an open-ended or defined number of forensic hospital beds for IPs;
2. A dedicated correctional system facility or a housing unit used for inpatient psychiatric care; and
3. A contract with a hospital system.

Many U.S. correctional systems, especially jails, do not have psychiatric inpatient care directly accessible for IPs. Indirect access may be available via the court system for IPs in need of treatment or via the forensic mental health system for evaluation of competency to stand trial or similar issues. Experience has demonstrated that the availability of CSUs and residential treatment beds has a direct bearing on the need for inpatient resources. No simple formula exists for reliably determining how many specialty psychiatric beds a system requires.

The treatment offered to prisoners in correctional inpatient psychiatric settings should meet the community standard of care, although how the treatment is delivered may be different due to safety and security concerns. In general, such IPs should be offered at least 4 hours per weekday of out-of-cell structured therapeutic activities (generally group therapy/activities) based on the psychosocial rehabilitation model and at least another 10 to 15 hours per day of out-of-cell unstructured activities (e.g., dayroom time, yard time). Exceptions to this principle should be based on the prisoner's clinical presentation (e.g., clinically too disorganized to appropriately participate). For maximum-security prisoners, the use of programming modules or other mechanisms such as partial restraint to a table may be needed for safety purposes.

Staffing and the use of telepsychiatry

Recruitment and retention of mental health staff, especially psychiatrists, to correctional mental health care services have been longstanding problems related to the rural location of many correctional facilities (especially prisons), the working conditions within the correctional facilities, noncompetitive salaries, and the lack of familiarity by most clinicians regarding correctional mental health systems. Such issues were exacerbated during the COVID-19 pandemic and were mitigated by the growing use of telepsychiatry. For a typical outpatient level of mental health care, the use of telepsychiatry is generally considered to be equivalent to services provided by an on-site psychiatrist if appropriate guidelines are followed, as summarized in Chapter 21.

The use of telepsychiatry for higher levels of care (e.g., residential, crisis, and/or inpatient), with some exceptions, is not considered to be equivalent to on-site coverage by a psychiatrist due to the significant difficulty in the following:

- Interacting with custody staff on a regular basis, which facilitates developing and maintaining a more therapeutic milieu within the higher level of care programs;
- Being aware of the current milieu issues and impacting such issues in a positive manner; and
- Establishing clinical leadership within the program.

The use of telepsychiatry is clearly better than having no access to a psychiatrist and should be permitted as a temporary measure until an on-site psychiatrist can be hired (APA, 2023). Under such circumstances, the guidelines summarized in Chapter 21 should be followed. As issues arise with tele-evaluations and treatment by mental health clinicians other than psychiatrists (e.g., psychologists, social workers), similar guidelines should be followed.

Summary

Meeting the needs of IPs with mental disorders requires access to a range of service levels, including outpatient, residential, crisis, and inpatient care. Factors such as system size may determine the availability of these services and the extent to which external resources or programs provide them. Nevertheless, each of these four components remains essential to meet prevailing standards of care and to provide appropriate mental health services to IPs. Telepsychiatry can be a useful tool in facilitating these services, but only when administered carefully and according to guidelines.

REFERENCES

American Psychiatric Association. (2016). *Psychiatric services in correctional facilities* (3rd ed.).

American Psychiatric Association. (2023). *Resource document on telepsychiatry for adults in jails and prisons.* https://www.psychiatry.org/getattachment/00e3f401-0792-4b78-90ba-5985dd791a4e/Resource-Document-on-Telepsychiatry-in-Jails-and-Prisons.pdf

Andrade, J. T. (2009). Psychopathy: Assessment, treatment, and risk management. In J. T. Andrade (Ed.), *Handbook of violence risk assessment and treatment: New approaches for mental health professionals* (pp. 241–290). Springer Publishing Company.

Appelbaum, K. L. (2009). Attention deficit hyperactivity disorder in prison: A treatment protocol. *Journal of the American Academy of Psychiatry and the Law, 37*(1), 45–49.

Appelbaum, K. L., Hickey, J. M., & Packer, I. (2001). The role of correctional officers in multidisciplinary mental health care in prisons. *Psychiatric Services, 52*, 1343–1347.

Bhaskara, S. M. (1999). Setting benchmarks and determining psychiatric workloads in community mental health programs. *Psychiatric Services, 50*, 695–697.

Cnaan, L. R., Blankertz, L., Messinger, K. W., & Gardner, J. R. (1988). Psychosocial rehabilitation: Toward a definition. *Psychosocial Rehabilitation, 11*(4), 62–78.

Community Mental Health Act of 1963, Pub. L. No. 88-164 (1963).

Condelli, W. S., Dvoskin, J. A., & Holanchock, H. (1994). Intermediate care programs for IPs with psychiatric disorders. *Bulletin of the American Academy of Psychiatry and the Law, 22*(1), 63–70.

Dvoskin, J. A., & Spiers, E. M. (2004). On the role of correctional officers in prison mental health. *Psychiatric Quarterly, 75*, 41–59.

Kalne, P. S., & Mehendale, A. M. (2022). The purpose of time-motion studies (TMSs) in healthcare: A literature review. *Cureus, 14*(10), e29869.

Lovell, D., Allen, D., Johnson, C., & Jemelka, R. (2001). Evaluating the effectiveness of residential treatment for prisoners with mental illness. *Criminal Justice and Behavior, 28*, 83–104.

Metzner, J. (1997). An introduction to correctional psychiatry: Part II. *Journal of the American Academy of Psychiatry and the Law, 25*(4), 571–579.

Metzner, J. L. (1998). An introduction to correctional psychiatry: Part III. *Journal of the American Academy of Psychiatry and the Law, 28*(1), 107–115.

Metzner, J., & Dvoskin, J. (2006). An overview of correctional psychiatry. *Psychiatric Clinics of North America, 29*, 761–772.

Metzner, J., & Hayes, L. (2006). Suicide prevention in jails and prisons. In R. Simon & R. Hales (Eds.), *Textbook of suicide assessment and management* (pp. 265–277). American Psychiatric Press.

National Commission on Correctional Health Care. (2015). *Standards for mental health services in correctional facilities.*

Smith, H., Sawyer, D. A., & Way, B. B. (2004). Correctional mental health services in New York: Then and now. *Psychiatric Quarterly, 75*, 21–39.

Smith, H., & Smith, L. D. (2006). Correctional-based mental health services: Designing a system that works. In M. Puisis (Ed.), *Clinical practice in correctional medicine* (pp. 292–305). Elsevier.

10

Restrictive housing and disciplinary infractions

Mary Perrien and Maureen L. O'Keefe

Introduction

Restrictive housing units (RHUs) function as the jail within a correctional system. Designed for the dangerous and violent individual who cannot be managed safely within the general carceral environment, RHUs are characterized by segregation from the general population, often in single-cell confinement with minimum time out of cell for showers and exercise (e.g., 5 hours per week). Other features include highly restricted movement, limited contact with others, and few privileges and services. Estimates suggest that 3% to 4% of incarcerated persons (IPs) may be held in RHUs on any given day, with 5% to 10% of IPs having spent at least 30 days in segregation over the prior year (Beck, 2015). However, inconsistent definitions of restrictive housing, varying conditions of confinement, and the fluidity of carceral placements make it difficult to accurately assess how widely the practice is used.

Restrictive housing has been criticized as an inhumane practice due to the degree of social isolation (Metzner & Fellner, 2010). Specifically, the lack of treatment, programs, and activities to engage the mind; restricted personal contact; lack of control over light and sound; lack of windows; and little or no access to the outdoors are considered more extreme than is required for the safe operation of correctional systems. The most significant issue is whether IPs can psychologically adapt to the austere conditions for long periods, particularly those with serious mental illness. Because IPs with serious mental illness may be more prone to rule infractions due to their symptoms and behavioral impairment, they are more likely to be placed in RHUs unless specific rules prohibit their placement.

Psychological impact of restrictive housing units

The psychological effect of RHUs is an area of concern that has received much attention in recent years. Scrutiny increased as the use of RHUs became widespread, and corrections administrators possessed little evidence to defend against claims of the harmful effects of RHUs or to support their assertions that RHUs made the rest of the correctional environment safer for staff and IPs. A constellation of symptoms became associated with such confinement, including perceptual changes, affective disturbances, cognitive difficulties, disturbing thought content, impulse control problems, psychological trauma, and other psychopathological features (Haney, 2018; Luigi et al., 2020). The National Commission on Correctional Health Care (NCCHC, 2016) issued a position statement noting that prolonged (more than 15 days) periods of confinement in RHUs are cruel, inhumane, degrading, and harmful. The United Nations Office on Drugs and Crime (2015) adopted the "Mandela Rules" forbidding prolonged and indefinite placement in RHUs (see Chapter 4). The international concerns around RHUs and its effects have created a growing need for empirical research.

Research into the impact of restrictive housing units

The negative effects of RHUs have been extensively documented by mental health professionals, advocacy groups, and media circuits (Kapoor & Trestman, 2016). However, these reports relied largely on qualitative or cross-sectional research designs, making it difficult to attribute the cause of those symptoms to restrictive housing. Longitudinal designs are better suited to examining change over time, although they are not without their limitations. Two longitudinal studies had strong research designs but were negatively affected by high attrition rates (40% to 94%) resulting from shorter stays in segregation than are typically encountered in the United States (Andersen et al., 2000; Zinger et al., 2001). These studies found conflicting results, making it even more difficult to draw conclusions relevant to RHUs as they operate today.

Access issues make rigorous research difficult, particularly within RHUs. These limitations include selection bias, response bias, nonexistent or inadequate comparison groups, single assessment periods, and longitudinal designs over short time periods. Keeping these issues in mind, the Colorado study (O'Keefe et al., 2010) was undertaken as a direct quasi-experimental study of the psychological effects of long-term segregation, designed to parse out the effects of RHUs from those of other carceral environments.

The Colorado study

Selection bias can occur when subjects are selected nonrandomly. Without randomization, a study runs the risk of not equally representing the population from which the sample is drawn. Small sample sizes, high refusal and attrition rates, and volunteer subjects are examples of selection bias that have characterized RHU research. In the Colorado study, approximately 150 IPs were targeted around the time of their segregation hearing to obtain baseline measures. RHU IPs were divided into two groups: no mental illness (NMI) and mental illness (MI). Comparison participants appeared to be matched across demographic, criminal history, treatment need, and institutional behavior measures.

Measurement of psychological change may be particularly susceptible to response bias, whereby subjects feel compelled to respond in a way consistent with what they think is expected. Subjective measures are generally more prone to response bias than objective measures because wording of questions or nonverbal cues can subtly lead the subject to respond in the hypothesized direction; subjective measures also require clinical judgment to interpret. For these reasons, the Colorado study selected standardized paper-and-pencil instruments. Measures were selected for their ease of administration to IPs in noncontact visiting booths and for their strong psychometric properties (i.e., reliability, validity, normative data). IPs completed 12 instruments (three measures assessing stable constructs were collected at baseline only), and clinical staff completed a 24-item assessment of psychological symptoms.

The Colorado study proposed to assess IPs at 3-month intervals over the course of 1 year. To limit attrition, IPs with fewer than 15 months remaining on their sentence were excluded, and subjects were kept in the study even if their conditions of confinement changed. Analyses using all cases and only "pure" cases (i.e., conditions of confinement remained constant) revealed similar patterns; therefore, all cases were used to increase statistical power.

Comparison groups enable researchers to distinguish the effects of RHUs from general carceral effects. Where comparison groups are absent or too dissimilar (i.e., volunteers, minimum-security IPs), it is impossible to rule out that IPs might worsen in correctional settings overall. In the Colorado study, IPs who had an RHU hearing but were returned to the general population served as comparison subjects. They met the same study criteria and selection procedures as RHU subjects but experienced less restrictive confinement. In addition, a third comparison group of behaviorally disruptive IPs with serious mental illness was enlisted to participate shortly after their placement into a special needs (SN) facility. Altogether, a total of 247 subjects across five groups were included: RHU MI, RHU NMI, comparison MI, comparison NMI, and SN MI.

Study hypotheses were that IPs in RHUs would exhibit psychological features consistent with previous research, that deterioration would be greater for MI subjects than NMI subjects, and that IPs in RHUs would experience greater deterioration over time than comparison IPs.

Test means for each group were compared to normative means of the nearest available reference group (e.g., nonclinical males, community adult samples) to test the first hypothesis. On average, compared to nonclinical norms, all groups except the comparison NMI group scored significantly higher than the normative means. These findings are consistent with extensive literature that reports serious psychopathology among RHU IPs. However, this psychopathology was present around the time of placement into RHUs and in the comparison groups, which suggests it was a preexisting condition and not unique to RHUs.

Composite scores were created from like scales across multiple instruments. For example, the anxiety composite score was derived from eight subscales across five instruments. The pattern of results showed improvement across all composites except withdrawal–alienation, with most change occurring between the first and second testing periods, followed by relative stability for the remainder of the time. Although there were differences between the RHU MI and NMI groups, they were not in the hypothesized direction; RHU MI improved more than RHU NMI. Comparison subjects followed the same pattern of improvement, which prevents one from concluding that RHUs cause psychological improvements. Nonetheless, the results did not support the third hypothesis that IPs in RHUs would deteriorate relative to comparison IPs.

The Colorado study joins a growing body of literature that suggests the effects of RHUs on psychological functioning are much smaller than originally believed (Gendreau & Labrecque, 2015). Because it was likely that some IPs in long-term RHU conditions would decompensate, additional analyses were conducted to identify the proportion who experienced negative change. Seven percent of segregated IPs appeared to change negatively over the study period based on IP and clinician ratings, but these declines were not associated with restrictive housing (O'Keefe et al., 2010; Walters, 2018). This finding is consistent with two independent meta-analytic studies that found small to moderate effects of segregation on IPs' psychological functioning, with substantially smaller effect sizes among studies having stronger research designs (Morgan et al., 2016). Taken together, the results suggest that serious psychopathology exists within RHUs at disproportionate rates, but psychological deterioration occurs less often than expected and at rates comparable to less restrictive confinement.

Implications of current research

Several factors limit the generalizability of the Colorado study. Due to eligibility criteria, these results should not be generalized to female, illiterate, or juvenile IPs. Second, subjects may have experienced an RHU previously, which could have affected their psychological functioning in this study. In fact, some may have sought an RHU for their own safety or preference and, thus, perceiving it as under their control, did not experience an exacerbation of symptoms. The conditions in RHUs vary from system to system; this study can only be generalized to other correctional settings to the extent that their confinement conditions are similar to those in Colorado at that time (see O'Keefe et al., 2010). Notably, RHU IPs had access to television and generally clean, quiet conditions, suggestive of positive IP–staff interactions that could be a powerful protective factor. Finally, without Colorado's SN facility, many diverted IPs would likely have been placed in RHUs, which could have proven detrimental to their well-being.

The Colorado findings neither dispute the disproportionately high rates of serious mental illness in RHUs nor promote the continued use of RHUs for IPs with serious mental illness. There is no evidence to suggest RHU placement is clinically appropriate. This study was intended to stimulate strong applied research within corrections, especially replication studies that can shed more light on IPs' mental health outcomes when conditions of confinement vary (Chadick et al., 2018). Correctional officials are encouraged to minimize the use of RHUs and to explore alternate means of housing offenders in less restrictive settings (NCCHC, 2016; United Nations Office on Drugs and Crime, 2015).

Mental health placements in restrictive housing units

There is a large consensus that IPs with serious mental illness should not be placed into RHUs, or if necessary, for no more than 2 weeks (NCCHC, 2016). However, there may be times when IPs with serious mental illness require a longer term high-security setting that is RHU-like. This would not be an RHU but would be a special housing unit that provides higher security while providing significant out-of-cell activity (e.g., recreation yard) and treatment (e.g., group therapy). Few would argue with the obligation to provide treatment to IPs with mental illness who are in RHU-like settings. Case law and correctional treatment standards have established that a minimum standard of care must be provided (American Psychiatric Association [APA], 2016; Cohen, 2008; NCCHC, 2015, 2018). Even IPs who are not believed to have a mental illness must be monitored at regular intervals for any signs of decompensation or development of symptoms of mental illness or suicidality (NCCHC, 2015, 2018).

The proportion of IPs with mental illness in RHUs and RHU-like housing can be an indicator of the overall quality of the mental health delivery system in a correctional system and signal deficiencies in the system (Cohen, 2008; Maszak-Prato & Graham, 2022; Metzner, 2002; Metzner & Fellner, 2010). Untreated or undertreated IPs with mental illness are more likely to act out, and undertrained custody staff are more likely to respond punitively to behaviors like self-harm (Maszak-Prato & Graham, 2022). Without appropriate housing, training, and treatment options, there is a greater likelihood that IPs who act out due to their mental illness will be treated punitively. While RHU placement may make it simpler for the system to manage the IP, it does not resolve the core issues; instead, it may cause further deterioration and limit access to care.

Many of the characteristics that make RHUs safer from a security perspective create challenges to providing care (Beven, 2005; Haney, 2018). The physical plant can present a physical barrier to adequate care, with little to no treatment space. Sometimes the culture can present obstacles to adequate care. Custody staff are trained with safety and security as their primary function. As a result, they may be reluctant to allow mental health staff to interview IPs alone, even handcuffed. Custody staff may insist on being present in treatment groups for safety reasons, despite the chilling effect on the therapeutic effectiveness of those groups. It becomes increasingly difficult to establish therapeutic rapport within the RHU environment. As described later in this chapter, many IPs can be treated safely and confidentiality maintained, even in the highest of security settings, when therapeutic and security staff collaborate equally.

Standards of care

Despite these difficulties, current standards assert that IPs in RHUs are expected to have available a full range of mental health services, including comprehensive assessment, suicide risk assessment, ongoing monitoring, crisis intervention, psychotropic medication management, group and individual psychotherapy, and access to inpatient treatment (American Bar Association, 2011; APA, 2016). These services are developed and coordinated by the treatment team and implemented according to an individualized treatment plan. When an IP is placed in an RHU, a timely screening review should be completed by trained, qualified health care staff and/or mental health staff to ensure there are no mental health conditions that would contraindicate such housing (NCCHC, 2015, 2018). When reviewing an IP's medical record, the focus is on psychiatric symptomatology and functioning that negatively impact placement in RHUs or require accommodation (NCCHC, 2015).

Mental health staff are expected to monitor all IPs in RHUs on a regular basis. The frequency and degree of monitoring increase based on the degree of isolation. For example, in an RHU where IPs experience extreme isolation with little to no social interaction, IPs would receive daily rounds by medical staff and at least weekly rounds by mental health (NCCHC, 2015). RHU rounds should include staff speaking to each IP, including those who are not currently receiving ongoing mental health treatment, although IPs with serious mental illness are also seen during other scheduled confidential clinical contacts throughout the week. RHU rounds serve a critical function in early identification of physical or psychological deterioration that should be followed by immediate intervention. Unfortunately, experience has shown that within RHUs and similar settings, rounds are often perfunctory, characterized by minimal interactions. Even the most skilled clinician cannot assess an individual and identify early decompensation from a brief glance into a darkened cell and a rushed greeting while moving down the tier. For rounds to meet their intended goals, contact must involve meaningful verbal interaction while observing the IP at the cell front. The conditions of the cell, as well as the person, should be noted. Unit security staff should also be consulted for their observations regarding each IP's functioning. Over time, these rounds and collateral data provide an invaluable source of information regarding IPs' mental status and functioning.

Treatment

When IPs identified as having serious mental illness are placed into RHUs, their regular mental health treatment, typically characterized by some combination of individual and group therapy and medication management, must be maintained. Due to the intense nature of the RHU setting, confidential treatment contacts should typically occur at least once or twice weekly, per modality. The treatment team determines the appropriate level of services based on the symptom presentation and functional level of the patient. The goal is to allow the IP to function as well as possible within the restricted environment and ultimately move to a less restrictive setting. For example, an IP with a serious mental illness and multiple functional impairments is expected to receive a minimum of 10 to 15 hours per week of structured therapeutic services out of cell (Metzner & Dvoskin, 2006). Mental health staff must immediately notify custody management of IPs who decompensate in RHUs and recommend that those IPs be placed in an alternative therapeutic setting (NCCHC, 2015).

Individual therapy can be logistically easier than group therapy in RHUs; a cuffed IP can meet with a clinician in a small room with windows, allowing supervision by custodial staff from outside while maintaining verbal confidentiality. Group treatment can be more challenging to deliver under conditions that still allow custody staff to maintain visual observation. Some facilities use programming modules similar to telephone booths with bars and Plexiglass. As many as 10 of those cubicles may be arranged in a semicircle. Other facilities secure the IP to a chain bolted to the floor or to a table or desk. There are advantages and disadvantages to each method. Clearly, programming modules take up a significant amount of space but allow IPs to be uncuffed inside and protected from each other. It is much easier and cheaper to configure a smaller space for group treatment by securing the IPs to the floor/desk. Clinical and custody staff should jointly review the options and available resources, considering the impact on both therapeutic milieu and correctional security before reaching consensus and proceeding.

Treatment services are provided based on individualized treatment plans that focus on current symptomatology, functional deficits, and behavior underlying the need for a restrictive setting. Group therapy typically includes anger management, stress management/relaxation, social skills/interpersonal relationships, criminal thinking, managing mental illness, medication management, and adjusting to incarceration.

Step-down programs

As correctional systems work to reduce the number of IPs held in RHUs, numerous systems have developed transitional units or step-down programs (Kline et al., 2018; Vanko, 2019). A step-down program has been defined as a program with an individualized structured review of IPs using established criteria to prepare them for transition to the general population setting following placement in RHUs (Vanko, 2019). These programs typically provide a pathway for IPs to work their way to a less restrictive setting using incentives or contingency management while maintaining the safety of the IP, their peers, and staff. Because existing RHUs have been constructed based on the policy of not releasing the IP to the general population until they are considered fully ready, IPs tend to have longer stays in this highly restrictive setting. Step-down programs allow IPs to progress through stages of increased privileges and fewer restrictions while demonstrating positive behavioral change.

Program outcomes

Vanko (2019) outlines critical components for step-down programs to be effective. There must be a clear path, and expectations should be communicated clearly and repeatedly to IPs. The programs should be voluntary, and IP placement should be based on individualized transparent reviews based on objective criteria. Conditions of confinement should differ significantly from RHUs through the use of step-down or progressive increases in out-of-cell time, meaningful programs and activities, and increasing privileges while decreasing restrictions. Individualized behavior plans, cognitive-behavioral treatment, and skill building should be prioritized.

Kupers and colleagues (2009) described such a program in Mississippi. When the IPs housed in RHUs were reclassified according to more objective standards, they found that approximately 80% did not meet the new restrictive housing criteria. This yielded a profound improvement in conditions of confinement and tremendous cost savings for the system. Kline et al. (2018) describe a step-down pilot program in the Virginia Department of Corrections (DOC). Utilizing a risk reduction model, the Virginia DOC was able to decrease its RHU population from 511 to 72 IPs, including a reduction in IPs with serious mental illness. The success of Virginia's step-down program highlighted the importance of non-RHU disciplinary sanctions following infractions. Approximately 80% of infractions in 2016 were addressed through non-RHU disciplinary sanctions. Most recently, Cloud et al. (2023) described RHU reform in the Oregon DOC that focused on IPs with serious mental illness whom staff perceived as the most challenging and who were housed in RHU-like conditions. The reforms were based on principles of dynamic security (fostering positive interpersonal relations between staff and IPs), normalization, and progression (transitioning IPs to the general population) adopted from the Norwegian Correctional Service practices. The Oregon DOC reforms resulted in reduced violence and use-of-force incidents, improved staff health and wellness, and improved sense of self and wellness for incarcerated participants. These studies support the positive impact of evidence-based interventions on the safety and security of a correctional facility and the well-being of IPs and staff.

Training of staff

Staff training is another critical component to a successful step-down program. Custody and other staff can provide critical support to mental health teams by reinforcing treatment principles and motivating IPs to participate in programming (Kline et al., 2018). To be effective, staff must gain the skills to accomplish this through adequate training. Training should cover the principles and goals of the program, communication skills, working with people with serious mental illness, motivational interviewing, de-escalation and conflict resolution, alternative sanction options, and basic behavioral principles so that consistency across shifts and staff can be reinforced.

It is recommended that custody, mental health, and nursing staff be trained together to facilitate cohesiveness and information sharing. There must be regular evaluation of program objectives and training as part of the overall quality improvement process. This facilitates a continuous evolution of the program and allows it to adapt to the different needs of the population over time. Treatment programs such as these are important because of their positive impact on facility safety (Cloud et al., 2023).

The disciplinary process

No discussion of RHUs would be complete without including the disciplinary process. Although violent misbehavior or consistent patterns of serious infractions may result in a reclassification determination resulting in RHU placement, there is also a formal disciplinary process that may result in a similar placement. The reader is directed to Cohen (2008) for a comprehensive legal review of the disciplinary process. Correctional mental health standards indicate that mental health professionals provide consultation in disciplinary proceedings (NCCHC, 2015). Most systems have a policy that defines the role of the clinician in the disciplinary process (Krelstein, 2002). This often includes a determination of whether the behavior was likely due to a mental illness or a cognitive disability and recommendations regarding the ability of the IP to understand the disciplinary process. The clinician also may recommend against imposing certain sanctions because they prevent decompensation of the IP (e.g., phone calls, visiting). These aspects distinguish this assessment process from formal forensic criminal responsibility evaluations that have a different threshold for positive findings.

Collaboration between mental health and custody staff is critical throughout all aspects of the disciplinary process and restrictive housing placement. Mental health staff can assist custody personnel in identifying effective alternative sanctions and behavioral concerns that can be included in treatment planning. As studies have shown, effective custody–mental health partnerships and implementation of meaningful programming increase safety and improve well-being for IPs and staff (Cloud et al., 2023).

Summary

The concern over the psychological impact of placing people in RHUs, particularly those with mental illness, remains a valid one. Although the Colorado study found that few IPs were negatively affected, it cannot be assumed that these findings translate to other correctional systems or even the same system over time or changing conditions. As this issue gains traction in the media and the courts, awareness of potential consequences from long-term restrictive housing is shaping society's "evolving standards of decency." While restrictive housing conditions vary from correctional system to system, those with more austere conditions tend to severely limit access to much-needed mental health services, when the opposite should be true. As systems exert greater control over IPs, they must escalate their monitoring and treatment services to help all IPs, particularly those with serious mental illness, to cope and progress to less restrictive environments.

REFERENCES

American Bar Association. (2011). *Treatment of prisoners* (3rd ed.).

American Psychiatric Association. (2016). *Psychiatric services in correctional facilities* (3rd ed.).

Andersen, H. S., Sestoft, D., Lillebaek, T., Gabrielsen, G., & Hemmingsen, R. (2003). A longitudinal study of prisoners on remand: Repeated measures of psychopathology in the initial phase of solitary versus nonsolitary confinement. *International Journal of Law and Psychiatry*, *26*, 165–177.

Beck, A. J. (2015). *Use of restrictive housing in U.S. prisons and jails, 2011–2012*. U.S. Department of Justice, Bureau of Justice Statistics.

Beven, G. (2005). Offenders with mental illness in maximum- and supermaximum-security settings. In C. Scott & J. Gerbasi (Eds.), *Handbook of correctional mental health* (pp. 209–228). American Psychiatric Publishing.

Chadick, C. D., Batastini, A. B., Levulis, S. J., & Morgan, R. D. (2018). The psychological impact of solitary: A longitudinal comparison of general population and long-term administratively segregated male inmates. *Legal and Criminological Psychology*, *23*, 101–116.

Cloud, D. H., Haney, C., Augustine, D., Ahalt, C., & Williams, B. (2023). The resource team: A case study of a solitary confinement reform in Oregon. *Public Library of Science One*, *18*(7), 1–25.

Cohen, F. (2008). *The mentally disordered offender and the law* (2nd ed.). Civic Research Institute.

Gendreau, P., & Labrecque, R. M. (2015). The effects of administrative segregation: A lesson in knowledge cumulation. In J. Wooldredge & P. Smith (Eds.), *Oxford handbook on prisons and imprisonment* (pp. 340–366). Oxford University Press.

Haney, C. (2018). Restricting the use of solitary confinement. *Annual Review of Criminology*, *1*, 285–310.

Kapoor, R., & Trestman, R. (2016). Mental health effects of restrictive housing. In M. Garcia (Ed.), *Restrictive housing in the US: Issues, challenges, and future directions* (pp. 199–232). National Institute of Justice.

Kline, B., Vanko, E., & Digard, L. (2018). *The safe alternatives to segregation initiative: Findings and recommendations for the Virginia Department of Corrections*. Vera Institute.

Krelstein, M. (2002). The role of mental health in the inmate disciplinary process: A national survey. *Journal of the American Academy of Psychiatry and the Law*, *30*(4), 488–496.

Kupers, T. A., Dronet, T., Winter, M., et al. (2009). Beyond supermax administrative segregation: Mississippi's experience rethinking prison classification and creating alternative mental health programs. *Criminal Justice and Behavior*, *20*(10), 2–14.

Luigi, M., Dellazizzo, L., Giguère, C. É., Goulet, M. H., & Dumais, A. (2020). Shedding light on "the Hole": A systematic review and meta-analysis on adverse psychological effects and mortality following solitary confinement in correctional settings. *Frontiers in Psychiatry*, *11*(840), 1–11.

Maszak-Prato, S., & Graham, L. (2022). Reducing the use of segregation for people with serious mental illness. *Prison Journal*, *102*(3), 283–303.

Metzner, J. L. (2002). Commentary: The role of mental health in the inmate disciplinary process. *Journal of the American Academy of Psychiatry and the Law*, *30*, 497–499.

Metzner, J., & Dvoskin, J. (2006). An overview of correctional psychiatry. *Psychiatric Clinics of North America*, *29*, 761–772.

Metzner, J. L., & Fellner, J. (2010). Solitary confinement and mental illness in U.S. prisons: A challenge for medical ethics. *Journal of the American Academy of Psychiatry and the Law*, *38*(1), 104–108.

Morgan, R. D., Gendreau, P., Smith, P., et al. (2016). Quantitative synthesis of the effects of administrative segregation on inmates' well-being. *Psychology, Public Policy, and the Law*, *22*(4), 439–461.

National Commission on Correctional Health Care. (2015). *Standards for mental health services in correctional facilities*.

National Commission on Correctional Health Care. (2016). *Position statement: Solitary confinement*. https://www.ncchc.org/wp-content/uploads/Solitary-Confinement-Isolation.pdf

National Commission on Correctional Health Care. (2018). *Standards for health services in prisons*.

O'Keefe, M. L., Klebe, K. J., Stucker, A., Sturm, K., & Leggett, W. (2010). *One-year longitudinal study of the psychological effects of administrative segregation*. Technical Report. Colorado Department of Corrections. https://www.ojp.gov/pdffiles1/nij/grants/232973.pdf

United Nations Office on Drugs and Crime. (2015). *United Nations standard minimum rules for the treatment of prisoners (the Nelson Mandela Rules)*. https://www.unodc.org/documents/justice-and-prison-reform/Nelson_Mandela_Rules-E-ebook.pdf

Vanko, E. (2019). *Step-down programs and transitional units: A strategy to end long-term restrictive housing*. Vera Institute. https://www.vera.org/downloads/publications/step-down-programs-and-transitional-units-strategy-to-end-long-term-restrictive-housing-policy-brief.pdf

Walters, G. (2018). Checking the math: Do restrictive housing and mental health need add up to psychological deterioration? *Criminal Justice and Behavior*, *45*(9), 1347–1362.

Zinger, I., Wichman, C., & Andrews, D. A. (2001). The psychological effects of 60 days in administrative segregation. *Canadian Journal of Criminology*, *43*, 47–88.

11

Funding of correctional health care and its implications

Robert L. Trestman and Jeremiah W. Burkhart

Introduction

Correctional health care is funded through a range of mechanisms that parallel fee-for-service and managed care models in the community. Like community health care, the use of health care in correctional settings is increasing. It is, however, often under more significant budgetary constraints and tighter management. This chapter includes a discussion of global capitation, per-incarcerated-person (IP) costs, at-risk contracting, and other contractual relationships.

Conceptual framework

Correctional expenditures made up an average of 2.5% of states' budgets in 2023, ranging between 1.2% and 6.8% (Sigritz, 2023). The combined state and federal expenditure on corrections in 2017 was approximately $81 billion (Buehler, 2021). The cost of incarceration fee for federal IPs in fiscal year 2022 who were housed in a Bureau of Prisons or non–Bureau of Prisons facility was $43,836; for IPs housed in residential reentry centers, the cost was $39,197 (Bureau of Prisons, 2023). This translates to $29,141 per state IP per year and slightly less for a federal IP, $28,283. Additionally, local governments spent $29.6 billion on corrections in 2017, which was 6% of their total expenditures (Buehler, 2021).

In turn, correctional health care is also expensive; it consumes between 9% and 18% of the total correctional budget, based on a large array of location-specific characteristics (Sridhar et al., 2018). Approximately one quarter of medical budgets are spent on mental health services (Schiff, 2017). Substantial political pressures exist to contain costs, with limited advocacy in the community or legislature. This is in tension with potential judicial oversight, consent agreements or decrees, the need to address health disparities, and the desire to deliver health care consistent with what should be community standards (American Psychiatric Association, 2015, pp. 1–3).

Funding of jail health care

In general, the county or city that it serves funds the jail. The only current exceptions are six states that have integrated jails into the state prison system: Alaska, Connecticut, Delaware, Hawaii, Rhode Island, and Vermont (Carson & Kluckow, 2023). Each of the 2,986 jails in the United States (Foudray et al., 2021), like the state and federal prison systems, has a constitutionally mandated responsibility to provide health care (*Bell v. Wolfish*, 1979; see Chapter 3). The system chosen for health care delivery typically varies by the size of the facility. Size is usually characterized simply as small, medium, or large, with respective bed capacities of 50 or fewer, 1,000 or fewer, and more than 1,000. Most small to medium facilities contract out care on a fee-for-service or hourly basis for nursing, mental health, and medical staff. Most connect closely with a local hospital for emergency, psychiatric, and medical care when needed. Large jails often have an internal health care system that more closely resembles a prison than a small jail, with substantial on-site staff and capacity for subacute care. The facility administrator, often the county sheriff, typically has responsibility for contract oversight and management.

Funding of prison health care

Prison health care is funded almost exclusively with state resources. In 2022, states spent over $64 billion in total to house over 1.2 million people (Carson & Kluckow, 2023; USA Facts, 2023). On average, states spend over $45,000 per year on each IP, but the expenditure per year for each IP in each state varies dramatically. In 2021, this ranged from a low of $23,000 in Arkansas to a high of $307,000 in Massachusetts (USA Facts, 2023). As noted previously, a state department of correction typically receives between 1.2% and 6.8% of the entire state budget and dedicates between 9% and 25% of that budget to health care (Sigritz, 2023). The administrator, typically titled secretary or commissioner, oversees this budget and the contract structure. In some states, the governor's office or the legislative branch gives guidance or direction. The norm for prison systems is to have contract arrangements for all health care through mechanisms that are discussed in more detail later in this chapter.

Medicaid, Medicare, and the Affordable Care Act

According to federal regulations that govern Medicaid and Medicare, the state may no longer bill Medicaid or Medicare for health care services while a person is incarcerated. The one exception to this rule has historically been overnight stays in a community hospital, other than emergency department visits and observational stays. Even with this opportunity for federal matching funds to pay (typically) 50% of the eligible expenses, many states have chosen not to exercise this option due to the complex billing process, which is structured on a per-IP basis, and the need to coordinate closely with the state Medicaid authority.

With the Patient Protection and Affordable Care Act in 2010 came the opportunity to initiate or maintain Medicaid enrollment for pretrial IPs in jails (Morrissey et al., 2016). The Patient Protection and Affordable Care Act does not allow for billing but does ease access to entitlements following release because more than 60% of jail IPs turn over on a weekly basis (Minton & Zeng, 2016). Some states have already worked to ease reentry by linking with the state Medicaid program to connect IPs to their entitlements immediately prior to release (Trestman & Aseltine, 2014). Further, as one element of the Patient Protection and Affordable Care Act requires coverage for children up to age 26 years by a parent's health care plan, this may allow for billing and cost recovery for off-site specialty care or overnight hospitalizations of such patients (Patient Protection and Affordable Care Act, 2010; Winkelman et al., 2017).

The newest addition to potential federal financial assistance is the Medicaid Reentry Section 1115 Demonstration Opportunity, implemented by the Centers for Medicare and Medicaid Services in 2023 (Lieber et al., 2024). This funding initiative allows state Medicaid programs to apply for a waiver to add key services for IPs during the 90 days prior to release. Allowable services that states may choose to apply for funding include the treatment of substance use disorders, mental illness, and other medical chronic conditions. The intent of this new program is to provide funding that links state correctional facilities to community providers, increasing the likelihood that treatment is available and provided during the critical reentry process.

Contract models

Prior to a period of rapid expansion of the incarcerated population in the early 1990s, most prison systems provided health care with their own employees or directly contracted for services. This changed, in most cases, with the dramatic increase in health care demands of a larger incarcerated population. States have pursued a range of approaches to meet the health care needs of their IPs. One extensive study of state prison systems examined factors that distinguished high- and low-cost systems, whose per-IP funding for health care ranged from $1,396 to $15,827 in 2015. The major findings, which accounted for 60% of the variability, suggested that it was not the range or number of services provided but rather the method of care delivery and the staffing mix that most affected per-capita costs (Schiff, 2017). Capitated contracts and increased use of midlevel practitioners (e.g., advanced practice nurses, physician's assistants) were two factors associated with decreased costs, while routine HIV screening at intake was associated with increased costs. A more recent study found that hepatitis C screening and linked treatment, where appropriate, increased costs for prison systems by $1,440 per person tested (Assoumou et al., 2020). The health benefits associated with this process were substantial and included a 23% higher cure rate and 54% reduced incidence of cirrhosis.

In-house providers versus outside providers

Most large jails and prison systems contract for health care provision. Some facilities, however, still manage health care in-house, either with their own employees or by directly subcontracting for specific services. This in-house approach survives as a legacy model, which may still be adequate in some settings. However, given the complexity of modern health care delivery and management, the use of outside providers and management systems has become the norm.

Outside vendor models

In by far the most common model, a jail or prison system contracts for health care services with an external partner or partners. For jails, such services often involve a local provider group. Large jails and prison systems usually go through a formal bidding process (often called a Request for Proposals) that specifies the requirements, service provisions, payment structure, oversight, and penalties for failure to deliver services or defined staffing levels. The provider of services may be a medical school or a for-profit company that specializes in correctional health care services. Contracts for health care services are typically time limited, ranging from 1 to 5 years; changes of vendor are not uncommon, which in theory puts pressure on the provider to provide high-quality and cost-effective care (Dober, 2014).

Global versus split contracting

The first decision a correctional administrator or contract manager must make is whether to contract for services as a whole or to carve out one or more services. Services that must be considered include acute, subacute, and chronic medical and surgical care; ambulatory through hospital-level care for mental health; dental care; nursing care; specialty care; diagnostic services; pharmacy services; medical records management; administrative oversight; and quality assurance. For example, general medical care might be contracted with one company, mental health treatment might be provided by a medical school's department of psychiatry, a pharmaceutical management firm might provide pharmacy services separately, and the correctional institution might do its own contract oversight.

There are advantages and disadvantages to each approach. The advantages to global contracting are simplicity and coordination of care delivery, administration, and oversight. One potential disadvantage is that the global care provider may have areas of weakness as well as strength. A split-service model allows for enhanced competition, selection of best-in-class providers, and the potential for optimized cost management. The negatives of such a model include the potential for redundant administrative structures, more difficult oversight, challenges in cross-disciplinary cooperation and collaboration, and the potential for cost or responsibility shifting between the different vendors.

Also, services may be divided by level of care and service line. For example, ambulatory services may be provided by one organization within the walls of the correctional institution, while a dedicated unit at a nearby hospital may provide acute care.

Liability

According to the U.S. Supreme Court, a government body remains responsible and, therefore, legally liable for providing correctional health care, whether the care is contracted or self-run. There are multiple considerations in practice that are based on the system (federal, state, or local) and on whether the care is contracted. In the federal prison system, the Supreme Court states that sovereign immunity does not apply to contracted providers (whether individuals or corporate entities) and interprets the Constitution to implicitly authorize an action for damages (known as a Bivens action) when a prisoner is harmed as the result of deliberate indifference to their medical needs (*Bivens v. Six Unknown Named Agents of Fed. Bureau of Narcotics*, 1971). Contracted providers in federal prisons remain subject to liability claims brought under state law and to licensure obligations (*Correctional Services Corporation v. Malesko*, 2001; Goldman, 2013; *Minneci v. Pollard*, 2012). *Minneci* (2012) said that in a privately run federal prison, Bivens does not apply, and IPs need to seek redress via state tort law. In other words, IPs in this situation have fewer legal protections.

In state or local correctional facilities, both the relevant government body and any involved contracted providers may be held accountable in federal court for an alleged violation of constitutional rights, with a standard of deliberate indifference (*Estelle v. Gamble*, 1976). The government body is always responsible for providing health care to IPs, whether government employees provide the care or not. Further, if the alleged deprivation was committed by contracted providers, the courts have determined that they were acting in lieu of a state employee and that they may also be held liable (Goldman, 2013; *West v. Atkins*, 1988). Depending on the alleged violation, suits may also be brought in state court for violation of state statutes, for negligence, and for violation of the state's constitution.

Funding models

Consistent with the panoply of arrangements for care delivery and reimbursement in the community, correctional health care has a similar diversity of funding mechanisms. These include such compensation structures as fee-for-service, cost based, capitation, high-cost carve-outs, hospital services, and specialty care. No model is perfect in all situations; each has specific benefits and risks. The traditional approach for health care provision is through fee-for-service arrangements. While this is still typical in small jail settings, larger jails and prison systems have generally moved away from this model to embrace some form of tighter health care cost management.

A cost-based model often includes divided oversight and care delivery. The correctional system negotiates a contract up front, with fixed unit costs for services, plus some defined percentage of compensation for administration and profit (typically 2% to 8% of care delivery costs). Once in place, correctional system employees or a third-party firm oversees utilization management, which allows for control over the costs generated. The tension in this approach is consistent with that of any fee-for-service model—the health care vendor may be motivated to generate more costs to create a greater profit. A burden of responsibility also rests on the correctional system to provide consistent and careful oversight.

Capitation models generally take two forms: global risk and per-IP capitation. As with any managed care contract, this can substantially shift the risk from the correctional system to the provider or vice versa based on the contract details. In the simplest situation, a global capitation contract guarantees a fixed amount of compensation for a defined array of service provision. This kind of contract will likely be used only in a stable, mature environment that has clear and adequate historical cost and utilization data. Here, the correctional system benefits by having a fixed, predictable budget. The contract must be structured carefully, with adequate oversight to ensure that all required care is delivered and that the care provider does not stay within budget by withholding needed services. The converse is also true, as the provider bears the risk of extraordinary costs, unless catastrophic limits are set. Such catastrophic limits typically take the form of a threshold cost per patient. An example would be contract language stating that when the annual cost of any individual patient exceeds a predetermined amount, say $40,000, the correctional system will absorb the excess cost. Another risk that the provider takes in this arrangement is an increase in the census of potential patients. The contract can address this risk by incremental modification of the compensation when the population increases by a given number, perhaps by a unit of 100 IPs, in any month. A more complicated financial arrangement involves per-IP capitation, where the average census on a monthly or quarterly basis determines compensation.

Inpatient hospital services may be funded in many ways. While some very large systems (e.g., Texas, California, and the Federal Bureau of Prisons) exclusively use prison-based hospitals, most systems contract with one or more hospitals for needed care. This generally saves the costs of correctional officer overtime compared to a system where patients occupy scattered beds in multiple hospitals and ensures public safety by negotiating for a secure unit within a specific hospital. In contrast with medical and surgical services, some states maintain their own psychiatric inpatient level of care within defined infirmary settings, with continuous nursing staff and psychiatrist coverage on-site or on call during evenings and weekends.

Similar to hospital care, systems need to contract for specialty services such as oncology, rheumatology, cardiology, and radiology. They typically do this either as part of an overall contract with the care provider or as a carve-out with individual or multispecialty groups. These may be on a fee-for-service basis (still quite common), by blocks of specified clinic time, or on a capitated basis. There may also be contractual carve-outs for transgender care and substance use disorder care. This is especially relevant for methadone treatment programs, which are easier to contract with than to achieve independent regulatory approval. Despite the regulatory hurdles, a few large jails, such as New York City's Rikers Island, have chosen to do so.

Performance measures

Contracts typically define performance measures and specify thresholds for clinical and operational targets. Where appropriate, they might also incorporate financial targets. Each of these areas may include process and outcome measures (Bellass et al., 2022). Examples of process measures include whether a given percentage threshold of staff training occurred (e.g., 100% of clinical staff certified in cardiopulmonary resuscitation in a biennial cycle) or a certain percentage of IPs received an intake screening (e.g., 98% within 4 hours of arrival). Outcome targets might include, for example, staff vacancy rates or the percentage of IPs with diabetes with a hemoglobin A1c below 7%. Specifically, as staffing levels are a critical component of contracted care delivery, a monetary penalty might exist for any month where nursing staffing has a vacancy rate greater than 5%. These measures are becoming more the norm in contracts and often are closely linked to key quality assurance initiatives (Tamburello et al., 2017).

Copays for health care

A tactic to reduce cost and moderate health care utilization, common in community settings too, is the expectation that IPs will be charged a copay for at least some of their medical care. For example, by 2022, IPs in all federal prisons and in 40 state prison systems were charged a copay when they sought medical care (Herring, 2022). The average charge is about $2. This may seem modest, but the financial reality for IPs is very different than in the world outside of prisons (American Civil Liberties Union, 2022). The typical prison job compensates IPs on average $0.14 per hour. All too often, such copays deter IPs from seeking care until they are already suffering substantial morbidity.

Summary

The funding of correctional health care is a complex enterprise, driven by constitutionally mandated care obligations on the one hand and resource constraints on the other. The costs of correctional health care are quite substantial, and the diversity of models of care delivery offers an administrative challenge, a financial challenge to the relevant jurisdiction, and a significant opportunity for cost effectiveness. Unfortunately, no comparative study of funding models has yet been done. As integrated electronic health and financial records are gradually introduced into correctional settings, opportunities for such studies, and the policy guidance provided by those results, may yield important information applicable to health care cost and outcome management in society more broadly.

REFERENCES

American Civil Liberties Union. (2022). *Captive labor: exploitation of incarcerated workers, ACLU and GHRC research report.* https://www.aclu.org/publications/captive-labor-exploitation-incarcerated-workers

American Psychiatric Association. (2015). *Psychiatric services in correctional facilities* (3rd ed.). American Psychiatric Publishing.

Assoumou, S. A., Tasillo, A., Vellozzi, C., et al. (2020). Cost-effectiveness and budgetary impact of hepatitis C virus testing, treatment, and linkage to care in US prisons. *Clinical Infectious Diseases: An Official Publication of the Infectious Diseases Society of America, 70*(7), 1388–1396.

Bell v. Wolfish, 441 U.S. 520 (1979).

Bellass, S., Canvin, K., McLintock, K., et al. (2022). Quality indicators and performance measures for prison health care: A scoping review. *Health & Justice, 10*(1), 1–19.

Bivens v. Six Unknown Named Agents of Fed. Bureau of Narcotics, 403 U.S. 388 (1971).

Buehler, E. (2021, July). *Justice expenditures and employment in the United States, 2017* (NCJ 256093). Bureau of Justice Statistics. https://bjs.ojp.gov/sites/g/files/xyckuh236/files/media/document/jeeus17.pdf

Bureau of Prisons. (2023). *Annual determination of average cost of incarceration fee (COIF)* [Notice]. 88 FR 655405. Department of Justice.

Carson, E. A., & Kluckow, R. (2023). *Prisoners in 2022—Statistical tables* (NCJ 307149). https://bjs.ojp.gov/document/p22st.pdf

Correctional Services Corporation v. Malesko, 534 U.S. 61 (2001).

Dober, G. (2014). Corizon needs a checkup: Problems with privatized correctional healthcare. *Prison Legal News, 25*(3), 1–15. https://www.prisonlegalnews.org/news/2014/mar/15/corizon-needs-a-checkup-problems-with-privatized-correctional-health care/

Estelle v. Gamble, 429 U.S. 97 (1976).

Foudray, C. M., Kramer, C., Rudes, D. S., Sufrin, C., Burr, E., & Parayil, T. (2021). The compendium of US jails: Creating and conducting research with the first comprehensive contact database of US jails. *Health & Justice, 9*(1), 12.

Goldman, J. (2013). Private provider liability in Eighth Amendment-based damages actions. *Correct Care, 27*(2), 18–30.

Herring, T (2022, February 1). *COVID looks like it may stay. That means prison medical copays must go.* Prison Policy Initiative. https://www.prisonpolicy.org/blog/2022/02/01/pandemic_copays/

Lieber, W. C., Zhang, J., & Brinkley-Rubinstein, L. (2024). Medicaid reentry section 1115 demonstration opportunity: Service funding for justice-involved populations. *JAMA Psychiatry, 81*(6), 537–538.

Minneci v. Pollard, 565 U.S. 118 (2012).

Minton, T. D., & Zeng, Z. (2016). *Jail inmates in 2015. Bureau of Justice statistical tables* (NCJ 250394). U.S. Department of Justice. https://bjs.ojp.gov/library/publications/jail-inmates-2015

Morrissey, J. P., Domino, M. E., & Cuddeback, G. S. (2016). Expedited Medicaid enrollment, mental health service use, and criminal recidivism among released prisoners with severe mental illness. *Psychiatric Services, 67*(8), 842–849.

Patient Protection and Affordable Care Act, Pub. L. No. 111–148, § 2701 (2010).

Schiff, M. (2017, October 18). *Prison health care costs and quality: How and why states strive for high-performing systems.* Pew Research Center. https://www.pewtrusts.org/en/research-and-analysis/reports/2017/10/prison-health-care-costs-and-quality

Sigritz, B. (2023). *2023 State expenditure report: Fiscal years 2021–2023.* National Association of Budget Officers.

Sridhar, S., Cornish, R., & Fazel, S. (2018). The costs of health care in prison and custody: Systematic review of current estimates and proposed guidelines for future reporting. *Frontiers in Psychiatry, 9*, 429610.

Tamburello, A., Kaldany, H., & Dickert, J. (2017). Correctional mental health administration. *International Review of Psychiatry, 29*(1), 3–10.

Trestman, R. L., & Aseltine, R. H., Jr. (2014). Justice-involved health information: Policy and practice advances in Connecticut. *Perspectives in Health Information Management, 11*(Winter), 1e.

USA Facts. (2023). *How much do states spend on prisoners?* https://usafacts.org/articles/how-much-do-states-spend-on-prisons/

West v. Atkins, 487 U.S. 42 (1988).

Winkelman, T. N., Choi, H., & Davis, M. M. (2017). The Affordable Care Act, insurance coverage, and health care utilization of previously incarcerated young men: 2008–2015. *American Journal of Public Health, 107*(5), 807–811.

SECTION III

Adapting psychiatric practice to correctional settings

12

Ethics in carceral mental health

Philip J. Candilis and Lindsay M. Poplinski

Can the imposition of this kind of suffering by an institution be morally justified? ... To propose or construct a correctional ethic would be an oxymoron, rather like presenting oneself as a married bachelor or a violent pacifist; or closer still, like constructing an ethic for slave-masters.

—Derek R. Brookes (2001, p. 40)

Introduction

The ethical analysis of health care in carceral settings suffers from the simplistic balance of care and security. Indeed, there are security limitations to clinical practice in these institutions because of the requirements to keep staff, incarcerated persons (IPs), and the community safe. Yet solutions that restrict the ethics of health care delivery do little to solve problems that result from the deprivation of liberty. In reviewing the legal, professional, and ethical standards of carceral practice, this chapter provides health care ethics as the model for solving the tensions inherent to penal life rather than as an adjunct to the security mission of the carceral institution.

This approach resonates strongly with the work of commentators who assert that health care professionals working with IPs should not be required to perform security functions (e.g., Kipnis, 2001). The work of health care professionals is protected by fundamental requirements of trust and resources, while deferring in general terms to institutional security. For health care professionals in a carceral setting, the problem arises in deciding how much deference must be given to security—a decision too frequently taken in favor of institutional policies that restrict health care delivery, limit formularies, curb confidentiality and time with IPs, and provide inadequate environments for treatment.

Mainstream policies that favor security over health are based on ideas of social role (Bradley, 1988) and the logic that clinicians wear "different hats" to manage the conflict between obligations toward an employer, a patient, and the public health of IPs in general (Brookes, 2001). Recent movement in the courts, professional societies, and the empirical literature demonstrates that social role approaches invite a simplistic deference to institutional security that at times still governs carceral ethics.

We begin by rejecting Brookes's nihilistic stance that positing a carceral ethic is an oxymoron—"a dangerous nonsense" serving to legitimize and entrench oppressive values (Brookes, 2001). The impulse to confine dangerous criminals is fundamental to the social contract and serves a legitimate purpose as long as it is carried out responsibly. However, the vulnerability of people in the control of a total institution (one that controls all aspects of personal behavior) does alter the ethical equation. Modern carceral ethics identifies obligations in numerous directions—to the individual, to the law, to the health professions, and to society as a whole—that call for a strengthening of health care values, attenuation of harms to those in detention, and rejection of a simplistic balance of duties.

Standard of care: legal, congressional, and organizational guidance

Prisoners do not have the freedom to seek and obtain their own medical treatment; rather, they rely on the institution to provide it for them. This reliance creates a legal duty to provide medical and psychiatric care (*Bowring v. Godwin*, 1977). In fact, IPs are the only class of American citizens who have a constitutionally protected right to receive health care through Eighth Amendment protections against cruel and unusual punishment (*Estelle v. Gamble*, 1976).

The minimum level of care constitutionally granted to IPs has become known as the "deliberate indifference" standard—a level near or above recklessness. However, based on this minimal standard alone, a facility could meet the "deliberate indifference" constitutional requirement yet still be found negligent in a medical malpractice suit for not providing the profession's standard of care (*Estelle v. Gamble*, 1976, p. 106). A medical malpractice lawsuit is based on a negligence standard, which is a higher standard than that of recklessness and brings common clinical standards into carceral ethics.

Subsequent cases have raised this minimal standard for some jurisdictions (see Chapter 3). IPs have been guaranteed access to mental health care (*Bowring v. Godwin*, 1977), and some federal courts have defined additional rights. *Ruiz v. Estelle* (1980), for example, required limits on seclusion alone as treatment, the need for trained mental health providers, reasonable medical records, and safety measures. *Madrid v. Gomez* (1995) further defined a person's right to speedy access to quality medical care and facilities; facilities must provide a quality assurance system and demonstrate measures to prevent suicides and respond to other emergencies. The high-profile extension of carceral health care to gender affirmation surgery was ultimately denied after initial progress through the Massachusetts courts. The First Circuit overturned the state court, and the U.S. Supreme Court declined to take it up (*Kosilek v. Spencer*, 2012; *Kosilek II En Banc*, 2014).

In addition to legal precedent, correctional facilities must meet standards set by other federal regulations (e.g., U.S. Department of Justice, National Institute of Corrections, 2001; U.S. Department of Justice, Office of the Inspector General, Evaluation and Inspections Division, 2024), individual state tort law requirements, and the individual state's department of corrections regulatory requirements. Given recent failures by the U.S. Bureau of Prisons in responding to medical emergencies and preventing suicide, anticipated challenges and lawsuits have the potential to expand existing obligations (U.S. Department of Justice, Office of the Inspector General, Evaluation and Inspections Division, 2024).

Professional organizations that govern corrections and mental health add their views to the appropriate standard of care. The National Commission on Correctional Health Care (NCCHC, 2014a, 2014b) Standards for Health Services in Jails and Prisons, for example, note that it is essential that IPs have access to care to meet their serious health needs (e.g., NCCHC, 2014b, p. 3); this reflects the U.S. Supreme Court standard of *Estelle v. Gamble* (1976). The NCCHC also sets specific standards, including that all IPs have a mental health evaluation within 14 days of admission to identify serious mental health needs (NCCHC, 2015).

The American Public Health Association (2003) has also published standards for carceral facilities. Their goal (p. 45) is that "mental health services, both diagnostic and therapeutic, must be made available to all incarcerated persons with acute and/or chronic psychiatric disorders including behavioral and emotional conditions, substance use disorders, and developmental disabilities." To meet these standards, a facility must have psychiatric services that are consistent with national community standards and written policies that ensure mental health screening at intake, acute care and suicide prevention programs, and appropriate staffing and mental health facilities.

The American Psychiatric Association (2016, p. 4) echoes this approach: "Timely and effective access to screening, evaluation, and mental health treatment is the hallmark of adequate mental health care." The guidelines further state:

> The fundamental policy goal for correctional mental health care is to provide the same quality of mental health services to each patient in the criminal justice system that *should be available* in the community. This policy goal is deliberately higher than the "community standard" that is called for in various legal contexts. (American Psychiatric Association, 2016, p. 5)

This policy goal effectively brings psychiatric services to a level that does not simply mirror what is available in a given community but provides services that should be available in any community.

In 2008, Congress passed the Mental Health Parity and Addiction Equity Act that required large group health insurance plans that provide benefits for mental health disorders to put that coverage on an equal footing with other physical illnesses. In March 2010, President Obama signed comprehensive health reform, the Patient Protection and Affordable Care Act (2010). One of the major tenets of this effort is that mental health and substance use disorder services achieve parity of access with that of other medical care. In 2016, parity rules were also applied to Medicaid managed care plans (Department of Health and Human Services, 2016). Despite persistent disparities, progress in this area is evident, and recent legal outcomes appear supportive (*E.W. v. Health Net Life Ins. Co.*, 2023). As the level of mental health care continues to rise in the community, so will the standard practiced in carceral settings.

Professionalism and human rights: ethical guidance

The traditional approach to forensic ethics is to apply an individualized ethical code to each setting. For example, if psychiatrists provide medicine or therapy to a patient, they are bound by the traditional rules of medical ethics, such as those propounded by the American Medical Association (2001). However, if psychiatrists engage in a forensic role such as that of a court expert, then a separate set of ethical guidelines apply. Here, the ethical code established by the American Psychiatric Association (2016) and the American Academy of Psychiatry and the Law (2005) holds sway. The physician attempts to negate any conflicts by remaining loyal to the code of the specific setting. The physician "wears the hat" based on the task at hand, attempting to choose one over the other (Strasburger et al., 1997).

However, carceral psychiatry requires the professional to assume more than one role simultaneously. Clinical disclosures, security, and public health concerns are so much the fabric of carceral interactions that they create a conflict far more acute than in many other health care environments. It is impossible to function under strict role requirements. One cannot simply be a treater or a forensic practitioner; the carceral psychiatrist is both. Ethical approaches from the standpoint of a robust professionalism acknowledge that an individual may be assigned unique duties that appear to operate under separate ethical principles based simply on the setting (Candilis et al., 2001, 2007; Martinez & Candilis, 2005). However, an evolving professional identity informed by a diverse group of professional practitioners whose ethnic, racial, gender, and other identities energize and define the profession cannot ignore fundamental ethical roots simply because they are working in a legal or carceral setting.

Individual values matter as well. Physicians invariably maintain a loyalty to their own internal values, duties, and ideals—standards essential for maintaining professional identity and integrity (Wynia et al., 1999). It is this consistency over time that anchors an individual or profession and helps resist the vagaries of social and situational forces. This is particularly true when these forces influence the professional to behave in ways contrary to historical values of medicine and psychiatry (Candilis et al., 2007).

Carceral psychiatry is a crucible of these conflicting personal and professional duties. There are traditional psychiatric services such as prescribing medication and psychotherapy, but carceral psychiatrists are sometimes asked to offer a psychiatric assessment for mitigating factors during disciplinary proceedings or to perform forensic assessment in smaller settings (Cervantes & Hanson, 2013). Nonetheless, physicians retain loyalties to patients, judicial bodies, the carceral facility, and even society. Under strict role requirements, it has been difficult to admit these values into the narrow view of carceral practice. However, a view of carceral professionalism that replaces narrow role theory with an integrated model of personal, professional, and community values may allow exactly that.

Richard Martinez couches professionalism in terms of the profession's social purpose, recognizing the importance of nondiscriminatory truth seeking, of addressing inequities, and of fairness—virtues or behaviors that apply across systems and services (Martinez, 2018). Unifying a profession's goals and purposes, whatever the setting, provides a far more integrated, less splintered ethics for carceral psychiatrists. More recently, Alec Buchanan has advocated forcefully for a related approach that places the inherent dignity or worth of all human beings at the foundation of forensic practice (Buchanan, 2014, 2015). He, and increasingly others, prioritizes human dignity as the highest ideal of medical, forensic, and professional ethics. The inherent worth of individuals has been a theme for philosophers since the time of Thomas Aquinas and Immanuel Kant (Rosen, 2012). Whether it comes from traditional religious origins (Aquinas) or secular thinking (Kant), respect for dignity is the touchstone for any human interaction.

Buchanan reminds the profession that even if forensic practice may harm someone, recognizing inherent worth frames the context of any encounter. This is essential for not objectifying others. Elevating human dignity, even in persons who have committed crimes and are incarcerated, protects values that are vulnerable in society (humanism, empathy) and vulnerable persons themselves (those incarcerated). This approach reminds psychiatrists that a relational encounter lies at the center of carceral practice as in any other corner of medical care.

It will not be lost on practitioners that dignity lies at the core of human rights theory. If people have inherent worth, they must have inalienable rights as described by celebrated documents like the U.S. Declaration of Independence (1776), the French Declaration of the Rights of Man (1789), the United Nations Universal Declaration of Human Rights (1948), and the African Charter on Human Rights (1981). It is a unifying idea that requires treating all persons with respect, thereby leveling the ethical playing field of jailers and jailed. In the same way that carceral care must meet community standards, IPs are due the same respect as those outside the wire. This expanded view of carceral practice recognizes the limits of strict "two-hat" thinking. Indeed, it minimizes damage to core beliefs when they conflict by drawing on values from outside the setting. If the requirements of a carceral institution appear onerous or punitive, comparison to community standards, organizational statements, or clinical training can have an important modifying influence. Developing a multidirectional perspective, rather than an insular one, allows ethical touchstones that may be unavailable otherwise. Moreover, the dynamic processes that exist among personal, professional, and community values are recognized not merely in the politics of correctional institutions and their communities but also in the contributions of practitioners. Prison suicides, assaults, escapes, and riots have far-reaching effects on staff and communities. They call on political, economic, and social solutions that extend beyond the carceral setting alone. All these elements encourage familiarity with a richer, more robust ethical framework.

Respect for the individual's perspective is borne out by attitude studies of coercion. Although it may seem intuitive that IPs hold predictable views of their confinement, the literature indicates otherwise. Studies spanning civil commitment, mandated outpatient treatment, jail diversion, and inpatient sex offender treatment indicate that fairness, transparency, and respect are among the factors that most influence individual perspectives. Even though they may be legally obligated to enter specific programs, most of these patients do not appear to view the pressure as unfair or coercive, even under conditions that meet all common definitions of compulsion (Cusack et al., 2010; Hoge et al., 1997; Munetz et al., 2014; Rigg, 2002).

Recent analyses of perceived coercion among persons convicted of sex offenses and among those in mandated treatment underscore the quality of informed consent and participation in decision-making in perceptions of coercion (Hachtel et al., 2019; Knack et al., 2020). Individuals' interests in being included in decision-making, following procedure, and being treated respectfully are consistent determinants of individual outlook and behavior (Lidz, 1997). Health care professionals can be particularly useful here in ensuring that discussion, consent, and understanding lead to engagement with treatment. For example, clinicians can acknowledge how cell-front evaluations may impact informed consent, confidentiality, and inclusion in decision-making. Reinforcing the move toward community standards can result in exactly the kind of behavioral conformity and treatment adherence jails and prisons try so assiduously to achieve.

Because contemporary ethics recognizes multiple perspectives or claims on the ethical behavior of the psychiatrist, the status of the individual under the control of the total institution cannot be minimized. The vulnerabilities of the individual have been recognized in the courts, in organizational statements, and in guidelines for carceral practice. When the individual comes up against the total institution, protections must be in place to account for that vulnerability.

This is crucial to understanding that *balancing* security and care can no longer serve as a tool for working with vulnerable, marginalized, or minoritized groups. Balancing competing interests instead of prioritizing vulnerable people and values maintains a status quo that arises from structural inequities that have yet to be resolved. Giving greater, rather than equal, attention to the experiences and narratives of institutionalized persons is far more sensitive to the history of societal imbalance and lack of resources that characterize carceral institutions. Public health and global mental health have already taken this stance against the criminalization of mental health (i.e., society's current position of having more persons diagnosed with mental illness in jails and prisons than in hospitals) in the same way that medicine and psychiatry have advanced the understanding of the social and racial determinants of health and forensic outcomes (American Public Health Association, 2018; Dvoskin et al., 2020; ten Have, 2015; Walker & Fox, 2018; World Health Organization, 2022).

Confronting bias: race, culture, and gender

Given the national overrepresentation of persons of color in the U.S. criminal legal system (Greenberg & Rosenheck, 2008; Trestman, 2018) and the differential treatment of minoritized groups in arrests, use of force, bail, and sentencing (Trestman, 2018), carceral institutions must develop a more sophisticated sensitivity to the bias inherent to practitioners and to the legal system. This means not only being aware of one's own biases—the American Bar Association and American Medical Association are among those recommending use of implicit bias assessment tools for practitioners open to examining their own beliefs (American Bar Association, 2023; American Medical Association, 2015)—but also practicing a kind of "thoroughness" that Ezra Griffith recommends for all cases that provoke bias or controversy (Griffith, 2018). Gathering information, reviewing cultural background, and acknowledging the individual's perspective are all elements of thoroughness and have been emphasized by commentators throughout forensic practice (i.e., Candilis & Griffith, 2021; Wills, 2011, 2025).

Similarly, data from carceral institutions recognize the presence of gender bias. Although women are less likely to be arrested and incarcerated than men (Friedman, 2015), women's experiences result in unique needs (see Chapter 55). Women in carceral settings more commonly experience abuse, poor physical and reproductive health, and higher rates of psychiatric disorders, substance use, and personality disorders than both women in the community and incarcerated men (Friedman, 2023; Friedman et al., 2019; MacDonald, 2013). Further, women are more likely to have been single parents than incarcerated men, which necessitates a broader societal recognition of the subsequent vulnerability of children from this context (Friedman et al., 2020). The unique medical requirements of women's perinatal care are "serious medical needs" as described in *Estelle v. Gamble* (1976) and thus must be provided for persons in the carceral setting.

Future empirical research aimed at overcoming bias and advancing health care in the carceral setting must consequently consider the representativeness of study samples and research teams alike to guard against perpetuating racial, cultural, and gender inequities. Evidence-based statements and recommendations made to inform policy and treatment should make clear the way in which study results generalize, the target population, and the assumptions that must hold for generalizations to be scientifically or statistically justifiable (Rudolph et al., 2023).

Summary

Simply balancing care and safety appears to be insufficient for psychiatrists who practice at the intersection of total institutions, their professions, and their incarcerated patients. It is not practical to parse out professional guidelines simply based on the specific task of the day. While one may hope to separate the tasks of clinical care, institutional safety, and forensic work, it is simply not possible in practice. Instead, carceral practice is based on ethics, law, professional guidance, and a research literature that identifies a series of requirements for daily practice.

The first concrete manifestation of this acknowledges the fundamental influence of health care values—of being physicians first. This means recognizing the inequities of a system that treats people differently from start to finish. It means having sufficient resources to offer mainstream treatments or appropriate alternatives when security-related limits are required. Rather than restricting formularies, this may mean having access to alternative therapies or medications that treat the common anxiety, sleep, or attention-deficit/hyperactivity problems that affect IPs. It may mean more mental health units to allay the human and financial costs of suicide watches, victimization of people diagnosed with mental illness, and assaults on staff. It almost certainly means developing diversionary alternatives to incarceration to address the vulnerability and treatment needs of persons with mental illness. It remains an extraordinary commentary on the state of mental health that the largest mental health institutions in the United States are jails and prisons (Torrey et al., 2010).

Acknowledging health care, individual, and professional values in a broad vision of humanism and professionalism means not participating in security functions except as needed to protect IPs and staff. It means advocating for clinical values and opposing mistreatment (Metzner & Fellner, 2010). Making the limits of confidentiality clear is a time-honored element of the informed consent process and need not be diluted in the carceral setting. Recognizing distinctions between treatment and forensic evaluation is both difficult and critical; confidentiality warnings and access to counsel require reminders that account for the cognitive, educational, cultural, and mental health vulnerabilities of patients.

Prioritizing vulnerable people and values and delivering clear descriptions of procedural requirements are the lessons of an evolution that supports the IP's perspective and can lead to more collaboration and less violence. Establishing a true carceral ethic promises exactly that.

REFERENCES

American Academy of Psychiatry and the Law. (2005). *Ethics guidelines for the practice of forensic psychiatry.* http://www.aapl.org/pdf/ETHICSGDLNS.pdf

American Bar Association. (2023, March 1). *Toolkits and projects. Best practices for promoting diversity, equity, and inclusion* [Webinar]. https://www.americanbar.org/groups/diversity/resources/toolkits

American Medical Association. (2001). *Code of medical ethics of the American Medical Association.* https://www.ama-assn.org

American Medical Association. (2015). *3 ways to battle unconscious bias.* https://www.ama-assn.org/deliveringcare/patient-support-advocacy/3-ways-battle-unconscious-bias

American Psychiatric Association. (2016). *Psychiatric services in correctional facilities* (3rd ed.).

American Public Health Association. (2003). *Standards for health services in correctional institutions.*

American Public Health Association. (2018). *Addressing law enforcement violence as a public health issue* (Policy Number 201811). https://www.apha.org/policies-and-advocacy/public-health-policy-statements/policy-database/2019/01/29/law-enforcement-violence

Bowring v. Godwin, 551 F.2d 44 (1977).

Bradley, F. H. (1988). *Ethical studies* (2nd ed.). Oxford University Press.

Brookes, D. R. (2001). The possibility of a correctional ethic. In J. Kleinig & M. L. Smith (Eds.), *Discretion, community, and correctional ethics* (pp. 39–68). Rowman & Littlefield Publishers.

Buchanan, A. (2014). Respect of dignity as an ethical principle in forensic psychiatry. *Legal and Criminological Psychology, 19*, 30–32.

Buchanan, A. (2015). Respect for dignity and forensic psychiatry. *International Journal of Law and Psychiatry, 41*, 12–17.

Candilis, P. J., & Griffith, E. E. H. (2021). Thoughtful forensic practice combats structural racism. *Journal of the American Academy of Psychiatry and the Law, 49*(1), 12–15.

Candilis, P. J., Martinez, R., & Dording, C. (2001). Principles and narrative in forensic psychiatry: Toward a robust view of professional role. *Journal of the American Academy of Psychiatry and the Law, 29*, 167–173.

Candilis, P. J., Weinstock, R., & Martinez, R. (2007). *Forensic ethics and the expert witness.* Springer.

Cervantes, N. C., & Hanson, A. (2013). Dual agency and ethics conflicts in correctional practice: Sources and solutions. *Journal of the American Academy of Psychiatry and the Law, 41*, 72–78.

Cusack, K. J., Steadman, H. J., & Herring, A. H. (2010). Perceived coercion among jail diversion participants in a multisite study. *Psychiatric Services, 61*, 911–916.

Department of Health and Human Services. (2016). *Final rule: Application of mental health and substance abuse disorder parity requirements to Medicaid managed care, CHIP, and benchmark coverage* (CMS-2333-F).

Dvoskin, J. A., Knoll, J. L., & Silva, M. (2020). A brief history of the criminalization of mental illness. *CNS Spectrum, 25*(5), 638–650.

Estelle v. Gamble, 429 U.S. 97 (1976).

E.W. v. Health Net Life Ins. Co., No. 21-4110 (10th Cir. 2023).

Friedman, S. H. (2015). Realistic consideration of women and violence is critical. *Journal of the American Academy of Psychiatry and the Law, 43*(3), 273–276.

Friedman, S. H. (2023). Searching for the whole truth: Considering culture in forensic psychiatric practice. *Journal of the American Academy of Psychiatry and the Law, 51*(1), 23–34.

Friedman, S. H., Kaempf, A., & Kauffman, S. (2020). The realities of pregnancy and mothering while incarcerated. *Journal of the American Academy of Psychiatry and the Law, 48*(3), 365–375.

Friedman, S. H., Tamburello, A. C., Kaempf, A., & Hall, R. C. (2019). Prescribing for women in corrections. *Journal of the American Academy of Psychiatry and the Law, 47*(4), 476–485.

Greenberg, G. A., & Rosenheck, R. A. (2008). Jail incarceration, homelessness, and mental health: A national study. *Psychiatric Services, 59*(2), 170–177.

Griffith, E. E. H. (2018). *Improving forensic performance through the pursuit of dignity*. Keynote address, Fifth Annual Forensic Conference, Saint Elizabeths Hospital, Washington, DC.

Hachtel, H., Vogel, T., & Huber, C. G. (2019). Mandated treatment and its impact on therapeutic process and outcome factors. *Frontiers in Psychiatry, 12*(10), 219.

Hoge, S. K., Lidz, C. W., Eisenberg, M., et al. (1997). Perceptions of coercion in the admission of voluntary and involuntary psychiatric patients. *International Journal of Law and Psychiatry, 20*, 167–181.

Kipnis, K. (2001). Health care in the corrections setting: An ethical analysis. In J. Kleinig & M. L. Smith (Eds.), *Discretion, community, and correctional ethics* (pp. 113–124). Rowman & Littlefield Publishers.

Knack, N., Chandler, J. A., & Fedoroff, J. P. (2020). A qualitative study of forensic patients' perceptions of quasi-coercive offers of biological treatment. *Behavioral Science and the Law, 38*(2), 135–151.

Kosilek II En Banc, 774 F.3d 63, 96, 1st Cir. (2014) (en banc), cert. denied, 135 S. Ct. 2059 (2015) (mem.).

Kosilek v. Spencer, 889 F. Supp. 2d 190 (2012).

Lidz, C. W. (1997). Coercion in psychiatric care: What have we learned from research? *Journal of the American Academy of Psychiatry and the Law, 26*(4), 631–637.

MacDonald, M. (2013). Women prisoners, mental health, violence and abuse. *International Journal of Law and Psychiatry, 36*(3–4), 293–303.

Madrid v. Gomez, 889 F. Supp. 1146 (1995).

Martinez, R. (2018). Professional identity, the goals and purposes of forensic psychiatry, and Dr. Ezra Griffith. *Journal of the American Academy of Psychiatry and the Law, 46*(4), 428–437.

Martinez, R., & Candilis, P. J. (2005). Commentary: Toward a unified theory of personal and professional ethics. *Journal of the American Academy of Psychiatry and the Law, 33*, 382–385.

Mental Health Parity and Addiction Equity Act (2008, updated November 13, 2013).

Metzner, J. L., & Fellner, J. (2010). Solitary confinement and mental illness in U.S. prisons: A challenge for medical ethics. *Journal of the American Academy of Psychiatry and the Law, 38*(1), 104–108.

Munetz, M. R., Ritter, C., Teller, J. L., & Bonfine, N. (2014). Mental health court and assisted outpatient treatment: Perceived coercion, procedural justice, and program impact. *Psychiatric Services, 65*(3), 352–358.

National Commission on Correctional Health Care. (2014a). *Standards for health services in jails*.

National Commission on Correctional Health Care. (2014b). *Standards for health services in prisons*.

National Commission on Correctional Health Care. (2015). *Standards for mental health services in correctional facilities*.

Patient Protection and Affordable Care Act, 42 U.S.C. § 18001 (2010).

Rigg, J. (2002). Measures of perceived coercion in prison treatment settings. *International Journal of Law and Psychiatry, 25*, 473–490.

Rosen, M. (2012). *Dignity*. Harvard University Press.

Rudolph, J. E., Zhong, Y., Duggal, P., Mehta, S. H., & Lau, B. (2023). Defining representativeness of study samples in medical and population health research. *BMJ Medicine, 2*(1), e000399.

Ruiz v. Estelle, 503 F. Supp. 1265 (1980).

Strasburger, L. H., Gutheil, T. G., & Brodsky, A. (1997). On wearing two hats: Role conflict in serving as both psychotherapist and expert witness. *American Journal of Psychiatry, 154*, 448–456.

ten Have, H. (2015). Respect for human vulnerability: The emergence of a new principle in bioethics. *Journal of Bioethical Inquiry, 12*(3), 395–408.

Torrey, E. F., Kennard, A. D., Eslinger, D., Lamb, R., Pavle, J., & Treatment Advocacy Center. (2010). *More mentally ill persons are in jails and prisons than hospitals: A survey of the states*. http://www.treatmentadvocacycenter.org/storage/documents/final_jails_v_hospitals_study.pdf

Trestman, R. L. (2018). Is justice really blind? Nondominant groups in the American justice system. *Journal of the American Academy of Psychiatry and the Law, 46*(4), 416–418.

U.S. Department of Justice, National Institute of Corrections. (2001). *Correctional health care: Guidelines for the management of an adequate delivery system*. http://static.nicic.gov/Library/017521.pdf

U.S. Department of Justice, Office of the Inspector General, Evaluation and Inspections Division. (2024). *Evaluation of issues surrounding inmate deaths in Federal Bureau of Prisons institutions*. https://oig.justice.gov/sites/default/files/reports/24-041.pdf

Walker, A. K., & Fox, E. L. (2018). Why marginalization, not vulnerability, can best identify people in need of special medical and nutrition care. *AMA Journal of Ethics, 20*(10), E941–E947.

Wills, C. (2011). Preparation. In A. Buchanan & M. A. Norko (Eds.), *The psychiatric report: Principles and practice of forensic writing* (pp. 22–34). Cambridge University Press.

Wills, C. D. (2025). Ethical facets of structural racism. In W. C. Darby & R. Weinstock (Eds.), *A practical guide to forensic psychiatric ethics in the 21st century*.

World Health Organization. (2022). *World mental health report: Transforming mental health for all*. https://www.who.int/publications/i/item/9789240049338

Wynia, M. K., Latham, S. R., Kao, A. C., Berg, J. W., & Emanuel, L. L. (1999). Medical professionalism in society. *New England Journal of Medicine, 341*(21), 1612–1616.

13

Working inside the walls

Cecilia Vigil and Anthony C. Tamburello[*]

Introduction

Walking into a correctional facility for the first time, much like the first moment on a mental health unit, is memorable. After having your belongings meticulously screened and then being subject to a pat-down search, you walk into an eerily quiet environment punctuated by the sound of closing mechanical doors. On the way to the clinic, you step aside as two correctional officers escort an incarcerated person (IP) down the hall. The marks on his face suggest that he was just in a physical altercation, and his loud protests indicate that he is unhappy about how this day is unfolding. For escorting officers, it looks like a typical day. While a carceral facility is an intimidating environment in which to live or work, it provided a temporary and sometimes permanent residence to 1,775,300 people in the United States in 2021 (Bureau of Justice Statistics, 2023), with many of them requiring mental health services.

The carceral psychiatrist must come to terms with the realities of the correctional setting to be secure, satisfied with the work, and clinically effective. For those interested in carceral mental health, this chapter examines the context in which the clinical work is done—that is, the physical environment and security, culture, personal safety, how to thrive in this setting, and personal liability.

In the United States, jails are short-term, local facilities that house people before arraignment or trial. They also house individuals serving sentences of less than 1 year. Prisons are state or federal facilities for adjudicated persons sentenced to more than 1 year. Most of what follows focuses on prisons and larger jails.

Physical environment and security

While most persons in the community are chiefly concerned with keeping IPs contained, it is equally important to keep the unauthorized out. Prisons are usually fortresslike structures intentionally placed away from large populations. They are surrounded by walls or fences topped with concertina (i.e., barbed) wire. Jails are smaller buildings, often in urban settings and cohoused with a courthouse or other public facilities.

There is typically a single point of entry for staff and visitors, with separate entries for IPs and commerce (i.e., deliveries). Staff and visitors are screened upon entry. Belongings are searched because many unauthorized items (i.e., contraband) are not allowed inside. Mobile phones, smart watches, other electronics, and unauthorized books are prohibited. Some facilities have entrances that lead directly to where IPs are housed. In those cases, anything potentially used as a weapon is prohibited, like a cup of hot coffee or an aluminum soda can. Most facilities will subject staff and visitors to a pat-down search and metal detector screening. Cameras are almost always forbidden unless approved for a specific purpose.

Entry is commonly protected by a heavily monitored entrance called a sally port, which is a system of two doors with a space between them. Only one door opens at a time so that those going through are temporarily trapped between the doors, limiting the opportunity for unauthorized transit. The sally port originates from the medieval tactic of using a secured doorway to harass a besieging force without endangering those within the fortress (McLean, 1998).

Many prisons have monotonous, empty, and colorless hallways, with a spartan, raw concrete design reminiscent of brutalist architecture. There is also a need to minimize hiding places, so the physical plant is typically basic. While some facilities are kept meticulously clean, others are less so. Movement within a prison can be time-consuming and is recognized by security staff as a high-risk period. Civilians may not be allowed to travel within the facility when large numbers of IPs are moving. Many prisons have mechanical gates that bar movement, and you must wait for an officer to grant you access.

Custody levels are an important organizing feature of carceral settings. They determine physical security measures, staffing models, access to different parts of the facility, the nature of staff escorts, privileges, permitted possessions, and even how medications are delivered. Each IP's custody level is determined by classification, which is essentially a risk assessment (see Chapter 8). Most classification systems generate a score based on the IP's charges, detainers/warrants, sentencing status, criminal history, escape history, institutional disciplinary history, substance use, and demographic variables (Federal Bureau of Prisons, 2019; Hardyman, Austin, & Tulloch, 2002). IPs with the highest risk are placed at the highest

*. The authors acknowledge the contributions of Bruce Gage, who authored this chapter in the textbook's first edition.

custody levels. Changes in classification level are primarily driven by rule infractions over time. Scores are typically updated following a serious negative event. Other classification considerations include the IP's needs, work assignments, and specific housing requirements (e.g., mental health or medical units). They may also incorporate formal/structured needs assessments, personality dimensions, and carceral history (Hardyman, Austin, Alexander, et al., 2002).

The highest custody settings, commonly designated maximum or supermaximum, often use sally ports for entry into housing units. The tiers are composed of single-occupancy cells with remote-controlled locks operated by an officer in a central and secured location. The cells have a built-in toilet, sink, bed, and sometimes a desk and stool. These areas are hardened, meaning that additional precautions are taken to ensure that prisoners cannot escape or readily destroy or weaponize anything. IPs typically cannot see each other, and even verbal communication can be difficult, as individuals are usually in their cells 23 hours per day. Supervision by custody staff is virtually always indirect—that is, the officers are not in the same physical space as the IPs but observe them visually or by camera. The observation is constant in that an officer can see a prisoner at any time. IPs are moved in security containment devices, such as a metal waist chain attached to wrist and ankle cuffs, with two or more staff directly controlling them. Visitation is limited to official visits, but some carceral settings allow noncontact family visits. IPs at the maximum custody level have few or no personal items and usually are not allowed to keep their own medications, except possibly vital medications needed in emergencies.

At intermediate custody levels—that is, high or medium—supervision by custody staff may be direct (with officers occupying the same space as unrestrained IPs) or indirect and is almost always constant. Cells may be individual or house small numbers of IPs with shared bathrooms. Escort practices are variable, but security containment devices are usually not required within the facility. Unescorted group movement between discrete areas occurs at specified times. IPs may eat in communal areas, go to activities and programs on or off the tier, and begin to hold jobs within the facility. Contact visits are common, although not universal. This is normally the least restrictive custody level in jails.

Minimum custody levels are still within facilities and have a secure perimeter. Dormitories are common in this setting, and supervision is typically direct but intermittent. Interaction between security and IPs is frequent. Escorting is rarely required within the facility. IPs may work outside of the secure perimeter while directly supervised by custody staff. Contact visits are the rule.

The lowest custody setting is prerelease or work release. These are typically transitional facilities sited in the community and have no perimeter security. Living arrangements vary widely. Supervision is direct and intermittent. IPs go into the community to work or engage in other specified activities during the day and return to the facility in the evening. Visiting is tracked but may not be controlled.

Carceral culture

While each carceral facility has its own culture, there are important themes that are widely applicable. Aspects of the subculture of IPs include the value of not "snitching" (sharing information about other prisoners with staff), "doing your own time" (not getting involved in others' business), respect, and avoiding an appearance of weakness. Incarcerated women also value respect and "doing your own time" and equally disdain snitching, though they develop more intimate, family-like relationships and place less emphasis on the solidarity of the community of IPs (Owen, 1998; Zaitzow, 2003; see Chapter 55).

The prison culture has a large body of cultural jargon, with only a few terms sampled here: a "bid" is a period of incarceration; a "cellie" or "bunkie" is a cellmate; a "fish" is a newly incarcerated person; a correctional officer is a "CO"; the "hole" is restrictive housing or solitary confinement; "to jail" is to do time well; a "duck" is a gullible person who can be manipulated; and a "kite" is a request for within-prison services (Prison Journalism Project, 2022). Terms may vary regionally and are context dependent. For example, a "kite" is also a contraband note passed to others secretly, such as in restrictive housing (Delgado, 2025).

Correctional staff are typically organized in a paramilitary hierarchical structure, much like community police. Good communication, respect, and following the chain of command in terms of addressing problems within the facility are expected. Regarding correctional staff, Higgins and colleagues (2021) discuss a culture of "us–them" that dehumanizes IPs as "others" who deserve whatever might befall them. Some may speak of "breaking" IPs rather than rehabilitating them (Weinstock, 1989). To assume that all correctional staff have these beliefs would be unfair. Staff culture also prioritizes the safety of coworkers (see Chapter 65). In 2022, the third highest rate of fatalities was among the protective service occupations, which includes correctional officers (Bureau of Labor Statistics, 2023).

Personal safety

A reasonable concern for those considering work in a prison is personal safety. The risk of workplace violence is a fact of life for physicians in any setting, from emergency departments and outpatient clinics to general and psychiatric hospitals (Caruso et al., 2022). A difference in carceral settings is that the workspace is shared with correctional officers who are principally tasked with keeping both staff and IPs safe. Part of the carceral clinician's job is to show an understanding and respect for security protocols. Correctional officers notice and appreciate this, as it implies a respect for their often thankless and dangerous job.

Carceral settings are dangerous for IPs and correctional officers alike. There were 120 homicides of state-sentenced incarcerated people during 2018, which was the highest number since 2001 (Bureau of Justice Statistics, 2021). A 2013 study of deaths and injuries among U.S. correctional officers over a 20-year period found an average of 11 work-related fatalities (most of which were from homicide) and over 12,000 nonfatal injuries requiring treatment in an emergency department per year (Konda et al., 2013).

Working in a carceral setting requires vigilance. Situational awareness and insight are critical. For example, it is important to be aware of one's situation, who is nearby, the location of means of egress, and how to call for help (e.g., panic buttons, intercoms, telephones). In particular, the scheduled movement times of IPs should be paid special attention. Clinical staff are wise to keep their distance in such a scenario unless their immediate help is requested (e.g., for de-escalation). Office supplies like pens, staplers, small metal objects, and scissors could be used as weapons and should be treated as such. For example, if staff interactions require the use of a writing implement (e.g., to complete forms or self-report instruments), providing a flexible safety pen is often advisable.

Maintaining proper boundaries promotes a safer environment for both staff and IPs. Doing an unapproved favor for an IP, or any action not consistent with the staff's professional duties, can place all persons at risk. Even something as innocuous as looking up a name, phone number, or location on the internet, when done for nonclinical reasons, can compromise a clinician. Staff in this situation may give an IP coercive power over them. In these situations, minor boundary crossings escalate over time and may culminate in extortion, high-risk boundary violations, and criminal behavior (e.g., sexual relationships, smuggling in contraband, or participation in escape attempts; Cooke et al., 2019). Besides the obvious violation of professional ethics of a doctor–patient sexual relationship, IPs do not have the capacity to consent to this.

Thriving as staff in a correctional environment

Clinical staff should be wary of identifying too strongly either with custodial staff or with IPs. Viewing IPs as "victims" of the penal system may make staff vulnerable to boundary violations. On the other hand, seeing patients who are incarcerated as an "inmate" or as an "other" limits one's ability to empathize with a human being in an extraordinary and stressful environment. Similarly, given the high rates of personality disorders and substance use disorders in these settings (American Psychiatric Association, 2016; Fazel & Danesh, 2002; Teplin, 1994), clinicians must guard against countertransference (see Chapter 37). Regardless, either of these extremes can compromise the care provided. Health care staff should appropriately empathize with their patients and advocate for their clinical needs. At the same time, they should be aware of potential nonclinical reasons for certain requests (such as medications at high risk for misuse; see also Chapter 30) and approach such requests with healthy skepticism. Obtaining collateral information (e.g., from outside records or other observers), with consent, can be helpful in such situations.

It is necessary to dress, speak, and behave professionally at all times. Staying calm in a crisis will help to defuse and de-escalate situations that may arise. Showing respect for others is essential, as both IPs and custody staff are sensitive to disrespect. Note that uniformed staff prefer to be referred to as officers rather than "guards," a term seen as demeaning. Staff must adapt to work without mobile phones, smartwatches, and other small electronics disallowed inside a secure perimeter, as smuggled phones may be used by IPs for criminal activity (Mooney, 2011). Alternatives include landline telephones, carrying reference books, and, if allowed, using computers to access online clinical resources.

Common challenges of the clinical work in jails and prisons include formulary restrictions, understaffing and high caseloads, older electronic or even paper medical record systems, and limited access to consultation. Psychiatrists can expect medication formulary restrictions to be in place in most correctional facilities, whether for cost or safety reasons, though typically there will be a process for ordering nonformulary medication when clinically justified (Morris et al., 2020; see also Chapter 27). Controlled medications, like benzodiazepines, stimulants, and medication for opioid use disorder, may also be nonformulary, limited, or unavailable (see Chapters 29 and 49). Hiring and retaining mental health professionals to work in correctional facilities is difficult and may be compounded by incomplete or inaccurate knowledge about the work (Morris & West, 2020).

A dilemma may be created when the carceral clinician witnesses excessive force against, or the abuse of, an IP. Speaking out may risk alienating custody staff, while failure to speak out raises ethical concerns. The American Psychiatric Association's *Principles of Medical Ethics With Annotations Especially Applicable to Psychiatry* (2013) sets as a guiding principle that "a physician shall be dedicated to providing competent medical care with compassion and respect for human dignity and rights" (p. 3). Thus, a psychiatrist should advocate for the best mental health interests of persons. In carceral settings, this likely amounts to a discussion with the supervisor(s) of the officers in question (Knoll, 2014), though individual jurisdictions may have specific procedures set by regulation or law. Correctional officers' supervisors will very likely want to know about these lapses, which could have negative consequences for everyone under their command. The problem of prison violence, including abuse of IPs, was the focus of the Commission on Safety and Abuse in America's Prisons (Gibbons & Katzenbach, 2006). The use of force in carceral settings, when absolutely necessary, must be balanced and humane (Specter, 2006). Knoll (2014) concluded that in response to witnessing clear and intentional abuse of an IP, the carceral clinician should "do the right thing."

Disruptive behavior by an IP can compromise the safety of the individual, as well as peers and staff. Lockdowns to manage such situations force other IPs to face interruptions to their scheduled activities. A psychiatrist may be called into such situations to intervene through de-escalation or to order emergency medication or therapeutic restraints (see Chapter 24). It is easy to place orders, but the adept psychiatrist will know when to act decisively and when to refrain because the risks of these interventions outweigh the benefits.

Relatively new to prison mental health care is gender-affirming care. Clark and colleagues (2017) expressed concern that "a lack of cultural and clinical competency, stemming from personal bias and lack of knowledge and experience, were the primary individual barriers resulting in inadequate and non-gender-affirming provision of care to transgender inmates" (p. 9). Clinicians must become comfortable working with transgender IPs and improve their knowledge of transgender health care as it relates to their work (see Chapter 56).

Personal liability

Though limited by the Prison Litigation Reform Act of 1996, IPs may bring frequent malpractice suits, civil rights suits (Appelbaum, 2010), and complaints to licensing boards against correctional clinicians. While prisons are higher risk settings for suits related to health care, psychiatrists are less likely to be sued than other medical practitioners there (Tamburello & Azuh-Showole, 2022). Whether frivolous or not, claims and suits often require some formal response. If a case becomes reportable, malpractice insurance may be denied or premiums may increase, even if the case is without merit and is ultimately dismissed.

The correctional psychiatrist needs to understand their malpractice coverage. Those who work for the public sector may be indemnified by the public entity or, less commonly, by a private carrier. Those who work for private companies that provide contractual services or who work under their own contract typically must provide their own malpractice coverage, although some companies and agencies provide indemnification. Before signing a contract to provide services, psychiatrists should look for "hold harmless" clauses that limit coverage or divert liability from the facility for certain outcomes (Knoll, 2010).

Correctional psychiatrists should consider carrying their own malpractice insurance, even when it is provided through their job. There are two reasons for this. First, a public agency may find that it is in its interest to settle a case rather than pay the costs of litigation or potentially lose a suit, leaving the psychiatrist with an adverse finding. Second, the interests of the public agency and the clinician may differ, in which case psychiatrists may find themselves in an adversarial relationship with the agency.

Suits for civil rights violations are not usually covered by malpractice insurance. Under 42 U.S.C. § 1983 (2012), clinicians are not automatically immune from civil rights litigation even if they follow statute, policy, or custom. However, *Estelle v. Gamble* (1976) set a standard of "deliberate indifference" that must be proven to show that an individual's Eighth Amendment rights were violated. Deliberate indifference is when a state actor knew of a serious medical need and failed to act. It is difficult to prove this, as most psychiatrists will act, whether adequately or not, when a need is recognized. A finding of a civil rights violation for deliberate indifference is more difficult to prove than negligence in a medical malpractice suit (Alsan et al., 2023). Deliberate indifference is a subjective standard, meaning that the state actor must have knowledge of the risk posed (*Farmer v. Brennan*, 1994). Protection is also provided by the Prison Litigation Reform Act of 1996, which requires that there be physical injury before money damages can be recovered for mental injuries. The Prison Litigation Reform Act of 1996 provides additional protections from civil suits by collecting filing fees from IPs and making cases easier for judges to dismiss. Another theory of liability can be found in the Americans With Disabilities Act, which applies to IPs (*Pennsylvania v. Yeskey*, 1998), who can then sue for money damages (*U.S. v. Georgia*, 2006).

Generally, courts grant deference to providers in jails and prisons, as long as the care is reasonable, professional judgment was used, and the clinician adheres to relevant laws and institutional policies (Tamburello & Azuh-Shawole, 2022). While the most common cause of liability in correctional settings is suicide, other and emerging concerns include inadequate care in restrictive housing, adverse medication reactions without adequate examination and informed consent, and failure to provide adequate discharge planning (Tamburello & Azuh-Showole, 2022). Emergency psychotropic treatment is permissible without informed consent when an IP is a danger to themselves or others (*Chambers v. Ingram*, 1988). The federal appellate case *Charles v. Orange County* (2019) held that providing an adequate supply of medication for IPs upon release from incarceration was part of "in-custody medical care." Another reason for rare malpractice findings is that clinical standards for carceral treatment are poorly articulated (Hoge et al., 2009).

Confidentiality is difficult to preserve in any setting with limited privacy, but it should still be respected and optimized to the extent consistent with safety in carceral settings. Failure to do this will likely impair therapeutic rapport, and it may subject the patient to risk from others or expose the psychiatrist to liability. A federal appellate court found that meetings with mental health staff within hearing of other IPs create a possible claim for violation of privacy (*Hunnicutt v. Armstrong*, 2005). Clinicians must also know whether their agency is considered a covered entity under the Health Insurance Portability and Accountability Act of 1996 (HIPAA), though many correctional systems are not. In addition, many states have exceptions and variations for carceral institutions by regulation or statute that allow or mandate release of information related to public safety. Carceral clinicians have no obligation to report past crimes other than legally mandated reporting requirements, such as child or elder abuse. However, there is an affirmative obligation to prevent future harm vis-à-vis the *Tarasoff* duty (Pinta, 2010). Any limitations of confidentiality should be disclosed prior to working with the patient.

Summary

Although there are many challenges in this work, psychiatric practice in jails and prisons can be highly rewarding. Carceral settings have a high prevalence of serious mental illness and complex comorbidities; the cases are interesting and challenging, and opportunities for skillful and creative management abound. While a carceral facility is not the treatment setting clinicians would prefer for people with mental illness, this is where many of them are, and it is a place where these individuals have both access to and a right to health care for both medical and psychiatric needs (*Bowring v. Godwin*, 1977; *Estelle v. Gamble*, 1976). Adequate discharge planning, including medication management when clinically appropriate, can have a lasting benefit for patients (Tamburello & Selhi, 2013). Carceral psychiatry is meaningful, important, and fulfilling.

REFERENCES

42 U.S.C. § 1983 (2012).

Alsan, M., Yang, C. S., Jolin, J. R., Tu, L., & Rich, J. D. (2023). Health care in U.S. correctional facilities—A limited and threatened constitutional right. *New England Journal of Medicine, 388*, 847–852.

American Psychiatric Association. (2013). *Principles of medical ethics with annotations especially applicable to psychiatry*. https://www.psychiatry.org/getmedia/3fe5eae9-3df9-4561-a070-84a009c6c4a6/2013-APA-Principles-of-Medical-Ethics.pdf

American Psychiatric Association. (2016). *Psychiatric services in jails and prisons* (3rd ed.).

Appelbaum, K. L. (2010). The mental health professional in a correctional culture. In C. Scott (Ed.), *Handbook of correctional mental health* (2nd ed., pp. 91–117). American Psychiatric Press.

Bowring v. Godwin, 551 F.2d 44 (1977).

Bureau of Justice Statistics. (2021). *Mortality in state and federal prisons, 2001–2018—Statistical tables*. https://bjs.ojp.gov/content/pub/pdf/msfp0118st.pdf

Bureau of Justice Statistics. (2023). *Correctional populations in the United States, 2021—Statistical tables*. https://bjs.ojp.gov/document/cpus21st.pdf

Bureau of Labor Statistics. (2023). *National census of fatal occupational injuries in 2022*. https://www.bls.gov/news.release/pdf/cfoi.pdf

Caruso, R., Toffanin, T., Folesani, F., et al. (2022). Violence against physicians in the workplace: Trends, causes, consequences, and strategies for intervention. *Current Psychiatry Reports, 24*(12), 911–924.

Chambers v. Ingram, 858 F.2d 351, 7th Cir. (1988).

Charles v. Orange County, No. 17-3506, 2d Cir. (2019).

Clark, K. A., Hughto, J. M. W., & Pachankis, J. E. (2017). "What's the right thing to do?" Correctional healthcare providers' knowledge, attitudes and experiences caring for transgender inmates? *Social Science & Medicine, 193*, 80–89.

Cooke, B. K., Hall, R. C. W., Friedman, S. H., Jain, A., & Wagoner, R. (2019). Professional boundaries in corrections. *Journal of the American Academy of Psychiatry and the Law, 47*(1), 91–98.

Delgado, A. (2025). *Prison slang: The complete guide*. https://communitylawfirm.com/prison-slang-guide

Estelle v. Gamble, 429 U.S. 97 (1976).

Farmer v. Brennan, 511 U.S. 825 (1994).

Fazel, S., & Danesh, J. (2002). Serious mental disorder in 23000 prisoners: A systematic review of 62 surveys. *Lancet, 359*, 545–550.

Federal Bureau of Prisons. (2019). *Inmate security designation and custody classification*. https://www.bop.gov/policy/progstat/5100_008cn.pdf

Gibbons, J. J., & Katzenbach, N. de B. (2006). *Confronting confinement: A report of the Commission on Safety and Abuse in America's Prisons*. https://www.vera.org/downloads/publications/Confronting_Confinement.pdf

Hardyman, P. L., Austin, J., Alexander, J., Johnson, K. D., & Tulloch, O. C. (2002). *Internal prison classification systems: Case studies in their development and implementation*. National Institute of Corrections.

Hardyman, P. L., Austin, J., & Tulloch, O. C. (2002). *Revalidating external prison classification systems: The experience of ten states and model for classification reform*. National Institute of Corrections.

Health Insurance Portability and Accountability Act, Pub. L. No. 104-191, § 264, 110 Stat. 1936 (1996).

Higgins, E. M., Smith, J., & Swartz, K. (2021). "We keep the nightmares in their cages": Correctional culture, identity, and the warped badge of honor. *Criminology, 60*, 429–454.

Hoge, S. K., Greifinger, R. B., Lundquist, T., & Mellow, J. (2009). Mental health performance measures in corrections. *International Journal of Offender Therapy and Comparative Criminology, 53*, 634–647.

Hunnicutt v. Armstrong, 152 Fed. Appx. 34 (2005).

Knoll, J. L. (2010). Suicide in correctional settings: Assessment, prevention, and professional liability. *Journal of Correctional Health Care, 16*(3), 188–204.

Knoll, J. L. (2014). The psychiatrist's obligation: Same as it ever was. *Correctional Mental Health Report, 15*(5), 69–70.

Konda, S., Tiesman, H., Reichard, A., & Hartley, D. (2013). U.S. correctional officers killed or injured on the job. *Corrections Today, 75*(5), 122–123.

McLean, A. (1998). *Medieval military engineering*. https://nicolaa5.tripod.com/articles/Hector/hist/HEngin.htm

Mooney, M. J. (2011, January 10). Cell phones in prison: A former inmate explains the real deal. *Broward Palm Beach New Times*. https://www.browardpalmbeach.com/news/cell-phones-in-prison-a-former-inmate-explains-the-real-deal-6459092

Morris, N. P., Hirschtritt, M. E., & Tamburello, A. C. (2020). Drug formularies in correctional settings. *Journal of the American Academy of Psychiatry and the Law, 48*(1), 2–6.

Morris, N. P., & West, S. G. (2020). Misconceptions about working in correctional psychiatry. *Journal of the American Academy of Psychiatry and the Law, 48*(2), 251–258.

Owen, B. (1998). *In the mix: Struggle and survival in a women's prison*. State University of New York Press.

Pennsylvania v. Yeskey, 524 U.S. 206 (1998).

Pinta, E. R. (2010). Tarasoff duties in prisons: Community standards with certain twists. *Psychiatric Quarterly, 81*, 177–182.

Prison Journalism Project. (2022). *A reporter's glossary of prison jargon*. https://prisonjournalismproject.org/a-reporters-glossary-of-prison-jargon/

Prison Litigation Reform Act, 42 U.S.C. § 1997e (1996).

Specter, D. (2006). Making prisons safe: Strategies for reducing violence. *Washington University Journal of Law & Policy, 22*, 125.

Tamburello, A., & Azuh-Showole, C. (2022). Correctional psychiatry. In P. Ash, R. L. Frierson, & S. H. Friedman (Eds.), *Malpractice and liability in psychiatry* (pp. 217–224), Springer.

Tamburello, A. C., & Selhi, Z. (2013). Commentary: Bridging the gaps for former inmates with serious mental illness. *Journal of the American Academy of Psychiatry and the Law, 41*, 510–513.

Teplin, L. A. (1994). Psychiatric and substance abuse disorders among male urban jail detainees. *American Journal of Public Health, 84*, 290–293.

U.S. Department of Justice Office of Public Affairs. (2024). *Justice Department files statement of interest in lawsuit concerning treatment for gender dysphoria in correctional settings*. https://www.justice.gov/opa/pr/justice-department-files-statement-interest-lawsuit-concerning-treatment-gender-dysphoria

U.S. v. Georgia, 546 U.S. 151 (2006).

Weinstock, R. (1989). Treatment of antisocial and other personality disorders in a correctional setting. In R. Rosner & R. B. Harmon (Eds.), *Correctional psychiatry* (pp. 41–59). Plenum Press.

Zaitzow, B. H. (2003). "Doing gender" in a women's prison. In B. H. Zaitzow & J. Thomas (Eds.), *Women in prison: Gender and social control* (pp. 21–38). Lynn Rienner Publishers, Inc.

14

Communicating with interdisciplinary professionals

Dean Aufderheide

Introduction

The art of communication is the language of leadership.

—James Humes

A national leader in corrections once told me that, of the myriad challenges he faced during his 30-year career, the most problematic were the result of poor communication. For problems and unwanted outcomes in health care settings, the origin is not dissimilar (O'Daniel & Rosenstein, 2008). In fact, most sentinel events occurring from medical errors in U.S. health care facilities result from breakdowns in communication (Grossman, 2011).

When the competing cultures and communication styles of correctional and health care professionals clash, communication efficacy is compromised, and the potential for problems and unwanted outcomes is compounded. Notwithstanding the inherent cultural differences among interdisciplinary staff (Vinokur-Kaplan, 1995), effective communication in a correctional setting is especially challenging for psychiatrists. Whether transitioning from the protective structure of a residency or moving from a private practice or other mental health setting, psychiatrists working in a jail or prison will likely experience their new environment as adversarial and replete with competing interests and priorities (Pinta, 2009). Also, unlike in a health care setting, where physicians are at the top of the hierarchy, psychiatrists working in a jail or prison are further down the totem pole in the organizational hierarchy. Since individuals on the lower end of a hierarchy tend to be uncomfortable speaking up about problems or concerns (Schyve, 2009), communication impediments in correctional psychiatry diminish the collaborative interactions necessary to ensure proper treatment is delivered. It is in such an environment that it becomes critically important for psychiatrists to develop communication strategies that create effective and sustainable working relationships not only with patients but also with the facility's leadership, security staff, treatment team members, and other interdisciplinary staff.

This chapter will discuss ways in which psychiatrists play a critical role in mission requirements that necessitate effective communication skills with interdisciplinary staff in jails and prisons. From identifying the variables in the correctional culture that shape communication to improving interdisciplinary collaboration, this chapter will explore the ways in which correctional psychiatrists can model effective communication styles and strategies that enhance professional credibility and improve treatment outcomes.

Defining communication

The two words "information" and "communication" are often used interchangeably, but they signify quite different things. Information is giving out; communication is getting through.

—Sydney J. Harris

A plethora of definitions attempt to describe the different communication modalities (verbal, nonverbal, etc.) and distinguishing variables for understanding communicative phenomena (Losee, 1999). A conventional way of thinking about communication may be that its purpose is to achieve a maximum level of accuracy and efficiency in a message. However, an organization's cultural identity and knowledge base play a role in framing a message and putting it into a context. For psychiatrists working in a correctional setting, therefore, it is critically important that their communication not only accurately conveys meaning but also creates a shared understanding among all the staff involved in the delivery of mental health services.

The importance of communication in correctional psychiatry

Communication works for those who work at it.

—John Powell

Just as the key to successful real estate transactions is said to be "location, location, location," the key to the successful practice of psychiatry in a correctional setting is "communication, communication, communication." Effective communication is at the heart of correctional psychiatry and involves the knowledge, motivation, and skills to interact effectively with all the interdisciplinary staff in the jail or prison environment. Communication competence, therefore, becomes the bridge between the distinct professional cultures and missions, creates shared values, and generates opportunities for interdisciplinary training. Whether through formal or informal interactions with staff, ongoing communication is critically important, as noted by Applebaum and colleagues (2001, p. 1346):

> Shared values and training bear fruit when security staff and mental health staff engage in ongoing communication and cooperation, both formally and informally and at the level of both line staff and administrators. Regular but informal interactions can help both groups move beyond preconceived notions and create an atmosphere of trust and communication. These casual interactions provide opportunities for mental health staff to become more sensitive to the concerns and perspective of security staff while they further inform officers about the nature and impact of mental disorders on inmate patients.

Whether in a patient interview, treatment team meeting, consultation with the facility's leadership, or discussion with security staff, there are opportunities for the correctional psychiatrist to communicate in such a way that builds credibility, strengthens cooperation, and generates collaboration. When psychiatrists model effective communication, they reinforce active participation by other members of the multidisciplinary treatment team. But when communication is constrained, distorted, fragmented, or misinterpreted, a vacuum is created. Misunderstandings multiply, and inaccurate information is perceived as fact. Ultimately, the psychiatrist loses credibility with facility leadership and other interdisciplinary staff, and the treatment delivery system becomes vulnerable to destabilization. Effective communication results in good treatment outcomes, and poor communication results in poor outcomes in the provision of psychiatric services in correctional settings.

Communicating in the corrections culture

> *Think like a wise man, but communicate in the language of the people.*
>
> —William Butler Yeats

It is imperative that psychiatrists are aware of the multicultural issues in the organization in which they work (Gaines, 1992; Kirmayer et al., 2003). An organizational culture consists of implicit and explicit assumptions to address its problems and is considered a valid way for its constituents to conceptualize and deal with those problems (Hampden-Turner & Trompenaars, 2004; Triandis, 1989). The basic assumption in correctional settings is the predominant supposition that the criminogenic characteristics of the carceral population present an omnipresent threat to the public, staff, and safety. The visible cues, including razor wire, uniformed officers, security restraints, and so forth, are constant reminders for psychiatrists that their communication style and strategy must be contextualized within the framework of the correctional culture. The correctional culture inculcates all staff with the primacy of safety and security, and as Hagberg and Heifetz (2000) discern, "The culture of an organization operates at both a conscious and subconscious level" (p. 2).

It is important, therefore, that psychiatrists understand the jail or prison culture, its mission, and its chain of command to be effective in their communications. Undermining organizational assumptions, displaying professional condescension, disregarding the chain of command, or being dismissive of input from others can destroy credibility in the correctional culture (Aufderheide, 2021). Consider the following case example of discrediting and counterproductive communication in a treatment team meeting.

CASE EXAMPLE 1: THE WRONG WAY TO BE RIGHT

It is Tuesday afternoon, and the treatment team is about to begin. Dr. Red, the prison psychiatrist, is already running late for the meeting and still has many patients to see before the end of the day. She generally finds treatment team meetings unhelpful and views them as an imposition on her time with patients. As usual, the other members of the treatment team are waiting for Dr. Red to arrive and are becoming increasingly irritated. They also have patients to see, Dr. Red is often late, and they feel she tends to take over the meeting and not listen to their viewpoints. In fact, some of the members have stopped offering their clinical input, preferring to adjourn the meeting as quickly as possible. Dr. Red finally arrives, and the first patient for discussion is Taylor, a 27-year-old man serving a life sentence. He has a history of treatment in prison for psychosis, as well as multiple disciplinary reports. Dr. Moore, a relatively new psychologist at the prison, has put Taylor on the list for discussion because the dorm sergeant expressed concerns about his deteriorating hygiene and behavior when he was conducting rounds this week. As Dr. Moore begins to share the concerns reported by security, Dr. Red interrupts; turns to Taylor's case manager, Mr. Hanky; and reproaches him, stating, "Isn't this the individual who was caught hoarding his medications several months ago? Aren't you aware he was probably planning to sell them?" Mr. Hanky does not always agree with Dr. Red but has learned over time that she interprets case discussion as a challenge to her professional authority during treatment team meetings. This tends to result in Dr. Red becoming more intransigent about her clinical opinion of the patient. Dr. Moore interjects that she reviewed the chart and, in fact, there appears to be a relationship between Taylor's deteriorating behavior and thought processes and the discontinuation of the medication. She turns to Nurse Jiminy, who has worked at the prison for years, and asks her opinion about Taylor. Nurse Jiminy feels put on the spot. She has to work directly with Dr. Red every day and wishes that Dr. Moore would leave her out of it. After all, she is a nurse, not a mental health expert like Dr. Red. Many of these individuals do manipulate the system, and Taylor does have a history of hoarding medication. As Nurse Jiminy is presenting pertinent information about Taylor's history of disciplinary reports, Dr. Red interrupts again, exclaiming, "You must have overlooked my progress note! Here it is in the chart. When I discontinued his medication, Taylor admitted that he is not really mentally ill. He is just trying to get his sentence reduced. I documented it right here. You are so naive. You have got to learn how to work with these individuals, or they are just going to manipulate you. Plus, you have never even met this individual." Dr. Moore feels her face beginning to turn red with embarrassment. She realizes that she still has a lot to learn and vows to be more prepared before she brings up a case again. While Mr. Hanky feels badly for Dr. Moore, he also surmises that Dr. Red's ego was injured when the sergeant didn't bring his concerns directly to her as the psychiatrist. Mr. Hanky is also worried about Taylor and has had more success discussing cases individually with Dr. Red in her office. Rather than publicly supporting Dr. Moore, he suggests they move on to the next patient and thinks to himself, "I'll talk to Dr. Red in private about this whole thing, and hopefully she will put Taylor back on his medication. These treatment team meetings sure are a waste of time!"

Conversely, psychiatrists must be aware of the pressures inherent in the correctional environment to "go along to get along." Pinta (2009, p. 150) warns:

> The adversarial nature of the prison environment and security needs can affect mental health care in a variety of ways. Balancing security and treatment needs can create role ambiguities and ethics-related concerns for psychiatrists and other correctional mental health professionals.

Engaging in idiomatic vernacular to describe behavior that is disparaging or demeaning to build an alliance with the security staff, for example, is professionally improper, unnecessary, and counterproductive. When this happens, a tendency to classify an individual's maladaptive behavior as "mad" or "bad" can emerge and subvert the diagnostic and treatment process, as Aufderheide (2004, p. 5) points out in the assessment of self-injurious behavior in correctional settings:

> Consequently, frustrated clinicians frequently resort to classifying self-injurious behavior into a taxonomy of intent, labeling behavior as "instrumental" or "manipulative" versus "truly suicidal" or "due to mental health reasons." This dichotomous taxonomy derives from the spurious assumption that self-harm threats and behavior associated with mental illness are "mad" behaviors, while risk with instrumental intent is manipulative and should be classified as "bad" behavior. Some correctional mental health experts have identified this tendency to classify disturbed behavior as "mad or bad" as a distinguishing characteristic of the correctional environment.

Discussions with colleagues, other mental health professionals, supervisors, and security staff can help in developing a perspective to sharpen awareness of the effects of the correctional culture on communication. Talking with others, either on a formal or informal basis, can also help to guard against the "go along to get along" proclivity. As increased awareness deepens insight, the psychiatrist's communication style and strategy can be capably contextualized within the framework of the correctional culture.

Communication to improve treatment efficacy

The single biggest problem in communication is the illusion that it has taken place.

—George Bernard Shaw

In much the same way that collaboration between health care professionals leads to improvement in decision-making, communication increases staff awareness of the importance of each other's type of knowledge and skills, which leads to improved treatment outcomes (O'Daniel & Rosenstein, 2008). With effective communication skills, correctional psychiatrists can use their expertise for input into the decision-making process and for the development of strategies to address the complexities associated with patient care and management. But psychiatrists must be acutely sensitive that when the content of their communication is not understood, it "falls on deaf ears" and results in a loss of credibility, as illustrated in the case example 2.

CASE EXAMPLE 2: PSYCHIATRIC PSYCHOBABBLE

After engaging in an act of self-injurious behavior, Smith was placed in a suicide-resistant cell. He continued being disruptive and threatening further self-harm unless his demands were met. De-escalation attempts by nursing staff were unsuccessful, and Smith was refusing to talk. After an emergency staff referral to mental health, the psychiatrist arrived at the cell and attempted to calm him down and conduct a risk assessment. As the crisis intervention continued, the warden, who had been notified of the escalating disruption, arrived on the mental health unit and asked the psychiatrist his assessment of the situation. "Well," the psychiatrist replied, "it appears this patient has symptomatology suggestive of a disruptive mood dysregulation disorder and instrumental self-harm tendencies associated with narcissism and selective mutism." "Thanks, Doc," replied the warden. "Now, tell me about the individual and what we're going to do."

This is an evident exaggeration of poor communication, but the example underscores that communication is only as effective as it is intelligible to the recipient. When communication is not understandable, psychiatric treatment may be unsupported or opposed by other staff. Aufderheide and Baxter (2010, p. 173) warn that "a failure to communicate regarding inmates in treatment, whether due to choice or benign neglect, results in less effective treatment." The solution is that, for psychiatrists working in a jail or prison, standardized communication tools should be used that are intelligible and effective, especially in crisis intervention situations. The SBAR (situation-background-assessment-recommendation) technique, for example, provides a framework for effective communication between health care staff, especially in circumstances that require immediate action (Institute for Healthcare Improvement, 2002). In similar environments, where highly trained professionals must use expert judgment in rapidly changing circumstances, the adoption of such standardized communication tools is an effective strategy to enhance collaboration and reduce risks (O'Daniel & Rosenstein, 2008).

Communication to improve interdisciplinary collaboration

If there is any great secret of success in life, it lies in the ability to put yourself in the other person's place and to see things from his point of view as well as your own.

—Henry Ford

There is a plausible explanation for the popularity of television reality programs about life in jails and prisons: Viewers seem mesmerized by the nonstop, frenzied activity and the constantly on-the-move correctional staff that are managing dangerous individuals. In these frenetic environments, where security precautions are implemented promptly, intake and interviews completed rapidly, and mental health interventions coordinated quickly, it is readily apparent that effective communication is the *sine qua non* of adroit interdisciplinary collaboration. If decisions about care are to be consequential for individuals with serious mental health needs, correctional psychiatrists must recognize that they are part of a team, understand their role on the team, and realize that problem solving and decision-making are most effective when communication underscores shared responsibility. Consider the following example of productive interdisciplinary communication in an interdisciplinary consultation with security staff in managing problematic individuals.

CASE EXAMPLE 3: WORKING TOGETHER WORKS

Dr. Marks is the primary psychiatrist at a prison inpatient unit. During the treatment team meetings, he often goes to great lengths to obtain input from everyone, including the security staff. He is aware that mental health staff and security staff often do not see eye to eye on how to handle incarcerated individuals because of their different experiences, training, and goals. He looks for moments where he can learn from security staff, as well as increase their knowledge and understanding of mental illness. One day, he is called during his lunch hour about a crisis occurring on the mental health unit. Although he is in the middle of his lunch, he knows how important it is to respond quickly and demonstrate that he is a member of the team. When he arrives a few minutes later, Nurse Charge and Lieutenant Bill explain that Jay has become agitated after receiving his lunch tray. He was insisting that his food had been tampered with, and even after Sergeant Sack told him he would try to obtain a different tray, he continued banging on the door and demanding to see the captain, whom he insisted he knew from a previous prison. He is now rapidly pacing in his cell, intermittently yelling and banging on the door. He has started to threaten to hurt staff. Dr. Marks has not previously treated Jay, who arrived over the weekend and has refused to see the treatment team this morning. However, he did note a history of impulsive aggression, particularly when Jay stops taking his medication. Lieutenant Bill asks Dr. Marks if he plans to write an order for emergency administration of medication, which will likely require a use of force. There are several staff at Jay's door, whose presence appears to be increasing his agitation, and other individuals are starting to react to the commotion as well. Aware of the prison hierarchy, Dr. Marks requests Lieutenant Bill's assistance, suggesting that he ask Sergeant Sack to select one officer to stay by Jay's door to monitor his behavior, while the remaining staff begin rounds in an effort to calm the other individuals. He also suggests a quick meeting to share information and formulate a plan. Dr. Marks listens intently and asks follow-up questions as Sergeant Sack describes Jay's loud, rapid speech and irrational demands, and how he even bent over backward by offering to obtain a different tray. Sergeant Sack also reports that Jay has a long history of disciplinary reports, including assaults on staff. Sergeant Sack added, "We really need to show Jay who runs this unit." Dr. Marks recognizes Sergeant Sack for his input and perspective, and he concurs that Jay is certainly a dangerous patient who needs to follow the rules on the unit. He explains that Jay appears to be experiencing an increase in racing, disorganized, and paranoid thoughts, likely due to his medication nonadherence. He also acknowledges the value of what he has learned from Lieutenant Bill: that in a highly agitated state, people will sometimes respond to simple commands from someone of a higher rank and/or a staff member that they know and trust. Lieutenant Bill quickly comments that, while he typically does not want to reinforce an individual's demands to speak with a particular staff member, all options at least need to be considered. A phone call to the captain reveals that he does indeed know the individual from a nearby prison where he previously worked. By the time he arrives, staff have done an excellent job of de-escalating the other individuals and getting them to remain on their bunks. The captain suggests Dr. Marks accompany him to the cell, and together they are able to convince Jay to cuff up so he can receive the injection of medication ordered by Dr. Marks. In a quick debriefing meeting, Dr. Marks thanks everyone, particularly Sergeant Sack and Lieutenant Bill, commenting, "Once again, talking together and working together has kept everyone safe."

This case example underscores the importance of reciprocal communication that breaks down barriers and builds a bridge of mutual respect and cooperation. Aufderheide and Baxter (2010) emphasize the importance of reciprocal communication in building collaborative working relationships.

Reciprocal communication is essential to the development of interdisciplinary collaboration. It is important that stereotypical labels that undermine the working relationship be addressed. For example, security officers may perceive the mental health staff as advocates or do-gooders. Mental health staff may see the officers as insensitive and unresponsive to the mental health needs of the incarcerated individuals and lacking professionalism. Whatever the source of friction, it is imperative that the two talk. Mental health staff need to educate the officers about what they do and the reasons they do it. Mental health staff should actively solicit opinions and insights from officers about the problems they deal with on a daily basis.

By communicating and modeling collaboration, individuals create opportunities for improvement in an organization (Lasker & Weiss, 2003). Accordingly, psychiatrists in correctional settings can improve treatment and patient management decisions by communicating and modeling collaboration with security staff and other members of the treatment team.

Summary

Communication—the human connection—is the key to personal and career success.

—Paul J. Meyer

Communication in psychiatry is important (Ditton-Phare et al., 2022; Novais et al., 2022). It involves basic skills, and there is no doubt that effective communication is at the heart of success for psychiatrists (Ditton-Phare et al., 2022). In fact, communication skills are important indicators of patients' quality of care, mental health measures (Ditton-Phare et al., 2017; Rotter & Hall, 1992), and even the psychiatrist's well-being (Cegala & Lenzmeier Broz, 2002). When working in a jail or prison setting, psychiatrists must be cognizant of the opportunities and barriers to effective communication existing at multiple levels. It is crucial, therefore, for psychiatrists to develop communication strategies that create sustainable working relationships both with their patients and with other interdisciplinary personnel, from front-line staff to the facility's leadership. As Aufderheide and Baxter (2010) exhort: "Communication from correctional mental health clinicians involved in treatment programs must be consistent and presented across a variety of facility settings" (p. 172).

Whether with the facility's leadership, security staff, or other members of the treatment team, the goal is to communicate in ways that engender understanding and involvement in support of treatment goals. Through an understanding of how the correctional culture impacts communication and by recognizing the importance of communication in interdisciplinary collaboration, correctional psychiatrists can model effective communication skills that preserve professional credibility and improve treatment outcomes.

REFERENCES

Applebaum, K. L., Hickey, J. M., & Packer, I. (2001). The role of correctional officers in multidisciplinary mental health care in prisons. *Psychiatric Services, 52*, 1343–1347.

Aufderheide, D. (2004). Assessing risk of suicide and self-injury in correctional settings. *National Psychologist, 13*, 5–6.

Aufderheide, D. (2021). Mental illness in America's prisons: An inconvenient truth ... The need for a public safety/public health model. *Advancing Corrections Journal, 12*, 75–90.

Aufderheide, D., & Baxter, J. D. (2010). Interdisciplinary collaboration in correctional practice. In T. Fagan & R. Ax (Eds.), *Correctional mental health: From theory to best practice* (pp. 169–186). Sage Publications.

Cegala, D. J., & Lenzmeier Broz, S. (2002). Physician communication skills training: A review of theoretical backgrounds, objectives and skills. *Medical Education, 36*(11), 1004–1016.

Ditton-Phare, P., Loughland, C., Duvivier, R., & Kelly, B. (2017). Communication skills in the training of psychiatrists: A systematic review of current approaches. *Australian and New Zealand Journal of Psychiatry, 51*(7), 675–692.

Ditton-Phare, P., Sandhu, H., Kelly, B., & Loughland, C. (2022). ComPsych communication skills training: Applicability of simulated patients in psychiatry communication skills training. *Australasian Psychiatry: Bulletin of Royal Australian and New Zealand College of Psychiatrists, 30*(4), 552–555.

Gaines, A. (1992). *Ethnopsychiatry: The cultural construction of professional and folk psychiatries.* State University of New York Press.

Grossman, D. (2011). *The cost of poor communication.* http://www.holmesreport.com/opinion-info/10645/The-Cost-Of-Poor Communications.aspx

Hagberg, J., & Heifetz, R. (2000). *Corporate culture/organizational culture: Understanding and assessment.* http://www.hegnet.com

Hampden-Turner, C., & Trompenaars, F. (2004). *Riding the waves of culture* (3rd ed.). Nicholas Brealey International.

Institute for Healthcare Improvement. (2002). *Guidelines for communicating with physicians using the SBAR process.* https://www.ihi.org/resources/tools/sbar-tool-situation-background-assessment-recommendation

Kirmayer, J. L., Gutder, J., Blake, C., & Jarius, E. (2003). Cultural consultation: A model of mental health services for multicultural societies. *Canadian Journal of Psychiatry, 4*, 145–153.

Lasker, R. D., & Weiss, E. S. (2003). Broadening participation in community problem solving: A multidisciplinary model to support collaborative practice and research. *Journal of Urban Health: Bulletin of the New York Academy of Medicine, 80*, 14–60.

Losee, R. (1999). Communication as complementary informative processes. *Journal of Information, Communication, and Library Sciences, 5*, 1–15.

Novais, F., Ganança, L., Barbosa, M., & Telles-Correia, D. (2022). Communication skills in psychiatry for undergraduate students: A scoping review. *Frontiers in Psychiatry, 13*, 972703.

O'Daniel, M., & Rosenstein, A. H. (2008). Professional communication and team collaboration. In R. Hughes (Ed.), *Patient safety and quality: An evidence-based handbook for nurses* (pp. 801–814). Agency for Healthcare Research and Quality.

Pinta, E. R. (2009). Decisions to breach confidentiality: When prisoners report violations of institutional rules. *Journal of the American Academy of Psychiatry and the Law, 37*, 150–154.

Rotter, D. L., & Hall, J. A. (1992). *Doctors talking with patients/Patients talking with doctors: Improving communication in medical visits.* Auburn House/Greenwood Publishing Group.

Schyve, P. (2009). Communication: The bond to patient safety. In *The Joint Commission guide to improving staff communication* (2nd ed.). Joint Commission Resources.

Triandis, H. C. (1989). The self and behavior in different cultural contexts. *Psychological Bulletin, 128*, 3–72.

Vinokur-Kaplan, D. (1995). Enhancing the effectiveness of interdisciplinary mental health treatment teams. *Administration and Policy in Mental Health, 22*, 521–530. https://doi.org/10.1007/BF02106536

15

Mental health screening and brief assessments

Daisy Ort, Michael P. Maloney, Joel Dvoskin, and Jeffrey L. Metzner

Introduction

An estimated 5 million individuals were under adult correctional supervision (i.e., jails, prisons, probation, and parole) in the United States at the end of 2021 (Carson & Kluckow, 2023). The number of incarcerated persons (IPs) with psychiatric symptoms is difficult to determine due to a variety of methodological challenges (Rukus & Kulkarni, 2019), including varying definitions of mental illness, severity thresholds, and diverse correctional settings. However, virtually every relevant study indicates that mental illness among IPs is widespread and increasing (Bronson & Berzofsky, 2017; Gottfried & Christopher, 2017; Maruschak et al., 2021; Mulvey & Schubert, 2017; Prins, 2014; Vogel et al., 2014).

Individuals with psychiatric symptoms are at a heightened risk for suicide (American Foundation for Suicide Prevention, 2024; Bolton et al., 2015; Moitra et al., 2021). This risk is substantially elevated in correctional settings (Dixon et al., 2020; see Chapter 51). There is great need to implement effective and timely mental health screenings and assessments in correctional settings to identify IPs who require mental health care and refer those identified to mental health and suicide prevention interventions (Hayes, 2017).

Implementing effective mental health screenings and evaluations in correctional settings is not only a matter of best practice but also a legal mandate established by the landmark ruling in *Ruiz v. Estelle* (1980), which described the identification of IPs in need of mental health care or suicide prevention as a component of a minimally adequate mental health treatment program. There is a strong consensus among health care professionals that universal screening and follow-up evaluation of positive screens are essential to facilitating treatment referrals and enhancing suicide prevention efforts (Fazel et al., 2016; Johnson et al., 2024; Konrad et al., 2007). The screening and evaluation process helps to identify individuals in need of immediate mental health interventions, ensure timely access to appropriate treatment, and prevent symptom exacerbation. It can also improve overall mental health outcomes and lead to lower rates of recidivism (Simpson, 2022).

Research also consistently indicates that implementing screenings and evaluations as part of suicide prevention efforts significantly contributes to reduced suicide rates (Stijelja & Mishara, 2022). The effectiveness of using screenings and evaluations as part of suicide prevention programming is reflected in the substantial decrease of jail suicide rates, which dropped from 107 per 100,000 in the mid-1980s to 38 per 100,000 by 2006, coinciding with the broader adoption of screening and assessment practices (Hayes, 2010). Hayes (2017) describes the foundational components of effective screening and assessment for suicidal ideation or behavior in correctional settings (p. 1):

> Intake screening and ongoing assessment of all inmates is critical to a correctional facility's suicide prevention efforts. It should not be viewed as a single event but as an ongoing process because inmates can become suicidal at any point during their confinement, including the initial admission into the facility; after adjudication when the inmate is returned to the facility from court; following receipt of bad news or after suffering any type of humiliation or rejection; confinement in isolation or segregation; and following a prolonged stay in the facility.

Intake screening

The initial admission screening serves as the first line of defense for identifying mental health needs among IPs. To guide this critical process, the National Commission on Correctional Health Care (NCCHC) has established specific mental health care standards to ensure effective and quality care. While these standards differ across various types of correctional settings (e.g., jails, prisons, juvenile detention centers, and corrections-based opioid treatment programs), consistent across all correctional settings is the need for immediate mental health screenings of all IPs upon admission (NCCHC, 2015, 2018a, 2018b).

Initial mental health screenings typically take place during the booking and admission process and are conducted by correctional or nursing staff trained in the administration of the screening instrument. One purpose is to identify IPs who require immediate and more comprehensive evaluation by a Qualified Mental Health Professional (QMHP), typically defined as a person who is licensed in a mental health profession such as psychiatry, psychology, clinical social work, psychiatric nursing, or counseling, who can assess for overt psychotic symptoms or potential danger to self or others. The screener should also obtain relevant information from the arresting officer with a focus on behavioral observations during arrest and transportation, and nursing staff should be provided with any available information about the IP's current medications. Ford and colleagues (2007) outlined the shared characteristics that should typically be considered and incorporated into screening processes:

1. *Brevity*: Large urban jails may process tens of thousands of new admissions each year. Because every new admission to a jail or prison must be screened, it is important that the screening process be brief.
2. *Clarity*: Admissions often occur at any time of the day or night, with many different people conducting admission screening. For any process to have validity, it must first have reliability (i.e., different evaluators should come to similar conclusions about each case). This can only be accomplished when definitions, thresholds, and criteria are clear.
3. *Trained screeners*: To attain consistency and reliability and because screeners usually lack advanced mental health training, every screener should be explicitly trained in the screening process and supervised to ensure competence and fidelity.
4. *Low false-negative rate*: False-negative findings could potentially result in an unnecessary and severe exacerbation of a mental illness or even in a preventable suicide. In other words, mental health and suicide screeners must always be trained to "err on the side of caution." It is especially important to identify those IPs who are at serious or imminent risk of suicide so that they may be kept safe pending a more comprehensive mental health and suicide risk assessment.
5. *Reasonable false-positive rate*: The consequences of a false-positive screen are relatively low, though an extremely high number of false-positive screens can result in many unnecessary assessments, thus wasting valuable clinical time that could otherwise be spent providing treatment.
6. *Documentation*: Every screen must be documented to enable administrators to track the process, ensure that every new admission is screened, and keep track of the percentage of positive versus negative screens. Adequate documentation of positive screens provides essential information to the QMHPs who will perform subsequent assessments.

In the authors' experience, with a well-designed and managed screening process, the initial screening and intake mental health evaluation should generally yield a combined positive referral rate of about 30%, necessitating a referral for a brief mental health assessment and potentially a comprehensive mental health evaluation conducted by a QMHP. When clinically appropriate (e.g., history or evidence of psychotic symptoms), an IP may be directly referred for a comprehensive mental health evaluation following the initial screening without undergoing a brief mental health assessment. In such cases, the brief mental health screening is unnecessary, as the result is assumed to be positive.

Several models have been implemented in jails and prisons for providing intake mental health screening. Options include screening by specially trained correctional officers, nurses, or QMHPs. Screening can also be administered by nurses as part of a health care (i.e., general medical) assessment (NCCHC, 2018a, 2018b). IPs who undergo a mental health evaluation due to screening positive on the initial admission screening do not require an intake mental health screening within 14 days, as they would have already been referred.

A positive screen on the initial admission screening or the intake mental health screening must result in a brief mental health assessment conducted by a QMHP, which in turn may lead to a referral for a comprehensive mental health evaluation. The brief mental health assessment typically includes a brief mental status exam and inquiry into the documented reasons for a positive screen. The assessment, on average, should take approximately 20 to 30 minutes to complete and document. Its purpose is to determine if there is an imminent risk of suicide or an urgent need for mental health treatment and to evaluate the likelihood of the IP requiring nonurgent mental health treatment during incarceration.

Comprehensive mental health evaluations must be performed by a QMHP. These evaluations typically result in mental health care for the IP and the development of a treatment plan, which becomes part of the IP's health care record. IPs who screen positive should receive a comprehensive suicide risk assessment before returning to the general population (see Chapter 51).

The mental health screenings and assessments described above should be conducted in a space (preferably an office) with adequate sound privacy, except when safety concerns (e.g., severe agitation) necessitate that the IP be accompanied by a correctional officer. Considering the spaces available and appropriate in each facility is essential, as IPs are unlikely to speak freely without some sense of privacy and confidentiality (NCCHC, 2019).

American Psychiatric Association guidelines

To supplement the standards set forth by the NCCHC, the American Psychiatric Association (2016) formulated additional guidelines for psychiatric services in correctional facilities. There are four distinct types of mental health screening and evaluation processes: reception mental health screening and referral, intake mental health screening and referral, brief mental health assessment, and comprehensive mental health evaluation.

1. *Reception mental health screening and referral* is initiated within 4 hours of the IP's arrival and consists of observation and structured inquiry into mental health history and present symptoms. Structured inquiry includes questions regarding suicide history, ideation, and potential; prior psychiatric hospitalizations and treatment; and current and past medications—both those prescribed and what is actually being taken (i.e., adherence).
2. *Intake mental health screening and referral* is a more comprehensive examination performed by a QMHP on each newly admitted IP within 14 days of arrival at an institution. It includes a review of the initial admission screening, behavioral observation, mental health history, assessment of suicide potential, and mental status examination. The intake mental health screening can reveal chronic medical and mental health problems that were not reported on entry into the facility and lead to referrals to chronic care clinics or mental health clinics.
3. *Brief mental health assessment* occurs within 72 hours of a nonurgent positive screening and includes a mental health

examination that is appropriate to the level of apparent need, with a written recommendation for a comprehensive mental health evaluation and treatment if indicated. In addition to a suicide risk assessment when appropriate, these assessments include a mental status examination, diagnostic formulation recommendations, and, if indicated, a treatment plan or a written recommendation for a comprehensive mental health evaluation.

4. *Comprehensive mental health evaluation* consists of a face-to-face interview with the IP and review of all reasonably available health records and collateral information. It concludes with a diagnostic formulation and, at a minimum, an initial treatment plan. A comprehensive mental health evaluation occurs when the brief mental health assessment is not adequate for diagnostic purposes or treatment planning purposes.

Facility-specific considerations

When tailoring mental health screening and assessment processes to meet the unique needs of each correctional facility, it is crucial to account for several factors, including the number of new bookings, the architectural layout of the jail or prison (e.g., adequacy of workspace), staffing and training, access to informational databases, history of previous arrests, and the prevalence and severity of mental illness. It is also important to consider overall differences between jails and prisons. As highlighted by Dvoskin and Brown (2015), jails often see a high turnover of IPs, leading to an increased acuity in mental illness, substance use disorders, and suicide risk and a heavier workload for initial assessments (see Chapter 7). In contrast, IPs in prisons typically face lengthy sentences, requiring a focus that extends beyond crisis response to more long-term treatment for serious and persistent mental illness. These differences reinforce the importance of a flexible and customized approach to accommodate the distinct demands of each facility type.

An example of differing approaches based on facility-specific considerations is that large correctional facilities with extensive mental health resources might opt for a screening process that prioritizes efficiency, accepting a higher rate of false-negative screens due to the availability of resources to address mental health disorders at a later stage. In contrast, facilities with limited mental health resources will need a more thorough screening process, selecting instruments with lower false-negative rates because the consequences for delayed recognition of serious mental illness are potentially greater. This approach prioritizes accuracy to ensure individuals with mental health needs receive proper attention despite resource and staffing constraints.

Another example of facility-based considerations involves the role of staff in health care screenings. Some correctional facilities have nursing staff perform health care screenings that also include mental health screening, while others separate medical and mental health screenings, allowing only mental health staff to conduct the screenings. Another variation is when nursing staff perform both medical and mental health screenings but use distinct instruments rather than a single instrument combining both. These variations reflect differences in resources, staffing, and training, influencing the design and implementation of the screening process and the specific instruments selected.

Mental health screenings and evaluations should be culturally sensitive. For instance, in Black and Latinx communities, heightened stigma and mistrust of providers may lead to underreporting during the screening and evaluation process (Eno Louden et al., 2023). To accurately address the mental health needs of individuals from diverse racial and ethnic groups, screenings and evaluations should have cross-cultural validity and be conducted by culturally competent professionals (Ricks & Eno Louden, 2015; see Chapter 22). Additionally, clinical observations and data, such as disengagement or avoidance of personal topics, should be conceptualized through a culturally and trauma-informed lens (Barber-Rioja, 2023). The culture and identities of examiners, which influence their language, choice of questions, and patience during evaluations, should also be considered to enhance multicultural competence (Heilbrun et al., 2021).

Structured screening and assessment instruments

In correctional settings, mental health personnel face a variety of challenges, including limited staffing, time and cost constraints, and perceived relevance to correctional goals, which often restrict the use of structured instruments during initial admissions and brief mental health assessments. Consequently, these tools are typically utilized during comprehensive assessments following a positive screen or when concerning behavioral observations, such as depression, argumentativeness, or self-harm, are noted.

A variety of mental health and suicide screening instruments have been developed to identify individuals with psychiatric symptoms and those who are at risk of suicide. Comprehensive studies on mental health screeners, such as those by Martin et al. (2013) and Gebbie et al. (2008), have thoroughly reviewed such instruments in correctional settings. Notably, the studies neither advocate for nor recommend a particular instrument. Similarly, the breadth of suicide risk assessment literature is extensive, including studies conducted by the Department of Veterans Affairs Evidence-Based Synthesis Program (Haney et al., 2012), which reviewed a wide array of self-harm and suicide risk assessment tools, citing over 100 references, as well as Brown's (2000) study, which evaluated 30 suicide risk assessment tools. Both large-scale studies concluded that existing data are insufficient to recommend a specific risk assessment tool. Findings from these comprehensive reviews of mental health screening instruments and suicide risk assessment tools reflect the consensus within the mental health field that a wide range of screening and assessment instruments can be similarly effective in detecting mental health disorders and evaluating suicide risk. There is strong agreement that clinically appropriate structured mental health and suicide risk assessment tools that are properly administered are critical components of correctional mental health and suicide prevention programs (Lurigio & Swartz, 2006).

When selecting appropriate instruments, particular attention should be given to high-risk groups, such as individuals with a history of suicide attempts (Moscicki, 2001). Mental health and suicide risk instruments are designed to be brief yet thorough, balancing the need for swift administration with the importance of accuracy and completeness. The screening process must be clear, consistent, and conducted by trained personnel to ensure reliability and minimize the chances of false negatives, which can have severe consequences, including the exacerbation of mental health symptoms or even death by suicide. Equally important is maintaining a reasonable false-positive rate to avoid unnecessary assessments and optimize clinical resources (Ford et al., 2007).

Most correctional mental health and suicide screening instruments are based on self-report; IPs are asked for information with little or no independent verification. Maloney et al. (2001) conducted a program analysis of some 16,000 new booking screens in the Los Angeles County jail system. To the question "Have you ever tried to hurt or kill yourself?," 3.5% responded "yes." An additional question querying whether the IP was "currently thinking about killing" themselves resulted in 0.65% responding "yes." However, during the same period, a sample of 1,000 newly booked IPs who participated in a personal interview during booking indicated that 14.5% of the men and 17.9% of the women reported previous suicide attempts, and about 5% of the men and 7.5% of the women acknowledged that they were currently suicidal. These findings suggest that the screening instrument failed to detect a considerable number of IPs with both a history of suicidal behavior and current suicidal ideation. Therefore, it is critical to evaluate continually the strengths and shortcomings of screening tools and to understand that they cannot substitute for a clinical assessment.

It is important to augment jail screens by using additional observational data (e.g., bizarre behavior) and collateral sources of information (e.g., reports from arresting officers, available electronic databases, past mental health records). In selecting or developing a correctional mental health screening tool, these should be designed to obtain data relevant to mental health diagnosis or history and to obtain information on the risk that an IP will experience serious mental health problems during their incarceration. There is a need for ongoing quality improvement studies to ensure that changes in population characteristics or other variables are appropriately considered in screening methods.

Example mental health instruments

The Brief Jail Mental Health Screen (BJMHS; *Figure 15.1*) requires approximately 3 minutes for administration and consists of eight items designed to assess for presenting symptoms, psychiatric hospitalization, and medication, with a yes/no response format. It does not contain any items that specifically query about suicide ideation, intent, or risk. The BJMHS has been used in jails across the United States and is recommended by the Substance Abuse and Mental Health Services Administration (2019) as an initial mental health screen for IPs.

Brief Jail Mental Health Screen

Section 1

Name: ____________	**Detainee #:** ____________	**Date:** __/__/____	**Time:** ________ AM
First MI Last			PM

Section 2

	Questions	No	Yes	General Comments
1.	Do you *currently* believe that someone can control your mind by putting thoughts into your head or taking thoughts out of your head?			
2.	Do you *currently* feel that other people know your thoughts and can read your mind?			
3.	Have you *currently* lost or gained as much as two pounds a week for several weeks without even trying?			
4.	Have you or your family or friends noticed that you are *currently* much more active than you usually are?			
5.	Do you *currently* feel like you have to talk or move more slowly than you usually do?			
6.	Have there *currently* been a few weeks when you felt like you were useless or sinful?			
7.	Are you *currently* taking any medication prescribed for you by a physician for any emotional or mental health problems?			
8.	Have you *ever* been in a hospital for emotional or mental health problems?			

Section 3 (Optional)

Officer's Comments/Impressions (check *all* that apply):		
☐ Language barrier	☐ Under the influence of drugs/alcohol	☐ Non-cooperative
☐ Difficulty understanding questions	☐ Other, specify: ____________	

Referral Instructions: This detainee should be referred for further mental health evaluation if he/she answered:

- **YES to item 7; OR**
- **YES to item 8; OR**
- **YES to at least 2 of items 1 through 6; OR**
- **If you feel it is necessary for any other reason**

☐ Not Referred

☐ Referred on __/__/____ to ____________

Person completing screen ____________

INSTRUCTIONS ON REVERSE

Figure 15.1 Brief Jail Mental Health Screen.

Correctional Mental Health Screen for Men (CMHS-M)

Name	Detainee #	Date _ _/_ _/_ _ _ _	Time ___:___
Last, First, MI		mm/dd/year	

QUESTIONS	NO	YES	COMMENTS
1. Have you ever had worries that you just can't get rid of?			
2. Some people find their mood changes frequently - as if they spend everyday on an emotional roller coaster. Does this sound like you?			
3. Do you get annoyed when friends or family complain about their problems? Or do people complain that you're not sympathetic to their problems?			
4. Have you ever felt like you didn't have any feelings, or felt distant or cut off from other people or from your surroundings?			
5. Has there ever been a time when you felt so irritable that you found yourself shouting at people or starting fights or arguments?			
6. Do you often get in trouble at work or with friends because you act excited at first but then lose interest in projects and don't follow through?			
7. Do you tend to hold grudges or give people the silent treatment for days at a time?			
8. Have you ever tried to avoid reminders, or to not think about, something terrible that you experienced or witnessed?			
9. Has there ever been a time when you felt depressed most of the day for at least 2 weeks?			
10. Have you ever been troubled by repeated thoughts, feelings, or nightmares about something you experienced or witnessed?			
11. Have you ever been in a hospital for non-medical reasons such as in a psychiatric hospital? (Do NOT include going to an Emergency Room if you were not hospitalized.)			
12. Have you ever felt constantly on guard or watchful even when you didn't need to, or felt jumpy and easily startled?			

TOTAL # YES: __________	**General Comments:**
Refer for further Mental Health Evaluation if the Detainee answered	
Yes to **6** or more items ***OR*** If you are concerned for any other reason	
○ **URGENT Referral** on _ _/_ _/_ _ _ _ to	
○ **ROUTINE Referral** on _ _/_ _/_ _ _ _ to	
○ **Not Referred**	
Person Completing Screen: ____________________	

Figure 15.2 Correctional Mental Health Screen for Men.

Recent studies have provided evidence supporting the efficacy and clinical usefulness of the BJMHS. One such study indicated that most IPs who screened positive on the BJMHS were in need of clinical care and that positive predictive values were up to 15% higher than previously reported (Gerritsen et al., 2022). Another study found that approximately 30% of the 695 jails surveyed utilized the BJMHS and considered it to be a valuable screening tool (Callahan & Noether, 2018).

The Correctional Mental Health Screen (CMHS) utilizes distinct questionnaires for men (CMHS-M; *Figure 15.2*) and women (CMHS-F; *Figure 15.3*) and is composed of 12 and eight staff-administered items, respectively. Like the BJMHS, the CMHS takes only a few minutes to administer and utilizes a yes/no response format. Both CMHS brief mental health screening instruments were found to be reliable, valid, feasible, and accurate measures that demonstrate good predictive validity for identifying IPs with psychiatric disorders (Ford et al., 2007, 2009).

A comparison of the data from both the BJMHS and the CMHS (male and female) suggest that the CMHS scales have slightly higher sensitivity (i.e., the proportion of true positives correctly identified) and specificity (i.e., the proportion of true negatives correctly identified; Martin et al., 2013). Positive scores on either scale should be considered as an entry point for further triage and evaluation. If an IP answers affirmatively to any screening question, they are generally interviewed and assessed for further clinical intervention and treatment. The CMHS has also been recommended as a screening instrument by the Substance Abuse and Mental Health Services Administration (2019).

Example suicide risk instruments

The Suicide Prevention Screening Guidelines Form (*Figure 15.4*), developed jointly by state and county agencies in New York (Sherman & Morschauser, 1989), is one of the first widely used

Correctional Mental Health Screen for Women (CMHS-W)

Name	**Detainee #**	**Date _ _/_ _/_ _ _ _**	**Time ___:___**
Last, First, MI		mm/dd/year	

Questions	**No**	**Yes**	**Comments**
1. Do you get annoyed when friends and family complain about their problems? Or do people complain you are not sympathetic to their problems?			
2. Have you ever tried to avoid reminders of, or to not think about, something terrible that you experienced or witnessed?			
3. Some people find their mood changes frequently-as if they spend everyday on an emotional rollercoaster. For example, switching from feeling angry to depressed to anxious many times a day. Does this sound like you?			
4. Have there ever been a few weeks when you felt you were useless, sinful, or guilty?			
5. Has there ever been a time when you felt depressed most of the day for at least 2 weeks?			
6. Do you find that most people will take advantage of you if you let them know too much about you?			
7. Have you been troubled by repeated thoughts, feelings, or nightmares about something terrible that you experienced or witnessed?			
8. Have you ever been in the hospital for non-medical reasons, such as a psychiatric hospital? (Do NOT include going to an Emergency Room if you were not hospitalized.)			

TOTAL # YES: ____________	**General Comments:**
Refer for further Mental Health Evaluation if the Detainee answered	
Yes to **5** or more items ***OR*** If you are concerned for any other reason	
○ **URGENT Referral** on _ _/_ _/_ _ _ _ to	
○ **ROUTINE Referral** on _ _/_ _/_ _ _ _ to	
○ **Not Referred**	
Person Completing Screen: ____________________	

Figure 15.3 Correctional Mental Health Screen for Women.

suicide prevention screeners in correctional facilities and has been implemented across jurisdictions throughout the United States. It is intended to be used within the first 72 hours of incarceration, and it is generally scored by the booking deputy (Daigle et al., 2006). The form consists of 17 questions: 11 examine suicide risk factors, five are specific to current behaviors that might be indicative of mental illness, and one examines criminal history. Responding "yes" to eight or more items results in a referral to the shift commander and eventually to a medical or mental health professional. In addition, responses to certain questions, such as endorsing suicidal thoughts or a past suicide attempt along with current feelings of hopelessness, will prompt an immediate referral.

The Columbia-Suicide Severity Rating Scale (CSSRS; *Figure 15.5*) is an interview-based assessment tool consisting of six items. The CSSRS is specifically designed to assess the frequency and intensity of suicidal thoughts and behaviors, differentiating between active and passive forms. It was developed by Posner et al. (2011), is utilized across a variety of settings, and has strong psychometric properties, including predictive validity, feasibility, and reliability. Findings from one study conducted in two prisons and six probation sites in New Zealand indicated that the CSSRS effectively increased the ability of receiving staff to assess both passive and active suicidal ideation and more accurately identify suicide risk among individuals under correctional supervision (Wilson, 2017).

Summary

The screening and assessment process is an essential foundation for ongoing intervention and treatment in correctional settings, where the prevalence of mental illness and the risk of suicide are exceptionally high. Through effective screening, resources can be allocated efficiently, ensuring that timely and necessary attention is given to those in need of intervention. Conducting screenings for every IP upon intake is mandatory. However, there is no universally accepted method for these screenings. Factors such as the facility type, size, architectural design, location, and availability of critical resources (including staffing, training, and informational databases) all contribute to the diversity of practices. Screening and assessment methods should be tailored to meet the unique requirements and needs of each facility in a culturally sensitive manner. Given the myriad differences and considerations across correctional facilities, screening and evaluation methods should be regarded as dynamic processes that necessitate ongoing quality improvement, with updates when necessary to maintain effectiveness.

Form 33<ill/> ADM (CC) (<ill/>)
State of New York
COMMISSION OF CORRECTION
Officer of Mental Health
SUICIDE PREVENTION SCREENING GUIDELINES

DETAINEE'S NAME	SEX	DATE OF BIRTH	MOST SERIOUS CHARGE(S)	DATE	TIME
NAME OF FACILITY		NAME OF SCREENING OFFICER		Detainee showed serious psychiatric problems during prior incarceration Yes_____ No_____	
Check appropriate column for each question					

	Column A YES	Column B NO	General Comments/Observations
OBSERVATIONS OF TRANSPORTING OFFICER			
1. Arresting or transporting officer believes that detainee may be a suicide risk. *If* **YES**, *notify Shift Commander.*			
PERSONAL DATA			
2. Detainee lacks close family or friends in the community.			
3. Detainee has experienced a significant loss within the last six months (e.g. loss of job, loss of relationship, death of close family member).			
4. Detainee is very worried about major problems other than legal situation (e.g., serious financial or family problems, a medical condition or fear of losing job).			
5. Detainee's family or significant other (spouse, parent, close friend, lover) has attempted or committed suicide.			
6. Detainee has psychiatric history. (*Note current psychotropic medications and name of most recent treatment agency.*)			
7. Detainee has history of drug or alcohol abuse.			
8. Detainee holds position of respect in community (e.g., professional, public official) and/or alleged crime is shocking in nature.			
If **YES**, *notify Shift Commander.*			
9. Detainee is thinking about killing himself.			
If **YES**, *notify Shift Commander.*			
10. Detainee has previous suicide attempt. (*Check wrists and note method.*)			
11. Detainee feels that there is nothing to look forward to in the future. (expresses feelings of helplessness or hopelessness).			
If **YES**, *to 10 and 11, notify Shift Commander.*			
BEHAVIOR/APPEARANCE			
12. Detainee shows signs of depression (e.g., crying, emotional <ill/>).			
13. Detainee appears overly anxious, afraid or angry.			
14. Detainee appears to feel unnaturally embarrassed or ashamed.			
15. Detainee is acting and/or talking in a strange manner (e.g., cannot focus attention, hearing or seeing things which are not there).			
16. A. Detainee is apparently under the influence of alcohol or drugs.			
B. If **YES**, is detainee incoherent, or showing signs of withdrawal or mental illness? *If* **YES** *to both A & B, notify Shift Commander.*			
CRIMINAL HISTORY			
17. This is detainees first arrest.			

TOTAL Column A ______________ ACTION
If total checks in Column A are B or more, notify Shift Commander.
Shift Commander notified: Yes _______ No _______ Supervision Instituted: Routine _______ Active _______ Constant _______
Detainee Referred to Medical/Mental Health: EMERGENCY NON-EMERGENCY If Yes: medical ______________________ medical ______________________ mental health ______________________ mental health ______________________ Medical/Mental Health Personnel Actions: (To be completed by medical/MH staff)

Figure 15.4 Suicide Prevention Screening Guidelines Form.

COLUMBIA-SUICIDE SEVERITY RATING SCALE
Screen Version - Recent

SUICIDE IDEATION DEFINITIONS AND PROMPTS	Past month	
Ask questions that are bolded and underlined.	**YES**	**NO**
Ask Questions 1 and 2		
1) *Have you wished you were dead or wished you could go to sleep and not wake up?*		
2) *Have you actually had any thoughts of killing yourself?*		
If YES to 2, ask questions 3, 4, 5, and 6. If NO to 2, go directly to question 6.		
3) *Have you been thinking about how you might do this?*		
E.g. "*I thought about taking an overdose but I never made a specific plan as to when where or how I would actually do it...and I would never go through with it*"		
4) *Have you had these thoughts and had some Intention of acting on them?*		
As opposed to "*I have the thoughts but I definitely will not do anything about them.*"		
5) *Have you started to work out or worked out the details of how to kill yourself? Do you intend to carry out this plan?*		

6) *Have you ever done anything, started to do anything, or prepared to do anything to end your life?*	**YES**	**NO**
Examples: Collected pills, obtained a gun, gave away valuables, wrote a will or suicide note, took out pills but didn't swallow any, held a gun but changed your mind or it was grabbed from your hand, went to the roof but didn't jump; or actually took pills, tried to shoot yourself, cut yourself, tried to hang yourself, etc.		
If YES, ask: Was this within the past three months?		

☐ Low Risk
☐ Moderate Risk
☐ High Risk

For inquiries and training information contact: Kelly Posner, Ph.D.
New York State Psychiatric Institute, 1051 Riverside Drive, New York, New York, 10032: posnerk@nyspl.columbia.edu

Figure 15.5 Columbia-Suicide Severity Rating Scale.

REFERENCES

American Foundation for Suicide Prevention. (2024). *Risk factors, protective factors, and warning signs*. https://afsp.org/risk-factors-protective-factors-and-warning-signs/

American Psychiatric Association. (2016). *Psychiatric services in correctional facilities* (3rd ed.).

Barber-Rioja, V., Garcia-Mansilla, A., & Rodriguez, E. (2023). Identification of mental illness in jails: Screening and assessment. In V. Barber-Rioja, A. Garcia-Mansilla, B. Subedi, & A. Batastini (Eds.), *Handbook of mental health assessment and treatment in jails* (pp. 21–37). Oxford University Press.

Bolton, J. M., Gunnell, D., & Turecki, G. (2015). Suicide risk assessment and intervention in people with mental illness. *BMJ (Clinical research ed.), 351*, h4978.

Bronson, J., & Berzofsky, M. (2017). *Indicators of mental health problems reported by prisoners and jail inmates, 2011–12*. https://bjs.ojp.gov/content/pub/pdf/imhprpji1112.pdf

Brown, G. K. (2000). *A review of suicide assessment measures for intervention research with adults and older adults* (Technical report submitted to NIMH under Contract No. 263-MH914950). National Institute of Mental Health.

Callahan, L. A., & Noether, C. D. (2018). Brief jail mental health screen utilization in U.S. jails. *Journal of Forensic Medicine Forecast, 1*(1), 1006.

Carson, E. A., & Kluckow, R. (2023). *Correctional populations in the United States, 2021—Statistical tables*. Bureau of Justice Statistics.

Daigle, M. S., Labelle, R., & Côté, G. (2006). Further evidence of the validity of the Suicide Risk Assessment Scale for prisoners. *International Journal of Law and Psychiatry, 29*(5), 343–354.

Dixon, K. J., Ertl, A. M., Leavitt, R. A., Sheats, K. J., Fowler, K. A., & Jack, S. P. D. (2020). Suicides among incarcerated persons in 18 U.S. states: Findings from the National Violent Death Reporting System, 2003–2014. *Journal of Correctional Health Care, 26*(3), 279–291.

Dvoskin, J., & Brown, M. C. (2015). Jails and prisons. In R. Trestman, K. Appelbaum, & J. Metzner (Eds.), *Oxford textbook of correctional psychiatry* (pp. 31–34). Oxford University Press.

Eno Louden, J., Adair, R., Romero, I., & Barber Rioja, V. (2023). Mental health screens used in U.S. corrections settings: Evidence of fairness with Black and Latinx people. *Psychology, Crime & Law*. https://doi.org/10.1080/1068316X.2023.2206657

Fazel, S., Hayes, A. J., Bartellas, K., Clerici, M., & Trestman, R. (2016). Mental health of prisoners: Prevalence, adverse outcomes, and interventions. *Lancet Psychiatry, 3*(9), 871–881.

Ford, J., Trestman, R. L., Osher, F., Scott, J. E., Steadman, H. J., & Robbins, P. C. (2007). *Mental health screens for corrections*. National Institute of Justice.

Ford, J. D., Trestman, R. L., Wiesbrock, V. H., & Zhang, W. (2009). Validation of a brief screening instrument for identifying psychiatric disorders among newly incarcerated adults. *Psychiatric Services, 60*(6), 842.

Gebbie, K. M., Larkin, R. M., Klein, S. J., et al. (2008). Improving access to mental health services for New York state prison inmates. *Journal of Correctional Health Care, 14*, 122–135.

Gerritsen, C., Adamo, V., Fulham, L., et al. (2022). Evidence for the ecological validity of the Brief Jail Mental Health Screen: Positive predictive value among remanded men and women. *Criminal Behaviour and Mental Health, 32*(4), 295–301.

Gottfried, E. D., & Christopher, S. C. (2017). Mental disorders among criminal offenders: A review of the literature. *Journal of Correctional Health Care, 23*(3), 336–346. https://doi.org/10.1177/1078345817716180

Haney, E. M., O'Neil, M. E., Carson, S., et al. (2012). *Suicide risk factors and risk assessment tools: A systematic review*. Department of Veterans Affairs.

Hayes, L. (2010). *National study of jail suicides: 20 years later*. https://info.nicic.gov/nicrp/system/files/024308.pdf

Hayes, L. M. (2017). *Guide to developing and revising suicide prevention protocols within jails and prisons*. National Center on Institutions and Alternatives. https://www.ncchc.org/wp-content/uploads/Suicide-Prevention-2017.pdf

Heilbrun, K., Kavanaugh, A., Grisso, T., Anumba, N., Dvoskin, J., & Golding, S. (2021). The importance of racial identity in forensic mental health assessment. *Journal of the American Academy of Psychiatry and the Law, 49*(4), 478–487.

Johnson, J. E., Ramezani, N., Viglione, J., Hailemariam, M., & Taxman, F. S. (2024). Recommended mental health practices for individuals interacting with U.S. police, court, jail, probation, and parole systems. *Psychiatric Services, 75*(3), 246–257.

Konrad, N., Daigle, M. S., Daniel, A. E., et al. (2007). Preventing suicide in prisons, part I: Recommendations from the International Association for Suicide Prevention Task Force on Suicide in Prisons. *Crisis, 28*(3), 113–121.

Lurigio, A. J., & Swartz, J. A. (2006). Mental illness in correctional populations: The use of standardized screening tools for further evaluation or treatment. *Federal Probation, 70*(2), 29–35.

Maloney, M. P., Reitz, E., & Ward, M. P. (2001). *Prevalence of risk factors for mental illness in a large county jail*. Unpublished manuscript.

Martin, M. S., Colman, I., Simpson, A., & McKenzie, K. (2013). Mental health screening tools in correctional institutions: A systematic review. *BMC Psychiatry, 13*, 275.

Maruschak, L., Bronson, J., & Alper, M. (2021). *Indicators of mental health problems reported by prisoners: Survey of prison inmates, 2016*. https://bjs.ojp.gov/sites/g/files/xyckuh236/files/media/document/imhprpspi16st.pdf

Moitra, M., Santomauro, D., Degenhardt, L., et al. (2021). Estimating the risk of suicide associated with mental disorders: A systematic review and meta-regression analysis. *Journal of Psychiatric Research, 137*, 242–249.

Moscicki, E. (2001). Epidemiology of completed and attempted suicide: Toward a framework of prevention. *Clinical Neuroscience Research, 1*, 310–323.

Mulvey, E. P., & Schubert, C. A. (2017). Mentally ill individuals in jails and prisons. *Crime and Justice, 46*, 231–277.

National Commission on Correctional Health Care. (2015). *Standards for mental health services in correctional facilities*.

National Commission on Correctional Health Care. (2018a). *Standards for health services in prisons*.

National Commission on Correctional Health Care. (2018b). *Standards for health services in jails*.

National Commission on Correctional Health Care. (2019). *Suicide prevention resource guide: National response plan for suicide prevention in corrections*. https://www.ncchc.org/wp-content/uploads/Suicide_Prevention_Resource_Guide.pdf

Posner, K., Brown, G. K., Stanley, B., et al. (2011). The Columbia-Suicide Severity Rating Scale: Initial validity and internal consistency findings from three multisite studies with adolescents and adults. *American Journal of Psychiatry, 168*(12), 1266–1277.

Prins, S. J. (2014). Prevalence of mental illnesses in US state prisons: A systematic review. *Psychiatric Services, 65*(7), 862–872.

Ricks, E. P., & Eno Louden, J. (2015). Slipping through the cracks: Is mental illness appropriately identified among Latino offenders? *Criminal Justice and Behavior, 43*(4), 525–538.

Ruiz v. Estelle, 503 F. Supp. 1265 (Southern District of Texas 1980).

Rukus, J., & Kulkarni, V. S. (2019). Easier said than done: Methodological challenges in exploring prevalence of mental health illness among rural jail inmates in the United States. *International Journal of Rural Criminology, 4*(2), 258–272.

Sherman, L. G., & Morschauser, P. C. (1989). Screening for suicide risk in inmates. *Psychiatric Quarterly, 60*, 119–138.

Simpson, A. I. F., Gerritsen, C., Maheandiran, M., et al. (2022). A systematic review of reviews of correctional mental health services using the STAIR framework. *Frontiers in Psychiatry, 12*, 747202.

Stijelja, S., & Mishara, B. L. (2022). Preventing suicidal and self-injurious behavior in correctional facilities: A systematic literature review and meta-analysis. *EClinicalMedicine, 51*, 101560.

Substance Abuse and Mental Health Services Administration. (2019). *Screening and assessment of co-occurring disorders in the justice system*. https://store.samhsa.gov/sites/default/files/pep19-screen-codjs.pdf

Vogel, M., Stephens, K. D., & Siebels, D. (2014). Mental illness and the criminal justice system. *Sociology Compass, 8*, 627–638.

Wilson, N. J. (2017). The Columbia-Suicide Severity Rating Scale: Validation for use as a screen for suicide risk in New Zealand prisons and probation settings. *Practice: The New Zealand Corrections Journal, 5*(2), 40.

16

Interviewing

*Anthony C. Tamburello**

Introduction

The psychiatric interview is the foundation for effective diagnosis and treatment of mental health disorders in any setting. The interview is also the necessary first step for clinical decision-making, including the need for treatment in general, the management of immediate and long-term safety concerns, the appropriate level and setting of care, and the specific treatments recommended. The core features of the psychiatric interview in a carceral setting will be familiar to any professional qualified to conduct one generally (American Psychiatric Association, 2006).

The base rate of mental health disorders in carceral settings, including serious mental illness, substance use disorders, and personality disorders, is high, and comorbidity is the rule (Tamburello et al., 2022; see Chapter 31). While many of these patients will come to the attention of the psychiatrist at intake, some may minimize their history on admission and present later, when symptoms or functional impairments develop (Trestman et al., 2007).

The intended audience for this chapter is any professional working in a carceral setting who is qualified to perform a general psychiatric evaluation. The objectives of this chapter are to describe the key elements of the general, nonemergent psychiatric interview in correctional settings; to examine important contextual factors; to discuss the value of collateral information; and to address concerns about deception, malingering, and countertransference. Screening examinations (Chapter 15), risk assessment (Chapters 51–54), psychological testing (Chapter 67), disciplinary evaluations (Chapters 10 and 66), and certain specialized examinations (e.g., the diagnosis of gender dysphoria; Chapter 56) are addressed elsewhere.

Especially in facilities with high patient turnover and precipitous discharges (e.g., jails), the prospect of conducting a psychiatric interview as described herein may seem daunting. An appropriate goal is for the psychiatrist to incorporate as many elements of the interview as possible, consistent with the time available. This may sometimes require conducting the interview over more than one session.

Contextual factors

An accurate and high-quality psychiatric interview in a jail or prison requires an appreciation of various contextual factors, including the referral source, the reason for the referral, active stressors experienced by the patient, the timing of the meeting in relation to these stressors, the setting of the interview, privacy and safety concerns, language and cultural considerations, current and historical symptoms and their relationship with substance use (if applicable), and the alignment of goals between the interviewer and interviewee, among others. Failure to recognize these factors may result in misdiagnosis or misattribution that may delay effective treatment.

Referral source and reason for consultation

A patient may come to the attention of the psychiatrist through numerous sources, such as mental health screeners, other health care providers, correctional officers, administrators, other civilian staff (e.g., social services), and self-referral. While requests received via staff may simply be another route of self-referral, the provenance of the request is helpful, as it may suggest a specific functional impairment (e.g., school or occupational) or a specific question to be answered (e.g., an internal affairs concern about an intercepted communication).

Especially if the referral source is a staff member who knows the patient and may have information about the patient's baseline level of function, recent behavioral changes, and relevant environmental factors, it is helpful for the first questions to be asked of this person. While a correctional officer will not ordinarily have the training, language, and experience of health care staff, they can reasonably be expected to know their duties and to observe behavior: Has the incarcerated person's (IP's) behavior changed recently, and have said changes presented a management problem for custody? While such questions provide useful information about emerging signs of mental illness and related functional impairment, they also convey respect for the role of the correctional officer, which promotes better collaboration, both now and later (see Chapter 14). Nevertheless, confidentiality requires that such communication be largely one-directional, unless the result of the interview includes a recommendation for safety or housing that must be acted upon by custody staff.

*. The author acknowledges the contributions of Li-Wen Lee, who was the author of this chapter in the textbook's first edition.

Setting and timing

Knowing where the patient is housed, both in general (e.g., lockup, jail, or prison) and specifically (e.g., the particular housing unit), is critically important. Someone newly arrested, remanded, or returning on a violation of conditional release is coming from outside the facility, with potential exposure to different stressors, traumas, influences, substances, and health care treatment (or lack thereof). Knowing how long it has been since the IP was in the community is especially relevant to assessing the risk of withdrawal from certain substances (see Chapter 46). The consequences of substance use include the more immediate effects of intoxication or withdrawal, as well as the production or exacerbation of psychiatric symptoms. While IPs with recent exposure to the community may be at higher risk for the influence of substances on mental health presentations, interviewers should be aware that contraband drugs and alcohol are also available within secure settings (see Chapter 45).

Anyone recently admitted to a correctional facility can be expected to experience stress from unresolved legal matters (e.g., new charges or a technical violation of conditional release), as well as from acute relational, occupational, and financial changes or losses. Any new environment will bring with it uncertainties about how one's needs will be met, including safety. Some facilities may have policies that institute safety protocols for any IP who has yet to have a formal suicide risk assessment. If such precautions are uncomfortable for the patient, this may lead to underreporting of symptoms. If transferred from another facility (e.g., from a jail to a prison), it is helpful to know how long the IP was at the previous facility; a brief stay at the local detention facility (e.g., for a parole violation) suggests that the same concerns for recent community exposure apply.

IPs referred from restrictive housing settings are anticipated to have stressors commonly experienced by those in isolated confinement, including the worsening or failure to improve of serious mental illness, as well as safety concerns (Metzner & Fellner, 2010; O'Keefe et al., 2013; see Chapter 10). While patients presently housed on a mental health unit likely have had some previous assessment in the facility, this usually suggests a more complicated history with impaired functioning observed in their previous treatment setting (see Chapter 9). Those housed in medical units, infirmaries, and hospice units likely have a greater burden of medical comorbidities, which may have direct or indirect relevance to their psychiatric presentation. In general population settings, the IP's security level (e.g., maximum, medium, minimum; see Chapter 13) can influence the level of structure provided in their housing unit and the risk of outside exposures, especially if the patient has access to furloughs, community work, or less supervised visitation. There can be notable cultural differences between facilities and even between housing units within a facility (Metzner, 1998), including differences in the level of crowding, gang presence, and the ways in which institutional rules are enforced. Whether the IP is housed alone, with one or more cellmates, or in a dorm setting has relevance for stressors, support, and safety (Zhong et al., 2021).

When the evaluation is to address a stressor, it is helpful to know if this is acute or more remote. For example, the interview technique, immediate safety concerns, and follow-up needs may be different for an IP who has just received a death notification or has just reported being sexually assaulted (see Chapter 70).

Privacy, safety, and confidentiality

In jails and prisons, safety and security requirements will supersede routine clinical matters. Correctional officers regulate entry, exit, and internal movement within the facility, and access to IPs is dictated by institutional policy and scheduling. Common examples include designated "count" times, meals, and staff shift changes. Scheduled recreation, education, work, and visitation times may or may not preclude a clinical interview but are best avoided because many IPs highly value these activities, and interfering with them may impact upon the patient's level of cooperation and future therapeutic alliance. Planning around institutional schedules may help ensure that adequate time is available for the interview, though this should not preclude exceptions for more urgent assessments.

Personal safety is important in any health care setting, and it is difficult to conduct a high-quality interview while feeling unsafe. It is essential for clinicians to be aware of their environment and to avoid exposure to vulnerable positions to the extent possible. While most IPs will see psychiatrists as helpful or potentially helpful to them, certain scenarios may be contentious (e.g., involuntary treatment, denial of requests for nonindicated medication). Clinicians should consider whether the interview location leaves them alone in a potentially dangerous situation and should be aware of how to exit the interview area should they feel threatened. In high-risk circumstances, it may be necessary to take more stringent security measures or to request that a correctional officer remain present during the interview. Though confidentiality is a priority, when in question, the safety of the patient, the examiner, and others is a higher priority. However, it is important to note that common correctional practices such as shackling IPs during mental health assessments or having an officer remain in the room can feel dehumanizing and deter patients from answering questions. Thus, security concerns must be balanced with the need for confidentiality and maintaining an IP's dignity.

The physical space where the interview is conducted should allow for as much confidentiality and clear communication as possible, consistent with safety. Especially in high-security settings such as restrictive housing, it may seem logistically simpler if the evaluation is conducted at the cell front. However, this is little different from conducting a psychiatric interview in public, especially when cellmates, nearby peers, or correctional officers are within earshot. Patients may view this as disrespectful, a rights violation, or uncaring, and such practices will reasonably result in withholding or modification of relevant clinical information. Interviews should occur in private, away from other IPs and, when possible, away from correctional officers (Blaauw & van Marle, 2007). As in any setting, it is not possible to guarantee confidentiality absolutely, with well-known exceptions for safety concerns and when required by law (Health Insurance Portability and Accountability Act, 1996). Additional limits on confidentiality in a carceral setting, such as information on potential security breaches, may apply as defined by law, regulation, or institutional policy. Interviewees should be informed at the outset of the interaction about the limits of confidentiality, with reminders when necessary.

Culture, language, and communication

The interviewee's ability to communicate effectively should be assessed; it is the responsibility of the interviewer to identify barriers to communication and to address them appropriately (American

Psychiatric Association, 2016). Professional interpreters certified to provide these services, with signed agreements of confidentiality, are preferred over noncertified health care staff. Outside of a true emergency, IPs and correctional officers should not be used for interpretation services, nor should clinicians without certified proficiency in the patient's language conduct interviews without the use of an interpreter. While in-person interpretation services are optimal, telephone interpreter services are an acceptable alternative. As in any health care setting, certified interpreters are expected to provide literal interpretations of what is said but are permitted to provide relevant cultural information (e.g., idioms) that may add value to the interview (Martinez-Gomez, 2014).

Hearing impairment affects approximately 6% of IPs (Bronson & Berzofsky, 2015), and correctional facilities must make reasonable accommodations for hearing impairment under the Americans With Disabilities Act (*Pennsylvania Department of Correction v. Yeskey*, 1998). Depending on the nature and extent of the hearing impairment, the use of a certified sign language interpreter with an appreciation for deaf culture may be required to conduct an adequate psychiatric assessment (Kuntz et al., 2023). In other cases, an assistive device such as a hearing aid or captioned telephone (i.e., CapTel) may be helpful.

In some instances, neurologic symptoms such as aphasia may be the source of the patient's communication barrier. Psychiatric symptoms such as thought disorder may also result in difficulty communicating. These problems may be misinterpreted by correctional staff as volitional, such as deliberately ignoring or defying instructions. Careful psychiatric interview and assessment can help clarify diagnoses and avoid misattribution of IPs' behaviors.

As addressed in Chapter 13, correctional culture in general values the appearance of strength and discourages the sharing of information with staff, which may manifest as withholding information during the interview (Rotter et al., 2005). Those who appear weak may be more vulnerable to victimization, and identification as a mental health patient, attendance at mental health appointments, or appearing at pill call may promote the perception of weakness, thereby motivating some IPs to avoid assessment or treatment. Furthermore, IPs may not trust mental health staff that they identify as being part of the system.

Thus, an interviewer's ability to establish trust is a key element of an effective interview. A better understanding of the patient's background and culture is helpful and can avoid misunderstandings. Psychiatrists are well advised to participate in cultural competence training and to make efforts to better understand the patient's specific culture (see Chapter 22).

Understanding jargon commonly used in the facility is helpful in correctly interpreting what the interviewee is saying and developing rapport with them, though the clinician should avoid presenting themselves disingenuously or in a manner that crosses boundaries. When the patient uses a term that is not familiar to the interviewer, this needs to be clarified. Even within a single carceral system, patients can use slang terminology differently from each other.

Psychiatrists should be clear about the purpose of the interview, their employer, and any limitations of their role. If IPs are reluctant or hostile when addressing their treatment needs, motivational interviewing may help overcome treatment resistance. Motivational interviewing has been used in forensic populations (McMurran, 2009) and has been promoted for use in correctional settings (Iarussi et al., 2016).

Interview elements

The structure of the psychiatric interview is similar in carceral and community settings (American Psychiatric Association, 2006, 2016), though the sequence of questions may vary based on context and interviewer style and preference. This section will address the core elements of the psychiatric interview.

Presenting illness

Also known as the history of presenting illness, this typically begins with understanding the patient's chief concern or the reason for referral. The history of presenting illness may be used as a starting point for gathering details that provide an understanding of how the IP's concerns are affecting their comfort, functioning, and risk. Open-ended and nonleading questions are most helpful for gathering accurate information, though progressively more directed questions may be necessary for clarification, especially when differentiating symptoms (e.g., depression or anxiety) from syndromes (e.g., major depressive disorder or panic disorder). A semi-structured interview, like the Quick Inventory of Depressive Symptomatology—Clinician Rating (Rush et al., 2003) is sometimes helpful. Formal psychological testing may also aid in clarifying diagnoses (see Chapter 67).

The history of presenting illness should always be considered in light of contextual factors. Is the IP presently subject to conflicts with peers (including gang activity) or correctional officers? Is the IP presently facing or anticipating a loss or change in the community or in the facility, especially one that negatively affects their relationships, freedom, health, or previously effective coping strategies? When did the symptoms begin, how long have they persisted, what makes them better or worse, and what is their relationship with stressors or with the use of substances? IPs may feel frustrated or guilty about stressors faced by their family in the community, as incarceration may reduce their ability to intervene directly. Incarceration can be a particular strain on long-term relationships; unlike in the community, marriage is a risk factor for suicide for IPs (Zhong et al., 2021).

Past psychiatric history

Important information related to past psychiatric history includes the onset and nature of mental health treatment; psychiatric hospitalizations, including when and where they occurred, the reason for admission, voluntary or involuntary status, duration, and treatment received; prior suicide attempts and deliberate self-harm; past psychiatric medications, including whether any were particularly helpful or harmful; and outpatient treatment, including the most recent provider in the community. A review of past mental health treatment can provide information about the trajectory of the illness, treatment options, and potential sources of collateral records. Prior nonadherence or involuntary treatment will often emerge from this history when told from the interviewee's perspective. When interviewing IPs who have been previously incarcerated, asking about prior symptoms and behavior during incarceration may help predict adjustment to their current circumstances and guide treatment.

Family, developmental, and psychosocial history

If known to the patient, the histories of blood relatives, including psychiatric illnesses, substance use disorders, hospitalizations, and suicide attempts and deaths by suicide, as well as effective interventions, may suggest genetic loading, risk factors, and insights into treatment options. Where the IP was born and raised provides biographical information that may lead to follow-up questions about their culture of origin. If known, exposure to substances in utero, birth trauma, developmental delays, and behavior problems may suggest a need for further inquiry about developmental, intellectual, and other disorders typically presenting in childhood. When persisting into adulthood, problems with impulse control, planning, or comprehension are relevant to an IP's ability to follow institutional rules. Besides biographical context, asking about the highest level of educational achievement, whether enrolled in special education (and why), behavior problems and serious disciplinary sanctions during school years, and the reason for not completing a course of study provides information about developmental functioning, conduct disorder, and sometimes opportunities for growth in the present. As IPs have high rates of exposure to adverse childhood events, it is essential to inquire about a history of childhood neglect or deprivation, physical abuse, and sexual abuse (see Chapter 36).

The relationship history includes gender identification and expression, sexual orientation and expression, marital status, the presence or absence of a current supportive (or contentious) relationship, previous marriages and long-term relationships, and any pattern of brief, intense relationships. The occupational history should include the patient's most recent employment status, longest job, trade union membership if applicable, typical reasons for terminating employment, and whether there is a pattern of quitting a job without another lined up, which may correlate with a diagnosis of antisocial personality disorder (Black & Blum, 2022). A basic military history, when applicable, includes the branch of service, years of service, highest pay grade and military occupational specialty, where stationed, any disciplinary hearings (i.e., Article 15 or Captain's Mast), combat experience, and type of discharge (e.g., honorable, other than honorable, dishonorable). Recent living situation, as well as any history of homelessness, may suggest supports in the community or lack thereof. Each of these elements suggests the IP's baseline functional capacity in the community and may assist in reentry planning.

Substance use history

In-depth inquiry into the patient's lifetime, recent, and current use of substances is critically important, including the substances used, and for each of these, the age of onset, route or method of use, frequency of use, and most recent use. It is helpful to ask about periods of abstinence and whether relevant psychiatric symptoms mentioned in the present illness and past psychiatric history were different or resolved during those periods. Whether the patient identifies as having a substance use disorder is worth noting, but more important is an accounting of the consequences of substance use, including medical (e.g., overdoses, medical complications, or withdrawal symptoms), relational, occupational, educational, financial, and legal problems. While substances may be more difficult to obtain in carceral settings, they often are accessible (see Chapter 45), and current use may cause interpersonal (e.g., debts) and institutional disciplinary problems. Treatment history and its effectiveness, especially prior prescription of medication for alcohol or opioid use disorders, may inform current and future treatment directions.

Medical history

While screening, assessment, and treatment of general medical conditions are typically the responsibility of other medical professionals, the psychiatrist is wise to note medical conditions that may present with mental health symptoms or complicate psychiatric management, including neurologic (e.g., traumatic brain injury and seizures), endocrine, rheumatologic, oncologic, cardiovascular, orthopedic, reproductive, nephrological, and gastroenterological conditions, among others. Collaboration with other medical professionals and specialists may be necessary.

Legal history

All IPs should be asked about their current legal entanglement, as well as their chronological history of arrest and convictions, including for violent or sexual offenses. If their reason for incarceration (whether an open charge or a violation of conditional release) is yet to be adjudicated, the interviewee may understandably be unwilling to disclose certain details for fear of compromising the ongoing case. It is important to remember the nonforensic (clinical) purpose of the interview and to limit questions to what is clinically relevant.

It is nevertheless appropriate to obtain information about the charges, the status of the case (including anticipated hearings and active appeals), and concerns the interviewee has about the pending case. If sentenced, it is helpful for reentry planning to know their anticipated release date and when they may be eligible for parole. Certain classes of offenses, such as sexual offenses, carry stigma within the correctional population and may make IPs more vulnerable to interpersonal stressors if their offenses become known. Persons arrested or sentenced for the first time, those with lengthy sentences, and those with high-profile or notorious cases in the community are particularly prone to adjustment difficulties. Understanding the role of mental illness in prior offenses may be helpful in foreseeing potential symptom manifestations in the correctional setting, so it is important to note prior forensic psychiatric evaluations of criminal matters, as well as current or prior case dispositions of not guilty by reason of insanity or guilty but mentally ill.

Mental status examination

As with other portions of the interview process, the components of the mental status examination are essentially the same as with a mental status examination conducted in the community, with attention to hygiene, affect, mood, thought process, hallucinations, delusions, suicidality, homicidality, insight, and judgment. The psychiatrist need not relegate the mental status examination to merely another subjective section of the interview, however. Objective observations, including appearance and behavior, examples of thought disorder, consistency between patient report and examination findings (e.g., mood and affect, subjective versus objective alertness, hyperactivity, inattention, and anxiety), and measured changes in weight, for example, are particularly helpful in making more confident diagnoses. Bedside cognitive screening is important whenever cognitive impairment is at issue or when age or medical infirmity suggests the need for a baseline assessment (Baillargeon et al., 2023; see Chapter 60).

Collateral information

As in community settings, collateral sources of information are important in interpreting interview findings. Prior treatment records, both during incarceration and in the community, should be obtained and reviewed. When possible, contacting family members or close friends may yield relevant information about the patient's personal and family psychiatric history and recent functioning. Requests for nonpublic collateral information, outside of an emergency situation, should be authorized by the patient consistent with applicable laws, regulations, and policies (Health Insurance Portability and Accountability Act, 1996).

Some collateral information may be publicly available, such as online judicial or correctional system databases that list information about the current offense and sentencing data. Other sources may not be public but are readily available to clinicians, such as institutional records that include the IP's criminal and disciplinary history or a state prescription monitoring program website, which authorized providers may use to confirm the past prescription of controlled medications in the community.

Managing countertransference, bias, and malingering

Countertransference is an occupational hazard of working in carceral settings. Some mental health professionals may see IPs as criminals primarily deserving punishment and not empathy; these individuals are likely better suited for work elsewhere. Conversely, clinicians may see IPs through a lens of unbridled advocacy, wishing to save them from the harms of a punitive and unjust carceral system. This type of countertransference can also be problematic if not discussed with mental health colleagues and actively managed.

More often, and quite naturally, the specific nature of an IP's instant or past offenses, especially those of a violent or sexual nature, may remind staff of negative personal experiences or otherwise kindle an emotional response. Patients with character pathology, those who present as demanding and entitled, and those who seek staff interventions that are outside their purview or potentially intended for nonmedical reasons may be off-putting. Negative countertransference may become apparent in patronizing, judgmental, avoidant, or dismissive attitudes or behavior by staff. Because IPs are sensitive to being judged or disrespected, this damages rapport and reduces the psychiatrist's ability to elicit necessary information.

Psychiatrists working in jails and prisons may be concerned about being deceived into providing services for persons who do not have a mental illness. The topic of malingering is addressed in detail in Chapter 20. Approaching a clinical interview through a lens of suspected malingering may bias the results. Clinicians should recall that, while malingering is a legitimate and serious concern, patients with mental illness may exaggerate or misattribute legitimate symptoms (e.g., partial malingering; Resnick, 1997). Just as concerning, those with a serious mental illness may minimize or deny symptoms entirely, either from a lack of insight or to avoid being perceived as weak. Interviewers should pay attention to internal (within the interview) and external (with previously documented interviews or collateral sources) historical inconsistencies, as well as inconsistencies between the history and objective observations. However, they should recall that deception is not mutually exclusive with having clinical needs.

Clinicians cannot always avoid emotional responses to an IP, but awareness enables them to manage countertransference appropriately and make the best possible assessment in the circumstances. During the interview, psychiatrists should maintain a nonjudgmental attitude. Countertransference may sometimes be a useful tool if clinicians recognize their own feelings as an opportunity to inform diagnosis and treatment (Colli et al., 2014).

Summary

Conducting a psychiatric interview in a jail or prison is a challenging task requiring an understanding of the patient's problem in its biographical, legal, cultural, structural, and situational context. A high-quality interview will be as thorough as possible within the time allowed and will consider objective signs, consistency of the data gathered, and relevant collateral information as well as management of countertransference and bias on the part of the interviewer. Accurate psychiatric interviewing promotes effective treatment for patients, which will improve outcomes, increase safety, and strengthen respect for psychiatric services by custody staff.

REFERENCES

American Psychiatric Association. (2006). *Practice guideline for the psychiatric evaluation of adults.*

American Psychiatric Association. (2016). *Psychiatric services in correctional facilities* (3rd ed.).

Baillargeon, J., Linthicum, L. C., Murray, O. J., et al. (2023). The prevalence of cognitive impairment and dementia in incarcerated older adults. *Journals of Gerontology: Series B, 78*(12), 2141–2146.

Blaauw, E., & van Marle, H. (2007). Mental health in prisons. In L. Moller, H. Stover, R. Jurgens, & A. Gatherer (Eds.), *Health in prison: A WHO guide to the essentials in prison health* (pp. 133–145). World Health Organization.

Black, D. W., & Blum, N. (2022). Clinical symptoms and assessment of antisocial personality disorder. In D. W. Black & N. J. Kolla (Eds.), *Textbook of antisocial personality disorder* (pp. 83–98). American Psychiatric Association Publishing.

Bronson, J., & Berzofsky, M. (2015). *Disabilities among prison and jail inmates, 2011–12.* https://bjs.ojp.gov/content/pub/pdf/dpji1112.pdf

Colli, A., Tanzilli, A., Dimaggio, G., & Lingiardi, V. (2014). Patient personality and therapist response: An empirical investigation. *American Journal of Psychiatry, 171*, 102–108.

Health Insurance Portability and Accountability Act, Pub. L. No. 104-191, § 264, 110 Stat. 1936 (1996).

Iarussi, M. M., Vest, R., Booker, A. T., & Powers, D. F. (2016). Motivational interviewing training in correctional education. *Journal of Correctional Education, 67*(1), 39–57.

Kuntz, L. A., Pratt, J., & Cotterell, M. (2023). Working with persons involved in the legal system who are deaf. *Journal of the American Academy of Psychiatry and the Law, 51*(2), 227–235.

Martinez-Gomez, A. (2014). Interpreting in prison settings: An international overview. *Interpreting, 16*, 233–259.

McMurran, M. (2009). Motivational interviewing with offenders: A systematic review. *Legal and Criminological Psychology, 14*, 83–100.

Metzner, J. L. (1998). An introduction to correctional psychiatry, part III. *Journal of the American Academy of Psychiatry and the Law, 28*(1), 107–115.

Metzner, J. L., & Fellner, J. (2010). Solitary confinement and mental illness in U.S. prisons: A challenge for medical ethics. *Journal of the American Academy of Psychiatry and the Law, 38*(1), 104–108.

O'Keefe, M. L., Klebe, K. J., Metzner, J., Dvoskin, J., Fellner, J., & Stucker, A. (2013). A longitudinal study of administrative segregation. *Journal of the American Academy of Psychiatry and the Law*, *41*(1), 49–60.

Pennsylvania Department of Correction v. Yeskey, 524 U.S. 206 (1998).

Resnick, P. J. (1997). Malingering of posttraumatic stress disorders. In R. Rogers (Ed.), *Clinical assessment of malingering and deception* (2nd ed., pp. 130–152). Guilford.

Rotter, M., McQuistion, H., Broner, N., & Steinbacher, M. (2005). Best practices: The impact of the "incarceration culture" on reentry for adults with mental illness: A training and group treatment model. *Psychiatric Services*, *56*(3), 265–267.

Rush, A. J., Trivedi, M. H., Ibrahim, H. M., et al. (2003). The 16-item Quick Inventory of Depressive Symptomatology (QIDS), Clinician Rating (QIDS-C), and Self-Report (QIDS-SR): A psychometric evaluation in patients with chronic major depression. *Biological Psychiatry*, *54*, 574–583.

Tamburello, A., Penn, J., Ford, E., et al. (2022). The American Academy of Psychiatry and the Law practice resource for prescribing in corrections. *Journal of the American Academy of Psychiatry and the Law*, *50*, S1–S62.

Trestman, R., Ford, J., & Zhang, W. W. (2007). Current and lifetime psychiatric illness among inmates not identified as acutely mentally ill at intake in Connecticut's jails. *Journal of the American Academy of Psychiatry and the Law*, *35*(4), 490–500.

Zhong, S., Senior, M., Yu, R., et al. (2021). Risk factors for suicide in prisons: A systematic review and meta-analysis. *The Lancet: Public Health*, 6(3), e164–e174.

17

Diagnostic review and revision

S. Ananya Yarrapureddy and Sohrab Zahedi

Introduction

The punishment of people with mental illness is not just a contemporary problem. Be it marginalization, confinement, or banishment, poor treatment of those with mental illness has been a pervasive theme throughout history (Dvoskin et al., 2020). To focus on the early United States, while there is not a clear understanding of colonial Americans' perception of mental illness, it is known that there were no available structured services for people with mental illness (Thompson, 1994). The responsibility to care for those afflicted with mental illness seems to have largely fallen upon individual families (Eldridge, 1996). When the illness was too severe or the situation too dangerous, afflicted individuals may have found themselves in almshouses and jails (Thompson, 1994; Truong et al., 2020). Throughout the 17th and 18th centuries, the concept of a diseased brain as the driver for mental illness evolved (Kendler et al., 2022), and some hospitals began opening wards to house individuals with mental illness. Many of the afflicted individuals still remained in prisons and poorhouses (Osborn, 2009).

In the early 1800s, on the shoulders of Enlightenment, a new philosophy of treating mental illness emerged. This was the concept of moral treatment—the idea that those with mental illness could recover if they were treated humanely and with compassion. Public asylums were developed, and by the end of the 1800s, asylums housed 75,000 individuals with mental illness (Osborn, 2009). As time went on and as the U.S. population continued to grow, asylums became overcrowded, housing nearly 560,000 patients at a peak in the 1950s (Bockoven, 1972). Around the same time, news reports brought the inhumane conditions in institutions to the public's consciousness.

In the post–World War II era, there was a renewed societal interest in understanding mental illness, which was reflected in the creation of the National Institutes of Mental Health. By the 1950s, chlorpromazine and other first-generation antipsychotics suddenly made the unlikely hope that people with mental illness could recover a real possibility. As financial constraints increased, state governments attempted to decrease utilization of asylums by developing community-based care. These factors, in combination with stronger public beliefs in rights for marginalized groups and new legislative restrictions on involuntary commitment, brought about the deinstitutionalization movement (Dvoskin et al., 2020; Osborn, 2009; see Chapter 2).

Unfortunately, the transition of care from asylums to community mental health centers was fraught with challenges. Too few in number and too limited in resources, outpatient centers failed to provide adequate care for the large numbers of individuals with moderate illness, let alone those with serious illness (Osborn, 2009). As a result, patients who previously might have been institutionalized found themselves in the community with limited support, sparse access to treatment, and the freedom to refuse treatment. These factors, in combination with an increasingly punitive societal view of substance use and a widespread "tough on crime" mentality, led individuals with mental illness to become incarcerated in unprecedented numbers (Dvoskin et al., 2020).

Today, individuals with mental illness are greatly overrepresented in carceral settings (Prins, 2014), and many more individuals with mental illness are housed in prisons and jails than in psychiatric hospitals. Approximately 100,000 psychiatric beds are available in the United States (American Psychiatric Association, 2022b), and the number of incarcerated persons (IPs) in jails and prisons hovers around 1.8 million (Carson & Kluckow, 2023). Prevalence estimates for mental illness within the correctional system vary, with one estimate indicating that 37% of individuals in prison and 44% of individuals in jail have had a history of at least one mental health problem (Bronson & Berzofsky, 2017).

Thus, although jails and prisons are far from the ideal setting to provide mental health treatment, there is no denying that the correctional system serves as a critical entry point for the diagnosis and treatment of individuals with mental illness (Prins, 2014). The diagnostic criteria delineated in the American Psychiatric Association's *Diagnostic and Statistical Manual of Mental Disorders*, 5th edition, text revision (American Psychiatric Association, 2022a), are intended to facilitate assessment in a "variety of clinical settings," including in carceral settings. Still, jail and prison settings raise several unique considerations that impact diagnosis. This chapter explores the process of diagnosis in carceral settings, as well as the importance and far-reaching impact of accurate diagnosis for incarcerated individuals.

The diagnostic process

The first step in establishing a diagnosis begins with a patient establishing care. An IP may enter into psychiatric care at any point during their incarceration. Some individuals may present with an established history, while others may enter the correctional setting in the throes of substance intoxication or withdrawal. Still others may develop behavioral and psychiatric symptoms, acute or nonacute, for the first time while incarcerated. All of these scenarios have community parallels. Correctional settings, however, have several unique considerations that can facilitate the establishment of psychiatric diagnoses.

Diagnostic assessment and revision over time

Psychiatric diagnoses are prone to shifting over time due to incorporation of new information, the impact of environmental support or stress, changes in a patient's symptoms, or the limitations imposed by our current understanding of psychiatric illness. One theoretical measure of diagnostic accuracy is diagnostic stability, which refers to the applicability of a diagnosis at subsequent evaluations. While multiple factors can influence the long-term stability of a diagnosis, one factor that may contribute to higher stability is diagnosis establishment while in the inpatient setting (Baca-Garcia et al., 2007). Inpatient settings allow for the closest observation of patients, lengthier observation periods, and collection of more collateral information than the typical outpatient assessment. Correctional settings afford the same opportunities; lengths of incarceration, even for some presentenced individuals, are longer than the typical inpatient hospital stay, which now averages around 7 days (American Psychiatric Association, 2022b). Moreover, prisons and jails have established procedures for supervision and documentation of observed events, providing readily accessible collateral information to clinicians. Correctional settings also limit the impact of diagnostic confounders, particularly substance use and treatment nonadherence. Perhaps because of these factors, diagnostic stability in the prison setting has been shown to be higher than in the community (Schilders & Ogloff, 2017).

Despite having greater diagnostic stability than in outpatient settings, diagnoses in corrections do change over time. In most cases, this is a result of clinicians observing a patient's longitudinal symptoms and revising the diagnosis based on new information. For example:

BR is a 26-year-old man admitted to the local jail for a charge of larceny. At booking, he appears agitated and is intrusive to other individuals. Officers become concerned when BR's peers begin posturing and yelling at him for violating their personal space. Even after being separated from others, BR is observed scanning the room frequently and at times appears to be speaking to himself. He denies any psychiatric history except for taking prescribed medications that help with sleep. A call to the local pharmacy reveals intermittent fills of a prescription for olanzapine, last prescribed by a local hospital and last dispensed several months ago as a 14-day supply. BR's urine toxicology screen is positive for phencyclidine (PCP).

BR is admitted to the infirmary, where he is observed, monitored for withdrawal, and treated with antipsychotic medications for his acute symptoms. His agitation disappears within a few days, and he no longer appears to be responding to internal stimuli. Once able to give a better history, he acknowledges using hallucinogens but continues to deny any substantial psychiatric history. He declines to provide permission to contact his family but agrees to continue taking prescribed antipsychotics for a period of time. Within weeks, while housed in a specialized mental health unit, he stops all follow-up visits and medications. Deemed no longer acutely psychotic and in better behavioral control, BR is eventually released to the general population. Six months later, he is again brought to clinical attention by concerned correctional officers due to his behaviors. They note that he has not been sleeping well, that he has been searching for food in the garbage can, and that he has not been showering or changing clothes. On interview, he is internally distracted, disorganized, confused, and intermittently laughing to himself. Correctional officers report a recent uptick in the smuggling of synthetic opiates on the housing unit and express a concern that BR may have had access to the substances. After an unremarkable evaluation at the local emergency department, BR is readmitted to the prison infirmary, where he refuses treatment and becomes subject to its involuntary application. This time, a notably longer period of treatment and observation is needed to remit his symptoms. BR is given a diagnosis of schizophrenia and monitored for a much longer period on a specialized unit before becoming eligible and appropriate for a return to the general population.

Given the high rate of drug use immediately before incarceration, the initial hours and days constitute a period of diagnostic uncertainty as lingering intoxication or withdrawal influence the clinical picture (Maruschak et al., 2021). Whether symptoms fully resolve or continue to persist after a reasonable period provides information regarding underlying diagnoses. Had this patient been managed solely in the community, he likely would have been admitted to an inpatient unit for several days. During that time, while a primary mood or psychotic illness may have been part of the differential, the working and discharge diagnosis would likely have been a substance-induced psychotic disorder, especially in the context of a positive urine toxicology screen and rapid symptom improvement. However, in the correctional setting, lengthier observation periods allow for enhanced diagnostic fine-tuning.

A second case example illustrates how collateral information from the correctional environment can be used to refine a patient's diagnosis and modify the treatment plan accordingly:

AC is a 30-year-old woman sentenced for assault and child endangerment who has already served 2 years of her 5-year sentence. She was admitted with diagnoses of schizophrenia and substance use disorders (cocaine and cannabis, in remission in a controlled environment). She has been maintained on an oral antipsychotic medication and has been functioning well. Yesterday, she began to sing loudly in her cell and tell people that if they have sex with her, she will "save them and make them holy." Known to correctional officers for her psychiatric condition, AC is brought to the infirmary for observation and to avoid incurring disciplinary charges for her behavior. A urine toxicology screen is negative for substances of abuse. A plasma level measurement of her prescribed antipsychotic reveals a lower than expected result, prompting suspicions of diversion.

Due to chronically poor insight and an established history of treatment nonadherence, the psychiatrist discusses with AC the possibility of changing her antipsychotic medication to a long-acting injectable formula. She agrees to make this change. With this approach, AC's stability is maintained until her end of sentence, avoiding the unnecessary polypharmacy or disciplinary infractions that may have occurred with a less careful approach to diagnosis and treatment planning.

As illustrated in the example above, the carceral system provides a unique means of obtaining input from others, which can influence and support diagnosis. In the community, these sources of collateral information may include local mental health authorities, pharmacies (see Chapter 18), family members, and medical records departments at hospitals. The carceral system offers additional sources, including an IP's arrest report, criminal history, behavior while in court or in their current housing unit, misconduct record, institutional movement history, and records from previous incarcerations. These additional sources may facilitate the establishment of a more accurate diagnosis.

In certain cases, response to treatment can guide diagnosis. In the community setting, where nonadherence rates hover around 50% (Semahegn et al., 2020), the inability to monitor medication administration can add an element of uncertainty, especially among those with severe mental illness or in cases where response to treatment is limited. In most correctional institutions, psychotropic medications are administered through direct observation, offering some assurance that the medication was ingested by the patient. While even direct observation can be circumvented by a motivated IP, it can still offer a degree of certainty regarding medication adherence and, subsequently, help inform diagnosis.

Impact of the carceral environment

Jails and prisons are high-stress environments, which may contribute to the emergence of psychiatric illness. Incarcerated individuals face the prospect of violence, a less-than-ideal living environment, restricted freedom, social isolation, and other pressures. While it is not clear to what extent corrections may potentiate psychiatric illness, it is known that stress exposure is a risk factor for the development of illnesses such as thought disorders, trauma-based diagnoses, and neurocognitive disorders (Armour, 2012; Cunha et al., 2023; Luo et al., 2023). Clinicians should keep in mind that characteristics of the correctional environment may independently influence onset of psychiatric symptoms or lead to the development of illness.

A discussion about diagnosis in corrections would not be complete without a discussion of feigning or exaggeration of illness. Concerns regarding secondary gain are valid and pervasive, with historical estimates showing rates of malingering as high as 32% in carceral settings (McDermott et al., 2013). While some external gain may be apparent (e.g., seeking a single cell, getting double meal portions, gaining access to medications with potential for abuse), it is important to remember that it is not unusual, when the system at large is inadequate or problematic, for an individual to exaggerate or feign symptoms for a variety of reasons that include housing issues, debts, and/or not receiving appropriate mental health treatment. It may be easy under such circumstances for the mental health clinician to focus on malingering or "manipulative behavior" and to dismiss the individual's mental health symptoms, which has the potential to lead to poor outcomes. Manipulation can prove to be an adaptive mechanism for individuals who are incarcerated. When this behavior is discussed with IPs in a nonjudgmental manner by clinicians, a safer and more effective means for IPs to interact within the correctional system can be promoted.

In the initial encounter with clinical staff, for individuals with the ability to provide a history and convey subjective symptoms, efforts should be made, especially when the clinical picture appears elusive, to objectively corroborate the history. Feigning or exaggerating symptoms for secondary gain is always a concern but should never lead to diagnostic cynicism. For example, the IP who reports thoughts of suicide may need close observational status. If actively engaging in self-harm, they may need placement in an infirmary with closer monitoring, restricted movement outside their cell, or provision of a safety garment and bedding material. Though difficult to use in attempted suicide, safety garments are both stigmatizing and uncomfortable. How an individual reacts to such a status may, at times, be diagnostic; however, assessments based on just the individual's reaction hold significant risk (see Chapter 51). IPs who simply seek single-cell housing or other privileges may stop their self-destructive behaviors when faced with the prospect of a safety gown and infirmary admission among individuals with severe mental illness. These IPs may be identified as malingerers or "behaviorally" disruptive. However, the possibility exists that someone truly at risk may behave in a similar fashion, placing themselves at further risk. Regardless, familiarity with an IP's behavioral responses to frustrations or triggers assists in maintaining safety. Such information requires a multidisciplinary team approach, including observation lasting weeks to months that can serve to guide the treatment plan once the individual is released back into the community.

Clinician factors

For practitioners, correctional health care environments are different from community environments. The day-to-day work can be quite isolating, as staff are unable to communicate with the outside world when they enter a facility (Hart, 2019). The nature of jails and prisons, with their primary focus on containment and control, can be antithetical to values central to medicine (Vandergrift & Christopher, 2021). Physicians may feel that they are unable to practice medicine optimally in such resource-anemic settings. Correctional work also takes place in a high-stress environment where physical or verbal aggression, or the perceived threat of it, can be a concern (Forman-Dolan et al., 2022). Essentially, the corrections environment contains a multitude of factors that can contribute to higher levels of stress and burnout (Forman-Dolan et al., 2022; see Chapter 65). For physicians, burnout can have significant consequences, including consequences that affect patient care, such as lower quality of care, diagnostic bias, and medical errors (De Hert, 2020).

Mental health professionals should also be aware that negative countertransference reactions such as fear, hatred, disgust, and mistrust may be common when working with individuals whose actions are viewed as morally or ethically off-putting. A proposed framework for managing these reactions includes consultation, collaboration, and supervision with other providers and a mindfulness of ethical guidelines in corrections (Mulay & Cain, 2018). Ultimately, as in any other setting, practitioners have a responsibility to manage their own countertransference and to minimize or mitigate its effects on diagnosis and treatment.

An institution's culture can, at times, interfere with clinical assessment, especially when individuals with serious mental illness are labeled as "behavioral." The term can be pejorative and attaches a manipulative motivation to behavioral dysfunction rather than attributing it to personality pathology, disinhibition secondary to traumatic brain injury, or intellectual disability (see Chapters 37, 57, and 58), all of which should be managed therapeutically. The treatment of these challenging individuals may include skill, deficit, and neuropsychological assessments, as well as limit setting to curb destructive behaviors when necessary. Treatment team planning that engages the individual will help to gain the patient's trust and cooperation (Appelbaum et al., 2001). A successful behavioral management approach hinges on a proper diagnosis (see Chapter 54).

The impact of diagnostic accuracy

Physicians who practice in correctional settings should be aware that diagnosis has impacts beyond what might be expected in the community. For incarcerated individuals with mental illness, accurate diagnosis and subsequent treatment may improve their quality of life in prison and impact their likelihood of reentering the criminal justice system.

Access to care

While in corrections, individuals with psychiatric illnesses are more likely to be victims of physical and sexual assault (Blitz et al., 2008; Canada et al., 2022), are at higher risk of suicide, are more likely to be involved in infractions and violent incidents (Fazel et al., 2016; Houser & Welsh, 2014; Schenk & Fremouw, 2012), and are more likely to spend time in restrictive housing (Remch et al., 2021). For the carceral psychiatrist, the proper identification and diagnosis of individuals with mental illness may prevent a vicious cycle of decompensation, punishment, and further decompensation. To this effect, some correctional facilities, in an effort to address concerns that restrictive housing units can exacerbate and propagate psychiatric illness, have turned instead to therapeutic diversion units, which are specially designed to provide care in a less punitive setting. Such units, when compared to restrictive housing units, have been shown to reduce infractions, use of inpatient-level psychiatric care, and self-injurious events (Remch et al., 2021). Admissions criteria for these units are multifactorial and typically initiated by behavioral health staff. This represents one example of how identification of those with mental illness has the potential to improve quality of life in corrections.

Reduction in recidivism

As a step further, better mental health while in prison has been associated with lower recidivism and better postrelease outcomes (Government Accountability Office [GAO], 2018; Wallace & Wang, 2020). For example, providing treatment for opioid use disorder in the form of medication (e.g., buprenorphine, naltrexone) and therapeutic communities has been shown to decrease rates of relapse postrelease and rates of recidivism (De Andrade et al., 2018). A 2018 GAO report found that individuals with serious mental illness are more likely to recidivate and emphasized the impact of proper treatment in mitigating such risk (GAO, 2018). Given that the vast majority of incarcerated individuals receive their first psychiatric diagnosis while incarcerated (Al-Rousan et al., 2017), the type of treatment that follows has the potential to reduce future arrest, incarceration, and decompensation. This places carceral clinicians in the unique position of being able to change the trajectory of dysfunction often seen with this population. For example, one study in the United Kingdom found that treatment delayed time to reoffense in individuals diagnosed with schizophrenia (Igoumenou et al., 2015).

Stigma and vulnerability

For IPs, stigma from self, correctional staff, or other IPs is a barrier to seeking psychiatric care and treatment (Canada et al., 2022). While such stigma can be present to a degree in the community, the negative consequences of receiving care are more pronounced in the correctional setting, where health care confidentiality may be inherently more limited. IPs with psychiatric diagnoses may worry that other IPs will perceive them as weak, making them vulnerable to harm. Receiving mental health treatment in corrections has also been linked to higher rates of victimization (Daquin & Daigle, 2018; Solbakken et al., 2024). Some psychiatric medications can weaken mental and physical faculties, which can also create a sense of unsafety (Canada et al., 2022). Those who are prescribed psychotropic medications may also become targets for coerced medication diversion. The carceral clinician should be mindful of these risks and their potential to impact diagnosis and treatment.

Systemic change and resource allocation

In an ideal correctional system, diagnosis would allow for unimpeded access to appropriate services, but in the current state, mental health care services in jails and prisons are not always sufficient to address patient needs. Keeping accurate records of IPs' diagnoses and analyzing these data as part of a quality improvement program can help decide how best to allocate scarce mental health resources. For example, data obtained in the federal prison system show that individuals with serious mental illness (broadly defined as individuals who currently or within the past year had a mental, behavioral, or emotional disorder as diagnosed by the DSM that has resulted in functional impairment), when compared to IPs without serious mental illness, are twice as likely to be incarcerated for violent offenses such as sex offenses, aggravated assault, homicide, and robbery, and half as likely to be incarcerated for drug or immigration offenses (GAO, 2018). Consistent with other sources of data, IPs with serious mental illness were found to be more likely to recidivate. IPs with a co-occurring substance use disorder are even more likely to recidivate, and mental health and substance use treatment was shown to decrease recidivism (GAO, 2018). Given that individuals with serious mental illness are disproportionately involved in the most serious offenses, identification and treatment of these patients has the potential to make a significant impact on recidivism. The same GAO analysis evaluated a variety of studies with programs designed to reduce recidivism risk in individuals with mental illness and found that programs that demonstrated success had multiple offered services, such as case management, employment assistance, housing, and release planning, in addition to substance use and mental health treatment. Thus, diagnosis is just one part of the puzzle of reducing recidivism.

Summary

Correctional facilities provide certain opportunities for diagnosis that are not readily found in community settings. While there are also certain drawbacks, the advantages are considerable and include opportunities for longitudinal observation, collection of collateral information, and limiting confounding variables. For psychiatrists, diagnostic reevaluation and reassessment to incorporate new information is a constantly occurring process. This process is crucial, as accurate diagnosis leads to more evidence-based treatments, decreases suffering, and reduces recidivism in individuals with mental illness.

REFERENCES

Al-Rousan, T., Rubenstein, L., Sieleni, B., Deol, H., & Wallace, R. B. (2017). Inside the nation's largest mental health institution: A prevalence study in a state prison system. *BMC Public Health*, *17*(1).

American Psychiatric Association. (2022a). *Diagnostic and statistical manual of mental disorders* (5th ed., text rev.).

American Psychiatric Association. (2022b). *The psychiatric bed crisis in the US: Understanding the problem and moving toward solutions.* https://www.psychiatry.org/getmedia/81f685f1-036e-4311-8dfc-e13ac425380f/APA-Psychiatric-Bed-Crisis-Report-Full.pdf

Appelbaum, K. L., Hickey, J. M., & Packer, I. (2001). The role of correctional officers in multidisciplinary mental health care in prisons. *Psychiatric Services, 52*(10), 1343–1347.

Armour, C. (2012). Mental health in prison: A trauma perspective on importation and deprivation. *International Journal of Criminology and Sociological Theory, 5*(2), 886–894.

Baca-Garcia, E., Perez-Rodriguez, M. M., Basurte-Villamor, I., Fernandez Del Moral, A. L., Jimenez-Arriero, M. A., Gonzalez De Rivera, J. L., Saiz-Ruiz, J., & Oquendo, M. A. (2007). Diagnostic stability of psychiatric disorders in clinical practice. *British Journal of Psychiatry, 190*(3), 210–216.

Blitz, C. L., Wolff, N., & Shi, J. (2008). Physical victimization in prison: The role of mental illness. *International Journal of Law and Psychiatry, 31*(5), 385–393.

Bockoven, J. S. (1972). Moral treatment in community mental health. *British Journal of Psychiatry, 121*(564), 569.

Bronson, J., & Berzofsky, M. (2017). *Indicators of mental health problems reported by prisoners and jail inmates, 2011–12.* Bureau of Justice Statistics, U.S. Department of Justice.

Canada, K., Barrenger, S., Bohrman, C., Banks, A., & Peketi, P. (2022). Multi-level barriers to prison mental health and physical health care for individuals with mental illnesses. *Frontiers in Psychiatry, 13.*

Carson, A. E., & Kluckow, R. (2023). *Correctional populations in the United States, 2021—Statistical tables.* Bureau of Justice Statistics, U.S. Department of Justice. https://bjs.ojp.gov/document/cpus21st.pdf

Cunha, O., Castro Rodrigues, A. D., Caridade, S., Dias, A. R., Almeida, T. C., Cruz, A. R., & Peixoto, M. M. (2023). The impact of imprisonment on individuals' mental health and society reintegration: Study protocol. *BMC Psychology, 11*(1).

Daquin, J. C., & Daigle, L. E. (2018). Mental disorder and victimisation in prison: Examining the role of mental health treatment. *Criminal Behaviour and Mental Health, 28*(2), 141–151.

De Andrade, D., Ritchie, J., Rowlands, M., Mann, E., & Hides, L. (2018). Substance use and recidivism outcomes for prison-based drug and alcohol interventions. *Epidemiologic Reviews, 40*(1), 121–133.

De Hert, S. (2020). Burnout in healthcare workers: Prevalence, impact and preventative strategies. *Local and Regional Anesthesia, 13,* 171–183.

Dvoskin, J. A., Knoll, J. L., & Silva, M. (2020). A brief history of the criminalization of mental illness. *CNS Spectrums, 25*(5), 638–650.

Eldridge, L. D. (1996). "Crazy brained": Mental illness in colonial America. *Bulletin of the History of Medicine, 70*(3).

Fazel, S., Hayes, A. J., Bartellas, K., Clerici, M., & Trestman, R. (2016). Mental health of prisoners: Prevalence, adverse outcomes, and interventions. *Lancet Psychiatry, 3*(9), 871–881.

Forman-Dolan, J., Caggiano, C., Anillo, I., & Kennedy, T. D. (2022). Burnout among professionals working in corrections: A two stage review. *International Journal of Environmental Research and Public Health, 19*(16), 9954.

Government Accountability Office. (2018). *Federal prisons: Information on inmates with serious mental illness and strategies to reduce recidivism.* https://www.gao.gov/assets/gao-18-182.pdf

Hart, D. (2019). Health risks of practicing correctional medicine. *AMA Journal of Ethics, 21*(6), E540–E545.

Houser, K. A., & Welsh, W. (2014). Examining the association between co-occurring disorders and seriousness of misconduct by female prison inmates. *Criminal Justice and Behavior, 41*(5), 650–666.

Igoumenou, A., Kallis, C., & Coid, J. (2015). Treatment of psychosis in prisons and violent recidivism. *BJPsych Open, 1*(2), 149–157.

Kendler, K. S., Tabb, K., & Wright, J. (2022). The emergence of psychiatry: 1650–1850. *American Journal of Psychiatry, 179*(5), 329–335.

Luo, J., Beam, C. R., & Gatz, M. (2023). Is stress an overlooked risk factor for dementia? A systematic review from a lifespan developmental perspective. *Prevention Science, 24*(5), 936–949.

Maruschak, L. M., Bronson, J., & Alper, M. (2021). *Alcohol and drug use and treatment reported by prisoners: Survey of prison inmates, 2016 (NCJ 252641).* Bureau of Justice Statistics, Office of Justice Programs, U.S. Department of Justice. https://bjs.ojp.gov/sites/g/files/xyckuh236/files/media/document/adutrpspi16st.pdf

McDermott, B. E., Dualan, I. V., & Scott, C. L. (2013). Malingering in the correctional system: Does incentive affect prevalence? *International Journal of Law and Psychiatry, 36*(3–4), 287–292.

Mulay, A. L., & Cain, N. M. (2018). Managing countertransference in correctional treatment settings: An updated perspective. *Journal of Forensic Psychology Research and Practice, 18*(1), 1–18.

Osborn, L. A. (2009). From beauty to despair: The rise and fall of the American state mental hospital. *Psychiatric Quarterly, 80*(4), 219–231.

Prins, S. J. (2014). Prevalence of mental illnesses in U.S. state prisons: A systematic review. *Psychiatric Services, 65*(7), 862–872.

Remch, M., Mautz, C., Burke, E. G., Junker, G., Kaniuka, A., Proescholdbell, S., Marshall, S. W., & Naumann, R. B. (2021). Impact of a prison therapeutic diversion unit on mental and behavioral health outcomes. *American Journal of Preventive Medicine, 61*(5), 619–627.

Schenk, A. M., & Fremouw, W. J. (2012). Individual characteristics related to prison violence: A critical review of the literature. *Aggression and Violent Behavior, 17*(5), 430–442.

Schilders, M. R., & Ogloff, J. R. P. (2017). Stability of life-time psychiatric diagnoses among offenders in community and prison settings. *Journal of Forensic Psychiatry & Psychology, 28*(1), 133–154.

Semahegn, A., Torpey, K., Manu, A., Assefa, N., Tesfaye, G., & Ankomah, A. (2020). Psychotropic medication non-adherence and its associated factors among patients with major psychiatric disorders: A systematic review and meta-analysis. *Systematic Reviews, 9*(1).

Solbakken, L. E., Bergvik, S., & Wynn, R. (2024). Breaking down barriers to mental healthcare access in prison: A qualitative interview study with incarcerated males in Norway. *BMC Psychiatry, 24*(1).

Thompson, J. W. (1994). Trends in the development of psychiatric services, 1844–1994. *Hospital & Community Psychiatry, 45*(10), 987–992.

Truong, A. H., Maguire, G. E., & Maguire, G. A. (2020). A history of psychiatry in the United States of America. *Taiwanese Journal of Psychiatry, 34*(2).

Vandergrift, L. A., & Christopher, P. P. (2021). Do prisoners trust the healthcare system? *Health & Justice, 9*(1).

Wallace, D., & Wang, X. (2020). Does in-prison physical and mental health impact recidivism? *SSM - Population Health, 11,* 100569.

18

Transition of pharmacology from community to corrections

Badr Ratnakaran and Robert L. Trestman

Introduction

Psychopharmacology, in general, is a challenging field that includes much art as well as science. Clinicians usually depend on self-report when making decisions regarding medication selection and dosing. When a patient becomes incarcerated, there are multiple potentially conflicting situations. Issues related to formularies, environmental stressors, changed support groups, and practice patterns all may contribute to medication management decisions. This chapter discusses both the clinical issues and pragmatic management opportunities that can lead to improved patient care and enhanced functioning.

There has been a substantial emphasis on continuity of care when people are released from correctional settings back to the community (see Chapters 23 and 50). However, much less has been written about the challenges regarding continuity of care when someone becomes incarcerated, particularly when psychotropic medications are involved. Psychotropic medications are often underutilized for treating mental illness in correctional facilities. Data from IQVIA National Sales from 2018 to 2020 show that the proportion of psychotropic medications distributed to jails and state prisons to treat depression and other severe mental illnesses was 0.36% and 0.48%, respectively (Curran et al., 2023). This shows a 4.1-fold relative disparity in the prescription of psychotropic medications compared to the relative burden of depression (1.46%) and other severe mental illnesses (1.97%) in the incarcerated population, according to data from the National Survey on Drug Use and Health from 2018 to 2020 (Curran et al., 2023).

Community management of psychotropic medication is of varying standards. A patient's medication regimen may be the result of thoughtful evaluation over several years of careful and incremental improvement and refinement. Conversely, it may have been compromised by a range of pragmatic issues or determined in a less formal manner, and the resulting treatment regimen may be inconsistent or inappropriate for the patient's diagnosis or diagnoses (Semahegn et al., 2020). A patient's medications may have been determined while their ongoing illicit drug use confounded the diagnostic picture. Collaboration between clinician and patient may have been poor, and subsequently, treatment adherence may have been marginal.

What, then, happens when a patient becomes incarcerated? The admission process is inherently stressful, filled with anxiety, uncertainty, and perhaps humiliation or fear. Such stressors may exacerbate underlying psychiatric symptoms. During this period, standard expectations include screening and an assessment interview, history taking, a release of information request, and confirmation of medications with the local pharmacy. The pharmacy will be able to confirm when and how regularly prescriptions were filled (albeit not how regularly they were taken). Contact with the treating community clinician or team, at least by obtaining copies of current, relevant treatment records (if not direct verbal communication), is very important. Unfortunately, in practice, such direct communication with the community care provider and information sharing are more often the exception than the rule. When integrated into standard practice, these combined steps help support continuity of care, particularly for patients with severe mental illness. Failures of the system through policy or implementation practices can compromise patient care (Morris & Zisman-Ilani, 2022). Factors to take into account at this stage of assessment include the nature and complexity of illnesses, medications being taken, co-occurrence of substance misuse, treatment adherence estimates, duration of treatment, severity of underlying illness, patients' insight into their mental illness and need for psychotropic medications, and patients' fragile clinical status.

Initial clinical considerations

First, clinical considerations need to drive decisions on whether to maintain the medications the patients took in the community. These clinical considerations include the accuracy of the community-based diagnosis, best estimates of adherence to medication in the community, the benefits versus side-effect burden of the medications, the existence of polypharmacy, the potential effects of detoxification on the diagnosis and effectiveness of the medication, and the appropriate duration of treatment for the underlying disorder.

The accuracy of the community-based diagnosis is a critical determinant in this process since the medications are intended to target signs and symptoms of psychiatric illness. Time pressures and constraints do not overrule the clinical and ethical obligation of the correctional psychiatrist to confirm the illness being treated. The ideal, as always, is to conduct a criterion-based assessment to determine whether specific psychiatric diagnoses, rather than non-specific isolated symptoms, exist. Everything else follows from this. One enormous advantage of correctional psychiatry is the opportunity rarely afforded psychiatrists in the community (since the drastic reduction of community-based inpatient psychiatric lengths of stay and elevated severity thresholds for admission to inpatient units) to observe the functioning of a patient in a safe, monitored environment (see Chapter 17). When diagnostic ambiguity exists, appropriate tapering of community medications can be conducted in many jail or prison settings with greater safety and collateral information than is achievable elsewhere. This ultimately may benefit the patient far more than simply maintaining community-based medications that may be inappropriate or unnecessary. Since 58% to 63% of correctional mental health patients have co-occurring substance misuse disorders (Bronson et al., 2017), eliminating ready access to illicit drugs may gradually resolve many of the anxiety, mood, and psychotic symptoms.

Adherence to medication in the community is always uncertain. Data clearly reflect that many psychiatric patients do not take their medications as prescribed. In a systematic review, 49% of patients with major psychiatric disorders were found to be nonadherent to their medications (Semahegn et al., 2020). Substance use, lack of social support, perceived stigma of mental illness and taking psychotropic medications, lack of insight, and medication costs were considered important risk factors for nonadherence to psychotropic medications (Semahegn et al., 2020). Lack of response to medications that the patient was supposed to be taking in the community may have occurred simply because the patient was not taking them as prescribed. Valuable information about psychotropic medications prescribed to a patient can be verified with community pharmacies or by requesting medical records from community-based treatment.

A common challenge for many people with severe mental illness is that often medications are given without a specific targeted disorder or symptom. A common response to questions about why each medication is being taken is, "I don't know." A typical scenario is that a patient may be given multiple medications, each of which is at a subtherapeutic dose. When multiple medications are used simultaneously without a clear clinical rationale and an intended purpose, the benefits diminish while the side-effect burden increases.

Polypharmacy, the simultaneous use of multiple medications, is increasing in frequency, and the prevalence of polypharmacy in psychiatry can range from 13% to 90% (Kukreja et al., 2013). One in three office visits to a psychiatrist results in three or more psychotropic prescriptions (Mojtabai & Olfson, 2010). While this may be justifiable when each medication has a specific indication or is being used as a clearly defined adjuvant, there is little research evidence to support polypharmacy (Sarkar, 2017)—but there is evidence of both attendant risks (Stassen et al., 2022) and financial costs (Kilian et al., 2018). This is notably the case where maximum therapeutic levels have not been achieved or the duration of treatment for a single medication has been insufficient (Kukreja et al., 2013). On admission to a correctional setting, an assessment of such polypharmacy is an important opportunity for therapeutic improvement and harm reduction.

Chronic, active substance use makes psychiatric diagnosis problematic at best. For example, combined opioid and cocaine abuse, with oscillating periods of intoxication and withdrawal, may readily mimic the presentation of bipolar disorder. Similarly, using psychiatric medications to treat such a presentation is very likely to be inadequate. The opportunity to observe someone, often for weeks or months, following detoxification from illicit substances may allow the clinician to make a substantially improved diagnostic assessment.

During assessment, urine drug tests (UDTs) might be relied upon by health care providers to detect substance use in incarcerated persons (IPs). Medications, including psychotropic medications, can cause false-positive results in UDTs (Moeller et al., 2017). Thus, a careful review of medications is needed before diagnosing an individual with a substance use disorder and initiating appropriate interventions. Important examples of psychotropic medications causing false-positive UDTs include lamotrigine causing a false-positive UDT for synthetic cannabinoids; sertraline causing a false-positive UDT for benzodiazepines; venlafaxine, lamotrigine, imipramine, and thioridazine causing a false-positive UDT for phencyclidine; and aripiprazole, bupropion, chlorpromazine, thioridazine, and trazodone causing a false-positive UDT for amphetamines (Moeller et al., 2017).

High rates of malingering can occur in jails and prisons, and inconsistencies between symptoms and behaviors must also be considered, as patients might be attempting to obtain psychotropic medications for diversion or abuse of prescription medications (American Academy of Psychiatry and the Law [AAPL], 2018; see Chapter 30). If malingering is suspected, a referral for psychological assessment may be appropriate (Glancy et al., 2015; see Chapter 67). Observations by the treatment team and nonclinical staff can help detect malingering and side effects of medications such as tremors; these observations can help make subsequent decisions about prescribing psychotropic medications.

Ensuring continuity of psychotropic medications is important in preventing deterioration of mental illness and adverse events like withdrawal symptoms from the medications. IPs may be transferred to an emergency department, an inpatient psychiatric unit in the community, or a state psychiatric hospital for management of a mental health crisis or for restoration of competency to stand trial. Upon their return, verbal doctor-to doctor communication and a written transfer document or discharge summary can help understand the treatment and changes in psychotropic medications prescribed for the patient (AAPL, 2018).

Pragmatic considerations

Multiple pragmatic considerations have an impact on continuity of care and the use of psychopharmacological agents. The first consideration may be a relatively limited formulary. Correctional settings frequently have formulary restrictions that are more restrictive than in many community-based environments. This may lead to a therapeutic substitution from a labeled medication to a generic that follows formulary limitations or to another agent in the same drug class upon clinical review by the psychiatrist. Virtually all institutions that have a restricted formulary do allow for nonformulary requests if the patient would clearly benefit only from a specific medication that is not on the formulary. This is particularly important for the unsentenced population who may rapidly, and unpredictably, return to the community. When an IP is sentenced, however, many facilities or systems will work to transition the patient to medications that are on the formulary.

Every effort must be made to provide appropriate treatment and prevent disruptions in the continuity of mental health care upon entry to correctional facilities. This can pose a challenge when IPs are admitted to a facility outside of normal business hours. The Continuity of Care provision of the Bureau of Prisons' national formulary addresses this issue (Federal Bureau of Prisons Health Services, 2022). The provision allows the continuation of nonformulary medications under certain circumstances: if there is no appropriate formulary substitute or if changing to a formulary substitute would not allow for proper monitoring until the next working day, *and* if withholding a specific medication would pose a significant risk to the patient. The provision allows dispensing nonformulary medication for 4 days under these circumstances. This allowance can be used while waiting for a nonformulary medication approval but cannot be used for initiating nonurgent nonformulary medications.

In contrast to the community, the near-universal standard in correctional settings is directly observed administration of psychiatric medications. In this context, either a nurse makes rounds with a medication cart to each housing unit or IPs present at a medication line. In either event, IPs take the medication under the observation of the nurse and/or an appropriately trained correctional officer who is expected to document whether the medication was taken and swallowed by the patient. In the community, this standard is typically met only in a hospital setting. The advantage is obvious—adherence is far more reliably determined and nonadherence may be addressed quickly. Directly observed medication administration may be compromised in practice settings that limit the ability of staff to observe the actions of the patient fully. One such example is in a restrictive housing unit, where medication may be administered at the cell through a small trap door. Directly observed administration is meaningful only when the cell door is opened to allow for full visibility of the patient. Directly observed administration, while admittedly reducing self-empowerment on the part of the patient, does make it far easier for the correctional psychiatrist to determine the effects and benefits of prescribed medication.

In the community, only limited attention is given to the frequency and timing of medications. Twice-daily and at-bedtime frequencies are commonly used in the community. However, their actual implementation in correctional settings may vary considerably from that in the community. Typical administration times in jails are driven by the practical needs of a facility linked to frequent court appearances. Morning medications may be administered well before 7 A.M.; bedtime medications may be administered at 6 P.M. Psychiatrists in such settings must work with custody staff to provide medications at clinically appropriate times. As-needed (PRN) medications may, in fact, rarely be administered in many correctional settings, given staff limits and the fact that the medications may be housed in a part of the facility well removed from the IP's cell. Care should be taken when prescribing psychotropic medications that rely on the intake of food (e.g., ziprasidone), as correctional settings may not adjust medication administration times based on food requirements (Burval et al., 2023). These factors may affect the patient's desire to take medications as prescribed and may also influence factors such as bioavailability and peak/trough timing.

The cost of psychotropic medications, particularly for patients with severe and persistent mental illness, is often ignored in the community, typically because the patient is on an insurance plan that traditionally covers most medications (e.g., Medicaid; Valuck et al., 2007). Often, there is a tendency in the community to use the newest branded medication at substantial incremental cost compared to older, generic medications. With rare exceptions, jails are funded entirely by the county and prisons by the state, typically with tight constraints. Given limited resources and frequently capped budgets, formulary restrictions may require that medications for a new IP undergo a review and potential replacement with generic medications of the same or a related drug class (see Chapter 27). Alternatively, IPs may be responsible for a copay. For example, although long-acting injectable antipsychotics can help in reducing the frequency of administration of antipsychotics, facilities may charge a fee for the administration of the medications (Burval et al., 2023).

Consistent with growing community concerns over the abuse of prescription medication, correctional settings present with significant abuse potential, in some ways consistent with the community and in other ways substantially divergent. The main psychopharmacological challenges have to do with stimulants and with sedative-hypnotics but also include medications rarely abused in the community. Beyond community concerns about potential overprescription of psychostimulants such as dextroamphetamine or methylphenidate, in jail or prison, there are concerns about diversion or extortion as well (Young & Cocallis, 2019). Sedative-hypnotics present similar concerns (see Chapter 30). Indeed, many correctional facilities and systems have policies prohibiting or severely limiting their use. Beyond these concerns are those consequent to the unique characteristics of jails and prisons, with the overall interdiction on illicit substances. As described in detail in Chapters 29 and 30, medications such as sedating antipsychotics (e.g., quetiapine) may be sought for their effects as sleep agents and bupropion (if crushed and inhaled nasally) for its effect as a stimulant (Aikoye et al., 2023). In contrast, there is a growing concern that precluding such agents as psychostimulants for the treatment of attention-deficit/hyperactivity disorder may lead to negative consequences (Young & Cocallis, 2019), including increased (rather than reduced) criminal behavior (e.g., Boland et al., 2020).

From jail to prison or from one prison to another

While the foregoing has focused on the initial admission from the community into a correctional setting, many similar issues apply when a patient transfers from a jail to a prison or from one prison to another. Preparation and review of transfer summary sheets and more detailed records are just as important in these situations and should be seen as the minimum standard in policy and in practice. Ideally, continuity of care and any concerns about diagnosis or treatment are best shared through direct communication. A telephone exchange between treating psychiatrists, in addition to review of documentation, is ideal.

Summary

Transition from the community to jail or prison or between correctional facilities is inherently stressful. It is also a time of significant risk of discontinuity in care management for people with serious mental illness. With thoughtful planning, however, correctional facilities and systems can develop and support policies and practices that not only minimize therapeutic disruption but also work to enhance therapeutic and functional outcomes.

REFERENCES

Aikoye, S., Basiru, T. O., Nwoye, I., Adereti, I., Asuquo, S., Ezeokoli, A., et al. (2023). Systematic review of abuse or overprescription of bupropion in American prisons and a synthesis of case reports on bupropion abuse in American prison and non-prison systems. *Cureus*, *15*(3), e36189.

American Academy of Psychiatry and the Law. (2018). Practice resource for prescribing in corrections. *Journal of the American Academy of Psychiatry and the Law*, *46*(2 Suppl.), S2–S50.

Boland, H., DiSalvo, M., Fried, R., Woodworth, K.Y., Wilens, T., Faraone, S.V., et al. (2020). A literature review and meta-analysis on the effects of ADHD medications on functional outcomes. *Journal of Psychiatric Research*, *123*, 21–30.

Bronson, J., Zimmer, S., & Berzofsky, M. (2017). *Drug use, dependence, and abuse among state prisoners and jail inmates, 2007–2009*. Bureau of Justice Statistics. https://www.bjs.gov/content/pub/pdf/dudaspji0709.pdf

Burval, J. K., Iuppa, C. A., Kriz, C. R., Lang, S.E., Nelson, L.A., Gramlich, N.A., et al. (2023). Barriers to access to psychiatric medications in Missouri county jails. *Mental Health Clinician*, *13*(5), 200–206.

Curran, J., Saloner, B., Winkelman, T. N. A., & Alexander, G. C. (2023). Estimated use of prescription medications among individuals incarcerated in jails and state prisons in the US. *Journal of American Medical Association Health Forum*, *4*(4), e230482.

Federal Bureau of Prisons Health Services. (2022). *National formulary part I*. https://www.bop.gov/resources/pdfs/2022_winter_formulary_part_1.pdf

Glancy, G. D., Ash, P., Bath, E. P., Buchanan, A., Fedoroff, P., Frierson, R.L., et al. (2015). AAPL practice guideline for the forensic assessment. *Journal of the American Academy of Psychiatry and the Law*, *43*(2 Suppl.), S3–53.

Kilian, R., Frasch, K., Steinert, T., Schepp, W., Weiser, P., Jaeger, S., et al. (2018). Cost-effectiveness of psychotropic polypharmacy in routine schizophrenia care. Results of the ELAN prospective observational trial. *Neurology, Psychiatry and Brain Research*, *30*, 47–55.

Kukreja, S., Kalra, G., Shah, N., & Shrivastava A. (2013). Polypharmacy in psychiatry: A review. *Mensa Sana Monographs*, *11*(1), 82–99.

Moeller, K. E., Kissack, J. C., Atayee, R. S., & Lee, K. C. (2017). Clinical interpretation of urine drug tests: What clinicians need to know about urine drug screens. *Mayo Clinic Proceedings*, *92*(5), 774–796.

Mojtabai, R., & Olfson, M. (2010). National trends in psychotropic medication polypharmacy in office-based psychiatry. *Archives of General Psychiatry*, *67*(1), 26–36.

Morris, N. P., & Zisman-Ilani, Y. (2022). Communication over incarceration: Improving care coordination between correctional and community mental health services. *Psychiatric Services*, *73*(12), 1409–1411.

Sarkar, S. (2017). Psychiatric polypharmacy, etiology and potential consequences. *Current Psychopharmacology*, *6*(1), 12–26.

Semahegn, A., Torpey, K., Manu, A., Assefa, N., Tesfaye, G., & Ankomah, A. (2020). Psychotropic medication non-adherence and its associated factors among patients with major psychiatric disorders: A systematic review and meta-analysis. *Systematic Reviews*, *9*(1), 17.

Stassen, H. H., Bachmann, S., Bridler, R., Cattapan, K., Herzig, D., Schneeberger, A., et al. (2022). Detailing the effects of polypharmacy in psychiatry: Longitudinal study of 320 patients hospitalized for depression or schizophrenia. *European Archives of Psychiatry and Clinical Neuroscience*, *272*(4), 603–619.

Valuck, R. J., Morrato, E. H., Dodd, S., Oderda, G., Haxby, D. G., Allen, R., & Medicaid Pharmacotherapy Research Consortium. (2007). How expensive is antipsychotic polypharmacy? Experience from five US state Medicaid programs. *Current Medical Research and Opinion*, *23*(10), 2567–2576.

Young, S., & Cocallis, K. M. (2019). Attention Deficit Hyperactivity Disorder (ADHD) in the prison system. *Current Psychiatry Reports*, *21*(6), 41.

19 Management of sleep complaints

Bernice S. Elger

Introduction

Incarcerated persons (IPs) often seek health care for sleep problems (Elger, 2004b; Kjelsberg & Hartvig, 2005; Nesset et al., 2011). More recently, there has been an increase in the number and quality of studies about sleep in incarcerated populations (Al-Khalil et al., 2024; Sfera et al., 2024; Sheppard & Hogan, 2022; Tussey et al., 2024). This includes work on the prevalence of insomnia and sleep complaints, as well as specific studies that explore treatment strategies using randomized controlled trials or mixed methods (An at al., 2019; Belleville et al., 2011; Dewa et al., 2015, 2017a, 2017b, 2018, 2024; Eichelman & Dorava, 2021; Elger, 2003; Elger & Sekera, 2009; Goudard et al., 2017; Lyu et al., 2015; Randall et al., 2019; Sylvia et al., 2021). This chapter will describe the relevant research and recommend best practices for the management of sleep complaints in correctional settings.

Community studies on insomnia management

According to studies on different continents, sleeplessness in the general population is common. Insomnia is reported in up to 50% of primary care patients and in nearly one third of the adult population worldwide (Boyle et al., 2022; Ellis et al., 2021; Ferini-Strambi et al., 2021; Mitchell et al., 2012; Perlis et al., 2021a, 2021b, 2022). In the United States, at least 10% of the population has been found to suffer from sleep problems (Kraus & Rabin, 2012; Sateia et al., 2000). The American College of Physicians advised to specifically screen and treat insomnia (Qaseem et al., 2016) in light of serious potential consequences such as increased risk of depression and hypertension (Cunnington et al., 2013). Impaired daytime functioning was reported by two thirds of persons suffering from insomnia (Ohayon & Lemoine, 2004a). Social, psychological, and medical conditions make some individuals more vulnerable than others. Insomnia complaints are more frequent in women; separated or divorced individuals; people who are less educated or unemployed; medically ill patients; those with recent stress; and those with depression, anxiety, or substance use (Elger, 2007; Hohagen et al., 1993; Ohayon & Lemoine, 2004b; Sateia & Nowell, 2004).

It is important to distinguish normal sleep variation from a sleep disorder. The American Sleep Disorders Association defines insomnia as "a repeated difficulty with sleep initiation, duration, consolidation, or quality that occurs despite adequate time and opportunity for sleep and results in some form of daytime impairment and lasting for at least one month" (Falloon et al., 2011). In the American Psychiatric Association's (APA's) *Diagnostic and Statistical Manual of Mental Disorders*, fifth edition, text revision (DSM-5-TR; APA, 2022), sleep–wake disorders encompass 10 conditions characterized by disturbed sleep and causing distress or impairment in daytime functioning: insomnia disorder, hypersomnolence disorder, narcolepsy, breathing-related sleep disorders, circadian rhythm sleep–wake disorders, non–rapid eye movement sleep arousal disorders, nightmare disorder, rapid eye movement sleep behavior disorder, restless legs syndrome, and substance/medication-induced sleep disorder. The DSM-5-TR allows for the diagnosis of sleep disorders even if they may be secondary to other mental or medical conditions (APA, 2022).

Experts generally agree that when managing insomnia complaints, physicians should seriously consider the patient's subjective perception of insomnia (Perlis et al., 2022; Sateia & Nowell, 2004). Acute (short-term) insomnia (less than 3 to 4 weeks) is often caused by situational stress, medical or psychological disorders, or circadian changes due to jet lag or shift work. Health care personnel should therefore discuss acute stress with patients and provide appropriate education. Short-term treatment strategies include sleep hygiene and the prescription of hypnotics, usually a benzodiazepine (BZD), if necessary (Cunnington et al., 2013; De Crescenzo et al., 2022).

In chronic insomnia (i.e., sleep problems that persist for more than 4 weeks), the dominant approach in the past has been pharmacological, most often with BZD receptor agonists (Morin & Benca, 2012; Sateia & Nowell, 2004). However, studies support that such medications alleviate symptoms only for a short time (De Crescenzo et al., 2022). After the first six weeks, the treatment effects of hypnotics degrade. Side effects of BZDs are well known and include the risks of habituation and tolerance, as well as paradoxical effects, falls, and cognitive impairment in the aging population (Champion et al., 2021; Ferini-Strambi et al., 2021; Markota et al., 2016; Mitchell et al., 2012; Perlis et al., 2022). Despite the shortcomings of pharmacological agents, nonpharmacological treatments remain insufficiently used. Cognitive-behavioral therapy (CBT) is effective and results in long-lasting and clinically significant improvement, whether used alone or in combination with pharmacological treatment. It has similar effect sizes to those of non-BZD hypnotics (Cunnington, 2013; Ferini-Strambi et al., 2021; Mitchell et al., 2012; Perlis et al., 2022;

Qaseem et al., 2016). Nonpharmacological treatments also benefit insomnia associated with medical or psychiatric illness. CBT does not necessarily require high personnel resources, as it can be used in individual or group therapeutic sessions or in the form of self-administered written or audiovisual material. Examples include stimulus control therapy, sleep restriction, sleep hygiene, paradoxical intention, progressive muscle relaxation, and cognitive therapy (Belleville et al., 2011; Mitchell et al., 2012; Morin & Benca, 2012; Qaseem et al., 2016; Sateia & Nowell, 2004).

Prevalence and causes of sleep problems in correctional settings

While most research about sleep disturbances in correctional settings is from Europe, similar findings have been reported elsewhere (Fakorede et al., 2023; Geng et al., 2021; Getachew et al., 2020; Li & Lai, 2019; Nkambule et al., 2023; Sheppard & Hogan, 2022). A recent review found prevalence rates that varied from 26% to 73% for insomnia and 43% to 88% for poor sleep quality in detention, with differences explained by methodology, geography, and gender (Sheppard & Hogan, 2022). A study of young detained persons in the United Kingdom demonstrated that while incarcerated, poor sleeping habits increased, and aggression correlated with reports of impaired quantity and quality of sleep (Ireland & Culpin, 2006). In a Swiss jail, 44% of patients seen in primary care consultations were diagnosed with insomnia, and only about half of them were substance users (Elger, 2004b). Among the non-substance-using insomnia patients, chronic forms of insomnia (longer than 3 weeks) were reported more often, so transitory adaptation difficulties were inadequate to explain their presentations. IPs who complained of insomnia were more often diagnosed with anxiety or depression than those without sleep complaints. Anxiety related to incarceration was the most frequently reported reason for sleep problems in various studies (Elger, 2004b; D'Aurizio et al., 2020; S. Zhang et al., 2023).

Jaeger and Monceau (1996) found high prescription rates for psychotropic drugs in French prisons, and two thirds were BZD and sedating antipsychotics. When comparing different French prisons, the authors showed significant variations in the quantity of psychotropic prescriptions. BZD and sedating antipsychotics were prescribed more often in jails than in posttrial detention centers, where IPs had access to more activities outside the cells, including work and opportunities to practice sports.

IPs often experience mental health disorders that are associated with insomnia. Posttraumatic stress disorder is common in IPs, whether preexisting or acquired (see Chapter 36). Other psychiatric morbidities, including depression, anxiety, and recent or current substance use, may develop or be exacerbated during incarceration.

However, sleep–wake disorders (in any setting) cannot simply be reduced to a secondary symptom of a mental disorder or substance use. Many consider chronic sleep problems in jails and prisons as a matter of injustice (Al-Khalil et al., 2024; Elumn et al., 2023, 2024; Leon-Jimenez, 2024; Sfera et al., 2024; Tussey et al., 2024; Yesuf et al., 2022). Other factors related to insomnia in IPs include excess time in cells, lack of physical activity, and daytime napping (Andersen et al., 2000; Bourgeois, 1997). Long periods of inactivity, especially at night when cells are closed early, may increase the subjective impression of a need to sleep longer than physiologically required (Jaeger & Monceau, 1996; Levin & Brown, 1975; Vasseur, 2001). A study by Rogers et al. (2003) suggests that conditions of confinement are a major reason for sleep disturbances, as detention may be associated with substantial fears about personal safety that in turn can cause hypervigilance. Those responsible for the management of sleep complaints in jails and prisons should thus keep in mind that, if the setting itself causes independent "situational" insomnia, treatment includes addressing the conditions of confinement wherever possible. Examples include offering sufficient activities outside the cell, such as work, education, and opportunities for physical activity.

Jaeger and Monceau's (1996) work interviewing both IPs and staff found that improving conditions of confinement in these ways led to decreased prescriptions of sleep medication. Staff observed IPs asking for more hypnotics and sedating medications in situations of increased stress, like anticipating sentencing, overcrowding, and interpersonal conflicts. About a third of the prison officers thought that hypnotic prescription led to more peaceful cohabitation. IPs reported that pharmacological interventions for sleep diminished suffering but also reduced feelings of aggression and dysphoria during the day. Ireland and Culpin's (2006) U.K. study replicated many of these findings.

Evidence-based management of sleep complaints in corrections

To be effective, management of sleep complaints in jails and prisons must take into account the causes of insomnia, including the conditions of confinement. The APA's (2016) practice guideline on psychiatric services in correctional settings proposes that IPs receive the care that *should be* available in the community, which echoes the equivalence principle set forth by the United Nations (1982). Medical ethics is to be respected independently of the legal status of a patient. IPs have the right to receive adequate treatment for serious medical needs (*Estelle v. Gamble*, 1975). The principle of equivalence of care also applies to insomnia evaluation and treatment. Perez-Sales (2019), taking a human rights–based approach, proposed an international standard of a minimum of 6 hours of continuous sleep per day in detention settings (Perez-Sales, 2019). Recent litigation over sleep deprivation has been observed in U.S. jails and prisons (Morris et al., 2021). However, the existing literature demonstrates that the evaluation of insomnia complaints in correctional settings often does not follow international standards of diligence. Various studies have shown benefit for nonpharmacological strategies (e.g., meditation, yoga, mindfulness, or CBT) for managing insomnia in correctional settings (An et al., 2019; Bartels et al., 2019; Ferszt et al., 2015; Griffiths & Hina, 2021; Kerekes et al., 2017; Nidich et al., 2016; Pralong et al., 2020; Sumter et al., 2009; J. Zhang et al., 2022), though CBT is underutilized (Randall et al., 2019).

Research suggests that the pharmacological management of insomnia complaints in non-substance-misusing IPs is insufficient (Elger, 2003, 2004a). A review of medical records indicated that most physicians did not question patients about sleep habits, sleep latency, and previous hypnotic use. Information about the daytime impact of insomnia was noted in only 7% of records. In most patients, insomnia improved only partially or not at all. Those whose insomnia did not respond or responded only partially to pharmacological treatment received the highest average number of hypnotic drugs (2.4 versus 1.4), suggesting that the medications selected were often ineffective.

Physicians working in correctional settings should respect the principles of medical ethics: beneficence, nonmaleficence, autonomy, and justice (see Chapter 12). In terms of beneficence, an adequate evaluation of insomnia complaints is necessary to make the right diagnosis and to provide adequate treatment (Qaseem et al., 2016). Nonmaleficence (i.e., the avoidance of harm) requires vigilant awareness that harm may result not only from side effects of pharmacological treatments but also from untreated insomnia (Aloni et al., 2021; Cunnington et al., 2013), including increased risks of self-harm, suicide, and aggression (Barker et al., 2016; Kerekes et al., 2017; Randall et al., 2019). In terms of autonomy, physicians should discuss potential harms and benefits with each patient (Elger, 2008). Such approaches respect patient rights and can increase adherence and improve treatment outcomes. From the perspective of justice, while overtreatment of insomnia complaints is medically and ethically problematic (Reeves, 2012), so is undertreatment, which includes both underprescription of medication and underutilization of evidence-based nonpharmacological treatments. Physicians may fear that IPs will misuse medication (Fay et al., 2024; Reeves, 2012). There is a tendency to ban BZDs from correctional settings and to instead use other agents (including antipsychotics and antidepressants), despite BZDs being recognized as the evidence-based treatment of acute insomnia in the community (Cunnington et al., 2013; De Crescenzo et al., 2022; Fay et al., 2024; Morin & Benca, 2012). Moreover, some alternative medications, especially neuroleptics, have important side effects, while their efficiency in various sleep disorders remains unclear (Maher & Theodore, 2012). If insomnia evaluation and treatment are not taken seriously in correctional settings, this is harmful to patients and may increase costs due to the possibly far-reaching consequences of undertreatment (Sateia & Nowell, 2004).

Evidence-based insomnia management in correctional institutions should include the following:

- *Sleep evaluation*: This includes a history of current and prior sleep complaints, previous medication intake, and a thorough review of symptoms and clinical examination to search for somatic or mental health comorbidities.
- *Improvement of the conditions of confinement*: Physicians have a duty to report public health problems (American Medical Association, 2016). They should inform prison and local public health authorities about inadequate prison conditions such as overcrowding, violence, qualitative and quantitative undernutrition (Wondimu et al., 2021), and lack of physical or other activities that, among other factors, contribute to insomnia in IPs. Health care personnel should also offer adequate therapies to help IPs cope with stress.
- *Nonpharmacological treatments*: Providing CBT and psychoeducation about sleep hygiene, relaxation techniques, and meditation to IPs may be the most cost-effective ways to promote healthy sleep patterns, as well as general mental health (Sumter et al., 2009). This may require training correctional physicians on CBT for insomnia and formally implementing education for IPs about sleep hygiene (Griffiths & Hina, 2021). Existing resources provide ready-to-use information about how to proceed and which material to use (Dewa et al., 2015, 2017a, 2017b, 2018, 2024; Falloon et al., 2011; Perlis et al., 2021b, 2022; Qaseem et al., 2016; Tamburello et al., 2022).
- *Pharmacological treatments*: Pharmacological treatment should be specific and address comorbidities associated with insomnia (Cameron et al., 2014; Eichelman & Dorava, 2021). Sedating antipsychotics and antidepressants should not be used routinely off-label for insomnia complaints. Patients must be informed about important side effects of alternative medications (e.g., non-BZD hypnotics and antihistamines) such as daytime sedation, weight gain, and anticholinergic side effects. Since sedating antidepressants are more toxic and less efficient than BZDs (Falloon et al., 2011), they are only justified if specific indications exist. In cases of acute insomnia, BZDs remain the first-choice medications. It is not justified to deny IPs appropriate pharmacological treatment because some of these drugs might be diverted. Different types of illicit substances enter correctional settings through many channels. Withholding medically indicated BZDs from IPs is often harmful because of the risk of using more dangerous alternatives available to them from the underground market (Elger, 2008). Given that the long-term efficacy of BZDs for insomnia is limited (De Crescenzo et al., 2022), short-term prescription with adequate follow-up is appropriate.

Summary

Sleep problems among IPs are common. Appropriate evaluation and treatment remain a challenge in correctional settings, but this is more a problem of adequate training than of resources. Correctional health professionals need appropriate education regarding insomnia evaluation and management. Guidelines should be based on the principle of equivalence of care and consider all evidence from research, both in the community and in correctional settings. Educational material from outside prisons exists and should be made available to IPs and health professionals. Priority should be given to improving the conditions of confinement and to nonpharmacological management strategies, but there is no evidence-based justification to replace BZD prescriptions with other agents like antipsychotics or antidepressants. The effective management of sleep complaints in correctional settings is consistent with ethical medical practice and will improve outcomes for patients and the facilities in which they reside.

REFERENCES

Al-Khalil, Z., Attarian, H., Dunietz, G. L., Gavidia Romero, R., Knutson, K., & Johnson, D. A. (2024). Sleep health inequities in vulnerable populations: Beyond sleep deserts. *Sleep Medicine X*, *7*, 100110.

Aloni, R., Levin, Y., Uziel, O., & Solomon, Z. (2021). Premature aging among trauma survivors—The longitudinal implications of sleep disruptions on telomere length and cognitive performance. *Journals of Gerontology: Series B, Psychological Sciences and Social Sciences*, *76*(2), 262–272.

American Medical Association. (2016). *Code of medical ethics—Chapter 8—Physician & the health of the community*. https://code-medical-ethics.ama-assn.org/chapters/physicians-health-community

American Psychiatric Association. (2016). *Psychiatric services in correctional facilities* (3rd ed.).

American Psychiatric Association. (2022). *Diagnostic and statistical manual of mental disorders* (5th ed., text rev.).

An, Y., Huang, Q., Zhou, Y., Zhou, Y., & Xu, W. (2019). Who can get more benefits? Effects of mindfulness training in long-term and short-term male prisoners. *International Journal of Offender Therapy and Comparative Criminology, 63*(13), 2318–2337.

Andersen, H. S., Sestoft, D., Lillebaek, T., Gabrielsen, G., Hemmingsen, R., & Kramp, P. (2000). A longitudinal study of prisoners on remand: Psychiatric prevalence, incidence and psychopathology in solitary vs. non-solitary confinement. *Acta Psychiatrica Scandinavica, 102*(1), 19–25.

Barker, L. F., Ireland, J. L., Chu, S., & Ireland, C. A. (2016). Sleep and its association with aggression among prisoners: Quantity or quality? *International Journal of Law and Psychiatry, 47*, 115–121.

Bartels, L., Oxman, L. N., & Hopkins, A. (2019). "I would just feel really relaxed and at peace": Findings from a pilot prison yoga program in Australia. *International Journal of Offender Therapy and Comparative Criminology, 63*(15–16), 2531–2549.

Belleville, G., Cousineau, H., Levrier, K., & St-Pierre-Delorme, M. E. (2011). Meta-analytic review of the impact of cognitive-behavior therapy for insomnia on concomitant anxiety. *Clinical Psychology Review, 31*(4), 638–652.

Bourgeois, D. (1997). Troubles du sommeil en milieu carcéral [Sleep disorders in prison]. *L'Encephale, 23*(3), 180–183.

Boyle, J. T., Vargas, I., Rosenfield, B., Grandner, M. A., & Perlis, M. L. (2022). Insomnia severity and degree of dysfunction: What is to be learned when these domains are discordant? *Behavioral Sleep Medicine, 20*(2), 164–172.

Cameron, C., Watson, D., & Robinson, J. (2014). Use of a synthetic cannabinoid in a correctional population for posttraumatic stress disorder-related insomnia and nightmares, chronic pain, harm reduction, and other indications: A retrospective evaluation. *Journal of Clinical Psychopharmacology, 34*(5), 559–564.

Champion, C., Novais, T., Dorey, J. M., Krolak-Salmon, P., & Lepetit, A. (2021). Réactions paradoxales aux benzodiazépines chez la personne âgée [Paradoxical reactions to benzodiazepines in the elderly]. *Geriatrie et Psychologie Neuropsychiatrie du Vieillissement, 19*(3), 305–312.

Cunnington, D. (2013). Non-benzodiazepine hypnotics: Do they work for insomnia? *BMJ, 346*, e8699.

Cunnington, D., Junge, M. F., & Fernando, A. T. (2013). Insomnia: Prevalence, consequences and effective treatment. *Medical Journal of Australia, 199*(8), S36–S40.

D'Aurizio, G., Caldarola, A., Ninniri, M., Avvantaggiato, M., & Curcio, G. (2020). Sleep quality and psychological status in a group of Italian prisoners. *International Journal of Environmental Research and Public Health, 17*(12), 4224.

De Crescenzo, F., D'Alo, G. L., Ostinelli, E. G., et al. (2022). Comparative effects of pharmacological interventions for the acute and long-term management of insomnia disorder in adults: A systematic review and network meta-analysis. *Lancet, 400*(10347), 170–184.

Dewa, L. H., Hassan, L., Shaw, J. J., & Senior, J. (2017a). Insomnia management in prisons in England and Wales: A mixed-methods study. *Journal of Sleep Research, 26*(3), 322–329.

Dewa, L. H., Hassan, L., Shaw, J. J., & Senior, J. (2017b). Trouble sleeping inside: A cross-sectional study of the prevalence and associated risk factors of insomnia in adult prison populations in England. *Sleep Medicine, 32*, 129–136.

Dewa, L. H., Hassan, L., Shaw, J., & Senior, J. (2018). Design of a treatment pathway for insomnia in prison settings in England: A modified Delphi study. *BMJ Open, 8*(8), e022406.

Dewa, L. H., Kyle, S. D., Hassan, L., Shaw, J., & Senior, J. (2015). Prevalence, associated factors and management of insomnia in prison populations: An integrative review. *Sleep Medicine Reviews, 24*, 13–27.

Dewa, L. H., Thibaut, B., Pattison, N., et al. (2024). Treating insomnia in people who are incarcerated: A feasibility study of a multicomponent treatment pathway. *Sleep Advances: A Journal of Sleep Research, 5*(1), zpae003.

Eichelman, B., & Dorava, A. (2021). Open outcome study of prazosin in a prison female population with traumatic dreams. *Journal of Correctional Health Care, 27*(4), 238–244.

Elger, B. S. (2003). Does insomnia in prison improve with time? Prospective study among remanded prisoners using the Pittsburgh Sleep Quality Index. *Medicine, Science, and the Law, 43*(4), 334–344.

Elger, B. S. (2004a). Management and evolution of insomnia complaints among non-substance-misusers in a Swiss remand prison. *Swiss Medical Weekly, 134*(3334), 486–499.

Elger, B. S. (2004b). Prevalence, types and possible causes of insomnia in a Swiss remand prison. *European Journal of Epidemiology, 19*(7), 665–677.

Elger, B. S. (2007). Insomnia in places of detention: A review of the most recent research findings. *Medicine, Science and the Law, 47*(3), 191–199.

Elger, B. S. (2008). Prisoners' insomnia: To treat or not to treat? Medical decision-making in places of detention. *Medicine, Science, and the Law, 48*(4), 307–316.

Elger, B. S., & Sekera, E. (2009). Prospective evaluation of insomnia in prison using the Pittsburgh Sleep Quality Index: Which are the factors predicting insomnia? *International Journal of Psychiatry in Clinical Practice, 13*(3), 206–217.

Ellis, J. G., Perlis, M. L., Espie, C. A., et al. (2021). The natural history of insomnia: Predisposing, precipitating, coping, and perpetuating factors over the early developmental course of insomnia. *Sleep, 44*(9), zsab095.

Elumn, J. E., Li, P., Lytell, M. S., Garcia, M., Wang, E. A., & Klar Yaggi, H. (2024). "What if that's your last sleep?" A qualitative exploration of the trauma of incarceration and sleep. *Sleep Advances: A Journal of the Sleep Research Society, 5*(1), zpad055.

Elumn, J. E., Saeed, G. J., Aminawung, J., et al. (2023). The sleep justice study—A prospective cohort study assessing sleep as a cardiometabolic risk factor after incarceration: a protocol paper. *BMC Public Health, 23*(1), 2107.

Estelle v. Gamble, 429 U.S. 97 (1976).

Fakorede, O. O., Onifade, P. O., Majekodunmi, O. E., & DadeMatthews, A. O. (2023). Nigerian prisoners' experience: Prison circumstances, family support and sleep quality. *International Journal of Prisoner Health, 19*(4), 524–535.

Falloon, K., Arroll, B., Elley, C. R., & Fernando, A., 3rd. (2011). The assessment and management of insomnia in primary care. *BMJ, 342*, d2899.

Fay, C., Bonsergent, M., Saillard, J., Huon, J. F., & Prot-Labarthe, S. (2024). Exploration of the barriers and enablers of benzodiazepines deprescribing in prisons: A qualitative study among health and social care professionals. *Basic & Clinical Pharmacology & Toxicology, 134*(1), 28–38.

Ferini-Strambi, L., Auer, R., Bjorvatn, B., et al. (2021). Insomnia disorder: Clinical and research challenges for the 21st century. *European Journal of Neurology, 28*(7), 2156–2167.

Ferszt, G. G., Miller, R. J., Hickey, J. E., Maull, F., & Crisp, K. (2015). The impact of a mindfulness based program on perceived stress, anxiety, depression and sleep of incarcerated women. *International Journal of Environmental Research and Public Health, 12*(9), 11594–11607.

Geng, F., Wang, J., Wen, C., Shao, Y., Wu, J., & Fan, F. (2021). Prevalence and correlates of sleep problems among Chinese prisoners. *Social Psychiatry and Psychiatric Epidemiology, 56*(4), 671–678.

Getachew, Y., Azale, T., & Necho, M. (2020). Poor sleep quality and associated factors among prisoners of the Diredawa

correctional facility in eastern Ethiopia. *Annals of General Psychiatry, 19*, 40.
Goudard, A., Lalande, L., Bertin, C., Sautereau, M., Le Borgne, M., & Cabelguenne, D. (2017). Sleep disorders and therapeutic management: A survey in a French population of prisoners. *Journal of Correctional Health Care, 23*(2), 193–202.
Griffiths, C., & Hina, F. (2021). Prisoner's insomnia prevalence, insomnia associated factors and interventions with sleep as an outcome: A review and narrative analysis. *International Journal of Prisoner Health, 18*(1), 27–42.
Hohagen, F., Rink, K., Kappler, C., et al. (1993). Prevalence and treatment of insomnia in general practice. A longitudinal study. *European Archives of Psychiatry and Clinical Neuroscience, 242*(6), 329–336.
Ireland, J. L., & Culpin, V. (2006). The relationship between sleeping problems and aggression, anger, and impulsivity in a population of juvenile and young offenders. *Journal of Adolescent Health: Official Publication of the Society for Adolescent Medicine, 38*(6), 649–655.
Jaeger, M., & Monceau, M. (1996). *La consommation des médicaments psychotropes en prison*. Ramonville Saint-Agne Editions Erès.
Kerekes, N., Fielding, C., & Apelqvist, S. (2017). Yoga in correctional settings: A randomized controlled study. *Frontiers in Psychiatry, 8*, 204.
Kjelsberg, E., & Hartvig, P. (2005). Can morbidity be inferred from prescription drug use? Results from a nation-wide prison population study. *European Journal of Epidemiology, 20*(7), 587–592.
Kraus, S. S., & Rabin, L. A. (2012). Sleep America: Managing the crisis of adult chronic insomnia and associated conditions. *Journal of Affective Disorders, 138*(3), 192–212.
Leon-Jimenez, F. E. (2024). Health in persons deprived of their liberty in South America: A painful reflection of our public health. *Annals of Global Health, 90*(1), 29.
Levin, B. H., & Brown, W. E. (1975). Susceptibility to boredom of jailers and law enforcement officers. *Psychological Reports, 36*(1), 190.
Li, M. R., & Lai, H. L. (2019). Insomnia and its associated factors in incarcerated adults: A cross-sectional study. *Nursing & Health Sciences, 21*(3), 330–335.
Lyu, S. Y., Chi, Y. C., Farabee, D., et al. (2015). Psychological distress in an incarcerated juvenile population. *Journal of the Formosan Medical Association = Taiwan yi zhi, 114*(11), 1076–1081.
Maher, A. R., & Theodore, G. (2012). Summary of the comparative effectiveness review on off-label use of atypical antipsychotics. *Journal of Managed Care Pharmacy: JMCP, 18*(5 Suppl. B), 1–20.
Markota, M., Rummans, T. A., Bostwick, J. M., & Lapid, M. I. (2016). Benzodiazepine use in older adults: Dangers, management, and alternative therapies. *Mayo Clinic Proceedings, 91*(11), 1632–1639.
Mitchell, M. D., Gehrman, P., Perlis, M., & Umscheid, C. A. (2012). Comparative effectiveness of cognitive behavioral therapy for insomnia: A systematic review. *BMC Family Practice, 13*(1), 40.
Morin, C. M., & Benca, R. (2012). Chronic insomnia. *Lancet, 379*(9821), 1129–1141.
Morris, N. P., Holliday, J. R., & Binder, R. L. (2021). Litigation over sleep deprivation in U.S. jails and prisons. *Psychiatric Services, 72*(10), 1237–1239.
Nesset, M. B., Rustad, A. B., Kjelsberg, E., Almvik, R., & Bjorngaard, J. H. (2011). Health care help seeking behaviour among prisoners in Norway. *BMC Health Services Research, 11*, 301.
Nidich, S., O'Connor, T., Rutledge, T., et al. (2016). Reduced trauma symptoms and perceived stress in male prison inmates through the transcendental meditation program: A randomized controlled trial. *Permanente Journal, 20*(4), 16–17.
Nkambule, E., Wella, K., & Mbakaya, B. C. (2023). Voice of incarcerated male youths in Malawi's semi-urban prisons: A qualitative study. *BMJ Open, 13*(10), e075925.
Ohayon, M. M., & Lemoine, P. (2004a). Daytime consequences of insomnia complaints in the French general population. *Encephale, 30*(3), 222–227.
Ohayon, M. M., & Lemoine, P. (2004b). Sleep and insomnia markers in the general population. *Encephale, 30*(2), 135–140.
Perez-Sales, P. (2019). The 6/24 rule: A review and proposal for an international standard of a minimum of six hours of continuous sleep in detention settings. *Torture, 29*(2), 1–10.
Perlis, M. L., Morales, K. H., Vargas, I., et al. (2021a). The natural history of insomnia: Does sleep extension differentiate between those that do and do not develop chronic insomnia? *Journal of Sleep Research, 30*(5), e13342.
Perlis, M. L., Pigeon, W. R., Grandner, M. A., et al. (2021b). Why treat insomnia? *Journal of Primary Care and Community Health, 12*, 21501327211014084.
Perlis, M. L., Posner, D., Riemann, D., Bastien, C. H., Teel, J., & Thase, M. (2022). Insomnia. *Lancet, 400*(10357), 1047–1060.
Pralong, D., Renaud, A., Secretan, A. D., et al. (2020). Nurse-led mind-body relaxation intervention in prison: A multiperspective mixed-method evaluation. *Nursing Outlook, 68*(5), 637–646.
Qaseem, A., Kansagara, D., Forciea, M. A., Cooke, M., Denberg, T. D., & Clinical Guidelines Committee of the American College of Physicians. (2016). Management of chronic insomnia disorder in adults: A clinical practice guideline from the American College of Physicians. *Annals of Internal Medicine, 165*(2), 125–133.
Randall, C., Nowakowski, S., & Ellis, J. G. (2019). Managing acute insomnia in prison: Evaluation of a "one-shot" cognitive behavioral therapy for insomnia (CBT-I) intervention. *Behavioral Sleep Medicine, 17*(6), 827–836.
Reeves, R. (2012). Guideline, education, and peer comparison to reduce prescriptions of benzodiazepines and low-dose quetiapine in prison. *Journal of Correctional Health Care, 18*(1), 45–52.
Rogers, R., Jackson, R. L., Salekin, K. L., & Neumann, C. S. (2003). Assessing Axis I symptomatology on the SADS-C in two correctional samples: The validation of subscales and a screen for malingered presentations. *Journal of Personality Assessment, 81*(3), 281–290.
Sateia, M. J., Doghramji, K., Hauri, P. J., & Morin, C. M. (2000). Evaluation of chronic insomnia. An American Academy of Sleep Medicine review. *Sleep, 23*(2), 243–308.
Sateia, M. J., & Nowell, P. D. (2004). Insomnia. *Lancet, 364*(9449), 1959–1973.
Sfera, A., Thomas, K. A., Ogunjale, I. A., Jafri, N., & Bota, P. G. (2024). Insomnia in forensic detainees: Is salience network the common pathway for sleep, neuropsychiatric, and neurodegenerative disorders? *Journal of Clinical Medicine, 13*(6), 1961.
Sheppard, N., & Hogan, L. (2022). Prevalence of insomnia and poor sleep quality in the prison population: A systematic review. *Journal of Sleep Research, 31*(6), e13677.
Sumter, M. T., Monk-Turner, E., & Turner, C. (2009). The benefits of meditation practice in the correctional setting. *Journal of Correctional Health Care, 15*(1), 47–57.
Sylvia, L. G., Chudnofsky, R., Fredriksson, S., et al. (2021). A pilot study of a stress management program for incarcerated veterans. *Military Medicine, 186*(11–12), 1061–1065.
Tamburello, A., Penn, J., Ford, E., et al. (2022). The American Academy of Psychiatry and the Law practice resource for prescribing in corrections. *Journal of the American Academy of Psychiatry and the Law, 50*, S1–S62.

Tussey, E. J., Perez, G. R., & Lynch, S. M. (2024). Sleepless behind bars: The connection between mental health, environment, and sleep among women in jail. *Sleep Advances*, *5*(1), zpae012.

United Nations. (1982). *Principles of Medical Ethics relevant to the role of health personnel, particularly physicians, in the protection of prisoners and detainees against torture and other cruel, inhuman or degrading treatment or punishment.* http://www.ohchr.org/EN/ProfessionalInterest/Pages/MedicalEthics.aspx

Vasseur, V. (2001). *Médecin chef à la prison de la santé.* Le Livre de Poche.

Wondimu, W., Girma, B., Sinaga, M., & Taye, A. (2021). Undernutrition and associated factors among incarcerated people in Mizan prison institute, southwest Ethiopia. *PLoS One*, *16*(5), e0251364.

Yesuf, Y. M., Birhan, A. A., Birara, A. G., Adimas, B. D., Bezabh, A. B., & Agmase, N. G. (2022). Prevalence and correlates of mental illness among inmates in North-western Ethiopia: A new look into the roles of rehabilitation service use. *Frontiers in Psychiatry*, *13*, 983355.

Zhang, J., Zheng, Z., Wang, L., et al. (2022). Effectiveness of a 4-day mindfulness-based intervention in a 2-month follow-up for Chinese Incarcerated people. *Behavior Therapy*, *53*(5), 981–994.

Zhang, S., He, J., Yang, Q., et al. (2023). Anxiety during the COVID-19 pandemic in prisoners who had high risks to suffer from mood disorders: A longitudinal study before and during the COVID-19. *Stress and Health*, *39*(1), 162–168.

20
Evaluation of malingering

James L. Knoll IV and Vikram Kumar

Introduction

Malingered mental illness in the carceral setting poses a complicated dilemma. Presentation may differ, detection strategies used elsewhere may not work in carceral settings, and inaccurate determinations may have serious consequences. Detection requires a thorough knowledge of genuine psychiatric illness characteristics, a systematic approach to evaluation, identification of objective indicators, and the use of scientifically validated psychological tests when necessary (Knoll & Resnick, 2017; Sweet et al., 2021). It is important that carceral clinicians investigate possibilities such as factitious disorder, dissimulation, and false imputation (Bellman et al., 2022). Carceral clinicians must be aware of their own misassumptions and biases about incarcerated persons' (IPs') response styles (Rogers et al., 2024), particularly in settings where IPs may have to convey their symptoms more forcefully to receive needed care.

Definition and differential diagnosis of malingering

The *Diagnostic and Statistical Manual of Mental Disorders*, fifth edition, text revision (DSM-5-TR) places malingering under "additional issues that require clinical attention" (American Psychiatric Association [APA], 2022). The DSM-5-TR defines malingering as the intentional production of false or grossly exaggerated physical or psychological symptoms, motivated by an external incentive (APA, 2022). In conditions such as wartime, where illnesses may be feigned, malingering is described as a potential adaptation mechanism. This phenomenon should be kept in mind when considering malingering in today's harsh carceral setting.

Malingering is not rare in carceral settings (Rogers, 2008a), but the prevalence rates of malingering are highly location driven and difficult to know with certainty (Fovet et al., 2024; Pierson et al., 2011). A study of individuals in jail found malingering in more than 66% of suspected cases (McDermott & Sokolov, 2009). Gottfried and colleagues (2017) estimated a 20% to 30% base rate of malingering in criminal forensic evaluations.

Malingering requires differentiation from factitious disorder, where illness is simulated with a motive to assume the sick role, also thought of as an internal (i.e., psychological) incentive (Kanaan & Wessely, 2010). In contrast to malingering, factitious disorders are always associated with an internal incentive. While the false or exaggerated symptoms are consciously reported, the internal incentive is assuming the sick role (Bass & Halligan, 2014). Malingering may be divided into three categories: pure malingering, partial malingering, and false imputation (Resnick & Knoll, 2018). In *pure malingering*, an individual feigns a nonexistent disorder. *Partial malingering* involves conscious exaggeration of actual symptoms. *False imputation* refers to ascribing genuine symptoms to a consciously recognized, unrelated cause. In comparison to pure malingerers who falsely report symptoms they have never experienced, false imputers understand how genuine symptoms are expressed and may be particularly difficult to detect (Bellman et al., 2022).

IPs with serious mental illness may exaggerate symptoms to avoid stressful environments like punitive isolation or to gain access to the protected environment of a mental health unit if being harassed by others. Motives beyond adaptation may include obtaining medications to misuse, avoiding disciplinary actions, or gaining transfers elsewhere. IPs who malinger may be transferred to carceral mental health units, where they are sometimes able to take advantage of IPs with genuine mental illness (Costopoulos et al., 2021).

Difficulties detecting malingering in carceral settings

Malingering assessment (McDermott, 2012) includes comprehensive clinical evaluation, testing, behavioral observation, collection of collateral information, and record review to avoid false-positive attribution (DeClue, 2002). Careful clinical evaluation is vital, and standardized testing can lend further validity (Vitacco & Rogers, 2010; see Chapter 67). Standardized instruments including the Structured Interview of Reported Symptoms, second edition, and the Minnesota Multiphasic Personality Inventory, second edition, may help in screening (Drob et al., 2009). A performance validity test (e.g., the Test of Malingered Memory [TOMM]) may be considered in challenging scenarios (Sweet et al., 2021). The Personality Assessment Inventory contains profile distortion indicators that have been found useful in forensic and carceral settings (Paulino et al., 2024). It is important to note that currently available tests cannot identify the motivation to feign or exaggerate symptoms and thus cannot definitively diagnose malingering; they are one part of a comprehensive clinical evaluation.

Table 20.1 Clinical factors warranting caution before diagnosing malingering in a carceral setting

- No clear external incentive
- Extensive history of psychiatric treatment
- Not self-referred
- Collateral information suggests psychiatric illness
- Is defensive, minimizes illness, or opposes treatment
- Shows improvement on psychiatric medication
- Does well or improves in a mental health unit
- Intellectual disability
- Frequently requires special observations
- High number of objective suicide risk factors
- History of serious traumatic brain injury

An incorrect diagnosis of malingering may have long-lasting detrimental effects for an IP with genuine mental illness and may lead to adverse outcomes such as improper placement, disciplinary sanctions, or treatment withdrawal. A finding of malingering in the carceral setting does not rule out the presence of genuine psychopathology. *Table 20.1* lists clinical factors to consider prior to reaching a conclusion of malingering (Knoll, 2006, 2009; Kupers, 2004).

Clinical assessment of malingering

Detection of malingering requires a thorough knowledge of genuine psychiatric symptoms and their presentations. This enables more accurate differentiation of malingered symptoms from genuine symptoms. Both genuine psychopathology and malingering can co-occur, and the clinician must delineate the relative presence of each (Sweet et al., 2021). Detection solely based on diagnostic criteria has resulted in low true-positive rates (Vitacco et al., 2007). The ideal approach includes a collaborative model to identify clear external incentives, serial unstructured assessments, observations over time, and select structured tests.

Psychosis

Hallucinations and delusions may both be part of a malingered presentation of psychosis. IPs should be questioned in detail about atypical hallucinations with nonleading questions about content, vividness, and other characteristics (Knoll & Resnick, in press). Being readily identifiable and therefore reproducible, hallucinations are the most widely reported symptoms in patients malingering psychosis (Bellman et al., 2022).

Genuine auditory hallucinations can be conversational or brief, and the content may be culturally dependent (Luhrman et al., 2015). Research suggests that many psychotic patients hear voices both internally and externally, so questioning whether the voices are inside or outside the head can lead to inconclusive findings (McCarthy-Jones & Resnick, 2014). Typical auditory hallucinations are experienced multiple times during the day and last seconds to hours. Individuals tend to report voices sounding unlike their own and usually belonging to someone recognizable. Up to 44% of individuals report having auditory hallucinations as "ideas inside their head" rather than voices heard from outside (McCarthy-Jones & Resnick, 2014). Upon receiving treatment, individuals report that auditory hallucinations become less distressing in about a month and less frequent and more controllable within 6 months (Schneider et al., 2011). Auditory hallucinations with atypical features are reported in less than 5% of patients (McCarthy-Jones & Resnick, 2014). Atypical voices include hearing a voice whose normal speaking tone is yelling, hearing just women's or children's voices, and never hearing the same voice twice. Other atypical presentations include claiming to hear voices of animals, robotic-sounding voices, voices that refer to the individual as "Mr." or "Mrs.," and voices heard whenever a window is opened (Stephane et al., 2006).

Persons experiencing genuine command auditory hallucinations frequently have noncommand hallucinations, as well as delusions (Thompson et al., 1992). Further, command hallucinations are rarely obeyed in the absence of other psychological variables (e.g., beliefs about the voices, coexisting delusions; Braham et al., 2004). Isolated command hallucinations without other psychotic symptoms should raise concerns about malingering. Up to 90% of persons who experience auditory hallucinations report having coping strategies such as taking extra medications, praying, sleeping, seeking company, or instructing the voices to go away (McCarthy-Jones & Resnick, 2014). Increased frequency of auditory hallucinations is reported by individuals when alone (McCarthy-Jones & Resnick, 2014). Malingerers may report hallucinations of implausible language or having themes that provide justification for illegal activity. For example, an IP charged with smuggling contraband claimed hearing voices that said, "Tell your girlfriend to smuggle in a cell phone." In a carceral setting, the possibility of genuine stress-induced psychotic symptoms should be carefully considered.

The most common symptom reported by individuals malingering psychosis are visual hallucinations (Bellman et al., 2022). Dramatic or otherwise atypical visual hallucinations should arouse suspicion (APA, 2022; Bellman et al., 2022). Malingerers report visual hallucinations more often than genuinely psychotic persons do (Cornell & Hawk, 1989). Visual hallucinations are usually of normal-sized people and seen in color, while malingerers may report monochromic or black-and-white images (Bellman et al., 2022; Green & Rosenfeld, 2011). Hallucinations of small people (i.e., Lilliputian hallucinations) may occur with alcohol use or central nervous system pathology (Cohen et al., 1994). Reports of visual hallucinations should prompt consideration of the possibility of substance use. Substance-induced visual hallucinations are seen better with the eyes closed or in darkened surroundings (Bellman et al., 2022). Unformed hallucinations, such as light flashes, shadows, or moving objects, are typically associated with neurologic disease or substance use (Cummings & Miller, 1987; Mitchell & Vierkant, 1991). Genuine olfactory hallucinations are present in 13% to 17% of persons with schizophrenia (Langdon et al., 2011) and are likely to be of unpleasant odors and tastes (Goodwin & Rosenthal, 1971). Olfactory hallucinations of pleasant odors or tastes are atypical and should arouse suspicion of malingering (McCarthy-Jones & Resnick, 2014).

Careful assessment of delusions is also necessary when considering malingering. Genuine delusions typically conform to the DSM-5-TR subtypes listed under delusional disorder (APA, 2022); they involve erotomanic, grandiose, jealous, or persecutory themes (Spitzer, 1992). The prevalence of delusional disorder among IPs is substantially greater than in the community, and persecutory delusions are among the most common subtype (Tamburello et al., 2015). Persecutory delusions are more likely to be acted on than the other types (Wessely et al., 1993). Genuine delusional systems reflect the intelligence level of the individual in terms of complexity and sophistication. Delusions of nihilism, poverty, disease, and guilt are commonly seen in depressive psychoses. Delusions with technical content (e.g., computer chips, electronic devices) occur 7 times more frequently in men than in women (Kraus, 1994). Malingerers are more likely to claim a sudden onset or disappearance of a delusion (Bellman et al., 2022). In contrast, genuine delusions usually take weeks to develop and much longer to resolve. The duration of existing delusions is also a potential indicator of treatment response time; longer held delusions may take longer to treat (Bellman et al., 2022). The resolution of genuine delusions follows a course of gradual surrender, along with the stabilization of the psychosis. First, the delusion will become less relevant. Later, the individual gradually relinquishes the belief after adequate treatment (Sacks et al., 1974).

Persons with genuine psychosis often demonstrate other symptoms such as disordered speech, odd behavior, or paranoia (Harrow et al., 2003). Observations of IPs' overall functioning in the carceral setting typically confirm this correlation, but there are exceptions. One exception is the patient with chronic schizophrenia who has grown accustomed to the delusions and may no longer behave in a corresponding manner. Another complicated scenario involves pure delusional disorders, where individuals may behave relatively normally except in regard to their circumscribed delusion. For example, an individual with somatic delusions may make frequent requests of the medical team (González-Rodriguez & Seeman, 2020), which can be easily misperceived as malingering if not carefully assessed. When questioned regarding delusional content, malingerers are more likely than others to show hypersensitivity, react confrontationally, or be defensive (Bellman et al., 2022).

Cognitive symptoms

Malingerers may feign intellectual deficits, giving incorrect answers to questions that an individual with a genuine, serious neurocognitive disorder could answer correctly (Sherman et al., 2020; Slick et al., 1999). They may claim impairments inconsistent with genuine memory impairment, such as long-term memory impairment that is worse than short-term impairment (Soliman & Resnick, 2010; Sweet et al., 2021). It is important to keep in mind that persons with genuine intellectual disabilities can exaggerate cognitive deficits, and persons of normal intellectual ability may successfully feign on intelligence tests (Graue et al., 2007). Multiple tests of effort are recommended for accuracy and to decrease false positives, in addition to obtaining collateral data (Victor & Boone, 2007). In particular, the TOMM has demonstrated a high rate of success in detecting malingering in groups of subjects with intellectual disabilities (Shandera et al., 2010).

The detection of malingering may prove challenging when IPs have genuine intellectual disabilities, and they may be falsely identified as showing poor effort on cognitive tests (Salekin et al., 2010; Salekin & Doane, 2009). Furthermore, there is considerable overlap between behaviors exhibited by individuals with intellectual disabilities and malingerers. For example, averted gaze, hesitancy in speech with long pauses, and abrupt and sparing answers can be seen in both groups (Everington et al., 2007). Therefore, careful consideration must be used when diagnosing malingering in IPs with intellectual disabilities (see Chapter 57). Collateral information such as past IQ testing and school records may be helpful when considering such cases.

Clinical indicators of malingering

Certain response styles during the clinical interview may help differentiate genuine from malingered mental illness (Walczyk et al., 2018). Malingerers may repeat questions, be evasive, or answer "I don't know" to straightforward questions (Knoll & Resnick, 2006). Malingerers are more likely to thrust forward or call attention to their illness, unlike individuals with genuine schizophrenia (Ritson & Forrest, 1970). Malingerers may thwart attempts at assessment by demonstrating extreme hostility or intimidation so that the assessment is prematurely terminated and detection is avoided. Malingerers are unlikely to imitate successfully the subtle signs of schizophrenia, such as negative symptoms (e.g., flat affect, alogia). Exceptions to this include IPs with a history of genuine schizophrenia or those who have become familiar with these symptoms by observing others with genuine psychosis.

Malingerers may be asked about improbable symptoms to see if they are endorsed (Rogers, 2018; Walczyk et al., 2018). For example, a suspected malingerer may be asked: "When people talk to you, do you see the words they speak spelled out?" (Miller, 2001). Malingerers may give a false or incomplete history, so it is critical to compare current self-reports with descriptions in health records (Soliman & Resnick, 2010; Sweet et al., 2021). Inconsistencies between self-report and behavioral observations require investigation and can be internal or external. Internal inconsistencies exist when an individual reports severe symptoms such as mental confusion or memory loss but can give multiple examples of the same. External inconsistencies occur between the self-reported level of functioning and others' observations. As noted above, caution is advised when observing behaviors of patients with intellectual disabilities, as there is considerable overlap in behaviors between those with genuine and malingered presentations.

Comprehensive malingering evaluation

Because of the complexities and potential consequences involved, a comprehensive evaluation is recommended when malingering is suspected (Resnick et al., 2017; Rogers et al., 2010; Sweet et al., 2021), the outline of which is given in *Table 20.2*. Records and collateral data should be reviewed prior to the interview, with careful consideration of supporting or refuting factors. The interview may need to be prolonged since fatigue diminishes the ability to maintain feigned symptoms (Anderson et al., 1959). Interview technique is critical in the detection of malingering, and it is important to refrain from verbal or nonverbal communications of suspicion (McDermott & Sokolov, 2009). The evaluation should begin with open-ended questions because asking directly about specific symptoms may provide clues (Soliman & Resnick, 2010). Evaluators can use questions about improbable or atypical symptoms to probe further (Knoll & Resnick, in press). Revisiting previously answered questions at a different time may elicit different responses in malingerers. Malingerers may employ different styles such as symptom exaggeration, reduced effort, and dissimulation (Rogers & Shuman, 2005). Atypical symptom reports must be considered contextually. In particularly difficult cases, evaluators can use a technique called "set shifting," which involves interspersing malingering detection questions with history taking, distractor questions, or even informal conversation. This may distract persons who are malingering and reveal important data (Drob & Berger, 1987). When questions are asked in a rapid fashion, individuals who are malingering may provide conflicting responses. Caution is advised when using this method in IPs with intellectual disabilities (Knoll & Resnick, in press).

Table 20.2 Comprehensive malingering evaluation in carceral settings

- Review psychiatric records
- Review relevant collateral information (e.g., offender files, staff observations)
- Conduct behavioral observations (over time and/or on inpatient unit)
- Conduct clinical interview(s) (may require several and/or extended length)
- Analyze clinical indicators of malingering
- Identify plausible external incentive(s)
- Conduct psychological testing if necessary (e.g., MMPI-2, SIRS-2, PAI, TOMM)
- Consider simultaneous presence of both malingering and genuine illness
- Meet with forensic clinician team to review and consolidate findings
- Support conclusion of malingering with multiple factual bases

Note. MMPI-2 = Minnesota Multiphasic Personality Inventory, 2nd edition; PAI = Personality Assessment Inventory; SIRS-2 = Structured Interview of Reported Symptoms, 2nd edition; TOMM = Test of Malingered Memory.

Challenging clinical scenarios

Two relatively common clinical challenges related to malingering in the carceral setting are feigned mental wellness (i.e., dissimulation) and so-called manipulative suicide threats.

Dissimulation

Dissimulation, or "faking good," is the concealment of genuine symptoms of mental illness to portray psychological health. In cases of malingering, a clear external incentive is apparent or identified through a comprehensive assessment. However, in cases of dissimulation, the incentives may be hard to recognize, even after thorough investigation (Bellman et al., 2022). The denial of psychiatric symptoms has been reported anecdotally in persons who have committed crimes (Diamond, 1994), but there is little research on individuals suppressing signs of mental illness (Rogers, 2008b). Some IPs may feel a greater sense of control by alleging that they faked past symptoms (Caruso et al., 2003). Other reasons IPs may dissimulate include avoiding the stigma and consequences of a mental illness diagnosis, fear of involuntary treatment, fear of harassment and coercion by peers, or a desire for more favorable housing or work assignments within the carceral system.

"Manipulation" versus suicide

Considering whether a patient is feigning suicidal intent is a common and necessary task for carceral clinicians, but it is also among the most difficult clinical challenges they face (Obegi, 2020; see also Chapters 51 and 52). Unfortunately, there is no evidence that feigned suicidal intent can be easily or reliably distinguished from genuine suicidal intent (Freedenthal, 2007). It is important that carceral clinicians be aware of the heterogeneity observed in individuals who attempt or complete suicide. Those who attempt suicide in a carceral setting are more likely to have a history of violent offending, trauma, substance use, and mental illness (Favril et al., 2020). Thus, when confronting possible feigned suicidality among IPs, an evidence-based, systematic suicide risk assessment is warranted, along with an approach following a stress–vulnerability model (Knoll, 2010; Scott et al., 2023).

The DSM-5-TR divides self-harm into "suicidal behavior" and "nonsuicidal self-injury" based on intent (APA, 2022). In nonsuicidal self-injury, there is intentional self-harming through gestures such as cutting to induce pain without suicidal intent. While psychiatry has tools for detecting feigned symptoms (Rogers, 2008a), there are no reliable tools for predicting low-base-rate behaviors such as suicide. This is precisely why the standard of care is to assess risk, not predict behavior (Simon, 2004). In carceral settings, self-harming behavior is a significant phenomenon and contributes to overall morbidity. Recent estimates place the prevalence of self-harm at 5% to 6% in male IPs and about 20% to 24% in female IPs. The carceral setting alone significantly raises suicide risk (Favril et al., 2020). Self-harm and suicidal behavior can impact carceral staff and overburden the system. From a clinical standpoint, self-injurious behavior in IPs is very challenging and raises concerns about suicide risk, personality disorder, and manipulative intent (see Chapter 52). These factors must be considered carefully to avoid making a premature conclusion of manipulation or malingering.

The term "deliberate self-harm" indicates self-harming behavior regardless of suicidal intent. An individual may simultaneously possess a desire to self-harm *and* a desire to commit suicide. Deliberate self-harm may risk accidental death or may transform into suicidal behavior over time. Avoidable risk may arise when persons who have previously engaged in instrumental suicidal behavior are erroneously dismissed as manipulative (Berman, 2006; Skeem et al., 2006). Self-mutilation and suicide attempts cannot be easily differentiated, even when patients are questioned about suicidal intent (Konrad et al., 2007). This fact underscores the importance of systematic suicide risk assessment on a case-by-case basis (see Chapter 51).

Summary

The detection of malingering in carceral settings is necessary to ensure the judicious use of limited treatment resources and to bring diagnostic accuracy to assessments. A comprehensive, systematic approach is required. The clinician must assemble evidence from a thorough evaluation, clinical records, collateral data, and psychological testing when necessary. A conclusion of malingering should be supported with multiple factual bases. The carceral setting provides many unique challenges to detecting malingered mental illness. The finding that an IP has malingered symptoms does not rule out the presence of true mental illness, and a determination of malingering should not exclude the individual from receiving needed mental health services.

REFERENCES

American Psychiatric Association. (2022). *Diagnostic and statistical manual of mental disorders* (5th ed., text rev.).

Anderson, E. W., Trethowan, W. H., & Kenna, J. C. (1959). An experimental investigation of simulation and pseudo-dementia. *Acta Psychiatrica Scandinavica Supplementum*, *34*(132), 1–42.

Bass, C., & Halligan, P. (2014). Factitious disorders and malingering: Challenges for clinical assessment and management. *The Lancet*, *383*(9926), 1422–1432.

Bellman, V., Chinthalapally, A., Johnston, E., Russell, N., Bruce, J., & Saleem, S. (2022). Malingering of psychotic symptoms in psychiatric settings: Theoretical aspects and clinical considerations. *Psychiatry Journal*, *2022*(1), 3884317.

Berman, A. L. (2006). Risk management with suicidal patients. *Journal of Clinical Psychology*, *62*(2), 171–184.

Braham, L. G., Trower, P., & Birchwood, M. (2004). Acting on command hallucinations and dangerous behavior: A critique of the major findings in the last decade. *Clinical Psychology Review*, *24*(5), 513–528.

Caruso, K. A., Benedek, D. M., Auble, P. M., & Bernet, W. (2003). Concealment of psychopathology in forensic evaluations: A pilot study of intentional and uninsightful dissimulators. *Journal of the American Academy of Psychiatry and the Law Online*, *31*(4), 444–450.

Cohen, M. A. A., Alfonso, C. A., & Haque, M. M. (1994). Lilliputian hallucinations and medical illness. *General Hospital Psychiatry*, *16*(2), 141–143.

Cornell, D. G., & Hawk, G. L. (1989). Clinical presentation of malingerers diagnosed by experienced forensic psychologists. *Law and Human Behavior*, *13*(4), 375–383.

Costopoulos, J. S., Proctor, D., Johnson, A. M., & Roberts, S. G. (2021). The impact of malingering on inpatient assault rates. *Acta Scientific Neurology*, *4*(6), 70–81.

Cummings, J. L., & Miller, B. L. (1987). Visual hallucinations: Clinical occurrence and use in differential diagnosis. *Western Journal of Medicine*, *146*(1), 46.

DeClue, G. (2002). Feigning malingering: A case study. *Behavioral Sciences & the Law*, *20*(6), 717–726.

Diamond, B. (1994). *The psychiatrist in the courtroom: Selected papers of Bernard L. Diamond* (M. D. J. Quen, Ed.). Analytic Press.

Drob, S. L., & Berger, R. H. (1987). Determination of malingering: A comprehensive clinical-forensic approach. *Journal of the American Academy of Psychiatry and the Law*, *15*, 519.

Drob, S. L., Meehan, K. B., & Waxman, S. E. (2009). Clinical and conceptual problems in the attribution of malingering in forensic evaluations. *Journal of the American Academy of Psychiatry and the Law*, *37*(1), 98–106.

Everington, C., Notario-Smull, H., & Horton, M. L. (2007). Can defendants with mental retardation successfully fake their performance on a test of competence to stand trial? *Behavioral Sciences & the Law*, *25*(4), 545–560.

Favril, L., Stoliker, B., & Vander Laenen, F. (2020). What differentiates prisoners who attempt suicide from those who experience suicidal ideation? A nationally representative study. *Suicide and Life-Threatening Behavior*, *50*(5), 975–989.

Fovet, T., Mundt, A. P., & Fazel, S. (2024). Psychiatry in prisons and corrections. In *Tasman's psychiatry* (pp. 4839–4866). Springer International Publishing.

Freedenthal, S. (2007). Challenges in assessing intent to die: Can suicide attempters be trusted? *OMEGA—Journal of Death and Dying*, *55*(1), 57–70.

González-Rodríguez, A., & Seeman, M. V. (2020). Addressing delusions in women and men with delusional disorder: Key points for clinical management. *International Journal of Environmental Research and Public Health*, *17*(12), 4583.

Goodwin, D. W., & Rosenthal, R. (1971). Clinical significance of hallucinations in psychiatric disorders: A study of 116 hallucinatory patients. *Archives of General Psychiatry*, *24*(1), 76.

Gottfried, E. D., Hudson, B. L., Vitacco, M. J., & Carbonell, J. L. (2017). Improving the detection of feigned knowledge deficits in defendants adjudicated incompetent to stand trial. *Assessment*, *24*(2), 232–243.

Graue, L. O., Berry, D. T., Clark, J. A., et al. (2007). Identification of feigned mental retardation using the new generation of malingering detection instruments: Preliminary findings. *Clinical Neuropsychologist*, *21*(6), 929–942.

Green, D., & Rosenfeld, B. (2011). Evaluating the gold standard: A review and meta-analysis of the structured interview of reported symptoms. *Psychological Assessment*, *23*(1), 95.

Harrow, M., O'Connell, E. M., Herbener, E. S., Altman, A. M., Kaplan, K. J., & Jobe, T. H. (2003). Disordered verbalizations in schizophrenia: A speech disturbance or thought disorder? *Comprehensive Psychiatry*, *44*(5), 353–359.

Kanaan, R. A., & Wessely, S. C. (2010). The origins of factitious disorder. *History of the Human Sciences*, *23*(2), 68–85.

Knoll, J. L. (2010). Correctional suicide: Assessment, prevention, & professional liability. *Journal of Correctional Healthcare*, *16*(3), 1–17.

Knoll, J. L. (2006). *Real world challenges in correctional psychiatry*. Presentation at the American Academy of Psychiatry and the Law 2006 Annual Meeting, Chicago, Illinois.

Knoll, J. (2009). Malingering—Are you really, really sure? *Correctional Mental Health Report*, *11*(2), 1–22, 30.

Knoll, J., & Resnick, P. J. (2006). The detection of malingered post-traumatic stress disorder. *Psychiatric Clinics of North America*, *29*(3), 629–647.

Knoll, J., & Resnick, P. (2017). Malingering and factitious disorder. In B. Puri & I. Treasden (Eds.), *Forensic psychiatry: Fundamentals and clinical practice* (pp. 229–236). CRC Press.

Knoll, J., & Resnick, P. (in press). Evaluation of malingered psychosis. *Behavioral Sciences & Law*.

Konrad, N., Daigle, M. S., Daniel, A. E., et al. (2007). Preventing suicide in prisons, part I: Recommendations from the international association for suicide prevention task force on suicide in prisons. *Crisis: The Journal of Crisis Intervention and Suicide Prevention*, *28*(3), 113.

Kraus, A. (1994). Phenomenology of the technical delusion in schizophrenics. *Journal of Phenomenological Psychology*, *25*(1), 51–69.

Kupers, T. (2004). Malingering in correctional settings. *Correctional Mental Health Report*, *5*(6), 81.

Langdon, R., McGuire, J., Stevenson, R., & Catts, S. V. (2011). Clinical correlates of olfactory hallucinations in schizophrenia. *British Journal of Clinical Psychology*, *50*(2), 145–163.

Luhrmann, T. M., Padmavati, R., Tharoor, H., & Osei, A. (2015). Hearing voices in different cultures: A social kindling hypothesis. *Topics in Cognitive Science*, *7*(4), 646–663.

McCarthy-Jones, S., & Resnick, P. (2014). Listening to voices: The use of phenomenology to differentiate malingered from genuine auditory verbal hallucinations. *International Journal of Law and Psychiatry*, *37*, 183–189.

McDermott, B. E. (2012). Psychological testing and the assessment of malingering. *Psychiatric Clinics of North America*, *35*, 855–876.

McDermott, B. E., & Sokolov, G. (2009). Malingering in a correctional setting: The use of the Structured Interview of Reported Symptoms in a jail sample. *Behavioral Sciences & the Law*, *27*(5), 753–765.

Miller, H. (2001). *M-FAST interview booklet*. Psychological Assessment Resources.

Mitchell, J., & Vierkant, A. D. (1991). Delusions and hallucinations of cocaine abusers and paranoid schizophrenics: A comparative study. *Journal of Psychology*, *125*(3), 301–310.

Paulino, M., Edens, J. F., Moniz, M., Moura, O., Rijo, D., & Simões, M. R. (2024). Personality assessment inventory (PAI) in forensic and correctional settings: A comprehensive review. *Journal of Forensic and Legal Medicine*, *103*, 102661.

Pierson, A. M., Rosenfeld, B., Green, D., & Belfi, B. (2011). Investigating the Relationship Between Antisocial Personality Disorder and Malingering. *Criminal Justice and Behavior*, *38*(2), 146–156. https://doi.org/10.1177/0093854810389292 (Original work published 2011)

Obegi, J. H. (2020). Differentiating genuine from feigned suicidality in corrections: A necessary but perilous task. *International Journal of Law and Psychiatry, 71*, 101573.

Resnick, P., & Knoll, J. (2018). Malingered psychosis. In R. Rogers & S. Bender (Eds.), *Clinical assessment of malingering and deception* (4th ed.), 98–121. Guilford Press.

Resnick, P. J., West, S., & Payne, J. W. (1997). Malingering of posttraumatic disorders. *Clinical Assessment of Malingering and Deception, 2*, 130–152.

Ritson, B., & Forrest, A. (1970). The simulation of psychosis: A contemporary presentation. *British Journal of Medical Psychology, 43*(1), 31–37.

Rogers, R. (2008a). *Clinical assessment of malingering and deception.* Guilford Press, 257–357.

Rogers, R. (2008b). Current status of clinical methods. In R. Rogers (Ed.), *Clinical assessment of malingering and deception* (3rd ed., p. 401). Guilford Press.

Rogers, R. (2018). Detection strategies for malingering. In R. Rogers & S. D. Bender (Eds.), *Clinical assessment of malingering and deception.* (4th ed., pp. 18–41) Guilford Press.

Rogers, R., Bender, S. D., & Hartigan, S. E. (2024). An overview of malingering and deception in neuropsychiatric cases. *Behavioral Sciences & the Law, 42*(1), 28–38.

Rogers, R., & Shuman, D. W. (2005). Malingering and deception in criminal evaluations. In *Fundamentals of forensic practice: Mental health and criminal law* (pp. 21–55). Springer.

Rogers, R., Vitacco, M. J., & Kurus, S. J. (2010). Assessment of malingering with repeat forensic evaluations: Patient variability and possible misclassification on the SIRS and other feigning measures. *Journal of the American Academy of Psychiatry and the Law, 38*(1), 109–114.

Sacks, M. H., Carpenter, W. T., Jr., & Strauss, J. S. (1974). Recovery from delusions: Three phases documented by patient's interpretation of research procedures. *Archives of General Psychiatry, 30*(1), 117.

Salekin, K. L., & Doane, B. M. (2009). Malingering intellectual disability: The value of available measures and methods. *Applied Neuropsychology, 16*(2), 105–113.

Salekin, K. L., Olley, J. G., & Hedge, K. A. (2010). Offenders with intellectual disability: Characteristics, prevalence, and issues in forensic assessment. *Journal of Mental Health Research in Intellectual Disabilities, 3*(2), 97–116.

Schneider, S. D., Jelinek, L., Lincoln, T. M., & Moritz, S. (2011). What happened to the voices? A fine-grained analysis of how hallucinations and delusions change under psychiatric treatment. *Psychiatry Research, 188*(1), 13–17.

Scott, R., Aboud, A., & Smith, T. (2023). Using the stress–vulnerability model to better understand suicide in prison populations. *Psychiatry, Psychology and Law, 30*(3), 299–333.

Shandera, A. L., Berry, D. T., Clark, J. A., Schipper, L. J., Graue, L. O., & Harp, J. P. (2010). Detection of malingered mental retardation. *Psychological Assessment, 22*(1), 50.

Sherman, E. M., Slick, D. J., & Iverson, G. L. (2020). Multidimensional malingering criteria for neuropsychological assessment: A 20-year update of the malingered neuropsychological dysfunction criteria. *Archives of Clinical Neuropsychology, 35*(6), 735–764.

Simon, R. I. (2004). *Assessing and managing suicide risk: Guidelines for clinically based risk management.* American Psychiatric Publishing.

Skeem, J. L., Silver, E., Appelbaum, P. S., & Tiemann, J. (2006). Suicide-related behavior after psychiatric hospital discharge: Implications for risk assessment and management. *Behavioral Sciences & the Law, 24*(6), 731–746.

Slick, D. J., Sherman, E. M., Iverson, G. L., Diagnostic criteria for malingered neurocognitive dysfunction: Proposed standards for clinical practice and research. *Clin Neuropsychol.* 1999; *13*(4), 545–561. doi:10.1076/1385-4046(199911)13:04;1-Y;FT545

Soliman, S., & Resnick, P. J. (2010). Feigning in adjudicative competence evaluations. *Behavioral Sciences & the Law, 28*(5), 614–629.

Spitzer, M. (1992). The phenomenology of delusions. *Psychiatric Annals, 22*(5), 252–259.

Stephane, M., Pellizzer, G., Roberts, S., & McClannahan, K. (2006). Computerized binary scale of auditory speech hallucinations (cbSASH). *Schizophrenia Research, 88*(1–3), 73–81.

Sweet, J. J., Heilbronner, R. L., Morgan, J. E., et al. (2021). American Academy of Clinical Neuropsychology (AACN) 2021 consensus statement on validity assessment: Update of the 2009 AACN consensus conference statement. *Clinical Neuropsychologist, 35*(6), 1053–1106.

Tamburello, A. C., Bajgier, J., & Reeves, R. (2015). The prevalence of delusional disorder in prison. *Journal of the American Academy of Psychiatry and the Law, 43*(1), 82–86.

Thompson, J. S., Stuart, G. L., & Holden, C. E. (1992). Command hallucinations and legal insanity. *Forensic Reports, 5*, 29–43.

Victor, T. L., & Boone, K. B. (2007). Identification of feigned mental retardation. In K. B. Boone (Ed.), *Assessment of feigned cognitive impairment: A neuropsychological perspective* (pp. 310–345). Guilford Press.

Vitacco, M. J., & Rogers, R. (2010). Assessment of malingering in correctional settings. In C. L. Scott (Ed.), *Handbook of correctional mental health* (2nd ed., pp. 255–276). American Psychiatric Publishing.

Vitacco, M. J., Rogers, R., Gabel, J., & Munizza, J. (2007). An evaluation of malingering screens with competency to stand trial patients: A known-groups comparison. *Law and Human Behavior, 31*, 249–260.

Walczyk, J. J., Sewell, N., & DiBenedetto, M. B. (2018). A review of approaches to detecting malingering in forensic contexts and promising cognitive load-inducing lie detection techniques. *Frontiers in Psychiatry, 9*, 700.

Wessely, S., Buchanan, A., Reed, A., et al. (1993). Acting on delusions: I. Prevalence. *British Journal of Psychiatry, 163*(1), 69–76.

21

Use of telepsychiatry

Ashley J. B. MacLean and Danielle B. Kushner

Introduction

Telepsychiatry, a branch of telemedicine, is being used increasingly for the remote diagnosis and treatment of incarcerated persons (IPs), as well as to conduct forensic evaluations. Telemedicine was first introduced to carceral settings in Florida in the 1980s (Ollove, 2016). With technological improvements and cost reductions, telemedicine spread in the 1990s to prisons, universities, and federal health systems (Shore, 2015). According to the National Survey on Prison Health Care, telepsychiatry was being used in at least 28 U.S. states by 2016, often in facilities in geographically remote areas (Maruschak et al., 2016). More recently, during the COVID-19 pandemic, there was a widespread increase in remote encounters, especially in jails and prisons to reduce the spread of illness, given the high COVID-19 rates noted in carceral settings (Burton et al., 2021).

Telepsychiatry has increased access to care for IPs, improved medical and carceral staff safety, and reduced costs (Ax et al., 2007; Edge et al., 2021). According to the U.S. Bureau of Justice Statistics, over half of IPs in jails and prisons were reported to have a mental illness in 2005 (James & Glaze, 2006). Yet, according to a later report, only about one third of IPs with a "mental health indicator" in 2011–2012 reported receiving treatment (Bronson & Berzofsky, 2017).

A shortage of psychiatrists has been a significant contributing factor to treatment barriers. With the evolution of telepsychiatry, many states, unable to recruit on-site psychiatrists, have turned to remote technology as an alternative way to increase accessibility to mental health and substance use treatment. While telepsychiatry addresses many of the challenges of understaffed jails and prisons, there may be limitations in its use for specific populations.

Access to care

Telepsychiatry has increased access to care for traditionally underserved areas such as jails and prisons. Prior to telepsychiatry, carceral facilities reported decreased assessments and treatment due to funding shortages, security priorities, and reduced access to on-site providers (Manfredi et al., 2005). A 2013 literature review concluded that telepsychiatry programs positively impacted carceral facilities by increasing access to effective psychiatric treatment and maintaining continuity of care (Deslich et al., 2013). Telemedicine has also decreased the time from referral to receiving care (Fox et al., 2007; Nacci, 2002).

Jails and prisons are often located in remote locations or distant areas of cities and states. Undesirable work locations and potentially long commutes may reduce recruitment of on-site psychiatrists and clinical staff, while the absence of a long daily commute can be an attractive benefit for telepsychiatrists (Edge et al., 2021). Upon arriving, challenging and time-consuming security procedures for entering and moving around the facilities may be an additional deterrent for on-site staff. Telepsychiatrists may be more efficient, due to having more time for patient documentation or other care-related activities because of less transport time (Deslich et al., 2013).

IPs requiring care not accessible at their carceral facility typically must be transported to off-site clinics or hospitals. However, stigmatization of wearing handcuffs during transport and the long travel times may deter IPs from agreeing to care. A 2021 review indicated that telepsychiatry reduced the inconvenience and stigma associated with transport to off-site appointments (Edge et al., 2021).

Safety

Psychiatrists may be apprehensive to work in jails or prisons due to concerns over safety (Fuehrlein et al., 2012; Kaftarian, 2019). The safety of both staff and the community may be improved by using telepsychiatry in carceral facilities. By removing the risk of physical contact with patients during appointments, telepsychiatry may help to ease safety concerns and increase physician recruitment (Deslich et al., 2013; Kaftarian, 2019). Furthermore, telepsychiatry may improve public safety by minimizing the risk of escape during IP transport to off-site appointments. The facilities that utilize telepsychiatry services within patient housing areas have reduced transport risks such as cuff injuries, assaults, escapes, and patient delays (Sales et al., 2018). However, due to the variability of telepsychiatry location and requirements within facilities, telepsychiatry does not reliably improve safety for IPs in carceral facilities.

Cost

Telepsychiatry has been shown to reduce overall administrative and staffing costs once established, although increased start-up costs associated with replacing and implementing the technology are an initial barrier (Larsen et al., 2004; Tian et al., 2021). With declining software, hardware, and video equipment prices, telepsychiatry has become more feasible (Lexcen et al., 2006).

Carceral facilities without on-site psychiatrists may require IPs to be transported to off-site clinics for care. Costs associated with these transports are not insignificant, requiring usually two correctional officers and a driver (Deslich et al., 2013). Telepsychiatry decreases the need, and associated costs, to transport IPs off-site; thus, telehealth has become a long-term strategy to reduce health care spending (Pew Charitable Trusts, 2014). For example, prisons in North Carolina estimated saving over $1 million in the first year following the implementation of telemedicine (Khairat et al., 2023). Additionally, some government agencies have provided incentives for the use of telemedicine (Deslich et al., 2013). Money saved using telepsychiatry ideally can be spent on expanding mental health resources.

Technology

Incorporating telepsychiatry into carceral settings may pose initial technological challenges. Carceral facilities are often old and may require additional infrastructure. Outdated computers may not support telepsychiatry software, and it may be necessary for facilities to purchase new hardware (Deslich et al., 2013). The telepsychiatrist's computer and software must also be compatible with that of the carceral facility, and they may need to work with the jail or prison's information technology department to circumvent firewalls. The jail and prison must regularly maintain their hardware/software, internet, and networking infrastructure. Moreover, protocols must be established for when equipment fails (Miller et al., 2005).

Certain telepsychiatry equipment in carceral settings may have safety features, such as protective casings, that can impact image and sound quality. This may further complicate the encounter if the IP completes the session in an area with loud background noise (Deslich et al., 2013). Staff may have varying levels of technical expertise, and those less familiar with technology may benefit from increased training (Perry et al., 2020).

Administrative issues and medical records

Successful telepsychiatry implementation requires on-site staff support (Edge et al., 2021). Given potential preexisting staff shortages, measures must be taken to accommodate additional staff demands associated with telepsychiatry in carceral facilities. One study showed that telemedicine in carceral facilities increased the administrative workload in scheduling appointments and coordinating tasks before the visits; however, staff became more efficient over time (Neuhaus et al., 2018). Results from a 2018 pilot study on the use of telemedicine in German carceral facilities revealed that 90% of respondents reported telemedicine increased nursing workload. Facilities need to be realistic about the administrative and clinical support required for successful telepsychiatry utilization, increasing staffing levels when needed (Colombo et al., 2023).

Facilities that still use paper medical records create challenges for the telepsychiatrist who does not have direct access to the patient chart. Record transmission can occur through mail, secure email, or fax, which may be time-consuming, be burdensome to staff, and affect patient care (Kaliebe et al., 2011). Digitalizing medical records would improve this process, as electronic medical records can be accessed off-site.

Understanding the setting and obtaining collateral information

Telepsychiatrists benefit from having a general understanding of prison or jail procedures and culture, along with the particular nuances of a facility. For example, having an awareness of the challenges related to facility alarms or transport issues will help telepsychiatrists better understand their patients' complaints or why they keep missing appointments or medications. Obtaining collateral information from on-site staff members can be more challenging when working remotely, as off-site providers are outside the conventional flow of information throughout the day. Thus, collaboration with on-site staff and developing procedures regarding communication are recommended (Kaftarian, 2019; Kaliebe et al., 2011).

Confidentiality, privacy, and informed consent

When using telepsychiatry in jails and prisons, maintaining confidentiality and privacy may be particularly challenging. For instance, carceral facilities prioritize security and generally require the presence of a chaperone during the session, which may be a nonclinical staff member, such as a correctional officer. This third-party presence may compromise the quality of the session due to privacy concerns (Antonacci et al., 2008; Myers et al., 2006) and may prevent truly informed consent being obtained if the IP does not have a choice regarding the presence of a third party in the room. Under such circumstances, the IP may not disclose certain information due to fears of retaliation or the spread of details about their alleged crime or health status, which could compromise their safety. In addition, other IPs could directly overhear the session if a private room is unavailable or if the room has poor soundproofing. These privacy concerns may decrease engagement during the session and potentially lead to treatment refusals. Alternatively, the use of headphones by IPs and correctional staff may improve privacy (Kaftarian, 2019).

The risk of privacy breaches due to interception of unencrypted video conferencing or hacking of encrypted lines is also a concern (Sullivan et al., 2008). Disclosure of the risks and benefits of telepsychiatry, including privacy and confidentiality issues, should be part of the informed consent process (Antonacci et al., 2008; Hyler & Gangure, 2003; Saleem et al., 2008; Sales et al., 2018). However, limited treatment options may compromise the noncoercive nature of informed consent (Hewson et al., 2021). Continued research on the legal and ethical issues of telepsychiatry in forensic settings is warranted, along with the need for guidelines for specific situations (Kister et al., 2023).

Establishing guidelines for missed appointments is necessary when working remotely, including rescheduling the session or assessing the need for in-person treatment. Missed appointments may be due to facility alarms or transport delays, or they may be due to patient refusal. When the IP does not attend their telepsychiatry session, obtaining collateral information from on-site staff may provide insight into their motivation for the refusal. Reasons for refusals include having another appointment, privacy issues, disinterest, hypervigilance, or other psychiatric symptoms. The appropriateness of telepsychiatry should be continually assessed, and another approach may be indicated if the modality is not working for an individual (Hewson et al., 2021).

Therapeutic rapport and efficacy

The current literature on the efficacy and effectiveness of telepsychiatry in carceral settings ranges from case reports to systematic reviews (Karachaliou et al., 2023; Tian et al., 2021). The studies vary in quality and patient populations, thus limiting generalization of outcomes, particularly in situations where higher levels of care are required. Concerns over building therapeutic rapport are one of the perceived barriers to the use of telepsychiatry in carceral settings, but the available literature suggests that telepsychiatry can positively or negatively impact therapeutic rapport depending on the scenario. Some individuals may feel more isolated with a remote provider, while others appreciate more reliable visits regardless of the technology. Furthermore, several studies have demonstrated telepsychiatry's effectiveness in carceral settings with regard to IP acceptance and satisfaction, provider alliance, and diagnostic reliability (Brodey et al., 2000; Morgan et al., 2008; Sharma & Devan, 2023).

A 2023 systematic review involving community populations revealed that the type of mental illness could impact the effectiveness of telepsychiatry and recommended the development of protocols related to diagnosis (Hagi et al., 2023). For depression, telepsychiatry was found to be more effective than in-person sessions, while for eating disorders, in-person treatment was found to be more effective (Hagi et al., 2023). Moreover, studies in carceral settings revealed that some IPs preferred telepsychiatry over in-person sessions to discuss sexual abuse issues, most likely due to confidentiality and privacy concerns (Carroll, 2020; Miller et al., 2008; Tucker et al., 2006). Conversely, for some IPs, the lack of an in-person provider further contributed to their feelings of isolation and stigma (Hewson et al., 2021).

Clinical use: levels of care

IPs receive care in various clinical settings depending on individual mental health needs. IPs should receive treatment that matches their needs and meets community standards of care (see Chapter 9). Except for an outpatient level of mental health care, telepsychiatry is generally not equivalent to receiving treatment by an on-site psychiatrist. For higher levels of care (e.g., mental health units, inpatient units), an on-site psychiatrist is better positioned to lead the IP's treatment and positively impact the milieu of the treatment setting, which includes developing relationships with the officers and nursing staff who have the most interaction with the IPs. However, the use of telepsychiatry in such settings is clearly better for the IPs than having no or very limited access to a psychiatrist. Under such circumstances, aggressive recruitment strategies should be implemented. Telepsychiatrists used in higher levels of care should periodically provide on-site coverage to become more familiar with the correctional and mental health staffs and the operations of the correctional facility (American Psychiatric Association, 2023). The level of care delivered remotely through telepsychiatry should match that of in-person treatment (Shore et al., 2018; Waller & Stotler, 2018). Research on the efficacy of telepsychiatry in jails and prisons, especially in higher level care settings, is still limited.

Practice guidelines for telepsychiatry in community populations do not specify any definitive contraindications (Shore et al., 2018). Still, due to the acuity of patient symptoms and the need for crisis interventions, IPs in mental health housing or crisis units may benefit from having an in-person psychiatrist. A California prison found that in-person care was used more often for persons who refused remote care or when it was deemed clinically appropriate (Burton et al., 2021). One source recommends that the use of telepsychiatry, compared to other treatment modalities, should be based on the provider's judgment (Shore et al., 2018).

IPs in administrative segregation housing generally have challenges accessing appropriate medical or psychiatric services due to enhanced security requirements, such as captain escort, spit mask, or ankle cuffs. These restrictions can make it challenging for these patients to be seen in a general psychiatric clinic, or even an area for telepsychiatry visits, due to the logistics of coordinating additional transport time. Commonly, an on-site psychiatrist conducts a clinical visit at a patient's cell, speaking through the door and, if available, visualizing the patient through the cell window. Due to audio-visual limitations, cell-side telepsychiatry may be challenging and is not recommended. Therefore, together with the lack of reliable escorts, in-person visits for this population may be more appropriate (American Psychiatric Association, 2023).

Telepsychiatry can be utilized in emergencies in carceral settings but requires the assistance of on-site health care providers, such as nursing or social work, and local medical capabilities to implement the plan of care. For some highly violent, uncooperative, or paranoid patients, telepsychiatry may be impractical and potentially delay treatment (Hewson et al., 2021; Saleem et al., 2008; Thrasher, 2023). High-risk individuals, including those with violent and aggressive behavior, may damage the equipment, requiring more staff for safety. Therefore, it is essential in the development of telepsychiatry policies and procedures to educate both on-site and remote staff of facility resources and capabilities for acute psychiatric emergencies.

Clinical use: special populations

Telepsychiatry outcomes may vary based on the distinct characteristics of specific populations. For example, telepsychiatry may be particularly advantageous for non-English-speaking or deaf patients by directly connecting them with language or American Sign Language interpreter services. However, accommodations such as headsets or large monitors with captioning may be required (Moreland et al., 2023). Local telepsychiatry monitors in the housing areas may be particularly useful due to potential transport challenges related to language barriers, visual impairment, or other medical issues.

Conversely, older IPs or those who have been incarcerated for long periods may be less familiar with technology. Additional assistance may be required to help these patients adapt to new procedures. Moreover, female or transgender individuals, especially those with particular trauma histories, may experience difficulty with telepsychiatry due to confidentiality concerns or security protocols requiring escort by staff of a particular gender. Some IPs may prefer in-person treatment for comfort and rapport.

As services for substance use disorders in jails and prisons continue to expand with more therapeutic and medication options (see Chapter 49), telepsychiatry can increase access to treatment, especially given increasing mortality rates due to overdose (Bureau of Justice Assistance, 2023). Despite the need for close collaboration with on-site nursing and medical staff for physical examination, vital signs, and possible emergency interventions, general evidence shows similar, if not better, treatment engagement using telepsychiatry for substance use disorders (Pham et al., 2025).

Legal and ethical considerations

Legal and ethical issues faced when using telepsychiatry with nonincarcerated populations include issues of licensure, liability, and security. These same concerns apply in carceral settings, with the addition of unique factors (Hyler & Gangure, 2003). The same ethical issues that affect in-person treatment in jails and prisons such as dual loyalty and informed consent are also applicable to carceral telepsychiatry (see Chapter 12). Privacy is also a significant concern in carceral settings, as discussed in the section on confidentiality. There is little case law on the topic currently, but with increased use, legal and ethical issues may reveal themselves over time (Caudill & Sager, 2015; Miller et al., 2008). IPs have a constitutional right to receive medical and mental health care, and inadequate mental health care is considered cruel and unusual punishment (*Bowring v. Godwin*, 1977; *Estelle v. Gamble*, 1976). Telepsychiatry is a key resource to help facilities meet this standard of care.

Forensic evaluations

In addition to providing direct clinical care, telepsychiatry is increasingly being used for forensic psychiatric evaluations, including competency to stand trial or mitigation evaluations. After the COVID-19 pandemic, self-reported use of telepsychiatry by forensic evaluators doubled (Bernhard et al., 2021). Initially, there were concerns about the admissibility of this technology to the courts under evidentiary standards outlined in *Daubert v. Merrill Dow Pharmaceuticals* (1993). However, following a number of studies supporting the efficacy of telepsychiatry in clinical treatment settings, additional research has demonstrated the reliability and validity of tele-evaluations compared to traditional in-person forensic evaluations (Manguno-Mire et al., 2007)

With ongoing court challenges due to delays and waitlists in certain states for competency to stand trial evaluations and treatment, video conferencing has provided an effective means to improve evaluation efficiency and decrease wait times (Luxton & Niemi, 2020). Furthermore, remote evaluations provide flexibility in rescheduling and an improved sense of security and safety for evaluators. Evidence suggests that telepsychiatry can enhance evaluator impartiality by providing increased access to evaluators outside available in-person resources (Gordon, 2016). Teleconferencing for defense lawyer conferences, court procedures, and testimony has also been used in recent years, but a discussion of these topics is beyond the scope of this chapter.

Summary

The expansion of telepsychiatry to jails and prisons has been a promising strategy to increase access to care for this historically underserved population. Telepsychiatry has been shown to reduce costs over time and improve provider safety, but concerns about privacy and confidentiality and its use in certain situations must be acknowledged. Guidelines on the appropriate use of telepsychiatry in carceral settings are needed to provide quality care and prevent overuse simply due to decreased costs or ease. Continued efforts should be made to recruit in-person psychiatrists to work in jails and prisons, especially in leadership and high-acuity settings. Further research on the use and limitations of telepsychiatry in carceral settings, especially for higher levels of care and specific populations, can help us understand and adequately serve the unique needs of this population.

REFERENCES

American Psychiatric Association. (2023). *Resource document on telepsychiatry for adults in jails and prisons.* https://www.psychiatry.org/getattachment/00e3f401-0792-4b78-90ba-5985dd791a4e/Resource-Document-on-Telepsychiatry-in-Jails-and-Prisons.pdf

Antonacci, D. J., Bloch, R. M., Saeed, S. A., Yildirim, Y., & Talley, J. (2008). Empirical evidence on the use and effectiveness of telepsychiatry via videoconferencing: Implications for forensic and correctional psychiatry. *Behavioral Sciences and the Law, 26*(3), 253–269.

Ax, R. K., Fagan, T. J., Magaletta, P. R., Morgan, R. D., Nussbaum, D., & White, T. W. (2007). Innovations in correctional assessment and treatment. *Criminal Justice and Behavior, 34*(7), 893–905.

Bernhard, P. A., McDowell, L., & Vincent, G. M. (2021). Forensic practitioners' use and perceptions of telepsychology before and during COVID-19. *Law and Human Behavior, 45*(5), 468.

Bowring v. Godwin, 551 F.2d 44 (4th Cir. 1977).

Brodey, B. B., Claypoole, K. H., Motto, J., Arias, R. G., & Goss, R. (2000). Satisfaction of forensic psychiatric patients with remote telepsychiatric evaluation. *Psychiatric Services, 51*(10), 1305–1307.

Bronson, J., & Berzofsky, M. (2017). Indicators of mental health problems reported by prisoners and jail inmates, 2011–12. *Bureau of Justice Statistics*, Special Issue, 1–16.

Bureau of Justice Assistance. (2023). *Leveraging telehealth for justice-involved populations with substance use disorders: Lessons learned and considerations for governors.* https://bja.ojp.gov/library/publications/leveraging-telehealth-justice-involved-populations-substance-use-disorders

Burton, P. R., Morris, N. P., & Hirschtritt, M. E. (2021). Mental health services in a US prison during the COVID-19 pandemic. *Psychiatric Services, 72*(4), 458–460.

Carroll, A. (2020). Forensic mental-health assessments after coronavirus disease 2019: Will telehealth lead us to trade psychological depth for convenience? *Medicine, Science and the Law, 60*(3), 169–171.

Caudill, R. L., & Sager, Z. (2015). Institutionally based videoconferencing. *International Review of Psychiatry, 27*(6), 496–503.

Colombo, M. G., Joos, S., & Koch, R. (2023). Implementing interprofessional video consultations with general practitioners and psychiatrists in correctional facilities in Germany: Results from a mixed-methods study. *BMC Health Services Research, 23*(1), 578.

Daubert v. Merrell Dow Pharmaceuticals, Inc., 509 U.S. 579 (1993).

Deslich, S. A., Thistlethwaite, T., & Coustasse, A. (2013). Telepsychiatry in correctional facilities: Using technology to improve access and decrease costs of mental health care in underserved populations. *Permanente Journal, 17*(3), 80.

Edge, C., Black, G., King, E., George, J., Patel, S., & Hayward, A. (2021). Improving care quality with prison telemedicine: The effects of context and multiplicity on successful implementation and use. *Journal of Telemedicine and Telecare, 27*(6), 325–342.

Estelle v. Gamble, 429 U.S. 97 (1976).

Fox, K. C., Somes, G. W., & Waters, T. M. (2007). Timeliness and access to healthcare services via telemedicine for adolescents in state correctional facilities. *Journal of Adolescent Health, 41*(2), 161–167.

Fuehrlein, B. S., Jha, M. K., Brenner, A. M., & North, C. S. (2012). Can we address the shortage of psychiatrists in the correctional setting with exposure during residency training? *Community Mental Health Journal, 48*, 756–760.

Gordon, S. (2016). Crossing the line: Daubert, dual roles, and the admissibility of forensic mental health testimony. *Cardozo Law Review, 37*, 1345–1399.

Hagi, K., Kurokawa, S., Takamiya, A., Fujikawa, M., Kinoshita, S., Iizuka, M., et al. (2023). Telepsychiatry versus face-to-face treatment: Systematic review and meta-analysis of randomised controlled trials. *British Journal of Psychiatry, 223*(3), 407–414.

Hewson, T., Robinson, L., Khalifa, N., Hard, J., & Shaw, J. (2021). Remote consultations in prison mental healthcare in England: Impacts of COVID-19. *British Journal of Psychiatry Open, 7*(2), e49.

Hyler, S. E., & Gangure, D. P. (2003). A review of the costs of telepsychiatry. *Psychiatric Services, 54*(7), 976–980.

James, D. J., & Glaze, L. E. (2006). *Mental health problems of prison and jail inmates* (NCJ 213600). U.S. Department of Justice, Office of Justice Programs, Bureau of Justice Statistics. https://bjs.ojp.gov/content/pub/pdf/mhppji.pdf

Kaftarian, E. (2019). Lessons learned in prison and jail-based telepsychiatry. *Current Psychiatry Reports, 21*, 1–7.

Kaliebe, K. E., Heneghan, J., & Kim, T. J. (2011). Telepsychiatry in juvenile justice settings. *Child and Adolescent Psychiatric Clinics, 20*(1), 113–123.

Karachaliou, E., Douzenis, P., Martinaki, S., Misouridou, E., Chatzinikolaou, F., & Douzenis, A. (2023). A systematic literature review on the application of telepsychiatry in correctional facilities/prisons: Necessity and modern challenges. *Journal of Technology in Behavioral Science*, 1–26.

Khairat, S., Zebrowski, A., Stabile, K., Bohlmann, A., Wallace, E., Yao, Y., ... Dorn, S. D. (2023). Assessment of stakeholder perceptions and cost of implementing a telemedicine specialty program at correctional facilities in North Carolina. *Permanente Journal, 27*(3), 49.

Kister, K., Laskowski, J., Dybała, E., & Makarewicz, A. (2023). Are we ready for Telepsychiatry? Benefits and challenges of digital psychotherapy. *Current Problems of Psychiatry, 24*.

Larsen, D., Hudnall Stamm, B., Davis, K., & Magaletta, P. R. (2004). Prison telemedicine and telehealth utilization in the United States: State and federal perceptions of benefits and barriers. *Telemedicine Journal and e-Health, 10*(Suppl. 2), S-81.

Lexcen, F. J., Hawk, G. L., Herrick, S., & Blank, M. B. (2006). Use of video conferencing for psychiatric and forensic evaluations. *Psychiatric Services, 57*(5), 713–715.

Luxton, D. D., & Niemi, J. (2020). Implementation and evaluation of videoconferencing for forensic competency evaluation. *Telemedicine and e-Health, 26*(7), 929–934.

Manfredi, L., Shupe, J., & Batki, S. L. (2005). Rural jail telepsychiatry: A pilot feasibility study. *Telemedicine Journal and E-Health, 11*(5), 574–577.

Manguno-Mire, G. M., Thompson, J. W., Jr, Shore, J. H., Croy, C. D., Artecona, J. F., & Pickering, J. W. (2007). The use of telemedicine to evaluate competency to stand trial: A preliminary randomized controlled study. *Journal of the American Academy of Psychiatry and the Law, 35*(4), 481–489.

Maruschak, L., Chari, K. A., Simon, A. E., & DeFrances, C. J. (2016). National survey of prison health care: Selected findings. *National Health Statistics Reports*, (96), 1–23.

Miller, T. W., Burton, D. C., Hill, K., Luftman, G., Veltkemp, L. J., & Swope, M. (2005). Telepsychiatry: Critical dimensions for forensic services. *Journal of the American Academy of Psychiatry and the Law, 33*(4), 539–546.

Miller, T. W., Clark, J., Veltkamp, L. J., Burton, D. C., & Swope, M. (2008). Teleconferencing model for forensic consultation, court testimony, and continuing education. *Behavioral Sciences and the Law, 26*(3), 301–313.

Moreland, C. J., Rao, S. R., Jacobs, K., & Kushalnagar, P. (2023). Equitable access to telehealth and other services for deaf people during the COVID-19 pandemic. *Health Equity, 7*(1), 126–136.

Morgan, R. D., Patrick, A. R., & Magaletta, P. R. (2008). Does the use of telemental health alter the treatment experience? Inmates' perceptions of telemental health versus face-to-face treatment modalities. *Journal of Consulting and Clinical Psychology, 76*(1), 158.

Myers, K., Valentine, J., Morganthaler, R., & Melzer, S. (2006). Telepsychiatry with incarcerated youth. *Journal of Adolescent Health, 38*(6), 643–648.

Nacci, P. L. (2002). *Implementing telemedicine in correctional facilities.* U.S. Department of Justice, Office of Justice Programs, National Institute of Justice. https://www.ojp.gov/pdffiles1/nij/190310.pdf

Neuhaus, M., Langbecker, D., Caffery, L. J., Taylor, M., Garner, L., Williams, G., ... Macdonald, G. A. (2018). Telementoring for hepatitis C treatment in correctional facilities. *Journal of Telemedicine and Telecare, 24*(10), 690–696.

Ollove, M. (2016). *State prisons turn to telemedicine to improve health and save money.* Huffington Post. https://www.huffpost.com/entry/state-prisons-telemedicine-health-money_n_56a10957e4b0404eb8f07a84

Perry, K., Gold, S., & Shearer, E. M. (2020). Identifying and addressing mental health providers' perceived barriers to clinical video telehealth utilization. *Journal of Clinical Psychology, 76*(6), 1125–1134.

Pew Charitable Trusts. (2014). *State health care prison spending.* https://www.pewtrusts.org/-/media/assets/2014/07/stateprisonhealthcarespendingreport.pdf

Pham, H., Lin, C., Zhu, Y., Clingan, S. E., Lin, L. A., Mooney, L. J., Murphy, S. M., Campbell, C. I., Liu, Y., & Hser, Y. I. (2025). Telemedicine-delivered treatment for substance use disorder: A scoping review. *Journal of Telemedicine and Telecare, 31*(3), 359–375. https://doi.org/10.1177/1357633X231190945

Saleem, Y., Taylor, M. H., & Khalifa, N. (2008). Forensic telepsychiatry in the United Kingdom. *Behavioral Sciences and the Law, 26*(3), 333–344.

Sales, C. P., McSweeney, L., Saleem, Y., & Khalifa, N. (2018). The use of telepsychiatry within forensic practice: A literature review on the use of videolink—A ten-year follow-up. *Journal of Forensic Psychiatry and Psychology*, *29*(3), 387–402.

Sharma, G., & Devan, K. (2023). The effectiveness of telepsychiatry: Thematic review. *BJPsych Bulletin*, *47*(2), 82–89.

Shore, J. (2015). The evolution and history of telepsychiatry and its impact on psychiatric care: Current implications for psychiatrists and psychiatric organizations. *International Review of Psychiatry*, *27*(6), 469–475.

Shore, J. H., Yellowlees, P., Caudill, R., Johnston, B., Turvey, C., Mishkind, M., ... Hilty, D. (2018). Best practices in videoconferencing-based telemental health April 2018. *Telemedicine and e-Health*, *24*(11), 827–832.

Sullivan, D. H., Chapman, M., & Mullen, P. E. (2008). Videoconferencing and forensic mental health in Australia. *Behavioral Sciences and the Law*, *26*(3), 323–331.

Thrasher, T. (2023). *Emergency psychiatry*. Oxford University Press.

Tian, E. J., Venugopalan, S., Kumar, S., & Beard, M. (2021). The impacts of and outcomes from telehealth delivered in prisons: A systematic review. *PLoS One*, *16*(5), e0251840.

Tucker, W., Olfson, M., Simring, S., Goodman, W., & Bienenfeld, S. (2006). A pilot survey of inmate preferences for on-site, visiting consultant, and telemedicine psychiatric services. *CNS Spectrums*, *11*(10), 783–787.

Waller, M., & Stotler, C. (2018). Telemedicine: A primer. *Current Allergy and Asthma Reports*, *18*, 1–9.

22

Cultural and structural competence

*Stephanie Eng, Harshit Sharma, Luca Pauselli, and Reena Kapoor**

Introduction

Cultural competence is an essential aspect of providing mental health care in any setting. An understanding of culture is even more important in correctional settings, as several unique factors may lead to conflict and misunderstanding if not adequately addressed. First, minority ethnic groups are vastly overrepresented in prisons and jails, so a familiarity with the predominant culture of those groups is necessary to engage incarcerated persons (IPs) in treatment and diagnose them accurately. Second, mental health clinicians may be unfamiliar with law enforcement culture, which heavily influences the practices of correctional officers and differs significantly from health care culture. Third, psychiatrists may bring their own cultural beliefs about crime and punishment to clinical encounters when providing health care in jails and prisons.

As complex and nuanced as understanding cultural factors can be, it is also only part of the picture. Correctional psychiatrists must also become familiar with the idea of structural competence, recognizing that health and illness are impacted by larger societal forces that persist outside of the clinical encounter such as poverty, racism, sexism, and homophobia. This chapter traces the development of cultural and structural competence, suggesting ways to apply those principles in jails and prisons and to improve patient care as a result.

Recognizing the importance of cultural and structural competence

The field of correctional psychiatry has formally acknowledged the importance of cultural awareness since the publication of the American Psychiatric Association's (APA's) standards for psychiatric services in jails and prisons in 2000 (APA, 2000); these principles were reaffirmed in the publication's most recent edition (APA, 2016). The APA standards highlight the need to provide training in important areas of cultural awareness, including ethnicity, gender, religious/spiritual beliefs, sexual orientation, and family factors, that influence expression of mental illness or psychological distress in correctional settings. The goals of this training are to improve tolerance of diverse populations, empathy for the minority experience, and understanding of ethnocentric bias and its potential effects.

Outside of corrections, psychiatry has experienced a massive growth of interest in cultural issues. The *Diagnostic and Statistical Manual of Mental Disorders* (DSM) first included guidance about the cultural formulation in its fourth edition, published in 1994 (APA, 1994). Since then, the field of cultural psychiatry has continued to expand, with an increased emphasis on the experience of minoritized groups in health care and the importance of practicing cultural humility in clinical encounters (Stubbe, 2020). The DSM, fifth edition, text revision (DSM-5-TR) carried this mission forward, revising the cultural formulation and providing clinicians with a semi-structured interview format to assess important cultural areas, such as definitions of the presenting problem, perceptions of the cause and context, and factors that affect coping and help seeking (APA, 2022).

As the field of cultural psychiatry has developed, scholars have applied its principles to the correctional setting (Kapoor et al., 2013; Ortega, 2011; Schar, 2023; Tseng et al., 2004). These resources provide guidance to correctional mental health clinicians on matters such as immigrant populations, language barriers, the validity of psychological testing in different ethnic groups, the stigma of mental illness in prison, religion's role in coping with the stress of incarceration, and many others.

Scholars have also begun to acknowledge that an understanding of culture alone is insufficient to explain many of the differences and disparities observed in health care settings. In the last decade, structural competence has emerged as a new framework to bring attention to the social drivers of mental health and illness. The concept of structural competence was introduced by Hansen and Metzl in 2014, describing the shift of U.S. medical education from a cross-cultural understanding of patients to an understanding of how larger social determinants of health affect individual health outcomes (Metzl & Hansen, 2014). Since that time, scholars have continued to expand on the concept and apply it to different health care settings, including in the postprison period (Metzl & Hansen, 2019; Treloar et al., 2021). Others have operationalized semi-structured interview questions that guide the assessment of how societal forces impact

*. The authors acknowledge the contributions of Ezra E. H. Griffith, who was a coauthor of this chapter in the first edition of the textbook.

patients' health (Bourgois et al., 2017). Correctional psychiatrists today have multiple resources at their disposal to educate themselves on how cultural and structural factors work synergistically to impact health and illness.

Current framework for cultural competence

Cultural competence is defined as congruent thoughts, actions, and policies that come together in a system or among people that enable effective work in cross-cultural situations (U.S. Department of Health and Human Services, 2013b). In health care, cultural competence is an ongoing process of striving to improve health professionals' capacities to adjust clinical practices to clients' cultural context and needs. There are many different models of cultural competence that have been studied empirically (Alizadeh & Chavan, 2016). A recent model proposed by Liu and colleagues (2021) attempted to synthesize the various models into three distinct domains: affective, cognitive, and behavioral. While these domains have not been studied directly in correctional settings, they provide a helpful framework that can be applied in prisons and jails, as well as in the community.

Affective domain

The affective domain emphasizes that clinicians should demonstrate humility, empathy, resilience, openness, and sensitivity to cultural differences. Correctional psychiatrists may recognize the difference in ethnic background and socioeconomic class between themselves, their patients, and other correctional staff. Additionally, they may recognize that medicine has its own culture, which is different from the law enforcement culture in which corrections professionals were educated. These differences should be navigated with cultural humility, which involves maintaining an open, self-exploratory, and self-critical stance about different cultural contexts and acknowledging that one's knowledge is always limited (Stubbe, 2020).

Cognitive domain

The cognitive domain emphasizes the continued acquisition of cultural knowledge and understanding. In prisons and jails, essential knowledge includes an understanding of the different norms and cultures of minority populations that are overrepresented in the criminal legal system. It also includes an understanding of special populations of prisoners such as women, juveniles, elderly persons, transgender and gender-nonconforming individuals, and immigrants.

Gaining such knowledge can allow psychiatrists and correctional staff to be aware of their implicit biases, which are unconscious preconceptualizations, attitudes, and stereotypes that can impact actions and decisions (Fitzgerald & Hurst, 2017). It is important to reflect openly and discuss issues of the patient's culture, including ethnicity and race, gender, age, class, education, religion, sexual orientation, and identification, as well as how they relate to characteristics of the treatment providers and custody staff. This reflection can reduce the impact of biases in the treatment of IPs.

Health care providers and custody staff should also be familiar with the cultural differences between their professions. Many correctional systems provide education about mental illness, such as Crisis Intervention Team training, to security officers so that they recognize signs and symptoms of illness and can respond appropriately (Hicks, 2011; see Chapter 24). In addition, mental health professionals must undergo training to understand the unique security aspects of the correctional setting—for example, use of force, searches, lockdowns, counts, and safety procedures (see Chapters 8 and 13).

Behavioral domain

The behavioral domain of cultural competence involves skills that ensure patient-centered care, such as respectful questioning, contextual inquiry, appropriate nonverbal communication, and use of interpreters when necessary. Applied to the correctional setting, this includes offering language assistance, including on-site or telephone interpreters, to IPs with limited English proficiency, even in remote facilities (U.S. Department of Health and Human Services, 2013a). It also includes providing written materials and facility policies to IPs in the primary languages of the communities served. Clinicians must also tailor communication to IPs' education levels and ask open-ended questions that uncover cultural nuances. Nonverbal communication must align with IPs' cultural context, while trauma-informed care helps ensure that clinical interactions are sensitive to previous traumatic experiences.

Health care systems are responsible for creating culturally appropriate goals and policies and for assessing how well these goals are being met over time. Correctional systems are no different; they must maintain a diverse workforce and analyze data about quality measures such as access to language assistance. When significant problems or disparities are identified, for example, delays in access to treatment for non-English speakers, systems must take steps to rectify these problems. These steps can include reallocation of resources, policy revision, grievance procedures, and other quality improvement measures (see Chapter 73). Finally, correctional systems are responsible for communicating the efficacy of these improvement efforts to all stakeholders, including IPs, custody staff, and health care providers.

Understanding cultural beliefs about the criminal legal system

Black and Hispanic individuals are significantly overrepresented in U.S. correctional settings compared to the general population. According to 2020 census data, Black individuals represented 13.6% of the U.S. population, Hispanic individuals 19.1%, and non-Hispanic White individuals 58.9% (U.S. Census Bureau, 2020). By contrast, data about prisons in the same year indicate that Black IPs made up 31.9% of the population, Hispanic IPs 20.6%, and non-Hispanic White IPs 28.1% (Bureau of Justice Statistics, 2021). According to the Bureau of Justice Statistics (2021), Black men were 5.7 times as likely to be imprisoned in 2020 as White men; Black males aged 18 to 19 were 12.5 times as likely to be imprisoned as White males of the same age. Furthermore, as of January 2023, 41.2% of IPs on death row were Black (Fins, 2023), and Black defendants were more likely to receive a death sentence if their victims were White (Paternoster et al., 2003, Pierce et al., 2017; U.S. General Accounting Office, 1990, Unah & Boger, 2001).

Black, Hispanic, and Native American communities have experienced the wide-ranging consequences of disparate criminal justice practices and mass incarceration, including disruptions to family life, perpetuation of income and wealth disparities, and undermining of political engagement. For example, the imprisonment of adult men leaves children without fathers. Children often seek sources of guidance, which, especially in urban environments, can be found in gang leaders who are respected by the community and influence the perception of incarceration as initiation instead of punishment (Morris, 2012). Mass incarceration also leaves many individuals of color disenfranchised due to felony convictions, diminishing the political power of their communities.

It is imperative for mental health professionals working with Black and Hispanic patients from impoverished or urban areas to understand cultural beliefs about the criminal legal system in these communities. Clinicians may misinterpret an IP's attitudes, labeling them as paranoid ideation or manifestations of antisocial personality disorder. These diagnoses might still be appropriate, but the patient's statements must be interpreted through a culturally informed lens to avoid misdiagnosis. This is particularly important given the historical context of psychiatric diagnoses being politicized and Black men being diagnosed with psychotic disorders at disproportionate rates (Metzl, 2009).

Understanding a patient's beliefs about the criminal legal system is also important when working with immigrant and refugee populations, which account for more IPs each year (see Chapter 62). In 2023, more than 170,000 immigrants were arrested by U.S. Immigrations and Customs Enforcement (2023). In 2022, 5.7% of the approximately 1 million people incarcerated in federal or state prisons in the United States, for whom citizenship data was available, were non-U.S. citizens (U.S. Department of Justice Office of Justice Programs, 2023). While most immigrants in detention are from Venezuela, Mexico, and Central America, detainees also include asylum seekers from nearly every country in the world (U.S. Immigrations and Customs Enforcement, 2023). Therefore, correctional mental health professionals are likely to encounter patients from many foreign cultures.

A common thread among many detained immigrants is that they come from countries in which the rule of law is not enforced consistently. In certain nations, corruption, bribery, political retaliation, and severe punishments are prevalent issues, and it may be difficult to find trustworthy professionals (e.g., judges, lawyers, or even doctors) who engage in their work independently from the government. This unfortunate reality may lead to immigrants losing faith in government agencies, including health care providers. As a result, mental health professionals may misdiagnose such guardedness or opposition as paranoia or antisociality. While it is impossible for a prison psychiatrist to become familiar with every country in the world, let alone their associated political problems, it is important to keep in mind that individuals from other cultures may have a very different understanding of the criminal legal system from that of the average White American.

Understanding the culture of prisons

Social scientists have long studied prison culture, describing a phenomenon called "prisonization" in which IPs adopt the norms and behaviors of the institution, characterized by harshness, predation, and a strict hierarchy of power (Clemmer, 1940). Two competing theories explain the development of this culture: the deprivation model (Sykes, 1958), which suggests it arises from deprivation of liberty, material goods, autonomy, heterosexual relationships, and security, and the importation model (Irwin & Cressey, 1962), proposing that IPs bring their preincarceration cultural norms into the prison environment.

Modern theorists have integrated these two models, stating that IPs' culture is influenced by both the shared experience of deprivation and individual characteristics such as stability of personality, the culture in which the IP was raised, and length of incarceration (Hochstetler & DeLisi, 2005). There is no one-size-fits-all culture of prisons, although the stereotype of prisons as hypermasculine environments in which power struggles are common still applies in some settings. The proliferation of women's prisons has further complicated matters, as women often approach the experience of incarceration differently from men, creating romantic relationships and pseudo-families rather than gang affiliations (Forsyth & Evans, 2003; see Chapter 55). Yet another complexity involves the growing population of transgender and gender-nonconforming IPs in a system that has traditionally viewed gender as binary (see Chapter 56). Thus, as prison populations have grown substantially since the 1980s, so too have the number of subcultures within prisons.

Once mental health clinicians have acquired a basic understanding of prison subcultures, they must assess the degree to which IPs have assimilated into one (or more) of these cultures. First, clinicians must inquire about a patient's culture outside of the correctional environment and then inquire about how their cultural beliefs and practices have changed since incarceration. In addition, clinicians should evaluate the extent to which a patient's adaptation to prison culture has been healthy or unhealthy. Has the patient found prosocial peers, or has behavior regressed in response to others? For example, some IPs learn maladaptive coping mechanisms such as smearing body fluids or engaging in self-injury from others whom they perceive as receiving more attention or care. Other IPs may react to prison culture in just the opposite way, seeing mental illness as a stigma and experiencing shame or fear about asking for help from mental health professionals.

Culturally and structurally competent practice in correctional settings

Considering the cultural context from which patients seek psychiatric care in correctional settings is crucial to combating marginalization and improving health outcomes. When mental health professionals better understand culture, they are less likely to pathologize patients' expressions of psychological distress that do not conform to Western conceptualizations of disease. For example, stigma about mental illness is common in the groups that are overrepresented in the U.S. prison system, including Black and Hispanic people, immigrants, refugees, and Native Americans. Stigma has been shown to lead to defensive behaviors, including avoidance, aggression, and fear responses (Moore et al., 2016). A culturally informed approach allows clinicians to understand how these behaviors might be adaptive in response to systemic marginalization, assess to what extent cultural factors play a role in the patient's presentation, and create an appropriate treatment plan.

Individuals involved with the criminal legal system are often treated with hostility, devalued, and dehumanized in prisons and broader society. Culturally competent care can foster respect and understanding in therapeutic relationships between mental health professionals and patients. For example, an IP may find the experience of speaking with a mental health professional stigmatizing or demeaning. Thus, regarding the IP as possessing both innate strength and dignity, particularly in front of others, is crucial. After establishing rapport and trust, one may then privately encourage the IP to speak freely and to be unashamed about asking for help (Ortega, 2011).

To be sure, culturally competent care has also been critiqued for inadvertently stereotyping patients of different racial and ethnic backgrounds. For example, understanding Asian patients as a monolithic group and assuming they uniformly somaticize psychiatric symptoms can lead clinicians to discount an individual patient's physical symptoms. Moreover, a purely cultural lens can be too narrow. It neglects to address how the societal context impacts patients' access to resources and behaviors in ways that result in poor health outcomes. The concept of structural competence better addresses how political, social, and economic forces have created systems of inequity based on race, gender, and other identity markers (Metzl & Hansen, 2014). For example, unequal food delivery systems, social service provisions, criminal justice practices, and residential zoning laws have produced and racialized health care inequities.

To build cultural and structural competence in psychiatric assessment and treatment, a checklist of steps to consider can be helpful. The DSM-5-TR provides a semi-structured cultural formulation interview that guides mental health professionals in obtaining culturally relevant information from the patient (APA, 2022). This cultural formulation can be adapted to the correctional context, as illustrated in Table 22.1.

Similarly, structural competence can be operationalized with clinical assessment tools that provide a framework to question how societal forces impact patients' health. Bourgois and colleagues (2017) created a "structural vulnerability" assessment tool to elucidate the pathways through which patients' health problems are exacerbated, which is illustrated in Table 22.2.

At first glance, Bourgois and colleagues' assessment tool may seem better suited to individuals in the community than in carceral settings, but the issues it raises are, in fact, relevant to prisons and

Table 22.1 Important areas of consideration for cultural formulation in correctional settings

Cultural identity before and after incarceration
- With what culture/subgroup(s) did the patient identify before entering the prison system?
- With what culture/subgroup(s) does the patient identify within the prison system?
- To what extent has the patient continued to associate with their culture of origin versus becoming assimilated with prison culture?
- How is the patient adjusting to the experience of isolation, loss, and deprivation common in all prisons?
- Does the patient's current cultural association represent an adaptive or maladaptive response to imprisonment?

Cultural beliefs about mental illness
- How is mental illness experienced/expressed/explained in the patient's culture of origin? To what degree is there stigma (or not)?
- How is mental illness perceived in the patient's prison subculture? By the custody staff?

Cultural beliefs about criminal legal system
- How are incarceration, the criminal legal system, and the patient's specific crime perceived in the patient's culture of origin? To what degree is there stigma (or not)?
- How is the patient's crime (such as sex offense, violence against child) perceived in the prison subculture? By the custody staff?

Cultural factors between patient and clinician
- What are the differences between the patient's cultural identity (both before and after prison) and the clinician's?
- What effect does the prison environment have on the clinician? Is the repeated exposure to the environment causing burnout in the clinician or perhaps adversely affecting perceptions of the patient?
- Is the clinician overidentifying with custody staff or with the patient (especially if one or the other is of the same culture as the clinician)?
- Is the physical plant or presence of other people such as custody officers affecting the patient's expression of symptoms or trust of the clinician?

Cultural factors affecting treatment planning
- Is the prison environment masking or exacerbating symptoms of mental illness? For example, is prolonged placement in restrictive housing exacerbating psychosis or depression?
- Can the clinician appreciate differences between the culture of the mental health staff and correctional officers?
- How can the clinician's understanding of cultural factors be translated into correctional language and made acceptable in a correctional culture? How can culturally aware treatment best be explained to officers focused on safety and security?
- To what extent can custody officers be involved in treatment planning, particularly when they share aspects of the patient's culture?

Note. Adapted from Kapoor, R., Dike, C., Burns, C., Carvalho, V., & Griffith, E. E. (2013). Cultural competence in correctional mental health. *International Journal of Law and Psychiatry, 36*(3–4), 273–280.

Table 22.2 Important areas of consideration for structural formulation

Financial security
- Did you have enough money to live comfortably—pay rent, food, and utilities?

Residence
- Did you have a stable and reliable place to sleep and store your possessions?

Food access
- Did you have adequate nutrition and access to healthy food?
- Did you have access to cooking facilities?

Social network
- What people make up your social network? Are these people healthy or unhealthy for you?
- Do you have enemies seeking to hurt you?

Discrimination
- Do you have friends or in-laws from different ethnic groups?
- Have you experienced discrimination based on your skin color, accent, place of origin, gender, or other identity markers?

Note. Adapted from Bourgois, P., Holmes, S., Sue, K., & Quesada, J. (2017). Structural vulnerability: Operationalizing the concept to address health disparities in clinical care. *Academic Medicine, 92*(3), 299–307.

jails. The carceral system itself creates structural problems that can adversely affect an individual's health. For example, access to healthy food is limited, housing assignments can change without warning, communication with friends and family is monitored, and exercise or outdoor recreation can be curtailed by staffing shortages. It is important for clinicians to understand the ways in which the correctional environment can be detrimental to mental health, even before considering the impact of the violence and trauma that often occur during incarceration. Inquiring about the patient's structural vulnerability factors prior to their incarceration is equally important, as it helps the clinician to understand all the societal forces that contributed to the patient's current presentation. Clinicians should also consider a patient's structural vulnerabilities upon release from prison, which will help create a reentry plan to better support the patient in the community (see Chapter 23).

Of course, correctional settings pose numerous challenges to providing culturally and structurally competent care. One barrier is that mental health professionals in correctional settings are overburdened and likely do not have the capacity to perform detailed cultural or structural formulation interviews. Second, despite mental health professionals' best intentions to provide culturally and structurally competent care, they are not entirely in control of how or when a treatment plan is implemented in a carceral setting. Mental health professionals face the challenge of including officers, whose primary concern is security, in treatment planning. This challenge can be met, but not without effort, communication, and goodwill among the parties.

When considering their role in carceral systems, clinicians must maintain humility and recognize that no one individual can overcome oppressive systems of power that have existed for centuries. Caring for patients can be done alongside advocating for systemic change, and both are an important part of a correctional psychiatrist's mission. All health professionals should work toward awareness of the extraclinical forces that negatively affect health outcomes in carceral settings, aligning with other stakeholders to promote systemic improvements, including through research, legislation, and community partnerships.

Summary

Some principles of cultural competence are common to all health care settings, including valuing diversity, communicating effectively, acquiring knowledge of different cultures, practicing cultural humility, and adapting to changes in the cultural environment. However, the correctional setting requires additional knowledge and skills. First, correctional mental health professionals must become familiar with cultural factors that affect the individual's experience of incarceration, such as ethnicity, gender, age, sexual orientation, and socioeconomic status. In addition, mental health professionals must learn about the culture of prisons. Mental health professionals in jails and prisons must be able to translate their ideas into correctional language so that security officers will understand and implement treatment plans. Finally, mental health professionals must become aware of how larger structural factors, including the criminal legal system itself, produce and racialize health inequities that contribute to poor health outcomes in jails and prisons. They must use this knowledge both to understand their patients' experiences and to advocate for systemic change.

REFERENCES

Alizadeh, S., & Chavan, M. (2016). Cultural competence dimensions and outcomes: A systematic review of the literature. *Health & Social Care in the Community*, *24*(6), e117–e130.

American Psychiatric Association. (1994). *Diagnostic and statistical manual of mental disorders* (4th ed.).

American Psychiatric Association. (2000). *Psychiatric services in jails and prisons* (2nd ed.).

American Psychiatric Association. (2016). *Psychiatric services in correctional facilities* (3rd ed.).

American Psychiatric Association. (2022). *Diagnostic and statistical manual of mental disorders* (5th ed., text rev.).

Bourgois, P., Holmes, S. M., Sue, K., & Quesada, J. (2017). Structural vulnerability: Operationalizing the concept to address health disparities in clinical care. *Academic Medicine*, *92*(3), 299–307.

Bureau of Justice Statistics. (2021). *Prisoners in 2020—Statistical tables.* https://bjs.ojp.gov/content/pub/pdf/p20st.pdf

Clemmer, D. (1940). *The prison community*. Christopher.

Fins, D. (2023). *Death row U.S.A., Winter 2023.* https://www.naacpldf.org/wp-content/uploads/DRUSAWinter2023.pdf

FitzGerald, C., & Hurst, S. (2017). Implicit bias in healthcare professionals: A systematic review. *BMC Medical Ethics*, *18*, 1–18.

Forsyth, C. J., & Evans, R. D. (2003). Reconsidering the pseudo-family/gang distinction in prison research. *Journal of Police and Criminal Psychology*, *18*(1), 15–23.

Hicks, E. (2011, August 10). *Crisis intervention in a correctional setting.* http://www.correctionsone.com/jail-management/articles/4206236-Crisis-intervention-in-a-correctional-setting/

Hochstetler, A., & DeLisi, M. (2005). Importation, deprivation, and varieties of serving time: An integrated-lifestyle-exposure model of prison offending. *Journal of Criminal Justice*, *33*, 257–266.

Irwin, J., & Cressey, D. (1962). Thieves, convicts, and the inmate subculture. *Social Problems*, *54*, 590–603.

Kapoor, R., Dike, C., Burns, C., Carvalho, V., & Griffith, E. E. (2013). Cultural competence in correctional mental health. *International Journal of Law and Psychiatry*, *36*(3–4), 273–280.

Liu, J., Gill, E., & Li, S. (2021). Revisiting cultural competence. *Clinical Teacher*, *18*(2), 191–197.

Metzl, J. M. (2009). *The protest psychosis: How schizophrenia became a black disease.* Beacon Press.

Metzl, J. M., & Hansen, H. (2014). Structural competency: Theorizing a new medical engagement with stigma and inequality. *Social Science & Medicine*, *103*, 126–133.

Metzl, J. M., & Hansen, H. (2019). *Structural competency in mental health and medicine: A case-based approach to treating the social determinants of health.* Springer.

Moore, K. E., Stuewig, J. B., & Tangney, J. P. (2016). The effect of stigma on criminal offenders' functioning: A longitudinal mediational model. *Deviant Behavior*, *37*(2), 196–218.

Morris, E. J. (2012). Respect, protection, faith, and love major care constructs identified within the subculture of selected urban African American adolescent gang members. *Journal of Transcultural Nursing*, *23*(3), 262–269.

Ortega, C. N. (2011). Issues in multicultural assessment and treatment. In T. J. Fagan & R. F. Ax (Eds.), *Correctional mental health: From theory to best practice* (pp. 125–144). Sage Publications.

Paternoster, R., Brame, R., Bacon, S., Ditchfield, A., Beckman, K., & Frederique, N. (2003). *An empirical analysis of Maryland's death sentencing system with respect to the influence of race and legal jurisdiction.* University of Maryland, College Park.

Pierce, G. L., Radelet, M. L., & Sharp, S. (2017). Race and death sentencing for Oklahoma homicides committed between 1990 and

2012. *Journal of Criminal Law and Criminology (1973–)*, *107*(4), 733–756.

Schar, C. H. (2023). A cultural competence framework for corrections in Hawai'i. In D. Moran, Y. Jewkes, K. L. Blount-Hill, & V. St. John (Eds.), *The Palgrave handbook of prison design*. Palgrave Macmillan, 603–619.

Stubbe, D. E. (2020). Practicing cultural competence and cultural humility in the care of diverse patients. *Focus*, *18*(1), 49–51.

Sykes, G. M. (1958). *The society of captives*. Princeton University Press.

Treloar, C., Schroeder, S., Lafferty, L., Marshall, A., Drysdale, K., Higgs, P., Baldry, E., Stoove, M., & Dietze, P. (2021). Structural competency in the post-prison period for people who inject drugs: A qualitative case study. *International Journal of Drug Policy*, *95*, 103261.

Tseng, W., Matthews, D., & Elwyn, T. S. (2004). *Cultural competence in forensic mental health*. Brunner-Routledge.

Unah, I., & Boger, J. C. (2001). *Race and the death penalty in North Carolina*. https://deathpenaltyinfo.org/resources/publications-and-testimony/studies/race-and-the-death-penalty-in-north-carolina

U.S. Census Bureau. (2020). *QuickFacts*. https://www.census.gov/quickfacts/fact/table/US/POP010220

U.S. Department of Health and Human Services. (2013a). *National standards for culturally and linguistically appropriate services (CLAS) in health and health care*. http://minorityhealth.hhs.gov/templates/browse.aspx?lvl=2&lvlID=15

U.S. Department of Health and Human Services. (2013b). *What is cultural competency?* http://minorityhealth.hhs.gov/templates/browse.aspx?lvl=2&lvlID=11

U.S. Department of Justice Office of Justice Programs. (2023). *Prisoners in 2022*. Bureau of Justice Statistics. https://bjs.ojp.gov/document/p22st.pdf

U.S. General Accounting Office. (1990). *Death penalty sentencing: Research indicates pattern of racial disparities*. http://www.gao.gov/assets/220/212180.pdf

U.S. Immigration and Customs Enforcement. (2023). *ICE releases fiscal year 2023 annual report*. https://www.ice.gov/doclib/eoy/iceAnnualReportFY2023.pdf

23

Community reentry preparation and coordination

*Henry A. Dlugacz**

Introduction

> *When the prison gates slam behind an inmate, he does not lose his human quality; his mind does not become closed to ideas; his intellect does not cease to feed on a free and open interchange of opinions; his yearning for self-respect does not end; nor is his quest for self-realization concluded. If anything, the needs for identity and self-respect are more compelling in the dehumanizing prison environment.*
>
> —*Procunier v. Martinez* (1974)

These words, written 50 years ago by Supreme Court Justice Thurgood Marshall, remind us that incarceration does not extinguish a person's humanity. Thirty years later, President George W. Bush brought Justice Marshall's insight to its logical conclusion: "We know from long experience that if released inmates can't find work, or a home, or help, they are much more likely to commit crime and return to prison" (Bush, 2004, para. 65).

All incarcerated persons (IPs) who do not die before release—approximately 97%—return to the community (Council of State Governments, 2002; Federal Bureau of Prisons, 2024). This simple reality makes it in society's enlightened self-interest to address the readiness of IPs to live a productive life. The criminal justice and correctional treatment systems affect an IP's behavior and opportunities upon release. Were they treated humanely? What skills did they acquire to enhance prosocial coping styles? Were they afforded educational or vocational opportunities? Was mental health treatment adequate? What linkages were made prior to release to address risk factors for recidivism and the need for continued treatment, housing, or employment?

Successful reentry planning considers these interrelated issues while building an individualized plan to address them. It begins at admission (or even sentencing) and continues after release (Petersilia, 2001); correctional mental health treatment is part of a continuum of care that extends to the community. Obtaining collateral information about preincarceration functioning and response to treatment aids in the accurate assessment of needs during incarceration and following release. Likewise, pertinent information from correctional treatment providers should be transmitted to the community programs that will provide ongoing care. This can be accomplished systematically, supplemented by clinician-to-clinician contact in specific circumstances. One study, noting the lack of sufficient staff in many correctional facilities, suggested improved, automated hand-offs of key information between correctional and community-based treatment providers (T. R. Miller et al., 2024). While promising, implementation of this approach is limited by the reality that, as of 2018, a mere 4.5% of state corrections departments had the infrastructure to utilize electronic medical records to share health information (Lieber et al., 2024). Even when pertinent information is conveyed by automated means, the exchanges of information can be enhanced by the nurturing of professional relationships through stakeholders' meetings, cross-training, and the creative use of technology (Dlugacz & Roskes, 2010). Reentry planning for people with serious mental illness should be a primary focus of correctional mental health care, not an afterthought to be considered only as release is imminent.

Scope of the problem

The United States incarcerates an immense number of people, inevitably leading to a large number of releases to the community. The U.S. Department of Justice reports that a combined 448,400 people were released from the Federal Bureau of Prisons and state prisons in 2022 (Carson & Kluckow, 2023). It is estimated that there are up to 7 million releases annually from local jails (Dumont et al., 2012). Among this group are a disproportionate number of people with severe mental illness (Dlugacz, 2014; Steadman et al., 2009). It is reported that 4.2% of the general adult population suffers from a serious mental illness, as compared to an estimated 20% to 26% of the jail population and 15% of the prison population (Garcia & Haskins, 2020).

*. The author thanks Emily Brouwer, Helen Haidemenos, Sophie Nettesheim, and Zachary Abu-Orf for their extensive and highly able assistance.

Despite the clear need for transitional services, they are not consistently available. A survey of U.S. jails found that about 20% of IPs with mental illness received discharge planning services (Hoge, 2007). One survey of New Jersey jails found a large variation in prerelease efforts among facilities, with some reporting that they provided aftercare plans for fewer than 10% of IPs with mental illness upon release and others reporting that they did so for between 75% and 100% of such IPs (Wolff et al., 2002). According to the Bazelon Center for Mental Health Law (2009), only one third of recently incarcerated persons receive assistance with accessing benefits. When these reentry services are provided, they vary considerably with respect to the population served, the approach used, and the locus of administrative authority. Rather than being based on empirical data, they tend to be localized in nature (Wilson & Draine, 2006).

One survey of reentry programs in the United States found that 74% were led by the criminal justice system and only 26% by the behavioral health system, with varying degrees of collaboration between the two. Those spearheaded by the criminal justice system were found to be more collaborative than those led by the behavioral health system (Wilson & Draine, 2006). This suggests that, despite an increased focus on breaking down service "silos," improved collaboration is needed (Dlugacz et al., 2007).

Even when reentry plans are provided, some community-based mental health organizations may be unwilling, unprepared, or unsure of how to best serve the justice-involved population. Some fall prey to stereotypes equating serious mental illness with potential violence, while others are not aware of the resources available to them (Shaffer et al., 2019). Further, the deteriorated state of the public mental health system in the United States can render even the most thoughtful plan meaningless.

Whatever the specific intervention indicated for any given individual, reentry planning should be considered a key aspect of the mental health treatment provided to IPs with mental disorders. This logical public health approach was supported on a federal constitutional basis in a recent opinion from the United States Court of Appeals for the Second Circuit: "Common sense and experience further support [the] theory that discharge planning is part of in-custody care" (*Charles v. Orange County*, 2019, p. 21). The "hub and spoke" approach encouraged by the Centers for Medicare and Medicaid Services in the substance use treatment context is also applicable to behavioral health treatment. In this model, the community-based treatment providers ("hub") assist in training and providing treatment in correctional settings (the "spoke"; Lieber et al., 2024). Some go further and promote the CommonSpirit community bank model, where community providers assist in funding some unreimbursed services in the carceral setting (Lieber et al., 2024). This could be supplemented by an approach where clinical staff have joint or hybrid assignments in community and correctional treatment settings, promoting continuity of care for specific patients upon release while bridging gaps in knowledge and breaking down misconceptions.

Obstacles to reentry

IPs with serious mental illness are at elevated risk across multiple domains when released. A recent study found that people released from jail, within the year, made up an estimated 19.9% of all adult deaths by suicide but only 2.8% of the adult population (T. R. Miller et al., 2024). Strikingly, the study concluded that "the nearly 7.1 million US adults released from jail in 2019 accounted for 1 in 5 adult suicides" (T. R. Miller et al., 2024, p. 10). Consistent with the need for comprehensive discharge planning, the authors advocated for focused public health suicide prevention measures to reduce this elevated risk of suicide among formerly incarcerated people, especially in the first year or two following release (T. R. Miller et al., 2024). The U.S. Department of Justice reported that "an estimated 68% of released prisoners were arrested within 3 years, 79% within 6 years, and 83% within 9 years" (Alper et al., 2018, p. 1). Furthermore, within 90 days of release, formerly incarcerated people are twice as likely as the general population to be hospitalized and/or die. In the case of death, they are more likely to die outside of the hospital, which suggests considerable barriers to health care access (Wang et al., 2013). One study found that IPs were almost 13 times more likely to die within the first 2 weeks of release than were other people with similar demographics (Binswanger et al., 2007a, 2007b).

Comorbid substance use disorders are also a significant problem, affecting about half of the prison population who have mental illness (Al-Rousan et al., 2017; Baranyi et al., 2022). IPs with co-occurring disorders are less likely to enroll and stay in treatment programs, more likely to relapse and recidivate, and more likely to face difficulty securing stable housing and social safety net program benefits (Fabian et al., 2021). Overall rates of homelessness are highly elevated in the correctional population. Unhoused IPs are more likely to have co-occurring mental health problems and substance use disorders and may be incarcerated for longer periods of time (Freudenberg et al., 2005; McNiel et al., 2005). Further, the criminal justice population overall has high levels of chronic medical conditions (Binswanger et al., 2012) and tends to have these conditions in more advanced stages than do age-adjusted comparators.

Approaches to reentry planning

The very nature of our correctional system, with its emphasis on punishment through the isolation of the individual from community support, poses a fundamental obstacle to successful reentry planning. The IP lives in a place that distorts human interactions (Dlugacz & Wimmer, 2013), dictating when to eat, when to go to sleep, even when to look up or look down. Patterns of interpersonal interactions that can save your life while incarcerated may be maladaptive in the free world (Rotter, 2010). This can have a direct impact on recidivism and treatment outcomes. One report found that "connectedness to the criminal community positively predicted recidivism during the first year post-release," whereas "connectedness to the community at large positively predicted community adjustment" (Folk et al., 2016, p. 353).

Better ways must be found to fulfill the custody and control functions of corrections while at the same time creating an environment that better prepares IPs to lead a productive, lawful life once released (Weinstein & Wimmer, 2010).

While the difficulties faced by recently incarcerated persons can be daunting, they also form a template for required interventions. The interplay between mental illness and recidivism is complex and requires attention in the reentry planning process (see Chapter 6). Noting the high rates of mental illness among the correctional population, practitioners assumed that linkage to treatment upon release would be a primary driver of improved criminal justice outcomes. While clinical interventions did improve clinical outcomes, they did not appear to significantly reduce recidivism. Studies show that the specific symptoms of serious mental illness are related to arrest in fewer than 10% of cases, suggesting that treatment as usual across the population will not have the desired effect on recidivism (Peterson et al., 2010; Rotter et al., 2014).

Other studies indicate that most people with mental illness have essentially the same risk factors for recidivism as do other people (Hall et al., 2012). This suggests that one primary focus of treatment in corrections and upon release should be on the types of cognitive-behavioral treatment that have been proven effective in reducing recidivism across the criminal justice population. Research related to the risk–need–responsivity model supports this approach (Bonta & Andrews, 2007). The risk–need–responsivity model uses risk assessment to identify a person's risk factors for criminal behavior so that they are specifically targeted by interventions individualized to the person's strengths, abilities, motivations, and learning style (Bonta & Andrews, 2007). In this approach, serious mental illness is only a minor risk factor (Bonta & Andrews, 2007).

However, just as the focus on standard treatment may have been overly simplistic, so too may be a rush to abandon it. Improving treatment outcomes has a value in and of itself and may serve to improve compliance with parole requirements. The episodic nature of psychosis may mask the relationship between mental illness and arrest (Hall et al., 2012). Because people with mental illness remain incarcerated longer than others, they may have a reduced chance to commit new crimes (Baillargeon et al., 2009; McNiel & Binder, 2007). One large study found that IPs with major psychiatric disorders had a substantially increased risk of multiple incarcerations over a 6-year period (Baillargeon et al., 2009).

However, other studies indicate that standard mental health treatment may indeed moderate recidivism. One found that routine outpatient treatment reduced the likelihood of arrest and that medication possession in the 90-day period following hospitalization appeared to provide further protection (Van Dorn et al., 2013). Treatment linkages are not a panacea and, in the absence of more comprehensive biopsychosocial interventions, are unlikely to single-handedly solve complex problems many decades in the making. Further study is required concerning the criminal justice population in general and with respect to the efficacy of specific approaches within subpopulations. A paltry 0.12% of projects funded by the National Institute of Health and 0.03% of those supported by the National Science Foundation since 1985 address incarceration (Lieber et al., 2024). Nonetheless, overall, "improved connections to services and better management of health conditions may also contribute to reduced rates of recidivism, particularly among individuals with health and substance [use] disorders" (Gates et al., 2014, p. 6).

Most studies on reentry programs report on successful linkage to services, not whether the service, intensity, or type was adequate (Draine & Herman, 2007). While released IPs may receive social or mental health services, one study showed that few get clinically meaningful levels of care during the first year of release (Lovell et al., 2002). Also, evidence-supported services (including integrated treatment for substance use disorder and mental illness; Kubiak et al., 2011) and the types of cognitive therapies risk–need–responsivity research recommends may not be widely available.

Some consumers make rational decisions to reject services that do not meet their needs, such as reentry planning that does not address housing. One study of jail detainees found that men listed employment and education as their top priorities, while women regarded treatment for substance use disorder as paramount. Both adult men and women regarded housing as a high priority (Freudenberg et al., 2005). The needs identified by these IPs hew closely to known strategies that reduce recidivism. While much is made of the population's lack of insight and misguided priorities, these IPs desired exactly the type of interventions that would help them avoid future incarcerations. A more recent study of released IPs with severe mental illness echoed these results, finding that housing and financial assistance were their top priorities. Only 12% of the group listed mental health treatment among their top two priorities for assistance following release (Wilson, 2013).

Successful reentry programs tend to have certain elements in common:

- Behavioral/cognitive treatment;
- Positive reinforcement;
- Intensive services that last 3 to 12 months and that occupy between 30% and 70% of the person's time;
- Use with high-risk IPs;
- Targeting of criminogenic needs;
- Use of actuarial assessments of risk;
- Interventions conducted in community rather than institutional settings; and
- Staffing skill sets matched to IPs' needs and learning styles (Cullen & Gendreau, 2000; Petersilia, 2004).

The focus on high-risk IPs is supported by research demonstrating that the placement of low-risk IPs in more intensive programs often increased their failure rates (Lowenkamp & Latessa, 2004).

Treatment and rehabilitation approaches that show promise for incorporation into successful reentry programs include peer mentoring (L. Miller, 2010), supported employment, and supportive housing (Draine & Herman, 2010). This approach is supported by the Centers for Medicare and Medicaid Services (Lieber et al., 2024). One study found that IPs with mental illness in a work-release program had higher success rates than other IPs in the program (Way et al., 2007), serving as a good reminder to challenge assumptions not based on empirical data or extensive real-world experience. A program to expand supportive housing in New York City proved to be cost-effective, resulting in fewer Medicaid costs, emergency service needs, and inpatient care expenditures (Gouse et al., 2023). The individuals placed in this supportive housing were ultimately more likely to start and remain in treatment for substance use disorder and spent less time in jail and shelters, further decreasing government spending (Gouse et al., 2023).

Another promising approach is Forensic Assertive Community Treatment, which is an adaptation of traditional assertive community treatment models (Cuddeback et al., 2013). Forensic Assertive Community Treatment attempts to close gaps in service between the mental health and treatment systems by including partnerships between the two and encouraging adherence to treatment through legal leverage (Lamberti & Weisman, 2010).

Brief motivational interviewing is an evidence-based counseling technique shown to improve motivation for treatment for several physical and emotional conditions (Rubak et al., 2005). Brief motivational interviewing is well suited to corrections because it can be used by a wide array of staff. The approach has utility for reentry planning because successful reentry and retention in aftercare go hand in hand. The sustained changes in behavior promoted by brief motivational interviewing make it conceptually similar to a public health intervention akin to a vaccine—a brief intervention with protective benefits extending well into the future.

A related resource developed in working with unhoused individuals—and more recently with the formerly incarcerated population—is Critical Time Intervention. It "provides several of the usual transitional services, such as vocational training, but there is a key focus on the critical factors of community and social support in reentry" (Galletta et al., 2021, p. 60). While no single approach is well suited to all IPs, these interventions are among those that should be considered when formulating an individualized, comprehensive reentry plan.

Access to benefits

No reentry plan is likely to succeed if not accompanied by the means to pay for it. Entitlements such as Medicaid, Medicare, Veterans Administration benefits, and Social Security Income help people to secure housing, mental health treatment, and sustenance (Bazelon Center for Mental Health Law, 2009). Because the period immediately following release poses particular risks, whenever possible, IPs should be assisted with applying for benefits before they are released. When this is not achievable, appointments can be made and required documents assembled so the person is well situated to follow through promptly following release.

Correctional systems can enter into prerelease agreements with the Social Security Administration that facilitate the submission of new applications for Social Security Administration benefits or the prompt reinstatement of suspended benefits upon an IP's release. Such agreements standardize communication between the Social Security Administration and correctional facilities by providing point persons in each organization and establishing procedures for the submission of applications and supporting documentation (Social Security, Program Operations Manual System, 2013). Training staff to complete applications for benefits improves success rates (McCormick & Perret, 2010).

Focused attention on benefits assistance can increase access to care. One study found that a program to help IPs with serious mental illness to enroll in Medicaid increased use of mental health services by 16% (Wenzlow et al., 2011). Most jurisdictions have developed mechanisms whereby Medicaid benefits are suspended rather than terminated during a person's incarceration. As of 2019, 43 states had opted to suspend Medicaid benefits rather than terminate them, and 23 states supported prerelease Medicaid enrollment programs that utilize automated electronic processes to resume benefits and access to treatment upon release (Kaiser Family Foundation, n.d.; National Conference of State Legislatures, 2023). At least three states (Wisconsin, Louisiana, and Ohio) have reported substantial increases in outpatient visits and even reductions in financial stress and recidivism for formerly incarcerated persons following the implementation of such reenrollment programs (National Conference of State Legislatures, 2023). Terminating Medicaid benefits upon incarceration can thwart the policy and fiscal goals of the states, as well the reentry plan for individuals released from corrections. The reenrollment process becomes burdensome, limiting individuals' willingness to reenroll and their access to adequate health care, while also limiting the state's receipt of federal funds for inpatient health care for IPs (National Conference of State Legislatures, 2023).

Even suspension of benefits, however, can disrupt continuity of care for IPs. Under some circumstances, jurisdictions may now apply to utilize Medicaid funding for a variety of covered treatments, including treatment for incarcerated juveniles (Mistak, 2023), treatment for substance use disorders and serious mental illness, and reentry planning services, by obtaining federal waivers from the Centers for Medicare and Medicaid Services (Traube & Guyer, 2021). Demonstration projects related to these expanded opportunities, referred to as 1115 waivers, offer "cautious hope relevant to addressing mental health issues among the justice-involved population" (Lieber et al., 2024, p. 537). Additionally, while not exclusively addressing formerly incarcerated populations, states can sometimes use Medicaid to provide housing services to individuals with disabilities, individuals with behavioral health conditions, and those at risk of homelessness (Chhean, 2023).

Many Western countries outside of the United States have more robust equivalence between prison and community health care (Exworthy et al., 2012; United Nations General Assembly, 1990). In countries such as the United Kingdom, universal health care reduces the concern that is so prevalent in the United States related to gaps in health coverage. Interestingly, released IPs in the United Kingdom face many of the same obstacles to successful reentry as do those in the United States, including lack of adequate community mental health care and difficulty securing employment and affordable housing (MacDonald, 2012). This demonstrates that while access to health benefits is a rate-limiting step in accessing needed services, it is only one part of the puzzle.

Practical suggestions

The scope of obstacles to successful reentry can be daunting. Stakeholder meetings to create the crucial buy-in (Dlugacz et al., 2007) and interagency meetings can foster collaboration and build informal networks that can be used once programs are operational (Dlugacz et al., 2007).

In-reach by community providers prior to an IP's release may improve the likelihood of follow-through after discharge. Where distances are prohibitive, video links can be used. IPs can be moved closer to home in the period leading up to their release to facilitate interaction with providers and family. Some providers are willing to meet the released IP at the institution's gate to assist with transportation; these so-called "warm hand-offs" can be highly beneficial in prompting a successful transition to community providers in the high-risk period directly following release. The same is true of ensuring release during daylight hours, when programs are open to connect with released IPs.

Unfortunately, approximately half of IPs who were taking medication for psychiatric conditions do not receive them while in prison (Lieber et al., 2024). For those who are prescribed psychotropic medications while incarcerated, a supply and/or prescription should be provided so that they can continue taking them until the time of their appointment with a community-based provider. Particularly for those who tend to be nonadherent with prescribed medications, correctional psychiatrists should consider transitioning the patient to long-acting medications as they approach a release date. A system that electronically sends a released IP's prescriptions to community pharmacies can be crucial to continuity of care (*Brad H. et al. v. City of New York et al.*, 2023).

Summary

Several factors will influence an IP's reentry plan: the person's illness, treatment while incarcerated, and ability to function in the community; the model of service delivery; and the correction facility's size, location, and function. Reentry planning cannot be divorced from the state of affordable housing and evidence-based treatment available in the community to which the person will return. Difficult though it may be, it is incumbent upon those working in corrections to address systemic problems and create plans that support people with mental illness in overcoming these formidable obstacles.

REFERENCES

Alper, M., Durose, M., & Marksman, J. (2018). *2018 update on prisoner recidivism: A 9-year follow-up period (2005-2014)*. U.S. Department of Justice, Office of Justice Programs, Bureau of Justice Statistics. https://bjs.ojp.gov/content/pub/pdf/18upr9yfup0514.pdf

Al-Rousan, T., Rubenstein, L., Sieleni, B., Deol, H., & Wallace, R. B. (2017). Inside the nation's largest mental health institution: A prevalence study in a state prison system. *BMC Public Health, 17*(1), 342.

Baillargeon, J., Binswanger, I. A., Penn, J. V., Williams, B. A., & Murray, O. J. (2009). Psychiatric disorders and repeat incarcerations: The revolving prison door. *American Journal of Psychiatry, 166*(1), 103–109.

Baranyi, G., Fazel, S., Langerfeldt, S. D., & Mundt, A. P. (2022). The prevalence of comorbid serious mental illnesses and substance use disorders in prison populations: A systematic review and meta-analysis. *Lancet Public Health, 7*(6), 492–493.

Bazelon Center for Mental Health Law. (2009). Linking to federal benefits for people exiting corrections. *Lifelines, 3*, 1–34. https://www.bazelon.org/wp-content/uploads/2017/01/Lifelines-All.pdf

Binswanger, I. A., Redmond, N., Steiner, J. F., & Hicks, L. S. (2012). Health disparities and the criminal justice system: An agenda for further research and action. *Journal of Urban Health: Bulletin of the New York Academy of Medicine, 89*(1), 98–107.

Binswanger, I. A., Stern, M. F., Deyo, R. A., et al. (2007a). Correction to release from prison: A high risk of death for former inmates. *New England Journal of Medicine, 356*, 536.

Binswanger, I. A., Stern, M. F., Deyo, R. A., et al. (2007b). Release from prison: A high risk of death for former inmates. *New England Journal of Medicine, 356*, 157–165.

Bonta, J., & Andrews, D. A. (2007). *Risk-Need-Responsivity model for offender assessment and rehabilitation*. https://www.publicsafety.gc.ca/cnt/rsrcs/pblctns/rsk-nd-rspnsvty/index-eng.aspx

Brad H. et al. v. City of New York et al., Index No. 117882/99, Urban Justice Center (2023, April), https://mhp.urbanjustice.org/wp-content/uploads/sites/10/2021/08/Brad_H_et_al_v_The_City_of_New_York_et_al_DECISION___ORDER_ON_76-002.pdf

Bush, G. W. (2004). *State of the Union address*. https://georgewbush-whitehouse.archives.gov/news/releases/2004/01/20040120-7.html

Carson, E. A., & Kluckow, R. (2023, November). *Prisoners in 2022—Statistical tables*. Bureau of Justice Statistics. https://bjs.ojp.gov/library/publications/prisoners-2022-statistical-tables

Charles v. Orange County, 17-3506-pr (2d Cir. 2019).

Chhean, E. (2023, October 2). *How states are using Medicaid authorities to cover housing-related services*. https://nashp.org/how-states-are-using-medicaid-authorities-to-cover-housing-related-services/

Council of State Governments. (2002). *Criminal Justice/Mental Health Consensus Project*. http://consensusproject.org/ downloads/Entire_report.pdf

Cuddeback, G. S., Wright, D., & Bisig, N. (2013). Characteristics of participants in jail diversion and prison reentry programs: Implications for forensic ACT. *Psychiatric Services, 64*, 1043–1046.

Cullen, F., & Gendreau, P. (2000). Assessing correctional rehabilitation: Policy, practice, and prospects. *Criminal Justice, 3*, 109–175.

Dlugacz, H. (2014). Correctional mental health in the United States. *International Journal of Prisoner Health, 10*, 3–26.

Dlugacz, H. A., Broner, N., & Lamon, S. (2007). Implementing reentry—Establishing a continuum of care of adult jail and prison releases with mental illness. In O. Thienhaus & M. Piasecki, *Correctional psychiatry: Practice guidelines and strategies* (pp. 12-1–12-37). Civic Research Institute.

Dlugacz, H. A., & Roskes, E. (2010). Clinically oriented reentry planning. In C. L. Scott (Ed.), *Handbook of correctional mental health* (2nd ed., pp. 395–431). American Psychiatric Publishing.

Dlugacz, H., & Wimmer, C. (2013). Legal aspects of administrating antipsychotic medications to jail and prison inmates. *International Journal of Law and Psychiatry, 36*, 213–228.

Draine, J., & Herman, D. (2007). Critical time intervention for reentry from prison for persons with mental illness. *Psychiatric Services, 8*, 1577–1581.

Draine, J., & Herman, D. (2010). Critical time intervention. In H. Dlugacz (Ed.), *Reentry planning for offenders with mental disorders: Policy and practice* (pp. 6–1–6–11). Civic Research Institute.

Dumont, D. M., Brockmann, B., Dickman, S., Alexander, N., & Rich, J. D. (2012). Public health and the epidemic of incarceration. *Annual Review of Public Health, 33*, 325–339.

Exworthy, T., Samele, C., Urquía, N., & Forrester, A. (2012). Asserting prisoners' right to health: Progressing beyond equivalence. *Psychiatric Services, 63*, 260–275.

Fabian, K., Shively, R., & Aufderheide, D. (2021). Co-occurring disorders in the incarcerated population: Treatment needs. *Corrections Today*. https://www.aca.org/common/Uploaded%20files/Publications_Carla/Docs/Corrections%20Today/2021%20Articles/CT_Jan-Feb_2021_Co-occurring%20Disorders.pdf

Federal Bureau of Prisons. (2024). *BOP statistics: Sentences imposed*. https://www.bop.gov/about/statistics/statistics_inmate_sentences.jsp

Folk, J. B., Mashek, D., Tangney, J., Stuewig, J., & Moore, K. E. (2016). Connectedness to the criminal community and the community at large predicts 1-year post-release outcomes among felony offenders. *European Journal of Social Psychology, 46*(3), 341–355.

Freudenberg, N., Daniels, J., Crum, M., Perkins, T., & Richie, B. E. (2005). Coming home from jail: The social and health consequences of community reentry for women, male adolescents, and their families and communities. *American Journal of Public Health, 95*, 1725–1736.

Galletta, E., Fagan, T. J., Shapiro, D., & Walker, L. E. (2021). Societal reentry of prison inmates with mental illness: Obstacles, programs, and best practices. *Journal of Correctional Health Care, 27*(1), 58–65.

Garcia, M., & Haskins, P. (2020, July 20). *Identifying needs related to managing seriously mentally ill individuals in corrections*. National Institute of Justice. https://nij.ojp.gov/topics/articles/

identifying-needs-related-managing-seriously-mentally-ill-individuals-corrections#1-0
Gates, A., Artiga, S., & Rudowitz, R. (2014, September 5). *Health coverage and care for the adult criminal justice-involved population*. https://www.kff.org/uninsured/issue-brief/health-coverage-and-care-for-the-adult-criminal-justice-involved-population/
Gouse, I., Walters, S., Miller-Archie, S., Singh, T., & Lim, S. (2023). Evaluation of New York/New York III Permanent Supportive Housing Program. *Evaluation and Program Planning*, *97*, 1–9.
Hall, D. L., Miraglia, R. P., Lee, L-W. G., Chard-Wierschem, D., & Sawyer, D. (2012). Predictors of general and violent recidivism among SMI prisoners returning to communities in New York State. *Journal of the American Academy of Psychiatry and the Law*, *40*, 221–231.
Hoge, S. K. (2007). Providing transition and outpatient services to the mentally ill released from correctional institutions. In R. B. Greifinger (Ed.), *Public health behind bars* (pp. 461–477). Springer.
Kaiser Family Foundation. (n.d.). *States reporting corrections-related Medicaid enrollment policies in place for prisons or jails*. https://www.kff.org/medicaid/state-indicator/states-reporting-corrections-related-medicaid-enrollment-policies-in-place-for-prisons-or-jails/?activeTab=map&currentTimeframe=0&selectedDistributions=medicaid-eligibility-suspended-rather-than-terminated-for-enrollees-who-become-incarcerated__prisons&sortModel=%7B%22colId%22%3A%22Location%22%2C%22sort%22%3A%22asc%22%7D
Kubiak, S. P., Essenmacher, L., Hanna, J., & Zeoli, A. M. (2011). Transitions between jail and community-based treatment for individuals with co-occurring disorders. *Psychiatric Services*, *62*, 679–681.
Lamberti, S. J., & Weisman, R. L. (2010). Forensic assertive community treatment: Origins, current practice, and future directions. In H. Dlugacz (Ed.), *Reentry planning for offenders with mental disorders: Policy and practice* (pp. 7–1–7–24). Civic Research Institute.
Lieber, W. C., Zhang, J., & Brinkley-Rubinstein, L. (2024). Medicaid reentry section 1115 demonstration opportunity. *JAMA Psychiatry*, *81*(6), 537.
Lovell, D., Gagliardi, G. J., & Peterson, P. D. (2002). Recidivism and use of services among persons with mental illness after release from prison. *Psychiatric Services*, *53*, 1290–1296.
Lowenkamp, C. T., & Latessa, E. J. (2004). *Understanding the risk principle: How and why correctional interventions can harm low-risk offenders, topics in community corrections*. National Institute of Corrections.
MacDonald, M. (2012). *Research report: United Kingdom*. http://www.throughcare.eu/partnerreports.html
McCormick, T. C., & Perret, Y. M. (2010). Accessing public benefits: More advocacy than entitlement. In H. Dlugacz (Ed.), *Reentry planning for offenders with mental disorders: Policy and practice* (pp. 3–2–3–20). Civic Research Institute.
McNiel, D. E., & Binder, R. L. (2007). Effectiveness of a mental health court in reducing criminal recidivism and violence. *American Journal of Psychiatry*, *164*, 1395–1403.
McNiel, D. E., Binder, R. L., & Robinson, J. C. (2005). Incarceration associated with homelessness, mental disorder, and co-occurring substance abuse. *Psychiatric Services*, *56*, 840–846.
Miller, L. (2010). Reentry as part of the recovery process. In H. Dlugacz (Ed.), *Reentry planning for offenders with mental disorders: Policy and practice* (pp. 10–2–10–8). Civic Research Institute.
Miller, T. R., Weinstock, L. M., Ahmedani, B. K., Carlson, N. N., Sperber, K., Cook, B. L., Taxman, F. S., Arias, S. A., Kubiak, S., Dearing, J. W., Waehrer, G. M., Barrett, J. G., Hulsey, J., & Johnson, J. E. (2024). Share of adult suicides after recent jail release. *JAMA Network Open*, *7*(5), 1–13.
Mistak, D. (2023, January 3). *Historic health changes in the omnibus appropriations bill*. https://cochs.org/omnibus-mistak-letter/
National Conference of State Legislatures. (2023, January 16). *Connecting recently released prisoners to health care: How to leverage Medicaid*. https://www.ncsl.org/civil-and-criminal-justice/connecting-recently-released-prisoners-to-health-carehow-to-leverage-medicaid
Petersilia, J. (2001). Prisoner reentry: Public safety and reintegration challenges. *Prison Journal*, *81*, 360–375.
Petersilia, J. (2004). What works in prisoner reentry? Reviewing and questioning the evidence. *Federal Probation*, *68*, 4–8.
Peterson, J., Skeem, J., Hart, E., Vidal, S., & Keith, F. (2010). Analyzing offense patters as a function of mental illness to test the criminalization hypothesis. *Psychiatric Services*, *61*, 1217–1222.
Procunier v. Martinez, 416 U.S. 396 (1974).
Rotter, M. (2010). A culturally competent approach to correctional adaptation. In H. Dlugacz (Ed.), *Reentry planning for offenders with mental disorders: Policy and practice* (pp. 8–1–8–6). Civic Research Institute.
Rotter, M., Carr, A., & Frischer, K. (2014). The premise of criminalization and the promise of offender treatment. In H. Dlugacz (Ed.), *Reentry planning for offenders with mental disorders: Policy and practice* (Vol. 2, pp. 1–1–1–11). Civic Research Institute.
Rubak, S., Sandbaek, A., Lauritzen, T., et al. (2005). Motivational interviewing: A systematic review and meta-analysis. *British Journal of General Practice*, *55*, 305–313.
Shaffer, J. S., Russo, J., Woods, D., & Jackson, B. A. (2019). *Managing the seriously mentally ill in corrections*. https://www.rand.org/pubs/research_reports/RR2698.html
Social Security, Program Operations Manual System. (2013). *Prerelease agreements*. https://secure.ssa.gov/apps10/poms.nsf/lnx/0500520910
Steadman, H. J., Osher, F. C., Robbins, P. C., Case, B., & Samuels, S. (2009). Prevalence of serious mental illness among jail inmates. *Psychiatric Services*, *60*(6), 761–765.
Traube, A., & Guyer, J. A. (2021, June 9). *States are leveraging Medicaid waivers to transform their behavioral health systems*. Manatt. https://www.manatt.com/insights/newsletters/manatt-on-health-medicaid-edition/states-are-leveraging-medicaid-waivers-to-transfor
United Nations General Assembly. (1990). *Basic principles for the treatment of prisoners*. http://www.un.org/documents/ga/res/45/a45r111.htm
Van Dorn, R. A., Desmarais, S. L., Petrila, J., Haynes, D., & Singh, J. P. (2013). Effects of outpatient treatment on risk of arrest of adults with serious mental illness and associated costs. *Psychiatric Services*, *64*, 856–962.
Wang, E. A., Wang, Y., & Krumholz, H. M. (2013). A high risk of hospitalization following release from correctional facilities in Medicare beneficiaries. *JAMA Internal Medicine*, *173*(17), 1621–1628.
Way, B., Abreu, D., Ramirez-Romero, D., Aziz, D., & Sawyer, D. A. (2007). Mental health service recipients and prison work release: How do the mentally ill fare compared to other inmates in prison work release programs? *Journal of Forensic Sciences*, *52*, 965–966.
Weinstein, J. B., & Wimmer, C. (2010). Sentencing in the United States. In H. Dlugacz (Ed.), *Reentry planning for offenders with mental*

disorders: Policy and practice (pp. 1-1–1-45). Civic Research Institute.

Wenzlow, A. T., Ireys, H. T., Mann, B., Irvin, C., & Teich, J. L. (2011). Effects of a discharge planning program on Medicaid coverage. *Psychiatric Services*, *62*, 73–78.

Wilson, A. B. (2013). How people with mental illness seek help after leaving jail. *Qualitative Health Research*, *23*, 1575–1590.

Wilson, A. B., & Draine, J. (2006). Collaborations between criminal justice and mental health systems for prisoner reentry. *Psychiatric Services*, *57*, 875–878.

Wolff, N., Plemmons, D., Veysey, B., & Brandli, A. (2002). Release planning for inmates with mental illness compared with those who have other chronic illnesses. *Psychiatric Services*, *53*, 1469–1471.

SECTION IV

Management of psychiatric emergencies

24

Crisis assessment and management

Reena Kapoor

Introduction

Crisis calls occur so frequently in correctional settings that they can begin to seem routine. Psychiatrists are regularly called away from scheduled assignments such as diagnostic interviews or medication clinics to respond to a wide array of concerns, including suicide attempts, acute changes in mental status or behavior, seizures, destruction of property, self-injury, smearing of bodily waste, fire setting, and flooding. Requests for urgent intervention can range from the informal request—"Doc, I need you to take a look at Jones"—to the formal system of color-coded emergency response after violence or suicide attempts. Regardless of the psychiatrist's formal work assignment, handling crises is an expected part of the job, almost always in collaboration with custody staff. This chapter reviews the pragmatics of evaluating and managing many common correctional events that lead to mental health crisis calls.

The crisis response system in correctional settings

Correctional psychiatrists receive requests for urgent consultations from many sources, including custody staff, other physicians, other mental health staff, and even persons outside the facility such as family members, court personnel, and attorneys. Table 24.1 lists common types of urgent evaluations in correctional settings.

Although psychiatrists can be asked to respond to crises anywhere within a correctional institution, some settings and subpopulations of incarcerated persons (IPs) are more likely to require crisis intervention. IPs who have a history of mental illness frequently use emergency care, as do IPs who are housed in high-security settings such as restrictive housing units (Knoll & Beven, 2010). A disproportionate number of self-harm and prison suicides occur in restrictive housing units (Luigi et al., 2020; Patterson & Hughes, 2008), and IPs are also more likely to display evidence of behavioral disturbances in those settings (Luigi et al., 2020; Lovell, 2008). Finally, psychiatrists in jails may be called to respond to suicide attempts more frequently than those assigned to prisons; both attempts and death by suicide are more common in jail settings, though this gap has narrowed in recent years (Bureau of Justice Statistics, 2021).

In contrast to other health care settings, a crisis response in prisons and jails often involves the use of chemical agents, riot gear, and video cameras. These paramilitary aspects of the emergency response can be intimidating and frightening. In addition, psychiatrists must adjust to the idea that they are not leading the response team but are instead collaborating with security staff. In recent years, many correctional systems have adapted the Crisis Intervention Team (CIT) model, first developed with police officers working in community settings, to prisons and jails (McNeeley & Donley, 2021). CIT involves a collaborative approach between security and mental health professionals. It is intended to enhance correctional officers' understanding of mental illness and to provide them with tools to communicate and intervene effectively with IPs (DuPont & Cochrane, 2000), The typical CIT training is 40 hours, consisting of both didactic instruction and role-playing exercises about mental illness. Studies indicate that CIT-trained police officers demonstrated better knowledge of mental illness, greater confidence in responding to crisis situations, and decreased use of force (Bonfine et al., 2014; Compton et al., 2015; Morabito et al., 2012).

Studies of CIT in corrections are more limited, but they generally indicate an improvement in correctional officers' self-reported knowledge and attitudes about mental illness immediately following the training (Canada et al., 2021; Comartin et al., 2020). Unfortunately, these improvements may decrease over time, with participants' skills returning to baseline in as little as 1 month after training (Davidson, 2016). Studies of CIT outcomes in corrections are mixed, showing that CIT-trained officers are more likely to make mental health referrals upon intervening in a crisis with an IP, but there is no reduction in use of force when compared with non-CIT-trained officers (McNeeley & Donley, 2021). Despite these mixed results, CIT has grown in use in jails and prisons, with the National Institute of Corrections now offering training to correctional systems across the country (National Institute of Corrections, 2022).

Even if not formally called CIT, collaboration between security, mental health, and sometimes medical professionals when responding to crises is common in correctional settings. When a "code" is called, multidisciplinary staff will often respond, with security personnel taking the lead to secure the scene. Depending on the acuity of the situation, mental health staff may be asked to help with verbal de-escalation, though they generally do not put hands on the IP. Such physical interventions are handled by security personnel. Depending on the circumstances, once the scene has been secured, mental health professionals may be asked to conduct a

Table 24.1 Common requests for urgent psychiatric evaluation

Requesting party	Type of evaluation
Security staff	• Suicide attempts or threats • Other self-injury • Clearance for placement in restricted housing • Evaluation after Prison Rape Elimination Act (PREA) allegation • Destruction of property • Smearing of bodily waste • Bizarre behavior observed in housing unit • Homicidal statements (usually in conjunction with other signs of mental illness)
Other physicians and medical providers	• Management of acute drug or alcohol intoxication or withdrawal • Refusal of medical care • Swallowing or insertion of foreign bodies • Mental status and capacity to engage in hunger strike
Nursing and other mental health professionals	• Refusal of psychiatric medication • Ordering of therapeutic restraints • Emergency medication • Discharge from treatment setting or transfer to less therapeutic environment • Referral for civil commitment or transfer to a psychiatric hospital
Courts	• Bizarre behavior observed during court appearance • Suicide risk assessment after imposition of long sentence
Families and attorneys	• Suicidal statements made during visit with family or attorney • Suicidal or threatening letters written by an incarcerated person

clinical assessment regarding the IP's need for acute psychiatric care, clinical restraints, or both, and medical staff may assess for physical injuries. This type of collaboration between mental health, medical, and security personnel may be followed by formal or informal debriefing procedures.

Approach to crisis assessment and management

Although crisis evaluations address a wide variety of problems, some features are common to all such assessments. Therefore, the correctional psychiatrist can use a relatively standardized approach to handling crises that serves to improve patient care and decrease the psychiatrist's anxiety in these challenging situations.

Maintaining a therapeutic role and appropriate boundaries

When collaborating with security staff in crisis situations, psychiatrists may feel pressure to conduct a cursory assessment or to "sign off" on the case so that disciplinary measures can be implemented. This pressure can be particularly acute when an IP has engaged in behavior that disturbs the officers, such as repeatedly banging on doors or smearing bodily waste. Custody staff often see punishment as the most effective method of stopping this behavior, and they seek the psychiatrist's approval or collaboration in moving forward with this plan. The psychiatrist may also feel exasperated by the IP's behavior, viewing it as an attempt to manipulate the conditions of confinement rather than as a symptom of mental illness.

Despite these pressures, psychiatrists must remember that their primary role is therapeutic, and therefore they must focus on the IP's best interest. Even if the IP displays evidence of antisocial traits, psychiatrists must complete a thorough and independent evaluation. When deciding on a course of action, they must not allow their desire to maintain collegial relationships with security staff to supersede their concern for the well-being of the patient. Furthermore, they must recognize their own feelings of frustration and ensure that they are not acting out against the patient or reflexively jumping to a diagnosis of malingering. Maintaining a therapeutic stance when working with severely disturbed individuals can be challenging but is nevertheless essential to creating an effective treatment relationship.

On the other hand, mental health professionals, including psychiatrists, may inadvertently distort the concept of a therapeutic relationship and place themselves at risk of engaging in boundary violations on behalf of the IP. For example, IPs often ask psychiatrists to intervene in areas that are traditionally managed by security staff, such as phone calls or housing decisions. In addition, some IPs make romantic overtures toward mental health professionals and may view the relationship as more than strictly professional. While psychiatrists should feel free to advocate for the health of their patients, they must also take care to maintain appropriate boundaries and avoid developing personal relationships with IPs. In crisis situations, psychiatrists should also be careful not to promise more assistance than they can provide. IPs may attempt to apply pressure on the psychiatrist by promising to end the crisis if their demands are met; such negotiations are usually counterproductive in the long term. Maintaining appropriate boundaries and clear role definitions between security and psychiatry is consistently a better approach.

Confidentiality and communication with the requesting party

In many correctional settings, psychiatrists will rarely be the first staff members to notice acutely dangerous behavior. These events tend to happen in housing units or other shared spaces in the facility, such as the recreation yard, health care unit, or vocational areas. To facilitate an effective emergency response, correctional facilities typically employ a "code" system to alert staff and summon them to the crisis. Some systems may also have other ways to request an urgent mental health evaluation at the request of an IP or of custody staff, such as by calling the on-call mental health clinician on a two-way radio.

By the time the psychiatrist arrives, other staff members have hopefully begun to gather necessary information from the IP, health record, and custodial electronic record-keeping system. In emergencies, rapid communication with security staff about the events leading up to the psychiatrist's intervention is essential. Psychiatrists should obtain information about who first identified the problem with the IP, what was observed, what steps were taken to address the matter, and what the IP's response was. In addition, psychiatrists should clarify what the party requesting the evaluation expects of the psychiatrist; this can range from informal assessments—"just take a look at him"—to involuntary medication and transfer to a psychiatric hospital.

Whenever possible, mental health and security staff should discuss this information in a private setting away from other IPs. Psychiatric emergencies, and sometimes just the presence of an unfamiliar face on the housing block, can attract many curious onlookers from other cells. As any information that IPs (or even other staff members) gain about the crisis may be used to taunt or harass the involved IP later, maintaining confidentiality should not be taken lightly.

In addition to the concern about future harassment by peers or officers, psychiatrists should evaluate the IP in a confidential setting whenever feasible for the usual therapeutic reasons; people are more likely to share their true feelings if not fearful of being overheard. Psychiatrists should make clear to the IP that they are there in a therapeutic capacity and are not trying to punish them. At the same time, psychiatrists should acknowledge the limits of confidentiality during an emergency evaluation, explaining that information about immediate threats to the safety and security of the facility must be shared with security staff. This may make an IP more reluctant to share, but a proactive advisement about limits of confidentiality is preferable to them feeling betrayed by the psychiatrist after the fact.

Environmental factors

During crises, correctional psychiatrists are often asked to evaluate IPs through the cell door, in a therapeutic module, or while being video recorded. The IP may be restrained with handcuffs, and in some instances, a chemical agent has already been sprayed in the area. All these environmental factors can influence the quality of the psychiatrist's assessment. A quiet, confidential setting is always preferable when conducting a psychiatric evaluation but cannot always be achieved in a crisis. In some situations, such as when an IP is acutely agitated or possesses a weapon, a psychiatrist would be foolish to interview them alone or without restraints. In other situations, IPs may simply refuse to come out of the cell. Although not ideal, a cell-front psychiatric evaluation may be required in these circumstances.

In addition to security concerns, recording devices can also play a role in shaping the psychiatrist's assessment during a crisis. In many emergencies, particularly those that are formally designated by a color-coded response system, corrections officers will video record the actions of staff and the IP for use in an operational review of the incident. Recently, correctional systems have required officers to carry body-worn cameras (BWCs) and activate them during crisis interventions (Welsh-Huggins, 2021). These programs are relatively new, and preliminary data indicate that correctional officers have negative perceptions of BWCs' ability to enhance safety or improve IPs' behavior, both before and after a year of experience with BWCs (Peterson et al., 2023). No data about the impact of BWCs on correctional officers' misconduct or use of force have yet been published (Peterson et al., 2023). Studies of BWCs in community-based police officers are not promising, indicating that they have no effect on use of force, arrests, assaults on officers, or officer injuries (Lum et al., 2020).

De-escalation

Psychiatrists responding to crises can use several de-escalation techniques to help IPs calm themselves and avoid the use of force (Richmond et al., 2012). First, psychiatrists should respect the personal space of the IP, trying to stand at least two arms' lengths away. When approaching the IP, psychiatrists should introduce themselves and state their role clearly. Multiple persons responding to a crisis can be perceived as threatening, so only one or two people at a time should talk to the IP to minimize fear and distress. Body language is important; psychiatrists should avoid gestures like clenched fists or crossed arms, which can be interpreted as provocative.

Psychiatrists and security officers should listen attentively and allow IPs to express the concerns that led to the crisis. Repeating the IP's words back to them and using statements such as "Tell me if I have this right ..." can help them to feel heard. If the IP is delusional, psychiatrists should avoid actively challenging the delusions, instead focusing on the emotions expressed by the IP in response to their beliefs. Similarly, psychiatrists should avoid making accusations of lying or malingering in the crisis, as these accusations can heighten tensions and prolong the incident. The goal is to allow the IP to express wishes and emotional distress without feeling attacked or demeaned.

To the extent possible, offering choices to the IP can also be helpful. For example, sometimes the IP can be allowed to choose which officer or mental health staff member attends to the crisis. This technique makes use of preexisting therapeutic alliances and can help the IP maintain some control over the situation. In another example, a choice between different forms of oral medication (liquid, pill, or dissolving strip) can be offered as an alternative to intramuscular injection. While de-escalation may not be successful in all cases, trying to avoid the use of force can be beneficial both in the short term and long term. IPs see that the psychiatrist is compassionate enough to help them avoid traumatic experiences such as cell extractions and restraints, and officers can learn more therapeutic and effective approaches to crisis management.

Elements of the psychiatric evaluation

While maintaining a relatively standardized approach is best, the specific elements of a psychiatric evaluation in a crisis can vary greatly based on the circumstances. For example, the assessment of an IP who has just attempted suicide can be very different in focus and duration from the assessment of one who has declared a hunger strike. In the former circumstance, the initial focus may be on getting the IP appropriate medical treatment for asphyxia or lacerations, and the psychiatrist may only briefly assess the patient before arranging for hospital transport. In the latter circumstance, the psychiatrist may conduct an extended evaluation, carefully documenting the IP's history of any mental illness and stated rationale for engaging in the hunger strike, performing a formal mental status exam, and determining the patient's capacity to refuse food. Both situations require urgent assessment, but the psychiatrist's approach is tailored to the needs of the IP and the requesting party.

In all cases, psychiatrists should conduct as thorough an evaluation as circumstances require, despite external pressures such as staff shift changes or desires to transfer the IP to another facility quickly. The IP's health and stability are the psychiatrist's primary concern. In general, psychiatrists should attempt to interview the IP, gather information from relevant collateral informants, perform necessary elements of the mental status exam, and discuss any changes to the treatment plan with the IP during a crisis evaluation. If any of these elements are omitted, psychiatrists should ensure that they are not neglected for the sake of convenience or because of inadequate resources. All elements of the assessment performed and the rationale for the chosen course of action must be documented.

Disposition options

When psychiatrists intervene in crisis situations, they are often asked to recommend a particular course of action to security staff.

If an IP has made a serious suicide attempt, the course of action is usually clear—stabilize the patient medically and then admit them to an intensive psychiatric treatment setting. However, many types of crises allow mental health and security staff to use more discretion to resolve the situation. Changes in housing placements, privilege levels, medication, and frequency or type of therapy are all possible. In some cases, transfer to a psychiatric or medical hospital may be necessary (see Chapter 26). With so many options, psychiatrists may find it difficult to make recommendations, particularly when facing time pressure.

Many correctional systems alleviate this confusion in nonemergency situations or after a crisis has stabilized by creating multidisciplinary teams to review decisions about IPs' mental health treatment and conditions of confinement. This approach can be helpful to ensure that all relevant factors are considered before deciding about disposition, including the IP's psychiatric stability, interpersonal relationships, history of violence, and coping skills. During the emergency, however, psychiatrists do not typically have the luxury of working through this supportive process and must reach a decision about immediate concerns quickly.

If the evaluating psychiatrist is concerned about the IP's safety, they should advocate for placing the patient in a secure and therapeutic setting such as an inpatient psychiatric unit or a psychiatric observation cell. This measure should be taken even if the IP engages in repetitive, nonlethal acts of self-injury and staff are growing tired of frequent transfers (see Chapter 52). If questioned about the need for emergency transfer, psychiatrists can refer to the literature about the high risk of completed suicide in patients who have made prior attempts, particularly by hanging, strangulation, or suffocation (Olfson et al., 2012; Runeson et al., 2010). Of course, crisis response is only one part of a comprehensive treatment plan for suicidal patients; psychiatrists should also advocate for a better long-term treatment plan for the IP to avoid repeated inpatient placements. However, in an emergency (in the absence of an existing long-term plan), psychiatrists should act cautiously and place the IP in a safe setting.

Restraint and seclusion

Guidelines from the National Commission on Correctional Health Care (NCCHC) state, "Mental health staff order clinical restraints and clinical seclusion only for patients exhibiting behavior dangerous to self or others *as a result of mental illness*" (NCCHC, 2015, p. 133, emphasis added). Although this guideline is clearly written, in a crisis, it can sometimes be difficult to tell whether an IP's violent or self-injurious behavior stems from mental illness. For example, if an IP climbs onto a ledge and threatens to jump if his TV or tablet computer is not returned to him, it may not be immediately apparent what the IP's underlying mental state is, and the acutely dangerous circumstances do not offer much opportunity for inquiry. In such circumstances, security personnel will generally need to secure the IP using approved security techniques, which may include chemical agents, physical holds, or security restraints. Once the IP and scene are secure, medical professionals should be called to assess acute medical needs (e.g., injuries), while mental health professionals should be called to assess the need for clinical restraint, emergency medication, seclusion, or hospitalization.

Restraint, seclusion, and emergency medication are discussed further in Chapter 25. When considering whether to order restraints, psychiatrists should use criteria consistent with the community standard—for example, is the patient an imminent danger to self or others, and have less restrictive interventions failed? (American Psychiatric Association, 2016; Metzner et al., 2007; NCCHC, 2015). When needed, four-point therapeutic restraints, like those found in the community, should be used. In almost all circumstances requiring therapeutic restraints, the IP should be transferred to a health care setting to be monitored (Metzner et al., 2007). Therapeutic restraints should be used for the shortest duration necessary to ensure the patient's safety (Metzner et al., 2007).

Many correctional systems use different types of restraints for security purposes, such as metal shackles, handcuffs, or belly chains (see Chapter 8). A psychiatrist should never order these for a therapeutic purpose. The use of custody restraints is governed by many factors unrelated to mental illness, such as seriousness of charge, gang affiliation, and history of institutional violence. The restraints are used to incapacitate IPs in a wide variety of circumstances, from recent assaultive behavior to routine transportation between areas of the facility. While some of these considerations may be relevant to an emergency psychiatric assessment, in general, they are less important than the IP's current mental status and intent for harm to self or others. The psychiatrist should focus on the IP's acute safety and health, using the same criteria and therapeutic techniques used in the community to respond to the dangerous behaviors of individuals with mental illness.

Documentation

After a crisis has been diffused, the psychiatrist must document the encounter in the medical record. Progress notes should contain all relevant information about the crisis and its resolution, including how the psychiatrist became involved in the situation, what information was obtained from collateral informants, the IP's version of events, their mental status, and the psychiatrist's assessment and plan. Psychiatrists should carefully articulate why they chose a particular course of action and why they rejected alternatives. In addition to protecting against litigation, this information guides mental health professionals who subsequently work with the IP to understand what triggered the crisis and what worked to diffuse it.

Depending on the nature and severity of the crisis, documentation in addition to the clinical record may also be required. Most correctional systems require documentation to keep track of serious incidents of self-injury, the use of restraints, and the use of cell extraction teams. In addition, a clinical review of every completed suicide and serious suicide attempt should be conducted, and recommendations about policy or procedure changes resulting from this review should be documented (NCCHC, 2015; see Chapter 74).

Crisis situations may also involve disciplinary actions against an IP, either as a precipitant to a mental health crisis or as a consequence of engaging in crisis-generating behavior. Psychiatrists frequently are asked to document their opinions regarding the IP's suitability for discipline in these situations. These evaluations are challenging, as psychiatrists are not trained to answer questions about how much punishment a person can or should endure. Nonetheless, psychiatrists play an important role in the IP disciplinary process, and their opinions are given considerable weight. Security staff typically ask two questions of psychiatrists: (a) Is the IP stable enough to proceed with the disciplinary process? (b) Did mental illness play a role in the events leading to the disciplinary infraction? Psychiatrists should consider these questions carefully and answer them honestly. A disciplinary evaluation is an opportunity to suggest alternative sanctions if appropriate, such as a treatment program specific to the IP's mental health- or substance-related needs (Tamburello & Haston, 2021).

Summary

Crisis calls are common in correctional settings, and psychiatrists play an integral role in crisis management. Requests for urgent psychiatric evaluations can come from many sources, including custody staff, nonpsychiatric physicians, mental health staff, courts, attorneys, and family members. Psychiatrists responding to these requests for evaluation may feel tremendous pressure to reach a conclusion that is consistent with the opinions of the requesting party. However, maintaining an independent and therapeutic stance when conducting crisis evaluations is crucial.

Some aspects of psychiatric evaluations in crisis situations are unique to the correctional environment, including cell-front evaluations, video recording, and leadership by security staff rather than medical professionals. Nonetheless, correctional psychiatrists should be guided by the same principles of medical ethics that apply to patient care in the community, placing the patient's well-being above all other concerns. They should strive, when possible, to conduct a thorough assessment in a confidential setting. In considering how best to resolve the crisis and care for the patient, psychiatrists should err on the side of caution and recommend placement in a safe and therapeutic setting, at least until a multidisciplinary team can consider other options. Finally, they should document the encounter carefully, articulating the rationale for the chosen course of action.

REFERENCES

American Psychiatric Association. (2016). *Psychiatric services in correctional facilities* (3rd ed.). American Psychiatric Publishing.

Bonfine, N., Ritter, C., & Munetz, M. R. (2014). Police officer perceptions of the impact of Crisis Intervention Team (CIT) programs. *International Journal of Law and Psychiatry*, *37*(4), 341–350.

Bureau of Justice Statistics. (2021). *Suicide in local jails and state and federal prisons, 2010–2019—Statistical tables.* https://bjs.ojp.gov/library/publications/suicide-local-jails-and-state-and-federal-prisons-2000-2019-statistical-tables

Canada, K. E., Watson, A. C., & O'Kelley, S. (2021). Utilizing crisis intervention teams in prison to improve officer knowledge, stigmatizing attitudes, and perception of response options. *Criminal Justice and Behavior*, *48*(1), 10–31.

Comartin, E. B., Wells, K., Zacharias, A., & Kubiak, S. (2020). The use of the crisis intervention team (CIT) model for corrections officers: Reducing incidents within a county jail. *Prison Journal*, *100*(5), 581–602.

Compton, M. T., Broussard, B., Reed, T. A., Crasafio, A., & Watson, A. C. (2015). Surveys of police chiefs and sheriffs and of police officers about CIT programs. *Psychiatric Services*, *66*, 760–763.

Davidson, M. L. (2016). A criminal justice system-wide response to mental illness: Evaluating the effectiveness of the Memphis Crisis Intervention Team training curriculum among correctional and law enforcement officers. *Criminal Justice Policy Review*, *27*, 46–75.

Dupont, R., & Cochrane, S. (2000). Police response to mental health emergencies: Barriers to change. *Journal of the American Academy of Psychiatry and the Law*, *28*, 338–344.

Knoll, J. L., IV, & Beven, G. E. (2010). Supermax units and death row. In C. L. Scott (Ed.), *Handbook of correctional mental health* (pp. 435–475). American Psychiatric Publishing.

Lovell, D. (2008). Patterns of disturbed behavior in a supermax prison. *Criminal Justice and Behavior*, *35*, 985–1004.

Luigi, M., Dellazizzo, L., Giguère, C. É., Goulet, M. H., & Dumais, A. (2020). Shedding light on "the Hole": A systematic review and meta-analysis on adverse psychological effects and mortality following solitary confinement in correctional settings. *Frontiers in Psychiatry*, *11*, 840.

Lum, C., Koper, C. S., Wilson, D. B., Stoltz, M., Goodier, M., Eggins, E., et al. (2020). Body-worn cameras' effects on police officers and citizen behavior: A systematic review. *Campbell Systematic Reviews*, *16*(3), e1112.

McNeeley, S., & Donley, C. (2021). Crisis Intervention Team training in a correctional setting: Examining compliance, mental health referrals, and use of force. *Criminal Justice and Behavior*, *48*(2), 195–214.

Metzner, J. L., Tardiff, K., Lion, J., et al. (2007). Resource document on the use of restraint and seclusion in correctional mental health care. *Journal of the American Academy of Psychiatry and the Law*, *35*, 417–425.

Morabito, M. S., Kerr, A. N., Watson, A. C., Draine, J., & Angell, B. (2012). Crisis intervention teams and people with mental illness: Exploring the factors that influence the use of force. *Crime & Delinquency*, *58*(1), 57–77.

National Commission on Correctional Health Care. (2015). *Standards for mental health services in correctional facilities.*

National Institute of Corrections. (2022). *Crisis intervention teams: A frontline response to mental illness in corrections.* https://nicic.gov/resources/nic-library/hot-topics/does-nic-have-information-crisis-intervention-teams-cit-2022

Olfson, M., Marcus, S. C., & Bridge, J. A. (2012). Emergency treatment of deliberate self-harm. *Archives of General Psychiatry*, *69*(1), 80–88.

Patterson, R. F., & Hughes, K. (2008). Review of completed suicides in the California Department of Corrections and Rehabilitation, 1999 to 2004. *Psychiatric Services*, *59*(6), 677–681.

Peterson, B. E., White, M. D., Cunningham, B., Lawrence, D. S., Lafferty, J., & Coldren, J. R., Jr. (2023). *Body-worn cameras in a correctional setting: Assessing jail deputy attitudes before, during, and after implementation.* CrimRxiv. https://www.crimrxiv.com/pub/sivy27p8/release/1

Richmond, J. S., Berlin, J. S., Fishkind, A. B., Holloman G. H., Jr., Zeller, S. L., Wilson, M. P., et al. (2012). Verbal de-escalation of the agitated patient: Consensus statement of the American Association for Emergency Psychiatry Project BETA de-escalation workgroup. *Western Journal of Emergency Medicine*, *13*(1), 17–25.

Runeson, B., Tidemalm, D., Dahlin, M., Lichtenstein, P., & Langstrom, N. (2010). Method of attempted suicide as predictor of subsequent successful suicide: National long term cohort study. *British Medical Journal*, *341*, c3222.

Tamburello, A. C., & Haston, L. (2021). Mischief, mayhem, and remediation. *Journal of the American Academy of Psychiatry and the Law*, *49*(3), 323–325.

Welsh-Huggins, A. (2021, October 29). *Prison systems adding body-worn cameras to security plans.* Courthouse News Service. https://www.courthousenews.com/prison-systems-adding-body-worn-cameras-to-security-plans/

25

Seclusion, restraint, and involuntary medication

Darren L. Lish[*]

Introduction

The use of seclusion and restraint (S/R) in mental health settings has long been fraught with legal and ethical concerns, as the practice can be dangerous. This is perhaps accentuated in the more punitive environment of jails and prisons within the United States. As a result, there is a national movement to reduce the use of S/R for mentally ill patients, both in the community and within jails and prisons. However, S/R remains a necessary intervention when less invasive options to maintain the safety of the incarcerated person (IP) and others have failed. For instance, in limited cases, S/R might be an appropriate option for acutely aggressive, agitated patients who require immediate intervention. The use of S/R preserves the safety of the patient, other IPs, and staff. This, in turn, supports a safer milieu.

In 1999, the Health Care Financing Administration, now the Centers for Medicare and Medicaid Services (CMS), defined rules for the use of S/R for facilities that participate in Medicare and Medicaid (42 C.F.R. § 482.13). While CMS regulations do not govern correctional facilities, these rules nevertheless heavily influenced subsequent guidelines, including the American Psychiatric Association's resource document (APA RD) on the use of S/R in correctional health care (Metzner et al., 2007) and that of the American Bar Association (2011).

The use of involuntary medication in jails and prisons refers to the practice of administering psychotropic medication to an individual against their will or without their consent. This topic often sparks debate among professionals, advocates, and policymakers, given the ethical dilemma involved. On the one hand, there is a duty of care to ensure the health and well-being of IPs, many of whom may have serious ongoing psychiatric symptoms that pose a risk to themselves or others. On the other hand, forcibly medicating individuals raises concerns about autonomy, consent, and human rights, and it may require the use of physical restraints or force, which can escalate tensions within a correctional facility, lead to allegations of abuse, and disrupt the relationship between the individual and their treatment providers.

Use of seclusion and restraint

Location

In jails and prisons, S/R may occur in corrections-based hospitals, infirmaries, or other special housing. If an IP is transferred out of a jail or prison into a community hospital for care, CMS rules typically guide the placement and monitoring of the individual in S/R. When S/R occurs in jail or prison, a health care setting with 24-hour nursing coverage, such as an infirmary, should be used, as specified by the APA RD (Metzner et al., 2007). It is not appropriate to use locked-down housing units for IPs with mental illness who require S/R for clinical reasons. Not only are these units typically not supportive or therapeutic, but also they likely will exacerbate the clinical condition for which the S/R is indicated in the first place. They also typically lack the health care staff necessary for treatment and monitoring.

Indications

There are several indications for S/R. They are appropriate when less restrictive forms of treatment have not proven effective or are not appropriate for the gravity of the clinical situation, as outlined in Table 25.1.

Just as there are indications for S/R, so too are there situations in which S/R is not appropriate: patients who have a marked fear of being restrained; patients who have marked claustrophobia in a seclusion room; lack of trained, qualified mental health and/or medical staff to monitor the S/R; lack of a seclusion room sufficiently free of ways in which a patient may self-injure; and staff requests for S/R that the ordering physician believes reflect neglect, abuse, or staff convenience. Health care staff should never order S/R for punitive purposes. Behaviors such as insolence, rudeness, or public masturbation are not reasons for S/R.

Prior to the use of S/R, less restrictive interventions (reflecting verbal, environmental, or pharmacological aspects) should be used when appropriate. Staff should be adequately trained to address the underlying psychopathology before and after S/R, and the patient's

---

*. The author would like to recognize the contributions of Gerard G. Gagné Jr., who authored this chapter in the first edition of this textbook.

Table 25.1 Indications for the use of seclusion and/or restraint in the correctional setting

- Signs and symptoms of significant danger to others that cannot be managed by less restrictive means
- Severe agitation for which emergency medication is inadequate or unavailable (e.g., allergy or known previous adverse effect) or has not yet taken effect
- Significant disruption of the clinical or residential milieu that threatens the rights or safety of patients or staff and for which less restrictive interventions are inadequate or not feasible
- Dangerous, agitated, or disruptive behavior whose origins are unclear and for which restraint and seclusion are likely to be safer than medication or other measures because of insufficient knowledge about the incarcerated person's medical condition

housing unit should have sufficient staffing and treatment programs to address the patient's mental illness.

Type of restraints

Custody restraints (usually metal handcuffs) should not be used for mental health purposes. Typically, soft, adjustable restraints are applied to both wrists and ankles. Another alternative is the restraint chair, which is a device that holds an individual in an upright, seated position, allowing them to face forward rather than up toward the ceiling like traditional four-point restraint. A review of the legal and medical literature on restraint chairs found that there was little to no medical risk and little legal liability when proper protocols and monitoring were followed (Castillo et al., 2015). Nurses in acute adult psychiatric settings have described benefits of the restraint chair compared to four-point restraint, noting that it is easier to use, more humane, and less traumatic for the individual (Visaggio et al., 2020). The restraint chair is an effective and safe alternative to four-point restraint. However, caution must be exercised in correctional settings because of the potential for its misuse for nontherapeutic purposes.

Seclusion room design

The safe practice of S/R includes design of the seclusion room. The National Association of Psychiatric Health Systems (Sine & Hunt, 2007) has published seclusion room design guidelines that address the type of fixtures, temperature controls, lighting, and patient visibility, among other factors. While these factors might sound inconsequential, they play a role both in treatment and in preventing self-injury or staff assault.

It is not uncommon to have constant, full-room lighting, particularly for several hours after the patient is placed in seclusion, to allow for easy staff visualization of the patient to assess ongoing aggressive behavior. The walls should be made of materials that cannot be picked apart or gouged for use in self-injury or as a weapon against staff. The room should be free of sharp corners and fixtures that jut out from the walls or ceiling. Windows should be made of shatterproof material, and the door should open outward so that the IP cannot barricade the room. Only staff should control locks. Furniture should be limited to a mattress. A toilet and sink, if included, should be of unitary metal construction with no sharp edges or ligature points. If not available in the room, toileting provisions must be made: A simple hole in the floor for toileting is inappropriate, as it is unsanitary and dehumanizing.

Restraint rooms are very similar in design to seclusion rooms, with the one major difference being the inclusion of a restraint bed. Given the limited resources in many jails and prisons, it is not uncommon for a single room to be used for both seclusion and restraint, in which case the restraint bed should be made of a resilient, durable material and should be a single, unitary platform; it should be secured to the floor. Recessed attachments for restraints should be an integral feature of a restraint bed.

Property

Unless specifically contraindicated, individuals who are being secluded and/or restrained should have access to clothing (preferably made of tear-resistant materials to prevent their use for new or additional self-injury), a blanket (also made of tear-resistant materials), and a mattress (preferably one made of foam, which is harder for patients to use for self-injurious behavior).

Time frame

CMS guidelines specify that S/R should be ordered by a physician or "licensed independent practitioner" (LIP) and that the initial face-to-face interview must occur within 1 hour of the order. The APA RD uses a 4-hour time frame, which may still be reasonable, as the correctional setting, in most cases, is not a hospital. The only exception is the need to protect the patient or staff from imminent, substantial harm (e.g., an acutely psychotic patient who is attempting to assault a custody officer). If the LIP is not a physician, consultation with the physician should occur within 4 hours. The physician's order for S/R should be obtained within 1 hour of the LIP initiating the S/R.

A face-to-face assessment during seclusion should occur no less frequently than every 12 hours after the initial assessment by a trained LIP, physician, or registered nurse. In certain cases, these face-to-face assessments should occur more frequently, particularly when patients present with comorbid medical conditions, dementia, significant intoxication, or withdrawal.

Prolonged restraint can lead to adverse events and even death from medical complications such as deep vein thrombosis and pulmonary embolism, even in healthy persons. This and other reasons dictate that time limits should be placed on S/R. Initial orders for S/R should be limited to 4 hours for adults and 2 hours for children and adolescents (aged 9 to 17 years). The APA RD requires consultation (at least by phone) with a physician, preferably a psychiatrist, when the face-to-face assessment is not performed by a physician. After the first set of orders, renewal orders for further S/R are required, which may be based on information conveyed by telephone or face-to-face evaluation. These renewal orders may, if required, be repeated for up to 24 hours. The duration of each renewal should follow the previously mentioned guidelines based on age (i.e., 4 hours for adults, 2 hours for children and adolescents).

Monitoring and patient protection

Once S/R is initiated, medical and mental health staff must carefully monitor the patient. During restraint, the IP is at risk for asphyxiation or compromised circulation, especially when the period of restraint is lengthy. The individual is also more vulnerable to abuse by other patients. Medical and mental health staff should consider continuous monitoring for patients who are intoxicated or withdrawing from substances, are actively engaged in self-injurious behavior, or are unfamiliar to staff.

Custody and medical/mental health staff should carefully document their observations of the IP during S/R. Notes should be taken at regular intervals. Staff may tend to complete observation checklists prematurely or to fill them in retrospectively, particularly during prolonged S/R; this practice must be eliminated.

During the first 2 hours of restraint, a nurse should repeatedly assess the condition of all four extremities, noting pulses, circulation, and evidence of injuries caused by the individual or the restraint. This ensures that the restraints were applied appropriately and that no injuries have been overlooked. Every 2 hours, the nurse should perform a more complete assessment of the patient that includes the circulation and integument examinations mentioned previously. In addition, the patient's behavior, general physical condition, and responses to interactions/treatment should be noted; this more complete examination should be documented. Every 2 hours, the nurse should perform range-of-motion exercises with each limb in sequence, ideally without the restraints in place on that limb, unless this is contraindicated. This assessment, like the previously mentioned assessments, should be performed based on the patient's level of cooperation to avoid unnecessary risks for staff or the patient. For example, if an individual remains highly agitated and threatening, safety dictates that range-of-motion exercises should not be performed. The rationale for the deferral of any portion of an assessment should be clearly documented.

Other staff responsibilities that are conducted at least every 2 hours include appropriate toileting and hygiene; nourishment needs should be addressed every 4 hours. Individuals can be escorted to nearby bathrooms if they are available and it is safe to do so. The alternative is to offer a urinal or bedpan (along with privacy). Vital signs should be assessed no less frequently than once every 8 hours, again assuming it is safe to do so. Fluids and meals should be offered regularly, the former more regularly than the latter. Mealtimes should be the same as the rest of the facility. Sharp utensils that could serve as a weapon or for self-injury must not be provided, so security utensils or finger foods should be offered instead. The use of the "nutraloaf" has been historically controversial and should be avoided. One study found that 14 states have banned the use of the nutraloaf as a disciplinary tool (Sobel et al., 2020). In addition to the concerns noted, careful attention should be paid to patients who are susceptible to exhaustion or patients at high risk of adverse reactions to S/R (e.g., obese patients, older patients, or medically compromised patients).

Policy

Written policies and procedures for S/R should be part of the institution's formal health care policy and procedures manual. Initial training and annual retraining of medical, mental health, and custody staff who are involved in S/R is essential. Where applicable, photographs and videotapes to augment regular training should be available. For example, the mechanical restraints typically used for medical restraint are not the same as those used for custody restraint. Staff should be familiar with the different types of restraints to optimize comfort and proper fit and to avoid injury or assaultive behavior. Training and retraining should focus on, but not be limited to, techniques of restraining IPs and the required follow-up assessments and interventions (e.g., range-of-motion exercises, vital signs checks, and observation of the patient's mental state). All staff should receive annual recertification. Ideally, training should include an experiential portion led by seasoned instructors so that techniques can be practiced and critiqued. Benefits of training include improved patient outcomes and decreased staff-related costs. Specifically, reduced staff and patient injuries result from the proper initiation and monitoring of S/R and training that reduces the need for S/R (Recupero et al., 2011).

Technique

Once the LIP or physician decides to initiate S/R, an S/R "leader" should be identified. The leader coordinates with custody staff to jointly inform the patient of the decision. To maximize efficiency and reduce potential harm, the team should present a simple, clear, and united statement to the patient in a calm, controlled manner. The S/R leader should clearly state the purpose of the S/R, identifying the target behaviors that are driving the decision to initiate S/R and that will need to stop before S/R is terminated. This interaction is not a time for psychodynamic formulation, negotiation, or decision reversal; to do so is not clinically indicated and can exacerbate an already fragile situation (see Chapter 24).

Just as important as the decision to initiate S/R is the decision to terminate it. When the patient has achieved the defined goals (e.g., agitation or aggression under control) and when the safety of the patient and staff is reasonably ensured, the patient should be released. This information is gathered through ongoing assessment and interaction with the patient (e.g., "How are you feeling right now? Do you feel in control of your behavior?") and can be inferred from direct observation (e.g., a once-agitated patient is no longer pacing the seclusion room, a once-threatening patient is calmly engaging staff and following directions).

Releasing S/R may be a graded process, titrated appropriately to follow the progressive improvement of a patient or to test a once highly threatening one. For example, it might be reasonable to release one or two extremities from a four-point therapeutic restraint to assess the patient's tolerance of gradually increasing levels of freedom. Likewise, while still being monitored closely by staff, an IP might remain in the seclusion room with the door ajar.

Following the placement of a patient on S/R, the staff should debrief as a group. This affords a review of the techniques used and allows staff to release tension and emotion related to initiating and completing the S/R process. A specific discussion of what interventions might have prevented the need for S/R should also be held. Follow-up with the patient is critical to review the rationale for S/R and the subsequent behavior that led to release. It is helpful to elicit the patient's impressions about the usefulness of the procedure, as this may provide insight into what they identify as triggers that led to the problematic behavior. This information can be incorporated into the patient's treatment plan. Naturally, the process of S/R should be well documented in the medical record.

Reducing the use of seclusion and restraint

Jails and prisons are being challenged to do more to limit the use of S/R as an intervention and to increase the therapeutic milieu of admittedly stark environments for patients with mental illness (Appelbaum, 2007; Champion, 2007; Metzner et al., 2007). Acknowledgment of the inherent risks associated with S/R as a tool for managing IPs with mental illness and the ethical dilemmas it poses have given momentum to the development of guidelines. Public health intervention models in the community have reduced the use of S/R by as much as 75%, with no increase in injuries to staff and patients (Lewis et al., 2009). Lion (2011) suggests that part of the solution to optimizing S/R is first acknowledging that it is an effective intervention that should be used in only rare situations and that it might require clinical certification.

Use of emergency and nonemergency involuntary medications

Individuals in correctional environments might refuse to take prescribed psychotropic medication for a variety of reasons, including concerns about side effects, lack of insight into their illness, stigma associated with psychotropic medication, and lack of an effective therapeutic relationship with prescribers. Medication nonadherence in jails and prisons can lead to worsening psychotic and mood symptoms that place patients and others at risk of harm. Examples include an inability to care for oneself by refusing to shower, eat, or sleep; aggression as a result of paranoia; self-injury or suicide attempts; and an inability to follow facility rules because of psychotic disorganization (APA, 2020).

The use of involuntary psychotropic medication in emergency situations is a well-recognized process in hospital settings when individuals present with serious psychiatric symptoms that put them at imminent risk of harm to themselves or others. Such situations can also arise in jail and prison settings. During such emergencies, it is generally acceptable, on a limited-time basis, to administer the minimum amount of psychiatric medication necessary to mitigate the immediate crisis, regardless of the patient's wishes (Burns, 2005). This is considered by the APA to be an essential part of mental health services in jails and prisons: "A full range of psychotropic medications, including involuntary medication, must be available, with the capacity to administer them in an emergency" (APA, 2000, pp. 38, 45). A recent survey of state and federal prison facilities found that 97% of prisons (35 out of 36) allowed for the involuntary use of psychotropic medication in emergency situations (Orta, 2023).

The use of nonemergency involuntary medication on a longer term basis is a clinical and legal process that differs from the use of such medications in the emergent situations described above. Usually, orders for administration of such medications involve individuals who are being treated in a hospital setting and require an order from a court of jurisdiction following a hearing on the matter. In general, a provider requesting an order for the use of nonemergent involuntary medication must show that the individual lacks capacity to make informed decisions about their psychiatric treatment, that they demonstrate an acute and/or chronic risk of dangerousness or grave disability as a result of their psychiatric symptoms, and that there are no less restrictive alternatives available.

In the landmark case *Washington v. Harper* (1990), the U.S. Supreme Court held that incarcerated individuals may be medicated in nonemergency situations without a court order. The case originated in Washington, where an individual named Brian Harper, who was incarcerated in a state prison, had been diagnosed with a serious mental illness and refused to take prescribed antipsychotic medication. Prison officials believed that Harper's untreated mental illness posed a danger to himself and others, and they sought to treat him with antipsychotic medication without his consent following an internal administrative hearing rather than a judicial hearing (that is required in the community when seeking such an involuntary medication order). The Supreme Court ruled in favor of Washington and upheld the prison's authority to involuntarily medicate Harper. The court's decision established several key principles: (a) prison officials can involuntarily administer antipsychotic medication to an IP if they can demonstrate that the medication is medically appropriate and necessary to maintain order and safety within the prison; (b) individuals are entitled to certain due process protections before being involuntarily medicated, including notice, a formal hearing before a panel of independent decision-makers, and the opportunity to present their objections; (c) the decision to medicate involuntarily must be based on a determination that the IP poses a danger to themselves or others due to their untreated mental illness, and (d) the decision should be made by a medical professional and should be based on sound medical judgment rather than for punitive or administrative reasons.

Harper addressed the use of involuntary medications in a prison setting, and there has been an ongoing question about whether the ruling could similarly be applied to jail detainees, particularly those pretrial defendants who have been found incompetent to stand trial based on an untreated serious mental illness. The issue of whether a defendant could be involuntarily medicated to render them competent to stand trial came before the U.S. Supreme Court in *Sell v. United States* (2003). The case involved Charles Sell, a dentist who faced federal charges for health care fraud and attempted murder and was found incompetent to stand trial. He was forcibly medicated with antipsychotic medication in a federal forensic psychiatric hospital following a judicial determination that he was dangerous. Dr. Sell appealed the decision to the U.S. Supreme Court, which found that there were not sufficient grounds to medicate based on dangerousness. However, the court articulated the conditions under which a pretrial detainee may be medicated over their objection for the strict purpose of restoring their competence to stand trial. The court found that four criteria must be met: (a) there is an important government interest in bringing the individual to trial, (b) the medication must be substantially likely to render the individual competent without undue side effects, (c) the medication is the least restrictive treatment option available to achieve the result of restoration, and (d) the medication is in the individual's best interest in light of their medical condition. Although *Sell* addressed involuntary medication only for pretrial individuals found incompetent to stand trial, it laid the foundation for the possibility of involuntarily medicating pretrial detainees more broadly.

The next major court ruling regarding the use of involuntary medications in the jail setting arose following the Ninth Circuit Court of Appeals' review of *United States v. Loughner* (2012). Jared Lee Loughner carried out a mass shooting in Tucson, Arizona, in 2011, killing six people and injuring numerous others, including then-U.S. representative Gabrielle Giffords. Loughner's mental health and the question of involuntary medication played a significant role in his legal proceedings. Following his arrest, Loughner was found incompetent to stand trial and involuntarily medicated utilizing a *Harper* order on the basis of dangerousness, though also with the purported purpose of restoring him to trial competence. Following a lengthy legal challenge, the Ninth Circuit Court of Appeals upheld the involuntary medication of Loughner under the *Harper* order, affirming that the standard in *Harper* applies equally to pretrial detainees as it does to sentenced prisoners. In its ruling, however, the court did not comment on the appropriateness of the setting where an involuntary medication order should be carried out (i.e., in a medical versus nonmedical facility). In effect, the ruling did not prohibit the use of involuntary medications in a (nonmedical) jail setting. There is ongoing debate about whether such a practice is in the best interest of the individual, with some scholars noting that a medical setting is the most appropriate location for such orders to be carried out (Felthous, 2012, 2013). However, given the lack of sufficient forensic psychiatric hospital beds in many states, which has led to long waitlists for inpatient restoration services and the increasing use of jail-based restoration programs (see Chapter 71), it is conceivable that jails may increasingly utilize involuntary medication orders, whether under *Harper* or *Sell*, for the treatment and restoration to competence of seriously mentally ill pretrial defendants. Accordingly, the APA's Council on Psychiatry and Law prepared a resource document to help guide clinicians with the process of using nonemergent involuntary medications in the jail setting (APA, 2020).

While there is no prohibition on jails adopting a *Harper*-type administrative review panel to make decisions about the administration of nonemergency involuntary medication, almost none seem to have done so. South Dakota is one state, however, that has adopted such a process in all its county jails (Torrey et al., 2014). In addition, in California, courts that have found a pretrial detainee incompetent to stand trial and unable to provide informed consent to prescribed medication may authorize the administration of involuntary medication if it is determined that the individual meets either *Harper* or *Sell* criteria (California Code, Penal Code § 1370, section (a)(2)(B), 2024). In jail-based competency restoration programs in California, these involuntary medication orders are often utilized within the jail environment to treat an individual's symptoms of serious mental illness, with the ultimate goal of restoring them to competency.

Summary

The judicious use of S/R can yield positive results for IPs who are at imminent risk of self-injury or injury to others and where other interventions have failed or are inappropriate. Before initiating S/R, the clinician must carefully weigh the clinical and ethical concerns of doing so. The ideal situation is one in which S/R is used as a tool of last resort as part of a more comprehensive, individualized treatment plan that seeks to ameliorate the behaviors and circumstances for which S/R is indicated.

The use of involuntary medication in correctional settings remains a divisive issue, with ethical, legal, and practical challenges. Balancing the duty of care with the protection of individual rights is an ongoing struggle. Providers practicing within jails and prisons must navigate this complex landscape carefully, ensuring that the use of involuntary medication is subject to stringent safeguards and continually evaluated to promote ethical and humane practices within these institutions. Whenever possible, alternatives to involuntary medication, such as therapeutic interventions, counseling, or de-escalation techniques, should be explored.

REFERENCES

American Bar Association. (2011). *Treatment of prisoners* (3rd ed.). http://www.americanbar.org/content/dam/aba/publications/criminal_justice_standards/Treatment_of_Prisoners.authcheckdam.pdf

American Psychiatric Association. (2000). *Psychiatric services in jails and prisons: A task force report of the American Psychiatric Association* (2nd ed.).

American Psychiatric Association. (2020). *Resource document on non-emergency involuntary medication for mental disorders in U.S. jails.*

Appelbaum, K. L. (2007). Commentary: The use of restraint and seclusion in correctional mental health. *Journal of the American Academy of Psychiatry and the Law, 35*, 431–435.

Burns, K. A. (2005). Psychopharmacology in correctional settings. In C. L. Scott & J. B. Gerbasi (Eds.), *Handbook of correctional mental health* (pp. 89–108). American Psychiatric Publishing.

California Code, Penal Code—PEN § 1370. (2024). *Inquiry into the competence of the defendant before trial or after conviction.* https://codes.findlaw.com/ca/penal-code/pen-sect-1370/

Castillo, E. M., Coyne, C. J., Chan, T. C., Hall, C. A., & Vilke, G. M. (2015). Review of the medical and legal literature on restraint chairs. *Journal of Forensic and Legal Medicine, 33*, 91–97.

Champion, M. K. (2007). Commentary: Seclusion and restraint in corrections—A time for change. *Journal of the American Academy of Psychiatry and the Law, 35*, 426–430.

Felthous, A. R. (2012). The involuntary medication of Jared Loughner and pretrial jail detainees in nonmedical correctional facilities. *Journal of the American Academy of Psychiatry and the Law, 40*, 98–112.

Felthous, A. R. (2013). The Ninth Circuit's *Loughner* decision neglected medically appropriate treatment. *Journal of the American Academy of Psychiatry and the Law, 41*, 105–113.

Lewis, M., Taylor, K., & Parks, J. (2009). Crisis prevention management: A program to reduce the use of seclusion and restraint in an inpatient mental health setting. *Issues in Mental Health Nursing, 30*, 159–164.

Lion, J. R. (2011). Commentary: On regulation, wishfulness, and denial. *Journal of the American Academy of Psychiatry and the Law, 39*, 477–479.

Metzner, J. L., Tardiff, K., Lion, J., Reid, W. H., Recupero, P. R., Schetky, D. H., Edenfield, B. M., Mattson, M., & Janofsky, J. S. (2007). Resource document on the use of restraint and seclusion in correctional mental health care. *Journal of the American Academy of Psychiatry and the Law, 35*, 417–425.

Orta, J., Barton, C., Ilao, P., & Apollonio, D. E. (2023). A review of policies on the involuntary use of psychotropic medications among persons experiencing incarceration in the United States. *Health & Justice, 11*, 9.

Recupero, P. R., Price, M., Garvey, K. A., Daly, B., & Xavier, S. L. (2011). Restraint and seclusion in psychiatric treatment settings: Regulation, case law, and risk management. *Journal of the American Academy of Psychiatry and the Law, 39*, 465–476.

Sell v. United States, 539 U.S. 166 (2003).

Sine, D. M., & Hunt, J. M. (2007). *Design guide for built environment of behavioral health facilities.* National Association of Psychiatric Health Systems.

Sobel, L., Stroud, K., & Weinstein, M. (2020). *Eating behind bars: Ending the hidden punishment of food in prison.* Impact Justice. https://impactjustice.org/impact/food-in-prison/#report

Torrey, E. F., Zdanowicz, M. T., Kennard, A. D., et. al. (2014). *The treatment of persons with mental illness in prisons and jails: A state survey.* Treatment Advocacy Center.

United States v. Loughner, 672 F.3d 731 (9th Cir. 2012).

Visaggio, N., Phillips, K. E., Milne, S., McElhinney, J., & Young, S. C. (2020). The restraint chair: A qualitative study of nurses' experience with the restraint chair versus four point restraint. *Archives of Psychiatric Nursing, 34*, 2–6.

Washington v. Harper, 494 U.S. 210 (1990).

26

Hospitalization

Michael A. Norko, Thomas Kocienda, and Charles Dike[*]

Introduction

In its report on psychiatric services in correctional facilities, the American Psychiatric Association (APA) noted the fundamental principle that "timely and effective access to mental health treatment is the hallmark of adequate mental health care" (APA, 2016, p. 4). Appropriate and adequate access to mental health care involves establishing an "atmosphere of empathy and respect for the dignity of the patient" that promotes privacy and patient engagement (APA, 2016, p. 20). Such a therapeutic milieu should include a sanitary and humane environment; adequate resources and mental health staff for observation, treatment, and supervision; social interactions that foster recovery; and transfer to a mental health unit or external facility when clinically indicated (APA, 2016, p. 20). This chapter explores the role of hospitalization in the design and operation of models of care across institutional boundaries, along with other relevant considerations for hospital-based care of incarceration persons (IPs).

Prevalence of mental illness in jails and prisons

The need for hospitalization of IPs is a product of the prevalence and acuity of mental illness and the limited scope of mental health services available in correctional environments. Studies have found that approximately 16% of IPs have serious mental illness and need psychiatric care (APA, 2016). Rates of serious mental illness for women in jails and prisons are significantly higher than for men (Gottfried & Christopher, 2017). A 1-day cross-sectional analysis of the IP population in Connecticut in 2022 found that nearly 32% of the population was assessed as needing some level of active treatment for a mental health disorder (Connecticut Sentencing Commission, 2022).

Data regarding the prevalence of serious mental illness in correctional settings span a wide range of findings because of varying methodologies among the studies and differences in IP population characteristics (Fazel et al., 2016; Prins, 2014). A 2012 review of 109 studies involving over 33,000 IPs in 24 countries concluded that 3.6% of men and 3.9% of women in prison had a psychotic illness, with higher prevalence in low-middle-income countries at 5.5% for men and women combined. That review also found that 10.2% of men and 14.1% of women had major depression (Fazel & Seewald, 2012). These percentages had not changed substantially over time, except that the prevalence of depression in U.S. studies increased from 1974 to 2005. By comparison, in the general population, the National Alliance on Mental Illness (NAMI) reported that, in the United States in 2023, the rate of serious mental illness was 5.5% and of any mental illness was 22.8% (NAMI, 2021). The Substance Abuse and Mental Health Services Administration reports similar results, with increases in both any mental illness and serious mental illness from 2008 to 2019 (Substance Abuse and Mental Health Services Administration, 2019).

The higher rates of serious mental illness in correctional settings may not be related so much to the direct effects of mental illness on criminal behavior (Peterson et al., 2010) as to a higher level of overlapping criminogenic needs and social determinants of behavioral health (e.g., adverse childhood experiences, employment and education challenges, housing instability, and neighborhood disorder) in this population (Ashekun et al., 2023; Rotter & Compton, 2022; see Chapter 6).

Given the prevalence of serious mental illness in correctional settings, the need for periods of psychiatric hospitalization can be anticipated. A Bureau of Justice Statistics report gives some indication of the percentages of IPs requiring such care: During incarceration, the rates of hospitalization were 2.7% for federal prisoners, 5.4% for state prisoners, and 2.2% for jail detainees (James & Glaze, 2006).

Prison and jail management of acute disorders

The IP experiencing acute psychiatric illness poses unique challenges. Given the number of IPs who have a history of psychiatric impairment, acute illness will frequently arise when they are in custody. We refer here to those IPs whose symptoms, dangerousness, or grave disability make them inappropriate for either the general population or a specialized housing unit for IPs with nonacute psychiatric illness (where available). Decisions for these IPs about whether

*. The authors acknowledge the contributions of Craig G. Burns, MD, who co-authored this chapter in the first edition of the textbook.

to seek outside hospitalization require consideration of potential advantages and risks in the correctional and hospital environments.

At any point within the criminal justice system—police lockup, jail, court, or prison—facility staff may identify IPs who are acutely ill. Each custodial environment or experience has its own stressors that can move otherwise dormant illness into manifest impairment. Unpredictable community-based events such as the death of loved ones, grave illness in family members, divorce, and loss of child custody can contribute to an IP's rapid decompensation. Some seriously ill IPs can remain undetected for most of an incarceration but come to the awareness of staff as the stress of returning to the community results in acute decompensation (Felthous, 2013b).

IPs experiencing acute decompensation may act out, generating disciplinary issues before being referred for mental health interventions. In such cases, the collaboration between mental health, security, and operational personnel yields the best outcomes regarding efforts to maintain safety and security while also attending to the health care needs of IPs. Operational and security staff will often mirror the approach demonstrated by mental health personnel when engaging with decompensated IPs, especially when mental health providers model good boundary management, coupled with a compassionate and respectful approach. It can be extremely validating for operational personnel if the mental health professional takes the time to solicit opinions from officers and to include these observations in mental health formulations. Such efforts often serve as the roots of mutual appreciation and collaboration (see Chapter 13). This supports the safe, effective management of IPs who are acutely ill; the crucial nature of this approach cannot be overstated.

Despite the stress inherent in carceral environments, the care of acute mental illness in jails and prisons may have some advantages over care in forensic psychiatric hospitals. The more secure correctional setting can frequently be more effective in managing the unpredictable and dangerous IP. Elements of the traditional correctional physical plant are part of this advantage. Correctional housing design routinely inhibits the open movement of IPs, which hospital settings cannot usually achieve, except for brief periods of emergency management. Correctional settings are able to monitor cells by camera, and security personnel can remotely operate locks and utilities. The safe delivery of medication and food to highly aggressive individuals who are acutely ill can be accomplished using cell door traps. Security personnel have extensive training and experience in secured movement, coordinated response to violent behavior, and crisis negotiation, and they operate within a clear chain of command that facilitates accountability and organization.

Even IPs who are severely impaired and potentially violent will often respond to the regulation and structure provided in the correctional setting. Set times for awakening, eating, hygiene, recreation, medication administration, and other interventions create predictability. Even an IP experiencing severe psychosis will often respond appropriately to uniformed officers and the presence of an officer in a leadership position who is directing interactions. These factors help manage dangerous IPs in acute decompensation of mental illness, if appropriately enhanced clinical care is equally available.

It is possible to generate enhanced psychiatric care in a correctional environment by following the standards and guidelines provided by the National Commission on Correctional Health Care (NCCHC) and APA, among others. For example, many relevant sections are presented in the NCCHC's *Standards for Mental Health Services in Correctional Facilities*, including those on safety, personnel and training, mental health care services and support, patient care and treatment, special mental health needs and services, and medical–legal issues (NCCHC, 2015).

Correctional systems that can offer both the essential and important elements described may have less need to rely on outside hospitals than those that struggle to meet even essential standards (see Chapter 73). However, even correctional systems that expend significant human and capital resources to approximate specialized hospital settings must acknowledge that, in the end, they are still jails and prisons. To provide a full range of services for IPs, correctional systems should develop collaborative relationships with area psychiatric hospitals with the ability to transfer IPs to those facilities for specialized care.

Collaboration with hospitals

Many states house more persons with mental illness in correctional institutions than in state psychiatric hospitals (Torrey et al., 2014). Among people who are incarcerated, those with mental illness, however, are more likely to have maladaptive responses to custody, often resulting in management problems, longer periods of incarceration secondary to disciplinary infractions (periodically rooted in untreated symptoms), and the loss of appropriate community supervision when full sentences are served. Mental illness is also a high-risk factor for suicide in IPs (Zhong et al., 2021; see Chapter 51).

Court orders for hospitalization (e.g., for competency restoration) early in the adjudication process can have a protective effect on IPs with mental illness. Movement to an inpatient hospital can provide a more supportive transition to custody while symptoms are remediated. Even when IPs are psychiatrically hospitalized for other than court-ordered reasons, they are still likely to return to prison, and adaptation to prison life remains an important goal.

Even with fully informed consent, voluntary transfers to psychiatric hospitals of IPs who are acutely ill can have unintended legal and clinical consequences. Prosecutors and defense attorneys may be wary of transferring pretrial detainees to psychiatric hospitals for reasons other than those ordered by the court for fear of influencing the trial process. Prosecutors may be concerned about generating mitigating factors that may weaken their case, and defense attorneys may be concerned about detecting malingered symptoms that may influence the court.

Treatment of pretrial detainees in psychiatric hospital settings other than a maximum-security hospital is challenging. As new patients improve, staff usually decrease restrictions placed on them and increase their privileges, interventions used to both demonstrate patients' improvement and assess their ability to self-regulate in different environments in the hospital. These interventions are problematic for pretrial detainees for whom the risk of elopement from the hospital is high, thereby placing clinicians in a bind. Ultimately, a physician's responsibility is to the needs of the patient, which should be the driving force that determines where an IP receives care (Vogel et al., 2013).

To assist with that determination, Vogel and colleagues (2013) proposed the concept of "fitness for imprisonment." They offered an algorithm for the decision about hospital transfer based on European prison experience that consists of assessments and analyses of whether the needed treatment is practicable in the correctional setting. They suggest evaluating four criteria, in this order: psychiatric diagnosis, acute need for treatment, danger to self and others, and inability to comply with treatment. In their suggested scheme, if all criteria are present, the IP is not "fit" for prison and should be transferred. If only some of the four criteria are present, additional factors should be reviewed, including first clinical manifestation of a psychological disorder, prognosis in prison versus hospital, need for special monitoring with the initiation of complex medication regimens, diagnostic uncertainty, and availability of trained staff (Vogel et al., 2013).

Another consideration is that other IPs may victimize IPs with mental illness (Daquin & Daigle, 2018). These vulnerabilities and risks may be temporarily better managed in a hospital. On a case-by-case basis, consideration of individual IPs' needs and risks, especially if formalized as protocols between correctional facilities and area psychiatric hospitals, will help clinical decision-makers choose the best place to meet IPs' needs.

Under British Columbia's temporary absence model, if a determination is made that an IP's clinical needs would be better served in a hospital, transfer to the hospital may be achieved through a temporary absence application (Olley et al., 2009). Another approach considers whether the IP can be ethically managed in prison. Such an analysis may consist of several considerations: the gravity of the IP's condition, the severity of the clinical and other risks involved, and the necessity of involuntary medication administration (Felthous, 2012).

Involuntary medication

An IP who is acutely psychiatrically ill may demonstrate a temporary risk of violence while symptoms remain untreated. In some circumstances, correctional facilities can more rapidly implement involuntary pharmacological interventions than hospitals, which require more complex or protracted procedural protections for involuntary treatment.

It is possible for some correctional settings to use a *Harper* panel process (*Washington v. Harper*, 1990) to administer psychiatric medication involuntarily to those who meet criteria. This involves an administrative hearing before a panel that includes a psychiatry provider not involved in the IP's care, as described in *Washington v. Harper* (see Chapter 25). The procedure also requires notice of the hearing, and rights to attend the hearing, present evidence and witnesses, cross-examine witnesses, have an advocate present, and file an appeal. The hearing must conclude that the individual has a serious mental illness and is "dangerous to self or others and the treatment is in the inmate's medical interest" (*Washington v. Harper*, 1990, p. 1040). The APA report notes that the *Harper* decision "does not require a lack of decisional competence or consideration of less intrusive means of intervention" (APA, 2016, p. 4).

In jurisdictions where the same procedural requirements apply equally between correctional and forensic hospital settings, however, the implementation of rapid pharmacological treatment is not a relevant consideration when deciding which setting would be preferred. For example, some county jails have no procedural mechanism for involuntary medication administration except in emergency situations (APA, 2020), and some state prison systems require the same type of court order for involuntary medication that would apply to patients in a hospital (e.g., Massachusetts). Clinicians working in correctional settings must be aware of the procedural requirements within their jurisdiction, recognizing that states may impose more restrictions on involuntary treatment than constitutionally required.

When involuntarily administering medications in prisons, some authors have argued that the treatment should occur in acute care psychiatric units to ensure safe and proper administration within a therapeutic milieu (Daniel, 2007; Felthous, 2013a). Involuntary medication use within nonmedical prison units can raise multiple concerns, including that medical staff may not be informed when medication is not administered, that compliance techniques used by correctional staff may result in harm, that there may be less balancing of patients' rights and jail regulations, and that clinical efforts to obtain the individual's cooperation with treatment may not be pursued vigorously (Felthous, 2012).

Laws and regulations regarding involuntary medication in emergency situations are similarly complex and varied across jurisdictions (28 C.F.R. 549.46, 2011; Dlugacz & Wimmer, 2013; NCCHC, 2015, MH-I-04). Emergency situations may not require *Harper* procedures but usually require a determination of dangerousness and mental illness. The NCCHC requires written administrative protocols for this purpose for a facility to achieve accreditation (NCCHC, 2015, MH-E-06). Interestingly, the federal code views seclusion and restraint as an alternative to consider before giving medications involuntarily (28 C.F.R. 549.46, 2011, 549.46(b)(1)(i)), although this is not generally how these procedures are ranked from a clinical perspective. For example, medical staff in a hospital would be unlikely to consider seclusion or restraint as a first alternative before administering involuntary medication in an emergency. Hospitals are restricted in the use of seclusion and restraint and have limits on staff's physical response and management of unpredictably violent individuals.

The need for involuntary medications may be one indication for hospital transfer in a subset of IPs (Felthous, 2012). Transferring IPs involuntarily to a psychiatric hospital requires the minimum due process articulated in *Vitek v. Jones* (1980), including effective and timely notice, a hearing with an independent decision-maker, the right to testify and examine other witnesses, and a written statement by the fact finder noting the reasons for a decision to transfer. This minimum due process will not be sufficient in jurisdictions that require other or more expansive procedures by statute or case law. A *Vitek* hearing may be used in some jurisdictions to facilitate an involuntary medication order; however, this may not provide sufficient procedure to accomplish that goal without further due process (Dlugacz & Wimmer, 2013; Metzner et al., 1998, p. 249). Even in a hospital setting, the evaluation of capacity to give informed consent requires careful consideration.

Hospitalization for acute or refractory disorders

Although some prisons offer a wide range of mental health services, this is not their primary mission. Further, prisons have no obligation to adhere to the provisions of the federal Patient Bill of Rights, which refer to persons "admitted to a program or facility for the purpose of receiving mental health services" (42 U.S.C. § 9501, § 9501 (1)). Because of their different primary goals, the milieu of mental health units in prisons is not the same as that of a hospital. While the provision of psychiatric care through telehealth services may mitigate workforce shortages and provide treatment that would otherwise be unavailable, it does not diminish the challenges of the prison milieu. For the most part, correctional institutions remain unable to provide care that is equivalent to a community or forensic hospital milieu. Special attention has been given to the design of the latter in recent years, including efforts to reduce the institutional feel of the facility, to enhance natural light and exposure to nature, to decrease noise, to create open spaces and wide hallways, and to eliminate blind spots (Dvoskin, 2002; Seppänen, 2018; Shaw, 2014). In contrast, prisons and jails remain bleak and security focused.

A supportive hospital milieu by itself fosters recovery. The milieu should, therefore, be part of the analysis in considering hospital transfer for IPs with serious acute or refractory illness or who are elderly or have other physical or emotional attributes that make them more vulnerable to victimization.

The discussion is further complicated by the observation that, for some individuals with mental impairments exhibiting dangerous behaviors, transfer to a hospital could lead to markedly increased restrictions in their freedom; hospital staff might feel they have to place these patients on close observation, sometimes by more than one staff member, for safety. These patients could require frequent use of restraints or seclusion to manage their aggressive behavior, despite current efforts to decrease the use of such practices (Wasser et al., 2023). In these highly restrictive situations, the hospital might not be the least restrictive environment for providing treatment to the patient who might be more easily managed in a standard prison cell. The U.S. Supreme Court has acknowledged similar concerns in concluding that prisoners retain a "residuum of liberty that would be infringed by a transfer to a mental hospital without complying with minimum requirements of due process" (*Vitek v. Jones*, 1980, p. 491).

The admission of prisoners to a forensic hospital unit is not without notable challenges. A major hurdle is getting front-line staff of the facility to view the transferred prisoners as they do other patients on the unit, not as criminals. The criminal history profile of many psychotic prisoners is similar to those of their nonpsychotic fellow prisoners (Coid & Ullrich, 2011); they are at higher risk of exhibiting behaviors associated with psychopathy and substance abuse and may be perceived to have a higher risk of escaping from the hospital. The presence of prisoners on a hospital unit may also disrupt the therapeutic program and place lower functioning hospital patients at risk of victimization (Phillips & Caplan, 2003).

Accordingly, these patients present significant safety and security risks that should be managed with as much care and attention as in a correctional facility. Areas of vulnerability for the hospital include access to materials that could be fashioned into sharp objects; exposure of the usual public sector patient population to potentially more dangerous individuals; safe and secure transportation of these patients to medical or other appointments outside of the hospital, necessitating careful and individualized assessment of risk (Dike et al., 2015; Wasser et al., 2022); and the inability of staff to monitor patient phone calls. Hospitalized patients have a right to converse with others privately, to have convenient and reasonable access to the telephone and mail, and to see visitors during regularly scheduled hours (42 U.S.C. § 9501). Hospital staff need to be particularly alert to the potential for some patients to conspire with accomplices outside or inside the hospital in an attempt to escape or to cause a disruption in the hospital. Careful attention should be paid to the increased staffing needs of hospitals that receive IPs for treatment and the need for other resources to engage them in appropriate and effective therapeutic and rehabilitation activities, relieving symptoms, providing structure, improving coping skills, and decreasing externalizing behaviors.

Management of IPs in a hospital would be nearly impossible without an easy process for their transfer back to prison when their aggressive or criminal behaviors overwhelm the hospital's resources. Therefore, interagency collaboration between the correctional agency and the psychiatric facility is key to successful management of IPs with mental illness.

Stigma and other challenges of the hospitalization decision

The U.S. Supreme Court has recognized that the consequences of involuntary hospitalization are "qualitatively different" from the usual effects of punishment (*Vitek v. Jones*, 1980, p. 493). But IPs are subject to stigma from other IPs (Edwards, 2000), whether they receive intensive mental health care in prison or a hospital. They are also subject to stigma from the public by both their imprisonment and their mental illness. Thus, prison officials and clinicians confronted with an IP in the midst of an acute psychiatric illness must choose between treatment environments that have advantages and disadvantages. Although such considerations may be aired in a *Vitek* hearing, the clinical principles described previously should drive decisions, taking into account the unique circumstances of each case. Clinical concerns must always be paramount in such decisions, but matters of security and safety cannot be ignored.

Another aspect of stigma especially relevant to correctional settings is the consideration of whether an IP's reported symptoms are malingered to obtain time away from the correctional environment. Accurate diagnosis can be challenging even in a hospital environment and requires careful observation, psychological assessment, and evaluation of intervention effectiveness. It is also important to note how stressful a correctional environment can be for someone experiencing psychiatric illness, and the transition to a therapeutic milieu can have ameliorative effects. Such effects, even if relatively rapid, should not lead to an automatic conclusion that the IP's complaints were malingered and the IP should, therefore, be returned quickly. Comprehensive assessment and treatment planning are warranted, including a plan for successful transition back to the correctional environment.

Finally, dwindling resources, especially of workforce in both types of institutions, and of psychiatric beds in hospitals, are additional burdens regarding transfer of IPs to psychiatric hospitals. Mental health professionals in leadership and administration must focus on effective advocacy for resources in both institutions.

Summary

A significant number of people with serious mental illness are found in correctional settings and must be provided with clinical care commensurate with their needs. Many of those needs may be met within the mental health care systems established in jails and prisons. When clinical conditions are more complex and require more intensive management, the availability of hospital-level care becomes important. While the decision to pursue hospitalization for an IP who is acutely ill is driven chiefly by clinical considerations, it is also influenced by security and safety concerns. These factors need to be considered on an individual basis, weighing the advantages and disadvantages of treatment in an outside hospital versus management in the prison or jail with available resources.

Involuntary medication and involuntary hospital transfer are situations that involve important legal rights, the protection of which requires due process established by federal and state laws and case precedents. Clinicians who work in correctional and hospital settings where sentenced individuals and pretrial detainees are treated must be aware of the relevant procedures required for these involuntary treatment modalities. In all jurisdictions, hospital-level care is necessary for a subset of sentenced individuals and jail detainees and must therefore be made available when appropriate.

REFERENCES

28 C.F.R. 549.46. (2011). *Procedures for involuntary administration of psychiatric medication.* http://federal.eregulations.us/cfr/section/title28/chapterv/part549/sect549.46?selectdate=11/1/2011

42 U.S.C. § 9501. (2006). *Mental health rights and advocacy—Bill of rights.* http://www.gpo.gov/fdsys/pkg/USCODE-2006-title42/pdf/USCODE-2006-title42-chap102.pdf

American Psychiatric Association. (2016). *Psychiatric services in correctional facilities* (3rd ed.).

American Psychiatric Association. (2020). *Resource document on non-emergency involuntary medication for mental disorders in U.S. jails.*

Ashekun, O., Zern, A., Langlois, S., & Compton, M.T. (2023). Adverse childhood experiences and arrest rates among individuals with serious mental illnesses. *Journal of the American Academy of Psychiatry and the Law, 51*, 329–336.

Coid, J., & Ullrich, S. (2011). Prisoners with psychosis in England and Wales: Diversion to psychiatric inpatient services. *International Journal of Law and Psychiatry, 34*, 99–108.

Connecticut Sentencing Commission. (2023). *Mental health disorders in Connecticut's incarcerated population.* https://ctsentencingcommission.org/wp-content/uploads/2023/03/Mental-Health-Disorders-in-Connecticuts-Incarcerated-Population-1.pdf

Daniel, A. E. (2007). Care of the mentally ill in prisons: Challenges and solutions. *Journal of the American Academy of Psychiatry and the Law, 35*, 406–410.

Daquin, J. C., & Daigle, L. E. (2018). Mental disorder and victimisation in prison: Examining the role of mental health treatment. *Criminal Behaviour and Mental Health, 28*, 141–151.

Dike, C. C., Nicholson, E., & Young, J. L. (2015). Transporting forensic psychiatric patients. *Journal of the American Academy of Psychiatry and the Law, 43*, 468–475.

Dlugacz, H., & Wimmer, C. (2013). Legal aspects of administrating antipsychotic medications to jail and prison inmates. *International Journal of Law and Psychiatry, 36*, 213–228.

Dvoskin, J. A., Radomski, S. J., Bennett, C., Olin, J. A., Hawkins, R. L., Dotson, L. A., & Drewnicky, I. N. (2002). Architectural design of a secure forensic state psychiatric hospital. *Behavioral Sciences and the Law, 20*, 481–493.

Edwards, K. A. (2000). Stigmatizing the stigmatized: A note on the mentally ill prison inmate. *International Journal of Offender Therapy and Comparative Criminology, 44*, 480–489.

Fazel, S., Hayes, A. Bartellas, K., Clerici, M., & Trestman R. (2016). Mental health of prisoners: Prevalence, adverse outcomes, and interventions. *Lancet Psychiatry, 3*, 871–881.

Fazel, S., & Seewald, K. (2012). Severe mental illness in 33 588 prisoners worldwide: Systematic review and meta-regression analysis. *British Journal of Psychiatry, 200*, 364–373.

Felthous, A. R. (2012). The involuntary medication of Jared Loughner and pretrial jail detainees in nonmedical correctional facilities. *Journal of the American Academy of Psychiatry and the Law, 40*, 98–112.

Felthous, A. R. (2013a). The Ninth Circuit's *Loughner* decision neglected medically appropriate treatment. *Journal of the American Academy of Psychiatry and the Law, 41*, 105–113.

Felthous, A. R. (2013b). Prisons and mental health: Introductory editorial: Hospitalizing mentally ill patients. *International Journal of Law and Psychiatry, 36*, 185–187.

Gottfried, E. D., & Christopher, S. C. (2017). Mental disorders among criminal offenders: A review of the literature. *Journal of Correctional Health Care, 23*, 336–346.

James, D. J., & Glaze, L. E. (2006). *Mental health problems of prison and jail inmates* (NCJ 213600). Department of Justice, Office of Justice Programs—Bureau of Justice and Statistics.

Metzner, J. L., Cohen, F., Grossman, L. S., & Wettstein, R. M. (1998). Treatment in jails and prisons. In R. W. Wettstein (Ed.), *Treatment of offenders with mental disorder* (pp. 211–264). Guilford Press.

National Alliance on Mental Illness. (2023). *Mental health by the numbers.* https://www.nami.org/about-mental-illness/mental-health-by-the-numbers/

National Commission on Correctional Health Care. (2015). *Standards for mental health services in correctional facilities.*

Olley, M. C., Nicholls, T. L., & Brink, J. (2009). Mentally ill individuals in limbo: Obstacles and opportunities for providing psychiatric services to corrections inmates with mental illness. *Behavioral Sciences and the Law, 27*, 811–831.

Peterson, J., Skeem, J., Hart, E., Vidal, S., & Keith, F. (2010). Analyzing offense patterns as a function of mental illness to test the criminalization hypothesis. *Psychiatric Services, 61*, 1217–1222.

Phillips, R. T. M., & Caplan, C. (2003). Administrative and staffing problems for psychiatric services in correctional and forensic settings. In R. Rosner (Ed.), *Principles and practice of forensic psychiatry* (2nd ed., pp. 505–512). Arnold.

Prins, S. J. (2014). The prevalence of mental illnesses in U.S. state prisons: A systematic review. *Psychiatric Services, 65*, 862–872.

Rotter, M., & Compton, M. (2022). Criminal legal involvement: A cause and consequence of social determinants of health. *Psychiatric Services, 73*, 108–111.

Seppänen, A., Törmänen, I., Shaw, C., & Kennedy, H. (2018). Modern forensic psychiatric hospital design: Clinical, legal and structural aspects. *International Journal of Mental Health Systems, 12*, 58.

Shaw, M. A. (2014). The secure residential psychiatric facility: Process, design, and results for behavioral healthcare. In E. C. Ritchie (Ed.), *Forensic and ethical issues in military behavioral health.* Office of the Surgeon General, Borden Institute.

Substance Abuse and Mental Health Services Administration. (2019). *Key substance use and mental health indicators in the United States: Results from the 2019 National Survey on Drug Use and Health.* https://www.samhsa.gov/data/sites/default/files/reports/rpt29393/2019NSDUHFFRPDFWHTML/2019NSDUHFFR090120.htm#ami

Torrey, E. F., Zdanowicz, M. T., Kennard, A. D., Lamb, H. R., Eslinger, D. F., Biasotti, M. C., & Fuller, D. A. (2014). *Treatment of persons with mental illness in prison and jails: A states survey.* Treatment Advocacy Center. https://www.treatmentadvocacycenter.org/reports_publications/the-treatment-of-persons-with-mental-illnes-in-prisons-and-jails-a-state-survey/

Vitek v. Jones, 445 U.S. 480 (1980).

Vogel, T., Lanquillon, S., & Graf. M. (2013). When and why should mentally ill prisoners be transferred to secure hospitals: A proposed algorithm. *International Journal of Law and Psychiatry, 36*, 281–286.

Washington v. Harper, 110 S. Ct. 1028 (1990).
Wasser, T., Strockbine, B. A., Hauser, L. L., Mathew, M. A., Gay, B., Smith, H. E., & Dike, C. C. (2022). An analysis of risk-assessment driven security restraint use during the transport of forensic patients. *Journal of the American Academy of Psychiatry and the Law, 50*, 74–83.
Wasser, T., Strockbine, B., Uyanwune, Y., & Kapoor, R. (2023). Restraint and seclusion practices and policies in U.S. forensic psychiatric hospitals. *Journal of the American Academy of Psychiatry and the Law, 51*, 566–574.
Zhong, S., Senior, M., Yu, R., Perry, A., Hawton, K., Shaw, J., & Fazel, S. (2021). Risk factors for suicide in prisons: A systematic review and meta-analysis. *Lancet Public Health*, 6(3), e164–e174.

SECTION V
Psychopharmacology

27

Formulary management

Nathaniel P. Morris and Paul R. S. Burton[*]

Introduction

Incarcerated populations tend to have high rates of mental illness, addiction, and other forms of mental health needs compared with broader populations (Fazel et al., 2016, 2017). No single treatment can adequately address the diverse mental health needs of incarcerated patients, and jails and prisons may need to offer a variety of mental health services, ranging from supportive psychotherapy to inpatient hospitalization, to meet the complex and evolving mental health needs of incarcerated patients. Psychiatric medications are just one component—although an essential one—of mental health services in many jails and prisons (Tamburello et al., 2022).

As with any patient population, clinicians must consider the risks and benefits when prescribing psychiatric medications to incarcerated patients. At the broader systems level, jail and prison authorities must also weigh competing pressures, including potential therapeutic benefits, safety risks, diversion concerns, financial costs, staff availability, and legal obligations, when determining the availability of each medication for patient care (Morris et al., 2020; Rucker & Schiff, 1990). The development of a psychiatric medication formulary, including a list of available medications and guidelines for their use, is an essential process for evaluating, balancing, and addressing these concerns (National Commission on Correctional Health Care [NCCHC], 2015). This chapter examines psychiatric medication formulary management in jails and prisons, including how pharmacy and therapeutics committees (P&TCs) can contribute to the development, implementation, monitoring, and refinement of such formularies, as well as help shape prescription practices. In addition, this chapter highlights how formularies should not just limit clinician use of and patient access to psychiatric medications but instead serve as a collaborative and guiding framework that supports safety, efficiency, and evidence-based practices in psychiatric medication prescribing in jails and prisons.

The importance of psychiatric medication formularies

Psychiatric medication formularies have become an integral part of mental health services in jails and prisons. Several trends have contributed to the growing importance of these formularies, of which this chapter explores just a few. First, over the last several decades, many jails and prisons have attracted scrutiny for providing inadequate health care, including mental health care. In a 1974 article, Goldsmith described the health care provided in many jails and prisons as unsafe and of poor quality, referring to the U.S. carceral system as the "barren wasteland of medical care" (Goldsmith, 1974, p. 575). Mental health care has not been exempted from such criticisms, with widespread concerns regarding the adequacy of staffing, suicide prevention, medication prescribing, and other aspects of mental health services behind bars (Metzner, 2002). Public attention to and litigation over inadequate care has led to efforts to improve the quality of and, to a certain extent, standardize mental health services offered to incarcerated patients (Metzner, 2002; NCCHC, 2015; Tamburello et al., 2022). The development of evidence-based psychiatric medication formularies offers one way to help achieve these goals.

Second, the incarceration of large numbers of people with mental health needs—and the growing responsibilities of jails and prisons to address these needs—means that these formularies now "play a significant and underrecognized role in the practice of psychiatry" (Morris et al., 2020, p. 2). According to a 2016 report, the "Los Angeles County Jail, Chicago's Cook County Jail, or the New York's Riker's Island Jail Complex each hold more mentally ill [people] than any remaining psychiatric hospital in the United States" (Treatment Advocacy Center, 2016, p. 1). Millions of people cycle through jails and prisons each year in the United States, and such formularies can shape the ways in which these individuals may receive (or not receive) specific psychiatric medications (Morris et al., 2020). As jails and prisons are left to provide the mental health services that are lacking in many communities, the medication formularies inside these carceral facilities may become the driving force behind the types and quality of care delivered in these locations.

Third, many jails and prisons have seen growing use of and financial costs related to psychiatric medications. In some jurisdictions, more than a quarter of incarcerated people are now receiving psychiatric medications (California Health Policy Strategies, 2020; Huh et al., 2017). A survey of state prison systems found that prescription drug spending consumed approximately 7% to 32% of prison health

*. The authors adapted this chapter from the work of Robert H. Berger, Robyn J, Wahl, and M. Paul Chaplin, who authored the chapter in the textbook's first edition.

budgets in 2015, and psychiatric medications often represent a considerable portion of such spending (Huh et al., 2017). Psychiatric medication formularies have emerged as a necessary tool in jails and prisons for managing the expanding availability of and costs related to different types of psychiatric medications (Ducate & Pondrom, 2003; Johnson & Friesen, 1998; Marcoux et al., 2012; Tamburello et al., 2017).

In recent years, psychiatric medication formularies in jails and prisons have drawn greater public attention. A number of jail and prison systems, such as the Federal Bureau of Prisons, now publish their medication formularies online and make them available to the public (Federal Bureau of Prisons Health Services, 2022). Academic journals related to medicine and criminal justice have published a number of articles related to formulary management (Kamath et al., 2013; Marcoux et al., 2012; Morris et al., 2020; Tamburello et al., 2012; Veysey et al., 2007). Professional organizations, such as the American Academy of Psychiatry and the Law, have released practice resources related to psychiatric prescribing to incarcerated patients (Tamburello et al., 2022). The NCCHC has integrated the need for and development of medication formularies into its standards for accreditation for carceral facilities (NCCHC, 2015). These findings reinforce that psychiatric medication formularies are assuming a key role in the delivery of mental health services behind bars and will likely continue to shape such care moving forward.

Pharmacy and therapeutics committees

Membership and organization

For some jails and prisons, particularly small ones with limited resources or staffing, decision-making regarding the availability of psychiatric medications may fall to just a few staff who are providing mental health services in these locations. Larger jail or prison systems, for example with multiple interconnected facilities in different locations, may choose to have a centralized psychiatric medication formulary process to standardize care across the jurisdiction's network. Regardless of the size of the system of care, psychiatric medication formularies in jails and prisons should be developed through an organized decision-making process (Ciccarello et al., 2021; NCCHC, 2015). As an example, P&TCs, also known as drug and therapeutics committees in some jurisdictions, are multidisciplinary decision-making bodies that oversee the development, implementation, monitoring, and refinement of such formularies (Ciccarello et al., 2021; Fijn et al., 2002; Loorand-Stiver, 2011; Tan et al., 2005). Integrating the roles and responsibilities of the P&TC into official jail or prison policies can be key for providing leadership support and ensuring buy-in from staff (Holloway & Green, 2003).

Regarding membership, a P&TC may have subcommittees related to different subspecialties, and a mental health P&TC is often chaired by psychiatric leadership (i.e., usually a mental health prescriber, such as chief of psychiatry, with appropriate medical training; Loorand-Striver, 2011; Quintiliani & Quercia, 2003). The multidisciplinary membership of a mental health P&TC often includes staff from psychiatry, pharmacy, nursing, or other disciplines with direct involvement and/or expertise in the prescription, dispensing, administration, or lab monitoring related to psychiatric medication prescribing (NCCHC, 2015; Tamburello et al., 2022). Membership in a P&TC is typically for a fixed time period (e.g., 1 or 2 years), and members should have familiarity with reviewing medical literature, including keeping up with peer-reviewed publications and evolving medical evidence (Quintiliani & Quercia, 2003). To avoid actual or perceived conflicts of interest, prospective members in a mental health P&TC should disclose financial or other relevant relationships with commercial interests prior to appointment and on a regular basis thereafter (Quintiliani & Quercia, 2003).

In addition to membership considerations, a mental health P&TC typically has a set of written policies to guide its functioning, including a schedule for regular meetings, voting procedures by members, and distribution of committee documents (e.g., formulary protocols, formulary updates, clinical practice guidelines, meeting minutes). These policies and publications should ideally be available to staff to support transparency, engagement with P&TC proceedings, and feedback from relevant parties (Holloway & Green, 2003). Some jail and prison systems require staff to work in multiple sites or locations separated by considerable distances; under these circumstances, advance planning for in-person meetings, or virtual meetings over tele- or videoconferencing, may be necessary (Hatton et al., 2005). In certain instances, for example, decision-making over complex or highly subspecialized treatment options, mental health P&TCs may also consider incorporating input from outside experts into the decision-making process (Hatton et al., 2005; Tamburello et al., 2022).

To summarize, as described in a 2003 World Health Organization publication, a P&TC should have "a multidisciplinary, transparent approach, technical competence and an official mandate" to function (Holloway & Green, 2003, p. 6).

Roles and responsibilities

As in community settings, P&TCs in jails and prisons have a wide range of roles and responsibilities (Lundquist & Becker, 2010). Beyond creating, implementing, and managing the psychiatric medication formulary (Tan et al., 2005), the P&TC must supervise prescribing practices to incarcerated patients on an ongoing basis, including evaluating the safety, effectiveness, ethical implications, and financial effects of medication use (Lundquist & Becker, 2010). A P&TC should review the latest evidence-based prescribing practices in jails and prisons to guide development of clinical protocols, including procedures for nonformulary requests, off-label prescribing, and other relevant treatment algorithms (Ciccarello et al., 2021; Kamath et al., 2013; Tamburello et al., 2022). Collecting and analyzing data in the jail or prison system enables the P&TC to monitor budgetary considerations, medication utilization, adherence to treatment protocols, and outcomes of committee initiatives, among other findings (Tamburello et al., 2022). To assist with risk mitigation, the P&TC may develop strategies for monitoring adverse effects related to medications, disseminating alerts to staff (e.g., pertinent changes to drug labeling, black box warnings), and following risk evaluation and mitigation strategy (REMS) requirements for specific medications (Loorand-Striver, 2011; Raber, 2010). Moreover, P&TCs must ensure that their procedures for medication use are consistent with administrative directives and recommended jail and prison policies at the county, state, or national level, depending on jurisdiction (Marcoux et al., 2012).

To meet its goals successfully, a P&TC must also engage with health professionals throughout the jail or prison system who are involved in the medication use process (Lundquist & Becker, 2010).

A comprehensive communication plan can facilitate bidirectional information sharing between P&TC members and broader jail and prison staff (Lundquist & Becker, 2010). Although the P&TC may help oversee and guide prescribing practices, health and custody staff working on the front lines play a key role in alerting the P&TC to clinical and operational concerns that arise during patient encounters (Fijn et al., 2002). In addition to receiving, considering, and integrating these concerns into formulary management, P&TC members in return also often provide education, supervision, and consultation in line with their expertise to front-line jail and prison staff (Ciccarello et al., 2021; Lindquist & Becker, 2010; Reeves, 2012). Examples of such education may include facility-specific case conferences, broader system-wide trainings, individual and group supervision, informational newsletters and emails, and disseminating new or pertinent medical literature (Ciccarello et al., 2021). Together, these initiatives may serve as opportunities not only for soliciting valuable feedback from broader jail and prison staff but also for supporting understanding of and adherence to evolving formulary guidelines, prescribing practices, and evidence-based treatment guidelines (Ciccarello et al., 2021; Reddan et al., 2004).

Principles of formulary management

Formulary development, additions, and deletions

Some jail and prison systems have existing medication formularies and will not require development of an entirely new psychiatric medication formulary (Federal Bureau of Prisons Health Services, 2022). On the other hand, certain situations, such as the establishment of new jail or prison systems, change in management of mental health services, or litigation, may require staff behind bars to create a new formulary. There is no one model psychiatric medication formulary that will adequately meet the needs of all different types of jail and prison systems (Morris et al., 2020). Staff overseeing formulary development, such as the P&TC, may wish to consult with colleagues from other jail and prison systems of similar sizes and patient populations. Doing so may offer lessons from existing formulary protocols about which medications may be useful to make available or restrict, as well as policy approaches to consider for individual medications or medication classes (Rosenheck et al., 2008). Some scholars have called for organizations, such as the American Psychiatric Association and the NCCHC, to collaborate on developing a series of model formularies that might apply to different jails and prisons, which might offer a framework for formulary development and help standardize access to psychiatric medications (Morris et al., 2020).

Determining which medications to add to or remove from the formulary list is a central function for staff overseeing formulary management, not only during initial formulary development but also on a regular basis thereafter. There should be protocols in place for the addition or removal of medications from the formulary, including how broader staff might request these changes (e.g., forms, online portal), the process and timelines for reviewing these requests, and the procedures by which the P&TC decides on whether to implement these suggestions (Fijn et al., 2002; Quintilani & Quercia, 2003). These protocols should be transparent to clinical staff working behind bars, offer opportunities for feedback, and provide timely updates, for example, through a regular newsletter or email update (Fijn et al., 2002; Holloway & Green, 2003; Rucker & Schiff, 1990; Quintilani & Quercia, 2003). Incarcerated patients may also provide valuable feedback on formulary availability of specific medications and often do so by discussing with their treating clinicians, communicating through local health care channels (i.e., medical slips), or pursuing legal recourse (e.g., grievances, litigation).

Different reasons may underlie decisions for psychiatric medication inclusion in or removal from the formulary. For example, new availability of generic versions of an existing psychiatric medication or new regulatory approval of a novel medication may offer reasons for adding a medication to the formulary, whereas excess costs, limited utilization by clinicians, or safety concerns might be reasons for removing a medication from a formulary (Holloway & Green, 2003; Raber, 2010). The P&TC, or staff overseeing the formulary if an official P&TC is not in place, should document the decision-making process behind changes to the formulary, including reasoning regarding why these changes were made (Raber, 2010).

Nonformulary requests

Overly restrictive formularies run the risk of cutting off incarcerated patients' access to clinically indicated psychiatric medications (Moffic, 2006; Morris et al., 2020). Medications that are designated "nonformulary" may be restricted to some degree or altogether unavailable in jails and prisons (Morris et al., 2020). For medications that are restricted but may be available in specific situations, the criteria for prescribing these medications and procedures for requesting such medications should be transparent and available to clinical staff (Fijn et al., 2002). For example, a prescribing clinician might submit a "nonformulary request" alongside a medication order detailing why an incarcerated patient is unable to tolerate or has previously tried preferred formulary medications without success, which may be approved or rejected by a reviewing pharmacist or psychiatric supervisor (Patel, 2003). In some situations, formulary protocol or the reviewing clinician might suggest a substitute medication available on the formulary, as opposed to a nonformulary medication, if the medication class and therapeutic intent are similar (Hoover et al., 1990).

Medication risk management

As with any patient population, medication diversion and misuse are concerns in jail and prison settings (Burns, 2009; Hilliard et al., 2013; McKee et al., 2014; Tamburello et al., 2012, 2022; see Chapter 30). Several reasons, such as high rates of substance use disorders among incarcerated people, harsh conditions of confinement, stress related to incarceration, and restricted access to substances, may explain why medication diversion and misuse remain pressing issues in many jails and prisons (McKee et al., 2014). According to medical literature and the authors' experiences caring for incarcerated patients, several psychiatric medications, including benzodiazepines (Reeves, 2012), quetiapine (Tamburello et al., 2012), bupropion (Hilliard et al., 2013), tricyclic antidepressants (McKee et al., 2014), and others (McKee et al., 2014; Tamburello et al., 2022), have diversion and misuse potential in jails and prisons. Controlled substances are generally restricted in jail and prison settings due to concerns regarding potential for diversion, misuse, and dependence, although a formulary may specify limited clinical circumstances (e.g., catatonia, seizures, acute pain, mania) in which use of controlled substances may be warranted (Burns, 2009; see Chapter 29). Medications for opioid use disorder treatment, such as buprenorphine or methadone, have also become more widely available in some jails and prisons, with emerging reports of diversion concerns related to such medications (Gryczynski et al., 2021).

Although medication diversion and misuse draw considerable attention when providing care behind bars, all medications, even when taken as prescribed and on the formulary, carry risks of adverse effects (McKee et al., 2014). A well-designed formulary should include guidelines for managing the risks related not only to diversion/misuse but also to common adverse effects. The formulary should also direct prescribers to other relevant decision support tools that guide safe and effective treatment choices (e.g., recommended monitoring guidelines, REMS requirements, dosing suggestions; McKee et al., 2014; Raber, 2010).

Off-label prescribing

Off-label prescribing, or the use of prescription medications for treatment purposes other than labeled indications approved by regulatory agencies, is common in many jails and prisons (Brown et al., 2018; Tamburello et al., 2022). Although potentially useful in some clinical situations, off-label prescribing in jail and prison settings raises several clinical, legal, and ethical concerns, such as the challenges of obtaining genuine informed consent when patients are incarcerated and may also have limited health literacy (Tamburello et al., 2022). Formularies should have guidelines to jail and prison clinical staff regarding off-label prescribing, for example, situations in which it may be allowable and situations in which it is prohibited (Ciccarello et al., 2021). Developing such guidelines may be particularly useful for medications (e.g., sleep and anxiety medications) that are commonly prescribed for off-label uses (Brown et al., 2018).

Supporting evidence-based practices

Supporting evidence-based practices should be a central goal of psychiatric medication formulary management in jails and prisons. Although formularies may be used to influence prescribing practices (Schumock et al., 2004), many of the research studies and surveys that drive health care practices, including mental health services, do not include people who are incarcerated or work behind bars (Wang et al., 2019). Still, evidence-based practices in formulary management refer not just to considering published medical literature to support formulary decisions but also to monitoring outcomes (e.g., medication utilization, treatment results) and using these findings to refine formulary policies on an ongoing basis (Ciccarello et al., 2021; Finnerty et al., 2002; Kamath et al., 2013). Medical literature may not always be directly applicable to individual carceral institutions or systems, and local knowledge (e.g., staff experiences, policies, outcomes) may not always reflect what is published in the medical literature. As a result, the P&TC, or staff otherwise responsible for formulary management, should integrate data from these different sources to guide the development of a therapeutic, safe, and efficient formulary (Ciccarello et al., 2021; Finnerty et al., 2002; Wang et al., 2019).

Even when clinicians and incarcerated patients choose approved or recommended formulary medications, these medications can be prescribed inappropriately (e.g., dosing, timing, frequency, combination with other treatments) without additional guidelines for broader clinical evaluation and management (Ciccarello et al., 2021; Lundquist & Becker, 2010). Outside of the formulary list of medications itself, the P&TC may play an important role in shaping broader clinical guidelines and recommended practices for psychiatric care in jail or prison settings (Lundquist & Becker, 2010). These practice guidelines must be shaped by current standards of psychiatric care in jails and prisons, involve input from psychiatric leadership with subject matter expertise and staff working directly with incarcerated patients, and undergo collaborative review within the multidisciplinary P&TC (Kamath et al., 2013; Lundquist & Becker, 2010; Reeves, 2012). Such guidelines should ideally be published in a clear and concise manner, as well as be easily accessible to clinical staff in jail and prison settings (Ciccarello et al., 2021; Lundquist & Becker, 2010). Periodic reviews and updates of these guidelines are essential in ensuring staff have access to current and relevant decision support tools. Finally, based on these guidelines and depending on the clinical issue, P&TCs may consider making informational handouts available to incarcerated patients or the broader public to support health literacy and broader understanding of psychiatric treatment considerations in the jail or prison setting.

Summary

Formularies are powerful and underrecognized tools that shape the mental health care of millions of people behind bars each year (Morris et al., 2020). Such formularies should not just be used by jail and prison administrators as rule-based frameworks to cut financial costs and restrict patient access to certain medications; instead, a well-designed formulary in jail or prison is developed in a manner that helps weigh the competing pressures of therapeutic benefits, safety risks, financial costs, legal obligations, and patient preferences (Morris et al., 2020). P&TCs offer a framework through which jail and prison staff can support such development in a transparent, multidisciplinary, and evidence-based manner (Holloway & Green, 2003). As jails and prisons have assumed the responsibility of front-line providers of mental health services in many places, these psychiatric medication formularies—and the processes behind their creation—will continue to draw attention from clinicians, patients, courts, and the broader public.

REFERENCES

Brown, G. P., Stewart, L. A., Rabinowitz, T., Boudreau, H., & Wright, A. J. (2018). Approved and off-label use of prescribed psychotropic medications among federal Canadian inmates. *Canadian Journal of Psychiatry*, *63*(10), 683–691.

Burns, K. A. (2009). The top ten reasons to limit prescription of controlled substances in prisons. *Journal of American Academy of Psychiatry and the Law*, *37*, 50–52.

California Health Policy Strategies. (2020). *The prevalence of mental illness in California jails is rising: An analysis of mental health cases & psychotropic medication prescriptions, 2009–2019*. https://calhps.com/wpcontent/uploads/2023/03/ Jail_MentalHealth_JPSReport_02-03-2020.pdf

Ciccarello, C., Leber, M. B., Leonard, M. C., et al. (2021). ASHP guidelines on the pharmacy and therapeutics committee and the formulary system. *American Journal of Health-System Pharmacy*, *78*(10), 907–918.

Ducate, S., & Pondrom, M. (2003). Ziprasidone reduces pharmacy costs in correctional in-patient psychiatric facilities. *International Congress on Schizophrenia Research*, *21*, 335.

Fazel, S, Hayes, A. J., Bartellas, K., Clerici, M., & Trestman, R. (2016). Mental health of prisoners: Prevalence, adverse outcomes, and interventions. *Lancet Psychiatry*, *3*(9), 871–881.

Fazel, S., Yoon, I. A., & Hayes, A. J. (2017). Substance use disorders in prisoners: An updated systematic review and meta-regression analysis in recently incarcerated men and women. *Addiction (Abingdon, England)*, *112*(10), 1725–1739.

Federal Bureau of Prisons Health Services. (2022). *National formulary part I*. https://www.bop.gov/resources/pdfs/2022_winter_formulary_part_1.pdf

Fijn, R., van Epnhuysen, L. S., Peijnenburg, A. J. M., Brouwers, J. R. B. J., & de Jong-van den Berg, L. T. W. (2002). Is there a need for critical ethical and philosophical evaluation of hospital drugs and therapeutics (D&T) committees? *Pharmacoepidemiology and Drug Safety*, *11*, 247–252.

Finnerty, M., Altmasberger, R., Bopp, J., Carpinello, S., Docherty, J. P., & Fisher, W. (2002). Using state administrative and pharmacy data bases to develop a clinical decision support tool for schizophrenia guidelines. *Schizophrenia Bulletin*, *28*(1), 85–94.

Goldsmith, S. B. (1974). The status of prison health care. A review of the literature. *Public Health Reports (Washington, D.C.: 1974)*, *89*(6), 569–575.

Gryczynski, J., Lee, J. D., Dusek, K., et al. (2021). Use of non-prescribed buprenorphine in the criminal justice system: Perspectives of individuals recently released from incarceration. *Journal of Substance Abuse Treatment*, *127*, 108349.

Hatton, R. C., Gonzolez-Rothi, R. J., Smith, W. D., & Knudsen, A. K. (2005). The use of virtual expert panels: Formulary decision-making in the 21st century. *Formulary*, *40*, 78–85.

Hilliard, W. T., Barloon, L., Farley, P., Penn, J. V., & Koranek, A. (2013). Bupropion diversion and misuse in the correctional facility. *Journal of Correctional Health Care*, *19*(3), 211–217.

Holloway, K., & Green, T. (2003). *Drug and therapeutics committees: A practical guide*. World Health Organization.

Hoover, S. E., White, L. J., & Weiner, J. (1990). Therapeutic substitution and formulary systems. *Annals of Internal Medicine*, *113*(2), 160–163.

Huh, K., Boucher, A., McGaffey, F., McKillop, M., & Schiff, M. (2017). *Pharmaceuticals in state prisons: How departments of corrections purchase, use, and monitor prescription drugs*. Pew Charitable Trusts. https://www.pewtrusts.org/-/media/assets/2017/12/pharmaceuticals-in-state-prisons.pdf

Johnson, J. A., & Friesen, E. (1998). Reassessing the relevance of pharmacoeconomic analysis in formulary decisions. *Pharmacoeconomics*, *5*(Pt. 1), 479–485.

Kamath, J., Zhang, W., Kesten, K., Wakai, S., Shelton, D., & Trestman, R. L. (2013). Algorithm-driven pharmacological management of bipolar disorder in Connecticut prisons. *International Journal of Offender Therapy and Comparative Criminology*, *57*(2), 251–264.

Loorand-Striver, L. (2011). Hospital-based pharmacy and therapeutics committees: Evolving responsibilities and membership. *Environmental Scan: Canadian Agency for Drugs and Technologies in Health*, *23*, 1–15.

Lundquist, T., & Becker, T. (2010). Medication management in correctional settings. In A. Ruiz, J. Dvoskin, C. Scott, & J. Metzner (Eds.), *Manual of forms and guidelines for correctional mental health* (pp. 83–111). American Psychiatric Publishing.

Marcoux, R. M., Simeone, J. C., Colavita, M., & Larrat, E. P. (2012). An innovative approach to pharmacy management in a state correctional system. *Journal of Correctional Health Care*, *18*(1), 53–61.

McKee, J., Penn, J. V., & Koranek, A. (2014). Psychoactive medication misadventuring in correctional health care. *Journal of Correctional Health Care*, *20*(3), 249–260.

Metzner, J. L. (2002). Class action litigation in correctional psychiatry. *Journal of the American Academy of Psychiatry and the Law*, *30*(1), 19–32.

Moffic, H. S. (2006). Ethical principles for psychiatric administrators: The challenge of formularies. *Psychiatry Quarterly*, *77*, 319–327.

Morris, N. P., Hirschtritt, M. E., & Tamburello, A. C. (2020). Drug formularies in correctional settings. *Journal of the American Academy of Psychiatry and the Law*, *48*(1), 2–6.

National Commission on Correctional Health Care. (2015). *Standards for mental health services in correctional facilities*.

Patel, N. N. (2023). A versatile prison psychiatric pharmacy program. *Journal of the American Pharmacists Association*, *63*(4), 1203–1210.

Quintiliani, R., & Quercia, R. A. (2003). How to create a therapeutics committee that is scientifically and economically sound. *Formulary*, *38*, 594–602.

Raber, J. H. (2010). The formulary process from a risk management perspective. *Pharmacotherapy*, *30*, 42S–47S.

Reddan, J. G., Sheehan, A. H., Eskew, J., & Elmes, G. (2004). Integration of a medication management infrastructure in a large, multihospital system. *American Journal of Health- System Pharmacists*, *61*, 2557–2561.

Reeves, R. (2012). Guideline, education, and peer comparison to reduce prescriptions of benzodiazepines and low-dose quetiapine in prison. *Journal of Correctional Health Care*, *18*(1), 45–52.

Rosenheck, R. A., Leslie, D. L., Busch, S., Rofman, E. S., & Sernyak, M. (2008). Rethinking antipsychotic formulary policy. *Schizophrenia Bulletin*, *34*(2), 375–380.

Rucker, T. D., & Schiff, G. (1990). Drug formularies: Myths-in-formation. *Medical Care*, *28*(10), 928–939.

Schumock, G. T., Walton, S. M., Park, H. Y., et al. (2004). Factors that influence prescribing decisions. *Annals of Pharmacotherapy*, *38*, 557–562.

Tamburello, A., Kaldany, H., & Dickert, J. (2017). Correctional mental health administration. *International Review of Psychiatry (Abingdon, England)*, *29*(1), 3–10.

Tamburello, A. C., Lieberman, J. A., Baum, R. M., & Reeves, R. (2012). Successful removal of quetiapine from a correctional formulary. *Journal of the American Academy of Psychiatry and the Law*, *40*, 502–508.

Tamburello, A., Penn, J., Ford, E., et al. (2022). The American Academy of Psychiatry and the Law practice resource for prescribing in corrections. *Journal of the American Academy of Psychiatry and the Law*, *50*(4 Suppl.), S1–S62.

Tan, E. L., Day, R. O., & Brien, J. E. (2005). Perspectives on drug and therapeutics committee policy implementation. *Research in Social and Administrative Pharmacy*, *1*, 526–545.

Treatment Advocacy Center. (2016). *Serious mental illness (SMI) prevalence in jails and prisons*. https://www.treatmentadvocacycenter.org/wp-content/uploads/2023/11/smi-in-jails-and-prisons.pdf

Veysey, B. M., Stenius, V., Mazade, N., & Schacht, L. (2007). Costs, control or just good clinical practice? The use of antipsychotic medications and formulary decision-making in large U.S. prisons and jails. *Journal of Offender Rehabilitation*, *45*(1–2), 189–206.

Wang, E. A., Macmadu, A., & Rich, J. D. (2019). Examining the impact of criminal justice involvement on health through federally funded, national population-based surveys in the United States. *Public Health Reports*, *134*(1 Suppl.), 22S–33S.

28

Medication administration and management

Catherine M. Knox

Introduction

The courts and professional organizations recognize access to clinically appropriate and timely treatment with psychotropic medication as an essential element of an adequate correctional mental health system (Morris et al., 2020; Tamburello et al., 2022). While receiving treatment, incarcerated persons (IPs) must be monitored and supervised clinically so that optimal patient outcomes are achieved. According to the U.S. Department of Justice, only 60% of state prisoners and 42% of federal prisoners surveyed in 2016 who experienced serious psychological distress in the last 30 days reported receiving mental health treatment. Of those with a history of mental health problems, 63% of state prisoners and 58% of federal prisoners reported receiving treatment while incarcerated (Maruschak et al., 2021). A more recent study found that the proportion of pharmaceuticals distributed to jails and prisons to treat depression and severe mental illness was lower than for nonincarcerated populations, with a fourfold disparity in treatment after correcting for the relative disease burden (Curran et al., 2023). Barriers to the identification and treatment of persons with mental illness in jails and prisons remain (Fazel et al., 2016). This chapter addresses the processes involved in the mechanics of pharmacotherapy in the correctional setting and discusses opportunities to enhance patient adherence.

Components of medication delivery

There are many steps, people, and processes involved in getting medication to the patient within a correctional facility. The major components and criteria for an adequate medication system are listed in Table 28.1. Psychiatrists should be familiar with the correctional facility's medication practices to make informed recommendations to patients for treatment (Tamburello et al., 2022). Correctional systems have been slow to adopt technology. What is considered the norm in health care settings, such as automated order entry, automated dispensing, or electronic medication administration records, is only beginning to be used in jails and prisons (Knox & Burrow, 2016; Rogers, 2020; Schiffner, 2017).

Prescribing

Collaboration with the patient to arrive at the best treatment decision possible is key to achieving patient cooperation and adherence with prescribed medication (Gault et al., 2013). While patients in the correctional setting have less voice in determining treatment (Tamburello et al., 2022), many studies show that considering the patient's perspective, preferences, expectations, and worries in arriving at decisions positively affects subsequent adherence with prescription medication (Bentley & Casey, 2017; Finnerty et al., 2018; Fiorillo et al., 2020; Gault et al., 2013; Townsend et al., 2022). This is especially challenging in correctional settings because of the propensity for patients to report symptoms for the purpose of obtaining certain desirable medications for diversion or misuse (Brink, 2018; Collins et al., 2017).

Medication formularies are used to control costs, guide clinical practice, and minimize medication diversion and misuse (Morris et al., 2020; see Chapter 27). Nevertheless, psychiatrists should have available several types of medications to treat various mental disorders. In addition, access to medications not on the formulary should be available upon request when it is clinically appropriate or in the case of newly admitted patients, until a suitable alternative is identified by the treating clinician (Tamburello et al., 2022; Trestman, 2015). A pharmacist should review each order in relation to the patient's medication profile to identify contraindications before medication is dispensed. Consultation with a pharmacist improves monitoring of patients with chronic conditions (including psychiatric disorders) and is becoming more available in correctional health care (American Society of Health-System Pharmacists, 2016; Griebe et al., 2016; Tamburello et al., 2022; Thompson et al., 2019).

Decisions about the choice of drug, dosing, and monitoring should also factor in the patient's program assignments and when medications are administered in the correctional facility (Tamburello et al., 2022). For example, sedating medication should not be given earlier than 8 p.m., long before the patient normally sleeps. Further, because a medication may have multiple uses, its indication or intended effect should be explained. This is especially helpful when other members of the health care team address patient concerns about the medication (Cuthbertson et al., 2017; Tariq et al., 2024).

Table 28.1 Components of an adequate medication delivery system

Prescribing	• The formulary includes several forms of each class of drug. • Medications not on the formulary are accessible via nonformulary request. • Orders for medication administration do not conflict with the patient's program and facility schedules. • Medication is administered consistently with the time it is ordered.
Dispensing	• Patients receive the first dose of new medications in a timely manner. • Medications are available if treatment must be administered before the pharmacy dispenses. • The physician and pharmacist jointly determine stock and starter medications.
Distributing	• Medications are delivered in a timely, safe, and clinically effective manner. • Security procedures prevent medication misuse. • Patient questions, absences, and refusals are addressed but do not delay medication delivery. • Medication administration is documented and used to guide clinical care.
Continuity	• Medication treatment is uninterrupted. • Problems that contribute to medication discontinuity are resolved. • Reminders for refills and renewals are used to prevent medication misses. • Medications are continued upon release from the facility in sufficient quantity until access to mental health treatment in the community is achieved.

Medication administration is costly in terms of nursing and correctional officer time. If the volume of medication prescribed exceeds the time available or staffing capacity, medications will be missed or given at inappropriate intervals. Use of evidence-based practice guidelines and strategies regarding dosage, strength, and frequency in prescribing are ways to manage the volume of medication to be administered each day (Knox & Burrow, 2016; Tamburello et al., 2022). For example, medications that can be administered once daily should preferentially be ordered this way, rather than as split dosing. If an order cannot be written to accommodate the patient's schedule or the staffing capacity, the psychiatrist should consider transferring the patient to a location that can carry out the intended treatment.

Orders to "crush and float" medication should be limited to patients who have diverted or misused medication recently, and the intervention should be included in their individualized treatment plan. Blanket policies (such as "crush and float" any administration of a particular medication) are discouraged since the impact on nursing time is significant and may result in untimely dosing. These policies should not be adopted in lieu of effective security practices, including drug surveillance programs and other structural solutions known to prevent misuse of drugs in correctional facilities (Collins et al., 2017; Knox & Burrow, 2016; Tamburello et al., 2022).

Dispensing and distribution

Prescribers should be mindful of the time needed to procure the first dose of medication after an order is written. Depending on the location and efficiency of the pharmacy, this may be less than an hour or as long as a week. Another potential delay is the time it takes for nursing staff to verify medications received from the pharmacy and to prepare them for administration. It may take another day or two before the medication is available to the patient, especially if large deliveries are received from the pharmacy and staffing levels are not adjusted to handle the influx. The pharmacy and physician should mutually determine clinically acceptable turnaround times and identify what stock medications need to be available in the interim or have an arrangement with a backup pharmacy (Collins et al., 2017; Knox & Burrow, 2016; Tamburello et al., 2022). In correctional facilities, psychotropic medications are usually administered to each patient dose by dose (i.e., directly observed therapy) because of concerns about the potential for self-harm and misuse (Collins et al., 2017; Tamburello et al., 2022). An unintended advantage of dose-by-dose administration is the ability to engage with the patient to support adherence and observe for side effects (Trestman, 2015). Some argue that directly observed therapy contributes to nonadherence if patients feel disempowered about when to take the medication, the time spent waiting in line is too long, or the medication is administered at an inconvenient time (Cuthbertson et al., 2017; Knox & Burrow, 2016). This is especially relevant if the medication is distributed in a place not protected from the elements or at a distance from the patient's housing unit.

Directly observed therapy medication is administered either by having patients come to a designated location (i.e., medication cart or pill window) or by delivering the medication to each individual in the housing unit or cell. On inpatient treatment units (i.e., mental health units or infirmaries), medication administration takes place on the unit. In restrictive housing units or other high-security areas, medication is administered at the cell or in the pod. Decentralized medication administration is staff intensive, and the physical plant can be difficult to navigate with medication carts. Centralized medication lines are challenging for correctional facilities to manage safely and can contribute to patient nonadherence (Collins et al., 2017; Knox & Burrow, 2016).

The facility health authority must advocate with the facility administrator so that the times, methods, and locations for medication delivery are timely, safe, and optimally therapeutic. Advocacy for enhanced nursing and security staffing may also be necessary to ensure proper medication administration. Other activities (e.g., IP movement, count times, officer shift changes) may impact the timeliness of medication administration and can affect the therapeutic effectiveness of the drug if doses are given too close or too far apart. The timing of administration must coincide with the intended purpose of the medication. For example, medication to be given at the hour of sleep should be given after 8 p.m. Arrangements must also be made to provide medications for patients who will be out to court or at a remote worksite when a dose is due (Knox & Burrow, 2016; Tamburello et al., 2022). Minimizing waiting times at a centralized pill call may reduce stigma and victimization (Cuthbertson et al., 2017; Tamburello et al., 2022).

Correctional officers manage movement of IPs to and from the medication area or escort health care personnel to administer medication in the unit. Officers also assist IPs to get ready to take their medications (e.g., getting off the bunk, getting water, being dressed appropriately) and eliminate distractions (e.g., loud television or games, crowding the medication area, interruptions). Both nursing and correctional staff should observe patients to ensure that medication is not "cheeked" or "palmed." This vigilance is especially important when the patient has misused medication previously or the diversion potential of the medication is high (Knox & Burrow, 2016; Tamburello et al., 2022).

Training for correctional officers should include the purpose of psychotropic medications, important precautions, and side effects. Officers with this knowledge can observe IPs and play a valuable role in the prevention, early identification, and management of negative side effects (Galanek, 2014; Knox & Burrow, 2016; Tamburello et al., 2022).

Questions, requests, and refusals can cause delays that contribute to untimely medication delivery. The nurse administering medication can answer simple questions, but if they are complicated or the patient is distressed, the patient should be asked to wait until after the distribution. If medication is not taken, the reason should be ascertained (e.g., the patient was at court or a medical appointment, had a visitor, was transferred, or was not let out of the cell). A patient who refuses a dose should be asked why to determine if there is a simple remedy to the problem. If patients miss pill call or refuse a dose, later administration of psychotropic medication should not be precluded if the dose can be given within a reasonable therapeutic time frame (Knox & Burrow, 2016).

During the COVID-19 pandemic, some correctional facilities were successful in having patients self-administer psychotropic medications with low risk for misuse or self-harm to reduce the potential for transmission of the virus (Tamburello et al., 2022). Individuals should also be given responsibility to self-administer medication during prerelease if they will be expected to do this when residing in the community (Knox & Burrow, 2016).

Distribution of medication should be periodically observed by a nursing supervisor for continuous quality improvement purposes. Examples of concerning practices include inadequate lighting, not observing for diversion, and inadequate and unhygienic practices such as slipping the pill container under the door. The review of video surveillance, if available, provides an impartial portrayal of medication administration at the facility.

Continuity

Continuity of medication administration is another challenge in correctional facilities. For example, when an IP is transferred to another housing location, their medication may not be moved to the corresponding medication cart or pill line. If the facility does not communicate such moves to the health care program, patients miss doses until the medication catches up or the pharmacy dispenses a new supply. Medication discontinuity can also occur when the pharmacy is not timely in processing refills or delivering supplies. The expiration of nonformulary approvals contributes to discontinuity when the expiration of the approval differs from the prescription's expiration date. Recommendations are to eliminate expiration dates for nonformulary approvals or ensure the expiration date coincides with the order's expiration. Obviously, discontinuity occurs if medication refills and renewals are not requested timely. Lapses should be reported, tracked, and reviewed to identify quality improvement opportunities (see Chapter 74).

Continuity of medication upon admission prevents potential crisis or relapse. Incarceration is also an opportunity to assess the medical necessity of medication prescribed by community providers (Trestman, 2015; see Chapter 18). Someone reporting taking psychotropic medication on admission should be referred to a psychiatrist to assess their need for medication at the next available appointment (or urgently, if clinically indicated). In the meantime, a prescriber should be contacted to determine whether bridge orders are needed. Intake staff should verify the prescription before the patient is seen by a provider (Knox & Burrow, 2016). Some correctional systems have joined a health information exchange or have a service to validate a prescription history electronically, greatly simplifying this task and improving accuracy.

The standard of care is to arrange for continuity of psychotropic medication during the transition to community mental health providers (Dlugacz, 2015; Tamburello et al., 2022; see Chapter 23). When informed of a pending release, the psychiatrist prescribes appropriate release medications. Patients are given a supply of medication at the time of release, or arrangements are made to fill the prescription in the community (Dlugacz, 2015). Stabilizing patients on medications prior to release, using medications that are available and affordable in the community, and using long-acting forms of medication increase the likelihood of continuity (American Psychiatric Association, 2016).

Medication adherence

A systematic review and meta-analysis of 35 studies regarding medication adherence among persons diagnosed with major mental illnesses reported that nonadherence was 49% across all diagnoses, with the highest rates in persons with schizophrenia (56%; Semahegen et al., 2020). A large study of veterans treated for posttraumatic stress disorder found that 34.6% discontinued their prescribed medication within 30 days, and 71.8% had discontinued medication within 6 months (Duek et al., 2020).

Adherence with psychotropic medication and reasons for nonadherence among IPs are similar to persons in the community, including side effects, stigma, lack of insight, and poor therapeutic relationships (Bentley & Casey, 2017; Cuthbertson et al., 2017; Duek et al., 2020; Fiorillo et al., 2020; Gault et al., 2013; Semahegen et al., 2020). Risks of nonadherence for IPs include relapse, victimization, violent behavior, suicidal behavior, recidivism, and increased frequency and duration of hospitalizations (Collins et al., 2017; Cuthbertson et al., 2017; Fazel et al., 2016; Muela et al., 2020). While 80% medication adherence is the threshold often mentioned in the literature (Knox, 2015), there is little evidence this level is sustainable for persons with mental illness (Semahegen et al., 2020). Excessive focus on adherence can be counterproductive and lead to more coercive interventions that ultimately cause the patient to withdraw from mental health treatment (Drake, 2018; Gault et al., 2013). Nevertheless, there is a growing body of evidence-based interventions that are worthy of consideration in working with IPs to improve adherence (Fazel et al., 2016). Methods to support adherence are listed in Table 28.2.

The quality of the patient–provider relationship influences medication adherence (Asher et al., 2023; Hamilton et al., 2022; Hsieh et al., 2022; Leiz et al., 2022). A collaborative working relationship contributed to medication adherence in a study of incarcerated women (Bentley & Casey, 2017). In another small study from Canada, IPs described "feeling understood" by health care providers as supporting medication

Table 28.2 Supporting medication adherence for incarcerated persons with mental illness

Treatment objective	Interventions
Devote time to address adherence as part of treatment	• Identify the patient's motivation and goals for treatment. • Link treatment interventions to the patient's motivation and goals. • Assess the patient's perspective about the importance , confidence in, and satisfaction with treatment. • Explore past and present reasons for nonadherence. • Use active listening and acknowledge the patient's experience, motivation, and goals for treatment. • Use structured interview tools to identify patients at high risk for poor adherence. • Use decision support protocols that assess adherence and promote patient involvement.
Facilitate development of insight and self-care	• Provide psychotherapy and psychoeducational programming. • Provide information and education about the medication, reasons it is prescribed, expected side effects, and self-care. • Increase visit frequency. • Use motivational interviewing techniques to discuss direct and indirect benefits of treatment in relation to the patient's goals and motivation for treatment. • Use cognitive-behavioral approaches to link adherence to symptom reduction. • Discuss reasons for nonadherence with the patient. • Embed medication taking into the patient's daily routine. • Provide the patient choice of time to take medication. • Provide reminders such as daily diaries, visual clues, and calendars. • Assign a medication buddy to help the patient remember to take medication.
Optimize treatment efficacy	• Monitor impact of medication on symptoms. • Anticipate side effects; provide guidance about how to manage them. • Acknowledge and explore the patient's distress with side effects. • Train staff in early identification and management of side effects. • Simplify or alter medication regimen to coincide with patient experience, motivation, and goals. • Consider missed-dose forgiving or long-acting formulas if clinically appropriate. • Eliminate or modify facility routines and culture that cause disruption or are disincentives to adherence (i.e., transfers, schedule conflicts, distance to walk, exposure to the elements, long waiting times at pill line, and administration times that conflict with programming or recreation).

Note. Adapted from Bentley and Casey (2017); Cuthbertson et al. (2017); Ehret et al. (2013); Gault et al. (2013); Knox and Burrow (2016); Mills et al. (2011); Muela et al. (2020); Tamburello et al. (2022).

adherence (Cuthbertson et al., 2017). A qualitative study conducted in England of persons ordered compulsory medication reported that adherence was achievable only after finding a professional willing to work collaboratively with them (Gault et al., 2013).

Duek and colleagues (2021) found that in veterans with posttraumatic stress disorder, factors associated with discontinuing pharmacotherapy were failure to engage in psychotherapy and a perception that their provider was indifferent or would not address side effects. A recent systematic literature review found that personal contact with a therapist was associated with increased adherence and that multifaceted interventions (e.g., personal contact and telehealth) were more powerful than single interventions (Leiz et al., 2022). Earlier follow-up after hospitalization was associated with increased medication adherence and outpatient utilization (Beadles et al., 2015).

In correctional settings, adherence is assessed simply by reviewing the patient's medication administration record. With electronic medication administration records, this review can be automated and the provider notified electronically, with follow-up scheduled as necessary (Knox & Burrows, 2016). As some patients strategically miss doses to minimize side effects while maintaining adequate efficacy, it is important to understand patients' perception of the medication's efficacy and side effects and the relative importance of each (Cuthbertson et al., 2017; Muiruri et al., 2023). Some patients with concerns about the medication have difficulty communicating these to their provider, and asking more open-ended questions about the treatment may help (Hamilton et al., 2022). Use of structured decision support tools, coupled with peer support, such as the CommonGround program (Ehret et al., 2013; Finerty et al., 2018; Fiorillo et al., 2020), improves adherence.

Some IPs report that they are not given enough information or explanation about medications and their side effects and purpose (Mills et al., 2011). In one study completed at a remand center in Canada, half of the participants reported not receiving an explanation of their illness or why the medication was prescribed. Even if explanation had been provided, these patients still perceived they lacked sufficient information. Helping IPs better understand their illness and treatment enhances medication adherence (Cuthbertson et al., 2017).

The routine and structure of the correctional setting can enable patients to take medication more regularly than they would on their own. However, the inflexibility of this environment can be a disincentive as well. Discussing reasons for nonadherence with the patient may identify problems such as long wait times or inappropriate timing that can be addressed systemically (Bentley & Casey, 2017; Cuthbertson et al., 2017; Ehret et al., 2013). For others, refusal to take medication may be an expression of self-determination in response to the loss of freedom (Tamburello et al., 2022).

Stigma is universally described as impacting adherence in IPs (Bentley & Casey, 2017; Cuthbertson et al., 2017; Gault et al., 2013), who perceive the loss of credible identity (i.e., being considered "crazy" or weak), feeling ashamed or embarrassed, and being disbelieved or mocked. At one women's facility, individuals with an external locus of control were more likely to experience stigma related to medications (Bentley & Casey, 2017). Townsend and colleagues (2022) found that experiencing side effects of antipsychotic medications was a significant source of embarrassment and shame, though when patients perceived themselves in a supportive environment, the sense of stigma was reduced and medication adherence improved. In a remand center in Canada, patients who were nonadherent were more likely to lack social support (Cuthbertson et al., 2017).

A patient's recovery is dependent upon gaining insight into their mental illness and developing the capacity for self-care. Qualitative studies described patients' development of insight as a series of phases evolving into stable conclusions about the role of medication each patient chooses to adopt. Some see medication as a protective factor that enhances recovery. Others will see it as a short-lived, temporary support when symptoms intensify (Asher et al., 2023; Gault et al., 2013). Reflective dialogue in psychotherapy facilitates the patient's recognition of how their attitudes and behaviors shape the choices made about medication. Motivational interviewing and cognitive-behavioral therapy can increase insight and help link adherence with symptom reduction (Ehret et al., 2013; Muela et al., 2020).

An advantage in treating mental illness in the correctional setting is the ability to observe the effects of prescribed medication closely. When correctional officers and nurses are trained to recognize symptoms and side effects associated with psychotropic medications, they can be more vigilant in referring patients promptly to the psychiatrist. Nursing staff can coach patients in self-care such as managing weight gain, addressing sedation, and coping with side effects (Knox & Burrow, 2016).

Adherence among prisoners who take psychotropic medication is strongly associated with patients' perception of treatment efficacy (Mills et al., 2011; Muela et al., 2020). Ehret and colleagues (2013) found that adherence improved as symptoms decreased among female prisoners with bipolar disorder. Bentley and Casey (2017) found this as well in another sample of incarcerated women treated with psychotropics.

The structural aspects of medication administration can also be altered to improve adherence (Ehret et al., 2013; Knox & Burrow, 2016; Mills et al., 2011). Examples are reducing medication burden by decreasing the number of doses each day, changing to a long-acting preparation, and administering medication at times and in ways that are more convenient for the patient but still clinically acceptable. Reducing episodes of medication discontinuity (e.g., transfers and schedule conflicts) improves adherence. It also reduces the incidence of adverse events and optimizes treatment efficacy (Knox & Burrow, 2016).

Summary

Psychopharmacology is a keystone in the treatment of mental illness. The prescription, preparation, delivery, and monitoring of psychotropics is a complex process and involves many personnel from nursing, mental health, and custody staff. In addition to the patient's clinical condition, the correctional environment and facility practices should be considered when making decisions about treatment. To support patient adherence, the psychiatrist should explain why medication has been prescribed, its intended effects, and how to address side effects. Adherence is assessed at each follow-up visit, and reasons for nonadherence explored with the patient. The psychiatrist provides information and education to other members of the treatment team so that they can assist the patient to optimize treatment.

In addition to prescribing, psychiatrists should be involved in the development of policies, procedures, and clinical guidelines concerning medications at the correctional facility, including decisions about medication formularies and the management of nonformulary requests. The accuracy, timeliness, and efficacy of medication treatment should be monitored as part of the facility's continuous quality improvement program. A comprehensive list of quality indicators concerning psychopharmacology in correctional settings developed by the American Academy of Psychiatry and the Law can be accessed online (Tamburello et al., 2022).

REFERENCES

American Psychiatric Association. (2016). *Psychiatric services in correctional facilities* (3rd ed.).

American Society of Health-Systems Pharmacists. (2016). ASHP guidelines on pharmacy services in correctional facilities. *American Journal of Health-Systems Pharmacists*, *73*, 1784–1790. https://www.ashp.org/-/media/assets/policy-guidelines/docs/guidelines/pharmacy-services-correctional-facilities.pdf

Asher, M., Roe, D., & Hasson-Ohayon, I. (2023). Attitudes toward and patterns of medication use among people with serious mental illness: There's more than meets the eye. *Frontiers in Psychiatry*, *14*, 1133140.

Beadles, C. A., Ellis, A., Lichstein, J. C., et al. (2015). First outpatient follow-up after psychiatric hospitalization: Does one size fit all? *Psychiatric Services*, *66*(4), 364–372.

Bentley, K. J., & Casey, R. C. (2017). Incarcerated women's experiences and beliefs about psychotropic medication: An empirical study. *Psychiatric Services*, *68*(4), 384–389.

Brink, J. (2018). Challenges in correctional psychiatry: Off-label prescribing. *Canadian Journal of Psychiatry*, *63*(10), 645–647.

Collins, T. N., Avondoglio, J. B., & Terry, L. M. (2017). Correctional psychopharmacology: Pitfalls, challenges, and victories of prescribing in a correctional setting. *International Review of Psychiatry*, *29*(1), 43–44.

Curran, J., Saloner, B., Winkelman, T. N., et al. (2023). Estimated use of prescription medications among individuals incarcerated in jails and prisons in the US. *JAMA Health Forum*, *4*(4), e230482.

Cuthbertson, L., Kowalewski, K., Edge, J., et al. (2017). Factors that promote and hinder medication adherence from the perspective of inmates in a provincial remand center: A mixed methods study. *Journal of Correctional Health Care*, *24*(1), 21–34.

Dlugacz, H. A. (2015). Community re-entry preparation/coordination. In R. L. Trestman, K. L. Applebaum, & J. L. Metzner (Eds.), *Oxford textbook of correctional psychiatry* (pp. 76–81). Oxford University Press.

Drake, R. E. (2018). Is treatment adherence the goal of shared decision making? *Psychiatric Services*, *69*(12), 1195.

Duek, O., Pietrzak, R. H., Petrakis, I., et al. (2021). Early discontinuation of pharmacotherapy in U.S. veterans diagnosed with PTSD and the role of psychotherapy. *Journal of Psychiatric Research*, *132*, 167–173.

Ehret, M. J., Shelton, D., Barta, W., et al. (2013). Medication adherence among female inmates with bipolar disorder: Results from a randomized controlled trail. *Psychological Services*, *10*(1), 106–114.

Fazel, S., Hayes, A. J., Bartellas, K., et al. (2016). Mental health of prisoners: Prevalence, adverse outcomes, and interventions. *Lancet Psychiatry*, *3*, 871–881.

Finnerty, M. T., Layman, D. M., Chen, Q., et al. (2018). Use of a web-based shared decision-making program: Impact on ongoing treatment engagement and antipsychotic adherence. *Psychiatric Services*, *69*(12), 1215–1221.

Fiorillo, A., Barlati, S., Bellomo, A., et al. (2020). Role of shared decision-making in improving adherence to pharmacological treatments in patients with schizophrenia: A clinical review. *Annals of General Psychiatry, 19*(43), 1–12. https://doi.org/10.1186/s12991-020-00293-4

Galanek, J. D. (2014). Correctional officers and the incarcerated mentally ill: Responses to psychiatric illness in prison. *Medical Anthropology Quarterly, 29*(1), 116–136.

Gault, I., Gallagher, A., & Chambers, M. (2013). Perspectives on medicine adherence in service users and carers with experience of legally sanctioned detention and medication: A qualitative study. *Patient Preference and Adherence, 7*, 787–799.

Griebe, K. M., Caniff, K. E., & Bostwick, J. R. (2016). Psychiatric pharmacists: Key allies to improve antipsychotic metabolic monitoring. *Psychiatric Services, 67*(4), 469–470.

Hamilton, J. E., Blanco, E., Selek, S., et al. (2022). Patient and provider perspectives on medication non-adherence among patients with depression and/or diabetes in diverse community settings—A qualitative analysis. *Patient Preference and Adherence, 16*, 1581–1594.

Hsieh, W. L., Yeh, S. T., Liu, W. I., et al. (2022). Improving medication adherence in community-dwelling patients with schizophrenia through therapeutic alliance and medication attitude: A serial multiple mediation model. *Patient Preference and Adherence, 16*, 1017–1026.

Knox, C. M. (2015). Medication administration and management: Directly observed therapy. In R. Trestman, K. Appelbaum, & J. Metzner (Eds.), *Oxford textbook of correctional psychiatry* (pp. 160–164). Oxford University Press.

Knox, C. M., & Burrow, G. F. (2016). *Medication management in the correctional setting (quick start for correctional nurses)*. Enchanted Mountain Press.

Leiz, M., Pfeuffer, N., Rehner, L., et al. (2022). Telemedicine as a tool to improve medicine adherence in patients with affective disorders—A systematic literature review. *Patient Preference and Adherence, 16*, 3441–3463.

Maruschak, L. M., Bonson, J., & Alper, M. (2021). *Indicators of mental health problems reported by prisoners: Survey of prison inmates, 2016*. Bureau of Justice Statistics. https://bjs.ojp.gov/library/publications/indicators-mental-health-problems-reported-prisoners-survey-prison-inmates

Mills, A., Lathlean, J., Forrester, A., et al. (2011). Prisoners' experiences of antipsychotic medication: Influences on adherence. *Journal of Forensic Psychiatry and Psychology, 22*(1), 110–125.

Morris, N. P., Hirschtritt, M. E., & Tamburello, A. C. (2020). Drug formularies in correctional settings. *Journal of the American Academy of Psychiatry and the Law, 48*(1), 2–6.

Muela, A., Aliri, J., Presa, B., et al. (2020). Randomised controlled trial of a treatment adherence programme for prisoners with mental health problems in Spain. *Criminal Behavior and Mental Health, 30*, 6–15.

Muiruri, C., van der Broek-Altenburg, E. M., Bosworth, H. B., et al. (2023). A quantitative framework for medication non-adherence: Integrating patient treatment expectations and preferences. *Patient Preference and Adherence, 17*, 3135–3145.

Rogers, D. (2020). Keeping tabs on meds. *Corrections Forum, 29*(3), 18–25, 41.

Semahegen, A., Torpey, K., Nanu, A., et al. (2020). Psychotropic medication non-adherence and its associated factors among patients with major psychiatric disorders: A systematic review and meta-analysis. *Systematic Reviews, 9*(17), 1–18. https://doi.org/10.1186/s13643-020-1274-3

Schiffner, B. (2017). The pill drill. *Corrections Forum, 26*(5), 34–38.

Tamburello, A., Penn, J., Ford, E., et al. (2022). The American Academy of Psychiatry and the Law practice resource for prescribing in corrections. *Journal of the American Academy of Psychiatry and the Law, 50*, S1–S62.

Tariq, R. A., Vashisht, R., Sinha, A., & Scherbak, Y., (2024). Medication dispensing errors and prevention. In *StatPearls*. StatPearls Publishing. https://pubmed.ncbi.nlm.nih.gov/30085607/

Thompson, C., Gunther, M., & Macek, P. (2019). Clinical pharmacists in correctional facilities: A literature review and future directions. *Journal of Correctional Health Care, 25*(3), 201–213.

Townsend, M., Pareja, K., Buchanan-Hughes, A., et al. (2022). Antipsychotic related stigma and the impact on treatment choice: A systematic review and framework synthesis. *Patient Preference and Adherence, 16*, 371–401.

Trestman, R. L. (2015). Transition of pharmacology from community to corrections. In R. Trestman, K. Appelbaum, & J. Metzner (Eds.), *Oxford textbook of correctional psychiatry* (pp. 99–101). Oxford University Press.

29

Prescribing hypnotic agents and controlled substances

*Rusty Reeves and Sadé D. Frazier**

Introduction

Any prescriber of a controlled substance in a correctional institution must recognize that most incarcerated persons (IPs) have used illicit substances, perhaps as many as 70% to 90% (Fazel et al., 2006, 2017; Maruschak et al., 2021; Mumola & Karberg, 2006), which is much higher than the rate in the general population, 42% (Substance Abuse and Mental Health Services Administration, 2023). With limited access to contraband, IPs often turn to the misuse of prescription medications.

IPs may exaggerate or feign symptoms to obtain controlled substances. Should intoxication occur, this poses a risk of overdose, disinhibition, suicide, and violence, and bad things can happen fast. Correctional officers, other staff, and IPs themselves may be injured. At year end 2020, 62% of all state IPs were serving sentences for a violent offense (Carson, 2022). Moreover, 31% of state prisoners and 25% of federal prisoners reported drinking alcohol at the time of the offense; similarly, 39% of state prisoners and 31% of federal prisoners reported using illicit substances at the time of the offense (Maruschak et al., 2021). According to the National Crime Victimization Survey (2006), 27% of victims of violence reported that the offender was using drugs or alcohol at the time of the offense.

The association of substance misuse and violence does not end at the prison gate. Aside from substance misuse, there is a culture among IPs of taking pills to relieve uncomfortable feelings. Then there is diversion of medications. Medications can be used as currency to buy or trade items or favors (Royal College of General Practitioners [RCGP] Secure Environments Group, 2019). IPs may intimidate or victimize vulnerable peers to obtain controlled substances (Tamburello et al., 2023). This inappropriate use of medications wastes staff time and resources in prison (Burns, 2009). Chapter 30 gives examples of prescribed medications at higher risk for misuse in correctional settings; these extend beyond hypnotics and controlled substances to ostensibly benign medications such as gabapentin, diphenhydramine, clonidine, and even ibuprofen (Tamburello et al., 2017). Numerous correctional resources consistently express the concern that sleep, opioid, and benzodiazepine medications can be misused or diverted (American Psychiatric Association, 2016; Friedman et al., 2019; RCGP Secure Environments Group, 2019; Tamburello et al., 2022, 2023).

Given this well-known misuse of medications in jails and prisons, sedative-hypnotics and other controlled substances are universally prescribed with caution, if at all, in correctional settings in the United States. Prescribers recognize they have a responsibility not only to treat the individual patient in the prison but also to protect the safety and security of the prison environment. State departments of corrections often have formularies and internal guidelines for the prescription of controlled substances, some of which are available online (Morris et al., 2020).

England has the most complete national psychotropic prescribing guidelines for correctional clinicians, published by the RCGP Secure Environments Group (2019). The RCGP offers specific recommendations for the treatment of insomnia, as well as substance use and misuse in corrections. These recommendations are offered in a red light–yellow light–green light hierarchy and are summarized and discussed below.

The United States does not offer a national guideline with explicit hierarchical instructions for psychotropic prescribing in corrections. However, standards have evolved, including with the publication of the first edition of this textbook in 2015. In the years since the American Academy of Psychiatry and the Law (AAPL) has developed a practice resource for prescribing psychiatric medications in adult corrections, first published in 2018 and then revised in 2022 (Tamburello, 2022). Although the practice resource was approved by the AAPL, the authors state that their recommendations do not constitute a practice guideline or establish the standard of care. Friedman and colleagues (2019) created a companion article offering adjunctive recommendations for prescribing psychotropics for women in corrections. Another companion article focused on prescribing psychotropics for justice-involved youth is available (Tamburello et al., 2023). These resources review the literature related to insomnia management and substance use disorder treatment but do not offer the explicit, hierarchical recommendations offered by the RCGP.

*. The authors acknowledge the contributions of Ingrid Li and Arthur Brewer, who were coauthors of this chapter in the first edition of this textbook.

Opioids

Opioids have been used for centuries and remain the most potent and reliable analgesic agents (Pasternak, 2011). They are used for the treatment of acute, chronic, and terminal pain. In time-limited circumstances, the efficacy of opioids has been extensively documented and broadly accepted (Fields, 2011). Opioids used long term, however, run the risk of misuse, diversion, and the development of an opioid use disorder. This section highlights the limited role of opioids in corrections and the caution that prescribers should exhibit when considering prescription of opioids. Complementary chapters in this textbook offer extensive discussions of pain management and pharmacotherapy for substance use disorders in correctional settings (see Chapter 40 and Chapter 49).

According to the National Commission on Correctional Health Care's (NCCHC's) position statement on chronic pain management (NCCHC, 2023), nonpharmacologic interventions are first-line treatment for patients with certain chronic pain conditions in accordance with evidence-based guidelines. Nonopioids are preferred over opioids when medications are used to treat chronic pain. The NCCHC position statement notes that if opioids are considered for treating noncancer pain, the Veterans Affairs and U.S. Department of Defense clinical practice guideline recommends buprenorphine instead of full agonist opioids (Sandbrink et al., 2023). The NCCHC also recommends that mental health and substance use disorders associated with chronic pain should be assessed and considered an essential element of the patient's treatment plan. The authors of this chapter commonly encounter patients with opioid use disorder who report experiencing pain and insist upon opioids or gabapentin, sometimes both. Gabapentin is misused in the community (Pittenger & Desan, 2007) and in corrections (Reccoppa et al., 2004; Soni & Walters, 2020). Gabapentinoids (e.g., gabapentin and pregabalin) are also associated with a higher rate of both hospitalization and opioid-related overdose mortality (Evoy et al., 2021). In the New Jersey Department of Corrections, where the authors work, both opioids and gabapentinoids are nonformulary medications.

The RCGP Secure Environments Group (2019), similarly to the NCCHC, states that nonpharmacological therapy is important in managing persistent pain. Nonsteroidal analgesics are the first line of pharmacological treatment of pain; opioids are to be used only when these treatments have failed. Opioids should be prescribed for as short a period as possible and at the lowest effective dose. Doses greater than 50 morphine milligram equivalents rarely provide further benefit or function but convey progressively increased risks (Dowell et al., 2022). The RCGP Secure Environments Group (2019) cautions that opioids have limited efficacy in persistent pain. Multidisciplinary collaboration is necessary for complex cases, especially when psychiatric or substance use disorders are comorbid.

The increasing use of buprenorphine in correctional settings for the treatment of opioid use disorder poses a new opportunity for IPs to divert opioids, even as buprenorphine might also save lives. Clinicians report that diversion is common despite directly observed administration; the literature supports their speculation (Monico et al., 2021; Tamburello & Martin, 2024; White et al., 2015). However, there is only one study that quantitatively assessed diversion, and this study found that buprenorphine was diverted more often (10%) than methadone (2%; Magura et al., 2009). The availability of liquid formulations of methadone is likely related to its lower observed incidence of diversion, though motivated persons may use an absorptive foreign object (like a cotton ball in the mouth) to avoid ingesting some of the medicine. Clever methods for diverting films of buprenorphine include placing it on an identification card, using dental hardware or even cavities, using sleight of hand, and using colored paper in the mouth as a decoy (Tamburello et al., 2022). There are as yet no published investigations of iatrogenic opioid use disorder associated with opioid substitution efforts in corrections.

There is no agreement, let alone an evidence-based agreement, about what to do when a patient is discovered to be diverting buprenorphine. The AAPL offers suggestions to reduce medication nonadherence in general, including formulary controls for higher risk medications, training of staff responsible for medication administration, and the promulgation of internal guidelines and peer review (Tamburello et al., 2022). Evans et al. (2022) offer suggestions to manage diversion of buprenorphine in a jail, including assessing reasons for the diversion, having standardized protocols for dosing, educating patients about the value of consistent adherence, and having a written policy for how diversion will be addressed. A study by Tamburello and Martin (2024) indicates that diversion of sublingual buprenorphine strips is more common when multiple strips are administered, rather than a single strip of a higher equivalent dose. Tamburello (2023) suggests that discontinuation should be an approach of last resort when buprenorphine diversion is identified. Crushing the tablet form of buprenorphine does not reduce bioavailability (Simojoki et al., 2010) and may also reduce diversion, though crushing consumes nursing time and may not be a viable option as a matter of facility-wide policy. An option is to discontinue the buprenorphine, especially if the patient's drug screen shows the total absence of buprenorphine. Another option is reducing the dose by the proportion of medication the patient is thought to divert. More frequent drug screens may encourage adherence. If methadone is available, liquid forms of this medication are more difficult to divert (Johnson & Richert, 2015). Yet another option is to offer an opioid antagonist (naltrexone) following discontinuation of the buprenorphine and a 1- to 2-week period of washout (American Society of Addiction Medicine, 2020). Depot buprenorphine may reduce diversion; however, the cost of such formulations is currently prohibitive, and there are few head-to-head studies comparing it to sublingual buprenorphine. Lee et al. (2021) found that patients openly randomized prerelease to extended-release buprenorphine had fewer in-jail medical visits and better retention in treatment postrelease than those getting sublingual buprenorphine. In any case, if the diverting patient is thought to have a genuine opioid use disorder, it is crucial to reassess the prescription or dosing of the buprenorphine before the patient is released.

Benzodiazepines

Benzodiazepines are controlled substances used to treat anxiety, agitation, insomnia, and withdrawal from alcohol. The correctional literature (Burns, 2010; National Institute for Health and Care Excellence, 2020; RCGP Secure Environments Group, 2019; Tamburello et al., 2022) confirms the authors' experience and opinion that benzodiazepines and their congener nonbenzodiazepine Z-drugs (e.g., zolpidem, zaleplon, eszopiclone) are subject to misuse and diversion and should not be prescribed as a first-line treatment of insomnia or anxiety in a correctional setting. Other chapters in this textbook address in detail the assessment and treatment of insomnia in corrections (see Chapters 19 and 35).

Safer first-line treatments of anxiety should initially be considered, including cognitive-behavioral therapy or selective serotonergic reuptake inhibitors; second-line options include venlafaxine, duloxetine, and buspirone (RCGP Secure Environments Group, 2019). A second-line agent for the autonomic manifestations of anxiety is propranolol (Lundquist & Becker, 2010; RCGP Secure Environments Group, 2019). Mirtazapine should be avoided for the treatment of anxiety, as it is associated with weight gain and diversion (RCGP Secure Environments Group, 2019; Tamburello et al., 2022).

Benzodiazepine prescribing in correctional psychiatry should generally be limited to detoxification from benzodiazepines or alcohol and to treatment of acute and severe agitation (as from psychosis or mania). Treatment should be for a short period, generally less than 2 weeks. The treatment of insomnia with benzodiazepines should be unusual. It should be reserved for severe and observed (i.e., documented by overnight nursing staff) insomnia, after an alternative lower risk medication has failed, and then only for a short period of time. Prior to prescribing benzodiazepines, the clinician should have a discussion with the patient that the medication is time limited and will be discontinued on a set date. Patients may develop physiological dependence with regular use in as little as 2 to 4 weeks of daily use (Peng et al., 2022), and doses should be tapered to discontinuation to avoid withdrawal (see Chapter 46).

Specific methods to reduce the potential for diversion of benzodiazepines include direct observation of pill administration by custody and nursing staff, prescribing medication in liquid form, or crushing and dissolving medication in liquid. Patients who are prescribed a benzodiazepine should have periodic toxicology screens to confirm that they are, in fact, taking the medication rather than diverting it.

Reduction in the prescriptions and dosages of benzodiazepines is an indirect opportunity to reduce diversion. Cabelguenne et al. (2018) showed in a 15-year study that correctional physicians' collaboration with pharmacists reduced both the dosages and proportion of patients on benzodiazepines. A practical and effective method used by Reeves (2012) to reduce the prescription of benzodiazepines in the New Jersey state prison system involved a physician-to-physician comparison of numbers of prescriptions, accompanied by a guideline for the treatment of insomnia that discouraged the routine use of benzodiazepines for sleep. Reeves then ranked each physician on a graph in the order of frequency of prescriptions. The ranking was done anonymously; each physician knew where they stood among colleagues but did not know the identities of the colleagues. Whether through effective education or healthy competition, this technique reduced the number of benzodiazepine prescriptions by 38% after 20 months.

Another, and perhaps more effective, way to reduce the prescription of benzodiazepines (or any medication for that matter) in a correctional setting is simply to make these medications nonformulary (see also Chapter 27). A clinician who wishes to prescribe a nonformulary medication must apply to a supervisor for permission. In addition to the "hassle" of applying, a nonformulary process reduces prescriptions by allowing a second review. The nonformulary process can also alleviate the burden of those prescribers who feel pressured to prescribe a marginally or nonindicated medication. The downside of making a medication nonformulary is that, unless an exception is made, it is not available for use in an emergency. Benzodiazepines are effective and can even be life-saving in cases of severe agitation, withdrawal, and seizures. Thus, the AAPL (Tamburello el., 2022) recommended that select benzodiazepines remain on a psychiatric formulary even as their routine use is discouraged.

Hypnotic medications

The quest for medications to address sleep complaints from IPs is ubiquitous, and anecdotes about the dubiousness of these complaints abound. A systematic review of 12 studies of insomnia in prison populations found that all 12 used self-report to ascertain insomnia (Sheppard & Lee, 2022). Prevalence rates for insomnia and poor sleep quality among these studies varied between 26% and 73%, and 43% and 88%, respectively.

At the same time, the disruptions to a good night's sleep in jails and prisons are real and well known, and insomnia has been associated with both mental health symptoms and poor medical health in IPs (Morris et al., 2021). Factors related to poor sleep in these settings include, but are not limited to, clanging doors, obstreperous cellmates, uncomfortable bedding, indoor lighting, a sedentary lifestyle, lack of exposure to a normal diurnal light cycle, damage to sleep architecture caused by the use of illicit drugs, social isolation, and anxiety over incarceration itself. Opioid users have long been known to experience disturbed sleep (Kay et al., 1981), which may not resolve when the opioid use stops (Staedt et al., 1996). Individuals with substance use disorders can have unrealistic expectations of sleep during periods of sobriety while incarcerated. Moreover, withdrawal from substances can cause insomnia (RCGP Secure Environments Group, 2019).

A review article by Elger (2007), noting that sleep medications did not relieve insomnia complaints in a sizable number of IPs, suggested that nonpharmacological treatments should be used more frequently to treat insomnia in prisons. This recommendation accords with general insomnia research in the community (see Chapter 19). Cognitive-behavioral therapy for insomnia (CBT-I) is effective and is a first-line treatment, preferred over short-term use of medications (Qaseem et al., 2016). Nevertheless, IPs with a history of substance use often prefer pharmacological rather than psychosocial interventions.

State correctional systems—at least several states with online formularies—vary in how they approach the management of insomnia with medication. California (California Correctional Health Services, 2024) offers keep-on-person melatonin for delayed sleep–wake phase disorder; however, oral hydroxyzine and diphenhydramine are nonformulary. Washington (Washington State Department of Corrections, 2023) places hydroxyzine and melatonin on its correctional formulary, though the latter is categorized as a "dietary supplement," and diphenhydramine is nonformulary for the treatment of insomnia. Texas (Texas Department of Criminal Justice Health Services Division et al., 2021) offers no hypnotics for adults but does offer melatonin for adolescents, even as nonpharmacological treatment explicitly remains first-line treatment. Oklahoma's formulary (Oklahoma Department of Corrections, 2022) does not mention the words "sleep" or "insomnia," though oral hydroxyzine is on-formulary for the treatment of anxiety. Rutgers University Correctional Health Care, the health care vendor for the New Jersey Department of Corrections, has a long-standing guideline for the treatment of insomnia, which recommends CBT-I as first-line treatment, including sleep hygiene, stimulus control, muscle relaxation, paradoxical intention, and sleep restriction. Rutgers University Correctional Health Care clinicians review explicit techniques with patients who present with insomnia symptoms. Brief (no more than 7 to 10 days) medication management of insomnia is the last line of treatment, and no specific medication is recommended. Antipsychotics, sedating antidepressants, and mood stabilizers are explicitly not recommended.

If an IP presents with the chief complaint of insomnia, the patient should be asked to complete a sleep diary or log. Better would be confirmation of the reported sleep pattern by correctional officers or nurses during rounds, if possible. Such observations may tax the limited resources of staff and, in any case, may be resisted by officers whose primary goal is to maintain safety and security. According to the RCGP Secure Environments Group (2019) and AAPL (Tamburello et al., 2022), the treatment of choice for insomnia in a correctional setting is CBT-I, which combines sleep hygiene (e.g., reduce caffeine, increase exercise during the day, avoid naps), stimulus control, sleep restriction, relaxation training, and cognitive restructuring. These skills can be taught in either individual or group sessions by mental health staff. Cognitive-behavioral treatments may lower health care costs, do not have the side effects of medications, avoid interactions with other prescribed medications, and avoid perpetuating drug misuse. The RCGP Secure Environments Group (2019) reports that sleep hygiene alone is effective in 30% of cases of primary insomnia. The authors of these resources acknowledge that implementation of these techniques may be difficult in corrections.

If a mental disorder is thought to be related to the reported insomnia, then a referral should be made to a psychiatrist. The psychiatrist should obtain a sleep history. An assessment should be taken of pertinent associated symptoms such as heightened arousal or excessive daytime sleepiness; sleep–wake schedule disorders; restless legs; snoring and other symptoms of obstructive sleep apnea; depression, anxiety, or other mental disorders; recent drug or alcohol use; and medical problems and current medications. If the psychiatrist suspects that another medical condition underlies the insomnia, the psychiatrist should make a referral to an internist.

According to the RCGP Secure Environments Group (2019), if the IP fails behavioral approaches for a primary sleep disturbance, then a brief trial of a sedating antihistamine (e.g., promethazine or diphenhydramine) is recommended as a first-line hypnotic, as antihistamines are less likely to be diverted than benzodiazepines or Z-drugs. Tolerance to the hypnotic effect of antihistamines may occur within 14 days, and short courses with breaks are recommended if treatment must be ongoing (RCRP Secure Environments Group, 2019). Z-drugs are a second-line hypnotic due to greater risk of diversion and misuse, but the risks exceed the benefits for benzodiazepines, tricyclic antidepressants, and sedating antidepressants prescribed for insomnia in prison (RCRP Secure Environments Group, 2019). The AAPL practice resource discusses various pharmacological interventions for insomnia, noting that low-dose doxepin may be useful (Tamburello et al., 2022). However, this practice resource was ultimately neutral about recommendations for pharmacotherapy of insomnia, stating that the literature does not support medication treatment for insomnia in corrections (Tamburello et al., 2022). In any case, hypnotic medications should be given under direct observation by nursing staff to prevent diversion or hoarding of the medication.

Morris and colleagues (2021) discuss recent litigation by IPs against their facilities related to conditions of confinement that disrupt healthy sleep patterns, speculating that restricting access to hypnotic medications could be a source of liability. However, they also cite case law that was skeptical of insomnia as a serious medical need for IPs (*Velasquez v. DiGugliemo*, 2012).

Summary

The misuse of substances is many times higher in the correctional population than in the general population. The literature has evolved regarding evidence-based recommendations regarding the prescription of hypnotics and controlled substances in jails and prisons. Hypnotics and controlled substances should be prescribed cautiously in these settings and should be avoided as first-line or long-term treatments. Just as in the community, CBT-I is the recommended first treatment. Guidelines, thoughtful use of formulary controls, and a measure of flexibility will assist in the appropriate prescription of these medications.

REFERENCES

American Psychiatric Association. (2016). *Psychiatric services in correctional facilities* (3rd ed).

American Society of Addiction Medicine. (2020). *National practice guideline for the treatment of opioid use disorder, 2020 focused update.* https://www.asam.org/quality-care/clinical-guidelines/national-practice-guideline

Burns, K. A. (2009). Commentary: The top ten reasons to limit prescription of controlled substances in prisons. *Journal of American Academy of Psychiatry and the Law*, *37*, 50–52.

Burns, K. A. (2010). Pharmacotherapy in correctional settings. In C. Scott (Ed.), *Handbook of correctional mental health* (2nd ed., pp. 321–344). American Psychiatric Publishing.

Cabelguenne, D., Picard, C., Lalande, L., et al. (2018). Benzodiazepine dose reduction in prisoner patients: 15 years' teamwork between psychiatrists and pharmacists. *Journal of Clinical Pharmacy and Therapeutics*, *43*(6), 807–812.

California Correctional Health Services. (2024). *Drug formulary.* https://cchcs.ca.gov/wp-content/uploads/sites/60/MS/CCHCS-CDCR-Formulary.pdf

Carson, E. A. (2022). *Prisoners in 2021—Statistical tables.* Bureau of Justice Statistics. https://bjs.ojp.gov/sites/g/files/xyckuh236/files/media/document/p21st.pdf.

Dowell, D., Ragan, K. R., Jones, C. M., Baldwin, G. T., & Chou, R. (2022). CDC clinical practice guideline for prescribing opioids for pain—United States. *MMWR Recommendations and Reports*, 71(RR-3), 1–95.

Elger, B. S. (2007). Insomnia in places of detention: A review of the most recent research findings. *Medicine, Science and the Law*, *47*, 191–199.

Evans, E. A., Pivovarova, E., Stopka, T. J., Santelices, C. S., Ferguson, W. J., & Friedman, P. D. (2022). Uncommon and preventable: Perceptions of diversion of medication for opioid use disorder in jail. *Journal of Substance Abuse Treatment*, *138*, 108746.

Evoy, K. E., Sadrameli, S., Contreras, J., Covvey, J. R., Peckham, A. M., & Morrison, M. D. (2021). Abuse and misuse of pregabalin and gabapentin: A systematic review update. *Drugs*, *81*(1), 125–156.

Fazel, S., Bains, P., & Doll, H. (2006). Substance abuse and dependence in prisoners: A systematic review. *Addiction, 101*, 181–191.

Fazel, S. A., Yoon, I. A., & Hayes, A. J. (2017). Substance use disorders in prisoners: An updated systematic review and meta-regression analysis in recently incarcerated men and women. *Addiction, 112*(10), 1723–1739.

Fields, H. L. (2011). The doctor's dilemma: Opiate analgesics and chronic pain. *Neuron, 69*(4), 591–594.

Friedman, S. H., Tamburello, A. C., Kaempf, A., & Hall, R. C. W. (2019). Prescribing for women in corrections. *Journal of the American Academy of Psychiatry and the Law, 47*, 476–485.

Johnson, B., & Richert, T. (2015). Diversion of methadone and buprenorphine by patients in opioid substitution treatment in Sweden: Prevalence estimates and risk factors. *International Journal on Drug Policy, 26*(2), 183–190.

Kay, D. C., Pickworth, W. B., & Neider, G. L. (1981). Morphine-like insomnia from heroin in nondependent human addicts. *British Journal of Clinical Pharmacology, 11*(2), 159–169.

Lee, J. D., Malone, M., McDonald, R., et al. (2021). Comparison of treatment retention of adults with opioid addiction managed with extended-release buprenorphine vs daily sublingual buprenorphine-naloxone at time of release from jail. *JAMA Network Open, 4*(9).

Lundquist, T., & Becker, T. (2010). Medication management in correctional settings. In A. Ruiz, J. Dvoskin, C. Scott, & J. Metzner (Eds.), *Manual of forms and guidelines for correctional mental health* (pp. 83–111). American Psychiatric Publishing.

Magura, S., Lee, J. D., Hershberger, J., et al. (2009). Buprenorphine and methadone maintenance in jail and post-release: A randomized controlled trial. *Drug and Alcohol Dependence, 99*(1–3), 222–230.

Maruschak, L. M., Bronson, J., & Alper, M. (2021, July). *Alcohol and drug use and treatment reported by prisoners: Survey of prison inmates, 2016*. Bureau of Justice Statistics. https://bjs.ojp.gov/library/publications/alcohol-and-drug-use-and-treatment-reported-prisoners-survey-prison-inmates

Monico, L. B., Gryczynski, J., Lee, J. D., et al. (2021). Exploring nonprescribed use of buprenorphine in the criminal justice system through qualitative interviews among individual recently released from incarceration. *Journal of Substance Abuse Treatment, 123*, 108267.

Morris, N. P., Hirschtritt, M. E., & Tamburello, A. C. (2020). Drug formularies in correctional settings. *Journal of the American Academy of Psychiatry and the Law, 48*(1), 2–6.

Morris, N. P., Holliday, J. R., & Binder, R. L. (2021). Litigation over sleep deprivation in U.S. jails and prisons. *Psychiatric Services, 72*(10), 1237–1239.

Mumola, C., & Karberg, J. (2006). *Drug use and dependence, state and federal prisoners, 2004*. Bureau of Justice Statistics. http://www.bjs.gov/content/pub/pdf/dudsfp04.pdf

National Commission on Correctional Health Care. (2023). *Position statement: Management of chronic pain*. https://www.ncchc.org/position-statements/

National Crime Victimization Survey. (2006). *Criminal victimization in the United States, 2005—Statistical tables*. Bureau of Justice Statistics. https://bjs.ojp.gov/content/pub/pdf/cvus06.pdf

National Institute for Health and Care Excellence. (2020). *Generalised anxiety disorder and panic disorder in adults: Management*. https://www.nice.org.uk/guidance/cg113

Oklahoma Department of Corrections. (2022). *Drug formulary*. https://oklahoma.gov/content/dam/ok/en/doc/documents/administration/medical-services/OK%20DOC%20Formulary%20JAN%202022.pdf.

Pasternak, G. W. (2011). *The opiate receptors*. Humana Press/Springer.

Peng, L., Meeks, T. W., & Blazes, C. K. (2022). Complex persistent benzodiazepine dependence—When benzodiazepine describing goes awry. *JAMA Psychiatry, 79*(7), 640.

Pittenger, C., & Desan, P. H. (2007). Gabapentin abuse and delirium tremens upon gabapentin withdrawal. *Journal of Clinical Psychiatry, 68*, 483–484.

Qaseem, A., Kansagara, D., Forciea, M. A., Cooke, M., & Denberg, T. D., Clinical Guidelines Committee of the American College of Physicians. (2016). Management of chronic insomnia disorder in adults: A clinical practice guideline from the American College of Physicians. *Annals of Internal Medicine, 165*(2), 125–133.

Reccoppa, L., Malcolm, R., & Ware, M. (2004). Gabapentin abuse in inmates with prior history of cocaine dependence. *American Journal of Addiction, 13*(3), 321–323.

Reeves, R. (2012). Guideline, education, and peer comparison to reduce prescriptions of benzodiazepines and low-dose quetiapine in prison. *Journal of Correctional Health Care, 18*, 45–52.

Royal College of General Practitioners Secure Environments Group. (2019). *Safer prescribing in prisons*. https://elearning.rcgp.org.uk/pluginfile.php/176185/mod_book/chapter/620/RCGP-safer-prescribing-in-prisons-guidance-jan-2019.pdf

Sandbrink, F., Murphy, J. L., Johansson, M., et al. (2023). The use of opioids in the management of chronic pain: Synopsis of the 2022 updated U.S. Department of Veterans Affairs and U.S. Department of Defense clinical practice guideline. *Annals of Internal Medicine, 176*(3), 388–397.

Sheppard, N., & Lee, H. (2022). Prevalence of insomnia and poor sleep quality in the prison population: A systematic review. *Journal of Sleep Research, 31*(6), e13677.

Simojoki, K., Lillsunde, P., Lintzeris, N., & Alho, H. (2010). Bioavailability of buprenorphine from crushed and whole buprenorphine (Subutex) tablets. *European Addiction Research, 6*(2), 85–90.

Soni, A., & Walters, P. (2020). A study of the reasons for prescribing misuse of gabapentinoids in prison including their co-prescription with opioids and antidepressants. *International Journal of Prisoner Health, 16*(1), 67–77.

Staedt, J., Wassmuth, F., Stoppe, G., et al. (1996). Effects of chronic treatment with methadone naltrexone on sleep in addicts. *European Archives of Psychiatry and Clinical Neuroscience, 246*, 305–309.

Substance Abuse and Mental Health Services Administration. (2023). *Table 1.6B—Illicit drug use in lifetime, past year, and past month*. https://www.samhsa.gov/data/report/2022-nsduh-detailed-tables

Tamburello, A. (2022). The case for medication for opioid use disorder during incarceration as standard of care. *Journal of the American Academy of Psychiatry and the Law, 50*(4), 502–508.

Tamburello, A. C., Kathpal, A., & Reeves, R. (2017). Characteristics of inmates who misuse prescription medication. *Journal of Correctional Health Care, 23*(4), 449–458.

Tamburello, A., Penn, J., Ford, E., et al. (2022). The American Academy of Psychiatry and the Law Practice resource for prescribing in corrections. *Journal of the American Academy of Psychiatry and the Law, 50*, S1–S62.

Tamburello, A., Penn, J., Negron-Munoz, R., & Kaliebe, K. (2023). Prescribing psychotropic medications for justice-involved juveniles. *Journal of Correctional Health Care, 2*, 94–108.

Tamburello, A., & Martin, T. L. (2024). Dosing and misuse of buprenorphine in the New Jersey Department of Corrections. *Journal of the American Academy of Psychiatry and the Law, 52*(4), 441–448.

Texas Department of Criminal Justice Health Services Division, the University of Texas Medical Branch Correctional Managed Care, and the Texas Tech University Health Sciences Center Office of Correctional Managed Health Care. (2021). *Correctional managed care formulary.* https://www.tdcj.texas.gov/divisions/cmhc/docs/CMC_Formulary_27th_Edition.pdf.

Velasquez v. DiGuglielmo, CIVIL ACTION No. 09-517 (E.D. Pa. Sep. 28, 2012).

Washington State Department of Corrections. (2023). *Pharmaceutical management and formulary manual.* https://www.doc.wa.gov/docs/publications/600-HA002.pdf

White, N., Ali, R., & Larance, B. (2015). The extramedical use and diversion of opioid substitution medications and other medications in prison settings in Australia following the introduction of buprenorphine–naloxone film. *Drug and Alcohol Review, 35*(1), 76–82.

30
Misuse of noncontrolled medications

Anthony C. Tamburello

Introduction

Opioids, benzodiazepines, and stimulants are controlled substances because they carry a higher risk for nonmedical use. Even if not classified as controlled by the U.S. Drug Enforcement Agency, certain other prescribed medications may also be misused. For this chapter, the word "misuse" is used to describe the taking of medication for reasons unintended by the prescriber (including recreational use), either without a prescription or by not following instructions in terms of dosing, timing, or route of administration.

Emergency room visits for nonsuicidal, nonmedical use of prescription medications, including antidepressants, anticonvulsants, and antipsychotics, rose 132% in the community between 2004 and 2011 (Substance Abuse and Mental Health Services Administration, Drug Abuse Warning Network, 2011), though federal monitoring of this has since become far less robust (Substance Abuse and Mental Health Services Administration, Drug Abuse Warning Network, 2023). Substance use disorders are common among incarcerated persons (IPs) and are not reliably interrupted by a period of incarceration. Misuse of medication occurs with some frequency in carceral settings and is a common concern for prescribers there (Tamburello et al., 2017). Although preferred by those with a substance use disorder, illegal drugs are difficult to obtain while incarcerated. When purchased from peers or staff, their cost (reflecting the time, effort, and risks associated with this criminal activity) is often prohibitive. By comparison, prescription medications are either stocked on-site within the jail or prison or obtained from pharmacies. IPs receive them at little or no cost when prescribed and can expect them to be dispensed in a reliable and timely manner. Even if caught using such medication inappropriately, the risk to the IP of legal consequences, beyond institutional sanctions, is remote.

While prescription medications are sometimes used to achieve a "high," they may also be sought to ease discomforts commonly experienced in a jail or prison (e.g., insomnia, subclinical anxiety, or simply boredom). Any medication with sedating properties may be considered by IPs for these purposes. Some may seek stimulating medications to counteract the effects of prescribed sedatives to allow them to be "on point" and alert enough to respond rapidly to real or perceived dangers in the facility. Stimulants may also be sought to manage real or perceived symptoms of attention-deficit/hyperactivity disorder. Institutional policies and the practice of individual prescribers may make it difficult to acquire medicines for attention-deficit/hyperactivity disorder through legitimate channels (see Chapter 38).

More subtle and medically concerning is the diversion of prescribed medications to a third party. Many prescribed medicines have a "street value" in carceral settings. They may be sold or bartered for items of interest. A patient with a legitimate need for medication, who may already have poor insight into their illness, may be enticed or coerced into transferring medication to a peer. This creates several dangerous problems. The source patient may worsen or fail to improve, which may lead to dose escalation, an incorrect conclusion about a treatment failure, poor functioning, and behavioral sequelae, including disruptive or violent conduct. Meanwhile, the recipient is exposed to medication risks without the benefits of informed consent or medical supervision.

Methods of medication misuse

Someone who intends to misuse medicine must obtain it without arousing suspicion from staff, move it to an unmonitored area, alter it if desired, then either transfer it to a third party or store it for later use. Psychiatric medications are most often administered by direct observation. Nevertheless, diversion of medication requires little sophistication. Common methods include "cheeking," where the medication is placed into the mouth but not swallowed, as well as "palming," where the medication is kept in the hand without putting it into the mouth. The powder from crushed tablets may be recovered by patients who hold it in the mouth between the jaw and an area of mucosa they have dried with cloth or tissue immediately prior to receiving the medication. Liquid forms of medication may be retrieved by placing a cotton ball in the mouth.

When staff are no longer directly observing, the patient may expectorate or vomit the pill (or fragments). A tablet may then be crushed using available hard objects and surfaces in preparation for intranasal (or intravenous) use, if desired. If a larger dose is required to achieve an anticipated effect, the product is accumulated over time and hidden to avoid detection.

Specific medications of concern

Antipsychotics

Quetiapine, a second-generation antipsychotic well known for its sedative and anxiolytic properties, has achieved notoriety as a misused medication, both in prison and in the community. Some have observed the practice of prescribing low-dose quetiapine to manage insomnia in prison (R. Reeves, 2012). Quetiapine is known colloquially as "quell," "Suzie Q," "Q," "squirrel," or "baby heroin" (Del Paggio, 2005; Waters & Joshi, 2007; Wen, 2009). Case reports in the community document misuse, including feigning or exaggerating serious psychiatric symptoms, preference for quetiapine versus an effective alternative agent, withdrawal and use to mitigate symptoms of withdrawal from other substances, tolerance, self-dosing, and combining with illicit substances to achieve a hallucinatory effect (Erdoğan, 2010). Some of the earliest case reports of quetiapine misuse involved prisoners, including descriptions of intranasal (Pierre et al., 2004), smoked (Haridas et al., 2010), and intravenous (Hussain et al., 2005) consumption. Psychiatric research and literature from the early 2000s suggested that quetiapine might be useful in persons with substance use disorders, resulting in initial confusion about its proper use (Knoll, 2008; Monnelly et al., 2004; Sattar et al., 2007).

These concerns have led to the removal of quetiapine from medication formularies in many carceral settings (Del Paggio, 2005; Tamburello et al., 2012). When quetiapine was removed from the medication formulary of the New Jersey Department of Corrections, nearly 45% of IPs whose quetiapine was stopped (n = 161) did not require an alternative antipsychotic medication at a 6-month follow-up (Tamburello et al., 2012).

Community case reports exist on the misuse of olanzapine for relaxing or euphoric effects (Kumsar & Erol, 2013; R. R. Reeves, 2007). Besides quetiapine, olanzapine was the only other antipsychotic that was repeatedly named as a psychotropic medication of concern by providers within the Santa Rita Jail (Del Paggio, 2005). According to a systematic review, higher doses of olanzapine than quetiapine may be required to achieve a recreational effect (Schifano et al., 2018).

Antidepressants

The misuse of tricyclic antidepressants (TCAs) in the community has been well reported (L. S. Anderson et al., 2017). Of 346 persons enrolled in a methadone program, 86 admitted to using amitriptyline for euphoric effects (Cohen, 1978). In a case series that informally reviewed 15 years of community hospital records, 14 cases of TCA misuse were identified. All of these were prescribed tertiary TCAs (e.g., amitriptyline, doxepin, or imipramine). Patients reported a sedative or euphoric effect from these medicines. All but one patient had a preexisting substance use disorder diagnosis, and only one had a current diagnosis of major depressive disorder. Four admitted to obtaining the TCA from a community drug dealer (Shenouda & Desan, 2013). TCAs are also prescribed by general medical practitioners for indications such as neuropathic pain. Most TCAs are inexpensive and, thus, may escape the attention of pharmacy and therapeutics committees. The likelihood of QT prolongation is considered higher with tertiary TCAs than with secondary TCAs (Goodnick et al., 2002). The greater anticholinergic and antihistaminergic properties of tertiary TCAs may explain both their greater toxicity and their greater incidence of misuse.

Bupropion has known stimulant properties that may be mildly comparable to methylphenidate. This is likely related to bupropion's inhibition of the reuptake of norepinephrine and dopamine (Chevassus et al., 2013). The misuse of bupropion in both the community and correctional systems is well known. According to the European Monitoring Agency, 10.8% of reports on adverse drug reactions, including seizures, were related to the misuse of buprenorphine (Schifano & Chiappini, 2018). Anecdotal reports suggest that a euphoric effect is more easily obtained when bupropion is crushed and then snorted, smoked, or injected, (R.R. Reeves & Ladner, 2013) which are routes of administration that bypass first-pass metabolism (McCabe et al., 2021), though chewing of buprenorphine tablets has also been described (Alnıak & Ulusoy, 2022). When removed from the formulary of the Texas correctional system, prescriptions for bupropion diminished from 1,966 to fewer than 100 between 2005 and 2013 (Hilliard et al., 2013).

Venlafaxine inhibits the reuptake of norepinephrine and serotonin and weakly inhibits the reuptake of dopamine. In community case reports, an "amphetamine-like" high was achieved by patients who took venlafaxine (Quaglio et al., 2008; Sattar et al., 2003). Higher doses (10 to 15 times higher than therapeutic doses), crushed and snorted tablets, and immediate-release forms of venlafaxine are purportedly more euphorigenic (Francesconi et al., 2015). Of note, venlafaxine was the second-generation antidepressant most likely to be associated with death in cases reported to the U.S. Poison Control Centers from 2000 to 2014, with bupropion being the second most likely (Nelson & Spyker, 2017). Dependence and withdrawal are reported more often for venlafaxine than bupropion (Schifano & Chiappini, 2018).

Mirtazapine is widely reported as being diverted and traded in prisons in Great Britain (Royal College of General Practitioners, 2019). It was also the most frequently found psychoactive substance in toxicology reports in medical examiner–investigated deaths in Finland, with 35 fatal poisonings identified to be related to its nonmedical use (Haukka et al., 2018). Anonymous surveys of patients on psychiatry or general medical services reported misuse of trazodone (35%) and quetiapine (30%; Slane et al., 2022). Community case reports of misuse of fluoxetine began to appear in the literature in 1987 when a woman with anorexia nervosa reported using high doses as an appetite suppressant (Wilcox, 1987). Since then, other reports indicate its recreational use and potential for dependence, apparently driven by the experience of euphoria from higher doses (Taïeb et al., 2004).

While approved by the U.S. Food and Drug Administration only for generalized anxiety disorder, buspirone is also used off-label as an antidepressant with a favorable side-effect profile (Wilson & Tripp, 2023). While generally considered to have low potential for misuse (Balster, 1990; Feighner & Boyer, 1989), reports of misuse of buspirone, usually by crushing and snorting, are found in the literature (Mezher et al., 2019; Raleigh, 1989; Swigart, 2021). References to the use of buspirone during incarceration, sometimes by "parachuting" (oral consumption of crushed pills wrapped in tissue paper), is described both in case reports and in social media posts (Mezher et al., 2019). In one such report, a psychiatrist resigned from a jail citing the challenge of correcting the overprescription of buspirone, as well as mirtazapine and olanzapine, which were frequently reported by custody staff as misused. As one example, a 5-day supply of buspirone was found in an IP's sock inside his cell (Berti, 2022).

Anticonvulsants

Anticonvulsants are prescribed by either psychiatrists or general medical providers for epilepsy, neuropathic pain, bipolar disorder, and various other indications. Community misuse of gabapentin is well established, with a rate of 1% of the entire general population, with much higher rates among those with prescriptions (40% to 65%) and those with opioid use disorders (15% to 22%; Smith et al., 2016). In a Florida prison intake facility, only 19 of 96 bottles of gabapentin remained with the person to whom it had been prescribed. Five of these patients acknowledged their recreational use of gabapentin, reporting a feeling of euphoria from it (Recoppa et al., 2004). Gabapentin was the most frequently misused medication in institutional charges in the New Jersey Department of Corrections from 2003 to 2013 (Tamburello et al., 2017). According to the Centers for Disease Control and Prevention, gabapentin is strongly linked with opioid-related overdoses, having been found in 85% to 90% of these in recent years (Mattson et al., 2022). Pregabalin is pharmacologically similar to gabapentin but is classified as schedule V by the U.S. Drug Enforcement Agency, has a higher liability for misuse, and is not a safer alternative to gabapentin (Schifano et al., 2018, Tambon et al., 2021). While opioid use and other psychiatric disorders are risk factors for misuse of gabapentinoids (e.g., gabapentin, pregabalin), primary cases have been reported (Tambon et al., 2021).

Occasional community reports describe misuse of carbamazepine for a euphoric effect, sometimes when combined with alcohol (Hosseini & Ahmadi, 2015; Stuppaeck et al., 1993; Sullivan & Davis, 1997). J. M. Mitchell and colleagues' (2012) placebo-controlled, randomized crossover trial linked levetiracetam to an increase in alcohol use for non–treatment seekers with previously lower levels of alcohol use. Animal studies suggest that levetiracetam may also augment the effects of cocaine (Guillama-Henríquez et al., 2020).

Anticholinergics and antihistamines

Case reports of the nonmedical use of anticholinergic medications like benztropine, including in patients with and without a mental illness, abound in the literature (Buhrich et al., 2020; Dilsaver, 1988; Land et al., 1991). Purported effects include euphoria, hallucinations, mood elevation, and relaxation. Some patients develop tolerance to the desired effects. Withdrawal symptoms of dysphoria and anxiety may be observed with abrupt discontinuation of anticholinergic medicines (Dilsaver, 1988). While less commonly prescribed today, several cases of misuse of trihexyphenidyl were reported in prisoners (Rouchell & Dixon, 1977).

Although its antihistaminergic properties have been speculated to counteract potentially reinforcing anticholinergic effects (Dilsaver, 1988), diphenhydramine misuse and dependence have been described in the community (Roberts et al., 1999; Thomas et al., 2009). Promethazine is an antiemetic with antihistaminic, anticholinergic, and weak antidopaminergic properties. In patients in a methadone clinic in San Francisco, 26% had a urine test positive for promethazine, with only 13% of these having a valid prescription for it (Shapiro et al., 2013). While promethazine is purported to augment an opioid high, its value in correctional settings may also be related to its sedating properties. When combined with codeine, it is referred to as "purple drank" or "lean," and it may have both sedating and euphoric effects (Miuli et al., 2020).

Antihypertensives

Clonidine was cited in over 6% of institutional charges of medication misuse in the New Jersey Department of Corrections (Tamburello et al., 2017). In a study of 90 nonhypertensive women in a methadone clinic, one third either admitted to misusing clonidine or had a positive urine test for it (F. Anderson et al., 1997). In a survey of 1,320 current or former intravenous drug users in Baltimore, 11% admitted to the "nonmedical" use of clonidine (Khosla et al., 2011). Users report desired effects including anxiolysis, sedation, and augmentation of the effects of other drugs (F. Anderson et al., 1997; Lauzon, 1992; Schaut & Schnoll, 1983; Schindler et al., 2013). Clonidine is known to increase and extend the effects of opioids and to reduce the amount of the latter needed for recreational use (B. G. Mitchell & Lee, 2021).

Muscle relaxants

The misuse of muscle relaxants has been reported in the community, particularly those with more sedating properties, such as baclofen (May, 1983; McDonald et al., 2001; Perry et al., 1998; Weißhaar et al., 2012). Baclofen overdose has been associated with serious morbidity and mortality, including coma and nonconvulsive status epilepticus (Weißhaar et al., 2012). Reports of misuse of and dependence involving carisoprodol were considerable enough for the U.S. Drug Enforcement Agency to reclassify it from noncontrolled to a schedule IV controlled substance in 2011 (Department of Justice, Drug Enforcement Administration, 2011).

Methods to reduce and manage misuse

Criminologists Duke and Trebilcock (2022) opined that conceptualizing the misuse of prescribed medications by IPs as a problem to be solved promotes doctor–patient distrust, ignores the legitimate needs IPs are trying to address, reassigns the responsibility for managing criminal behavior from custodial to health care staff, and discourages appropriate medical care. Whenever possible, health care staff should support and promote adequate health care services, including those relevant to substance use disorders (Gunter & Antoniak, 2010), as well as recreational, occupational, and educational opportunities for IPs. Concerns about the misuse or diversion of medications should never prevent the treatment of legitimate medical and mental illnesses. Nevertheless, an approach to prescribing that balances clinical acumen and environmental sensitivity is both necessary and appropriate when providing health care services in a jail or prison.

Accurate diagnosis promotes appropriate prescribing and nonprescribing. While symptom reporting is an essential component of psychiatric formulation, providers should not feel stymied when reported subjective symptoms are inconsistent with objective signs of illness (e.g., weight measurement, psychomotor retardation, psychomotor agitation, cognitive screening), dysfunction, or collateral information (e.g., staff observations, family reports, outside records). Awareness of and sensitivity to a patient's history of substance use disorders or reliable history of medication misuse is important. If the diagnosis is unclear and the situation is nonemergent, providers may consider delaying pharmaceutical intervention to allow time for further observation and data collection. As a further clinical aid, clinician-rated symptom scales can be used, as well as referral to a mental health tier or referral for psychological testing, to aid in diagnostic clarification (see also Chapters 16, 20, and 67).

It is generally prudent to consider evidence-based psychotherapies as first-line treatment for primary insomnia, uncomplicated adjustment disorders, and subclinical depression or anxiety symptoms. When pharmacotherapy is required, certain prescribing strategies may reduce, although not eliminate, the risk for misuse or diversion. Whenever appropriate, choose lower risk medications. Do not prescribe medication without an indication, avoid prescribing off-label, and avoid prescribing sedating medications on a PRN (i.e., as needed) basis. Prescribe the lowest effective dose. If a patient requires repeated dose escalation, carefully reevaluate the diagnosis and treatment. When prescribing despite an unclear indication, more frequent psychiatric follow-up may be necessary, along with additional history and examination to improve the prescriber's diagnostic clarity.

Although some IPs may defeat these strategies, prescribing medication in liquid form or crushing tablets and "floating" them in water will increase the difficulty of diverting medications and may reduce the demand. Although both reviewing a current "do not crush" list (Pharmacist's Letter, 2023) and consulting with a pharmacist is advisable, most pills can be dispensed in crushed form (with extended-release formulations being notable exceptions). If available, serum levels may show evidence of nonadherence or partial adherence. Screening of the urine or blood is of limited value for the detection of unauthorized use of noncontrolled prescription medication, although testing for a specific substance may be appropriate on a case-by-case basis. For patients who require antipsychotic medication, a long-acting injectable virtually eliminates the risk of covert nonadherence. Anticholinergic medication is not always required for the prophylaxis of extrapyramidal symptoms, even for those prescribed first-generation agents (World Health Organization, 2012). If prescribed as a precaution for a patient on antipsychotic medication, consider a taper of anticholinergic medication to establish its necessity.

Systematic approaches to this problem include staff training, medication administration policy, and formulary controls. Anyone responsible for administering or monitoring medication, including nursing and custody staff, should receive training on the detection of cheeking, palming, and similar techniques. Physicians and physician extenders, regardless of discipline, should receive orientation and ongoing in-service training on this matter. Whether controlled or noncontrolled, medications at higher risk for misuse are best administered as directly observed therapy. If institutional policy requires that a higher risk medication be dispensed as keep-on-person, the smallest practicable quantity should be allowed. As medical or mental health providers may prescribe higher risk medications, interdisciplinary collaboration and communication are important. Pharmacy and therapeutics committees should preferentially include medications with lower risk for misuse and diversion on the formulary, and they should promulgate guidelines to limit requests for higher risk medicines to clinically appropriate cases (see Chapter 27).

Summary

Prescription medication misuse is common and potentially dangerous in carceral settings. This concern is dynamic and likely to change as new medications become available and there is increased availability of established medications (as may follow a patent expiration). Experimentation by IPs in terms of methods of misuse will certainly always play a role. Prescribers must therefore have an "ear to the ground" and make reports to peers and health care supervisors on developments in this regard. Pharmacy and therapeutics committees should solicit and respond to information regarding emerging trends in prescription medication misuse.

REFERENCES

Alnıak, İ., & Ulusoy, S. (2022). Bupropion use disorder by chewing. *Journal of Addiction Medicine*, *16*(4), 492–494.

Anderson, F., Paluzzi, P., Lee, J., Huggins, G., & Svikis, D. (1997). Illicit use of clonidine in opiate-abusing pregnant women. *Obstetrics and Gynecology*, *90*(5), 790–794.

Anderson, L. S., Bell, H. G., Gilbert, M., Davidson, J. E., Winter, C., Barratt, M. J., Win, B., Painter, J. L., Menone, C., Sayegh, J., & Dasgupta, N. (2017). Using social listening data to monitor misuse and nonmedical use of bupropion, a content analysis. *JMIR Public Health Surveillance*, *3*(1), e6.

Balster, R. L. (1990). Abuse potential of buspirone and related drugs. *Journal of Clinical Psychopharmacology*, *10*(3 Suppl.), 31S–37S.

Berti, D. (2022). *"Unethical and dangerous": Psychiatrist resigns amid "rampant" prescription drug abuse at jail.* Corrections1. https://www.corrections1.com/correctional-healthcare/articles/unethical-and-dangerous-psychiatrist-resigns-amid-rampant-prescription-drug-abuse-at-jail-o0i5qUBi9FHSe9Pq/

Buhrich, N., Weller, A., & Kevans, P. (2000). Misuse of anticholinergic drugs by people with serious mental illness. *Psychiatric Services*, *51*(7), 928–929.

Chevassus, H., Farret, A., Gagnol, J. P., et al. (2013). Psychological and physiological effects of bupropion compared to methylphenidate after prolonged administration in healthy volunteers. *European Journal of Clinical Pharmacology*, *69*(4), 779–787.

Cohen, M. J. (1978). Abuse of amitriptyline. *Journal of the American Medical Association*, *240*(13), 1372–1373.

Del Paggio, D. (2005). Psychotropic medication abuse in correctional facilities. *Bay Area Psychopharmacology Newsletter*, *8*, 1–6.

Department of Justice, Drug Enforcement Administration. (2011). Schedules of controlled substances: Placement of carisoprodol into schedule IV. *Federal Register*, *76*(238), 77330–77360.

Dilsaver, S. C. (1988). Antimuscarinic agents as substances of abuse: A review. *Journal of Clinical Psychopharmacology*, *8*(1), 14–22.

Duke, K., & Trebilcock, J. (2022). "Keeping a lid on it": Exploring the "problematisations" of prescribed medications in prisons in the UK. *International Journal of Drug Policy*, *100*(103515), 1–10.

Erdoğan, S. (2010). Quetiapine in substance use disorders, abuse and dependence possibility: A review. *Turk Psikiyatri Derg*, *21*(2), 167–175.

Feighner, J. P., & Boyer, W. F. (1989). Serotonin-1A anxiolytics: An overview. *Psychopathology*, *22*(Suppl. 1), 21–26.

Francesconi, G., Orsolini, L., Papanti, D., Corkery, J. M., & Schifano, F. (2015). Venlafaxine as the "baby ecstasy"? Literature overview and analysis of web-based misusers' experiences. *Human Psychopharmacology*, *30*(4), 255–261.

Goodnick, P. J., Jerry, J., & Parra, F. (2002). Psychotropic drugs and the ECG: Focus on the QTc interval. *Expert Opinion on Pharmacotherapy*, *3*(5), 479–498.

Guillama-Henríquez, A., Hernandez-Huerta, D., & Alonso-Sánchez, E. B. (2020). Levetiracetam-Related Alcohol Abuse in a

Postencephalitic Patient. *Journal of clinical psychopharmacology, 40*(6), 632–634.

Gunter, T. D., & Antoniak, S. K. (2010). Evaluation and treating substance use disorders. In C. L. Scott (Ed.), *Handbook of correctional mental health* (2nd ed., p. 170). American Psychiatric Publishing.

Haridas, A., Kushon, D., Gurmu, S., & Oluwabusi, O. (2010). Smoking quetiapine: A "Maq Ball"? *Primary Psychiatry, 17*(9), 38–39.

Haukka, J., Kriikku, P., Mariottini, C., Partonen, T., & Ojanperä, I. (2018). Non-medical use of psychoactive prescription drugs is associated with fatal poisoning. *Addiction, 113*, 464–472.

Hilliard, W. T., Barloon, L., Farley, P., Penn, J. V., & Koranek, A. (2013). Bupropion diversion and misuse in the correctional facility. *Journal of Correctional Health Care, 19*, 211–217.

Hosseini, S. H., & Ahmadi, A. (2015). Abuse potential of carbamazepine for euphorigenic effects. *Drug Research, 65*(4), 223–224.

Hussain, M. Z., Waheed, W., & Hussain, S. (2005). Intravenous quetiapine abuse. *American Journal of Psychiatry, 9*, 1755–1756.

Khosla, N., Juon, H. S., Kirk, G. D., Astemborski, J., & Mehta, S. H. (2011). Correlates of non-medical prescription drug use among a cohort of injection drug users in Baltimore City. *Addictive Behaviors, 36*, 1282–1287.

Knoll, J. L. (2008). Psychopharm news. *Correctional Mental Health Report, 10*(1), 5–6.

Kumsar, N. A., & Erol, A. (2013). Olanzapine abuse. *Journal of Substance Abuse, 34*, 73–74.

Land, W., Pinsky, D., & Salzman, C. (1991). Abuse and misuse of anticholinergic medications. *Hospital and Community Psychiatry, 42*(6), 580–581.

Lauzon, P. (1992). Two cases of clonidine abuse/dependence in methadone-maintained patients. *Journal of Substance Abuse Treatment, 9*, 125–127.

Mattson, C. L., Chowdhury, F., & Gilson, T. P. (2022). *Trends in gabapentin detection and involvement in drug overdose deaths—23 states and the District of Columbia, 2019–2020*. https://www.cdc.gov/mmwr/volumes/71/wr/pdfs/mm7119a3-H.pdf

May, C. R. (1983). Baclofen overdose. *Annals of Emergency Medicine, 12*(3), 171–173.

McCabe, D. J., McGillis, E., & Willenbring, B. A. (2021). Clinical effects of intravenous bupropion misuse reported to a regional poison center. *American Journal of Emergency Medicine, 47*, 86–89.

McDonald, N. J., Festa, M. S., & Wilkins, B. (2001). Instructive case: Teenage coma. *Journal of Paediatrics and Child Health, 37*, 395–396.

Mezher, A. W., McKnight, C. A., & Caplan, J. P. (2019). Buspirone abuse: No safe haven. *Psychosomatics, 60*(5), 534–535.

Mitchell, B. G., & Lee, J. (2021). Case report: Concurrent clonidine abuse and opioid use disorder. *Journal of Psychoactive Drugs, 53*(4), 373–377.

Mitchell, J. M., Grossman, L. E., Coker, A. R., & Messing, R. O. (2012). The anticonvulsant levetiracetam potentiates alcohol consumption in non-treatment seeking alcohol abusers. *Journal of Clinical Psychopharmacology, 32*(2), 269–272.

Miuli, A., Stigliano, G., Lalli, A., Coladonato, M., D'Angelo, L., Esposito, F., Cappello, C., Pettorruso, M., Martinotti, G., Schifano, F., & Di Giannantonio, M. (2020). "Purple drank" (codeine and promethazine cough syrup): A systematic review of a social phenomenon with medical implications. *Journal of Psychoactive Drugs, 52*(5), 453–462.

Monnelly, E. P., Ciraulo, D. A., Knapp, C., LoCastro, J., & Sepulveda, I. (2004). Quetiapine for treatment of alcohol dependence. *Journal of Clinical Psychopharmacology, 24*(5), 532–535.

Nelson, J. C., & Spyker, D. A. (2017). Morbidity and mortality associated with medications used in the treatment of depression: An analysis of cases reported to U.S. poison control centers, 2000–2014. *American Journal of Psychiatry, 174*(5), 438–450.

Perry, H. E., Wright, R. O., Shannon, M. W., & Woolf, A. D. (1998). Baclofen overdose: Drug experimentation in a group of adolescents. *Pediatrics, 101*(6), 1045–1048.

Pharmacist's Letter. (2023). *Meds that should not be crushed*. https://pharmacist.therapeuticresearch.com/Content/Segments/PRL/2014/Aug/Meds-That-Should-Not-Be-Crushed-7309

Pierre, J. M., Shnayder, I., Wirshing, D. A., & Wirshing, W. C. (2004). Intranasal quetiapine abuse. *American Journal of Psychiatry, 9*, 1718.

Quaglio, G., Schifano, F., & Lugoboni, F. (2008). Venlafaxine dependence in a patient with a history of alcohol and amineptine misuse. *Addiction, 103*, 1572–1574.

Raleigh, F. R. (1989). Buspirone: Potentials for abuse? *DICP: Annals of Pharmacotherapy, 23*(12), 1035.

Recoppa, L., Malcolm, R., & Ware, M. (2004). Gabapentin abuse in inmates with prior history of cocaine dependence. *American Journal on Addictions, 13*, 321–323.

Reeves, R. (2012). Guideline, education and peer comparison to reduce prescriptions of benzodiazepines and low-dose quetiapine in prison. *Journal of Correctional Health Care, 18*(1), 45–52.

Reeves, R. R., & Ladner, M.E. (2013). Additional evidence of the abuse potential of bupropion. J Clin Psychopharmacol, *33*(4), 584–585.

Reeves, R. R. (2007). Abuse of olanzapine by substance abusers. *Journal of Psychoactive Drugs, 39*(3), 297–299.

Roberts, K., Gruer, L., & Gilhooly, T. (1999). Misuse of diphenhydramine soft gel capsules (Sleepia): A cautionary tale from Glasgow. *Addiction, 94*(10), 1575–1578.

Rouchell, A. M., & Dixon, S. P. (1977). Trihexyphenidyl abuse. *American Journal of Psychiatry, 134*(11), 1315.

Royal College of General Practitioners. (2019). *Safer prescribing in prisons*. https://elearning.rcgp.org.uk/pluginfile.php/176185/mod_book/chapter/620/RCGP-safer-prescribing-in-prisons-guidance-jan-2019.pdf

Sattar, S. P., Grant, K. M., & Bhatia, S. C. (2003). A case of venlafaxine abuse. *New England Journal of Medicine, 348*(8), 764–765.

Sattar, S. P., Schultz, S. K., Arndt, S., Soundy, T., & Petty, F. (2007). Long-term adjunctive quetiapine may reduce substance use—A preliminary retrospective study. *South Dakota Medicine: Journal of the South Dakota State Medical Association, 60*(11), 437–439.

Schaut, J., & Schnoll, S. H. (1983). Four cases of clonidine abuse. *American Journal of Psychiatry, 140*(12), 1625–1626.

Schifano, F., & Chiappini, S. (2018). Is there a potential of misuse for venlafaxine and bupropion? *Frontiers in Pharmacology, 9*, 239.

Schifano, F., Chiappini, S., Corkery, J. M., & Guirguis, A. (2018). Abuse of prescription drugs in the context of novel psychoactive substances (NPS): A systematic review. *Brain Sciences, 8*(4), 73.

Schindler, E. A. D., Tirado-Morales, D. J., & Kushon, D. (2013). Clonidine abuse in a methadone-maintained clonazepam-abusing patient. *Journal of Addiction Medicine, 7*(3), 218–219.

Shapiro, B. J., Lynch, K. L., Toochinda, T., Lutnick, A., Cheng, H. Y., & Kral, A. H. (2013). Promethazine misuse among methadone maintenance patients and community-based injection drug users. *Journal of Addiction Medicine, 7*, 96–101.

Shenouda, R., & Desan, P. H. (2013). Abuse of tricyclic antidepressant drugs: A case series. *Journal of Clinical Psychopharmacology, 33*(3), 440–442.

Slane, A., Robert, S., Rarrick, C., & Weeda, E. (2022). Survey of noncontrolled medication misuse patterns. *Mental Health Clinician, 12*(3), 199–204.

Smith, R. V., Havens, J. R., & Walsh, S. L. (2016). Gabapentin misuse, abuse and diversion: A systematic review. *Addiction (Abingdon, England), 111*(7), 1160–1174.

Stuppaeck, C. H., Whitworth, A. B., & Fleischhacker, W. W. (1993). Abuse potential of carbamazepine. *Journal of Nervous and Mental Disease, 181*(8), 519–520.

Substance Abuse and Mental Health Services Administration, Drug Abuse Warning Network. (2011). *National estimates of drug-related emergency department visits* (HHS Publication No. [SMA] 13-4760, DAWN Series D-39).

Substance Abuse and Mental Health Services Administration, Drug Abuse Warning Network. (2023). *Findings from drug-related emergency department visits, 2022* (Publication PEP23-07-03-001). Center for Behavioral Health Statistics and Quality, Substance Abuse and Mental Health Services Administration. https://www.samhsa.gov/data

Sullivan, G., & Davis, S. (1997). Is carbamazepine a potential drug of abuse? *Journal of Psychopharmacology, 11*(1), 93–94.

Swigart, A. (2021). Buspirone abuse by insufflation: A case report. *Journal of Clinical Psychopharmacology, 41*(1), 89–90.

Taïeb, O., Larroche, C., Dutray, B., Baubet, T., & Moro, M. R. (2004). Fluoxetine dependence in a former amineptine abuser. *American Journal of Addictions, 13*(5), 498–500.

Tambon, M., Ponté, C., Jouanjus, E., Fouilhé, N., Micallef, J., Lapeyre-Mestre, M., & French Addictovigilance Network (FAN). (2021). Gabapentinoid abuse in France: Evidence on health consequences and new points of vigilance. *Frontiers in Psychiatry, 12*, 639780.

Tamburello, A. C., Kathpal, A., & Reeves, R. (2017). Characteristics of inmates who misuse prescription medication. *Journal of Correctional Health Care, 23*(4), 449–458.

Tamburello, A. C., Lieberman, J. A., Baum, R., & Reeves, R. (2012). Successful removal of quetiapine from a correctional formulary. *Journal of American Academy of Psychiatry and the Law, 40*(4), 502–508.

Thomas, A., Nallur, D. G., Jones, N., & Deslandes, P. N. (2009). Diphenhydramine abuse and detoxification: A brief review and case report. *Journal of Psychopharmacology, 23*(1), 101–105.

Waters, B. M., & Joshi, K. G. (2007). Intravenous quetiapine-cocaine use ("Q-ball"). *American Journal of Psychiatry, 164*(1), 173–174.

Weißhaar, G. F., Hoemberg, M., Bender, K., et al. (2012). Baclofen intoxication: A "fun drug" causing deep coma and nonconvulsive status epilepticus—A case report and review of the literature. *European Journal of Pediatrics, 171*(10), 1541–1547.

Wen, P. (2009, July 13). Psychiatric drug sought on streets. *Boston Globe.*

Wilcox, J. A. (1987). Abuse of fluoxetine by a patient with anorexia nervosa. *American Journal of Psychiatry, 144*(8), 1100.

Wilson, T. K., & Tripp, J. (2013). *Buspirone.* https://www.ncbi.nlm.nih.gov/books/NBK531477/

World Health Organization. (2012). *Role of anticholinergic medications in patients requiring long-term antipsychotic treatment for psychotic disorders.* http://www.who.int/mental_health/mhgap/evidence/resource/psychosis_q6.pdf

SECTION VI

Disorders and syndromes

31

Diagnostic prevalence and comorbidity

Stuart D. M. Thomas

Introduction

Prisons and jails remain a growth industry, with many countries having to increase correctional services to cope with the ever-burgeoning population. Up-to-date statistics on the prison population are made available through a World Prison Brief series, published and regularly updated by the Institute for Crime & Justice Policy Research at the University of London in the United Kingdom. The most recent statistics indicate that the world prison population has increased by 24% since 2000, although there are substantial differences across and within different continents, relative to population growth across the same time frame (Fair & Walmsley, 2021). More than 30 million individuals cycle through prisons per year (Fazel et al., 2016); of the estimated 10.77 million people in prison at any one time worldwide, the vast majority are men, with around 740,000 (6.9%) being female (Fair & Walmsley, 2022). One long-standing issue in the literature and popular press across many jurisdictions has been the prevalence of mental disorders found in prisons. This chapter outlines the best available evidence pertaining to the correctional prevalence of common mental disorders and considers the key challenges involved in ascertaining accurate estimates of the rates of different diagnoses.

Setting the scene

Studies of the rates of mental disorders in prisons and jails have been reported in the literature for more than 4 decades. Early commentators argued that people with mental disorders were overrepresented in the criminal justice system because behaviors exhibited by these individuals were being criminalized, largely due to the lack of viable community-based treatment options (e.g., Gunn et al., 1991; Teplin, 1984). However, other commentators have asserted that a range of factors, including the many social disadvantages that accompany mental disorders, and not the mental disorders per se lead to imprisonment (e.g., Draine, 2002; Engel & Silver, 2001).

A review of the international literature on diagnostic prevalence reveals considerable heterogeneity, with considerable study-to-study variability. Much of the heterogeneity of the prevalence estimates has been attributed to a higher prevalence of disorders being reported in low- and middle-income countries (e.g., Fazel & Seewald, 2012). Increases in the prevalence of mental disorders in prisons have commonly been associated with decreases in the availability of psychiatric beds in the community (e.g., Gabrysch et al., 2019). Systematic reviews have synthesized the published literature over sustained periods of time; these reviews provide compelling evidence, with pooled prevalence estimates spanning multiple jurisdictions and time periods, that fewer hospital beds are associated with higher rates of mental illness in prisons. What they are less clear in providing is detailed information about trends in prisoner populations over time. Pooled estimates are also potentially misleading when prevalence estimates between countries vary considerably (Fazel et al., 2016).

Identifying trends and changes over time is an important part of being able to effect service delivery reform in response to changing profiles of need. Recent Canadian research has helped bridge this knowledge gap, suggesting that increases in the prison population, attributable in the Canadian context to legislative changes and harsher sanctions, have led to changes in prisoner demographics and concomitant increases in the prevalence of mental and substance use disorders (Butler et al., 2022). By contrast, while there have been decreases in the rates of incarceration in Scandinavian countries over the last decade, the proportion identified as having a diagnosed mental disorder has increased (Bukten et al., 2024).

Apart from untangling the reasons behind the apparent discrepancies in the published literature, it is also necessary to consider with whom or where comparisons are being made to assert that mental disorders are over- or underrepresented. For example, a control/comparison population should ideally be as similar to those (in this case) in the prison setting where mental disorders are being assessed (with respect to age, gender, and other characteristics) and to those who have been assessed for the presence of mental disorders using the same approach—whether that be a standardized screening instrument, assessment, or diagnostic test. This helps to ensure that any comparisons being made are comparing "like with like." Therefore, to make and/or substantiate the claim that mental disorders (and more specifically individual mental illnesses) are disproportionally represented in prison settings, a comparison needs to be made between the estimated rates of these disorders in prison and those found in the general community.

Research findings report either point prevalence (i.e., the number of people with the disorders of interest as a proportion of the total number of individuals being considered) or period prevalence (i.e., the number of "cases" counted/identified over a specified time frame). Other studies contrast "current" rates of mental disorder (cross-sectional at one point in time, in the last month, or over the last 12 months) with lifetime histories of mental disorder. The latter approach has the advantage of not only capturing a snapshot of the current psychiatric morbidity but also considering a broader vulnerability for those not currently symptomatic. This is important, as the latter group may potentially require a different approach, now or in the future, to support their rehabilitative and psychosocial needs and to aid in successful community reintegration.

To contextualize the available data on rates of mental disorders in prisons, and noting that there are some differences in prevalence estimates between different countries, there is a broad consensus that around one in five people in the community will experience a mental illness over a 12-month period, and about half of all people in the community will experience a mental illness across their lifetime (Australian Institute of Health and Welfare, 2024; National Alliance on Mental Illness, 2024). The most commonly diagnosed disorders, affecting more than one third of people across their lifespan, are anxiety disorders, mood disorders, and substance use disorders. As prisoners are part of the general community, a reasonable starting point would be to assume that these rates would be similar among prison populations. The evidence, however, shows that the prevalence of mental disorders is higher in prison populations.

There is also strong evidence from the United States and Canada that rates of mental and substance use disorders have increased over the last 20 years (Butler et al., 2022). A recent Australian study supports these findings, comparing self-reported rates of mental illness from three cross-sectional surveys of adult prisons in the state of New South Wales conducted in 2001, 2009, and 2015 (Browne et al., 2023). The authors reported that "those reporting any mental health diagnosis steadily increased … from 39.1% in 2001 to 63.1% in 2015" (Browne et al., 2023, p. 554); they also noted that there were significant increases found across all diagnoses, with the exception of personality disorders. Possible explanations for these findings are multiplicitous.

How common are mental disorders in prisons?

While there have been several persuasive commentaries documenting the rise of mental disorders in prisons (e.g., Torrey et al., 2010), a very poignant observation, made more than 50 years ago, has considerable contemporary significance. It stated that prisons have been left to deal with incarcerated persons whose behavior, while being "marked enough to interfere with discipline and communication," was not sufficient to satisfy admission criteria to psychiatric services (Walker & McCabe, 1973). This powerful statement has been reinforced multiple times since. One of the core questions, therefore, relates to prison health care service provision and the degree to which prisons can adequately cater to the needs of those with different mental disorders. While it is now undisputed that prisoners should have access to the same quality and range of mental health services as they would be able to access in the community (McCall-Smith, 2016; Reed, 2003) and that prisons have a legal obligation to provide these services (Steadman et al., 2005; see Chapter 3), research has consistently found that prisoners present with significant ongoing needs across a wide range of domains (Thomas et al., 2008). Many prisoners also present with symptoms best treated in mental health settings (Earthrowl et al., 2003; Torrey et al., 2010). Due to the high admission thresholds for public mental health services, challenges with throughput, and inadequate community mental health services provision leading to bottlenecks, the opportunity for transfer for the purposes of treatment remains limited.

An additional consideration when interpreting the literature is that studies operationalize and/or report their prevalence estimates according to idiosyncratic, practical, or financial reasons, which leads to the inclusion and/or exclusion of various mental disorders. There are further complications by virtue of the variability evident between different countries' systems to facilitate mental health service delivery (Aboaja et al., 2023), different approaches to how the police and the courts respond to people with mental illness, and variability in rates of incarceration for different types of offenses (Fazel et al., 2016). Collectively, these factors have an impact on prevalence estimates; this helps to explain some of the variability reported across studies and the higher rates reported in low- and middle-income countries.

One of the most extensive publications in the area remains a systematic review that pooled 62 studies from 12 countries to estimate rates of serious mental disorders among approximately 23,000 prisoners (Fazel & Danesh, 2002). The authors included studies that captured diagnoses in the last 6 months, while personality disorders were considered across the lifespan. They found that personality disorder (predominantly antisocial personality disorder) was the most common mental disorder among prisoners, accounting for 65% of male and 42% of female prisoners. Estimated rates of psychosis were 3.7% for male and 4.0% for female prisoners, while major depressive disorders were found among 10% of male and 12% of female prisoners. The authors concluded that the rates of psychosis and major depression were several times higher than those found in the general community but that antisocial personality disorder had the most marked overrepresentation—roughly 10 times higher among prisoners than in the general community. These findings were replicated a decade later (Fazel & Seewald, 2012), with a subsequent publication noting "little change in rates over the last three decades" (Fazel et al., 2016, p. 3).

Substance use problems have long dominated the correctional mental disorder literature; the association with criminal activity is noted at all stages of the justice system. An early Australian study by Heffernan and colleagues (2003) found that, at the front end, 86% of police arrestees had at least one substance use disorder, many had multiple disorders, and 80% were classified as substance dependent. Similar proportions of their sample had significant psychological distress, with rates proportionate to the number of substance-related disorders. A British study of remand and sentenced prisoners published around the same time reported similarly high rates of substance use prior to imprisonment, with high rates of comorbidity between mental illness and substance abuse disorders. Furthermore, those who were dependent on stimulants or opioids were more than 6 times more likely to also present with a personality disorder (Singleton et al., 2003).

A systematic review that examined the prevalence of substance dependence and abuse (now called substance use disorders) among male and female prisoners reported substantial heterogeneity between studies; estimated point prevalence rates for alcohol abuse and dependence varied between 18% and 30% for male prisoners and between 10% and 24% for female prisoners (Fazel et al., 2006). The authors commented that the rates were dramatically higher than those found in the general population and particularly high with respect to the female prisoner population. There is evidence that rates of diagnosed drug or alcohol problems or dependence have increased over time too, although rates of self-reported regular use of drugs in the 12 months prior to custody have decreased (Brown et al., 2023). These findings are similar to patterns in substance use found in the general population. The consistently high prevalence estimates have led some commentators to press for prison to be considered as a distinct "treatment opportunity" (Baranyi et al., 2022; Brooke et al., 2002).

While the majority of the published literature has focused on rates of mental disorder in male prisons, several studies that solely focused on female prisoners have also been reported. For example, Parsons and colleagues (2001) found that more than half of a sample of women remanded to prison had at least one mental disorder (which did not include those with substance dependence) and that 11% were diagnosed with psychotic disorders. An Australian study (Tye & Mullen, 2006) reported similar rates but highlighted the dramatic increase in prevalence (up to 84%) when substance use and dependence were included. This study found that more than one third of the female prisoners were diagnosed with drug-related disorders, major depression, and posttraumatic stress disorder. The recent Australian study by Browne and colleagues (2023) noted that self-reported lifetime rates of mental health diagnoses for women in prison rose from 52.6% to 76.8%, comparing self-report data from 2001 and 2015. The authors noted that the women surveyed "reported higher rates of most psychiatric diagnoses, psychiatric hospitalization, prescribed medication and self-harm" (Browne et al., 2023, p. 559). Further, the odds of reporting mental health and/or drug and alcohol comorbidity were 2 times higher (OR = 2.07, 95% CI 1.43–2.99) for women in prison in 2015 than in 2001. In addition, the rate of posttraumatic stress disorder reported in the 2015 survey was more than 2 times higher for female than male prisoners (20.1% versus 9.7%).

Comorbidity of disorders

Studies have long suggested that comorbid mental illnesses and substance use disorders are common (e.g., DiCataldo et al., 1995) and of particular concern (Brinded et al., 2001). The added complexity of the increased rates of comorbid mental disorders found among prisoners serves to define a significant prison subgroup that places additional demands on prison health care services (Thomas et al., 2008). One of the core challenges here, identified in a 2015 report by the Substance Abuse and Mental Health Services Administration, is what was described as the "failure to comprehensively examine one or more of the disorders [and] inadequate staff training to identify and assess the disorders" (Substance Abuse and Mental Health Services Administration, 2015, p. 11). Put simply, individuals are not being adequately screened for the presence of comorbid disorders and therefore are not being afforded a treatment opportunity and have worse outcomes. A recent systematic review of 50 studies reinforced this, arguing for the need for better screening of comorbid disorders and noting that these individuals are characterized as having more significant criminal histories, worse treatment responses, and more negative outcomes upon release from prison (Baranyi et al., 2022). Their review helpfully provides more contemporaneous estimates of the extent of comorbidity in prisons. Based on their pooled analysis of just under 25,000 people, they reported that "around half of the prison population with non-affective psychosis or major depression have a comorbid substance use disorder" (Baranyi et al., 2022, p. e557).

As noted above, of real concern is the compelling evidence that prisoners with comorbid mental health and substance-related disorders have worse criminal justice outcomes (Baillargeon et al., 2009; Forsythe & Gaffney, 2012; Trestman et al., 2007). It is well established that their treatment and support needs are likely to remain for a lengthy period, well beyond incarceration, and the adverse postrelease outcomes of those with a mental disorder are well documented (Bukten et al., 2024). For example, an Australian report by the New South Wales Bureau of Crime Statistics and Research found that prisoners diagnosed with both mental health and substance-related disorders (in excess of 40% of a sample of 1,208 prisoners) reoffended at a higher rate than those who were diagnosed with solely a substance use disorder or a non–substance use mental disorder (Smith & Trimboli, 2010).

Over 20 years ago, Abram and colleagues (2003) specifically highlighted the importance of screening for comorbid substance-related disorders and contended that prisons must facilitate pathways into treatment for this group. Not much has changed since. Extending the earlier argument, Baranyi and colleagues (2022) bring into question the effectiveness of current treatment models in prison, which traditionally separate out mental health and substance misuse services, calling for research into the efficacy of an integrated screening and treatment model to better meet people's needs and improve outcomes.

How are mental disorders identified?

A central explanation for the variability in the estimated prevalence of mental disorders relates to the means and methods used for case ascertainment. As noted by Fazel and colleagues (2016), the means of identification can lead to both under- and overestimation of different disorders. Many studies have sought to consider mental disorders through very general means such as through answers to simple questions from the broad health screens routinely administered upon reception to prison (see Chapter 15). Such screening questions record self-reported histories of contacts with mental health services and/or self-reported diagnoses, and they are generally used upon entry to prison to screen for placements associated with identified vulnerability. Large-scale prison surveys that have been reported commonly in the literature typically adopt a similar approach, with relatively generic questions about mental health used to gain a general sense about the extent of psychiatric morbidity (among other things) in prison. These studies are useful in that they can provide a cost-efficient "snapshot" of the rates of psychiatric morbidity in prisons; however, they are also limited in detailing the extent, nature, and severity of the presenting conditions.

While there are strong human rights and public health arguments about the need to adequately identify and treat incarcerated persons with mental disorders, there is ample evidence that the reception screening process continues to miss a considerable proportion of those with mental illnesses (e.g., Martin et al., 2013; Teplin, 1990). A number of more detailed screening tools have been developed (see Chapter 15). While they have shown some promise in related environments (Baksheev, Ogloff, & Thomas, 2012), their utility, as tested through replication studies, remains limited. A systematic review of studies published up to 2011 revealed that six of the 22 screening tools identified in the review had replication studies available. Overall, the authors noted that the available tools do not perform as well with female as with male prisoners (Martin et al., 2013).

How confident can we be with estimated prevalence rates?

As with any diagnostic screen, test, or checklist, there is an inherent degree of error. While there is always the potential for bias associated with self-report, the very nature and purpose of the assessment tool/screen/instrument needs to be considered. For example, some screening tools are designed to be overly inclusive so as to catch as many of the target group as possible, thus leading to a number of false positives. While many authors have highlighted the sometimes significant limitations with the standard brief prison health screening processes (e.g., Steadman et al., 2005; Teplin, 1990), others have questioned the validity of using standardized diagnostic screens and tests in correctional environments (e.g., Andersen, 2004). For example, Heffernan and colleagues (2003) note the validity of the Composite International Diagnostic Interview (Kessler et al., 1998) with respect to substance-related disorders, yet Falissard and colleagues (2006) point to some potential pitfalls with making valid and reliable mental health diagnoses in jails and prisons, suggesting that the standardized measures underestimate the true prevalence of mental disorders. By comparing diagnoses identified through use of the Mini-International Neuropsychiatric Interview (Sheehan et al., 1998) with clinician assessments (using an open-ended clinical interview), Falissard and colleagues (2006) reported that the rates of all mental disorders were consistently higher when using the open-ended clinical interview method. This finding supports earlier research in other contexts that concluded that the administration of diagnostic measures by trained lay interviewers represented a conservative case ascertainment method compared to detailed clinical assessment (Murphy et al., 2000). Authors have suggested that the impact of the correctional environment itself on the individual (e.g., Baksheev, Thomas, & Ogloff, 2012) may contribute to the lower levels of agreement found when individual disorders are considered (Falissard et al., 2006). This stance is supported by Martin and colleagues (2013), whose systematic review noted the importance of contextual factors when considering the utility of a screening/assessment tool. As aptly demonstrated by Bradley-Engen and colleagues (2010), there is real value (where practicable) in using multiple data sources in combination to attain a more comprehensive picture of the rates of mental disorder. This is especially the case with capturing and recording the presence of comorbid substance use disorders.

Summary

While a great deal of international research has been conducted on the prevalence of mental disorders in prisons, a synthesis of this evidence demonstrates substantial heterogeneity. Due to the varying methodologies used, it is necessary to drill down beyond the headline findings of individual studies to understand the basis on which mental disorders are determined and what inclusion/exclusion criteria are used. What is apparent across many, if not all, jurisdictions is that the need for mental health care is far greater than is currently being provided. The result is that many prisoners are being held in suboptimal treatment and rehabilitation environments. The available evidence shows that substance use disorders (both primary and comorbid) are common and that there is a pressing need for more effective treatment for prisoners during and immediately after incarceration to help tackle adverse outcomes. The common comorbidity of substance use and personality disorders found in prison populations certainly complicates standard treatment approaches and suggests that a different suite of strategies may need to be considered. Finally, the overrepresentation of more severe disorders, especially psychotic disorders, among prisoners continues to present a challenge for already overburdened and overstretched correctional health services.

We must continue to focus on improving the responsiveness and cohesion of multiagency service responses to fulfill our public health obligations to people detained in our prison systems, as well as evidencing the effectiveness of interventions and supports. Prisons continue to represent an excellent treatment opportunity and a chance to connect individuals with a wide range of supports and services to help foster community connectedness and reintegration. While we must continue to exercise caution in assigning mental health diagnoses to individuals (Taylor & Gunn, 2008), we are also obliged to identify psychiatric vulnerability as early as possible and to provide timely, quality assessment and treatment to help improve experiences and outcomes.

REFERENCES

Aboaja, A., Pangurangi, P., Almeida, S., Castelletti, L., Rivera-Arroyo, G., Optiz-Welke, J., & Barlow, S. (2023). Six nations: A clinical scenario comparison of systems for prisoners with psychosis in Australia, Bolivia and four European nations. *BJPsych International*, *20*(1), 13–17.

Abram, K., Teplin, L., & McClelland, G. (2003). Comorbidity of severe psychiatric disorders and substance use disorders among women in jail. *American Journal of Psychiatry*, *160*(5), 1007–1010.

Andersen, H. S. (2004). Mental health in prison populations: A review—With special emphasis on a study of Danish prisoners on remand. *Acta Psychiatrica Scandinavica*, *424*, 5–59.

Australian Institute of Health and Welfare. (2024). *Mental health*. https://www.aihw.gov.au/mental-health/overview/prevalence-and-impact-of-mental-illness

Baillargeon, J., Binswanger, I. A., Penn, J. V., Williams, B. A., & Murray, O. J. (2009). Psychiatric disorders and repeat incarcerations: The revolving prison door. *American Journal of Psychiatry*, *166*(1), 103–109.

Baksheev, G. N., Ogloff, J., & Thomas, S. (2012). Identification of mental illness in police cells: A comparison of police processes, the Brief Jail Mental Health Screen and the Jail Screening Assessment Tool. *Psychology, Crime and Law*, *18*(6), 529–542.

Baksheev, G. N., Thomas, S. D. M., & Ogloff, J. R. P. (2012). Psychopathology in police custody: The role of importation, deprivation and interaction models. *International Journal of Forensic Mental Health*, *11*(1), 24–32.

Baranyi, G., Fazel, S., Langerfeldt, S. D., & Mundt, A. P. (2022). The prevalence of comorbid serious mental illness and substance use disorders in prison populations: A systematic review and meta-analysis. *Lancet Public Health*, *7*, e557–e568.

Bradley-Engen, M. S., Cuddeback, G. S., Gayman, M. D., Morrissey, J. P., & Mancuso, D. (2010). Trends in state admission of offenders with serious mental illness. *Psychiatric Services, 61*(12), 1263–1265.

Brinded, P. M. J., Simpson, A. I. F., Laidlaw, T. M., Fairley, N., & Malcolm, F. (2001). Prevalence of psychiatric disorders in New Zealand prisons: A national study. *Australian and New Zealand Journal of Psychiatry, 35*, 166–173.

Brooke, D., Taylor, C., Gunn, J., & Maden, A. (2002). Substance misusers remanded to prison: A treatment opportunity. *Addiction, 93*(12), 1851–1856.

Browne, C. C., Korobanova, D., Yee, N., Spencer, S. J., Ma, T., Butler, T., & Dean, K. (2023). The prevalence of self-reported mental illness among those imprisoned in New South Wales across three health surveys, from 2001 to 2015. *Australian and New Zealand Journal of Psychiatry, 57*, 550–561.

Bukten, A., Virtanen, S., Hesse, M., Chang, Z., Lehmann Kvame, T., Thylstrup, B., Tverborgvik, T., Skjarvo, I., & Stavseth, M. R. (2024). The prevalence and comorbidity of mental health and substance use disorders in Scandinavian prisons 2019–2019: A multi-national register study. *BMC Psychiatry, 24*, 95.

Butler, A., Nicholls, T., Samji, H., Fabian, S., & Lavergne, M. R. (2022). Prevalence of mental health needs, substance use, and co-occurring disorders among people admitted to prison. *Psychiatric Services, 73*, 737–744. https://doi.org/10.1176/appi.ps.202000927

DiCataldo, F., Greer, A., & Profit, W. E. (1995). Screening prison inmates for mental disorder: An examination of the relationship between mental disorder and prison adjustment. *Bulletin of the American Academy of Psychiatry and the Law, 23*(4), 573–585.

Draine, J. (2002). Where is the "illness" in the criminalization of mental illness? In W. H. Fisher (Ed.), *Community-based interventions for criminal offenders with severe mental illness, research in community and mental health* (pp. 9–21). Emerald Group Publishing.

Earthrowl, M., O'Grady, J., & Birmingham, L. (2003). Providing treatment to prisoners with mental disorders: Development of a policy. *British Journal of Psychiatry, 156*, 40–45.

Engel, R. S., & Silver, E. (2001). Policing mentally disordered suspects: A re-examination of the criminalization hypothesis. *Criminology, 39*(2), 225–252.

Fair, H., & Walmsley, R. (2021). *World prison population list* (13th ed.). Institute for Crime & Justice Policy Research.

Fair, H., & Walmsley, R. (2022). *World female imprisonment list (5th ed.): Women and girls in penal institutions, including pre-trial detainees/remand prisoners.* Institute for Crime & Justice Policy Research.

Falissard, B., Loze, J. Y., Gasquet, I., Duburc, A., de Beaurepaire, C., Fagnani, F., & Rouillon, F. (2006). Prevalence of mental disorders in French prisons for men. *BMC Psychiatry, 6*, 33.

Fazel, S., Bains, P., & Doll, H. (2006). Substance abuse and dependence in prisoners: A systematic review. *Addiction, 101*, 181–191.

Fazel, S., & Danesh, J. (2002). Serious mental disorder in 23000 prisoners: A systematic review of 62 surveys. *Lancet, 359*, 545–550.

Fazel, S., Hayes, A. J., Bartellas, K., Clerici, M., & Trestman, R. (2016). Mental health of prisoners: Prevalence, adverse outcomes, and interventions. *Lancet Psychiatry, 3*, 871–881.

Fazel, S., & Seewald, K. (2012). Severe mental illness in 33588 prisoners worldwide: Systematic review and meta regression analysis. *British Journal of Psychiatry, 200*, 364–373.

Forsythe, L., & Gaffney, A. (2012, July). *Mental disorder prevalence at the gateway to the criminal justice system* (Trends and Issues in Crime and Criminal Justice, 438). Australian Institute of Criminology.

Gabrysch, C., Fritsch, R., Priebe, S., & Mundt, A. P. (2019). Mental disorder and mental health symptoms during imprisonment: A three-year follow-up study. *PLoS ONE, 14*(3), e0213711.

Gunn, J., Maden, A., & Swinton, M. (1991). Treatment needs of prisoners with psychiatric disorders. *British Medical Journal, 303*, 338–341.

Heffernan, E. B., Finn, J., Saunders, J. B., & Byrne, G. (2003). Substance use disorders and psychological distress among police arrestees. *Medical Journal of Australia, 179*, 408–411.

Kessler, R. C., Andrews, G., Mroczek, D., Ustun, T. B., & Wittchen, H-U. (1998). The World Health Organization Composite International Diagnostic Interview Short Form (CIDI-SF). *International Journal of Methods in Psychiatric Research, 7*(4), 171–185.

Martin, M. S., Colman, I., Simpson, A., & McKenzie, K. (2013). Mental health screening tools in correctional institutions: A systematic review. *BMC Psychiatry, 13*, 275.

McCall-Smith, K. (2016). United Nations standard minimum rules for the treatment of prisoners (Nelson Mandela Rules). *International Legal Materials, 55*, 1180–1205.

Murphy, J. M., Monson, R. R., Laird, N. M., Sobol, A. M., & Leighton, A. H. (2000). A comparison of diagnostic interviews for depression in the Stirling County study: Challenges for psychiatric epidemiology. *Archives of General Psychiatry, 57*, 230–236.

National Alliance on Mental Illness. (2024). *Mental health by the numbers.* https://www.nami.org/mhstats

Parsons, S., Walker, L., & Grubin, D. (2001). Prevalence of mental disorder in female remand prisoners. *Journal of Forensic Psychiatry, 12*, 194–202.

Reed, J. (2003). Mental health care in prisons. *British Journal of Psychiatry, 182*, 287–288.

Sheehan, D. V., Lecrubier, Y., Harnett Sheehan, K., Amorim, P., Janavs, J., Weiller, E., Hergueta, T., Baker, R., & Dunbar, G. C. (1998). The Mini-International Neuropsychiatric Interview (M.I.N.I.): The development and validation of a structured psychiatric interview for DSM-IV and ICD-10. *Journal of Clinical Psychiatry, 59*(Suppl. 20), 22–33.

Singleton, N., Farrell, M., & Meltzer, H. (2003). Substance misuse among prisoners in England and Wales. *International Review of Psychiatry, 15*, 150–152.

Smith, N., & Trimboli, L. (2010). *Comorbid substance and non-substance mental health disorders and re-offending among NSW prisoners* (Contemporary Issues in Crime and Justice). BOCSAR, NSW Bureau of Crime Statistics and Research.

Steadman, H. J., Scott, J. E., Osher, F., Agnesa, T. K., & Robbins, P. C. (2005). Validation of the Brief Mental Health Screen. *Psychiatric Services, 56*, 816–822.

Substance Abuse and Mental Health Services Administration. (2015). *Screening and assessment of co-occurring disorders in the justice system* (HHS Publication No. PEP19-SCREEN-CODJS).

Taylor, P., & Gunn, J. (2008). Diagnosis, medical models and formulations. In K. Soothill, P. Rogers, & M. Dolan (Eds.), *Handbook of forensic mental health* (pp. 237–243). Willan Publishing.

Teplin, L. A. (1984). Criminalizing mental disorder: The comparative arrest rate of the mentally ill. *American Psychologist, 39*, 794–803.

Teplin, L. (1990). Detecting disorder: The treatment of mental illness among jail detainees. *Journal of Consulting and Clinical Psychology, 58*, 233–236.

Thomas, S., McCrone, P., & Fahy, T. (2008). How do psychiatric patients on prison healthcare centres differ from inpatient in secure psychiatric inpatient units? *Psychology, Crime and Law, 15*(8), 729–742.

Torrey, E. F., Kennard, A. D., Eslinger, D., Lamb, R., & Pavle, J. (2010). *More mentally ill persons are in jails and prisons than hospitals: A survey of the states.* Treatment Advocacy Center and National Sheriffs' Association.

Trestman, R., Ford, J., Zhang, W. W., & Wiesbrock, V. (2007). Current and lifetime psychiatric illness among inmates not identified as acutely mentally ill at intake in Connecticut's jails. *Journal of the American Academy of Psychiatry and the Law*, *35*(4), 490–500.

Tye, C. S., & Mullen, P. E. (2006). Mental disorders in female prisoners. *Australian and New Zealand Journal of Psychiatry*, *40*(3), 266–271.

Walker, N., & McCabe, S. (1973). *Crime and insanity in England* (Vol. 2). Edinburgh University Press.

32

Psychotic disorders

Todd Tomita and Rakesh Lamba

Introduction

Psychotic disorders are several times more prevalent in correctional settings than in the community. Clinicians working in different correctional settings will assess and treat incarcerated persons (IPs) with psychotic disorders. Rates of serious mental illness, including schizophrenia, are higher in U.S. correctional settings (e.g., prisons, jails, police lockups, detention facilities) than in the general population (Keepers et al., 2020). A meta-analysis of 33,588 prisoners from 24 countries found a prevalence of psychosis of 3.6% in male prisoners and 3.9% in female prisoners (Fazel & Seewald, 2012). Another meta-analysis of 13,135 prisoners from 13 low- and middle-income countries found that the 1-year prevalence rate for psychosis was 6.2% (Baranyi et al., 2019).

The correctional setting is not the community. There is wide variability in psychiatric care provision between jails and prisons and across different jurisdictions. Further, an IP's time in the correctional system is not dictated by treatment needs. Short periods in custody may provide little opportunity for treatment of psychotic disorders. Conversely, long custodial terms may provide the opportunity for optimal treatment. Thus, correctional rather than clinical time frames may determine what types of treatment intervention can be implemented.

Psychotic disorders in corrections

Psychosis may present in various forms and can be the product of medical and psychiatric etiologies. Schizophrenia spectrum disorders and substance-induced psychotic disorders are common conditions that psychiatrists in corrections will diagnose and treat. As observed prototypically in the schizophrenia spectrum disorders (schizophrenia, schizophreniform psychosis, delusional disorder, schizoaffective disorder, and schizotypal personality disorder), psychosis is characterized by abnormalities in one or more of the following five domains: delusions (fixedly held false beliefs), hallucinations (perception-like experiences that occur without an external stimulus), disorganized thinking (off the point, tangential, illogical, or unintelligible statements or responses to questions), grossly abnormal behavior (e.g., childlike silliness, catatonia, stupor, or mutism), and negative symptoms (e.g., diminished emotional expression, diminished speech output, anhedonia and asociality; American Psychiatric Association, 2022).

The differential diagnosis of psychotic disorders will vary depending on the stage of incarceration. Recently incarcerated individuals, for example, are at greater risk of substance-induced psychotic conditions than those serving long-term sentences, where the diagnosis of a primary psychotic disorder might be made more confidently. The expressed behavior and symptomatology of psychotic disorders may vary in duration from a few days to weeks (e.g., in most substance-induced psychotic states and the time-limited regression into psychosis seen in persons with severe personality disorder with few coping strengths and in crisis), months, or years (schizophreniform psychosis, schizophrenia, and delusional disorder; American Psychiatric Association, 2022; World Health Organization, 2021).

Chronic use of certain illicit substances (e.g., methamphetamine) may result in prolonged and even permanent psychosis, thus rendering problematic the unambiguous distinction between substance-induced psychosis and schizophrenia (Arunogiri et al., 2020; Glasner-Edwards & Mooney, 2014; Lecomte et al., 2013; Ujike & Sato, 2004). The psychotic features may be indistinguishable, and it may only be the retrospective pattern of recovery that clarifies the psychotic disorder diagnosis (Arunogiri et al., 2020; Sekeguchi et al., 2021). Transient psychotic symptoms, especially nonbizarre persecutory delusions, have been observed in prisoners and may be a function of environmental stressors or exposure to trauma (Glancy et al., 2020; Tamburello et al., 2022). Malingering of psychotic symptoms, particularly for individuals with previous incarceration experience, presents challenges that are not found in the community (see Chapter 20). Malingering and genuine psychotic disorders may coexist. Malingering requires a comprehensive assessment as a cursory assessment that concludes an IP is malingering may have long-lasting adverse effects for someone with an untreated psychotic disorder. Malingering is a label that is easy to apply but difficult to remove.

Assessment

Identification and proper diagnosis are the foundational components, as the presence of a major mental disorder will often influence the operational management of disruptive IPs. Psychosis-related functional impairment with withdrawn, disorganized, or disruptive behaviors can upset the operational mission of security and prompt a disciplinary approach. Of course, not all disruptive acts and other impairments are the product of psychotic illness. Consequently, identification and proper diagnosis of a psychotic disorder are critical care components, particularly as comorbidities such as substance use disorders and personality disorders are common (Baranyi et al., 2022; Fazel & Danesh, 2002). Often, comorbidity seems more the rule than the exception. Therefore, the psychiatrist is frequently tasked with differentiating volitional disruption from psychosis-related impairment.

Correctional officers can be an invaluable source of collateral information about the behavior and functioning of an IP being evaluated for a psychotic disorder. Officers have the most contact with IPs and are well situated to observe changes in behavior and functional impairments, both new and ongoing. A collaborative approach with officers focused on aligned priorities, such as helping a disruptive IP settle, is optimal (see Chapter 14; Glancy et al., 2020; Tamburello et al., 2022). While correctional officers can make important contributions to the interdisciplinary management and treatment of IPs (Appelbaum et al., 2001), they are often not in a position to differentiate volitionally produced problem behaviors from those produced by psychotic illness (e.g., undiagnosed schizophrenia may be misidentified as intentional mischief making, particularly in IPs with comorbid personality disorders). Experienced clinicians can help identify treatable cases such as the ostensibly personality-disordered IPs with a missed underlying delusional disorder who respond well to treatment once identified.

A meta-analysis of 21 studies in 15 countries showed that for individuals with schizophrenia spectrum disorders, there is a threefold increase in violence risk, which rises to 10-fold with comorbid substance use (Whiting et al., 2022). IPs with symptoms of psychosis should be treated, as studies of correctional populations indicate that there is a small but significant minority of people who commit sometimes unpredictable, psychotically motivated crimes (Skeem et al., 2015). Psychosis has a strong effect on offending behavior in prison, with paranoid thinking the best predictor of violent offenses (Felson et al., 2012). Psychotropic medications relieve many of the manifestations of mental illness; therefore, disruptive behaviors are most likely to occur when individuals with psychotic disorders are nonadherent with medication (O'Keefe & Schnell, 2007).

Correctional treatment settings

While key elements of optimal treatment of psychotic disorders in the correctional setting can be drawn from clinical practice guidelines, the health care resources available within a particular correctional system and the legal provisions and resources for involuntary treatment may limit treatment possibilities. High-income countries with reasonable correctional health care levels, access to psychiatric hospital beds, and, if necessary, legal provisions for involuntary treatment can obviously adhere to evidence-informed treatment better than middle- or low-income countries that lack these resources (Aboaja et al., 2023). The evidence regarding the impact of restrictive housing units (RHUs) on IPs with major mental illness remains inconsistent (see Chapter 10). The proportion of IPs with mental illness in RHUs can be an indicator of the overall quality of a correctional system, as untreated or undertreated IPs are more likely to act out due to their mental illness. IPs with schizophrenia may behave in a disruptive manner, resulting in disciplinary infractions and RHU placement. The American Psychiatric Association's Guideline for the Treatment of Patients With Schizophrenia recommends avoiding RHU placement for behaviors that are directly related to schizophrenia because such an intervention is likely to exacerbate rather than reduce psychotic symptoms, as well as increase rather than reduce disruptive behaviors (Keepers et al., 2020).

For individuals with severe forms of psychotic disorder, tenure in a correctional environment may provide more opportunities for stabilizing treatment than if the individual remained in the community. Longer tenures in custody can provide an opportunity for clarifying diagnosis and optimizing treatment. For example, a Canadian study followed remand prisoners with serious mental illness, the majority with psychosis, for up to 1 year; all showed improvement with a reduction in illness severity (Jones et al., 2023). The structure of the prison itself may help diminish positive psychotic symptoms (Adams & Ferrandino, 2008; Blaauw et al., 2007). The positive outcomes that flow from incarceration might be attributable to factors such as safety, structure, reduced drug and alcohol consumption, and consistent access to medication and health care services (Blaauw et al., 2007; Gabrysch et al., 2020; Hassan et al., 2011; Taylor et al., 2010).

Pharmacological interventions

Treatment of psychotic disorders in correctional settings should be guided by general clinical practice standards, with modifications as needed for the correctional context. Evidence-based clinical practice guidelines offer a scientific and clinically sound basis for making treatment decisions consistent with the evolving community standard of care (Scott, 2010). The independence of prescribers may be challenged by the desires and concerns of other staff about the potential for violent behavior in certain IPs, as there may be pressure to prescribe more sedating drugs to reduce a perceived risk. The response of operational staff to disruptive behavior that they see as mentally disordered may create unique pressures within the health care system in a correctional institution (Adams & Ferrandino, 2008). While correctional staff may understandably be searching for a way to settle a disruptive IP, a sound decision to treat will be based on an assessment that there is an underlying treatable psychotic condition or a clear rationale for off-label antipsychotic medication (Collins et al., 2017). The issue for correctional prescribers is the lack of guidance regarding adapting clinical practice guidelines for prescribing to their correctional context. American and Canadian practice resources for prescribing in corrections are available that provide a guide for prescribers on health care operations related to medication in correctional institutions and, specifically, on evidence-based prescribing practice for schizophrenia and other psychotic disorders in these settings (Glancy et al., 2020; Tamburello et al., 2022).

Antipsychotic medications are the primary treatment for IPs with psychotic disorders. The following section addresses some general principles related to antipsychotic medication prescribing in correctional settings. A full review of the pharmacotherapy for psychotic disorders is beyond the scope of this chapter. Most prescribers will be able to practice within their institutional correctional formulary, as there is no definitive evidence that either first-generation antipsychotic or second-generation antipsychotic medications differ in efficacy; the only clear differences relate to their side-effect profiles (Barnes et al., 2020; Keepers et al., 2020; National Institute for Clinical Excellence [NICE], 2014; Remington et al., 2017). It is, however, important that correctional policy permits access to nonformulary medications on a case-by-case basis to ensure access to appropriate treatment for serious mental illness (Scott, 2010).

Patients with psychotic disorders need closer monitoring in the acute phase of treatment. Generally, 4 to 6 weeks is an adequate trial for antipsychotic medication. Still, a lack of minimal improvement on an antipsychotic medication after 2 to 4 weeks should prompt reassessment, including for overt or covert nonadherence and possible change of antipsychotic medication (Keepers et al., 2020). After a response, patients with a confident diagnosis of chronic psychotic illness should continue antipsychotic medication to reduce the risk of relapse (Barnes et al., 2020; Keepers et al., 2020; NICE, 2014; Remington et al., 2017).

The only efficacy exception is clozapine, which is more effective. Clinical practice guidelines recommend clozapine for treatment-resistant patients who have failed two adequate trials of antipsychotic medications (Barnes et al., 2020; Keepers et al., 2020; NICE, 2014; Remington et al., 2017). Clozapine may be particularly efficacious for patients with treatment-resistant schizophrenia and persistent suicidality and aggression (Barnes et al., 2020; Keepers et al., 2020; Remington et al., 2017). While recommended, in practice, clozapine treatment is only possible if health care in the correctional setting can meet the clozapine monitoring and reporting requirements (Glancy et al., 2020; Tamburello et al., 2022). Clozapine treatment for IPs with psychotic disorders is more effective compared to other antipsychotic medications in improving institutional adjustment and delaying time to reoffending (Balbuena et al., 2010; Mela & Depiang, 2016).

Clozapine is effective in treating IPs with treatment-resistant schizophrenia with high rates of comorbid substance use disorder and personality disorder (Martin et al., 2008). A Swedish national registry study showed substantial reductions in violent offending for people with schizophrenia after they started taking clozapine (Bhavsar et al., 2020). There are, however, patient and prescriber barriers around perceived dangers of adverse effects and difficulty of monitoring in the prison setting (Martin et al., 2008). Successful implementation of clozapine treatment often requires a systematic approach rather than relying on the individual prescriber. For example, the North Carolina prison system successfully implemented a consultative system for clozapine initiation with the local university's school of medicine, which led to increased treatment access and a 390% increase in the number of IPs using clozapine over a 5-year period (Pruette et al., 2023).

Treatment with long-acting injectable antipsychotic medication is an important consideration in patients with poor or uncertain adherence and treatment nonresponse with oral antipsychotic medication (Barnes et al., 2020; Keepers et al., 2020; NICE, 2014; Remington et al., 2017). Real-world observational studies show advantages for long-acting injectable antipsychotic medication compared to oral preparations in preventing relapse, but randomized control trials show equivalent efficacy (Barnes et al., 2020; Keepers et al., 2020). Practically, long-acting injectable antipsychotic medications are often underutilized, given that they make provision of treatment, monitoring, and promoting adherence in the correctional setting much simpler. A long-acting injectable antipsychotic medication can be of particular benefit for IPs who have had multiple psychotic episodes and, at release, may be at risk of a gap in treatment and nonadherence (Keepers et al., 2020).

Guidelines focus on specific psychiatric disorders. In correctional settings, however, other psychotic disorders (e.g., delusional disorder) and intermittent psychotic symptoms that may accompany certain personality disorders may be the focus of treatment. Further, transient psychotic symptoms, especially nonbizarre persecutory delusions, may occur due to environmental stressors or exposure to trauma (Glancy et al., 2020; Tamburello et al., 2022). Potential treatment benefit needs to be weighed against the risk of adverse effects of antipsychotic medication. A treatment plan that flows from a well-reasoned diagnosis based on adequate assessment is the best approach to managing the risk of unnecessary prescribing of antipsychotic medication (Glancy et al., 2020; Tamburello et al., 2022).

Treatment guidelines generally recommend continuation of antipsychotic medication for every patient diagnosed with schizophrenia and suggest that it be maintained for at least 2 years (Barnes et al., 2020; NICE, 2014; Remington et al., 2017). For other psychotic disorders, the longitudinal course of the patient's psychotic episode and the certainty of the diagnosis will guide decisions about treatment continuation. Treatment adherence reduces violent recidivism. Two Swedish national population registry studies showed that adherence to antipsychotic medication reduced rates of violent reoffending. In one study, the rates of violent crime were reduced by 45% in patients receiving antipsychotic medication, with notable reductions in patients receiving long-acting injectable antipsychotics (Fazel et al., 2014). The other study examined the association between the prescription of antipsychotic medication and violent reoffending after release from prison. Rates of violent reoffending were lower when individuals were being dispensed antipsychotic medication (Chang et al., 2016).

Polypharmacy and high-dose antipsychotic medication prescribing practices have been identified in correctional settings (Griffiths et al., 2012; Hervás et al., 2019). Polypharmacy may be the product of high rates of off-label prescribing of antipsychotic medications, which is common in correctional settings (Carey & Barlow, 2022; Pelizza et al., 2022). Off-label prescribing may reflect appropriate correctional clinical practices. For example, a Canadian prison study found that rates of prescribing off-label psychotropic medication were not elevated relative to rates cited in the community (Brown et al., 2018). With psychotic disorders, a categorical recommendation against antipsychotic medication polypharmacy may be unwarranted. An extensive nationwide cohort study showed that rehospitalization rates for patients with schizophrenia may be reduced for patients receiving combination therapy with two antipsychotic medications, including combining an oral and long-acting injectable formulation, as compared to monotherapy (Tiihonen et al., 2019). Additionally, there is no evidence that combining antipsychotic medications is any more harmful than using a single medication beyond the common side effects of each drug (Keepers et al., 2020). In regard to high-dose prescribing of antipsychotic medication, the available evidence suggests no benefit for treatment-resistant schizophrenia, and side effects are likely to be increased (Barnes et al., 2020; Keepers et al., 2020; Remington et al., 2017). When prescribing in the correctional context, clinicians should be attentive to the risk of prescription medication abuse, especially quetiapine (see Chapter 30).

Psychosocial interventions

Psychosocial interventions in correctional settings for IPs with psychotic disorders can be broadly divided into three groups: (a) mental health recovery interventions focused on treating psychotic disorders that mirror community treatment interventions such as psychiatric rehabilitation, (b) correctional treatment programs that are designed for people without serious mental illness that address criminogenic factors to reduce recidivism, and (c) interventions designed for IPs with serious mental illness that address both mental health recovery and recidivism. Evidence indicates that this third group of interventions is required to reduce recidivism in IPs with psychotic disorders. Psychosocial interventions must address the co-occurring issues of mental illness and criminal risk (Bewley & Morgan, 2011; Morgan et al., 2012, 2020; Parisi et al., 2022). The scientific literature indicates that treatment programs for IPs demonstrate the highest efficacy in reducing recidivism when interventions are designed in accordance with the risk–need–responsivity (RNR) principles and use cognitive-behavioral therapy components that target criminogenic needs (Andrews, Bonta, & Hoge, 1990; Andrews, Zinger, et al., 1990; Bonta & Andrews, 2016; Douglas et al., 2008; Gendreau & Goggin, 1996; Gendreau et al., 1996).

RNR principles align the results of assessment with interventions to reduce reoffending behaviors. The risk principle maintains that higher risk individuals should be offered more intense services, and the need principle directs that services should target identified criminogenic needs—that is, dynamic risk factors that, when changed, decrease the probability of recidivism. The responsivity principle holds that treatment should be matched to the abilities and learning styles of the individual (Bonta & Andrews, 2016). Untreated psychotic disorder or persisting illness-related functional impairments can be viewed as responsivity factors. It is the criminogenic risk factors in IPs with serious mental illness that predict recidivism (Bonta et al., 2014; Carr et al., 2021; Lund et al., 2013; Skeem et al., 2014; Wilson et al., 2020). The criminogenic risk factors drawn from the RNR principles are the eight central risk and need factors: (a) criminal history, (b) pro-criminal companions, (c) pro-criminal attitudes and cognitions, (d) antisocial personality pattern, (e) education/employment, (f) family/marital, (g) substance abuse, and (h) leisure/recreation (Bonta & Andrews, 2016).

RNR-informed treatments adopt cognitive-behavioral therapy–based approaches such as cognitive skills training (e.g., identifying and addressing maladaptive, overly simplistic, judgmental, or pro-criminal thinking styles), emotional dysregulation (e.g., anger management), problem-solving skill development (internalized prosocial conflict resolution), and realignment of dysfunctional behavioral styles with prosocial norms. Behavior modification through reinforcement, modeling, or role rehearsal is a typical component. These programs are usually offered in group-based, psychoeducational formats and may be supplemented with more specific programs that target other common criminogenic needs such as substance use (Douglas et al., 2008).

In comprehensive reviews (Bewley & Morgan, 2011; Morgan et al., 2012), researchers evaluated 26 studies of treatment programs for 1,649 incarcerated men with mental illness in North American correctional institutions to examine the effectiveness of correctional interventions that adhered to the RNR principles of effective programming. The review found that effective programming addressed the co-occurring issues of mental illness and criminal recidivism. Effective treatments were intensive in nature and structured, often with a formal treatment manual, and incorporated cognitive-behavioral models with homework components and targeted criminogenic needs. Results suggest that these treatment interventions with incarcerated men with mental illness effectively reduced symptoms of distress, improving their ability to cope with their problems, and resulted in improved behavioral markers including institutional adjustment and reduced recidivism.

Another systematic review examined 21 studies of treatment programs for 1,175 IPs with serious and persistent mental illness (Parisi et al., 2022). All interventions targeted criminogenic risk factors, were group based, and used cognitive-behavioral therapy strategies. Results indicated that these treatment interventions reduced violence and recidivism. The review found that the most common treatment approach was to adapt and modify an existing evidence-based correctional intervention for those without serious mental illness to accommodate the needs of those with serious mental illness. This is consistent with the responsivity principle, which emphasizes the need to tailor evidence-based interventions to specific populations' learning and treatment needs. The challenges of implementing evidence-based practices are well articulated in a review of treatment services for persons with mental illness in the U.S. criminal justice system (Brandt, 2012). Indeed, the problems posed by high prevalence rates of mental illness, uneven availability and implementation of evidence-based programs, dearth of trained staff, difficulties in establishing and sustaining a therapeutic milieu and program fidelity, and fiscal constraints present barriers to the provision of evidence-based care in many, if not most, countries' correctional systems.

Summary

The clinical presentation of IPs with psychotic symptoms can be complex. Consequently, establishing a well-reasoned diagnosis of a psychotic disorder is the foundation for treatment. Clinical assessment in the correctional setting requires appropriate physical space to conduct interviews, adequate time, and privacy. Critical components of the diagnostic database are access to collateral information such as previous treatment records and behavioral observations from officers. Assessment should identify empirically derived criminogenic risk factors, including comorbid substance use disorders and personality disorders.

Although correctional resources, as well as security and administrative obstacles, can pose treatment challenges, there are clear evidence-informed treatment approaches drawn from the scientific and clinical literature that can help clinicians lead the way to optimal treatments for IPs with psychotic disorders. Psychopharmacological treatments should adhere to clinical practice guidelines. Provisions to prescribe clozapine and access nonformulary medications when needed should be available. Access to nonpharmacological psychiatric treatments such as electroconvulsive therapy should be available to address treatment-resistant psychosis, mania, and depression. Psychosocial interventions to address recidivism should follow the RNR principles and address both mental health recovery and criminogenic factors such as substance use disorder and personality disorder. Treatment should incorporate release planning, as IPs with psychotic disorders are at increased risk of gaps in treatment and relapse after release from a correctional setting. Coordination with reentry services is needed to maintain continuity of care and reduce the likelihood of recidivism.

REFERENCES

Aboaja, A., Pandurangi, P., Almeida, S., et al. (2023). Six nations: A clinical scenario comparison of systems for prisoners with psychosis in Australia, Bolivia and four European nations. *BJPsych International*, *20*(1), 13–17.

Adams, K., & Ferrandino, J. (2008). Managing mentally ill inmates in prisons. *Criminal Justice and Behavior*, *35*, 913–927.

American Psychiatric Association. (2022). *Diagnostic and statistical manual of mental disorders* (5th ed., text rev.).

Andrews, D. A., Bonta, J., & Hoge, R. D. (1990). Classification for effective rehabilitation: Rediscovering psychology. *Criminal Justice and Behavior*, *17*, 19–52.

Andrews, D. A., Zinger, I., Hoge, R. D., Bonta, J., Gendreau, P., & Cullen, F. T. (1990). Does correctional treatment work? A clinically relevant and psychologically informed meta-analysis. *Criminology*, *28*, 369–404.

Appelbaum, K. L., Hickey, J. M., & Packer, I. (2001). The role of correctional officers in multidisciplinary mental health care in prisons. *Psychiatric Services*, *52*, 1343–1347.

Arunogiri, S., McKetin, R., Verdejo-Garcia, A., & Lubman, D. I. (2020). The methamphetamine-associated psychosis spectrum: A clinically focused review. *International Journal of Mental Health and Addiction*, *18*(1), 54–65.

Balbuena, L., Mela, M., Wong, S., Gu, D., Adelugba, O., & Tempier, R. (2010). Does clozapine promote employability and reduce offending among mentally disordered offenders? *Canadian Journal of Psychiatry*, *55*, 50–56.

Baranyi, G., Fazel, S., Langerfeldt, S. D., & Mundt, A. P. (2022). The prevalence of comorbid serious mental illnesses and substance use disorders in prison populations: A systematic review and meta-analysis. *Lancet Public Health*, *7*(6), e557–e568.

Baranyi, G., Scholl, C., Fazel, S., Patel, V., Priebe, S., & Mundt, A. P. (2019). Severe mental illness and substance use disorders in prisoners in low-income and middle-income countries: A systematic review and meta-analysis of prevalence studies. *Lancet Global Health*, *7*(4), e461–e471.

Barnes, T. R., Drake, R., Paton, C., et al. (2020). Evidence-based guidelines for the pharmacological treatment of schizophrenia: Updated recommendations from the *British Association for Psychopharmacology*. *Journal of Psychopharmacology*, *34*(1), 3–78.

Bewley, M. T., & Morgan, R. D. (2011). A national survey of mental health services available to offenders with mental illness: Who is doing what? *Law and Human Behavior*, *35*, 351–363.

Bhavsar, V., Kosidou, K., Widman, L., et al. (2020). Clozapine treatment and offending: A within-subject study of patients with psychotic disorders in Sweden. *Schizophrenia Bulletin*, *46*(2), 303–310.

Blaauw, E., Roozen, H. G., & Marle, H. G. C. (2007). Saved by structure? The course of psychosis within a prison population. *International Journal of Prisoner Health*, *3*, 248–256.

Bonta, J., & Andrews, D. A. (2016). *The psychology of criminal conduct* (6th ed.). Routledge.

Bonta, J., Blais, J., & Wilson, H. A. (2014). A theoretically informed meta-analysis of the risk for general and violent recidivism for mentally disordered offenders. *Aggression and Violent Behavior*, *19*(3), 278–287.

Brandt, A. L. S. (2012). Treatment of persons with mental illness in the criminal justice system: A literature review. *Journal of Offender Rehabilitation*, *51*, 541–558.

Brown, G. P., Stewart, L. A., Rabinowitz, T., Boudreau, H., & Wright, A. J. (2018). Approved and off-label use of prescribed psychotropic medications among federal Canadian inmates. *Canadian Journal of Psychiatry*, *63*(10), 683–691.

Carey, L., & Barlow, S. (2022). Review of antipsychotic prescribing at HMP/YOI Low Newton. *BJPsych Bulletin*, *46*(1), 26–32.

Carr, W. A., Baker, A. N., & Cassidy, J. J. (2021). Diagnostic moderators of the risk-recidivism relationship for offenders with mental illness. *International Journal of Offender Therapy and Comparative Criminology*, *65*(16), 1756–1774.

Chang, Z., Lichtenstein, P., Långström, N., Larsson, H., & Fazel, S. (2016). Association between prescription of major psychotropic medications and violent reoffending after prison release. *JAMA*, *316*(17), 1798–1807.

Collins, N., Avondoglio, J. B., & Terry, L. M. (2017). Correctional psychopharmacology: Pitfalls, challenges, and victories of prescribing in a correctional setting. *International Review of Psychiatry*, *29*(1), 34–44.

Douglas, K. S., Nicholls, T. L., & Brink, J. (2008). Psychological/behavioural treatment of the potentially violent patient. In P. Kleespies (Ed.), *Evaluating and managing behavioral emergencies: An evidence-based resource for the mental health practitioner* (p. 290). American Psychiatric Association Books.

Fazel, S., & Danesh, J. (2002). Serious mental disorder in 23 000 prisoners: A systematic review of 62 surveys. *The Lancet*, *359*, 545–550.

Fazel, S., & Seewald, K. (2012). Severe mental illness in 33 588 prisoners worldwide: Systematic review and meta-regression analysis. *British Journal of Psychiatry*, *200*(5), 364–373.

Fazel, S., Zetterqvist, J., Larsson, H., Långström, N., & Lichtenstein, P. (2014). Antipsychotics, mood stabilisers, and risk of violent crime. *The Lancet*, *384*(9949), 1206–1214.

Felson, R. B., Silver, E., & Remster, B. (2012). Mental disorder and offending in prison. *Criminal Justice and Behavior*, *39*, 125–143.

Gabrysch, C., Sepúlveda, C., Bienzobas, C., & Mundt, A. P. (2020). "Maybe it is only in prison that I could change like this": The course of severe mental illnesses during imprisonment—A qualitative 3-year follow-up study from Chile. *Frontiers in Psychology*, *11*, 514611.

Gendreau, P., & Goggin, C. (1996). Principles of effective programming with offenders. *Forum on Corrections Research*, *8*, 38–40.

Gendreau, P., Little, T., & Goggin, C. (1996). A meta-analysis of the predictors of adult recidivism: What works! *Criminology*, *34*, 401–433.

Glancy, G., Tomita, T., Waldman, J., et al. (2020). *Practice resource for prescribing in corrections*. Canadian Academy of Psychiatry and the Law. http://www.capl-acpd.org/wp-content/uploads/2020/03/CAPL-Rx-Guide-Corrections-FIN-EN-Web.pdf

Glasner-Edwards, S., & Mooney, L. J. (2014). Methamphetamine psychosis: Epidemiology and management. *CNS Drugs*, *28*, 1115–1126.

Griffiths, E. V., Willis, J., & Spark, M. J. (2012). A systematic review of psychotropic drug prescribing for prisoners. *Australian and New Zealand Journal of Psychiatry*, *46*, 407–421.

Hassan, L., Senior, J., Edge, D., & Shaw, J. (2011). Continuity of supply of psychiatric medicines for newly received prisoners. *The Psychiatrist*, *35*, 244–248.

Hervás, G., Ruano, C., Sanz-Alfayate, G., Algora, I., Celdran, M. A., & Mur, M. A. (2019). Analysis of the management of antipsychotics in a group of prisons. *Revista espanola de sanidad penitenciaria*, *21*(2), 88–94.

Jones, R. M., Gerritsen, C., Maheandiran, M., Penney, S., & Simpson, A. I. (2023). Change in severity of mental disorder of remand prisoners: An observational group-based trajectory study. *Canadian Journal of Psychiatry*, *68*(6), 418–425.

Keepers, G. A., Fochtmann, L. J., Anzia, J. M., et al. (2020). The American Psychiatric Association practice guideline for the treatment of patients with schizophrenia. *American Journal of Psychiatry*, *177*(9), 868–872.

Lecomte, T., Mueser, K. T., MacEwan, W., et al. (2013). Predictors of persistent psychotic symptoms in persons with methamphetamine abuse receiving psychiatric treatment. *Journal of Nervous and Mental Disease*, *201*, 1085–1089.

Lund, C., Hofvander, B., Forsman, A., Anckarsäter, H., & Nilsson, T. (2013). Violent criminal recidivism in mentally disordered offenders: A follow-up study of 13–20 years through different sanctions. *International Journal of Law and Psychiatry*, *36*(3–4), 250–257.

Martin, A., O'Driscoll, C., & Samuels, A. (2008). Clozapine use in a forensic population in a New South Wales prison hospital. *Australian and New Zealand Journal of Psychiatry*, *42*, 141–146.

Mela, M., & Depiang, G. (2016). Clozapine's effect on recidivism among offenders with mental disorders. *Journal of the American Academy of Psychiatry and the Law*, *44*, 82–90.

Morgan, R. D., Flora, D. B., Kroner, D. G., Mills, J., Varghese, F., & Steffan, J. S. (2012). Treating offenders with mental illness: A research synthesis. *Law and Human Behavior*, *36*, 37–50.

Morgan, R. D., Scanlon, F., & Van Horn, S. A. (2020). Criminogenic risk and mental health: A complicated relationship. *CNS Spectrums*, *25*(2), 237–244.

National Institute for Clinical Excellence. (2014). *Psychosis and schizophrenia in adults: prevention and management. NICE guidelines.*

O'Keefe, M. A., & Schnell, M. J. (2007). Offenders with mental illness in the correctional system. *Journal of Offender Rehabilitation*, *45*, 81–104.

Parisi, A., Wilson, A. B., Villodas, M., Phillips, J., & Dohler, E. (2022). A systematic review of interventions targeting criminogenic risk factors among persons with serious mental illness. *Psychiatric Services*, *73*(8), 897–909.

Pelizza, L., Davide, M., Giuseppina, P., & Pietro, P. (2022). Prevalence and appropriateness of antipsychotic prescribing in an Italian prison: Is everything always really overprescribed? *Journal of Clinical Psychopharmacology*, *42*(1), 31–36.

Pruette, M. E., Zarzar, T. R., & Sheitman, B. B. (2023). Expanding clozapine use in state prisons: A review of the North Carolina experience. *Journal of Correctional Health Care*, *29*(2), 109–114.

Remington, G., Addington, D., Honer, W., Ismail, Z., Raedler, T., & Teehan, M. (2017). Guidelines for the pharmacotherapy of schizophrenia in adults. *Canadian Journal of Psychiatry*, *62*(9), 604–616.

Scott, C. L. (2010). *Handbook of correctional mental health* (2nd ed.). American Psychiatric Publishing.

Sekiguchi, Y., Okada, T., & Okumura, Y. (2021). Treatment response distinguishes persistent type of methamphetamine psychosis from schizophrenia spectrum disorder among inmates at Japanese medical prison. *Frontiers in Psychiatry*, *19*(12), 629315.

Skeem, J. L., Steadman, H. J., & Manchak, S. M. (2015). Applicability of the risk-need-responsivity model to persons with mental illness involved in the criminal justice system. *Psychiatric Services*, *66*(9), 916–922.

Skeem, J. L., Winter, E., Kennealy, P. J., Louden, J. E., & Tatar, J. R., II. (2014). Offenders with mental illness have criminogenic needs, too: Toward recidivism reduction. *Law and Human Behavior*, *38*(3), 212–224.

Tamburello, A., Penn, J., Ford, E., et al. (2022). The American Academy of Psychiatry and the Law practice resource for prescribing in corrections. *Journal of the American Academy of Psychiatry and the Law*, *50*(4), 636–637.

Taylor, P. J., Walker, J., Dunn, E., Kissell, A., Williams, A., & Amos, T. (2010). Improving mental state in early imprisonment. *Criminal Behaviour and Mental Health*, *20*, 215–231.

Tiihonen, J., Taipale, H., Mehtälä, J., Vattulainen, P., Correll, C. U., & Tanskanen, A. (2019). Association of antipsychotic polypharmacy vs monotherapy with psychiatric rehospitalization among adults with schizophrenia. *JAMA Psychiatry*, *76*(5), 499–507.

Ujike, H., & Sato, M. (2004). Clinical features of sensitization to methamphetamine observed in patients with methamphetamine dependence and psychosis. *Annals of the New York Academy of Sciences*, *21*, 279–287.

Whiting, D., Gulati, G., Geddes, J. R., & Fazel, S. (2022). Association of schizophrenia spectrum disorders and violence perpetration in adults and adolescents from 15 countries: A systematic review and meta-analysis. *JAMA Psychiatry*, *79*(2), 120–132.

Wilson, A. B., Ishler, K. J., Morgan, R., Phillips, J., Draine, J., & Farkas, K. J. (2020). Examining criminogenic risk levels among people with mental illness incarcerated in US jails and prisons. *Journal of Behavioral Health Services & Research*. Advance online publication. https://doi.org/10.1007/s11414-020-09737-x

World Health Organization. (2021). *International statistical classification of diseases and related health problems* (11th ed.).

33

Mood disorders

*Jayesh Kamath and Brian Wasicek**

Introduction

Mood disorders have long been a part of humanity's historical narrative; more than 2,000 years ago Hippocrates wrote, "If fear or distress last for a long time it is melancholia." Mood disorders refer to a broad category that encompasses unipolar depressive disorders and bipolar disorders (BDs; American Psychiatric Association, 2022). Decades of research conducted in community and correctional settings have shown close but controversial relationships between mood disorders, aggression, and criminality. This chapter reviews some of these relationships and presents best practice and evidence-based approaches to the correctional management and treatment of mood disorders.

Epidemiology

A systematic review summarizing 28 studies conducted in state prison settings found wide variations in prevalence estimates of mood disorders (Prins, 2014). The prevalence of major depressive disorder (MDD) ranged between 9% and 29%, and that of BD ranged between 5.5% and 16% (Prins, 2014). The variations in prevalence estimates were due to heterogeneity of sampling strategies, data collection, study designs, diagnostic instruments used, operationalization of mental illness, and other methodological differences. Despite these variations, the review confirmed that the prevalence rates for mood disorders were substantially higher in U.S. state prisons compared to community settings (Prins, 2014). The 2011–2012 National Inmate Survey conducted in state and federal prisons and jails used self-reports gathered from 106,532 incarcerated persons (IPs). It revealed that 24% of IPs in prison and 30% of IPs in jail reported having MDD, and 17% of IPs in prison and 24% of IPs in jail reported having BD (Bronson & Berzofsky, 2017). Cassau and Goodwin (2012) found high rates of moderate to severe depression (41.7%) in German pretrial detainees using psychometric instruments, though the authors cautioned that some items like "loss of libido" and "loss of interest" were confounded by their situation and that most subjects (76.1%) improved in a second assessment 3 weeks later.

Studies suggest a higher prevalence of MDD in female IPs than male IPs (Fazel & Seewald, 2012). High rates and severity of depression have also been found in pregnant and postpartum women who gave birth in prison (Howland et al., 2021). Gunter and colleagues (2008) reported no gender-based differences for other major mood disorders (e.g., dysthymia, BDs). Compared to their counterparts in community settings, elderly IPs have 2.8 times higher rates of depression and 4.9 times higher rates of BD (Di Lorito et al., 2018). Domalanta and colleagues (2003) reported high rates of depressive symptoms (47%) and MDD (9.8%) in incarcerated youths (Domalanta et al., 2003).

A persistent and bidirectional relationship exists between mood disorders and incarceration (Fovet et al., 2015; Schnittker et al., 2012). The 12-month prevalence of MDD and BD was much higher in individuals with a history of incarceration compared to those without (MDD, 9.2% versus 6.4%; BD, 5.8% versus 2.5%; Schnittker et al., 2012). Conversely, incarceration was associated with a 45% increase in the odds of lifetime MDD (Schnittker et al., 2012). Incarceration also showed strong associations with other mood disorders, especially dysthymia and BD (Schnittker et al., 2012). Schnittker and colleagues (2012) also reported that incarceration was related to a higher risk of subsequent mood disorders, and these disorders in turn were strongly related to increased disability. A recent national longitudinal cohort study confirmed these findings, with individuals with prior incarceration having higher rates of depression and lower quality of life at age 50 (Bovell-Ammon et al., 2023).

The consequences of confinement related to social determinants of health play a critical role in the close, bidirectional relationship between incarceration and depression (Turney et al., 2012). Results from the Fragile Families and Child Wellbeing Study indicate that the association between the two is also related to the well-known consequences and negative impact of incarceration on socioeconomic status, family functioning, and social and economic integration (Turney et al., 2012).

Mood disorders may also play an important role in recidivism. The frequency of criminal acts is higher in patients with BD, especially when comorbid with substance use disorders (SUDs; Fovet et al., 2015). Baillargeon, Binswanger, and colleagues (2009) reported that IPs with BD were 3.3 times more likely to have had four or more

*. The authors acknowledge the contributions of Ajay Shah, MD, who coauthored this chapter in the textbook's first edition.

previous incarcerations compared with IPs who had no major psychiatric disorders. Zgoba and colleagues (2020) found that 55% of IPs with mood disorders were rearrested within 3 years of release, but differences were only significant when SUDs were comorbid. Regardless, other research suggests that each period of incarceration increases the risk for and severity of subsequent mood disorders (Schnittker et al., 2012).

Comorbidities

SUDs represent the most common comorbidity in IPs with mood disorders. Baranyi and colleagues (2022), in a systematic review and meta-analysis, reported that the prevalence of MDD and comorbid SUDs (9.1%) was about twice as high in prison populations as in community samples. Studies have also consistently shown higher rates of SUDs in IPs with BDs compared with those with other mood disorders or other serious mental illness. In male detainees, rates of co-occurring SUDs were higher among persons with BD than those with unipolar depression (Abram & Teplin, 1991).

Anxiety disorders and impulse control disorders are also highly comorbid with mood disorders. Lifetime prevalence of an anxiety disorder was seen in 86.7% of bipolar I patients and 89.2% of bipolar II patients. Compared to the general population, patients with bipolar I disorder have more than a sevenfold increase in lifetime prevalence of intermittent explosive disorder (38.1% compared to 5.2%; Kessler et al., 2005; Merikangas et al., 2007). In general, patients with BDs also have high rates of comorbid personality disorders, specifically antisocial and borderline personality disorder (Lenzenweger et al., 2007).

Coexistence of personality and impulse control disorders with mood disorders, especially BD, can present unique management challenges in the correctional setting. Inadequate symptom control, combined with difficulties adapting to the correctional environment, can exacerbate maladaptive behaviors, including aggression (toward peers, correctional officers, and other staff; see Chapter 53) or self-injurious behaviors, both with and without suicidal intent (see Chapter 52). Consequently, IPs with serious mental illness are more likely to be charged with facility rule violations or infractions and, as a result, serve longer sentences (James & Glaze, 2006). The relationship between mood disorders and violent behaviors is complex (Lamb & Weinberger, 2011). While it is generally accepted that most persons with serious mental illness are no more dangerous than the general population, a subgroup of patients with certain co-occurring disorders (e.g., BD combined with recent substance use) are at greater risk for violence (Fovet et al., 2015). This is especially concerning when symptoms are inadequately controlled in a stressful environment such as a correctional setting (Lamb & Weinberger, 2011).

Individuals with serious mental illness and an incarceration history are much more vulnerable to traumatic life experiences than the general population. Social instability and other socioeconomic challenges increase the likelihood of traumatic experiences, including physical abuse, violent assaults, and sexual victimization (Gunter et al., 2012; Reed et al., 2009). Studies conducted in correctional settings further suggest a close relationship between traumatic experiences, mood disorders, and criminal behavior (Green et al., 2016; Gunter et al., 2012; Özsoy et al., 2022; Reed et al., 2009). Posttraumatic stress disorder (PTSD) is also highly comorbid with mood disorders in incarcerated individuals, again especially women (Binswanger et al., 2010; Gunter et al., 2012; see Chapter 36).

IPs with mood disorders have frequent medical comorbidities (Binswanger et al., 2010). These are partially the result of socioeconomic factors such as social instability and poor nutrition. Antipsychotics and mood stabilizers used in the management of mood disorders are known to increase the risk of weight gain and metabolic syndrome (Vancampfort et al., 2013). Conversely, Murdoch and colleagues (2008) found higher rates of depression in IPs with chronic medical conditions (Murdoch et al., 2008).

Although not a comorbidity per se, socioeconomic disadvantages have major and direct contributions to the management and prognosis of mood disorders in the correctional setting (Fontanarosa et al., 2013). Addressing problems like homelessness, unemployment, underemployment, inadequate education, and access to entitlements can lead to improved outcomes during transition to the community (see Chapter 23).

Suicide risk

Studies conducted with both men and women in correctional settings have shown a strong association between depression and near-lethal suicide attempts (Marzano et al., 2010; Rivlin et al., 2010). Related individual factors include recent life events; past trauma; childhood abuse; family history of suicide; high scores on measures of depression, anxiety, aggression, impulsivity, and hostility; and low levels of self-esteem and social support (Lekka et al., 2006; Marzano et al., 2011). Prison-related factors include being returned to custody from parole or probation, being housed alone, and negative prison experiences (Marzano et al., 2011; Reeves & Tamburello, 2014). Baillargeon, Penn, and colleagues (2009) reported an elevated risk of completed suicide in patients with MDD and BD in the Texas prison system. See Chapter 51 for a more extensive discussion of suicide risk and management.

Assessment

IPs with mood disorders present diagnostic challenges like those in the community, such as differentiating between unipolar and bipolar depression and between primary and secondary (e.g., substance-induced) mood disorders. IPs may have diagnostic confounders not seen elsewhere, most often in the first months after arrest. Use of substances prior to and withdrawal from substances early during incarceration may cause or exacerbate mood and anxiety symptoms. Similarly, distress associated with incarceration, disappointments with court decisions, guilt, feelings of abandonment toward loved ones in the community, and adjustment to the correctional environment can cause or exacerbate mood symptoms. Loss of freedom, in some cases indefinitely, can lead to grieving with prominent anger and despair. When transient and subsyndromic, these symptoms may be better characterized as adjustment disorder (see Chapter 34). Withdrawal from substances can present with mood lability, which may lead to a misdiagnosis of BD. Given the overlap between negative feelings in MDD and PTSD, extensive traumatic histories may complicate a mood disorder diagnosis. Some of these confounders, like PTSD and SUDs, are not mutually exclusive (American Psychiatric Association, 2022).

These unique diagnostic challenges require correctional clinicians to adapt their assessment and management strategies. Like the community setting, differentiating between primary and secondary disorders is the key first step. A single cross-sectional clinical interview is frequently inadequate and can lead to misdiagnosis. Critical elements of appropriate correctional diagnostic assessments include comprehensive and longitudinal evaluation of past mood episodes; evidence of mood episodes during substance-free periods; typical symptoms experienced during substance withdrawal; prior therapeutic trials and estimates of adherence to treatment; and contribution of psychiatric and medical comorbidities to current mood symptoms, including the impact of traumatic experiences. Assessment of psychosocial factors and their contribution to presenting symptoms is crucial in any diagnostic assessment.

It is frequently necessary to consider other sources such as past medical or psychiatric records; reports from community providers; and information from family, friends, or other loved ones. Communication with a community pharmacy regarding recent medications and dates of refills can provide valuable data (see Chapter 18). Laboratory assessments such as substance screens, metabolic panels, and thyroid function tests are also helpful at intake to consider substance-related and medical disorders in the differential diagnosis. Like psychiatric medications, inadequate access to medications used to treat medical comorbidities (e.g., insulin, antihypertensives) and nonadherence with these medications are common problems in the community (Kini & Ho, 2018), so these may be relevant concerns for IPs coming from the community. Furthermore, many IPs do not have primary care physicians or may miss medical appointments. Exacerbation or inadequate control of medical conditions may present as symptoms of mood disorders (see Chapter 39).

Reassessment of symptoms at every visit, especially in the first few months of incarceration, enhances diagnostic accuracy. As above, the clinical picture frequently evolves over weeks to months, often for the better, as symptoms of substance withdrawal resolve and the IP adjusts to the environment.

Assessment of mood disorders in IPs should consider factors that may complicate treatment and prognosis. The Systematic Treatment Enhancement Program for Bipolar Disorder study showed that in community samples, comorbid anxiety can increase severity, negatively impact recovery, increase suicide risk, and significantly worsen the prognosis of a mood episode (Simon et al., 2007). BD patients with mixed features, compared with those with classic presentations, are more difficult to manage, have worse prognoses, and are significantly more likely to have an early age of onset, rapid cycling in the past year, bipolar I subtype, history of suicide attempts, and more days in the preceding year with irritability or mood elevation (Goldberg et al., 2009). In this context, it is notable that IPs with BD, especially incarcerated men, frequently present in mixed states with high comorbid anxiety (Kamath et al., 2013). Irritability and agitation are commonly seen in IPs who present with depression. Such "agitated depression," whether unipolar or bipolar in nature, is frequently resistant to treatment, with higher behavioral risks, including an increased risk of suicidal behaviors (Swann, 2013).

Use of standardized assessments in correctional settings is helpful given the complexities discussed. Such assessments are rarely used there in practice due to lack of resources, funding, and time (Easton et al., 2008). The Structured Clinical Interview for DSM-5-TR (*Diagnostic and Statistical Manual of Mental Disorders*, fifth edition, text revision) is considered the gold standard for diagnostic assessment (American Psychiatric Association, 2022). It is a useful research tool but often too time-consuming for clinical use. Prison studies have evaluated structured instruments such as the Mini-International Neuropsychiatric Interview (MINI) or the MINI-Plus (Falissard et al., 2006; Gunter et al., 2008). Butcher and colleagues (2021) found that the Patient Health Questionnaire-9 may overdiagnose depressive episodes in prisoners (Butcher et al., 2021). In another study, a brief version of the Center for Epidemiological Studies–Depression scale was useful for detecting depression in a group of IPs in jail (Juarros-Basterretxea et al., 2021). Screening tools should be used to complement a comprehensive interview and not as a substitute for it.

Management

Like the management of mood disorders in the community, both pharmacotherapy and psychotherapy play critical roles in the treatment of mood disorders in correctional settings (Tamburello et al., 2022). Treatment planning should account for psychiatric comorbidities (e.g., PTSD, SUDs), medical comorbidities (including the possibility of pregnancy), and other complicating factors (e.g., psychosocial; Friedman et al., 2019). Other considerations include the individual's psychotropic medication regimen in the community, including any medications with withdrawal risks (e.g., selective serotonin reuptake inhibitors) and drug–drug interactions. IPs with diagnosed mood disorders who are withdrawing from substances or experiencing a significant exacerbation of symptoms might require short-term, heightened symptomatic management with anxiolytics and in some cases mood stabilizers. Substance withdrawal protocols should be implemented when required (see Chapter 46). As above, the symptomatology might change as symptoms related to adjustment or substance withdrawal resolve. Continuous symptom and diagnostic reevaluation should drive optimization of medication regimens, considering both risks and benefits.

In a study conducted in the Connecticut Department of Correction, algorithm-driven treatment of BD demonstrated significant benefits, including improved clinical outcomes, improved quality of life, and reduced polypharmacy by optimizing utilization of evidence-based medications (Ehret et al., 2013; Kamath et al., 2013). Correctional formularies are frequently restricted to manage costs, enhance consistency of care, and, at times, prevent the risk of misuse and diversion of prescribed medications (Morris et al., 2020; see Chapter 27). Correctional clinicians can have access to nonformulary medications with special approval but are generally expected to work within formulary restrictions. Kamath and colleagues (2013) reported the effectiveness and benefits of algorithm-driven treatment of BD while working within formulary restrictions. During the implementation process, researchers had to accommodate certain variations to the algorithm to be consistent with formulary restrictions (Kamath et al., 2010). The implementation was successful despite restrictions, partially because the algorithm included several medication options. While not a practice guideline, interested readers are referred to the American Academy of Psychiatry and the Law's Practice Resource for Prescribing in Corrections for a discussion of community practice guidelines on pharmacotherapy for mood disorders as applied to these settings (Tamburello et al., 2022).

Psychotherapy, either as monotherapy or adjunctive treatment, can play a critical role in managing mood disorders in the correctional setting. Individual or group psychotherapy can be very helpful in managing the despair of incarceration and in improving coping skills. Psychotherapies such as cognitive-behavioral therapy, interpersonal psychotherapy, and dialectical behavioral therapy have been adapted to treat offenders with serious mental illness (Johnson et al., 2019; Yoon et al., 2017; see Chapters 42 and 43).

Discharge planning

Mood disorders are often recurrent and sometimes chronic or even lifelong. Planning for transition to the community upon release is critical to ensure successful reentry and integration of IPs with mood disorders, and thus to reduce recidivism (see Chapter 23). Crucial aspects of release planning include arranging continuity of clinical care via appointments with providers in the community, ensuring access to medications immediately after release, and addressing socioeconomic needs (including access to health insurance) in a comprehensive manner.

Summary

IPs with mood disorders present significant diagnostic and treatment challenges to correctional clinicians due to higher severity of symptoms, complex psychiatric and medical comorbidities, complicated psychosocial challenges, higher risk of suicidality, and frequent involvement in the criminal justice system. Brief but structured diagnostic assessments and the use of evidence-based treatments including pharmacotherapy and psychotherapy can significantly improve management and outcomes for IPs with mood disorders.

REFERENCES

Abram, K. M., & Teplin, L. A. (1991). Co-occurring disorders among mentally ill jail detainees. Implications for public policy. *American Psychologist*, *46*(10), 1036–1045.

American Psychiatric Association. (2022). *Diagnostic and statistical manual of mental disorders* (5th ed., text rev.).

Baillargeon, J., Binswanger, I. A., Penn, J. V., Williams, B. A., & Murray, O. J. (2009). Psychiatric disorders and repeat incarcerations: The revolving prison door. *American Journal of Psychiatry*, *166*(1), 103–109.

Baillargeon, J., Penn, J. V., Thomas, C. R., Temple, J. R., Baillargeon, G., & Murray, O. J. (2009). Psychiatric disorders and suicide in the nation's largest state prison system. *Journal of the American Academy of Psychiatry and the Law*, *37*(2), 188–193.

Baranyi, G., Fazel, S., Langerfeldt, S. D., & Mundt, A. P. (2022). The prevalence of comorbid serious mental illnesses and substance use disorders in prison populations: A systematic review and meta-analysis. *Lancet Public Health*, *7*(6), e557–e568.

Binswanger, I. A., Merrill, J. O., Krueger, P. M., White, M. C., Booth, R. E., & Elmore, J. G. (2010). Gender differences in chronic medical, psychiatric, and substance-dependence disorders among jail inmates. *American Journal of Public Health*, *100*(3), 476–482.

Bovell-Ammon, B. J., Fox, A. D., & LaRochelle, M. R. (2023). Prior incarceration is associated with poor mental health at midlife: Findings from a National Longitudinal Cohort Study. *Journal of General Internal Medicine*, *38*(7), 1664–1671.

Bronson, J., & Berzofsky, M. (2017). *Special report: Indicators of mental health problems reported by prisoners and jail inmates, 2011–12.* U.S. Department of Justice. https://bjs.ojp.gov/content/pub/pdf/imhprpji1112.pdf

Butcher, E., Packham, C., Williams, M., et al. (2021). Screening male prisoners for depression and anxiety with the PHQ-9 and GAD-7 at NHS Healthcheck: Patterns of symptoms and caseness threshold. *BMC Psychiatry*, *21*(1), 446.

Cassau, J. S., & Goodwin, D. E. (2012). The phenomenology and course of depressive syndromes in pre-trial detention. *International Journal of Law and Psychiatry*, *35*(3), 231–235.

Di Lorito, C., Vollm, B., & Dening, T. (2018). Psychiatric disorders among older prisoners: A systematic review and comparison study against older people in the community. *Aging & Mental Health*, *22*(1), 1–10.

Domalanta, D. D., Risser, W. L., Roberts, R. E., & Risser, J. M. H. (2003). Prevalence of depression and other psychiatric disorders among incarcerated youths. *Journal of the American Academy of Child and Adolescent Psychiatry*, *42*(4), 477–484.

Easton, C. J., Devine, S., Scott, M., & Wupperman, P. (2008). Commentary: Implications for assessment and treatment of addictive and mentally disordered offenders entering prisons. *Journal of the American Academy of Psychiatry and the Law*, *36*(1), 35–37.

Ehret, M. J., Shelton, D., Barta, W., et al. (2013). Medication adherence among female inmates with bipolar disorder: Results from a randomized controlled trial. *Psychological Services*, *10*(1), 106–114.

Falissard, B., Loze, J. Y., Gasquet, I., et al. (2006). Prevalence of mental disorders in French prisons for men. *BMC Psychiatry*, *6*, 33–40.

Fazel, S., & Seewald, K. (2012). Severe mental illness in 33,588 prisoners worldwide: Systematic review and meta-regression analysis. *British Journal of Psychiatry*, *200*(5), 364–373.

Fontanarosa, J., Uhl, S., Oyesanmi, O., & Schoelles, K. M. (2013). *Interventions for adult offenders with serious mental illness.* Agency for Healthcare Research and Quality. https://www.ncbi.nlm.nih.gov/books/NBK158915/

Fovet, T., Geoffroy, P. A., Vaiva, G., Adins, C., Thomas, P., & Amad, A. (2015). Individuals with bipolar disorder and their relationship with the criminal justice system: A critical review. *Psychiatric Services*, *66*(4), 348–353.

Friedman, S. H., Tamburello, A. C., Kaempf, A., & Hall, R. C. W. (2019). Prescribing for women in corrections. *Journal of the American Academy of Psychiatry and the Law*, *47*(4), 476–485.

Goldberg, J. F., Perlis, R. H., Bowden, C. L., et al. (2009). Manic symptoms during depressive episodes in 1,380 patients with bipolar disorder: Findings from the STEP-BD. *American Journal of Psychiatry*, *166*(2), 173–181.

Green, B. L., Dass-Brailsford, P., Hurtado de Mendoza, A., et al. (2016). Trauma experiences and mental health among incarcerated women. *Journal of Psychological Trauma*, *8*(4), 455–463.

Gunter, T. D., Arndt, S., Wenman, G., et al. (2008). Frequency of mental and addictive disorders among 320 men and women entering the Iowa prison system: Use of the MINI-Plus. *Journal of the American Academy of Psychiatry and the Law*, *36*(1), 27–34.

Gunter, T. D., Chibnall, J. T., Antoniak, S. K., McCormick, B., & Black, D. W. (2012). Relative contributions of gender and traumatic life experience to the prediction of mental disorders in a sample of incarcerated offenders. *Behavioral Sciences and the Law*, *30*(5), 615–630.

Howland, M. A., Kotlar, B., Davis, L., et al. (2021). Depressive symptoms among pregnant and postpartum women in prison. *Journal of Midwifery & Women's Health*, *66*(4), 494–502.

James, D. J., & Glaze, L. E. (2006). *Special report: Mental health problems of prison and jail inmates*. U.S. Department of Justice. https://www.loc.gov/item/2023692130/.

Johnson, J. E., Stout, R. L., Miller, T. R., et al. (2019). Randomized cost-effectiveness trial of group interpersonal psychotherapy (IPT) for prisoners with major depression. *Journal of Consulting and Clinical Psychology*, *87*(4), 392–406.

Juarros-Basterretxea, J., Escoda-Menéndez, P., Vilariño, M., Rodríguez-Díaz, F. J., & Herrero, J. (2021). Using the CES-D-7 as a screening instrument to detect major depression among the inmate population. *International Journal of Environmental Research and Public Health*, *18*(3), 1361.

Kamath, J., Temporini, H., Quarti, S., et al. (2010). Best practices: Disseminating best practices for bipolar disorder treatment in a correctional population. *Psychiatric Services*, *61*(9), 865–867.

Kamath, J., Zhang, W., Kesten, K., Wakai, S., Shelton, D., & Trestman, R. (2013). Algorithm-driven pharmacological management of bipolar disorder in Connecticut prisons. *International Journal of Offender Therapy and Comparative Criminology*, *57*(2), 251–264.

Kessler, R. C., Berglund, P., Demler, O., Jin, R., Merikangas, K. R., & Walters, E. E. (2005). Lifetime prevalence and age-of-onset distributions of DSM-IV disorders in the National Comorbidity Survey Replication. *Archives of General Psychiatry*, *62*(6), 593–602.

Kini, V., & Ho, P. M. (2018). Interventions to improve medication adherence: A review. *JAMA*, *320*(23), 2461–2473.

Lamb, H. R., & Weinberger, L. E. (2011). Meeting the needs of those persons with serious mental illness who are most likely to become criminalized. *Journal of the American Academy of Psychiatry and the Law*, *39*(4), 549–554.

Lekka, N. P., Argyriou, A. A., & Beratis, S. (2006). Suicidal ideation in prisoners: Risk factors and relevance to suicidal behaviour. A prospective case-control study. *European Archives of Psychiatry and Clinical Neuroscience*, *256*(2), 87–92.

Lenzenweger, M. F., Lane, M. C., Loranger, A. W., & Kessler, R. C. (2007). DSM-IV personality disorders in the National Comorbidity Survey Replication. *Biological Psychiatry*, *62*(6), 553–564.

Marzano, L., Fazel, S., Rivlin, A., & Hawton, K. (2010). Psychiatric disorders in women prisoners who have engaged in near-lethal self-harm: Case-control study. *British Journal of Psychiatry*, *197*(3), 219–226.

Marzano, L., Hawton, K., Rivlin, A., & Fazel, S. (2011). Psychosocial influences on prisoner suicide: A case-control study of near-lethal self-harm in women prisoners. *Social Science and Medicine*, *72*(6), 874–883.

Merikangas, R. C., Akiskal, H. S., Angst, J., et al. (2007). Lifetime and 12-month prevalence of bipolar spectrum disorder in the National Comorbidity Survey Replication. *Archives of General Psychiatry*, *64*(5), 543–552.

Morris, N. P., Hirschtritt, M. E., & Tamburello, A. C. (2020). Drug formularies in correctional settings. *Journal of the American Academy of Psychiatry and the Law*, *48*(1), 2–6.

Murdoch, N., Morris, P., & Holmes, C. (2008). Depression in elderly life sentence prisoners. *International Journal of Geriatric Psychiatry*, *23*(9), 957–962.

Özsoy, F., Taşcı, G., & Atmaca, M. (2022). Investigating the association of criminal behavior with childhood traumas, impulsivity, and dominant temperaments in bipolar I disorder. *Primary Care Companion for CNS Disorders*, *24*(4), 21m03103.

Prins, S. J. (2014). Prevalence of mental illnesses in US state prisons: A systematic review. *Psychiatric Services*, *65*(7), 862–872.

Reed, E., Raj, A., Falbo, G., et al. (2009). The prevalence of violence and relation to depression and illicit drug use among incarcerated women in Recife, Brazil. *International Journal of Law and Psychiatry*, *32*(5), 323–328.

Reeves, R., & Tamburello, A. (2014). Single cells, segregated housing, and suicide in the New Jersey Department of Corrections. *Journal of the American Academy of Psychiatry and the Law*, *42*(4), 484–488.

Rivlin, A., Hawton, K., Marzano, L., & Fazel, S. (2010). Psychiatric disorders in male prisoners who made near-lethal suicide attempts: Case-control study. *British Journal of Psychiatry*, *197*(4), 313–319.

Schnittker, J., Massoglia, M., & Uggen, C. (2012). Out and down: Incarceration and psychiatric disorders. *Journal of Health and Social Behavior*, *53*(4), 448–464.

Simon, N. M., Zalta, A. K., Otto, M. W., et al. (2007). The association of comorbid anxiety disorders with suicide attempts and suicidal ideation in outpatients with bipolar disorder. *Journal of Psychiatric Research*, *41*(3–4), 255–264.

Swann, A. C. (2013). Activated depression: Mixed bipolar disorder or agitated unipolar depression? *Current Psychiatry Reports*, *15*(8), 376.

Tamburello, A., Penn, J., Ford, E., et al. (2022). The American Academy of Psychiatry and the Law practice resource for prescribing in corrections. *Journal of the American Academy of Psychiatry and the Law*, *50*(4), 636–637.

Turney, K., Wildeman, C., & Schnittker, J. J. (2012). As fathers and felons: Explaining the effects of current and recent incarceration on major depression. *Journal of Health and Social Behavior*, *53*(4), 465–481.

Vancampfort, D., Vansteelandt, K., Correll, C. U., et al. (2013). Metabolic syndrome and metabolic abnormalities in bipolar disorder: A meta-analysis of prevalence rates and moderators. *American Journal of Psychiatry*, *170*, 265–274.

Yoon, I. A., Slade, K., & Fazel, S. J. (2017). Outcomes of psychological therapies for prisoners with mental health problems: A systematic review and meta-analysis. *Journal of Consulting and Clinical Psychology*, *85*(8), 783–802.

Zgoba, K. M., Reeves, R., Tamburello, A., & Debilio, L. (2020). Criminal recidivism in inmates with mental illness and substance use disorders. *Journal of the American Academy of Psychiatry and the Law*, *48*(2), 209–215.

34 Adjustment disorders

Graham D. Glancy[*]

Introduction

Becoming incarcerated and the physical, social, and psychological challenges associated with incarceration typically constitute major life stressors for incarcerated persons (IPs). The development of acute adjustment disorder (AD) is common in these settings. This chapter discusses the prevalence, presentation, assessment, and management of AD in jails and prisons.

Prevalence of adjustment disorders in corrections

Although there are few epidemiological studies of AD, prevalence estimates in the general population have been found to be less than 1% (Patra & Sarkar, 2013). Among patients in primary care settings with psychiatric disorders, studies have indicated prevalence rates to be between 11.7% and 17.9% (Casey, 2006; Patra & Sarkar, 2013). Prevalence estimates in correctional settings are also scarce and are subject to the same diagnostic pitfalls that complicate the identification of AD in other populations. A few studies have attempted to determine prevalence rates among IPs. In a longitudinal study of mental disorders in a cohort of male IPs on remand, AD was estimated to be present in 17 newly received remand prisoners (11.48%) who had been identified as having a mental disorder (n = 148; Birmingham et al., 1996). In a larger study that used data on IPs in the New Jersey correctional system, 237 IPs (7.7%) with an Axis I mental disorder diagnosis were identified as having AD (n = 3,073; Pogorzelski & Blitz, 2005). Another study compared the incidence of psychiatric morbidity during remand imprisonment between solitary confinement (i.e., restrictive housing) and nonsolitary confinement settings in a large Danish remand prison. AD was found to be the most common incident disorder in both settings, with 81% (n = 30/37) in the solitary confinement group and 93% (n = 13/14) in the nonsolitary confinement group (Andersen et al., 2000).

Due to a weak research foundation, and what some experts perceive as a lack of scientific interest in AD (Jager et al., 2012), current incidence and prevalence estimates of the disorder may not accurately reflect the prison environment, especially considering that each correctional facility houses divergent populations of IPs at different stages of the judicial process and may be governed by a different set of rules and practices (Andersen, 2004). These factors are particularly relevant when AD is measured in populations of IPs remanded in custody compared to populations of long-term convicted prisoners; the two groups may have different patterns of occurrence. Factors that influence the differences between remand and convicted prisoners may operate at the institutional level, such as access to psychiatric treatment, availability of programs and services, length of sentence, and exposure to serious offenders. At the psychological level, feelings associated with conviction, acceptance of the sentence, recent losses, and coping with the prison environment may all play a role in AD variations. Regardless, incarcerated patients with AD represent a significant portion of those referred to psychiatric services, especially within the jail setting.

Complexity of diagnosis and identification

Given its broad classification criteria, AD has been subject to various criticisms related to validity and reliability (Jager et al., 2012). Some have challenged the classification as a "wastebasket" diagnosis (Casey, 2006), while others have pointed out the inability of the classification to appropriately distinguish cases that require psychiatric intervention from normal adaptive reactions to stressors (Andersen, 2004; Bachem & Casey, 2018; Casey, 2006; Walsh & Corcoran, 2011). The revised International Classification of Diseases-11 now recognizes AD as a standalone disorder, but only a few studies have examined its distinctive features and risk factors under the new diagnostic definition (e.g., see Zelviene et al., 2020). O'Donnell and colleagues (2019) note that AD has been reclassified to be positioned with acute stress disorder and posttraumatic stress disorder in the fifth edition of the *Diagnostic and Statistical Manual of Mental Disorders* (DSM-5). They note that a key diagnostic criterion is the patient's apparently excessive or disproportionate response in relation to the severity of the stressor. They note that the International Classification of Diseases-11 considers AD's cardinal feature to be a failure to adapt to the stressor, as evidenced by continuing symptoms and preoccupation with the situation. This would seem to be an advance in the understanding of this disorder, and it opens

*. The author acknowledges the contributions of Stefan R. Treffers, who was a coauthor of this chapter in the textbook's first edition.

up a pathway for treatment. Treatment would then be directed to facilitating the process of adaptation.

Diagnosis of AD becomes further complicated by symptomatology that overlaps with other disorders, specifically mood and anxiety disorders (Andersen, 2004). Casey (2006), for example, emphasizes the difficulty in adequately distinguishing AD from major depression, especially depression of mild to moderate severity. While both disorders share a similar set of diagnostic criteria, the latest revision of the DSM precludes a diagnosis of AD when the criteria for major depression are satisfied (American Psychiatric Association, 2022). Although some researchers have contended that the AD diagnosis has been subordinated to the diagnosis of other mental disorders (Jager et al., 2012), Casey (2006) suggests that research efforts have favored disorders for which specific treatments are available, thus excluding AD from more extensive clinical and academic consideration.

Despite these criticisms, individuals diagnosed with AD were seen as a distinct group compared to those without a diagnosis (Despland et al., 1995). These diagnosed patients tended to share symptomatology with depressive disorders but were marked by differences related to age, treatment length, and type of stressor (Casey, 2006; Despland et al., 1995; Patra & Sarkar, 2013). Individuals with AD had higher quality-of-life scores than those with major depressive disorder (Patra & Sarkar, 2013). Regarding the reliability and stability of the diagnosis, studies have yielded mixed results, with varying degrees of interrater and predictive reliability (Casey, 2006; Jager et al., 2012; Patra & Sarkar, 2013). Detailed clinical interviews have suggested that major depressive disorder can be conceptualized as an intense shutdown and relative unresponsiveness to life events. In contrast, AD can be seen as a more dynamic reaction to stressful events, with a variable course of symptoms corresponding to the impact of life stressors (Zapata-Ospina & Jiménez-Benítez, 2023).

Comorbidity

Diagnostic obstacles also extend to findings of comorbidity. Studies have found comorbidity rates to be relatively high. In a representative community sample of elderly residents in Zurich, 46.1% of patients were found to have one or two other mental disorders, with major depression and posttraumatic stress disorder the most common comorbidities (Maercker et al., 2008). Jager and colleagues (2012) discovered that 47.3% of patients had one or more comorbid mental disorders using International Classification of Diseases-10 criteria. Of those patients with comorbid diagnoses, 29.6% had a mental disorder resulting from psychotropic substance use and 15.4% from a personality disorder (Jager et al., 2012). It seems likely that comorbidity is even more extensive in correctional populations. Yet another layer of complexity is the relationship between subthreshold symptoms of mood and anxiety disorders and a diagnosis of AD.

Guidelines for psychological treatment

Treatments for AD in the general population consist mainly of brief interventions (Casey, 2009), involving three broad components: removing or reducing the stressor, facilitating adaptation to the stressor, and altering the response to the stressor. Specific psychological therapies may include supportive, psychoeducational, cognitive, and psychodynamic approaches.

While none of these therapies have demonstrated superiority in treating AD, cognitive-behavioral therapy (CBT) has become generally accepted as a treatment for a wide range of mental health problems. The clarity and brevity of this treatment make it suitable for use in a variety of settings, including correctional ones (Regehr & Glancy, 2020).

Landenberger and Lipsey (2005) have suggested that treatment effectiveness and recidivism reduction depend on the quality of the CBT provided. In environments where psychiatric resources are strained, such as prisons and especially jails, programmed treatment approaches may not be possible, although psychological therapies may be more viable in long-term correctional facilities. With high turnover and a large proportion of IPs assigned to clinicians, the fast-paced nature of jails often demands the symptomatic treatment and management of mental illness with limited psychiatric consultation.

Roberts (2000) describes a seven-stage model based on preexisting work in crisis intervention:

Initial assessment

The initial assessment includes a psychiatric history and mental state examination, with an emphasis on whether the patient is actively suicidal (see Chapter 16). Appropriate measures are indicated for suicidal patients (see Chapter 51). For patients who are not actively suicidal, a psychiatric history would cover data that would assist in the differentiation of a mood or anxiety disorder, a personality disorder, or a substance use disorder and withdrawal.

Establish rapport

Establishing rapport is perhaps one of the most important skills in carceral psychiatry. It is necessary to develop the ability to be an empathic, nonjudgmental clinician. Being empathic does not necessarily mean that the therapist is easily manipulated into doing things that would be unethical or outside the therapeutic envelope. Nevertheless, by demonstrating concern and interest, and by assisting with basic needs, it is surprising how quickly therapeutic rapport can be developed. Although the therapist's services are generally strictly rationed, the therapist is nevertheless an important figure for the patient, possibly the only person to whom they can express emotions safely.

Identify the major problems

It is important to attempt to delineate the various dimensions related to the patient's distress. These often involve not only the stresses of being in a carceral environment but also absence of one's usual social supports, imminent marital separation, possible job loss, financial strain, and loss of reputation. Some of these problems may be chronic, likely exacerbated by the current incarceration, and others may be new. The purpose of enumerating these problems is so that the patient and therapist can clarify and work on each one in turn; the therapist should guard against becoming overwhelmed in this process.

Process feelings and provide support

The therapist uses active listening techniques to explore the relevant issues. This includes considering previous coping strategies and instilling hope. Positive coping strategies should be delineated and reinforced. Sometimes these are as simple as suggesting a distraction, perhaps playing cards or exercising, to reduce stress and increase involvement with others. In addition, it may be helpful to delineate supports on the outside that the patient can contact and mobilize. Some patients are ashamed to approach people; however, if encouraged to do so, friends and relatives may be accepting and supportive. Nothing is lost by the initial approach.

Explore alternatives

Some patients have limited or rigid coping strategies. Substance use and acting out may have been familiar, though maladaptive, strategies. More adaptive strategies can be suggested and developed with guidance. It is sometimes necessary to point out that gains may be incremental, and more ambitious goals may be considered for the long term. Assisting the patient with finding acceptable, flexible alternatives is necessary, while always maintaining proper boundaries and paying attention to security provisions.

Formulate an action plan

Formulating an action plan might involve specific tasks such as exercising daily and taking advantage of daily yard privileges. Suggestions such as contacting family and friends and requesting support from appropriate sources may be helpful. Referrals to chaplaincy, social workers, and outside agencies may be considered. It may be necessary to focus on anticipated losses and better clarify their true nature. For example, whereas an IP may have heard that he was facing 2 to 4 years in jail, his lawyer may have negotiated the possibility of a plea bargain involving just a few months. Spouses, family, and friends who were initially rejecting may eventually resolve their own anger and become more accommodating to the patient.

Establish follow-up plans

The initial interventions for AD may include seeing and working with patients on a regular basis. This can be quite reassuring to them. It is possible that after the initial period of crisis, they are restored to normal equilibrium and do not require long-term support or treatment. In other cases, referrals to programs and agencies should be considered to work on long-term goals that relate to substance use disorders, antisocial peer groups, and other criminogenic factors.

In the correctional setting, CBT has reduced recidivism rates among individuals released to the community (Landenberger & Lipsey, 2005; Lipsey & Landenberger, 2001). These therapies incorporate strategies designed to manage anger, have IPs take responsibility for their behavior, improve problem-solving skills, develop life skills, and set goals (Lipsey & Landenberger, 2001). In a meta-analysis of studies that examined group-oriented CBT programs, Wilson and colleagues (2005) found that reductions in recidivism rates ranged from 20% to 30% for treated IPs compared to control groups. CBT intervention that focuses on finding meaning in life after a stressful event may be particularly helpful (Quero et al., 2023).

Other approaches include stress inoculation training (Meichenbaum, 1993), mindfulness-based stressed reduction (Kabat-Zinn, 1982), and mindfulness-based cognitive therapy (Segal et al., 2002). These latter approaches incorporate Eastern approaches with relaxation techniques. They have been demonstrated to be useful in various populations, and some research has suggested their utility in correctional settings (Samuelson et al., 2007).

In response to these constraints, some jails and prisons have adopted variations of crisis intervention to deal with IPs who cannot cope with a particular event and have high levels of fear, tension, confusion, or subjective discomfort (Dass-Brailsford, 2007). The cumulative effect of imprisonment, family disruption, strains on marriage, and the uncertainty of one's fate may cause excessive stress, leading to a crisis. Crisis intervention strategies used in a correctional context have evolved from more traditional forms practiced by front-line emergency personnel (see Chapter 24). These strategies have been tailored to deal with altercations among IPs, instances of self-harm, suicidal ideation, and personal life events that can lead to conflict while in custody (French, 1981; Kulic, 2005). Research in this area has provided evidence that individuals who experience crises are somewhat more open to suggestions than they would be normally (Kulic, 2005). Crisis intervention is intended to be a short-term approach where clinicians help the individual to identify coping skills and restore precrisis functioning (Dass-Brailsford, 2007; Kulic, 2005). Through prevention and stabilization, these interventions are geared toward management of crises rather than full-fledged treatment (Dass-Brailsford, 2007; French, 1981).

Psychopharmacological approaches

In the real world of correctional psychiatry, a psychopharmacological approach to treating AD is intended to treat severe symptoms (e.g., anxiety, insomnia, acute stress reactions) for a short duration. Another factor to be taken into consideration is that many patients may already be taking medications prior to incarceration. These previous medication regimens may or may not be optimal (see Chapter 18). It is not uncommon to see patients who have gradually accumulated an irrational polypharmacy regimen in the community, including redundant medications or questionable combinations of medications. Often, the first task of the correctional psychiatrist is to begin to rationalize treatment. Certain types of medications and obviously inappropriate polypharmacy should be addressed immediately, especially the chronic use of benzodiazepines, opiates, and psychostimulants given without clear indication. Correctional institutions tend to have restrictions on the use of these medications for a variety of reasons (see Chapter 29). It must be kept in mind that most IPs have substance use disorders, and certain medications may promote aggression (Glancy & Knott, 2003). The diversion and circulation of these medications may increase the potential for misuse and acute adverse reactions (see Chapter 30).

When depressive symptoms coexist with anxiety and insomnia, sedating antidepressants may be a suitable option. These include mirtazapine or trazodone (Glancy & Knott, 2003). Selective serotonin reuptake inhibitors and serotonin–norepinephrine reuptake inhibitors may also be considered for the management of anxiety. In practice, these medications appear to be useful even in the absence of rigorous or evidence-based research. Buspirone, an anxiolytic 5-HT 1 agonist with significant antiaggressive effects, also appears helpful in practice (Glancy & Knott, 2003). These medications are generally well tolerated and helpful in the crisis period. Given that AD is typically short-lived when treated, the need for continuing pharmacological treatment should be reassessed at regular intervals.

Medications should ideally be given in conjunction with psychological treatments, as described previously. The crisis model is particularly applicable and can be combined with CBT on an informal or formal basis. CBT can also be given in a group format, where this is possible. Mindfulness strategies have been useful in a variety of settings, including incarceration, and should be considered if feasible given institutional resources.

Suicide risk

Many patients in correctional settings are young men, close in age to adolescence. In a study of suicidality among outpatient adolescents diagnosed with AD, Pelkonen and colleagues (2005) discovered that 25% showed suicide attempts, threats, or ideation. They also suggested that risk factors such as previous psychiatric treatment and severe psychosocial impairment at entry to treatment were commonly present in suicidal adolescents with major psychiatric disorders. Other findings in the adolescent sample included dysphoric mood and depressive symptoms associated with continued suicidal ideation; these symptoms were common in completed suicides by adolescents with AD (Pelkonen et al., 2005). In differentiating between suicide risk in AD patients versus those with major depression, Carta and colleagues (2009) suggested that the AD group presents a lower risk for suicide, a shorter-lived interval of suicidality, and a lower likelihood of planned suicide compared to the group with major depression.

Reported rates of suicide have varied given the diversity that exists in populations of IPs (see Chapter 51). Way and colleagues (2005) suggest that AD, as a risk factor for suicide in correctional settings, should be given more attention. This is supported by their finding that 28% of suicide victims in a sample of IPs who had contact with mental health services had a diagnosis of AD. Common acute precursors to suicide included conflict with other IPs, recent disciplinary action, overall fear, physical illness, and adverse news related to one's personal circumstances (Way et al., 2005).

Clinicians must carefully assess suicidality, not only during the initial assessment period but also on an ongoing basis, especially as patients' circumstances change. Such changes may involve an adverse turn in legal proceedings (such as receiving new charges) or a change in personal circumstances (such as news that a spouse is filing for divorce or restricting access to children). Adverse life events such as these may precipitate a new crisis and decompensation, requiring the therapist to reappraise the approach to treatment and reassess suicide risk.

Summary

AD is frequently seen among IPs and can represent a complex diagnostic picture. With these complexities in mind, it is important for clinicians to use sound clinical judgment, taking into consideration the patient's personal circumstances and the context in which their symptoms are being presented (Casey, 2009). This chapter gives guidance to clinicians who are on the front lines in difficult circumstances. They are often dealing with patients who are overwhelmed with significant adverse life events, whose history reveals that they have dealt with emotional disturbances by acting out, or who have struggled with substance use for many years. These patients present with comorbidities, often complicated by substance use disorder and withdrawal. Clinicians may have very little information at their disposal, yet they will have to make difficult decisions under pressure. Clinicians must take an empathic approach while maintaining clear boundaries and keeping in mind the security constraints of the institution. Treatment of AD in correctional settings requires a keen application of a variety of complementary clinical skills.

REFERENCES

American Psychiatric Association. (2022). *Diagnostic and statistical manual of mental disorders* (5th ed., text rev.).

Andersen, H. S. (2004). Mental health in prison populations. A review with special emphasis on a study of Danish prisoners on remand. *Acta Psychiatrica Scandinavica, 424*(Suppl.), 5–59.

Andersen, H. S., Sestoft, D., Lillebaek, T., Gabrielsen, G., Hemmingsen, R., & Kramp, P. (2000). A longitudinal study of prisoners on remand: Psychiatric prevalence, incidence and psychopathology in solitary vs. non-solitary confinement. *Acta Psychiatrica Scandinavica, 102*, 19–25.

Bachem, R., & Casey, P. (2018). Adjustment disorder: A diagnosis whose time has come. *Journal of Affective Disorders, 227*, 243–253.

Birmingham, L., Mason, D., & Grubin, D. (1996). A follow-up study of mentally disordered men remanded to prison. *Criminal Behavior and Mental Health, 8*(3), 202–213.

Carta, M. G., Balestrieri, M., Murru, A., & Hardoy, M. C. (2009). Adjustment disorder: Epidemiology, diagnosis and treatment. *Clinical Practice and Epidemiology in Mental Health, 5*(15), 1–15.

Casey, P. (2006). The "afterthought" diagnosis: Rehabilitating adjustment disorders. *Expert Review of Neurotherapeutics, 6*(2), 145–151.

Casey, P. (2009). Adjustment disorder: Epidemiology, diagnosis and treatment. *CNS Drugs, 23*(11), 927–938.

Dass-Brailsford, P. (2007). Crisis interventions. In P. Dass-Brailsford (Ed.), *A practical approach to trauma: Empowering interventions* (pp. 93–114). Sage.

Despland, J. N., Monod, L., & Ferrero, F. (1995). Clinical relevance of adjustment disorder in DMS-III-R and DSM-IV. *Comprehensive Psychiatry, 36*(6), 454–460.

French, L. (1981). Clinical perspectives on crisis intervention in jails. *Prison Journal, 61*(1), 43–54.

Glancy, G. D., & Knott, T. F. (2003). Psychopharmacology of violence—Part IV. *American Academy of Psychiatry and the Law Newsletter, 28*(1), 12–13.

Jager, M., Burger, D., Becker, T., & Frasch, K. (2012). Diagnosis of adjustment disorder: Reliability of its clinical use and long-term stability. *Psychopathology, 45*(5), 305–309.

Kabat-Zinn, J. (1982). An outpatient program in behavioral medicine for chronic pain patients based on practice of mindfulness meditation: Theoretical considerations and preliminary results. *General Hospital Psychiatry, 4*, 33–47.

Kulic, K. R. (2005). The Crisis Intervention Semi-Structured Interview. *Brief Treatment and Crisis Intervention, 5*(2), 143–157.

Landenberger, N. A., & Lipsey, M. W. (2005). The positive effects of cognitive-behavioral programs for offenders: A meta-analysis of factors associated with effective treatment. *Journal of Experimental Criminology, 1*(4), 451–476.

Lipsey, M. W., & Landenberger, N. A. (2001). Cognitive-behavioral programs for offenders. *Annals of the American Academy of Political and Social Science, 578*, 144–157.

Maercker, A., Forstmeier, S., Enzler, A., et al. (2008). Adjustment disorders, posttraumatic stress disorder, and depressive disorders in old age: Findings from a community survey. *Comprehensive Psychiatry, 49*(2), 113–120.

Meichenbaum, D. (1993). Stress inoculation training: A twenty year update. In L. Woolfolk & P. Lehrer (Eds.), *Principles and practice of stress management* (2nd ed., pp. 373–406). Guilford.

O'Donnell, M., Agathos, J., Metcalf, O., Gibson, K., & Lau, W. (2019). Adjustment disorder: Current developments and future directions. *International Journal of Environmental Research and Public Health*, *16*(14), 2537.

Patra, B. N., & Sarkar, S. (2013). Adjustment disorder: Current diagnostic status. *Indian Journal of Psychological Medicine*, *35*(1), 4–9.

Pelkonen, M., Marttunen, M., Henriksson, M., & Lonngvist, J. (2005). Suicidality in adjustment disorder: Clinical characteristics of adolescent outpatients. *European Child & Adolescent Psychiatry*, *14*(3), 174–180.

Pogorzelski, W., & Blitz, C. L. (2005). Behavioral health problems, ex-offender reentry policies, and the "Second Chance Act." *American Journal of Public Health*, (10), 1718–1724.

Quero, S., Palau-Batet, M., Tur, C., Mor, S., Campos, D., Rachyla, I., Grimaldos, J., & Marco, J. H. (2023). Effect of an internet-based intervention for adjustment disorder on meaning in life and enjoyment. *Current Psychology*, *42*(24), 20543–20555.

Regehr, C., & Glancy, G. (2020). *Mental health social work practice in Canada*. Oxford University Press.

Roberts, A. R. (2000). *Crisis intervention handbook: Assessment, treatment, and research*. Oxford University Press.

Samuelson, M., Carmody, J., Kabat-Zinn, J., et al. (2007). Mindfulness-based stress reduction I. Massachusetts Correctional Facilities. *Prison Journal*, *87*(2), 254–268.

Segal, Z. V., Williams, J. M. G., & Teasdale, J. D. (2002). *Mindfulness-based cognitive therapy for depression: A new approach to relapse prevention*. Guilford Press.

Walsh, J., & Corcoran, J. (2011). A social work perspective on the adjustment disorders. *Social Work in Mental Health*, *9*(2), 107–121.

Way, B. B., Miraglia, R., Sawyer, D. A., Beer, R., & Eddy, J. (2005). Factors related to suicide in New York state prisons. *International Journal of Law and Psychiatry*, *28*(3), 207–221.

Wilson, D. B., Bouffard, L. A., & Mackenzie, D. L. (2005). A quantitative review of structured, group-oriented, cognitive-behavioral programs for offenders. *Criminal Justice and Behavior*, *32*(2), 172–204.

Zapata-Ospina, J. P., & Jiménez-Benítez, M. (2023). "I was very sad, but not depressed": Phenomenological differences between adjustment disorder and a major depressive episode. *Frontiers in Psychiatry*, *14*, 1291659.

Zelviene, P., Kazlauskas, E., & Maercker, A. (2020). Risk factors of ICD-11 adjustment disorder in the Lithuanian general population exposed to life stressors. *European Journal of Psychotraumatology*, *11*(1), 1–9.

35
Anxiety disorders

Catherine F. Lewis

Introduction

Excessive worry or fear that causes impairment in an individual's daily life characterizes anxiety disorders. While some degree of anxiety can be adaptive, when stress levels become too high, impairment results. Symptomatology can persist beyond normal developmental periods, be excessive in response to a stimulus, be persistent (i.e., lasting more than 6 months), or be excessive (i.e., worry in response to normal concerns). Anxiety disorders are often comorbid with other disorders and heighten risk for increased service utilization, morbidity, and mortality (Blanco et al., 2013; Kessler et al., 1999; Saha et al., 2020). Individuals with anxiety disorders present early and often to health care providers outside of psychiatry because of somatic symptoms and, in doing so, frustrate providers and themselves, as well as drive up health care costs. Untreated anxiety disorders increase morbidity and mortality, including risk for suicidal behavior (Kessler et al., 1999; Scheer et al., 2020).

This chapter examines the anxiety disorders using case vignettes and discusses best practices for treatment. Research on anxiety disorders within correctional settings has been sparse. Posttraumatic stress disorder (PTSD), categorized as an anxiety disorder before the publication of the *Diagnostic and Statistical Manual of Mental Disorders*, fifth edition (DSM-5; American Psychiatric Association [APA], 2013), emerged as a topic for correctional research during the 25 years prior to its publication. Little emphasis was placed on the "lesser siblings" of PTSD (e.g., panic disorder, agoraphobia, generalized anxiety disorder, social phobia). The arrival of the DSM-5 and the DSM, fifth edition, text revision (DSM-5-TR; APA, 2022) has forced a reconceptualization of PTSD and a focus on developmental aspects of anxiety disorders, as well as a "lifespan" approach. Anxiety disorders confer substantial risk for worse psychiatric and medical outcomes if left untreated, including in correctional populations; for this reason, they should not be discounted. Correctional practitioners should screen for and treat anxiety disorders effectively. Table 35.1 includes lifetime prevalence data for clinical populations of men and women with anxiety disorders in community and correctional settings (Black, 2004; Collins & Bailey, 1990; Gunter & Weisman, 2008; Jordan et al., 1996; Kessler et al., 1994, 2012; Lewis, 2005, 2010; Powell et al., 1997).

Selective mutism

HD is an 18-year-old man with an unknown history admitted to a large regional urban jail on charges of trespassing, breach of peace, resisting arrest, and assault on a police officer. Since his arrest a week ago, he has not spoken to staff or other incarcerated men. Initially placed in a double cell, he got into a fight and went into restrictive housing. The cellmate explained that HD was "weird, staring at me, and I thought he was going to snap." HD would not speak to anyone about what happened. He next went to the mental health infirmary for observation. Staff saw him talking to himself when he did not know he was being watched and at one point singing a rap song. When they confronted him about this, he looked away. He began to communicate by nodding and gesturing. Staff gave him paper, and he wrote responses. He directed them to his sister, who lived out of state. The sister explained he had an eighth-grade education. A severely anxious child, he stopped talking at age 5. He would become mute intermittently and had received special services (i.e., an Individualized Education Program) in school. His anxiety worsened as he aged, and he received medications. He began using cannabis and alcohol in seventh grade and often skipped class. He ultimately dropped out and lived an itinerant lifestyle. They have stayed in touch intermittently. She described him as an intelligent child whose anxiety held him back from being able to achieve. He repeated multiple grades because of truancy.

Discussion of case

Selective mutism typically has its onset in early childhood and is a rare disorder with a prevalence between 0.2% and 1.9% and equal distribution in males and females (Viana et al., 2009). Most studies on prevalence have been on child and adolescent populations. Core symptoms of the disorder include the failure to speak in social situations where there is the expectation to speak despite speaking in other situations. The disorder cannot be attributable to psychosis or a communication disorder. In a correctional setting, particularly a jail setting with an unknown patient, psychosis must be ruled out, as well as medical issues like delirium that can cause patients to be unable to respond verbally. Evaluators must also ensure HD does not have a hearing disorder and that he speaks and understands English. HD attempts to communicate with them by gesturing and writing. At that point, they may assume he is malingering, but the

Table 35.1 Prevalence of anxiety disorders

	Community			Incarcerated		
	Male	**Female**	**Both**	**Male**	**Female**	**Both**
Specific phobia						
Black (2004)						4.0%
Gunter and Weisman (2008)						4.7%
Kessler et al. (2012)	9.9%	17.5%	13.8%			
Kessler et al. (1994)	6.7%	15.7%	11.3%			
Lewis (2005)					4.9%	
Social anxiety disorder						
Black (2004)						6.0%
Gunter and Weisman (2008)						10.4%
Kessler et al. (2012)	11.8%	14.7%	13.0%			
Kessler et al. (1994)	11.1%	15.5%	13.3%			
Lewis (2010)					10.0%	
Lewis (2005)					1.2%	
Panic disorder						
Black (2004)						12.0%
Gunter and Weisman (2008)						4.2%
Jordan (1996)					4.7%	
Kessler et al. (2012)	3.3%	7.0%	5.2%			
Kessler et al. (1994)	2.0%	5.0%	3.5%			
Lewis (2010)					3.8%	
Lewis (2005)					6.2%	
Powell et al. (1997)				5.1%		
Agoraphobia						
Black (2004)						16.0%
Gunter and Weisman (2008)						16.6%
Kessler et al. (2012)	2.0%	3.2%	2.6%			
Kessler et al. (1994)	3.5%	7.0%	5.3%			
Lewis (2010)					3.8%	
Generalized anxiety disorder						
Black (2004)						4.0%
Collins and Bailey (1990)				3.4%		
Gunter and Weisman (2008)						19.1%
Jordan (1996)					1.4%	
Kessler et al. (2012)	4.6%	7.7%	6.6%			
Kessler et al. (1994)	3.6%	6.6%	5.1%			
Lewis (2010)					4.6%	
Lewis (2005)					1.2%	
Powell et al. (1997)					5.1%	
Separation anxiety disorder	**Adults**					
Kessler et al. (2012)	4.6%	8.2%	6.6%			

information gathered from his sister proves critical in the diagnosis of selective mutism.

Treatment of selective mutism in an adult should include pharmacotherapy and cognitive-behavioral psychotherapy (Steains et al., 2020). The most robustly studied and supported medications for the treatment of selective mutism have been selective serotoninergic reuptake inhibitors (SSRIs; Kaakeh & Stumpf, 2008; Manassis et al., 2015). They would also treat potential comorbid social phobia, should it be present. Because selective mutism in this case has been a pervasive and enduring diagnosis, medications should not be viewed as an episodic or short-term intervention.

Selective mutism, though rare, is important for jails. Silent incarcerated persons (IPs) pose difficult challenges. They cannot be assessed easily, and this poses problems in secure settings. HD's cellmate noted his belief he might be attacked. The police charged HD with assault in part because he would not communicate with them. Staff initially believed HD might be psychotic, then thought he was faking (i.e., first overestimated then underestimated his pathology). Ultimately, correct diagnosis hinges upon communication; selective mutism challenges diagnostic abilities.

Social anxiety disorder

TR is a 42-year-old man who is incarcerated for the first time after being arrested for his third driving under the influence charge. He is married, is employed as a financial analyst, and has no other legal history. Correctional officers make a mental health referral because they notice he is using the bathroom at odd times; he is in a dorm and makes requests to use the bathroom at night. At first, the officers believed this happened because of fears of assault, but they observe him moving freely throughout the dorm, participating in pickup basketball games, and eating in a group at the end of the bench in the communal dining area. He is quiet but well liked within the dorm because he reads well, is bilingual, and helps fellow incarcerated men with letters from home. When asked why he requests to use the bathroom at odd times, he blushes and becomes silent. He does agree to see a mental health practitioner. When officers ask the mental health practitioner about whether he has been seen, they note he has not showed up for three appointments. The officers walk him to the fourth appointment to ensure he gets evaluated.

Once TR is evaluated, he describes having no history of mental health treatment. He denies having any issues, but when questioned specifically about the bathroom, he gets embarrassed. He discloses that he cannot urinate in front of other people. This difficulty began in middle school, and he has avoided public bathrooms since. He has difficulty going to the bathroom in unfamiliar settings, including friends' houses, restaurants, and rest stops. This has limited his ability to socialize and travel, and it has affected his employment opportunities. He began to drink in his late 20s before going to parties with his wife and found this relieved his anxiety. He describes the public dormitory-style bathrooms in the prison as a "nightmare" and feels panicked when he enters them. He worries about what other men think when he tries to urinate and becomes increasingly panicky when he tries to urinate—to the point it becomes impossible. He describes his heart racing, getting sweaty and lightheaded, feeling flushed, and becoming nauseous as he attempts to urinate. He knows this is not reasonable and he has nothing physically wrong with him; he has seen more than one urologist who has ruled out any medical issue. Despite not having anything wrong with him, he cannot quell his anxiety when he is in a bathroom with other people and must urinate; he cannot do it.

Discussion of case

Social anxiety disorder is among the most prevalent psychiatric disorders. Although social anxiety has an early onset (i.e., around 13 years of age), it tends to have a chronic course (Leichsenring & Leweke, 2017). The defining characteristic of social anxiety disorder is a fear of scrutiny by others in social situations (e.g., social interactions, being observed eating or drinking, performing in front of others). Paruresis or "shy bladder syndrome" has been recognized as a subtype of social anxiety disorder characterized by difficulty urinating in front of other people, which results in avoidance of public restrooms (Hammelstein et al., 2005; Vythilingum et al., 2002). The lifetime prevalence of paruresis, a subtype of social anxiety disorder, was found to be 6.6% in males in the National Comorbidity Study (Kessler et al., 1998). A more recent, smaller study specifically assessing the issue using a self-report checklist found a point prevalence of 2.8% in a sample of males (Hammelstein et al., 2005). Paruresis has higher prevalence in males and is associated with significant comorbid psychopathology, including major depression, alcohol use disorder, and obsessive-compulsive disorder (Vythilingum et al., 2002).

Despite TR reporting no prior mental health history, he should be screened carefully for symptoms of depression, alcohol use disorder, and other subtypes of social anxiety disorder. He has multiple charges of driving under the influence, and it is likely that he meets criteria for alcohol use disorder. Paruresis tends to be undertreated and underdiagnosed because those suffering from it believe their symptoms are medical (Hammelstein et al., 2005). Common symptoms, as with TR, include difficulty urinating in situations where others are present, including public restrooms with a line, a busy public restroom, or a quiet public restroom (Vythilingum et al., 2002). The paniclike symptoms experienced by TR, including trembling (44.4%), sweating (38%), shortness of breath (34.9%), blushing (34.9%), and nausea (17.5%), have been noted (Vythilingum et al., 2002). Despite not seeking mental health treatment, men with paruresis, like TR, have significant impairment and report avoidance of fluids (15.9%), traveling (38.1%), sports events/parties (36.5%), social invitations (36.5%), and dating (33.5%; Vythilingum et al., 2002). More than half have turned down job offers based on symptoms (Vythilingum et al., 2002). The lag time in diagnosis is typical in cases of paruresis; the average time to diagnosis is 13.8 ± 1.1 years until a diagnosis is made (Vythilingum et al., 2002). This delay occurs because of shame and a belief the symptoms are medical; TR's course is consistent with this trajectory. In diagnosing and managing TR, comorbid depression needs to be ruled out. His alcohol use disorder must also be treated. Cognitive-behavioral interventions, including graded exposure therapy with relaxation work, have shown efficacy in treating paruresis (Hambrook et al., 2016; Kuoch et al., 2019). Medications such as SSRIs are useful for longer term treatment of social anxiety, including paruresis (Blanco et al., 2003; Hambrook et al., 2016).

Panic disorder

CD is a 37-year-old woman with insulin-dependent diabetes mellitus who is HIV positive and hepatitis C positive. She has a strongly positive family history of coronary artery disease and a history of polysubstance use, including intravenous heroin and cocaine, cannabis, and alcohol. She has had trauma in childhood including sexual abuse, but she refuses to engage in mental health services. She takes medications for HIV and has been stable with respect to infectious disease for years. She has well-controlled asthma and diabetes in the correctional environment. She presents multiple times for emergent medical appointments complaining of chest pain and shortness of breath. During these episodes, she is tachycardic, hyperventilates, and expresses fears she is having a heart attack and will die. She has had episodes in her cell causing medical codes. During the codes, she is rushed to the infirmary and ruled out for a heart attack. Multiple workups, including one at an outside hospital by a cardiologist, have been negative. When she sees the mental health practitioner, she reports similar episodes on the "outside" that began in her 20s. She describes these as times of "fear" that caused her to go to the emergency room. She self-medicates with cannabis or alcohol. These episodes have worsened without the ability to self-medicate since she has been incarcerated.

Discussion of case

Panic disorder confers elevated risk for suicide attempts (OR 5.6 [2.9–10.7]) and suicidal ideation (OR 3.9 [2.8–5.3]) in noncorrectional populations (Kessler at al., 1999). The 3-year prevalence of suicide attempts in people with panic disorder is 4.6% (Scheer et al., 2020). The risk would be expected to be higher in correctional populations, where comorbidity and disease burden exceed that in clinical populations (Lewis, 2005, 2010; Warren et al., 2002; Zlotnick, 1999). This should prompt a careful evaluation of CD for comorbid depression, including past episodes and their severity. Her history, despite her use of substances, is consistent with likely panic disorder with onset in the late teens or early 20s. Given her trauma history, she should also be assessed for PTSD, which confers risk for suicide when present with major depression (Brodsky et al., 2001).

The case warrants an integrated approach to CD's treatment. She perceives her symptoms as purely physical; thus, medical and psychiatric staff should see CD contemporaneously (i.e., preferably proximate in time as part of a team assessment). This facilitates integrated assessment with team feedback to CD that her symptoms are not cardiac in origin and offers a consistent treatment plan. It also assures her she is safe. The APA provides guidelines for treating panic disorder, which include basics such as ruling out medical conditions causing symptomatology and suicidality (APA, 2009). CD should be prescribed medication to treat her panic disorder; the best option for her would be an SSRI with minimal interactions with her other medications. A critical consideration with panic disorder is starting low and titrating slowly upward to a dose high enough to adequately treat (i.e., often higher than that required to treat major depression; APA, 2009). The psychiatrist, along with the primary care provider, can schedule nonemergent appointments with CD to explain that the medication is safe and ensure compliance. This integrated treatment assuages concerns regarding side effects and minimizes somatization and misperceptions about potential side effects. CD should also receive cognitive-behavioral therapy, which is the most robustly validated treatment for panic disorder (APA, 2009); it can be in either a group or an individual setting. The therapy could be presented as specifically for panic disorder or as therapy for women with chronic illness aimed to decrease anxiety and panic symptoms.

Agoraphobia

JP is an 18-year-old Latina woman incarcerated for the first time as an adult on a charge of larceny in the first degree. Her correctional counselor refers her to the mental health department because of concerns that she will not leave her cell to go to the communal dining area. She is eating food primarily from commissary and items brought back from the communal dining area by her cellmate. JP is known to the mental health department already; she was prescribed venlafaxine twice daily upon admission for depression and anxiety because she had been receiving it in the community for depression diagnosed at age 14. A review of the medication administration records shows she takes the medication in the morning when nurses administer medications at her cell, but she does not attend the medication line, which requires an exit from her cell and standing to wait in line at a more distant location. When a mental health practitioner formally evaluates JP, she tells them that, ever since about age 15, she has been fearful of standing in lines or being in a crowd. She avoids these situations. She also fears bridges and will not drive across them, often altering routes or insisting that her family alter routes. She struggles being a passenger in a car, even with her family. She cannot explain these worries beyond saying that she cannot tolerate the belief that she will be unable to get out of the situation or get help if she had a problem with her anxiety. She avoids situations to mitigate her anxiety, and although she finds it depressing, the relief has been worth it to her. She leads a solitary life, is unemployed, and was receiving mental health treatment for depression and PTSD before her admission. She notes that the twice-daily venlafaxine she took had helped her, but she cannot overcome her anxiety to get to the medication line in person.

Discussion of case

The DSM-5 for the first time categorized agoraphobia as a standalone disorder, distinct from panic disorder. Agoraphobia has a lifetime prevalence of 1.5% and a 12-month prevalence of 1.0% (Roest et al., 2018). Symptoms of agoraphobia tend to emerge early (i.e., at around age 14), as in this case, and result in significant impairment (Roest et al., 2018; Wittchen et al., 1998). Among respondents in one large study, nearly half (43.3%) reported severe impairment because of agoraphobia symptoms, and the subjects reported an average of 40.3 days missed from work or school during of the previous year (Roest et al., 2018). JP reports a solitary life where she stays at home most days and does not attend school or work or date. This is consistent with significant psychological and social impairment. Although her depressive symptoms have been treated, her agoraphobic symptoms limit her in the community and in corrections.

In approaching this case, JP needs to be screened for depressive symptoms to ensure that, because she is not taking all her venlafaxine, she does not have recurrent symptoms. Because agoraphobia has a high degree of comorbidity with other anxiety disorders (84.1%), disruptive disorders (26.3%), substance use disorders (31.5%), and affective disorders (59.6%), the latter of which she has already been diagnosed with, careful screening of this young woman is warranted (Roest et al., 2018). Although she reports a good response with venlafaxine for her depressive symptoms, she still has significant problems with agoraphobic symptoms. It would be important to know how much venlafaxine she was taking. To adequately treat agoraphobic symptoms, the dose needs to be higher than that for depressive symptoms; she also needs to confirm she was consistently taking her medication. If she was consistently taking the venlafaxine at an adequate dose and it had not worked, she could then attempt a trial of an SSRI along with a trial of cognitive-behavioral therapy to treat her agoraphobia.

Generalized anxiety disorder

BT is a 41-year-old Black woman referred to the mental health department by her correctional counselor because of a letter from her attorney, who noted increasing difficulty with her focusing on her case because she cannot sleep. Medical providers already treat her for migraines, peptic ulcers, and hypertension. They have noted increased visits over the past 3 months and difficulty controlling her headaches, along with complaints of stomach upset they cannot explain medically. When the mental health practitioner sees her, she complains of anxiety about her case and being separated from her three elementary school-aged children, one of whom has special needs. She worries about them at night, when her mind races and she cannot sleep. She then is tired, irritable, and restless during the day. She is exhausted, cannot concentrate, and finds herself daydreaming when she should be paying attention in court. These difficulties have been happening throughout her incarceration (i.e., for 9 months). She has struggled with similar problems since her early 20s; she ruminates about issues and describes herself as a worrier. She has lost weight, worries to the point of nausea, and feels a lump in her throat when she tries to eat. She finds that cannabis relieves her insomnia and when home will smoke a blunt at night to alleviate her anxiety. She does not think that drug use has caused issues for her and does not drink alcohol.

Discussion of case

BT describes many symptoms consistent with generalized anxiety disorder (GAD), including difficulty concentrating, fatigue, irritability, and sleep disturbance. Many of these symptoms overlap with depressive symptoms, and BT should be carefully screened for depression, which is often comorbid with GAD (Goodwin & Stein, 2021). She should also be screened for any potential medical issues that cause her anxiety, though these are less likely given its chronicity with onset in her teenage years. GAD has a higher likelihood of comorbidity with personality disorders and with externalizing disorders (e.g., attention-deficit/hyperactivity disorder, pathological gambling, and all substance use disorders except alcohol use disorder) than major depression (Blanco et al., 2013). It would be important, therefore, to complete a careful and thorough diagnostic assessment of BT. Most individuals with comorbid depression and GAD develop depressive symptoms before GAD (Beesdo, 2010), so a longitudinal history with life history onset of symptomatology would be important for BT. Among patients with medical issues, psychiatrists frequently diagnose GAD; when present, it increases health utilization (Davidson et al., 2008). Untreated GAD increases risk for complications including development of major depression, substance use disorder, and risk for suicide (Davidson et al., 2008). Primary treatment for BT should include pharmacotherapy with either a selective SSRI or serotonin–norepinephrine reuptake inhibitor. She should also receive cognitive-behavioral therapy to assist her with abstinence from substances and to help manage her anxiety symptoms. Because her symptoms have been persistent and enduring, she will likely need maintenance therapy on medication.

Summary

Correctional populations, like their clinical counterparts, have a high prevalence of anxiety disorders. Anxiety disorders confer risk for comorbid disease, suicidal behavior, and higher health service utilization. Anxiety disorders themselves are often comorbid and have an early age of onset. Individuals with a greater disease burden (i.e., greater number of diagnoses, higher symptom count) have worse outcomes than those with uncomplicated disorders. These impaired outcomes include deteriorating trajectory of illness, increased health service utilization, a worse prognosis, and an increased likelihood of morbidity and mortality (Kessler et al., 1999; Wu et al., 1999). Thus, while anxiety disorders may not be the primary focus of the correctional system, their importance must be recognized. Unrecognized anxiety disorders can result in behavior that is disruptive and may appear to be volitional. They can also lead to overuse of health services that are already facing substantial demands. Appropriate, available, and consistent assessment, diagnosis, and treatment that are well integrated can successfully intervene in the range of anxiety disorders that present in correctional settings.

REFERENCES

American Psychiatric Association. (2009). *Treating panic disorder: A quick reference guide.* https://psychiatryonline.org/pb/assets/raw/sitewide/practice_guidelines/guidelines/panicdisorder-guide-1410457202640.pdf

American Psychiatric Association. (2013). *Diagnostic and statistical manual of mental disorders* (5th ed.).

American Psychiatric Association. (2022). *Diagnostic and statistical manual of mental disorders* (5th ed., text rev.).

Beesdo, K., Pine, D. S., Lieb, R., et al. (2010). Incidence and risk patterns of anxiety and depressive disorders and categorization of generalized anxiety disorder. *Archives of General Psychiatry, 67*(1), 47.

Black, D. (2004). Use of the Mini International Neuropsychiatric Interview (MINI) as a screening tool in prisons: Results of a preliminary study. *Journal of the American Academy of Psychiatry and the Law, 32*(32), 156–162.

Blanco, C., Raza, M., Shneier, R., et al. (2003). The evidence-based pharmacological treatment of social anxiety disorder. *International Journal of Neuropsychopharmacology, 6*(4), 427–442.

Blanco, C., Bragdon, L. B., Schneier, F. R., et al. (2013). The latent structure and comorbidity patterns of generalized anxiety disorder and major depressive disorder: A national study. *Depression and Anxiety, 31*(3), 214–222.

Brodsky, B. S., Oquendo, M., & Ellis, S. P. (2001). The relationship of childhood abuse to impulsivity and suicidal behavior in adults with major depression. *American Journal of Psychiatry, 158*(11), 1871–1877.

Collins, J. J., & Bailey, S. L. (1990). Relationship of mood disorders to violence. *Journal of Nervous and Mental Disease, 178*(1), 44–47.

Davidson, J. R., Zhang, W., Connor, K. M., et al. (2008). Review: A psychopharmacological treatment algorithm for generalised anxiety disorder (GAD). *Journal of Psychopharmacology, 24*(1), 3–26.

Goodwin, G. M., & Stein, D. J. (2021). Generalised anxiety disorder and depression: Contemporary treatment approaches. *Advances in Therapy, 38*(S2), 45–51.

Gunter, T. D., & Weisman, G. (2008). Frequency of mental and addictive disorders among 320 men and women entering the Iowa prison system: Use of the MINI Plus. *Journal of the American Academy of Psychiatry and the Law, 36*, 27–34.

Hambrook, D., Taylor, T., & Bream, V. (2016). Cognitive behavioural therapy for paruresis or "shy bladder syndrome": A case study. *Behavioural and Cognitive Psychotherapy, 45*(1), 79–84.

Hammelstein, P., Pietrowsky, R., Merbach, M., et al. (2005). Psychogenic urinary retention ("paruresis"): Diagnosis and epidemiology in a representative male sample. *Psychotherapy and Psychosomatics, 74*(5), 308–314.

Jordan, B. K. (1996). Prevalence of psychiatric disorders among incarcerated women. *Archives of General Psychiatry, 53*(6), 513.

Kaakeh, Y., & Stumpf, J. L. (2008). Treatment of selective mutism: Focus on selective serotonin reuptake inhibitors. *Pharmacotherapy: Journal of Human Pharmacology and Drug Therapy, 28*(2), 214–224.

Kessler, R. C., McGonagle, K. A., Zhao, S., et al. (1994). Lifetime and 12-month prevalence of DSM-III-R psychiatric disorders in the United States. *Archives of General Psychiatry, 51*(1), 8.

Kessler, R. C., Petukhova, M., Sampson, N. A., et al. (2012). Twelve-month and lifetime prevalence and lifetime morbid risk of anxiety and mood disorders in the United States. *International Journal of Methods in Psychiatric Research, 21*(3), 169–184.

Kessler, R. C., Borges, G., & Walters, E. E. (1999). Prevalence of and risk factors for lifetime suicide attempts in the National Comorbidity Survey. *Archives of General Psychiatry, 56*(7), 617.

Kessler, R. C., Stein, M. B., & Berglund, P. (1998). Social phobia subtypes in the National Comorbidity Survey. *American Journal of Psychiatry, 155*(5), 613–619.

Leichsenring, F., & Leweke, F. (2017). Social anxiety disorder. *New England Journal of Medicine, 376*(23), 2255–2264.

Lewis, C. F. (2005). Post-traumatic stress disorder in HIV-positive incarcerated women. *Journal of the American Academy of Psychiatry and the Law, 33*(4), 455–464.

Lewis, C. F. (2010). Childhood antecedents of adult violent offending in a group of female felons. *Behavioral Sciences & the Law, 28*(2), 224–234.

Manassis, K., Oerbeck, B., & Overgaard, K. R. (2015). The use of medication in selective mutism: A systematic review. *European Child & Adolescent Psychiatry, 25*(6), 571–578.

Powell, T. A., Holt, J. C., & Fondacaro, K. M. (1997). The prevalence of mental illness among inmates in a rural state. *Law and Human Behavior, 21*(4), 427–438.

Roest, A. M., de Vries, Y. A., Lim, C. C., et al. (2019). A comparison of DSM-V and DSM-IV agoraphobia in the World Mental Health Surveys. *Depression and Anxiety, 36*(6), 499–510.

Saha, S., Lim, C. W., Cannon, D. L., et al. (2020). Co-morbidity between mood and anxiety disorders: A systematic review and meta-analysis. *Depression and Anxiety, 38*(3), 286–306.

Scheer, V., Blando, C., Olfson, M., et al. (2020). A comprehensive model of predictors of suicide attempt in individuals with panic disorder: Results from a national 3-year prospective study. *General Hospital Psychiatry, 67*, 127–135.

Schneider, S., Blatter-Meunier, J., Herren, C., et al. (2011). Disorder-specific cognitive-behavioral therapy for separation anxiety disorder in young children: A randomized waiting-list-controlled trial. *Psychotherapy and Psychosomatics, 80*(4), 206–215.

Steains, S. Y., Malouff, J. M., & Schutte, N. S. (2021). Efficacy of psychological interventions for selective mutism in children: A meta-analysis of Randomized Controlled Trials. *Child: Care, Health and Development, 47*(6), 771–781.

Viana, A. G., Beidel, D. C., & Rabian, B. (2009). Selective mutism: A review and integration of the last 15 years. *Clinical Psychology Review*, *29*(1), 57–67.

Vythilingum, B., Stein, D. J., & Soifer, S. (2002). Is shy bladder syndrome a subtype of social anxiety disorder? A survey of people with paruresis. *Depression and Anxiety*, *16*(2), 84–87.

Warren, J. I., Hurt, S., Loper, A. B., et al. (2002). Psychiatric symptoms, history of victimization, and violent behavior among incarcerated female felons. *International Journal of Law and Psychiatry*, *25*(2), 129–149.

Wittchen, H.-U., Nelson, C. B., & Lachner, G. (1998). Prevalence of mental disorders and psychosocial impairments in adolescents and young adults. *Psychological Medicine*, *28*(1), 109–126.

Wu, L. T., Kouzis, A. C., & Leaf, P. J. (1999). Influence of comorbid alcohol and psychiatric disorders on utilization of mental health services in the National Comorbidity Survey. *American Journal of Psychiatry*, *156*(8), 1230–1236.

Zlotnick, C. (1999). Antisocial personality disorder, affect dysregulation and childhood abuse among incarcerated women. *Journal of Personality Disorders*, *13*(1), 90–95.

36

Posttraumatic stress disorder and trauma-informed care

Nancy Wolff and Catherine F. Lewis

Introduction

Prison and jail populations have dense and patterned concentrations of childhood and adult trauma (Wolff, 2022). The maturing effects of childhood trauma have been extensively studied for decades, with robust evidence documenting that exposure to trauma, especially during childhood, increases the likelihood of behavioral health disorders such as depression, anxiety, posttraumatic stress disorder (PTSD), and substance use disorders (SUDs; Anda et al., 2006). Related behavioral problems, including aggression and violence, may culminate in criminality (Altintas & Bilici, 2018; Widom, 1989). The connection between trauma and criminality explains, in part, the high concentrations of trauma and behavioral health disorders within incarcerated populations, but it also suggests that trauma is being criminalized (Simkins & Katz, 2002; Thordarson & Rector, 2020; Wolff, 2022). Although the interdependencies between trauma, behavioral disorders, and criminality are well established in the literature, in practice, incarcerated persons (IPs) are treated less as people in need of therapeutic help and more as threats to society. With predictability, correctional settings, replicating the traumatic stressors of childhood (Wolff, 2022), instigate criminogenic behaviors and pathologies that immediately challenge corrections management and eventually are exported back into the community upon release (Listwan et al., 2011). The cycle of violence and victimization risk continues because, when in the presence of trauma and its hydra-headed effects, the perceived threat response of IPs overrides and dominates their need for therapeutic intervention.

This chapter provides a blueprint that recognizes the reluctance of the correctional system to address trauma, the lack of funding and staffing expertise to support and sustain a therapeutically sensible response to trauma, and the superseding public health imperative to treat and rehabilitate trauma in cost-effective ways. The blueprint for action identifies promising trauma-focused interventions and recommends access and allocation principles for rationing scarce resources. It furthermore addresses principles of engagement that serve to establish and sustain the therapeutic bond between those in need and those promoting the voluntary use of available services. For the purposes of this chapter, the term "prison" refers to any correctional setting.

Trauma concentrations

Definitionally, trauma includes physical, sexual, and emotional abuse, as well as neglect and adversity, experienced directly or vicariously. It may occur in childhood or adulthood while residing in either community or correctional settings. There are high concentrations of all types of traumas in IPs (i.e., trauma concentrations). Epidemiologic research has consistently found higher rates of childhood trauma among IPs when compared to community samples (Karlsson & Zielinski, 2020; Liu et al., 2021; Messina & Schepps, 2021; Wolff, 2022). A recent meta-analysis of prison-based victimization estimated prevalence rates of 18.8% for physical victimization and 12.4% for sexual victimization (Caravaca-Sánchez et al., 2022). History of past trauma is a consistently strong predictor of future trauma in prison settings (Wolff et al., 2023) and the community (Papalia et al., 2021; Widom et al., 2008).

Trauma events and symptoms often culminate in stressor-related disorders (Liu et al., 2021). An international meta-analysis estimated a point prevalence of PTSD at 6.2% for incarcerated men (5 times higher than the general population) and 21.1% for incarcerated women (8 times higher than the general population), with lifetime rates of 18% in incarcerated men and 40% in incarcerated women (Baranyi et al., 2018). In a meta-analysis conducted by Tolin and Foa (2006), women were found to have more exposure to early childhood sexual abuse, which likely explains their higher prevalence of adult PTSD. However, when boys and girls were exposed to similar sexual abuse in childhood, they developed PTSD at the same rates (Tolin & Foa, 2006), suggesting that the virulence and timing of the abuse, rather than the gender of the child, are the critical factors.

Exposure to trauma in childhood increases the likelihood of experiencing behavioral health problems in adulthood (McKay et al., 2021). Prison-based rates of major depression, anxiety, and SUDs are 3 to 10 times higher than in the general population (Fovet et al., 2023) and have often been shown to be comorbid in IPs with PTSD (Facer-Irwin et al., 2019). When PTSD and depression are comorbid, the risk of suicide rises (Brodsky et al., 2001).

Trauma and criminality

Researchers have found a strong and consistent association between childhood trauma and antisocial behavior (Altintas & Bilici, 2018; Burke et al., 2023). Emotional reactions to and behavioral dyscontrol associated with trauma in childhood begin early (Ford et al., 2010). Specifically, children exposed to maltreatment are more likely to display externalizing behaviors (Ford & Delker, 2018) and are in turn more likely to engage in lawbreaking (Loeber & Burke, 2011).

Other researchers have focused on the connection between trauma, antisocial behavior, and incarceration (Kerig & Becker, 2015). Adults with more severe childhood trauma are significantly more likely to commit violent behavior (Horan & Widom, 2015). Another study of a large sample of incarcerated men found a strong association between traumas (experienced either in childhood or in adulthood) and interpersonal problems, difficulty with self-regulation, and aggressive behavior (Wolff & Shi, 2012). Overall, histories of childhood trauma—and related impaired self-regulation—have been associated with violent behavior, aggression, and hostility in adolescence and adulthood (Altintas & Bilici, 2018; Fox et al., 2015; Messina & Schepps, 2021).

Many people enter prison with coping styles that have been conditioned by their trauma histories. In addition to having a diminished capacity to regulate impulsivity, trauma survivors often have well-practiced fight-or-flight responses (van der Kolk, 2014) combined with predispositions for risk taking (Briere, 2019). This means that when trauma survivors are faced with abuse of authority or power; fear incited by bullying, harassment, or abuse; and loss of privacy or safe boundaries, they often reflexively seek refuge in conduct that reflects powerlessness: substance use, promiscuity, self-harm, and abusive relationships. They may also rebel through defiant and deviant behaviors like drug dealing, gambling, crime, and fighting (Wolff, 2022). In this way, people with trauma histories arrive to prison primed to react pathologically. Traditional prison environments with their hierarchical power structures; harsh, restrictive, rigid, and inconsistently enforced rules; tight control over privacy and movement; and impersonal authority figures serve as the perfect triggers (Levenson & Willis, 2019). Prison confinement, for many, is a flashback to their traumatic childhoods, where they are "in a position of both psychological and material weakness, and their dependency leaves them ... unable to contest [their] parents' untrammeled power" (Sparks et al., 1996, p. 46). Prison settings, in this way, can retraumatize vulnerable people by triggering memories of harmful treatment and abuse (and related protective reactions), with the risk of new experiences to rival those of their past (Wolff, 2022).

Posttraumatic stress disorder in correctional settings

While still a research diagnosis, "complex PTSD," or disorders of extreme stress not otherwise specified, has potential relevance in incarcerated populations. Complex PTSD includes pervasive, enduring personality disturbance (e.g., affective modulation difficulties, impulsive behavior, impaired relationships), persistent somatization, depression, and dissociative symptoms (Herman, 1992). Survivors with complex PTSD have been exposed, typically, to multiple traumas, often with onset early in childhood (Herman, 1992). Complex PTSD occurs in survivors of childhood physical and sexual abuse, chronic spousal abuse, and even combat-related trauma (Newman et al., 1997; Roth et al., 1997).

IPs often have intensive and extensive exposure to multiple traumas over their lifetimes (Wolff, 2022), including repetitive childhood sexual abuse, poverty, neglect, exposure to street violence resulting in deaths, exposure to domestic violence within the home, sexual assaults, and violent partnerships. An IP with this type of history may exhibit violent conflict with a cellmate, report multiple somatic symptoms, or engage in self-harming behavior, with or without lethal intent. A simple diagnosis of PTSD may not do justice to this multidimensional clinical presentation, while the concept of complex PTSD informs a starting point for treatment of at-risk, high utilizers of health services.

Awareness of trauma concentrations and appreciation for the complex histories and presentations of IPs with PTSD better enable health care staff to provide relief and rehabilitation to people who have suffered the lifetime consequences of trauma, to destress prison environments and reduce their breeding potential for violence and victimization, and to improve public health and safety by returning people to the community with healthier coping, thinking, and prosocial skills. Optimizing this opportunity requires, first, seeing the majority of people in prison as trauma-sensitized people in need of therapeutic help and as threats to society only if trauma remains unaddressed, and second, using the available evidence base (Grady et al., 2023; Malik et al., 2023) and cost-effective principles to develop, implement, evaluate, and fund a comprehensive therapeutic response to trauma concentrations inside prisons (Wolff, 2022).

Blueprint for trauma-informed care in correctional settings

Principle #1: Universal screening and assessment of trauma

Given the trauma concentrations in prisons, screening must be universal. For it to be cost-effective, the procedures for screening must be easy to implement, while the instruments must be valid, reliable, suitable for low literacy levels, and easy to administer and score. Table 36.1 shows frequently used, brief, self-administered trauma screening instruments for adults with moderate to strong psychometric properties. Table 36.2 shows validated screening instruments and a semi-structured interview instrument that may be progressively used to aid in making a PTSD diagnosis.

Since IPs with PTSD may present with complex psychopathology including SUDs, suicidal behavior, externalizing personality pathology, and affective disorders including major depression (Lewis, 2010; Warren et al., 2002; Zlotnick, 1999), screening for and treating comorbid affective conditions (e.g., major depression) is an essential component of risk management for IPs with PTSD. If left untreated, depressive symptoms are synergistic with PTSD symptoms and can result in suicidal behavior (Brodsky et al., 2001). Because of the high prevalence of antisocial personality disorder in the correctional system and the ease with which PTSD can be malingered (Matto et al., 2019), collateral data should be gathered and nonleading questions utilized.

Because of the scarcity of behavioral health resources in correctional settings, targeted trauma treatment considers the severity

Table 36.1 Trauma screening instruments for adults

- **Brief Trauma Questionnaire (BTQ)** assesses 10 traumatic events using a yes/no format, followed by probes about level of danger and injury (Schnurr et al., 2002). https://www.ptsd.va.gov/professional/assessment/documents/BTQ.pdf
- **Life Events Checklist (LEC)** screens for 17 traumatic events over the life course and probes direct or vicarious experiencing, severity, and distress (Gray et al., 2004). https://www.ptsd.va.gov/professional/assessment/documents/LEC5_Standard_Self-report.PDF
- **Stressful Life Events Screening Questionnaire (SLESQ)** assesses 13 traumatic events including direct and witnessed trauma using a yes/no format followed by questions about severity (Goodman et al., 1998). http://ctc.georgetown.edu/339952.html
- **Trauma History Questionnaire (THQ)** assesses 24 types of events with yes/no responses, followed by questions about frequency and age at occurrence (Hooper et al., 2011). https://www.ptsd.va.gov/professional/assessment/te-measures/thq.asp
- **Trauma History Screen (THS)** screens for 13 events using a yes/no format followed by questions about frequency and level of distress (Carlson et al., 2011). https://www.ptsd.va.gov/professional/assessment/documents/THS.pdf

Table 36.2 Posttraumatic stress disorder instruments for adults

- **Primary Care PTSD Screen for DSM-5 (PC-PTSD-5)**, a five-item screen designed to identify people with probable PTSD in primary care settings that can be added to intake forms (Bovin et al., 2021; Prins et al., 2016). https://www.ptsd.va.gov/professional/assessment/screens/pc-ptsd.asp
- **PTSD Checklist for DSM-5 (PCL-5)**, a 20-item self-administered rating scale that can be used for those who screen positive on the PC-PTSD-5. The PCL-5 measures symptoms regarding a patient's worst experience (Weathers et al., 2013). https://www.ptsd.va.gov/professional/assessment/documents/PCL5_Standard_form.PDF
- **PTSD Symptom Scale Interview for DSM-5 (PSS-I-5)**, a 24-item semi-structured interview to assess the intensity and frequency of DSM-5 PTSD symptoms over the previous month; may be used to confirm a positive screen (Foa et al., 2016). http://www.advanced-counseling.com/dl/PSSI-5.pdf

of the symptoms relative to the recovery capital (White & Cloud, 2008). Severity captures the extent to which trauma-related symptoms are hindering functioning and quality of life, whereas recovery capital (often referred to as "resilience") is the "breadth and depth of internal and external resources that can be drawn upon to initiate and sustain recovery" (White & Cloud, 2008, p. 22). Personal recovery capital includes a person's problem-solving capabilities, self-awareness, self-esteem, self-efficacy, sense of optimism, interpersonal skills, and healthy coping skills. Assigning people to levels of trauma-focused treatment by severity of need alone ignores personal recovery capital that can hinder or foster recovery trajectories. People with high personal recovery capital may benefit from less intensive treatment interventions, while those with low recovery capital may need more intensive treatment even if the severity is lower.

Principle #2: Evidence-based trauma-focused interventions

The American Psychological Association's (2017) practice guideline strongly recommends four treatment modalities for adults with PTSD: cognitive-behavioral therapy, cognitive processing therapy, prolonged exposure, and cognitive therapy. The guideline conditionally recommends three others: brief eclectic psychotherapy, eye movement desensitization therapy, and narrative exposure therapy. All these except for eye movement desensitization therapy are phase 2 trauma-processing (usually individual) therapies that focus on

Table 36.3 Phase 1 trauma-stabilizing interventions

- **Seeking Safety** (men and women): An integrated intervention for trauma and substance use that is strengths based, manualized (25 topics), incorporates cognitive-behavioral and psychoeducational techniques, and is delivered in group settings (two 90-minute sessions per week; Najavits, 2002).
- **Beyond Trauma** (women): An intervention that is strengths based and integrates cognitive-behavioral, expressive arts, guided imagery, and relational therapy to women's trauma treatment; manualized (12 sessions); was adapted for women and girls; is delivered in group settings (two 2-hour sessions per week; Covington, 2016).
- **Healing Trauma** (women) and **Exploring Trauma** (men): A brief intervention adapted from Beyond Trauma, for both women and men; manualized (six sessions); available in Spanish (Covington, 2016).
- **Trauma Affect Regulation: Guide for Education and Therapy (TARGET)** (women): A manualized, strengths-based, trauma-focused psychotherapy (twelve 75-minute therapy sessions with homework assignments) that can be delivered in group settings (Ford et al., 2013).

Table 36.4 Phase 2 trauma-processing interventions

- **Traumatic Incident Reduction** (women): Includes one-on-one therapy with a trained "facilitator"; sessions are highly structured and meet weekly for 60 to 90 minutes, with the number of sessions dependent on need (Valentine & Smith, 2001).
- **Expressive Writing Exercises With Dialectical Behavior Therapy** (DBT, men and women): Includes 2.5-hour group biweekly sessions for 9 weeks, with nine DBT-modeled education-based sessions and nine sessions on structured writing assignment (Bradley & Follingstad, 2003).

revisiting and reexamining intrusive traumatic memories. Phase 1 therapies, by contrast, are present-focused, skills-based group interventions that attempt to reduce and stabilize symptoms and establish a sense of safety. Phase 1 and phase 2 therapies studied in correctional populations are summarized in Tables 36.3 and 36.4, respectively.

The evidence base for prison-based trauma-focused interventions is small, methodologically diverse in design and rigor, inclusive of mostly phase 1 trauma-stabilizing interventions delivered to incarcerated women (Grady et al., 2023; Hidayati et al., 2023; Malik et al., 2023), and without reference to cost-effectiveness. Nevertheless, evidence shows that it is feasible to deliver trauma-focused treatment to incarcerated men and women (Wolff, 2022) and that both phase 1 and phase 2 trauma-focused treatments can improve symptoms (Malik et al., 2023).

Several cognitive therapies for PTSD have shown preliminary efficacy for IPs with PTSD, including manualized interventions addressing PTSD, substance use, and externalizing behavior (e.g., Seeking Safety, Trauma Affect Regulation: Guide for Education and Therapy, Male-Trauma Recovery Empowerment Model; Ford et al., 2013; Najavits et al., 2007; Wolff et al., 2015; Zlotnick et al., 2003).

Other research has focused on the use of stress reduction interventions to support trauma recovery. Yoga and mindfulness meditation programs provided to IPs modestly improve psychological well-being and behavioral function (Auty et al., 2017). A pilot study of a corrections-adapted version of the Mindfulness-Based Stress Reduction intervention found significant reductions in prison stress, PTSD symptoms, and depression, with improved coping and self-efficacy in men with above-average levels of prison stress (Wolff, 2018).

Medication management may be a useful adjunct for treating PTSD, with most support in community guidelines for selective serotonin reuptake inhibitors and serotonin–norepinephrine reuptake inhibitors (Management of Posttraumatic Stress Disorder and Acute Stress Disorder Work Group, 2023; Tamburello et al., 2022). Research involving medication for IPs with PTSD is limited, though it is important to consider the side-effect profile and patient characteristics when selecting an agent (Management of Posttraumatic Stress Disorder and Acute Stress Disorder Work Group, 2023; Tamburello et al., 2022). Older agents have shown efficacy in treating PTSD (e.g., tricyclic antidepressants, monoamine oxidase inhibitors), but their potential lethality if hoarded and adverse side-effect profile render them not front-line choices for correctional or clinical populations. Benzodiazepines have not shown robust benefit in treating PTSD (Braun et al., 1990; Gelpin et al., 1996) and are not recommended by guidelines (Management of Posttraumatic Stress Disorder and Acute Stress Disorder Work Group, 2023). Long-term use in populations with high risk for SUDs is problematic.

Atypical antipsychotics as monotherapy do not have robust support in PTSD, and their metabolic side effects are concerning for a population that already struggles with obesity, hypertension, and heightened risk for diabetes and heart disease (Wang et al., 2017). They may be considered in refractory cases to augment treatment for comorbid disorders (e.g., major depression, psychotic symptoms) and have shown some benefit in those cases (Crapanzano et al., 2023; Pae et al., 2008). The alpha-adrenergic antagonist prazosin has shown efficacy for decreasing nightmares (Reist et al., 2021; Zhang et al., 2020) but not for improving overall symptoms of PTSD, so its use should be targeted accordingly (Management of Posttraumatic Stress Disorder and Acute Stress Disorder Work Group, 2023). Alpha-adrenergic antagonists may cause rebound hypertension if not taken consistently.

Principle #3: Match treatment intensity to patient needs

Phase 2 interventions, while they may be more effective for some, are more costly because they require specialized training, more staff time, and more clinical supervision compared to group-based, manualized trauma-stabilizing (phase 1) interventions. Given the variable but concentrated behavioral health needs within resource-constrained jails and prisons, the therapeutic impact would most likely be optimized by designing an incremental approach that matches need to levels of care and is deployed in multiple integrated steps:

- **Step 1: Trauma education.** Develop educational materials on trauma and its hydra-headed impacts on well-being. Distribute this material to all IPs at admission and all staff as part of their hiring orientation, as well as through public service announcements on the facility's education channels.
- **Step 2: Screening for trauma distress.** Implement universal screening for trauma, related symptoms, and recovery capital at admission and at crisis points during incarceration to identify levels of need.
- **Step 3: Stabilize those with moderate to high need.** Provide lower cost phase 1 trauma-stabilizing interventions. This might include trauma-focused therapy integrated with SUD treatment, given their comorbidity, and the use of peer facilitators (see Chapter 44). Consider a psychiatric referral whenever symptoms impair functioning or the individuals' capacity to participate in psychotherapy.
- **Step 4: Trauma recovery.** Provide phase 2 trauma-processing interventions to those who have not sufficiently recovered from phase 1 treatment, with a goal of reducing trauma symptoms sufficiently to allow adequate functioning. This might include creating a separate housing unit analogous to corrections-based residential programs for SUD treatment.
- **Step 5: Intensive case management.** For those seriously wounded people who are struggling with complex PTSD, treatment needs may be best met on a mental health housing unit or in a hospital setting.
- **Step 6: Maintenance.** Provide stress reduction programming to support stabilization and healing from trauma with the use of peer and volunteer facilitators. This might include mindfulness-based programming, such as yoga and mindfulness-based stress reduction (Wolff, 2018).

Principle #4: Interventions delivered efficiently and with fidelity

In real-world settings, evidence-based interventions are ineffective if they are delivered absent some critical active ingredient and may not be cost-effective if produced or delivered inefficiently. Behavioral health interventions are socially complex (Wolff, 2000). Group and individual therapies draw on the relational attributes of the professionals delivering the treatment and the environmental conditions supporting their efforts. These "active ingredients" complement the content of the intervention and are essential to reproduce the therapeutic effects attributed to them through experimental investigations. The expected effectiveness of evidence-based interventions may not materialize in practice if key elements are missing. Moreover, the presence of toxic environmental factors (e.g., traumagenic conditions of confinement) may nullify, offset, or diminish the expected impact of these interventions. Similarly, resources are wasted when staff are insufficiently trained or supervised or when services are provided by overly specialized, higher cost professionals.

Productive mental health professionals optimize their use of resources, materials, and technologies in ways that decrease waste and increase the quality of services provided. Their productivity is enhanced by a trauma-informed environment that values a positive work culture and a safe work environment that is respectful and supportive. Similarly, to perform optimally, these professionals must have access to materials for evidence-based interventions and receive high-quality training and supervision that develops and supports their competencies to forge healthy therapeutic relationships with patients. Their productivity increases when they are provided with the tools, training, resources, and environmental conditions to deliver high-value services. Most phase 1 trauma-stabilizing interventions can be competently delivered by social workers or peer facilitators who receive high-quality training and continuous supervision (Messina & Schepps, 2021). Higher cost staff should be reserved for the delivery of phase 2 interventions.

Trauma-informed care

A trauma-informed environment promotes and supports healing and recovery and is complementary to the production of trauma-focused interventions. A trauma-informed organization "recognizes the signs and symptoms of trauma in clients, families, staff, and others involved with the system, and responds by fully integrating knowledge about trauma into policies, procedures, and practices, and seeks to actively resist re-traumatization" (Substance Abuse and Mental Health Services Administration, 2014, p. 9). The California Corrections Health Care Services embraces trauma-informed care (Messina & Schepps, 2021). Interested readers are referred to guidance by the National Institute of Corrections (2023) on becoming trauma informed and a related article by Levenson and Willis (2019). A trauma-informed environment requires engagement of and educational efforts for all staff that interact with IPs, not just health care professionals.

The effectiveness of trauma-focused interventions depends critically on the willingness of IPs to seek and engage with treatment. People are more inclined to seek treatment if they value the expected benefits and if they trust and feel safe with the professionals delivering the care (Wolff, 2022). The therapeutic alliance between client and provider has been deemed the "quintessential integrative variable" of behavioral health interventions (Wolfe & Goldfried, 1988). Fovet and colleagues (2023) advanced three principles for delivering behavioral health services in correctional settings: Behavioral health providers are exclusively confidential, respectful, nonjudgmental, and empathic healers (i.e., they are not involved with any security or forensic activities of the prison); confidentiality standards for IPs are equivalent with community standards with exceptions (e.g., imminent safety concerns or plans to cape) disclosed prior to and during treatment; and IPs have the right to consent to and discontinue treatment. These principles assure patients that their private information will be treated confidentially and their preferences respected. When taken together, they support the process of therapeutic engagement necessary to provide effective trauma-informed care.

Summary

Correctional settings have high concentrations of individuals with trauma histories, and cost-effective interventions can be delivered there. Correctional systems should be incentivized to adopt recovery-oriented systems of trauma-informed care as part of their behavioral health mission. Trauma recovery efforts should follow the path of SUD recovery by seeking dedicated funding to build and sustain a cost-effective tiered system of care that is scaled to the needs of patients. Trauma-informed care works best when provided in an integrated trauma-informed setting. Not just health care providers but all staff who interact with IPs need to be engaged to improve both the conditions of confinement and the conditions of the workplace. Strategically investing in the environment, screening and treatment resources, technology, and workforce development, as well as adopting and implementing economically informed principles to produce and deliver trauma-focused services, then emerges as a value proposition consistent with the behavioral health mission of correctional systems and their obligations to the welfare of the individual and society.

REFERENCES

Altintas, M., & Bilici, M. (2018). Evaluation of childhood trauma with respect to criminal behavior, dissociative experiences, adverse family experiences and psychiatric backgrounds among prison inmates. *Comprehensive Psychiatry, 82*, 100–107.

American Psychological Association. (2017). *Clinical practice guideline for the treatment of PTSD*. https://www.apa.org/ptsd-guideline/ptsd.pdf

Anda, R. F., Felitti, V. J., Bremner, J. D., et al. (2006). The enduring effects of abuse and related adverse experiences in childhood: A convergence of evidence from neurobiology and epidemiology. *European Archives of Psychiatry and Clinical Neuroscience, 256*(3), 174–186.

Auty, K. M., Cope, A., & Liebling, A. (2017). Systematic review and meta-analysis of yoga and mindfulness meditation in prison. *International Journal of Offender Therapy and Comparative Criminology, 61*(6), 89–710.

Baranyi, G., Cassidy, M., Fazel, S., Priebe, S., & Mundt, A. P. (2018). Prevalence of posttraumatic stress disorder in prisoners. *Epidemiologic Reviews, 40*(1), 134–145.

Bovin, M. J., Kimerling, R., Weathers, F. W., et al. (2021). Diagnostic accuracy and acceptability of the Primary Care Posttraumatic Stress Disorder Screen for the Diagnostic and Statistical Manual of Mental Disorders (Fifth Edition) among US veterans. *JAMA Network Open, 4*(2), e2036733.

Bradley, R., & Follingstad, D. (2003). Group therapy for incarcerated women who experienced interpersonal violence: A pilot study. *Journal of Traumatic Stress, 16*(4), 337–340.

Braun, P., Greenberg, D., Dasberg, H., & Lerer, B. (1990). Core symptoms of posttraumatic stress disorder unimproved by alprazolam treatment. *Journal of Clinical Psychiatry, 51*(6), 236–238.

Briere, J. (2019). *Treating risky and compulsive behavior in trauma survivors*. Guilford Press.

Brodsky, B. S., Oquendo, M., Ellis, S. P., Haas, G. L., Malone, K. M., & Mann, J. J. (2001). The relationship of childhood abuse to impulsivity and suicidal behavior in adults with major depression. *American Journal of Psychiatry, 158*(11), 1871–1877.

Burke, C., Ellis, J. D., Peltier, M. R., et al. (2023). Adverse childhood experiences and pathways to violent behavior for women and men. *Journal of Interpersonal Violence, 38*(3–4), 4034–4060.

Caravaca-Sánchez, F., Aizpurua, E., & Wolff, N. (2022). The prevalence of prison-based physical and sexual victimization in males and females: A systematic review and meta-analysis. *Trauma, Violence, and Abuse, 24*(5), 3476–3492.

Carlson, E. B., Smith, S. R., Palmieri, P. A., et al. (2011). Development and validation of a brief self-report measure of trauma exposure: The Trauma History Screen. *Psychological Assessment, 23*, 463–477.

Covington, S. (2016). *Beyond trauma. A healing journey for women* (2nd ed.). Hazelden Publishing.

Crapanzano, C., Damiani, S., Casolaro, I., & Amendola, C. (2023). Quetiapine treatment for post-traumatic stress disorder: A systematic review of the literature. *Clinical Psychopharmacology and Neuroscience, 21*(1), 49–56.

Facer-Irwin, E., Blackwood, N. J., Bird, A., et al. (2019). PTSD in prison settings: A systematic review and meta-analysis of comorbid mental disorders and problematic behaviours. *PLoS One, 14*(9), e0222407.

Foa, E. B., McLean, C. P., Zang, Y., et al. (2016). Psychometric properties of the Posttraumatic Stress Disorder Symptom Scale Interview for DSM-5 (PSSI-5). *Psychological Assessment, 28*(10), 1159–1165.

Ford, J. D., Chang, R., Levine, J., & Zhang, W. (2013). Randomized clinical trial comparing affect regulation and supportive group therapies for victimization-related PTSD with incarcerated women. *Behavior Therapy, 44*(2), 262–276.

Ford, J. D., & Delker, B. C. (2018). Polyvictimization in childhood and its adverse impacts across the lifespan: Introduction to the special issue. *Journal of Trauma & Dissociation, 19*(3), 275–288.

Ford, J. D., Elhai, J. D., Connor, D. F., & Frueh, B. C. (2010). Polyvictimization and risk of posttraumatic, depressive, and substance use disorders and involvement in delinquency in a national sample of adolescents. *Journal of Adolescent Health, 46*(6), 545–552.

Fovet, T., Mundt, A. P., & Fazel, S. (2023). Psychiatry in prisons and corrections. In A. Tasman, M. Riba, R. D. Alarcon, et al. (Eds.), *Tasman's psychiatry* (5th ed., pp. 1–28). Springer.

Fox, B. H., Perez, N., Cass, E., Baglivio, M. T., & Epps N. (2015). Trauma changes everything: Examining the relationship between adverse childhood experiences and serious, violent, and chronic juvenile offenders. *Child Abuse & Neglect, 46*, 163–173.

Gelpin, E., Bonne, O., Peri, T., Brandes, D., & Shalev, A. Y. (1996). Treatment of recent trauma survivors with benzodiazepines: A prospective study. *Journal of Clinical Psychiatry, 57*(9), 390–394.

Goodman, L., Corcoran, C., Turner, K., Yuan, N., & Green, B. (1998). Assessing traumatic event exposure: General issues and preliminary findings for the Stressful Life Events Screening Questionnaire. *Journal of Traumatic Stress, 11*(3), 521–542.

Grady, M. D., Tripodi, S., Herod, L., & Rudzinski, M. (2023). Behavioral health interventions for incarcerated adults with histories of trauma: A scoping review. *Research on Social Work Practice, 34*(4), 415–432.

Gray, M., Litz, B., Hsu, J., & Lombardo, T. (2004). Psychometric properties of the Life Events Checklist. *Assessment, 11*, 330–341.

Herman, J. L. (1992). Complex PTSD: A syndrome in survivors of prolonged and repeated trauma. *Journal of Traumatic Stress, 5*(3), 377–391.

Hidayati, N. O., Suryani, S., Rahayuwati, L., Fitrasanti, B. I., & Ahmad, C. (2023). A scoping review of correctional-based interventions for women prisoners with mental health problems. *Social Sciences, 12*(8), 452.

Hooper, L., Stockton, P., Krupnick, J., & Green, B. (2011). Development, use, and psychometric properties of the Trauma History Questionnaire. *Journal of Loss and Trauma, 16*, 258–283.

Horan, J. M., & Widom, C. S. (2015). Cumulative childhood risk and adult functioning in abused and neglected children grown up. *Development and Psychopathology, 27*(3), 927–941.

Karlsson, M. E., & Zielinski, M. J. (2020). Sexual victimization and mental illness prevalence rates among incarcerated women: A literature review. *Trauma, Violence, & Abuse, 21*(2), 326–349.

Kerig, P. K., & Becker, S. P. (2015). Early abuse and neglect as risk factors for the development of criminal and antisocial behavior. In J. Morizot & L. Kazemian (Eds.), *The development of criminal and antisocial behavior* (pp. 181–199). Springer.

Levenson, J. S., & Willis, G. M. (2019). Implementing trauma-informed care in correctional treatment and supervision. *Journal of Aggression, Maltreatment & Trauma, 28*(4), 481–501.

Lewis, C. F. (2010). Childhood antecedents of adult violent offending in a group of female felons. *Behavioral Sciences & the Law, 28*(2), 224–234.

Listwan, S., Sullivan, C., Agnew, R., Cullen, F., & Colvin, M. (2011). The pains of imprisonment revisited: The impact of strain on inmate recidivism. *Justice Quarterly, 30*(1), 144–168.

Liu, H., Li, T. W., Liang, L., & Hou, W.K. (2021). Trauma exposure and mental health of prisoners and ex-prisoners: A systematic review and meta-analysis. *Clinical Psychology Review, 89*, 102069.

Loeber, R., & Burke, J. D. (2011). Developmental pathways in juvenile externalizing and internalizing problems. *Journal of Research on Adolescence, 21*(1), 34–46.

Malik, N., Facer-Irwin, E., Dickson, H., Bird, A., & MacManus, D. (2023). The effectiveness of trauma-focused interventions in prison settings: A systematic review and meta-analysis. *Trauma, Violence, & Abuse, 24*(2), 844–857.

Management of Posttraumatic Stress Disorder and Acute Stress Disorder Work Group. (2023). *VA/DoD clinical practice guideline*. U.S. Government Printing Office. https://www.healthquality.va.gov/guidelines/MH/ptsd/

Matto, M., McNiel, D. E., & Binder, R. L. (2019). A systematic approach to the detection of false PTSD. *Journal of the American Academy of Psychiatry and the Law, 47*(3), 325–334.

McKay, M. T., Cannon, M., Chambers, D., et al. (2021). Childhood trauma and adult mental disorder: A systematic review and meta-analysis of longitudinal cohort studies. *Acta Psychiatrica Scandinavica, 143*(3), 189–205.

Messina, N. P., & Schepps, M. (2021). Opening the proverbial "can of worms" on trauma-specific treatment in prison: The association of adverse childhood experiences to treatment outcomes. *Clinical Psychology & Psychotherapy, 28*(5), 1210–1221.

National Institute of Corrections. (2023). *Becoming trauma informed: An essential element for justice settings*. https://nicic.gov/series/becoming-trauma-informed-essential-element-justice-settings

Najavits, L. M. (2002). *Seeking safety: A treatment manual for PTSD and substance abuse*. Guilford Press.

Najavits, L. M., Rosier, M., Nolan, A. L., & Freeman, M. C. (2007). A new gender-based model for women's recovery from substance abuse: Results of a pilot outcome study. *American Journal of Drug and Alcohol Abuse, 33*(1), 5–11.

Newman, E., Riggs, D. S., & Roth, S. (1997). Thematic resolution, PTSD, and complex PTSD: The relationship between meaning and trauma-related diagnoses. *Journal of Traumatic Stress, 10*(2), 197–213.

Pae, C. U., Lim, H. K., Peindl, K., et al. (2008). The atypical antipsychotics olanzapine and risperidone in the treatment of posttraumatic stress disorder: A meta-analysis of randomized, double-blind, placebo-controlled clinical trials. *International Clinical Psychopharmacology, 23*(1), 1–8.

Papalia, N., Mann, E., & Ogloff, J. R. P. (2021). Child sexual abuse and risk of revictimization: Impact of child demographics, sexual abuse characteristics, and psychiatric disorders. *Child Maltreatment, 26*(1), 74–86.

Prins, A., Bovin, M. J., Smolenski, D. J., et al. (2016). The primary care PTSD screen for DSM-5 (PC-PTSD-5): Development and evaluation within a veteran primary care sample. *Journal of General Internal Medicine, 31*(10), 1206–1211.

Reist, C., Streja, E., Tang, C. C., Shapiro, B., Mintz, J., & Hollifield, M. (2021). Prazosin for treatment of post-traumatic stress disorder: A systematic review and meta-analysis. *CNS Spectrums, 26*(4), 338–344.

Roth, S., Newman, E., Pelcovitz, D., van der Kolk, B., & Mandel, F. S. (1997). Complex PTSD in victims exposed to sexual and physical abuse: Results from the DSM-IV field trial for posttraumatic stress disorder. *Journal of Traumatic Stress, 10*(4), 539–555.

Schnurr, P. P., Spiro, A., III, Vielhauer, M. J., Findler, M. N., & Hamblen, J. L. (2002). Trauma in the lives of older men: Findings from the normative aging study. *Journal of Clinical Geropsychology, 8*(3), 175–187.

Simkins, S., & Katz, S. (2002). Criminalizing abused girls. *Violence Against Women, 8*(12), 1474–1499.

Sparks, R. J., Bottoms, A. E., & Hay, W. (1996). *Prisons and the problem of order*. Oxford University Press.

Substance Abuse and Mental Health Services Administration. (2014). *TIP 57: Trauma-Informed care in behavioral health services.* http:// store. samhsa.gov/shin/content//SMA14-4816/SMA14-4816.pdf

Tamburello, A., Penn, J., Ford, E., et al. (2022). The American Academy of Psychiatry and the Law practice resource for prescribing in corrections. *Journal of the American Academy of Psychiatry and the Law*, *50*(4), 636–637.

Thordarson, H., & Rector, T. (2020). From trauma-blind to trauma-informed: Re-thinking criminalization and the role of trauma in persons with serious mental illness. *CNS Spectrums*, *25*(5), 577–583.

Tolin, D. F., & Foa, E. B. (2006). Sex differences in trauma and posttraumatic stress disorder: A quantitative review of 25 years of research. *Psychological Bulletin*, *132*(6), 959–992.

Valentine, P., & Smith, T. (2001). Evaluating traumatic incident reduction therapy with female inmates: A randomized controlled clinical trial. *Research on Social Work Practice*, *11*(1), 40–52.

van der Kolk, B. A. (2014). *The body keeps the score: Brain, mind, and body in the healing of trauma.* Penguin Books.

Wang, E. A., Redmond, N., Dennison Himmelfarb, C. R., et al. (2017). Cardiovascular disease in incarcerated populations. *Journal of the American College of Cardiology*, *69*(24), 2967–2976.

Warren, J. I., Hurt, S., Loper, A. B., Bale, R., Friend, R., & Chauhan, P. (2002). Psychiatric symptoms, history of victimization, and violent behavior among incarcerated female felons: An American perspective. *International Journal of Law and Psychiatry*, *25*(2), 129–149.

Weathers, F. W., Litz, B. T., Keane, T. M., Palmieri, P. A., Marx, B. P., & Schnurr, P. P. (2013). *The PTSD Checklist for DSM-5 (PCL-5)–Standard* [Measurement instrument]. https://www.ptsd.va.gov/

White, W., & Cloud, W. (2008). Recovery capital: A primer for addictions professionals. *Counselor*, *9*(5), 22–27.

Widom, C. S. (1989). Child abuse, neglect, and violent criminal behavior. *Criminology*, *27*(2), 251–271.

Widom, C. S., Czaja, S. J., & Dutton, M. A. (2008). Childhood victimization and lifetime revictimization. *Child Abuse & Neglect*, *32*(8), 785–796.

Wolfe, B. E., & Goldfried, M. R. (1988). Research on psychotherapy integration: Recommendations and conclusions from an NIMH workshop. *Journal of Consulting and Clinical Psychology*, *56*(3), 448–451.

Wolff, N. (2000). Using randomized controlled trials to evaluate socially complex services: Problems, challenges and recommendations. *Journal of Mental Health Policy & Economics*, *3*(2), 97–109.

Wolff, N. (2018). Improving wellness and reducing stress among incarcerated men with mindfulness-based stress reduction programming. *Journal of Yoga & Physiology*, *5*(3), 555665.

Wolff, N. (2022). *The shadow of childhood harm behind the prison wall.* Oxford University Press.

Wolff, N., Aizpurua, E., & Peng, D. (2023). Reducing the methodological heterogeneity ("noise") in the literature predicting in-prison interpersonal harm in male populations. *Trauma, Violence, & Abuse*, *25*(2), 1315–1334.

Wolff, N., Huening, J., Shi, J., Frueh, B. C., Hoover, D. R., & McHugo, G. (2015). Implementation and effectiveness of integrated trauma and addiction treatment for incarcerated men. *Journal of Anxiety Disorders*, *30*, 66–80.

Wolff, N., & Shi, J. (2012). Childhood and adult trauma experiences of incarcerated persons and their relationship to adult behavioral health problems and treatment. *International Journal of Environmental Research and Public Health*, *9*(5), 1908–1926.

Zhang, Y., Ren, R., Sanford, L. D., et al. (2020). The effects of prazosin on sleep disturbances in post-traumatic stress disorder: A systematic review and meta-analysis. *Sleep Medicine*, *67*, 225–231.

Zlotnick, C. (1999). Antisocial personality disorder, affect dysregulation and childhood abuse among incarcerated women. *Journal of Personality Disorders*, *13*(1), 90–95.

Zlotnick, C., Najavits, L. M., Rohsenow, D. J., & Johnson, D. M. (2003). A cognitive-behavioral treatment for incarcerated women with substance abuse disorder and posttraumatic stress disorder: Findings from a pilot study. *Journal of Substance Abuse Treatment*, *25*(2), 99–105.

37

Personality disorders

Donald E. McLawhorn and Daniel Jackson

Introduction

The *Diagnostic and Statistical Manual of Mental Disorders*, fifth edition, text revision (DSM-5-TR) defines personality traits as "enduring patterns of perceiving, relating to, and thinking about the environment and oneself that are exhibited in a wide range of social and personal contexts" (American Psychiatric Association [APA], 2022). A personality (or "character" in earlier literature) is "the sum of the consistently displayed personality traits and habitual modes of response an individual uses" to navigate the world (Chessick, 1993). Personality disorder (PD) is considered to be present when these traits and modes of response deviate "markedly from the norms and expectations of the individual's culture," having become "inflexible and maladaptive and [causing] significant functional impairment or subjective distress" (APA, 2022). The DSM-5's Personality and Personality Disorders Work Group defined PD as "the failure to develop a sense of self-identity and the capacity for interpersonal functioning that are adaptive in the context of the individual's cultural norms and expectations" (APA, 2010; Millon, 2011).

This class of disorders comprises an important aspect of correctional psychiatry, as they co-occur frequently with the primary mental disorders of the DSM, substance use disorders, and criminal recidivism (Black et al., 2007, 2010). They also account for significant portions of violence and suicide (Sarchiapone et al., 2009). Given the limitations of this complex topic to a single chapter, only the PDs causing the most difficulties in correctional settings are discussed in detail: borderline, antisocial, narcissistic, and paranoid PDs.

Classification and epidemiology of personality disorders

The DSM-5-TR clusters PDs as indicated in Table 37.1. This arrangement follows neither etiological nor treatment models but was based on what appeared to be symptomatologic similarities of the odd/eccentric, dramatic/emotionally erratic, and anxious/fearful presentations of the disorders in the respective clusters.

Among the system's disadvantages is that diagnoses are constituted as discrete, categorical entities according to a descriptive phenomenology offered in a checklist of criteria, some of which are explicit behaviors. Some personality traits of particular interest to forensic practice are excluded from the diagnostic nosology, such as the construct of psychopathy (Hare, 2004).

Alternative classifications of PDs rely on additional features of interest, such as degree of impairment (Hopwood et al., 2019). The DSM-5's alternative model for personality disorders (AMPD; (APA, 2013) and the International Classification of Diseases-11 (ICD-11; World Health Organization [WHO], 2022) are part of a trend toward a dimensional model of PDs (Jackson et al., 2023), which may assist with differential diagnosis. For example, personality traits can be placed on a continuum of mild to extreme disturbance, where movement toward one pole is associated with deficits in reality testing, as illustrated in Figure 37.1. Such a continuum assists with differentiating transient episodes of psychotic experience in personality pathology from primary psychotic disorders that share persistently impaired reality testing (Jackson et al., 2023). Similarly, a range from introversion (internalizing) to extroversion (externalizing) suggests an array of externalizing disorders, with higher levels of extroversion associated with increased violence (Kernberg, 2001).

Borderline personality disorder (BPD), antisocial personality disorder (ASPD), narcissistic personality disorder (NPD), and paranoid personality disorder (PPD) have been shown to have the highest prevalence in corrections and are associated with violence and suicidality. Incarcerated persons (IPs) with Cluster B disorders have greater deficits in the ability to reflect on others' mental states and have more dismissive attachment than personality disordered persons who are not incarcerated (Levinson & Fonagy, 2004). Psychopathy as a manifestation of personality pathology is also conceptualized as being organized on a borderline level of personality (Gacono & Smith, 2021a, 2021b), and its relationship to challenges in corrections is well known. The following sections discuss BPD,

Table 37.1 DSM-5-TR personality disorders

Cluster A	Cluster B	Cluster C
Paranoid	Antisocial	Avoidant
Schizoid	Borderline	Dependent
Schizotypal	Histrionic	Obsessive-compulsive
	Narcissistic	

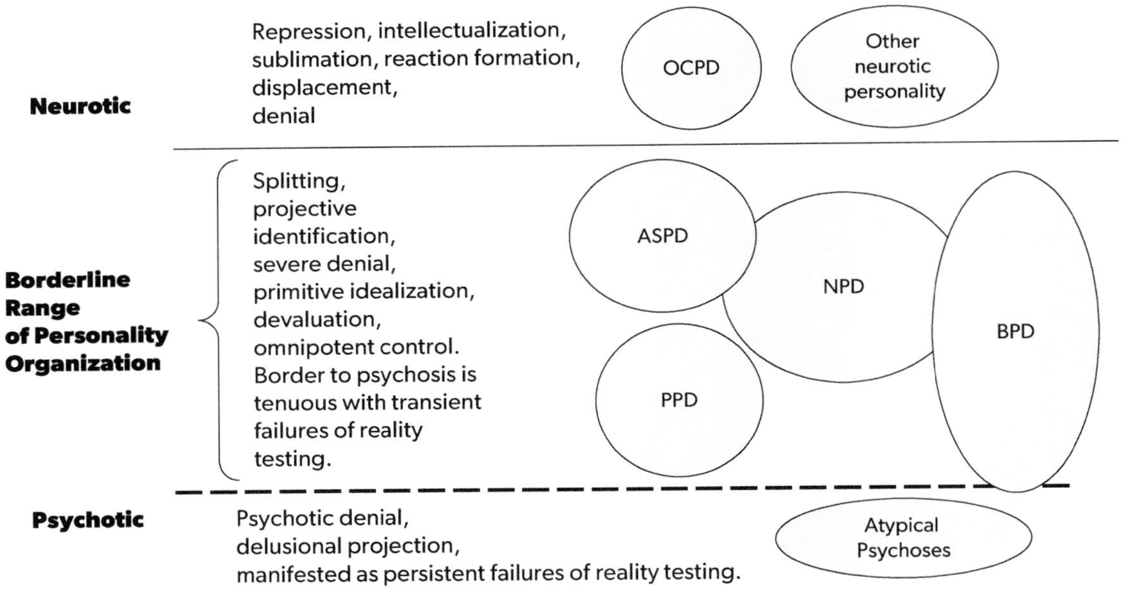

Figure 37.1 Levels of personality organization. ASPD = antisocial personality disorder; BPD = borderline personality disorder; NPD = narcissistic personality disorder; OCPD = ; PPD = paranoid personality disorder.

ASPD, NPD, and PPD with these issues in mind, though data for the latter two are lacking. Each section describes what is known about epidemiology and treatment. First, however, a brief comment on epidemiology is fitting.

Attempts to characterize the epidemiology of PDs in correctional settings must acknowledge severe limitations. Accurate prevalence figures are challenged by PDs not being amenable to the exigency of brief, sensitive screens for newly incarcerated individuals. Thus, typical screenings tend to stress nonspecific psychotic and affective symptoms, violence, and suicidality (see Chapter 15). Furthermore, the correctional setting itself may confound accurate diagnosis, given the "code of conduct" adopted by many IPs (Rotter et al., 2002) and the often comorbid, nonspecific symptoms utilized in categorical psychiatric diagnoses (Becker et al., 2000). Incarceration stereotypes may also lead to false demographic proportions for a given diagnosis (e.g., antisocial) or the assumption that "a crime was associated with a mental illness simply because it was horrific, deviant, or bizarre" (Knoll & Dietz, 2023). Finally, there are potential ramifications for service connection levels should a PD diagnosis be made rather than, for example, a mood or psychotic disorder diagnosis, leading to ethical conflicts for psychiatrists.

Keeping in mind the epidemiological challenges in any attempt to describe the accurate prevalence of PDs in correctional settings, current data reflect some patterns. Prevalence of any PD is much higher in correctional samples than in general population or civil clinical samples. Among those in short-term incarceration in Quebec, 18% were diagnosed with any PD, 14.8% of whom were men and 47% women. In England and Wales, prevalence among remanded men was as high as 78% for having any PD, with 68% for sentenced men and 50% for women (Singleton et al., 1998). Among incarcerated English and Welsh men aged 60 and older, 30% were diagnosed with any PD (Fazel et al., 2001). Comparatively, prevalence of any PD was found to be 7.8% globally (Winsper et al., 2020) and 12.16% in Western countries (Volkert et al., 2018).

Borderline personality disorder

The DSM-5-TR describes BPD's essential feature as "a pervasive pattern of instability of interpersonal relationship, self-image, and affects, and marked impulsivity that begins by early adulthood and is present in a variety of contexts" (APA, 2022). This is consistent with the task force's focus on the failure to develop a sense of self-identity and impaired relational capacity (APA, 2010). The behavioral indicators of these deficits manifest in various ways and are less important than the underlying psychology; this is one reason abandonment fear, suicidal behavior, and self-mutilation are not necessary criteria for diagnosis. Rather, affective instability and poorly integrated and distinct mental representations of self and important others, particularly in the "area of close interpersonal involvement" (Kernberg, 1995), are the disorder's core aspects. Patients "split" internal representations or concepts of self and important others into dichotomous good or bad psychological models or heuristic frameworks, manifesting in idealization and devaluation of others as the patient projects a representation onto the other.

The unstable sense of self, impulsivity, and difficulties with anger make for displays of temper and fighting. There is some evidence that among correctional populations, "experiences of anger and emotion dysregulation may be more strongly reflective of BPD than ASPD" (McGonigal & Dixon-Gordon, 2020). This is consistent with affective neuroscience models that differentiate "cold" aggression (predatory and calculating) from "hot" (reactive and impulsive; Panksepp & Biven, 2012). Finally, the term "borderline" refers to the range of organization between neurotic and psychotic, implying that more severe borderline pathology will likely manifest with episodes of failed reality testing—the DSM's criterion 9, "paranoid ideation." The ICD goes a step further, noting that the "borderline pattern" may share "transient dissociative symptoms or psychotic-like features (e.g., brief hallucinations, paranoia) in situations of high affective arousal" (WHO, 2022). In severe pathology, BPD's psychotic symptoms are not uncommon and presage worse outcomes (Jackson et al., 2023).

Several difficulties arise in the care of patients with BPD. First is the risk of misattributing symptoms to a primary or affective psychosis, accompanied by the potential for unnecessary and ineffective pharmacological treatment, side-effect burdens, and potentially unhelpful behavioral interventions (Jackson et al., 2023). Second, BPD can be expected to predict aggression and institutional misconduct (Moore et al., 2018). Disordered interpersonal relating leads to triangulation and splitting of prison staff, conflict with other IPs, and risk of self-harm behavior and suicidality. Elevated expressions of emotional dysregulation, anger (McGonigal & Dixon-Gordon, 2020), and impulsivity combine to exacerbate tension and impending adverse events in an incarcerated environment.

Epidemiology

The prevalence of BPD in noncorrectional settings varies broadly by population. Morgan and Zimmerman (2018) reviewed 22 studies published from 1985 to 2010 and found prevalence rates of 0% to 3.9%, with a median of 1.1%. Other recent studies estimate that 0.7% to 2.7% of adults in the general population are affected (Ellison et al., 2018; Leichsenring et al., 2023). Numbers are higher among outpatients (11%) and psychiatric inpatients (22%; Ellison et al., 2018), and the DSM-5-TR reports that approximately 75% of those diagnosed with BPD are female (APA, 2022). However, there is reason to believe that prevalence does not differ markedly between genders (Sansone & Sansone, 2011). Suicide, metabolic disorders, respiratory disorders, infectious disease, and life expectancy are all significantly worse in those with BPD compared to the general population (Leichsenring et al., 2023).

The prevalence of BPD in jails and prisons is estimated to be higher than the general population. A sample of participants in Iowa revealed that 29.5% of new IPs met criteria for BPD. The difference between men and women was considerable: 54.5% of women met criteria, whereas only 26.8% of men did (Black et al., 2007). Conn et al. (2010) used the Personality Assessment Inventory (Morey, 2007) pre- and posttrial in a county jail, finding that 44.7% of the sample met criteria for BPD, including a statistically significant gender difference between participants meeting the criteria (women, 52.1%; men, 41.6%).

Pharmacotherapy

There are no randomized controlled trials (RCTs) of pharmacotherapy for BPD in correctional settings. Nevertheless, such treatments are commonplace and include antidepressants, mood stabilizers, and antipsychotics to target mood stabilization and agitation. In community samples, psychotropic treatment for BPD has little to no effect on overall symptom severity, self-harm, suicide-related outcomes, psychosocial functioning, and interpersonal problems (Stoffers-Winterling et al., 2022). Cochrane reviews conclude that "use of medications in BPD is still not reflected or supported by the current evidence" (Stoffers-Winterling et al., 2020). Systematic review and meta-analysis have similarly demonstrated that "the efficacy of pharmacotherapies to improve BPD is limited to improvement of individual symptoms but not the condition overall. Even for the improvement of symptoms, the certainty of evidence is low" (Gartlehner et al., 2021). Despite the common clinical practice of prescribing lamotrigine for mood stability, empirical evidence for the practice is lacking (Pahwa et al., 2020). While similar statements can be made about the common prescription of second-generation antipsychotics, some systematic reviewers conclude there "may be a role for clozapine in treating severe treatment refractory BPD, especially for those patients at high risk of suicide and frequent hospitalisations" (Han et al., 2023).

Psychotherapy

Contrasted with pharmacological approaches, BPD-specific psychotherapy modalities have more support concerning their efficacy for numerous types of outcomes compared to control groups. These therapeutic modalities include, but are not limited to, mentalization-based treatment, dialectical behavior therapy (DBT), transference-focused psychotherapy, dynamic deconstructive psychotherapy, schema-focused therapy, and systems training for emotional predictability and problem solving (STEPPS). Most RCTs focus on DBT, followed by mentalization-based treatment (Storebø et al., 2020). A growing research base demonstrates robust support for long-term psychodynamic treatment of PDs, including BPD, in the community setting (Leichsenring & Rabung, 2011; Thor Cornelius, 2017), but there are no RCTs of its use in correctional settings. Clinical guidelines around dynamic treatment suggest that "the patient's cognitive style and capacity for introspection" inform whether a patient is a suitable candidate for psychodynamic or cognitive-behavioral therapy (CBT; Stone, 2019). Advocates for the role of psychodynamic therapies in corrections may lead future research efforts (Mea et al., 2022; Mulay et al., 2017).

For BPD in correctional settings, the number of studies, kinds of interventions, and generalizability of treatments are significantly limited compared to the general population and are largely relegated to STEPPS and DBT. Black and colleagues (2008, p. 883) describe STEPPS as

> a manual-based group-treatment program for persons with BPD that combines cognitive-behavioral elements with skills training, but does not include individual therapy. The program consists of 20, 2-hour weekly sessions with facilitators who follow detailed lesson plans. Subjects receive a packet of materials each week, including an agenda and homework assignments.

Data were collected for up to 20 weeks for 10 women with BPD in the Iowa Department of Corrections (Black et al., 2008), showing statistically significant results with large effect sizes for various symptom ratings. A larger study produced similar findings, also demonstrating efficacy of the treatment in individuals with comorbid BPD and ASPD (Black et al., 2013, 2016).

DBT is a type of CBT combining behavioral and mindfulness approaches in a dialectical process aimed at integrating difference and enabling acceptance and change. In correctional settings, DBT aims to reduce aggressive behavior and impulsive outbursts and reduce suicidal and nonsuicidal self-injurious behavior. Nee and Farman (2008) evaluated two DBT programs for women with BPD in the United Kingdom that utilized year-long and 16-week programs. The study yielded statistically significant results with large effect sizes for various symptom ratings and encouraging results from the 16-week program. Difficulties with implementation included lack of appropriately trained and follow-up staff, delivery team attrition, dropout and prison transfer, and general costs (Nee & Farman, 2008).

Antisocial personality disorder

Essential for the diagnosis of ASPD is a "pervasive pattern" of both the disregard for and violation of the rights of others (APA, 2022). To be diagnosed, an individual must be 18 or older and have exhibited behavior patterns severe enough, before age 15, to indicate conduct disorder. These categorical criteria conceptualize ASPD as having its origins in whatever underlies the early disruptive phenomena of conduct disorder and therefore considers them somehow continuous. This preserves the idea that the problem being diagnosed involves aberrant and dysfunctional personality development. Someone with no indication of adolescent conduct disorder who only developed antisocial behavior after a midlife substance use disorder or prison sentence should be conceptually distinguished from someone with a long history of empathic deficits, callousness, and disregard for others. That is, the population of those with antisocial behaviors is not homogenous, and alternative diagnoses can be applied for those without the relevant adolescent/childhood history.

In the spirit of dimensional models "representing spectra of personality dysfunction on a continuum with other mental disorders" (APA, 2022), psychodynamic and object relations theory, informed by neuroscience, have conceptualized ASPD along a continuum including malignant narcissism, borderline psychopathology, and psychopathy (Kernberg, 1995; Meloy, 1992). ASPD is seen as a particularly severe borderline condition, with its most severe form manifesting in ASPD patients who also have traits consistent with psychopathy as measured by the Hare Psychopathy Checklist (Gacono & Smith, 2021a, 2021b). Given the DSM-5's AMPD, the categorical system of diagnosing should lead to findings of PD comorbidity, especially disorders with common traits. Regarding BPD and ASPD, multiple investigators have highlighted such comorbidity and attempts at differentiation (e.g., Anderson et al., 2022; Becker et al., 2000; Black et al., 2007, 2016). From a dimensional perspective, rather than claim comorbidity, it makes more sense to acknowledge a group of phenomena coalescing around a borderline personality organization, with personalities failing to mirror the diagnostic manual in a homogenous way. Particular deficits in functioning (e.g., empathy, intimacy) and pathological traits may predominate (e.g., impulsivity, risk taking, hostility) in a manner that appears comorbid from a categorical perspective. Space limitations prevent full delineation; future editions of the DSM may tackle this matter in earnest.

An obvious question arises regarding antisocial behavior within IPs diagnosed with psychotic disorders. By definition, if ASPD and psychopathy are conceptualized as borderline conditions, then it makes no sense to diagnose a persistently psychotic patient (excluding affective and substance-induced psychoses) with any of the PDs described here. The DSM makes a similar clarification with exclusion criteria. It is conceivable, however, that someone with the underlying biological contributions to underarousal and diminished empathic capacity could eventually develop a schizophrenia spectrum illness. In fact, many clinicians in correctional settings would attest that this combination of psychosis and antisocial traits exists. In such a situation, the patient would probably receive comorbid diagnoses, but an alternative view would acknowledge a psychotic personality with antisocial or psychopathic traits.

Epidemiology

ASPD and BPD are the most researched and prevalent PD diagnoses found in correctional populations. Morgan and Zimmerman's (2018) review of 22 studies published from 1985 to 2010 found prevalence rates for ASPD of 0% to 4.1%, with a median of 1.2%. The prevalence of ASPD among those newly incarcerated was 35% in an American sample, with no statistically significant difference between men and women (Black et al., 2010). Similar prevalence figures have been found (37%) among men in a Dutch prison (Bulten et al., 2009). In an inpatient correctional psychiatric facility in central New York, 26.4% of the sample was diagnosed with ASPD, and 39% of men received a diagnosis of any PD compared to 16% of women. Among the satellite outpatient facilities in the study, 13.9% of the sample was diagnosed with ASPD (Rotter et al., 2002). From a categorical perspective, comorbidity with BPD was reported at 26% in one civilian setting (Becker et al., 2000).

Pharmacotherapy

There are no medications approved specifically for the treatment of ASPD. The United Kingdom's National Institute for Health and Clinical Excellence (2013) published guidelines for the assessment and treatment of the disorder, but it discourages routine use of medications as treatment. Rather, medications should target comorbid symptoms of anxiety or depression in accord with other guidelines. Expert review has highlighted that although "psychosocial interventions are the first option" (Sesso & Masi, 2023), medications are still used to target symptoms. Antiepileptics, lithium, second-generation antipsychotics, selective serotonin reuptake inhibitors, tricyclic antidepressants, and dopamine agonists are not uncommonly used, for example (Khalifa et al., 2020; Sesso & Masi, 2023). Cochrane review, however, indicates that current data are insufficient to draw any meaningful conclusions for practice (Khalifa et al., 2020).

Psychotherapy

Despite some promising studies, an updated Cochrane review suggests "very limited evidence available" for "psychological interventions" as of 2020 (Gibbon et al., 2020). However, some efforts are worth noticing. Saradjian and colleagues (2013) conducted a 5-year treatment program for 18 British men who carried the categorical diagnosis of ASPD or prominent psychopathy. They found high comorbidity with BPD, NPD, and PPD. Individual psychotherapy and cognitive interpersonal group therapy lasted the entire 5-year period, including individual affect regulation skills training and numerous therapy groups focused on schema, affect, addictive behaviors, offense, and interpersonal relationships. The treatment response was characterized by good attendance and reduction in restrictive housing placement due to violence or other management problems. Some participants were moved to low-security units. During the first 2 years of treatment, the average number of violent incidents dropped from 18.4 to 2.4 per person (Saradjian et al., 2013).

Bernstein and colleagues (2023) conducted an RCT of schema therapy versus treatment as usual for 103 men sentenced for majority violent offenses in the Netherlands. Sixty percent met criteria for ASPD, 21% for NPD, and 17.1% for BPD. The remainder had PPD or Cluster B traits. Those who were randomized to schema therapy were more likely to attain supervised or unsupervised leave (the outcome measures for rehabilitation) and more favorable outcomes on PD scales (Bernstein et al., 2023).

In Wilson's (2014) meta-analysis reviewing effects of treatment on recidivism for those with ASPD, one study (McKendrick et al., 2006) showed that a modified therapeutic community reduced recidivism in incarcerated men with ASPD, as indicated by follow-up data from 1 year after prison release.

Narcissistic personality disorder

NPD is characterized by "a pervasive pattern of grandiosity, need for admiration, and lack of empathy that begins by early adulthood and is present in a variety of contexts" (APA, 2022). Those with NPD may carry a stereotype of nearly bombastic grandiosity. Alternatively, "grandiose beliefs about the self as superior and special" may be camouflaged by "a vulnerable presentation of humility, self-doubt, shame proneness, and inferiority" (Diamond et al., 2021). Theoretical models of personality development are robust and plentiful, placing NPD in the class of "borderline" conditions arising from early formative experiences inadequate to engrain healthier interpersonal relating, a sense of self, and more mature defenses (Campbell & Miller, 2011; Diamond et al., 2021; Kernberg, 1995).

Given the lack of empathy and propensity for exploitation often seen in NPD, clinicians may be inclined to diagnose ASPD instead (Caligor et al., 2015). Similarly, "reference to others for self-definition" (APA, 2022) can vacillate between idealization and devaluation in a manner reminiscent of BPD. Even the belief that others envy the narcissistic individual may carry a paranoid quality with equivocal reality testing suggestive of PPD. However, the narcissistic person lacks "pervasive distrust or search for hidden motives," instead viewing others' envy as the motivation for nefarious actions (Ronningstam & Weinberg, 2013). When distinguishing whether the PD is predominantly characterized by traits of narcissism or antisociality, it is helpful to recall that

> even at the more severe end of the spectrum, individuals with narcissistic personality disorder do not demonstrate the total breakdown of moral functioning and absence of any capacity for loyalty that typifies antisocial personality disorder, nor is narcissistic personality disorder typically associated with the history of childhood conduct disorder that is common in antisocial personality disorder. (Caligor et al., 2015, p. 419)

Those with NPD tend to project the negative aspects of the self onto others, while "ideal representations of self and others (i.e., what one aspires to be through identification with admired others) overshadow the real self (i.e., a realistic sense of actual abilities and potential)" (Diamond et al., 2021, p. 16). Therefore, it would be unsurprising for a patient to remain relatively stable in the idealization of a psychiatrist, whereas with BPD, alterations in idealization and devaluation are expected.

The sense of entitlement and grandiosity in NPD may foster antagonistic interactions with peers and clinicians and contribute to threatening behavior, bullying, and rule breaking. While IPs with NPD may be thought not to account for as much violence or other behavioral concerns as those with ASPD or BPD, meta-analyses not specific to correctional settings have demonstrated that narcissism is related to both aggression and violence regardless of gender, and those scoring high in narcissism traits are particularly prone to aggression when they believe they have experienced a provocation (Kjærvik & Bushman, 2021). A study of female IPs in Greece revealed that narcissistic traits positively correlated with aggression, while criminal offense type did not (Kalemi et al., 2019). The underlying fragility of these persons, and the shame and humiliation they may be vulnerable to, increases their risk for depression and suicide (Caligor et al., 2015; Ronningstam & Weinberg, 2013).

Epidemiology

Morgan and Zimmerman's (2018) review of 22 studies published from 1985 to 2010 found NPD prevalence rates of 0% to 5.7%, with a median of 0.4%. Writing a systematic review in 2008, Dhawan and colleagues (2010) estimated a mean community prevalence of 1.06%. The same year, Stinson and colleagues (2008) sought nationally representative prevalence data from participants of the Wave 2 National Epidemiologic Survey on Alcohol and Related Conditions; they reported lifetime prevalence of NPD at 6.2%.

One study of British IPs revealed a prevalence of NPD of 7% (Ullrich et al., 2008), yet overall, there is a dearth of prevalence data for categorical diagnoses of NPD in correctional settings. This may be because some studies elect to investigate outcomes from traits or dimensional aspects of narcissism such as "pathological narcissism" or "grandiose narcissism" rather than the prevalence of PD itself (Kalemi et al., 2019; Velotti et al., 2020).

Pharmacotherapy

There are no medications approved by the U.S. Food and Drug Administration for NPD, nor has any standardized pharmacological treatment demonstrated utility (Mitra & Fluyau, 2023; Yakeley, 2018). Data are further limited because studies tend to measure comorbid symptomatology rather than measures specific to NPD (Dhawan et al., 2010). As a result, "psychopharmacologic intervention is symptom driven" (Caligor et al., 2015) and targets various symptoms such as depressed mood, impulsivity, and aggression.

Psychotherapy

The mainstay of treatment for NPD is psychological therapy, and modalities are normally divided into psychodynamic or CBT approaches. Historically, psychodynamically oriented authors have produced a much larger literature on the conceptualization and treatment of pathological narcissism. In recent years, transference-focused psychotherapy, mentalization-based treatment, schema-focused therapy, DBT, and meta-cognitive interpersonal therapy have been commonly used in community settings (Choi-Kain et al., 2022; Crisp & Gabbard, 2020; Diamond et al., 2021; Yakeley, 2018). No RCTs specific to NPD exist. Data on psychotherapy involving NPD are addressed in the psychotherapy section of ASPD above.

Paranoid personality disorder

PPD entails "pervasive distrust and suspiciousness of others such that their motives are interpreted as malevolent" (APA, 2022). The primary traits constituting personality functioning in PPD are mistrust/suspiciousness, antagonism/aggressiveness, introversion/excessive autonomy, hypersensitivity, hypervigilance, and rigidity (Carroll, 2009). These traits are known to manifest variously, including extreme distrust, holding grudges, intolerance of feeling slighted, preoccupation with suspicions of intended harm from others, reluctance to confide in others, misinterpretation of innocent events as carrying malign ulterior meaning, querulous litigation, and regular suspicions of infidelity on the part of romantic partners (Carroll, 2009). Descriptions of paranoid personalities date at least to Kraepelin (1921), and differentiating the nature of paranoid ideas from frank delusion has been a perennial challenge.

The conditions most likely to confound diagnosis are delusional disorder and schizophrenia. Both show persistent manifestations of failed reality testing, with ideas held despite contrary evidence. The PPD patient, however, is expected at least to tolerate the possibility that their interpretation of the world is an overreaction or that there may be alternative ways to view matters (Carroll, 2009). The paranoid hermeneutical frame that colors the life of PPD patients can be idiosyncratic in nature, or it may make them susceptible to the seemingly delusional thought content encountered in those who hold an "extreme overvalued idea." The distinction is that "true delusions are generally unshareable and are associated with a disintegration of personality, while overvalued ideas are shareable and occur in an intact personality without such disintegration" (Rahman et al., 2019, p. 2).

PPD appears to be among the more neglected of severe PDs in psychiatric research. However, Lee (2017) studied a civilian sample of 115 adults diagnosed with PPD, 208 diagnosed with BPD, and 417 normal controls. Those diagnosed only with PPD met on average more than two criteria for BPD. The reverse was not true: Those meeting criteria for BPD on average only met 1.5 criteria for PPD. Comparison of suicide attempts and self-injurious behavior demonstrated that risk was higher for the BPD group than for the PPD group. Meeting criteria for both PPD and BPD led to higher risk than PPD alone, but not higher risk for BPD alone; that is, those exhibiting traits at the diagnostic threshold for both conditions may be at a higher risk of self-harm than those PPD patients that have fewer BPD traits. Scales of aggression and impulsivity similarly demonstrated that meeting criteria for both disorders was associated with greater impulsivity and aggression compared to controls. PPD was significantly more aggressive than BPD, while BPD was more impulsive and self-injurious than PPD (Lee, 2017).

Violence by those with PPD may be more of a concern in correctional settings. While caution against unduly attributing excess risk of violence to persons with PPD must be exercised, "paranoid traits do indeed increase the risk of violence" (Carroll, 2009). Furthermore, the externalizing dimension is another risk factor for aggression (Knoll & Dietz, 2023), germane to externalized antagonism in paranoia (Krueger et al., 2021). The sensitivity to provocation, challenges to social status, and distrust of authority (Carroll, 2009) are descriptive features of PPD that are relevant to violence in correctional settings.

Epidemiology

Morgan and Zimmerman's (2018) review of 22 studies published from 1985 to 2010 found prevalence rates of 0.4% to 5.1%, with a median of 1.1%. Lee (2017) described a prevalence of 1.21% to 4.4% in the general population. Ullrich and colleagues' (2008) study of British IPs revealed a prevalence of 23%, the same figure given by the DSM-5 (APA, 2013). Estimates of PPD in correctional settings require qualification given the nature of the correctional context (Rotter et al., 2002) and lower reliability of diagnosis among clinicians (Lee, 2017). Therefore, level of functioning and personality traits should be ascertained for the time period before incarceration, and the use of dimensional models (i.e., AMPD's personality disorder–trait specified; APA, 2022) may aid diagnosis (Lee, 2017).

Pharmacology

Data regarding pharmacotherapy for PPD is scant (Koch et al., 2016). A case series with nonforensic patients (Birkeland, 2013) revealed little that is helpful other than that antipsychotics may be well tolerated. That said, as with other disorders in this chapter, pharmacotherapy to target particular symptoms is common but should not be expected to result in the patient no longer meeting diagnostic criteria for PPD.

Psychotherapy

A variety of psychotherapeutic modalities have been used in PPD, including psychodynamic (Crisp & Gabbard, 2020; Gabbard & Crisp, 2018) and CBT treatments. A major barrier to treatment recognized in the literature is that "the nature of their disturbance is not conducive to perceiving their own pathology, and their treatment may ultimately be burdened by their mistrust of physicians" (Vyas & Khan, 2016, p. 10). One example of this difficulty is described in a 5-year study of changes in global functioning scales among PPD patients in Norway who were treated with a combination of group and analytic therapy. PPD patients and avoidant PD patients were among those with "low change" (Kvarstein & Karterud, 2012). A similar study of CBT and psychodynamic group therapy in Norway found that Cluster A disorders improved less than other PDs (Karterud et al., 2003).

Summary

This chapter introduces the constellation of conditions that stem from a borderline level of personality organization and are most likely to create difficulties in the correctional setting in terms of interpersonal discord, conflict with other IPs and treatment staff, risk for suicide and self-injurious behavior, and risk for aggression and violence. These borderline conditions similarly rely on "primitive psychological mechanisms ... resulting in reliance upon the primitive defenses of splitting, projective identification, denial, primitive idealization, devaluation, and omnipotent control" to varying degrees recognizable by the predominance of particular PD traits and styles (Kernberg, 2016, p. 150). Studies indicate that PDs are more prevalent in correctional settings than in the general population, though evidence of effective treatment remains sparse. The unique challenges posed by PDs in correctional settings call for ongoing research efforts in this vast and complex field.

REFERENCES

American Psychiatric Association. (1980). *Diagnostic and statistical manual of mental disorders* (3rd ed.).

American Psychiatric Association. (2010). *American Psychiatric Association DSM-5 development.* https://www.psychiatry.org:443/psychiatrists/practice/dsm

American Psychiatric Association. (2013). *Diagnostic and statistical manual of mental disorders* (5th ed.).

American Psychiatric Association. (2022). *Diagnostic and statistical manual of mental disorders* (5th ed., text rev.).

Anderson, J. L., et al. (2022). Differentiating borderline and antisocial personality disorders in forensic settings. *Psychology, Crime & Law, 28*(2), 132–152.

Becker, D. F., et al. (2000). Comorbidity of borderline personality disorder with other personality disorders in hospitalized adolescents and adults. *American Journal of Psychiatry, 157*(12), 2011–2016.

Bernstein, D. P., et al. (2023). Schema therapy for violent PD offenders: A randomized clinical trial. *Psychological Medicine*, *53*(1), 88–102.

Birkeland, S. F. (2013). Psychopharmacological treatment and course in paranoid personality disorder: A case series. *International Clinical Psychopharmacology*, *28*(5), 283–285.

Black, D. W., et al. (2007). Borderline personality disorder in male and female offenders newly committed to prison. *Comprehensive Psychiatry*, *48*(5), 400–405.

Black, D. W., et al. (2008). STEPPS: Systems Training for Emotional Predictability and Problem Solving in women offenders with borderline personality disorder in prison—A pilot study. *CNS Spectrums*, *13*(10), 881–886.

Black, D. W., et al. (2010). Antisocial personality disorder in incarcerated offenders: Psychiatric comorbidity and quality of life. *Annals of Clinical Psychiatry: Official Journal of the American Academy of Clinical Psychiatrists*, *22*(2), 113–120.

Black, D. W., et al. (2013). Systems Training for Emotional Predictability and Problem Solving (STEPPS) group treatment for offenders with borderline personality disorder. *Journal of Nervous & Mental Disease*, *201*(2), 124–129.

Black, D. W., et al. (2016). Do people with borderline personality disorder complicated by antisocial personality disorder benefit from the STEPPS treatment program? *Personality and Mental Health*, *10*(3), 205–215.

Bulten, E., Nijman, H., & Van Der Staak, C. (2009). Psychiatric disorders and personality characteristics of prisoners at regular prison wards. *International Journal of Law and Psychiatry*, *32*(2), 115–119.

Caligor, E., Levy, K. N., & Yeomans, F. E. (2015). Narcissistic personality disorder: Diagnostic and clinical challenges. *American Journal of Psychiatry*, *172*(5), 415–422.

Campbell, W. K., & Miller, J. D. (2011). *The handbook of narcissism and narcissistic personality disorder: Theoretical approaches, empirical findings, and treatments.* John Wiley & Sons.

Carroll, A. (2009). Are you looking at me? Understanding and managing paranoid personality disorder. *Advances in Psychiatric Treatment*, *15*(1), 40–48.

Chessick, R. D. (1993). *A dictionary for psychotherapists: Dynamic concepts in psychotherapy*. J. Aronson.

Choi-Kain, L. W., Simonsen, S., & Euler, S. (2022). A mentalizing approach for narcissistic personality disorder: Moving from "me-mode" to "we-mode." *American Journal of Psychotherapy*, *75*(1), 38–43.

Conn, C., et al. (2010). Borderline personality disorder among jail inmates: How common and how distinct? *Corrections Compendium*, *35*(4), 6–13.

Crisp, H., & Gabbard, G. O. (2020). Principles of psychodynamic treatment for patients with narcissistic personality disorder. *Journal of Personality Disorders*, *34*(Suppl.), 143–158.

Dhawan, N., et al. (2010). Prevalence and treatment of narcissistic personality disorder in the community: A systematic review. *Comprehensive Psychiatry*, *51*(4), 333–339.

Diamond, D., et al. (2021). *Treating pathological narcissism with transference-focused psychotherapy*. Guilford Publications.

Ellison, W. D., et al. (2018). Community and clinical epidemiology of borderline personality disorder. *Psychiatric Clinics of North America*, *41*(4), 561–573.

Fazel, S., et al. (2001). Hidden psychiatric morbidity in elderly prisoners. *British Journal of Psychiatry*, *179*(6), 535–539.

Gabbard, G., & Crisp, H. (2018). *Narcissism and its discontents: Diagnostic dilemmas and treatment strategies with narcissistic patients.* American Psychiatric Publishing.

Gacono, C. B., & Smith, J. M. (2021a). A psychodynamic model of psychopathy: Using Gullhaugen et al. (2021) as a reference. *Archives of Assessment Psychology*, *11*(1), 113–126.

Gacono, C. B., & Smith, J. M. (2021b). Understanding the psychopath from a psychodynamic perspective: A Rorschach study. *Archives of Assessment Psychology*, *11*(1), 77–93.

Gartlehner, G., et al. (2021). Pharmacological treatments for borderline personality disorder: A systematic review and meta-analysis. *CNS Drugs*, *35*(10), 1053–1067.

Gibbon, S., et al. (2020). Psychological interventions for antisocial personality disorder. *Cochrane Database of Systematic Reviews*, *9*(9), CD007668.

Han, J., et al. (2023). A systematic review of the role of clozapine for severe borderline personality disorder. *Psychopharmacology*, *240*(10), 2015–2031.

Hare, R. D. (2004). *Hare Psychopathy Checklist-Revised* (2nd ed.). MHS, Multi-Health Systems.

Jackson, D., McLawhorn, D. E., & Pal, S. (2023). Borderline personality organization as an aid in differential diagnosis. *Journal of Nervous and Mental Disease*, *211*(7), 479–485.

Kalemi, G., et al. (2019). Narcissism but not criminality is associated with aggression in women: A study among female prisoners and women without a criminal record. *Frontiers in Psychiatry*, *10*, 21.

Karterud, S., et al. (2003). Day treatment of patients with personality disorders: Experiences from a Norwegian treatment research network. *Journal of Personality Disorders*, *17*(3), 243–262.

Kernberg, O. F. (1995). *Borderline conditions and pathological narcissism*. Jason Aronson.

Kernberg, O. F. (2001). Borderline personality disorder. In N. J. Smelser & P. B. Baltes (Eds.), *International encyclopedia of social & behavioral sciences*. Elsevier Science.

Kernberg, O. F. (2016). What is personality? *Journal of Personality Disorders*, *30*(2), 145–156.

Kernberg, O. F. (2022). *Hatred, emptiness, and hope: Transference-focused psychotherapy in personality disorders.* American Psychiatric Publishing.

Khalifa, N. R., et al. (2020). Pharmacological interventions for antisocial personality disorder. *Cochrane Database of Systematic Reviews*, *2020*(9), CD007667.

Kjærvik, S. L., & Bushman, B. J. (2021). The link between narcissism and aggression: A meta-analytic review. *Psychological Bulletin*, *147*(5), 477–503.

Knoll, J., & Dietz, P. (2023). Mass violence and the complex spectrum of mental illness and mental functioning. *JAMA Psychiatry*, *80*(2), 186.

Koch, J., et al. (2016). Review of pharmacologic treatment in cluster A personality disorders. *Mental Health Clinician*, *6*(2), 75–81.

Kraepelin, E. (1921). *Manic-depressive insanity and paranoia*. E. & S. Livingstone.

Krueger, R. F., et al. (2021). Validity and utility of Hierarchical Taxonomy of Psychopathology (HiTOP): II. Externalizing superspectrum. *World Psychiatry*, *20*(2), 171–193.

Kvarstein, E. H., & Karterud, S. (2012). Large variations of global functioning over five years in treated patients with personality traits and disorders. *Journal of Personality Disorders*, *26*(2), 141–161.

Lee, R. (2017). Mistrustful and misunderstood: A review of paranoid personality disorder. *Current Behavioral Neuroscience Reports*, *4*(2), 151–165.

Leichsenring, F., et al. (2023). Borderline personality disorder: A review. *JAMA*, *329*(8), 670–679.

Leichsenring, F., & Rabung, S. (2011). Long-term psychodynamic psychotherapy in complex mental disorders: Update of a meta-analysis. *British Journal of Psychiatry: Journal of Mental Science*, *199*(1), 15–22.

Levinson, A., & Fonagy, P. (2004). Offending and Attachment: The relationship between interpersonal awareness and offending in a prison population with psychiatric disorder. *Canadian Journal of Psychoanalysis/Revue Canadienne de Psychanalyse*, *12*(2), 225–251.

McGonigal, P. T., & Dixon-Gordon, K. L. (2020). Anger and emotion regulation associated with borderline and antisocial personality features within a correctional sample. *Journal of Correctional Health Care*, *26*(3), 215–226.

McKendrick, K., et al. (2006). Modified therapeutic community treatment for offenders with MICA disorders. *Journal of Offender Rehabilitation*, *44*(2–3), 133–159.

Mea, E., Nappi, G., & Latorre, V. (2022). Psychodynamic approaches to treating violent offenders in psychiatric wards and clinics. In C. Martin, V. R. Preedy, & V. B. Patel (Eds.), *Handbook of anger, aggression, and violence* (pp. 1–21). Springer International Publishing.

Meloy, R. J. (1992). *The psychopathic mind: Origins, dynamics, and treatment*. Jason Aronson.

Millon, T. (2011). *Disorders of personality: Introducing a DSM/ICD spectrum from normal to abnormal*. John Wiley & Sons.

Mitra, P., & Fluyau, D. (2023). Narcissistic personality disorder. In *StatPearls*. StatPearls Publishing.

Moore, K. E., et al. (2018). The relation of borderline personality disorder to aggression, victimization, and institutional misconduct among prisoners. *Comprehensive Psychiatry*, *84*, 15–21.

Morey, L. C. (2007). *Personality Assessment Inventory (PAI): Professional manual*. Psychological Assessment Resources.

Morgan, T. A., & Zimmerman, M. (2018). Epidemiology of personality disorders. In *Handbook of personality disorders: Theory, research, and treatment* (2nd ed., pp. 173–196). Guilford Press.

Mulay, A. L., Kelly, E., & Cain, N. M. (2017). Psychodynamic treatment of the criminal offender: Making the case for longer-term treatment in a longer-term setting. *Psychodynamic Psychiatry*, *45*(2), 143–173.

National Institute for Health and Care Excellence. (2013). *Antisocial personality disorder: Prevention and management*. http://www.ncbi.nlm.nih.gov/books/NBK555205/

Nee, C., & Farman, S. (2008). Treatment of borderline personality disorder in prisons: Findings from the two dialectical behaviour therapy pilots in the UK. In J. Hagen & E. Jensen (Eds.), *Personality disorders: New research*. Nova Science Publishers.

Pahwa, M., et al. (2020). Efficacy and tolerability of lamotrigine in borderline personality disorder: A systematic review and meta-analysis. *Psychopharmacology Bulletin*, *50*(4), 118–136.

Rahman, T., Meloy, J. R., & Bauer, R. (2019). Extreme overvalued belief and the legacy of Carl Wernicke. *Journal of the American Academy of Psychiatry and the Law Online* [Preprint] .

Ronningstam, E., & Weinberg, I. (2013). Narcissistic personality disorder: Progress in recognition and treatment. *FOCUS*, *11*(2), 167–177.

Rotter, M., Steinbacher, M., & Smith, H. (2002). Personality disorders in prison: Aren't they all antisocial? *Psychiatric Quarterly* [Preprint].

Sansone, R. A., & Sansone, L. A. (2011). Gender patterns in borderline personality disorder. *Innovations in Clinical Neuroscience*, *8*(5), 16–20.

Saradjian, J., Murphy, N., & McVey, D. (2013). Delivering effective therapeutic interventions for men with severe personality disorder within a high secure prison. *Psychology, Crime & Law*, *19*(5–6), 433–447.

Sarchiapone, M., et al. (2009). Risk factors for attempting suicide in prisoners. *Suicide and Life-Threatening Behavior*, *39*(3), 343–350.

Sesso, G., & Masi, G. (2023). Pharmacological strategies for the management of the antisocial personality disorder. *Expert Review of Clinical Pharmacology*, *16*(3), 181–194.

Singleton, N., et al. (1998). *Psychiatric morbidity among prisoners: Summary report* (591872010-001).

Stinson, F. S., et al. (2008). Prevalence, correlates, disability, and comorbidity of DSM-IV narcissistic personality disorder: Results from the wave 2 National Epidemiologic Survey on Alcohol and Related Conditions. *Journal of Clinical Psychiatry*, *69*(7), 1033–1045.

Stoffers-Winterling, J., Storebø, O. J., and Lieb, K. (2020). Pharmacotherapy for borderline personality disorder: An update of published, unpublished and ongoing studies. *Current Psychiatry Reports*, *22*(8), 37.

Stoffers-Winterling, J. M., et al. (2022). Pharmacological interventions for people with borderline personality disorder. *Cochrane Database of Systematic Reviews*, *2022*(11).

Stone, M. H. (2019). Borderline personality disorder: Clinical guidelines for treatment. *Psychodynamic Psychiatry*, *47*(1), 5–26.

Storebø, O. J., et al. (2020). Psychological therapies for people with borderline personality disorder. *Cochrane Database of Systematic Reviews*, *2020*(11).

Thor Cornelius, J. (2017). The case for psychoanalysis: exploring the scientific evidence. In *Core competencies of relational psychoanalysis: A guide to practice, study and research*. Routledge.

Ullrich, S., et al. (2008). Detecting personality disorders in the prison population of England and Wales: Comparing case identification using the SCID-II screen and the SCID-II clinical interview. *Journal of Forensic Psychiatry & Psychology*, *19*(3), 301–322.

Velotti, P., Rogier, G., & Sarlo, A. (2020). Pathological narcissism and aggression: The mediating effect of difficulties in the regulation of negative emotions. *Personality and Individual Differences*, *155*, 109757.

Volkert, J., Gablonski, T.-C., & Rabung, S. (2018). Prevalence of personality disorders in the general adult population in Western countries: Systematic review and meta-analysis. *British Journal of Psychiatry*, *213*(6), 709–715.

Vyas, A., & Khan, M. (2016). Paranoid personality disorder. *American Journal of Psychiatry Residents' Journal*, *11*(1), 9–11.

Wilson, H. A. (2014). Can antisocial personality disorder be treated? A meta-analysis examining the effectiveness of treatment in reducing recidivism for individuals diagnosed with ASPD. *International Journal of Forensic Mental Health*, *13*(1), 36–46.

Winsper, C., et al. (2020). The prevalence of personality disorders in the community: A global systematic review and meta-analysis. *British Journal of Psychiatry*, *216*(2), 69–78.

Wong, S. C. P., et al. (2012). The effectiveness of violence reduction treatment for psychopathic offenders: Empirical evidence and a treatment model. *International Journal of Forensic Mental Health*, *11*(4), 336–349.

World Health Organization. (2022). *Personality disorders and related traits, ICD-11 for mortality and morbidity statistics*. https://icd.who.int/browse11/l-m/en#/http%253a%252f%252fid.who.int%252ficd%252fentity%252f37291724

Yakeley, J. (2018). Current understanding of narcissism and narcissistic personality disorder. *BJPsych Advances*, *24*(5), 305–315.

38

Attention deficit disorders

Todd Tomita and Michael K. Champion[*]

Introduction

Few disorders in correctional settings present the degree of diagnostic challenge and treatment controversy as does attention-deficit/hyperactivity disorder (ADHD). The nature of the condition, its assessment, and its management in these settings combine to create a perfect storm of potentially vexing challenges for the correctional psychiatrist.

The core symptoms of adult ADHD—difficulties in sustaining attention or impulsivity and persistent overactivity—are neither pathognomonic nor specific. Most incarcerated persons (IPs) with ADHD have comorbid psychiatric disorders, including affective disorders, anxiety disorders, substance use disorders, and personality disorders. Because the mainstay of evidence-informed adult ADHD treatment is stimulant medication, assessment can be further complicated, as IPs may seek controlled prescriptions for diversion or misuse.

Potential risks and benefits of stimulant treatment need to be balanced at an individual and correctional institution level. A treatment approach with clear criteria is necessary to provide treatment access to those who need it and to defuse time-consuming lobbying, grievances, and complaints from those who seek stimulants for nonmedical reasons. This chapter concludes with an ADHD correctional treatment model that balances risks and needs.

Prevalence

ADHD occurs at far higher rates among justice-involved populations than in the community. A recent global systematic review and meta-analysis found that the rate of childhood ADHD persisting into adulthood was 2.6%, with 6.8% of adults having ADHD symptoms regardless of a childhood diagnosis (Song et al., 2021). Prevalence estimates among IPs range from 9% to 50% (Tamburello et al., 2022). Although this broad prevalence range may accurately reflect diverse settings, significant methodological shortcomings exist in these prevalence studies: nonrepresentative correctional samples, use of adolescent rather than adult populations, reliance on single sources of information, exclusive use of self-reports, use of community-based screening tools not validated in correctional settings, and overreliance on simplistic symptom counts on screening instruments. IPs often present with complex psychiatric histories and multiple comorbidities that make it challenging for even seasoned diagnosticians to identify ADHD in such patients reliably, especially without a more comprehensive diagnostic evaluation. One screening tool, for example, consists of six questions, including "How often are you distracted by activity or noise around you?" Given the typically crowded, cacophonous, and often hazardous environment in jails and prisons, a positive response to this question has little discriminatory value.

One meta-analysis addressed methodological shortcomings by only reviewing studies that assessed ADHD by diagnostic interview in unselected adult prison samples (Fazel & Favril, 2024). This review found that the prevalence rate of ADHD in men was 8.3%, or one in 12. While this prevalence rate will accord with the clinical experience of most seasoned correctional psychiatrists, it is considerably lower than most previous reviews and highlights the importance of using clear and consistent inclusion criteria in meta-analyses.

Assessment in correctional settings

Accurate diagnosis generally requires obtaining a thorough clinical history by a qualified professional; reliably establishing a childhood onset of symptoms; gaining input from collateral informants who know the patient well; inspecting objective records such as school report cards, teacher comments, prior clinical evaluations, and special education records for evidence of past ADHD-like symptoms and impairments; using current *Diagnostic and Statistical Manual of Mental Disorders* (DSM)–based diagnostic criteria; and ruling out alternative explanations for the symptoms (Bolea-Alamañac et al., 2014; Canadian ADHD Resource Alliance [CADDRA], 2020; Murphy & Gordon, 2006; National Institute for Clinical Excellence [NICE], 2019).

*. The authors acknowledge the contributions of Kenneth L. Appelbaum and Kevin R. Murphy, who were the coauthors of this chapter in the first edition of this textbook.

Most correctional systems do not have the time and resources to conduct such rigorous assessments, which compromise the reliability of making accurate ADHD diagnoses in these settings. For a confident diagnosis of ADHD, an adequately comprehensive assessment is needed to establish these three essential diagnostic elements (CADDRA, 2020; Murphy & Gordon, 2006; NICE, 2019): ongoing chronic ADHD core symptoms that cause demonstrable functional impairment, documented childhood onset of ADHD core symptoms, and symptoms and impairments that are not explainable by comorbid conditions.

Although commonly thought of as a disorder of childhood, most individuals with ADHD have symptoms persisting into adulthood, especially inattention, restlessness, poor planning, and impulsivity (Faraone et al., 2006; Fayyad et al., 2007; Turgay et al., 2012). Regardless of age, however, ADHD remains challenging to diagnose for several reasons (Murphy & Gordon, 2006). Inattention and impulsivity, the hallmark symptoms of ADHD, are part of the universal human experience, which leads to diagnostic dimensional uncertainty. These symptoms also occur with many other psychiatric disorders and thus lack categorical specificity. Conditions that share symptoms with ADHD include affective disorders; personality disorders; anxiety disorders; intermittent explosive disorder; substance use disorders; neurocognitive impairment due to head injury, delirium, or dementia; psychotic disorders; and medication side effects (American Psychiatric Association [APA], 2022). Inaccurate or poor recall of childhood symptoms and impairment, lack of available collateral informants who know the IP well, and inability to obtain corroborating data or historical records complicate the validation of childhood onset of core symptoms required to meet the DSM, fifth edition, text revision (DSM-5-TR) criteria for an ADHD diagnosis as an adult.

The high rates of comorbidity in IPs with ADHD are probably the most vexing diagnostic challenge; comorbidity is the rule rather than the exception. Mood disorders, anxiety disorders, substance use disorders, and personality disorders are common in correctional populations. Community epidemiological data from the United States showed in persons with ADHD a fivefold increase in any mood disorder, a fourfold increase in any anxiety disorder, and a sevenfold increase in substance use disorders (Kessler et al., 2006). A meta-analysis showed in IPs with ADHD a fivefold increase in affective disorders, a threefold increase in anxiety disorders, and a twofold increase in both substance use disorders and personality disorders (Young, Sedgwick, et al., 2015).

The clinical expression of ADHD and comorbidities is highly heterogeneous. Establishing that ADHD rather than comorbid psychiatric conditions is causing relevant symptoms requires adequate information and clinical judgement supplemented by collateral information; screening measures or a self-reported diagnosis will not suffice. For example, are problems with concentration and attention limited to an active mood episode, or are such symptoms more longstanding in this patient?

Optimal diagnosis of ADHD relies on a well-documented, lifelong history of problems, ideally with third-party corroboration. Diagnostic complexities routinely arise because adult recall of childhood symptoms tends to be unreliable (APA, 2022). Clinicians in correctional settings often need to treat ADHD based on some degree of diagnostic uncertainty; an incomplete database is the norm. There will likely be some missing elements from the evaluation, such as inadequate time for a comprehensive clinical interview, an unreliable or unduly prolonged process to obtain historical records or data from collateral informants, or difficulties in communication with officers and other staff to obtain needed behavioral observations. If there are too many missing elements, it may be impossible to establish whether a diagnosis of ADHD is present or not with reasonable clinical certainty. It is especially difficult to identify bona fide ADHD among IPs, as these patients routinely present with complex histories that may include multiple comorbidities, trauma and traumatic brain injuries, and longstanding substance use. A further challenge is that some IPs may seek stimulant medication for nonclinical reasons, including cognitive benefits, energizing effects, euphoric mood effects, or to obtain a divertible prison commodity.

The most important component in an evaluation for ADHD focuses on the degree and chronicity of impairment caused by ADHD symptoms. ADHD is a neurodevelopmental condition that can persist throughout the lifespan. At its core is a persistent and pervasive pattern of inattention or impulsivity and persistent overactivity. The diagnosis in older adolescents and adults requires at least five symptoms of inattention or hyperactivity and impulsivity that result in clinically significant impairment in social, academic, or occupational functioning and that several of these symptoms have been present since prior to age 12 (APA, 2022). Individuals with fewer symptoms, brief or episodic symptoms, or symptoms that do not result in significant functional impairment do not qualify for a DSM-5-TR ADHD diagnosis.

Few, if any, individuals go through life without experiencing moments of inattention to details, poor organization of tasks and activities, restlessness, or impulsive decisions. With ADHD, however, symptoms have been readily apparent, persistent, and severe, resulting in significant disruption and underachievement in major life activities, including social, academic, and vocational areas (Barkley et al., 2008). A reliable ADHD diagnosis in adults requires objective evidence of clinically significant dysfunction, not merely self-perceptions of underachievement.

Rating scales can aid in screening for the possible presence of an ADHD diagnosis. Some standardized self-report measures for ADHD include the Conners' Adult ADHD Rating Scale, the Brown Attention Deficit Disorder Scale, the Barkley Adult ADHD Rating Scale (BAARS-IV), and the Adult ADHD Self-Report Scale v1.1 Symptom Checklist (ASRS-V1.1). A shorter version of the ASRS-V1.1, the Adult ADHD Self-Report Scales v1.1 Screener, consists of only six items and can be used as a starting point to determine whether a more thorough assessment for ADHD is warranted. Murphy and Adler (2004) describe these rating scales in more detail. Caution is needed when using and interpreting community instruments that are not standardized for correctional settings. For example, one study of men in Swedish high-security prisons found that the Brown Attention Deficit Scale but not the ASRS-V1.1 differentiated between those with ADHD and those with antisocial personality disorder (Etterlid-Hägg et al., 2023). Young and colleagues (2016) compared the BAARS-IV against clinical diagnosis and found that it had high specificity (96.3%) but low sensitivity (37.9%). The authors noted that a briefer version of the BAARS-IV was better for screening purposes. Rating scales can complement but not replace a comprehensive clinical evaluation, which remains the diagnostic "gold standard" (NICE, 2019).

Offending, institutional adjustment, and recidivism

Adult male IPs with ADHD have been shown to be younger at first offense and to receive multiple convictions, and their ADHD symptoms are strongly associated with institutional aggression (Mohr-Jensen & Steinhausen, 2016; Young et al., 2011). Other studies show an association between ADHD symptoms and both violent and nonviolent breaches of prison discipline (Gordon et al., 2012; Young et al., 2009). Some studies, however, find no association between ADHD and offending (Crowley et al., 1998; Grieger & Hosser, 2012).

Stimulant medication treatment for adults with ADHD may reduce the risk of further criminality. One Swedish national registry study found that current treatment with ADHD medication was associated with reduced criminal convictions in men and women (Lichtenstein et al., 2012). Another Swedish national registry study showed that rates of violent reoffending in released male prisoners were lower during periods when stimulant medication was being dispensed (Chang et al., 2016).

The scientific literature indicates that criminogenic risk factors identified in the risk–needs–responsivity model, such as substance use and antisocial personality patterns, are the best predictors of recidivism in IPs with mental illness (Bonta et al., 2014; Carr et al., 2021; Wilson et al., 2020). The responsivity principle holds that treatment should be matched to the abilities and learning styles of the IP (Bonta & Andrews, 2016). The current conceptualization of responsivity in the risk–needs–responsivity treatment model does not include specific psychiatric disorders. However, while an ADHD diagnosis is not explicitly considered in the risk–needs–responsivity model, ADHD clinical symptoms such as short attention span and poor frustration tolerance are seen as responsivity factors. The clinical logic of viewing untreated ADHD symptoms as a responsivity factor is straightforward, as inattention or impulsivity and persistent overactivity can interfere with participation in treatment programs (McCormick et al., 2015; Skeem et al., 2014; Young et al., 2011). Research provides indirect evidence for ADHD as a responsivity factor. Huntley and Young (2014) found significantly higher rates of substance use in those whose ADHD symptoms persisted over time, whereas those whose symptoms were fully remitted showed substance use rates similar to normal controls.

Pharmacological and psychotherapeutic interventions

Given the numerous diagnostic challenges in correctional settings, a well-reasoned probable diagnosis of ADHD may be sufficient to precede an empirical trial of medication. Community ADHD treatment guidelines provide evidence-informed recommendations for pharmacological and psychotherapeutic interventions for adults with ADHD (Bolea-Alamañac, 2014; CADDRA, 2020; NICE, 2019). The evidence-informed treatment of adult ADHD is uncomplicated: A combination of stimulants and cognitive-behavioral therapy is optimal (CADDRA, 2020; NICE, 2019). The challenge is translating community-based recommendations into the correctional setting. Psychotherapy specifically for ADHD is unlikely to be a commonly available intervention in correctional settings. Instead, correctional treatment programs or psychiatric rehabilitation interventions may provide cognitive-behavioral therapy that, while not specifically focused on ADHD, still effectively addresses impairments (e.g., cognitive-behavioral therapy strategies using "stop and think" techniques to reduce impulsivity and diaries and time schedules to improve organizational skills).

Prescribing stimulants requires balancing efficacy against risks of misuse and diversion. Deciding between sustained-release or immediate-release formulations of stimulant medication is an important consideration. Community guidelines for the treatment of adult ADHD recommend long-acting stimulants, including lisdexamfetamine and methylphenidate (Bolea-Alamañac, 2014; CADDRA, 2020; NICE, 2019). Lisdexamfetamine and atomoxetine have shown lower abuse liability in community studies (Bolea-Alamañac, 2014), and both are recommended in community guidelines for adult ADHD treatment. Lisdexamfetamine is a dextroamphetamine prodrug that needs to be metabolized to the active drug after ingestion. Atomoxetine is a nonstimulant norepinephrine reuptake inhibitor with a delayed onset of action and may be the first-line choice for patients with substance use disorders (Bolea-Alamañac, 2014; NICE, 2019). In the correctional setting, community recommendations may need to be modified. Specifically, crushing short-acting stimulant medications reduces the risk of diversion (APA, 2016; Appelbaum, 2009; see Chapter 29).

Treatment data from children and adolescents indicate the relative treatment efficacy of ADHD medications. In a comprehensive guideline review, stimulant medications were found to have an effect size (Cohen's *d*) of around 1.0. Among nonstimulant medications, the selective norepinephrine reuptake inhibitor atomoxetine and two selective α-2 adrenergic agonists (extended-release guanfacine and extended-release clonidine) had an effect size of around 0.7 for all three (Wolraich et al., 2019). Assuming this data holds for adults, all medications work, but nonstimulant medications are less robust than stimulant medications. Of course, there are different risk considerations for adults. For example, cardiovascular risks always need to be considered when prescribing stimulants to adult patients (NICE, 2019).

Almost all randomized controlled trials of stimulant treatment in correctional settings show positive results for men with ADHD (Asherson et al., 2016; Ginsberg & Lindefors, 2012; Ginsberg et al., 2012, 2015; Kostenius et al., 2014). Only one, though recent, trial showed no benefit for stimulant treatment, possibly related to a strong placebo response, low levels of adherence in the treatment arm, and underdosing of the study medication (Asherson et al., 2023).

Prescribing considerations in correctional settings

Stimulant medications have substantial economic value among IPs, which may lead to diversion, sometimes involuntarily through threats or extortion. Falsified or exaggerated symptom presentations in an effort to obtain medication can consume precious psychiatric time (see Chapter 20). IPs may file grievances, board of licensure or registration complaints, or legal actions against psychiatrists who fail to provide a desired prescription. Disparate prescribing thresholds increase the likelihood of complaints against more conservative psychiatrists, especially when a decision is made to discontinue a medication started in the community or elsewhere in the correctional system. Most practitioners would rather avoid such adversarial encounters.

Nursing staff often face equally vexing challenges. The special handling, monitoring, and documentation required for controlled substances demand substantial time, potentially overwhelming an institution's capacity as the number of patients on these medications mounts. Custody staff also have valid concerns about the consequences of substance availability and misuse within correctional facilities (Tamburello et al., 2022).

The high prevalence of substance-related disorders among IPs leads many correctional staff to question the wisdom of introducing controlled substances into the environment. These concerns have merit, but correctional staff also want disruptive individuals to settle and engage in assigned work and programs. If ADHD treatment can lead to better collaboration and communication between clinical and operational staff, this adds value and may justify the inevitable diversion risks (Tamburello et al., 2022).

Although it remains difficult to form clear conclusions about the specific connections between ADHD and offending, institutional adjustment, and recidivism, the balance of the scientific evidence supports the pharmacological treatment of IPs with ADHD. Treatment advocacy without nuance, however, can be counterproductive. The challenge is determining which patients need treatment. ADHD is most often interwoven with comorbidities, and some behaviors may reflect normative reactions to experiences of incarceration. Not all ADHD symptoms can or need to be treated in the correctional setting, as may be the case in the community too.

A balanced approach

In the absence of a complete ban on access to stimulant medications—an option that is neither recommended nor necessary—correctional facilities need an approach that balances access to treatment while mitigating adverse effects on staffing resources, security, and litigation risk. A carefully implemented protocol for stimulant prescriptions can go a long way toward achieving this goal. Such an approach enhances diagnostic consistency in a multiprovider environment and helps support psychiatrists when they make treatment decisions. A good example was implemented in the Massachusetts prison system (Appelbaum, 2009), and key aspects thereof are recommended by the APA's guideline on psychiatric services in correctional facilities (2016).

A balanced approach to ADHD treatment recognizes that correctional settings are different than the community. Clinical and operational needs align best when treatment goals are pragmatic and utilitarian. Custodial staff's primary interests include reducing disruptive behavior, optimizing participation in programming and activities, and generally having facility operations run as smoothly as possible. In this light, efforts targeted toward providing ADHD assessments and treatment only to substantially impaired IPs with persistent difficulties in their daily activities will likely be supported by all. If IPs with bona fide ADHD respond positively to treatment by exhibiting fewer functional problems, everybody wins. Although this approach results in the treatment of fewer patients with stimulant medications, it has the advantage of ensuring them for those who need it most, while minimizing administrative and monitoring responsibilities, reducing risks of diversion and misuse, and diminishing disability for some individuals (Applebaum, 2009).

Whether to use stimulants for an IP whose only significant problem involves disruptive behavior presents a dilemma. As previously noted, impulsivity and other ADHD symptoms could contribute to institutional maladjustment, and related behaviors might improve with effective treatment. If this is the sole basis for prescribing, however, some IPs might intentionally misbehave to gain access to stimulants. This can become an especially dangerous situation if it encourages self-injury, assaults, or other harmful acts. For this reason, prudence would suggest that the functional justification for treatment with stimulants requires more than just transient serious misbehavior. Legitimate ADHD results in a chronic and pervasive pattern of impairment rather than a sudden onset in a circumscribed situation associated with secondary gain.

Other than making an accurate diagnosis, the single most important consideration when deciding whether to treat an IP with stimulant medications concerns current functioning and activities. Unless ADHD symptoms significantly interfere with an IP's active engagement, or attempts to engage, in work assignments, educational activities, or other programming, the benefits of stimulants do not warrant the cost in resources or risks. Difficulties with leisure or recreational activities by themselves would not meet this functional threshold (Appelbaum, 2009).

The importance of active and observable impairment before initiating treatment is relevant regardless of setting. A diagnosis of ADHD requires functional impairment (APA, 2022). Impairment can be measured by a combination of methods, including observations by custody and program staff, documented behavioral problems, input from family members or significant others when possible, and the use of brief, easily administered rating scales that survey the presence of ADHD symptoms and associated functional impairments (Barkley & Murphy, 2006), some of which allow others (e.g., correctional officers, work supervisors, family members, treatment providers) to rate an IP's symptoms and impairments. While collateral sources include work assignment supervisors, programming staff, continuing education teachers, and health care providers, the richest sources are correctional and program officers who have regular contact with IPs during these activities and in their housing units (Tamburello et al., 2022).

The special risks and challenges associated with the prescription of controlled substances in correctional facilities support an initial preference for nonstimulants, absent contraindications or previously adequate but unsuccessful trials. When stimulants prove necessary, the shorter acting agents are crushable and thus less susceptible to diversion and misuse. The corollary disadvantage of more frequent administration lessens if dosing occurs only when needed for important activities. Community guidelines generally recommend long-acting stimulant formulations, but risk considerations can take precedence, and crushed short-acting agents provide the least diversion potential (CADDRA, 2020). If long-acting stimulants are used, capsule formulations that can be opened and dispersed in liquid are the preferred option.

Continuing prescriptions for IPs who misuse or divert their medications makes little sense. As part of informed consent, IPs should be advised that misuse or diversion will result in discontinuation of stimulant medication. Access to medications should also require engagement in appropriate nonpharmacological interventions. Patients not meaningfully participating in recommended ADHD educational and psychotherapeutic activities also risk discontinuation of stimulant medication. In the event that stimulant medications must be discontinued, prescribers may consider offering lower risk options.

This approach to the assessment and treatment of ADHD in correctional settings appropriately limits the number of IPs who receive stimulant medications while allowing access to those who truly need them. Some may view this approach as unjustifiably restrictive, and others may see it as injudiciously permissive (Appelbaum, 2009; Burns, 2009). The approach strikes a reasonable balance between the competing interests, needs, and risks in the correctional environment (Applebaum, 2009). When implemented in the Massachusetts prison system over a 2-year period, this approach resulted in a manageable statewide stimulant treatment prevalence of about 1% (Appelbaum, 2011).

Summary

Pharmacotherapy is the mainstay of treatment for ADHD in most correctional settings. The balanced approach reviewed in this chapter is recommended to address the risks of prescribing stimulants in a way that still ensures treatment for appropriate patients. The practical consequence of this approach is a reduction in unnecessary diagnostic assessments. The approach fits with the reality of scarcity of time and resources. The key recommendations include (APA, 2016; Appelbaum, 2009):

- Assess and treat only IPs who have current and persistent functional impairments that impede active participation in programming, educational activities, and work assignments;
- Whenever practical, conduct a comprehensive diagnostic assessment that includes clinical examination, history of symptoms, record reviews, observations of third parties, and symptom rating scales;
- Treat with nonstimulants and nonpharmacological interventions whenever practical and effective;
- Do not initiate or continue the use of stimulant medications for IPs who do not meaningfully participate in recommended educational and nonpharmacological therapies;
- When stimulants are necessary, use shorter acting, crushable stimulant medication to lessen the risk of diversion;
- Lessen the needed frequency of medication administration by timing the use of shorter acting stimulants to coincide with important activities; and
- Discontinue stimulants for IPs who misuse or divert their medications and consider offering lower risk options.

REFERENCES

American Psychiatric Association. (2016). *Psychiatric services in correctional institutions* (3rd ed.). American Psychiatric Publishing.

American Psychiatric Association. (2022). *Diagnostic and statistical manual of mental disorders* (5th ed., text rev.).

Appelbaum, K. L. (2009). Attention deficit hyperactivity disorder in prison: A treatment protocol. *Journal of the American Academy of Psychiatry and the Law*, *37*, 45–49.

Appelbaum, K. L. (2011). Stimulant use under a prison treatment protocol for attention-deficit/hyperactivity disorder. *Journal of Correctional Health Care*, *17*, 218–225.

Asherson, P. J. E., Evans, C., & Young, S. J. (2016). *A pilot study of Concerta XL in adult offenders with ADHD.* https://kclpure.kcl.ac.uk/portal/files/97264393/ADHD_CIAO_final_report_28.2.2016.3.pdf.

Asherson, P. J., Johansson, L., Holland, R., et al. (2023). Randomised controlled trial of the short-term effects of osmotic-release oral system methylphenidate on symptoms and behavioural outcomes in young male prisoners with attention deficit hyperactivity disorder: CIAO-II study. *British Journal of Psychiatry: Journal of Mental Science*, *222*(1), 7–17.

Barkley, R. A., & Murphy, K. R. (2006). *Attention-deficit hyperactivity disorder: A clinical workbook*. Guilford Press.

Barkley, R. A., Murphy, K. R., & Fischer, M. (2008). *ADHD in adults: What the science says*. Guilford Press.

Bolea-Alamañac, B., Nutt, D. J., Adamou, M., et al. (2014). Evidence-based guidelines for the pharmacological management of attention deficit hyperactivity disorder: Update on recommendations from the British Association for Psychopharmacology. *Journal of Psychopharmacology*, *28*(3), 179–203.

Bonta, J., & Andrews, D. A. (2016). *The psychology of criminal conduct* (6th ed.). Routledge.

Bonta, J., Blais, J., & Wilson, H. A. (2014). A theoretically informed meta-analysis of the risk for general and violent recidivism for mentally disordered offenders. *Aggression and Violent Behavior*, *19*(3), 278–287.

Burns, K. A. (2009). The top ten reasons to limit prescription of controlled substances in prisons. *Journal of the American Academy of Psychiatry and the Law*, *37*, 50–52.

Canadian ADHD Resource Alliance. (2020). *Canadian ADHD practice guidelines, 4.1 edition.* https://adhdlearn.caddra.ca/wp-content/uploads/2022/08/Canadian-ADHD-Practice-Guidelines-4.1-January-6-2021.pdf

Carr, W. A., Baker, A. N., & Cassidy, J. J. (2021). Diagnostic moderators of the risk-recidivism relationship for offenders with mental illness. *International Journal of Offender Therapy and Comparative Criminology*, *65*(16), 1756–1774.

Chang, Z., Lichtenstein, P., Långström, N., Larsson, H., & Fazel, S. (2016). Association between prescription of major psychotropic medications and violent reoffending after prison release. *Journal of the American Medical Association*, *316*(17), 1798–1807.

Crowley, T. J., Mikulich, S. K., MacDonald, M., Young, S. E., & Zerbe, G. O. (1998). Substance-dependent, conduct-disordered adolescent males: Severity of diagnosis predicts 2-year outcome. *Drug and Alcohol Dependence*, *49*(3), 225–237.

Etterlid-Hägg, V., Pauli, M., & Howner, K. (2023). A comparative study of prison inmates with and without ADHD: Which neuropsychological and self-report measures are most effective in detecting ADHD within correctional services? *Journal of Attention Disorders*, *27*(7), 721–730.

Faraone, S. V., Biederman, J., & Mick, E. (2006). The age-dependent decline of attention deficit hyperactivity disorder: A meta-analysis of follow-up studies. *Psychological Medicine*, *36*(2), 159–165.

Fayyad, J., De Graaf, R., Kessler, R., et al. (2007). Cross-national prevalence and correlates of adult attention-deficit hyperactivity disorder. *British Journal of Psychiatry*, *190*, 402–409.

Fazel, S., & Favril, L. (2024). Prevalence of attention-deficit hyperactivity disorder in adult prisoners: An updated meta-analysis. *Criminal Behaviour and Mental Health*, *34*(3), 339–346.

Ginsberg, Y., Hirvikoski, T., Grann, M., & Lindefors, N. (2012). Long-term functional outcome in adult prison inmates with ADHD receiving OROS-methylphenidate. *European Archives of Psychiatry and Clinical Neuroscience*, *262*(8), 705–724.

Ginsberg, Y., Långström, N., Larsson, H., & Lindefors, N. (2015). Long-term treatment outcome in adult male prisoners with attention-deficit/hyperactivity disorder: Three-year naturalistic follow-up of a 52-week methylphenidate trial. *Journal of Clinical Psychopharmacology*, *35*(5), 535–543.

Ginsberg, Y., & Lindefors, N. (2012). Methylphenidate treatment of adult male prison inmates with attention-deficit hyperactivity disorder: A randomized, double-blind placebo-controlled trial with open-label extension. *British Journal of Psychiatry: Journal of Mental Science*, *200*(1), 68–73.

Gordon, V., Williams, D. J., & Donnelly, P. D. (2012). Exploring the relationship between ADHD symptoms and prison breaches of discipline amongst youths in four Scottish prisons. *Public Health*, *126*, 343–348.

Grieger, L., & Hosser, D. (2012). Attention deficit hyperactivity disorder does not predict criminal recidivism in young adult offenders: Results from a prospective study. *International Journal of Law and Psychiatry*, *35*, 27–34.

Huntley, Z., & Young, S. (2014). Alcohol and substance use history among ADHD adults: The relationship with persistent and remitting symptoms, personality, employment, and history of service use. *Journal of Attention Disorders*, *18*, 82–90.

Kessler, R. C., Adler, L., Barkley, R., et al. (2006). The prevalence and correlates of adult ADHD in the United States: Results from the National Comorbidity Survey Replication. *American Journal of Psychiatry*, *163*, 716–723.

Konstenius, M., Jayaram-Lindström, N., Guterstam, J., Beck, O., Philips, B., & Franck, J. (2014). Methylphenidate for attention deficit hyperactivity disorder and drug relapse in criminal offenders with substance dependence: A 24-week randomized placebo-controlled trial. *Addiction (Abingdon, England)*, *109*(3), 440–449.

Lichtenstein, P., Halldner, L., Zetterqvist, J., et al. (2012). Medication for attention deficit-hyperactivity disorder and criminality. *New England Journal of Medicine*, *367*, 2006–2014.

McCormick, S., Peterson-Badali, M., & Skilling, T. A. (2015). Mental health and justice system involvement: A conceptual analysis of the literature. *Psychology, Public Policy, and Law*, *21*(2), 213.

Mohr-Jensen, C., & Steinhausen, H. C. (2016). A meta-analysis and systematic review of the risks associated with childhood attention-deficit hyperactivity disorder on long-term outcome of arrests, convictions, and incarcerations. *Clinical Psychology Review*, *48*, 32–42.

Murphy, K. R., & Adler, L. A. (2004). Assessing attention-deficit/hyperactivity disorder in adults: Focus on rating scales. *Journal of Clinical Psychiatry*, *65*(Suppl. 3), 12–17.

Murphy, K. R., & Gordon, M. (2006). Assessment of adults with ADHD. In R. A. Barkley (Ed.), *Attention–deficit hyperactivity disorder: A handbook for diagnosis and treatment* (3rd ed., pp. 425–452). Guilford Press.

National Institute for Clinical Excellence. (2019). *Attention deficit hyperactivity disorder: Assessment and management*. https://www.nice.org.uk/guidance/ng87

Skeem, J. L., Winter, E., Kennealy, P. J., Louden, J. E., & Tatar, J. R., II. (2014). Offenders with mental illness have criminogenic needs, too: Toward recidivism reduction. *Law and Human Behavior*, *38*(3), 212–224.

Song, P., Zha, M., Yang, Q., Zhang, Y., Li, X., & Rudan, I. (2021). The prevalence of adult attention-deficit hyperactivity disorder: A global systematic review and meta-analysis. *Journal of Global Health*, *11*, 04009.

Tamburello, A., Penn, J., Ford, E., et al. (2022). The American Academy of Psychiatry and the Law practice resource for prescribing in corrections. *Journal of the American Academy of Psychiatry and the Law*, *50*(4), 636–637.

Turgay, A., Goodman, D. W., Asherson, P., et al. (2012). Lifespan persistence of ADHD: The life transition model and its application. *Journal of Clinical Psychiatry*, *73*, 192–201.

Wilson, A. B., Ishler, K. J., Morgan, R., Phillips, J., Draine, J., & Farkas, K. J. (2020). Examining criminogenic risk levels among people with mental illness incarcerated in US jails and prisons. *Journal of Behavioral Health Services & Research*. Advance online publication. https://doi.org/10.1007/s11414-020-09737-x

Wolraich, M. L., Hagan, J. F., Allan, C., et al. (2019). Clinical practice guideline for the diagnosis, evaluation, and treatment of attention-deficit/hyperactivity disorder in children and adolescents. *Pediatrics*, *144*(4), e20192528.

Young, S. J., Adamou, M., Bolea, B., et al. (2011). The identification and management of ADHD offenders within the criminal justice system: A consensus statement from the UK Adult ADHD Network and criminal justice agencies. *BMC Psychiatry*, *11*, 1–14.

Young, S., Moss, D., Sedgwick, O., Fridman, M., & Hodgkins, P. (2015). A meta-analysis of the prevalence of attention deficit hyperactivity disorder in incarcerated populations. *Psychological Medicine*, *45*(2), 247–258.

Young, S., González, R. A., Mutch, L., et al. (2016). Diagnostic accuracy of a brief screening tool for attention deficit hyperactivity disorder in UK prison inmates. *Psychological Medicine*, *46*(7), 1449–1458.

Young, S., Gudjonsson, G. H., Wells, J., et al. (2009). Attention deficit hyperactivity disorder and critical incidents in a Scottish prison population. *Personality and Individual Differences*, *46*, 265–269.

Young, S., Sedgwick, O., Fridman, M., et al. (2015). Co-morbid psychiatric disorders among incarcerated ADHD populations: A meta-analysis. *Psychological Medicine*, *45*(12), 2499–2510.

39

General medical disorders with psychiatric implications

Jennifer S. Bradford and Erik J. Garcia[*]

Introduction

Medical conditions that have psychiatric symptoms represent a significant diagnostic dilemma, particularly in the correctional health setting. More than half of incarcerated persons (IPs) in the United States have symptoms of a major mental illness (James & Glaze, 2006). However, the pervasiveness of substance use disorders, the increasing prevalence of elderly IPs (Carson & Sabol, 2012), and limited access to a patient's past medical and psychiatric records all contribute to the challenge of discerning when a psychiatric presentation results from an underlying medical condition. One early study underscored this challenge, noting that 46% of the patients admitted to community psychiatric wards had an unrecognized medical illness that either caused or exacerbated their psychiatric illness (Hall et al., 1981). A more recent study observed that 55 of 1,340 admissions (2.8%) to inpatient psychiatry settings were due to unrecognized medical conditions (Reeves et al., 2010).

Another challenge to recognizing medical illnesses that present with psychiatric features is the term "medically clear." This term is ambiguous because there is no universal standardization of the phrase, which impacts patient care (Thrasher et al., 2019) in several ways, including decreased communication between the psychiatric and medical teams, lack of clarity about the assessment completed to determine "medical clearance," and uncertainty if the clearance is for psychiatric evaluation or transfer to a psychiatric inpatient facility (Wilson et al., 2023). Nonetheless, the standard emergency room medical clearance of patients who present for psychiatric admission has revealed an increased risk for such underlying medical conditions among patients with any of the following five characteristics: advanced age, a history of substance use disorder, no prior history of mental illness, lower socioeconomic status, or significant preexisting medical illnesses (Gregory et al., 2004).

This chapter examines several of these risk groups and focuses on the presenting symptoms of delirium, mood disorders, and psychosis and the underlying medical conditions that can mimic or exacerbate them.

High-risk association

IPs share many risk factors, especially substance use and low socioeconomic status, associated with higher incidence of psychiatric presentation of medical illnesses. Patients recently incarcerated may experience untimely identification of withdrawal symptoms from prescribed or illicit substances following admission (Bureau of Justice Assistance) with symptoms ranging from depression and anxiety to frank psychosis (Chapter 46). The increase in the abuse of substances like cocaine, methamphetamine, and cannabis is leading to an increase of substance-induced psychosis that has short- and long-term mental health consequences (Fiorentini et al., 2021). Traumatic brain injury (TBI), seen in 48% to 72% of IPs (McKinlay et al., 2013), is closely associated with substance use and low SES and may present with delirium and dementia, depression, mood lability, and impulsivity (see Chapter 58). Finally, elderly patients, particularly those with multiple significant medical conditions, have a higher risk for a psychiatric presentation of medical issues. With almost 10% of IPs already over 55 years of age and the prison population aging (Carson & Sabol, 2012), this scenario will become more prevalent (see Chapter 60). Records of prior medical and mental health evaluations should be obtained whenever possible to help assess the etiology of current psychiatric symptoms. Lack of prior mental health diagnoses should prompt a particularly thorough evaluation.

Delirium and dementia

Delirium is an acute state of confusion or disturbance of consciousness caused by an underlying medical condition and characterized by rapid onset and fluctuating severity (Lipowski, 1989; Sood & McStay, 2009). Features include inability to sustain attention, global disruption of cognition, and disruption of the sleep–wake cycle, with symptoms often worse at night. The most common causes of delirium are substance use and withdrawal in younger patients and medication side effects in older patients. Anticholinergic medications are most associated with delirium in the elderly, but nonsteroidal anti-inflammatory

*. The authors acknowledge the contributions of Warren J. Ferguson, who was a coauthor of this chapter in the textbook's first edition.

drugs, diuretics, antihypertensives, and cimetidine have also been implicated (Lipowski, 1989). Infections, especially urinary tract and pulmonary infections, also commonly cause delirium in the elderly, while central nervous system (CNS) infection (encephalitis) can cause delirium in all age groups. Patients with HIV have a significant risk for delirium because of HIV CNS infection, CNS encephalitis (often due to cytomegalovirus or herpes simplex virus), and mass lesions (commonly lymphoma or toxoplasmosis). Other conditions associated with delirium include metabolic derangements such as hepatic failure and uremia, hyponatremia, hypokalemia, hypocalcemia, and hypoglycemia. Hyperosmolar states, as seen in severe hyperglycemia, can also present with delirium. Vitamin B_{12} deficiency caused by malabsorption, proton pump inhibitor use, or bariatric surgery (also a risk for thiamine [vitamin B_1] deficiency) can present with acute delirium or dementia (Kibirige et al., 2013).

In the *Diagnostic and Statistical Manual of Mental Disorders*, fifth edition, text revision, dementia is grouped among neurocognitive disorders, which also include cognitive changes from TBI or HIV (American Psychiatric Association, 2022). Dementia more commonly describes cognitive decline in the elderly. As with delirium, dementia can present with global cognitive impairment, affecting memory, thought process, and orientation. Unlike delirium, however, dementia has a slow and insidious onset; stable, instead of fluctuating, symptoms; and no alteration of consciousness or attention. Language skills are often minimally affected, which may delay early recognition of the disorder.

In younger patients, neurocognitive disorder most commonly occurs with TBI, a condition suffered by more than half of the current prison population (McKinlay et al., 2013). The emergence of fentanyl in the street opioid supply has led to an exponential rise in drug overdose over the past 5 years, with over 80% being nonfatal (Chang et al., 2020) and with varying states of neurocognitive dysfunction as a result (Mahoney et al., 2023; Winstanley et al., 2021). Prolonged alcohol use, particularly in patients with poor nutritional intake, is associated with Korsakoff dementia. Although less frequent now that highly active antiretroviral therapy is available, HIV-associated cognitive impairment remains common, with direct and immunologically mediated pathology implicated (Ellis et al., 2023). HIV encephalopathy, progressive multifocal leukoencephalopathy, and toxoplasmosis may all present as dementia (Garvey et al., 2011). Other infections such as Lyme disease and neurosyphilis should also be considered in the evaluation (Miklossy, 2008). The incidence of syphilis rose 28% in 2021 and continues to rise (Dyer, 2022), and neurosyphilis remains a relatively common complication that can occur at any stage of syphilis (Chow, 2021). The clinical presentation can be variable and may be expressed as psychosis, depression, personality change, or nondescript progressive dementia (Ropper, 2019). In older patients, Alzheimer's dementia and multi-infarct (vascular) dementia remain the most common causes of neurocognitive disorder, but the differential diagnosis includes mass-occupying lesions (particularly with focal neurological findings), Parkinson's disease, frontotemporal neurocognitive disorder, Lewy body dementia, and prion-associated disease (Manning & Ducharme, 2010).

Medical conditions presenting as mood disorders

A strong association exists between many medical conditions and major depressive disorder (MDD). Between 10% and 15% of patients with a recent myocardial infarction or stroke, especially of the left middle carotid artery, have symptoms of MDD (Gadalla, 2008). MDD occurs at a rate 1.2 to 2 times higher in adults with type 2 diabetes (Anderson et al., 2001; Markowitz et al., 2011). Depression is the most common comorbidity found in patients who have one or more chronic diseases (Sinnige et al., 2013). While the causality of debilitating medical illness and major depression is complex and multifactorial, several medical conditions present with symptoms of MDD, which often resolve with treatment.

Endocrine disorders, which are frequently unrecognized, often present with symptoms of depression. These disorders include hypothyroidism, hyperadrenalism (Cushing syndrome), adrenal insufficiency (Addison's disease), hyperparathyroidism, and hypoparathyroidism. Other presenting symptoms can include slowed mental processing and impaired memory with hypothyroidism, as well as irritability and mental slowing with hyperparathyroidism (resulting in hypercalcemia) and hypoparathyroidism (Levenson, 2006; O'Brien et al., 2006). Each condition has associated physical and laboratory hallmarks that can aid in recognition, but they are often detected in routine lab tests (see Patient Evaluation section). New research indicates that prolonged sequelae of COVID-19 infection—"long COVID"—can present with symptoms of insomnia, anxiety, posttraumatic symptoms, and mood disorders for up to 6 months (Badenoch et al., 2021) or more. Finally, with the growing prevalence of obesity, obstructive sleep apnea is an important consideration. A clear link has been established between obstructive sleep apnea and major depression (Schroder & O'Hara, 2005; Vanek et al., 2020).

Between 38% and 45% of patients with HIV have depression (Rabkin, 2008). Incarcerated persons infected through intravenous drug use may have an even higher prevalence, given the independent association between intravenous drug use and depression (Mackesy-Amiti et al., 2012). Of particular concern, depression in patients with HIV may indicate an underlying opportunistic infection (e.g., toxoplasmosis), a mass-occupying lesion (e.g., CNS lymphoma), or HIV-related cognitive decline (e.g., HIV encephalopathy, progressive multifocal leukoencephalopathy; Cohen et al., 1999).

Anxiety and panic attacks can be associated with many medical conditions, presenting a diagnostic challenge. The new or sudden onset of anxiety or panic should prompt a rapid evaluation for several serious physiological causes such as hypoxemia and hypoglycemia. Hypoglycemia is nearly always iatrogenic. Atrial fibrillation, congestive heart failure, myocardial infarction, asthma, and use of beta-agonist inhalers (the mainstay of treatment for bronchospasm) may present with symptoms of anxiety. Anxiety can also occur with endocrine disorders such as hypothyroidism, hyperthyroidism, and pheochromocytoma; the latter two are associated with tremor and tachycardia. In addition, hyperthyroidism can potentiate or present as bipolar disorder (Woesner et al., 2014). As with depression, anxiety may accompany chronic medical conditions, most notably TBI, Parkinson's disease, and chronic obstructive pulmonary disease (Lavery & White, 2009).

Medical conditions presenting with psychosis or mania

Delusions or hallucinations caused by medical illness are most frequently a component of delirium and dementia seen in patients aged 65 years or older (Patkar et al., 2004; Rabins et al., 1982). Up to 40% of patients with Alzheimer's disease have auditory or visual hallucinations (Paulsen et al., 2001). Hallucinations and paranoia commonly occur with Parkinson's disease and its treatment with dopamine agonists; they typically occur in conjunction with the characteristic rigidity and ataxia. In Huntington's disease, psychosis often precedes the characteristic choreiform movements seen in the disorder (Shiwach, 1994). Psychotic symptoms or mania may occur with systemic lupus erythematous (Rogers, 1996) and multiple sclerosis (Torales, 2018), but depression is more common. Refractory epilepsy has been associated with an increased prevalence of schizophrenia (Fruchter et al., 2014), and some seizures can cause hallucinations. For example, nondominant hemisphere temporal lobe seizures happen with mania and psychoses, while isolated auditory hallucinations occur with dominant temporal lobe seizures (Mula, 2014).

Metabolic and endocrine abnormalities such as thyrotoxicosis and, rarely, hypothyroidism (Prasad's syndrome) can present with mania and psychosis (Mula, 2014). Adrenal insufficiency (Addison's disease) and, more commonly, Cushing syndrome can also present with depression, mania, and psychosis (Kelly, 1996; Leigh & Kramer, 1984). In addition, treatment with high doses of corticosteroids may produce psychotic symptoms such as hallucinations or behavior that may be confused with mania.

Olfactory or gustatory hallucinations suggest underlying seizures, while tactile hallucinations suggest substance intoxication or withdrawal. Auditory hallucinations, while more commonly seen in schizophrenia, may be a feature of medically related psychosis.

Patient evaluation

Repeated psychiatric presentations to the emergency room may lead to overlooking patients' medical concerns under the assumption that symptoms are solely psychiatric (Wilson et al., 2017). Some features should raise the suspicion that a psychiatric presentation is the result of an underlying medical condition. As noted previously, the elderly IP, those with multiple medical conditions, and patients with HIV and substance use disorders are at particular risk. Patients with a well-established history of major mental illness and documented response to appropriate treatment are unlikely to have a causative medical illness, though accurate records are rarely available in the correctional setting. Conversely, the new or abrupt onset of psychiatric symptoms should prompt further evaluation, especially when accompanied by somatic complaints or physical findings such as tachycardia, tremor, or alteration in cognitive function.

Clinical evaluation should include vital signs with oximetry and finger-stick blood sugar, if available. In addition to a mental status evaluation, physical exam should include thyroid palpation, vascular exam (carotid bruits and pulse), cardiac and respiratory exam, and a thorough neurological exam. If there is suspicion of dementia, the Montreal Cognitive Assessment is particularly useful for diverse populations, as it has been validated in many languages (Montreal Cognitive Assessment, n.d.).

Preliminary lab testing should include renal and hepatic functions, thyroid-stimulating hormone and free T_4, vitamin B_{12}, electrolytes, glucose, and serum calcium. Urinalysis or dipstick analysis is especially important for elderly patients with delirium. HIV and syphilis tests and toxicology screens should be obtained. Further lab evaluation might include testing for systemic lupus erythematous. Although nonspecific, elevated C-reactive protein and erythrocyte sedimentation rate can suggest an active infectious or inflammatory process.

Focal neurologic changes; evidence of a CNS infection such as meningeal signs, fever, and headache; and new onset of psychosis or delirium all merit prompt referral for further evaluation and care.

Summary

IPs have a high prevalence of mental illness, substance abuse, and chronic medical conditions that are often untreated prior to incarceration. The aging of incarcerated populations, frequent histories of TBI, and lack of access to thorough medical evaluations further complicate systematic evaluation of behavioral health symptoms. Priority should be given to assessing patients for treatable, serious medical conditions that can mimic mental illness. Chief among these are metabolic derangements, conditions that lead to hypoxemia, acute substance withdrawal, CNS infections or space-occupying lesions, and iatrogenic side effects of prescribed medications.

REFERENCES

American Psychiatric Association. (2022). *The diagnostic and statistical manual of mental disorders* (5th ed., text rev.).

Anderson, R. J., Freedland, K. E., Clouse, R. E., & Lustman, P. J. (2001). The prevalence of comorbid depression in adults with diabetes: A meta-analysis. *Diabetes Care*, *24*, 1069–1078.

Badenoch, J. B., Rengasamy, E. R., Watson, C., et al. (2021). Persistent neuropsychiatric symptoms after COVID-19: A systematic review and meta-analysis. *Brain Communications*, *4*(1), fcab297.

Carson, E. A., & Sabol, W. J. (2012). *Prisoners in 2011* (NCJ 239808). Bureau of Justice Statistics, U.S. Department of Justice.

Chang, L., Eisenberg, M., Ferris, L., et al. (2020). The impact of various risk assessment time frames on the performance of opioid overdose forecasting models. *Medical Care*, *58*(11), 1013–1021.

Chow, F. (2021). Neurosyphilis. *Continuum (Minneapolis, Minn.)*, *27*(4), 1018–1039.

Cohen, P. T., Sande, M. A., & Volberding, P. (1999). *The AIDS knowledge base: A textbook on HIV disease from the University of California* (3rd ed.). Lippincott-Raven.

Dyer, O. (2022). Syphilis and gonorrhoea cases soar in US. *BMJ (Clinical Research Ed.)*, *378*, o2355.

Ellis, R. J., Marquine, M. J., Kaul, M., Fields, J. A., & Schlachetzki, J. C. M. (2023). Mechanisms underlying HIV-associated cognitive impairment and emerging therapies for its management. *Nature Reviews Neurology*, *19*(11), 668–687.

Fiorentini, A., Cantù, F., Crisanti, C., Cereda, G., Oldani, L., & Brambilla, P. (2021). Substance-induced psychoses: An updated literature review. *Frontiers in Psychiatry*, *12*, 694863.

Fruchter, E., Kapara, O., Reichenberg, A., et al. (2014). Longitudinal association between epilepsy and schizophrenia: A population-based study. *Epilepsy and Behavior*, *31*, 291–294.

Gadalla, T. (2008). Association of comorbid mood disorders and chronic illness with disability and quality of life in Ontario, Canada. *Chronic Diseases and Injuries in Canada*, *28*, 148–154.

Garvey, L., Winston, A., Walsh, J., et al. (2011). HIV-associated central nervous system diseases in the recent combination antiretroviral therapy era. *European Journal of Neurology*, *18*, 527–534.

Gregory, R. J., Nihalani, N. D., & Rodriguez, E. (2004). Medical screening in the emergency department for psychiatric admissions: A procedural analysis. *General Hospital Psychiatry, 26*, 405–410.

Hall, R. C., Gardner, E. R., Popkin, M. K., Lecann, A. F., & Stickney, S. K. (1981). Unrecognized physical illness prompting psychiatric admission: A prospective study. *American Journal of Psychiatry, 138*, 629–635.

James, D., & Glaze, L. (2006). *Mental health problems of prison and jail inmates* (NCR 213600). U.S. Department of Justice, Office of Justice Programs, Bureau of Justice Statistics.

Kelly, W. F. (1996). Psychiatric aspects of Cushing's syndrome. *QJM, 89*, 543–551.

Kibirige, D., Wekesa, C., Kaddu-Mukasa, M., & Waiswa, M. (2013). Vitamin B12 deficiency presenting as an acute confusional state: A case report and review of literature. *African Health Sciences, 13*, 850–852.

Lavery, L. L., & White, E. M. (2009). Other cognitive and mental disorders due to a general medical condition. In B. J. Sadock, V. A. Sadock, & P. Ruiz (Eds.), *Kaplan & Sadock's comprehensive textbook of psychiatry* (9th ed., p. 1226). Lippincott Williams & Wilkins.

Leigh, H., & Kramer, S. I. (1984). The psychiatric manifestations of endocrine disease. *Advances in Internal Medicine, 29*, 413–445.

Levenson, J. L. (2006). Psychiatric issues in endocrinology. *Primary Psychiatry, 13*, 27–30.

Lipowski, Z. J. (1989). Delirium in the elderly patient. *New England Journal of Medicine, 320*, 578–582.

Mackesy-Amiti, M. E., Donenberg, G. R., & Ouellet, L. J. (2012). Prevalence of psychiatric disorders among young injection drug users. *Drug and Alcohol Dependence, 124*, 70–78.

Mahoney, J. J., 3rd, Winstanley, E. L., Castillo, F., et al. (2023). A pilot study investigating cognitive impairment associated with opioid overdose. *Drug and Alcohol Dependence, 247*, 109865.

Manning, C. A., & Ducharme, J. K. (2010). Dementia syndromes in the older adult. In P. A. Lichtenberg (Ed.), *Handbook of assessment in clinical gerontology* (2nd ed., pp. 155–178). Academic Press.

Markowitz, S. M., Gonzalez, J. S., Wilkinson, J. L., & Safren, S. A. (2011). A review of treating depression in diabetes: Emerging findings. *Psychosomatics, 52*, 1–18.

McKinlay, A., Corrigan, J., Horwood, L. J., & Fergusson, D. M. (2013). Substance abuse and criminal activities following traumatic brain injury in childhood, adolescence, and early adulthood. *Journal of Head Trauma Rehabilitation, 29*(6), 498–506.

Miklossy, J. (2008). Biology and neuropathology of dementia in syphilis and Lyme disease. *Handbook of Clinical Neurology, 89*, 825–844.

Montreal Cognitive Assessment. (n.d.). https://mocacognition.com

Mula, M. (2014). Epilepsy-induced behavioral changes during the ictal phase. *Epilepsy and Behavior, 30*, 14–16.

O'Brien, R. F., Kifuji, K., & Summergrad, P. (2006). Medical conditions with psychiatric manifestations. *Adolescent Medicine Clinics, 17*, 49–77.

Patkar, A. A., Mago, R., & Masand, P. S. (2004). Psychotic symptoms in patients with medical disorders. *Current Psychiatry Reports, 6*, 216–224.

Paulsen, J. S., Ready, R. E., Hamilton, J. M., Mega, M. S., & Cummings, J. L. (2001). Neuropsychiatric aspects of Huntington's disease. *Journal of Neurology, Neurosurgery and Psychiatry, 71*, 310–314.

Rabins, P. V., Mace, N. L., & Lucas, M. J. (1982). The impact of dementia on the family. *Journal of the American Medical Association, 248*, 333–335.

Rabkin, J. G. (2008). HIV and depression: 2008 review and update. *Current HIV/AIDS Reports, 5*, 163–171.

Reeves, R., Parker, J., Loveless, P., et al. (2010). Unrecognized physical illness prompting psychiatric admission. *Annals of Clinical Psychiatry, 22*(3), 180–185.

Rogers, M. (1996). Psychiatric aspects. In P. H. Schur (Ed.), *The clinical management of systemic lupus erythematosus* (2nd ed.). Lippincott-Raven.

Ropper, A. H. (2019). Neurosyphilis. *New England Journal of Medicine, 381*(14), 1358–1363.

Schroder, C. M., & O'Hara, R. (2005). Depression and obstructive sleep apnea (OSA). *Annals of General Psychiatry, 4*, 13.

Shiwach, R. (1994). Psychopathology in Huntington's disease patients. *Acta Psychiatrica Scandinavica, 90*, 241–246.

Sinnige, J., Braspenning, J., Schellevis, F., Stirbu-Wagner, I., Westert, G., & Korevaar, J. (2013). The prevalence of disease clusters in older adults with multiple chronic diseases—A systematic literature review. *PLoS One, 8*, e79641.

Sood, T. R., & McStay, C. M. (2009). Evaluation of the psychiatric patient. *Emergency Medical Clinics of North America, 27*, 669–683, ix.

Thrasher, T. W., Rolli, M., Redwood, R. S., et al. (2019). "Medical clearance" of patients with acute mental health needs in the emergency department: A literature review and practice recommendations. *WMJ: Official Publication of the State Medical Society of Wisconsin, 118*(4), 156–163.

Torales, J., González, I., Barrios, I., Ventriglio, A., & Bhugra, D. (2018). Manic episodes due to medical illnesses: A literature review. *Journal of Nervous and Mental Disease, 206*(9), 733–738.

United States, Department of Justice, Office of Justice Programs, Bureau of Justice Assistance. *Managing Substance Withdrawal in Jails: A Legal Brief. Feb. 2022, NCJ 304066*

Vanek, J., Prasko, J., Genzor, S., et al. (2020). Obstructive sleep apnea, depression, and cognitive impairment. *Sleep Medicine, 118*(4), 156–163.

Wilson, M. P., Hamrick, E., Stiebel, V., & Nordstrom, K. (2023). Contemporary practices for medical evaluation of the psychiatric patient in the emergency department. *Focus (American Psychiatric Publishing), 21*(1), 28–34.

Wilson, M. P., Nordstrom, K., Anderson, E. L., et al. (2017). American Association for Emergency Psychiatry task force on medical clearance of adult psychiatric patients. Part II: Controversies over medical assessment, and consensus recommendations. *Western Journal of Emergency Medicine, 18*(4), 640–646.

Winstanley, E. L., Mahoney, J. J., 3rd, Castillo, F., & Comer, S. D. (2021). Neurocognitive impairments and brain abnormalities resulting from opioid-related overdoses: A systematic review. *Drug and Alcohol Dependence, 226*, 108838.

Woesner, M. E., Marsh, J., & Kanofsky, J. D. (2014). The assertive community treatment team: An appropriate treatment for medical disorders that present with prominent psychiatric symptoms. *Primary Care Companion for CNS Disorders, 16*(4), 10.4088/PCC.14br01639.

Woody, D. M., Chen, C., & Parker, J. (2023). Catatonia in a patient with bipolar affective disorder and hypothyroidism: A diagnostic and therapeutic challenge. *Cureus, 15*(10), e46989.

40

Psychiatric assessment and management of chronic pain

Robert L. Trestman and Anthony C. Tamburello

Introduction

Pain is a subjective experience arising from injury, illness, deformity, or physiologic derangement, and sometimes from unknown sources. Chronic pain differs from acute pain in many ways. First, by definition, the pain has become enduring and goes beyond the expected period of healing, whether in the context of trauma or surgery or as part of a degenerative or progressive disease. The typical time frame used for defining chronic pain is longer than 6 months (Turk & Okifuji, 2001), though time frames of more than 6 weeks have been described (Gill et al., 2019). Another characteristic that distinguishes chronic from acute pain is the emotional element of perceived suffering (Turk & Okifuji, 2001). In this context, suffering is the experiential component distinct from nociceptive activity that typically defines the experience of acute pain (Turk & Okifuji, 2001). This component of chronic pain makes it potentially relevant to psychiatric assessment and intervention. Chronic pain is generally considered maladaptive (Gill et al., 2019) and is an independent risk factor for suicide (Racine, 2018).

The National Commission on Correctional Health Care (NCCHC) revised their position statement on the management of chronic pain for incarcerated persons (IPs; NCCHC, 2023). The NCCHC supports evidence-based assessment, individualized treatment planning, availability of evidence-based nonpharmacologic treatment options, appropriate assessment and treatment of comorbid mental health and substance use disorders, and a preference for nonopioid over opioid medications when pharmacotherapy is indicated (NCCHC, 2023).

Chronic pain management in a carceral setting is challenging due to a host of factors. First, most IPs being treated have a history of substance use disorders, with even higher rates in jails, women, and persons with comorbid mental health problems (Tamburello et al., 2022). Further, the population of incarcerated adults has a disproportionate prevalence of significant chronic medical and psychiatric conditions (Skarupski et al., 2018). The aging population in carceral settings has increased the burden of medical problems and accumulating functional disabilities (Barry et al., 2020). Finally, access to illicit drugs is limited in carceral settings. Persons who may have relied on illegal substances in the community for pain management may shift to prescription medication use or misuse.

To date, there are no studies on the prevalence of chronic pain conditions in IPs in the United States. Croft and Mayhew (2015) reviewed charts in two prisons in the United Kingdom and found evidence of chronic noncancer pain, defined as receiving daily analgesia for at least 3 months prior to review, in 20% of IPs there.

This chapter addresses the psychiatric assessment and management of chronic pain in carceral settings. Apropos of the assessment, information is provided regarding the factors to be elicited in a chronic pain interview, the methods used to assess chronic pain, and the assessment factors appropriate to integrate into a management plan. Subsequently, the methods used to manage chronic pain from a psychiatric perspective in the carceral setting are discussed. The need for consistent communication and interdisciplinary coordination, which are key elements of successful pain management, is reviewed. The factors involved in a management plan and various methods for tracking the outcomes of treatment, some unique to carceral settings, are also described.

Assessment of chronic pain

Biological factors

Though it is unusual for a psychiatrist to have primary responsibility to assess a pain concern in a carceral environment, an appropriate assessment of chronic pain will include a comprehensive history, physical examination, and review of any available prior records. Documentation should include the character of current pain and other associated physiological symptoms, as well as current and past medications and relevant laboratory and imaging data. It is helpful to document the specific characteristics of the pain problem, such as the nature, location, and frequency of symptoms, as well as any recent changes, such as precipitating events that elicited the referral (e.g., increased pain, decreased function, contemplation of surgery). Any needed referrals and diagnostic tests should be ordered and conducted to rule in or out treatable underlying conditions.

Psychiatric comorbidities

Many psychiatric conditions, including mood disorders, anxiety disorders, personality disorders, somatic symptom disorders, and factitious disorders, may present with complaints of pain, may co-occur with the disorder causing the pain, or may exacerbate the pain. Treatment for primary disorders of mood, anxiety, and personality would proceed as per standard practice and are addressed elsewhere in this text (see Chapters 33, 35, and 37). Complaints of pain secondary to or exacerbated by these conditions would be expected to improve with treatment of the psychiatric comorbidity. Numerous studies using various methodologies have found high rates of depression and anxiety in chronic pain patients, especially those prescribed opioids or with an opioid use disorder (van Rijswijk et al., 2019).

Somatic symptom disorder

A focused pain complaint that cannot be entirely attributed to a specific medical disorder but causes genuine suffering and distress is the core characteristic of somatic symptom disorder with predominant pain (American Psychiatric Association [APA], 2022, p. 352). This was previously known as pain disorder (APA, 2022). A diagnosis of somatic symptom disorder with predominant pain requires disproportionate and persistent thoughts about the seriousness of one's pain, persistently high levels of anxiety about the pain, or excessive time and energy invested in pain symptoms, and symptoms must be persistent, usually for more than 6 months (APA, 2022). A somatic symptom disorder does not by itself exclude another medical condition. No prevalence studies on somatic symptom disorder have been done since the publication of the *Diagnostic and Statistical Manual of Mental Disorders*, fifth edition (DSM-5); however, the prevalence in the community is estimated to be around 5% based on previous research of somatization disorder (Park et al., 2022).

Factitious disorder

Factitious disorder imposed on self involves physical or psychological symptoms that are intentionally produced or feigned to assume the sick role (APA, 2022). The three key criteria for this disorder are falsification of symptoms or signs or intentional induction of illness or injury; presentation by the patient as being ill, impaired, or injured; and the occurrence of the behavior in the absence of obvious external rewards (APA, 2022, p. 368). Typically, there are subjective symptoms such as complaints of acute abdominal pain in the absence of objective evidence of such pain. There may be self-inflicted conditions, which might include the production of abscesses by injection of saliva or feces into the skin. There may also be exaggeration or exacerbation of preexisting general medical conditions. This situation might present as, for example, feigning of a grand mal seizure by an individual with a previous history of seizure disorder. A defining characteristic of a factitious disorder is that external incentives for the behaviors, such as economic gain or avoiding legal responsibility, are absent. Factitious disorder with mostly physical symptoms is commonly referred to as Munchausen's syndrome, named for an 18th-century German officer known to embellish his life story (Asher, 1951).

Malingering

Malingering is defined as the "intentional production of false or grossly exaggerated physical or psychological symptoms, motivated by external incentives such as avoiding military duty, avoiding work, obtaining financial compensation, evading criminal prosecution, or obtaining drugs" (APA, 2022, p. 836). Malingering is not a mental disorder but is considered a problem that may be a focus of clinical attention. Clues that raise suspicion include a medicolegal context, inconsistencies between expressed complaints and objective observations, poor cooperation with diagnosis and treatment efforts, and a diagnosis of antisocial personality disorder (APA, 2022, p. 836). The presence of a clear external motivation differentiates malingering from factitious disorder.

Correctional settings clearly set the stage for malingering behavior, since opportunities to manage and control the environment by the offender are typically otherwise very limited. However, caution must be exercised in making a diagnosis of malingering (see Chapter 20). The risk of inappropriately withholding appropriate treatment is a major concern. Also, once someone is labeled as a malingerer, their concerns or threats (e.g., of suicide) may be ignored, with potentially serious consequences. Malingering is not mutually exclusive with a serious medical or mental illness. Malingering behavior may be employed by a patient to bring attention to their actual needs (Rogers & Bender, 2018). In general, it is clinically appropriate to assume a patient is not malingering until given good reason to believe otherwise (Gill et al., 2019).

> **CASE EXAMPLE**
>
> A patient with low back pain in a medium-security facility was repeatedly observed ambulating with a walker by program personnel. On one occasion, when he was unaware that he was being observed, he was seen casually carrying his walker over his shoulder while ambulating with appropriate body posture and gait. Staff conducted an assessment, considering possible motives including securing the walker to use as a weapon, to conceal contraband, to support obtaining pain medication, or to secure disability benefits upon return to the community

Assessing malingering of chronic pain is particularly challenging (Tuck et al., 2019). Formal psychological tests to assess for feigning do exist (McDermott & Feldman, 2007), such as the Structured Interview of Reported Symptoms–2 (Rogers et al., 2010), but this is not specific for the feigning of pain complaints. Two psychometric tests validated for chronic pain patients include the Minnesota Multiphasic Personality Inventory and the Life Assessment Questionnaire (Tearnan, 2020). Beyond formal assessment, identification of a pattern of inconsistencies (historical, subjective reports versus examination findings, observations by clinical or custody staff, etc.) is helpful to support a suspicion of malingering. Reported complaints might be inconsistent with physiology—for example, a midline split of sensation (Stone et al., 2005). Malingering is a possible consideration when the symptoms do not improve with appropriate treatment or when test results dispute information provided by the patient (Aronoff et al., 2007). Additional patient behaviors that are consistent with malingering include accurately predicting physical deteriorations, providing selective or misleading information, refusing to sign appropriate releases of information for collateral information (e.g., family or community providers), and focusing on "victimization" by medical personnel (McDermott & Feldman, 2007). Conclusions about the malingering of pain should be made with caution. Pain is a subjective experience, and neither psychometric tests nor clinical methods are yet validated specifically for the detection of malingered chronic pain (Tuck et al., 2019).

Differential diagnosis

In contrast to factitious disorders and malingering, somatic symptom disorders are not under voluntary (conscious) control. Illness anxiety disorder is like somatic symptom disorder in that the patient is excessively worried about having an illness but differentiated from somatic symptom disorder by symptoms (e.g., pain) being either mild or absent (APA, 2022).

The clinical interview

Elements of a comprehensive psychiatric assessment of chronic pain include a clinical interview, medical history, substance use history, pain history, relevant psychosocial histories (family, work, educational), legal history in the context of civil litigation, and specific assessment of pain-coping skills. Key elements of the pain history include the characteristics of the pain, circadian variability, and activities that may increase or diminish the experience of pain.

The initial history should focus on functional impairment rather than solely subjective reports of how strong the pain is. Use of a structured tool to assess coping strategies may also prove valuable (Harland & Georgieff, 2003). Other helpful information includes how well the patient understands the pain problem; the expected course of treatment; and the patient's attitude toward health, illness, and health care providers. The accumulation of adverse childhood experiences (as is often the experience of IPs) is associated with a 20% to 30% increased risk of chronic pain conditions (You et al., 2019).

Establishing the extent and prominence of substance use is key in the assessment. The degree to which the patient turns to medication or drugs as a solution to problems (as opposed to self-motivation, effort, and active participation in treatment) may inform the expected complexity and prognosis of therapy. For example, while a history of opioid misuse does not absolutely rule out opioid pain management, it does complicate treatment because the patient may have tolerance levels that will require high-dose treatment.

Observation is a critical tool for clinical assessment of chronic pain. Pain behaviors should be noted, including grimacing, moaning, limping, limitations in range of motion, rubbing the affected area, use of mobility assistive devices, and avoidance of certain activities, as well as consistency of these behaviors with pain reports. The patient bringing up pain in nonmedical contexts, such as with other staff and peers, may support the validity of these concerns. The correctional environment offers something that outpatient evaluation in the community does not: opportunities for round-the-clock observation by custody staff, when the patient is not aware that they are being observed.

Also important is assessment of functional impairment, including limitations to activities of daily living such as self-care, exercise, or interpersonal skills. The pattern of general health care utilization by the patient should be characterized, including the nature, frequency, and pattern of past contacts with the health care team. Adherence with medication, scheduled appointments, and follow-up with recommendations will suggest the patient's ability and motivation to participate in treatment of chronic pain.

A patient's incarcerated status should never invalidate their expressed medical or psychiatric concern. However, environmental challenges, high rates of substance use disorders, and the underground market for diverted medications demand that attention be paid to the potential for ulterior motives in presenting with chronic pain. Substance use disorders are common in this population and should be assessed and diagnosed on intake (or as new information becomes available) using criteria from the most recent version of the DSM (APA, 2022). Research suggests that higher scores for pain catastrophizing and disability and lower scores for mindfulness predicted misuse of opioids. Pain intensity was not associated with opioid misuse (Paschali et al., 2019). An earlier study found that a prior history of opioid or sedative–hypnotic misuse, family history of substance misuse, history of heavy tobacco use, and age younger than 50 years were associated with current opioid misuse (Sehgal et al., 2012). Medication may be diverted for sale or barter or because of extortion by peers (see Chapters 29 and 30). Some IPs reporting chronic pain and impaired mobility may wish to be moved to a more comfortable housing unit or to receive a medical order for a bottom bunk.

> **CASE EXAMPLE**
>
> Mr. Smith had been disabled for 1 year after a low-back injury during his arrest. The patient had undergone a variety of diagnostic tests that did not identify likely pain generators. Although he complained of extreme pain, the physical findings did not explain his level of suffering and disability. During incarceration, Mr. Smith was placed in a lower bunk in a preferred housing unit with accommodations for those with disabilities.

Psychiatric management of chronic pain in a correctional setting

Successful psychiatric management of chronic pain requires a coordinated team effort. Close collaboration with the treatment team, which should include primary or specialty care physicians, nurses, clinical therapists, and, where appropriate, custody staff, begins with a review of the treatment plan, a definition of everyone's roles, and the sequence of interventions. Physical and occupational therapists may not be available in a correctional setting, but if they are available, they should be included as key members of the team.

Existing medical conditions must be identified and treated. Psychiatric conditions such as depression or anxiety should be treated aggressively. Existing substance use disorders should also be treated (see Chapters 47 to 49). Otherwise, the underlying pathology, both physiological craving and psychological dependence, will complicate the treatment of chronic pain (Garland et al., 2013).

Initiating treatment

Following the assessment, an important next step is to engage the patient in a review of findings and recommendations. A clearly written treatment plan should be drafted and reviewed carefully with the patient. The plan should specify the nature of treatment and the responsibilities of the patient for adherence. If opioids are to be used, directly observed therapy is a near-universal requirement in correctional settings (see Chapter 29). Consequences for violations should be specified. Diversion of medication, failure of random urine drug testing (if indicated), falsification of continued disability, and similar actions should have clearly staged consequences, up to and including tapering to discontinuation of opioid medication.

Pain medication

While a detailed review of the risks of pharmacologic pain management is outside the scope of this chapter, it is important to recognize the limitations of medications in the management of chronic pain, particularly opioid medications (Chou et al., 2009; van Tulder & Koes, 2012). Their lack of clearly demonstrated effectiveness in chronic noncancer pain and their adverse side effects (Manchikanti et al., 2010), coupled with the risks of use in correctional settings, should make their use the exception rather than the rule. A treatment algorithm offered by Gill and colleagues (2019) for chronic pain in carceral facilities suggests the following sequence for somatic or visceral pain: acetaminophen, nonsteroidal anti-inflammatory drugs, cyclooxygenase-2 inhibitors, muscle relaxants, then opioids. For neuropathic pain, the sequence would be anticonvulsants (e.g., gabapentin or oxcarbazepine), serotonin–norepinephrine reuptake inhibitors, tricyclic antidepressants, add-on treatment with nonsteroidal anti-inflammatory drugs for mixed pain, then opioids. Attention should be paid to medications' decreasing benefit over time and their increasing side-effect burden (van Tulder & Koes, 2012). Medical and psychiatric prescribers should coordinate to avoid lithium toxicity when coprescribed with nonsteroidal anti-inflammatory drugs (Gill et al., 2019). Careful monitoring and documentation of ongoing benefit, potential dose escalation, and treatment adherence are critical to effective management of chronic pain with medications in the correctional setting.

Management of co-occurring psychiatric disorders

Any co-occurring psychiatric disorder, depression and anxiety being the most common of these, should be treated aggressively to improve the response to chronic pain management. Dual modality antidepressants like serotonin–norepinephrine reuptake inhibitors and tricyclic antidepressants may be useful both for chronic pain and for depression and anxiety (Gill et al., 2019). Duloxetine has specific U.S. Food and Drug Administration indications for chronic musculoskeletal pain, diabetic peripheral neuropathic pain, and fibromyalgia ("Duloxetine Prescribing Information," 2010).

The treatment of somatic symptom disorder with predominant pain is often complicated, and there is little consensus in the field. There is conflicting evidence that cognitive-behavioral therapy (CBT) alone (Kroenke, 2007), CBT in combination with an antidepressant such as a selective serotonin reuptake inhibitor (Kroenke, 2007), or a selective serotonin reuptake inhibitor alone (Fishbain et al., 1998; Luo et al., 2009) may each prove effective in reducing the severity of the symptoms and enhancing daily function. Because these studies have not been conducted in correctional settings, the clinician and patient will likely be best served by an individually adapted approach that considers local resources and patient acceptance. A discussion of procedural interventions, from site-specific steroid injections to corrective surgeries, is beyond the scope of this chapter.

Psychotherapeutic options

Miller and Rollnick (1991) developed an approach called motivational interviewing for use with patients with substance use disorders. It has found extensive use over the intervening decades and is very relevant in the treatment of chronic pain (Kerns & Rosenberg, 2000). The concepts of rolling with resistance, change talk, self-efficacy, and ambivalence bring flexibility and often enhance engagement in the treatment process (Miller & Rollnick, 1991).

As noted previously, chronic pain incorporates substantial psychological components beyond pure physiological nociceptive stimulation. These psychological elements have generally been most successfully addressed with variants of CBT to target coping skills, self-regulation, and perceived functional limitations (Morley, 2011; Turk & Okifuji, 2002; Turk et al., 2008). One study that used CBT for patients with chronic pain and co-occurring substance use disorders found that 50% of patients were functioning well and were opioid-free at 12 months following the intervention (Currie et al., 2003). CBT is well suited to the correctional environment, as its various manualized versions allow for ease of learning, use, and monitoring, and it can generally be adapted to the specific facility requirements. While typically group based, CBT can be delivered to an individual patient. It is highly structured and has integrated defined exercises to reinforce learning and generalizability to the specific problems being addressed. In CBT, patients are expected to take an active role rather than be passive recipients of information. Thoughts have an impact on affective and physiological arousal, both of which may serve to change behavior.

A core component of many forms of CBT is functional analysis, wherein the patient is taught to deconstruct an event and then restructure it to allow for a positive outcome when a similar situation arises in the future (Rummel et al., 2012). The basic outline follows an easily remembered ABC format: (a) clearly describe the Activating event (e.g., back pain), (b) recognize the Belief associated with that event ("I can't cope with this"), and (c) identify the Consequent emotion(s) (hopelessness, fear, anger). The intervention consists of guided development of alternative, positive beliefs and consequent emotions to minimize distress (Rummel et al., 2012).

Other nonpharmacologic treatment

Education about adaptive coping strategies for chronic pain is low risk and often of benefit. Examples include regular appropriate exercise, positive self-statements (e.g., "I will deal with the pain,") directly addressing stressors that make the pain worse, and using religious beliefs or behaviors to promote endurance in adversity (Peres & Lucchetti, 2010). Pacing of physical activity—in other words, not doing too much or too little—is an important balance that patients must learn (Gill et al., 2019). Setting specific, reasonable goals, such as walking the recreation yard five circuits a day, 3 days a week, is a useful way to promote coping strategies (Gill et al., 2019). The benefits of modern relaxation therapy techniques are well established (Jacobson, 1938), though they have evolved substantially and include a variety of breathing techniques, progressive muscle relaxation, visualization exercises, meditation, and various forms of guided imagery (Chen & Francis, 2010). Practiced twice daily at times of relative quiet while in a comfortable position, relaxation techniques have been demonstrated to be a useful element of chronic pain management (Chen & Francis, 2010). Lower quality evidence also supports tai chi and yoga as adjuvant treatment for chronic pain (Gill et al., 2019).

Monitoring progress

Monitoring pain symptoms and functioning within the facility is important. While daily diaries and scales maintained by the patient to record pain severity and functional activity may be useful, observations by clinical and custodial staff are equally, if not more, valuable.

Summary

Chronic pain is among the more challenging conditions to address in any setting. Management of these problems in carceral settings can be complicated by limited access to modalities like physical and occupational therapy, as well as environmental differences (e.g., physical plant) that may make assessment and treatment more difficult. There can also be advantages in terms of limited access to illegal substances and more opportunities for staff observation to facilitate assessment and monitoring of the patient's response to the treatment plan. Effective treatment requires a multidisciplinary approach, addressing any relevant medical and psychiatric comorbidities; evidence-based psychotherapeutic work; and engagement by the patient.

REFERENCES

American Psychiatric Association. (2022). *Diagnostic and statistical manual of mental disorders* (5th ed., text rev.).

Aronoff, G. M., Mandel, S., Genovese, E., et al. (2007). Evaluating malingering in contested injury or illness. *Pain Practice, 7*(2), 178–204.

Asher, R. (1951. Munchausen's syndrome. *Lancet, 257*, 339–341.

Barry, L. C., Coman, E., Wakefield, D., et al. (2020). Functional disability, depression, and suicidal ideation in older prisoners. *Journal of Affective Disorders, 266*, 366–373.

Chen, Y. L., & Francis, A. J. (2010). Relaxation and imagery for chronic, nonmalignant pain: Effects on pain symptoms, quality of life, and mental health. *Pain Management Nursing, 11*, 159–168.

Chou, R., Fanciullo, G. J., Fine, P. G., et al. (2009). Clinical guidelines for the use of chronic opioid therapy in chronic noncancer pain. *Journal of Pain, 10*(2), 113–130.

Croft, M., & Mayhew, R. (2015). Prevalence of chronic non-cancer pain in a UK prison environment. *British Journal of Pain, 9*(2), 96–108.

Currie, S. R., Hodgins, D. C., Crabtree, A., Jacobi, J., & Armstrong, S. (2003). Outcome from integrated pain management treatment for recovering substance abusers. *Journal of Pain, 4*(2), 91–100.

Duloxetine prescribing information. (2010). https://www.accessdata.fda.gov/drugsatfda_docs/label/2010/022516lbl.pdf

Fishbain, D. A., Cutler, R. B., Rosomoff, H. L., & Rosomoff, R. S. (1998). Do antidepressants have an analgesic effect in psychogenic pain and somatoform pain disorder? A meta-analysis. *Psychosomatic Medicine, 60*, 503–509.

Garland, E. L., Froeliger, B., Zeidan, F., Suveg, K., & Howard, M. O. (2013). The downward spiral of chronic pain, prescription opioid misuse, and addiction: Cognitive, affective, and neuropsychopharmacologic pathways. *Neuroscience and Biobehavioral Reviews, 37*(10 Pt. 2), 2597–2607.

Gill, T., Metts, J., & Ugwueze, G. (2019). The evaluation and management of chronic pain in the correctional setting. *Journal of Correctional Health Care, 25*(4), 382–393.

Harland, N. J., & Georgieff, K. (2003). Development of the Coping Strategies Questionnaire 24, a clinically utilitarian version of the Coping Strategies Questionnaire. *Rehabilitation Psychology, 48*(4), 296.

Jacobson, E. (1938). *Progressive relaxation*. University of Chicago Press.

Kerns, R. D., & Rosenberg, R. (2000). Predicting responses to self-management treatments for chronic pain: Application of the pain stages of change model. *Pain, 84*(1), 49–55.

Kroenke, K. (2007). Efficacy of treatment for somatoform disorders: A review of randomized controlled trials. *Psychosomatic Medicine, 69*, 881–888.

Luo, Y. L., Zhang, M. Y., Wu, W. Y., Li, C. B., Lu, Z., & Li, Q. W. (2009). A randomized double-blind clinical trial on analgesic efficacy of fluoxetine for persistent somatoform pain disorder. *Progress in Neuro-Psychopharmacology and Biological Psychiatry, 33*(8), 1522–1525.

Manchikanti, L., Benyamin, R., Datta, S., Vallejo, R., & Smith, H. (2010). Opioids in chronic noncancer pain. *Expert Review of Neurotherapeutics, 10*(5), 775–789.

McDermott, B. E., & Feldman, M. D. (2007). Malingering in the medical setting. *Psychiatric Clinics of North America, 30*(4), 645–662.

Miller, W. R., & Rollnick, S. (1991). *Motivational interviewing: Preparing people to change addictive behavior*. Guilford Press.

Morley, S. (2011). Efficacy and effectiveness of cognitive behaviour therapy for chronic pain: Progress and some challenges. *Pain, 152*(3), S99–S106.

National Commission on Correctional Health Care. (2023). *Position statement on management of chronic pain, amended August 2023*. https://www.ncchc.org/wp-content/uploads/Management-of-Chronic-Pain-9-2023.pdf

Park, J. H., Kummerlowe, M., & Leal, J. (2022). Somatic symptom disorder with predominant pain treated by electroconvulsive therapy: A case report. *American Journal of Geriatric Psychiatry, 30*(4), S106–S107.

Paschali, M., Lazaridou, A., Dorado, K., et al. (2019). Screening for current opioid misuse and associated risk factors among patients with chronic pain prescribed opioids. *Journal of Pain, 20*(4), S58.

Peres, M. F., & Lucchetti, G. (2010). Coping strategies in chronic pain. *Current Pain and Headache Reports, 14*, 331–228.

Racine, M. (2018). Chronic pain and suicide risk: A comprehensive review. *Progress in Neuro-psychopharmacology and Biological Psychiatry, 87*(Pt. B), 269–280.

Rogers, R., & Bender, S. D. (2018). *Clinical assessment of malingering and deception* (4th ed.). Guilford Press.

Rogers, R., Sewell, K. W., & Gillard, N. D. (2010). *Structured Interview of Reported Symptoms (SIRS), 2nd edition: Professional manual*. Psychological Assessment Resources.

Rummel, C., Garrison-Diehn, C., Catlin, C., & Fisher, J. E. (2012). Clinical functional analysis: Understanding the contingencies of reinforcement. In W. O'Donahue & J. S. Fisher (Eds.), *Cognitive behavior therapy: Core principles for practice* (pp. 13–36). J. Wiley & Sons.

Sehgal, N., Manchikanti, L., & Smith, H. S. (2012). Prescription opioid abuse in chronic pain: A review of opioid abuse predictors and strategies to curb opioid abuse. *Pain Physician, 15*, ES67–ES92.

Skarupski, K. A., Gross, A., Schrack, J. A., Deal, J. A., & Eber, G. B. (2018). The health of America's aging prison population. *Epidemiologic Reviews, 40*(1), 157–165.

Stone, J., Carson, A., & Sharpe, M. (2005). Functional symptoms in neurology: Management. *Journal of Neurology, Neurosurgery & Psychiatry, 76*(Suppl. 1), i13–i21.

Tamburello, A. C., Penn, J., Ford, E., et al. (2022). The American Academy of Psychiatry and the Law practice resource for prescribing in corrections. *Journal of the American Academy of Psychiatry and the Law, 50*(4 Suppl.), S1–S62.

Tearnan, B. H. (2020). Psychometrics for detecting pain-related malingering. In M. Incayawar & S. M. Bouchard (Eds.), *Overlapping pain and psychiatric syndromes: Global perspectives* (pp. 106–120). Oxford University Press.

Tuck, N. L., Johnson, M. H., & Bean, D. J. (2019). You'd better believe it: The conceptual and practical challenges of assessing malingering in patients with chronic pain. *Journal of Pain*, *20*(2), 133–145.

Turk, D. C., & Okifuji, A. (2001). Pain terms and taxonomies. In D. Loeser, S. H. Butler, J. J. Chapman, et al. (Eds.), *Bonica's management of pain* (3rd ed., pp. 18–25). Lippincott Williams & Wilkins.

Turk, D. C., & Okifuji, A. (2002). Psychological factors in chronic pain: Evolution and revolution. *Journal of Consulting and Clinical Psychology*, *70*(3), 678–690.

Turk, D. C., Swanson, K. S., & Tunks, E. R. (2008). Psychological approaches in the treatment of chronic pain patients—When pills, scalpels, and needles are not enough. *Canadian Journal of Psychiatry*, *53*(4), 213–223.

Van Rijswijk, S. M., van Beck, M. H. C. T., Schoof, G. M., et al. (2019). Iatrogenic opioid use disorder, chronic pain and psychiatric comorbidity: A systematic review. *General Hospital Psychiatry*, *59*, 37–50.

van Tulder, M., & Koes, B. (2012). International guidelines for the diagnostics and treatment of acute, subacute, and chronic back pain. In M. I. Hasenbring, A. C. Rusu, & D. C. Turk (Eds.), *From acute to chronic back pain: Risk factors, mechanisms, and clinical implications* (pp. 419–432). Oxford University Press.

You, D. S., Albu, S., Lisenbardt, H., et al. (2019). Cumulative childhood adversity as a risk factor for common chronic pain conditions in young adults. *Pain Medicine*, *20*(3), 486–494.

SECTION VII

Psychotherapy and other nonpharmacologic treatments

41

Applying the recovery model in prisons and jails

Joel T. Andrade and Debra A. Pinals

Introduction

Mental health professionals and substance use treatment providers have worked with "recovery" concepts for many years (Onken et al., 2007). The President's New Freedom Commission on Mental Health (2002) spoke to important aspects of mental health care systems that were challenged, recognizing that "care must focus on increasing consumers' ability to successfully cope with life's challenges, on facilitating recovery, and on building resilience, [and] not just on managing symptoms" (p. 5). The report also stated that "recovery will be the common, recognized outcome of mental health services" (p. 4). These words now are decades old, but they highlight principles that would become integral to general mental health services.

Correctional settings are also recognized as a place where mental health services are needed and delivered, but they are built around confinement and the general principles of sentencing that include retribution, deterrence, incapacitation, and rehabilitation (Appelbaum & Zaitchik, 1995). Thus, it might seem that there is such a fundamental distinction between a prison or jail and a place of treatment that a "recovery" orientation seems inappropriate or unrealistic.

In this chapter, we address recovery, describing ways of defining this construct. We also review considerations related to recovery-oriented services that may be feasible and even helpful in correctional environments and describe some of the tensions between recovery and responsibility when working with an incarcerated population. Finally, we present recommendations for and examples of recovery-oriented programs in correctional settings.

Recovery: shared definitions

According to the U.S. Substance Abuse and Mental Health Services Administration (SAMHSA, 2014), recovery from mental disorders and/or substance use disorders can be defined as "a process of change through which individuals improve their health and wellness, live a self-directed life, and strive to reach their full potential" (p. 3). The historical conceptualization of recovery in the treatment of substance use disorders has followed a different trajectory from recovery from mental disorders, although these are increasingly becoming integrated concepts. Regarding substance use, for example, the framework of engaging in a 12-step model with a "sponsor" stems from the origins of Alcoholics Anonymous in the 1930s (Alcoholics Anonymous, 2014), with a goal of abstinence defining recovery. Recovery from mental disorders is a more recent concept. In the 1990s, conceptualizations of psychiatric rehabilitation and recovery, and how these relate to the treatment of mental disorders, were refined and expanded. This resulted in a shift in thinking from mental disorders as lifelong conditions to disorders from which individuals can recover and for which services can be brought to assist individuals to live productive, meaningful lives, even if some symptoms persist.

Ideas behind recovery in psychiatric services have been viewed as a vision, a process, and a potential outcome (Onken et al., 2007). Recovery involves individuals but equally and necessarily has affected systems of services that have become "recovery oriented." Although symptom reduction can be a critical element of a recovery story, social determinants of health (e.g., discrimination, access to entitlements and rehabilitative services) also may become part of a recovery journey and can affect the process of recovery. Onken and colleagues (2007) further delineated elements of recovery to include personal narratives that encompass stories of coping, healing, wellness, and thriving. SAMHSA (2012) has established 10 principles of recovery:

- Hope;
- Person driven;
- Many pathways;
- Holistic;
- Peer support;
- Relational;
- Culture;
- Addresses trauma;
- Strengths/responsibility; and
- Respect.

These guideposts, taken in turn, can help managers of behavioral health services in a correctional setting identify what might and might not be suitable for system care delivery.

Criminogenic focus of treatment

Correctional mental health populations present with unique characteristics, including higher rates of personality disorder, psychopathy (Hare, 1991/2003), violence, and substance use. Research finds that treatment interventions that address criminogenic factors and risk–need–responsivity (RNR) principles are more effective in reducing criminal recidivism than treatments that do not (Andrews et al., 1990; Andrews & Bonta, 2010). How do recovery tenets fit into a system that is geared to treat individuals with mental illness who may have propensities toward criminal conduct? It is first important to understand basic elements of RNR treatment to see how it can all fit together.

The three areas—risk, need, and responsivity—are each made up of certain principles. The risk principle calls for matching an individual's risk level with the intensity of intervention: High-risk individuals should receive the most intense treatment interventions, followed by their medium-risk and low-risk counterparts. The need principle calls for specific interventions aimed at addressing these criminogenic needs (Andrews et al., 2006). The responsivity principle calls for the specific characteristics of an individual's ability to engage in treatment, such as cognitive ability and motivation for treatment, to be addressed. This principle can also include the treatment provider's ability to address the individual's needs. Research on responsivity finds that the most effective treatments for addressing criminal recidivism are based on cognitive-behavioral, behavioral, and social learning techniques (Smith et al., 2009). Meta-analyses have found a 28% reduction in recidivism when programs adhere to RNR principles (Andrews & Bonta, 2010). A study that compared incarcerated persons (IPs) with serious mental illness to those without found that antisocial attitudes and criminal thinking patterns were similar between these two groups (Morgan et al., 2010). Such findings support adherence to RNR principles in the treatment of IPs with mental illness to decrease recidivism and problematic behavior while incarcerated.

Rehabilitation

Correctional environments have historically been thought of as places where an individual could be rehabilitated from criminal behavioral patterns (Bosworth, 2010). In some ways, current RNR-framed treatment programs are a developmental next step toward this type of criminal rehabilitation and, as noted, are geared toward identifying and confronting antisocial attitudes and behaviors as a focus of treatment (Osher et al., 2012).

According to Anthony (1993), the rehabilitation model for severe mental illness includes a recognition that psychiatric illness includes impairments, such as those seen with active symptoms; dysfunction, which may mean that as a result of such symptoms the person cannot perform certain functions or tasks otherwise considered "normal"; disability, which reflects that because of dysfunction and impairment a person may not be able to perform in a certain role; and disadvantage, which reflects that opportunities for individuals with serious mental illness may be limited. Psychiatric rehabilitation is an important concept that helps clinicians approach individuals with these challenges separate from their antisocial cognitions and behaviors.

In mental health services, rehabilitation and recovery become intermingled concepts. Deegan (1988) noted important distinctions between them. Specifically, rehabilitation refers to "services and technologies made available to persons with disabilities so that they might learn to adapt to their world" (Deegan, 1988, p. 11). Recovery relates more to the person's individualized process of change as they overcome their disabilities. As Deegan (1988) notes, rehabilitation services that do not consider the individual's personal motivations, abilities, and readiness, as well as symptoms, may be of no use. Thus, recovery processes become the frame of reference for rehabilitation efforts.

Systems and recovery "readiness"

Individual recovery can affect systems and services, and these can affect recovery. As such, increased attention has been paid to elements in a system that make it recovery oriented. Anthony (2000) outlined initial standards one might consider in examining whether a system is recovery oriented. Key themes include using language that supports recovery, integrating consumers of services into all levels of service planning and feedback, identifying where recovery can be incorporated into policy, and recognizing that one of the missions of the service system is to improve role functioning, quality of life, and empowerment and satisfaction with services.

There may be significant barriers for a correctional system as it adopts some of these elements, and the need for institutional security cannot be overlooked. That said, programming for IPs with substance use and mental health disorders could be supported by recovery principles. This requires a careful understanding of how, given the value of self-determination and personal choice in the recovery construct, recovery principles must be balanced by important safety considerations and the legal realities of an individual's situation. These matters may need to be continually revisited for both individuals and the correctional system. There should not be confusion about recovery from symptoms, or improved functioning and social integration even with residual symptoms, and recovery from all of life's complexities and problems.

Recovery versus safety in a correctional setting

Individuals in correctional environments have been either charged with criminal conduct (pretrial detainees) or adjudicated guilty of a criminal offense (sentenced IPs). Unique clinical aspects of this population require special attention. For example, among IPs, the base rate of antisocial personality disorder has been found to be between 60% (Côté & Hodgins, 1990) and 80% (Hare, 1991/2003). The construct of psychopathy is much more discriminant, and findings indicate that 15% to 25% of incarcerated individuals meet criteria for psychopathy (Hare, 1991/2003). Psychopathic individuals engage in significantly more institutional violence than their nonpsychopathic peers. This has been shown in incarcerated samples (Hill et al., 1996) and civil psychiatric samples (Heilbrun et al., 1998; see Chapter 37). Instrumental/calculated self-injurious behavior, which can be challenging with this population, can also compromise institutional safety. Therefore, recovery orientation may need to be more circumspect with some individuals by helping to motivate positive behavioral choices (rather than verbal attestations that they are willing and ready to change) that may move them toward improved outcomes.

Complicated questions have been raised about recovery and personal responsibility for individuals whose criminal behavior may be related to mental illness (Pouncey & Lukens, 2010). Mental health, administration, and security personnel have important obligations to maintain institutional safety and to provide care and treatment for IPs. Recovery does not give permission for individuals to do whatever they want to support their independence. Autonomy and personal choice cannot override the social contract that requires public safety. Correctional mental health services may have administrative and clinical obligations to lessen the risk of harm to self or others that an individual with mental illness (or substance use issues) might pose.

Thus, although a recovery framework emphasizes shared decision-making, with the patient at the center, there may also be a need to balance competing institutional needs and public safety concerns. Provisions to override treatment refusal, for example, have been considered permissible under the U.S. Constitution when institutional safety is at risk (*Washington v. Harper*, 1990). However, the laws of some states do not allow such overrides for IPs in nonemergencies (see Chapter 25). Safety and security may subjugate an individual's wishes and self-determination in some situations and jurisdictions. Correctional providers are typically familiar and experienced with these constructs in service delivery, more so than treatment providers in the community. That said, even when coercion in care is needed, how one perceives services vis-à-vis coercion can affect outcomes. For example, increased perceptions of coercion were negatively correlated with perceptions of recovery and predictive of subsequent criminal involvement in one criminal justice sample (Pratt et al., 2013). Research continues to emerge; over time, we may learn more about how conversations with IPs can foster a sense of autonomy, even when providers have legal and/or institutional mandates to act in ways that contradict IPs' wishes. When dialogue and person-centered care occur in a correctional environment, individuals may have more prominent voices in their behavioral and other treatment interventions that could lead to improved outcomes.

Examples of institutional efforts to support recovery goals

Trauma-informed services

Trauma histories among IPs are common (Blair-Lawton et al., 2020; N. A. Miller & Najavits, 2012), including witnessing prior violence and experiencing physical and sexual abuse. These histories can contribute to aggressive behavior (Sarchiapone et al., 2009) and behavioral health treatment needs. For example, justice-involved men and women showed high rates of childhood trauma, which contributed to more significant behavioral health challenges and needs, especially in cases of early sexual trauma (Wolff & Shi, 2012).

Correctional systems can be traumatizing. The Prison Rape Elimination Act of 2003 (2003) reflects this reality, recognizing that the prevalence of sexual assault among prisoners needed further attention and mandating protections for the IP population (see Chapter 70). N. A. Miller and Najavits (2012) point out several elements in the correctional environment that can be traumatizing or can serve as a trigger for individuals with trauma histories, such as shackling, overcrowding, lighting, lack of privacy, security personnel operating to maintain order, pat-downs, strip searches, restricted movement, and disciplinary actions (see also Owens et al., 2008). Institutions with a trauma-informed perspective recognize the practices that may inadvertently create additional challenges for individuals who have trauma histories, and they seek to minimize retraumatization.

To promote recovery, trauma-informed strategies are strongly recommended (see Chapter 36). Trauma-specific interventions such as Seeking Safety (Najavits, 2002) and Trauma Recovery and Empowerment (Harris, 2014) have been used effectively (Fallot & Harris, 2002; Lynch et al., 2012; Najavits, 2006). Other models also exist and have been made readily accessible through SAMHSA's website, the Center for Health Care Strategies (2024), and the National Strategy for a Trauma Informed Care Operating Plan (Interagency Task Force on Trauma Informed Care, 2018).

Peer support

In recent years, there has been growing awareness of the importance of individuals with lived experience with mental illness supporting others in their recovery. Even in correctional settings, programs have been designed to demonstrate the impact of IPs helping IPs (see Chapter 44). For example, Loeb and colleagues (2013) described how IPs can assist other IPs who are facing terminal illness by providing support and companionship to the dying. In the mental health context, peer support helps individuals move through their illness, inspires hope and meaning, and provides a sense of social connectedness. Similarly, forensic peers, which include individuals with a history of criminal justice involvement and behavioral health challenges, are increasingly recognized as an important source of support for persons with co-occurring disorders in the justice system (Davidson & Rowe, 2008). These peers become part of the workforce. When peer supporters are hired to come into correctional institutions, there may be challenges to overcome, including appropriate screening and vetting of criminal backgrounds prior to hire (Bureau of Justice Assistance, 2022; L. D. Miller & Massaro, 2008).

Consumer-guided services

It is crucial to obtain consumer viewpoints about service delivery in a recovery-oriented system (Clossey & Rheinheimer, 2013). Correctional institutions may do this through special meetings between IPs and the leadership of the institution, allowing IPs to have a regular process and forum where their voices can be heard to help improve services. In addition to these meetings, general IP surveys and reviews of medical and mental health services can help identify shortfalls or even abuses. There may be the risk of unfounded IP complaints; however, routine reviews of IPs' perspectives of treatment services, especially those delivered in restrictive housing and specialized treatment units, can provide helpful data to inform system improvements.

Fostering hope and creating meaning

Hope in a correctional setting may seem elusive, especially for individuals serving lengthy or life sentences. However challenging, finding hope while incarcerated will foster positive outcomes and lead to reduced institutional infractions and lower rates of recidivism (Dekhtyar et al., 2012). Working with IPs to help support their ability to find meaning can be an important contribution to making the institution more recovery oriented. This support can, in turn, help individuals "give back" as appropriate, where there may be opportunities for personal narrative or sharing of recovery journeys to help others find similar hope and meaning.

Evidence-based treatment for substance use disorders

Over the past decade, prisons and jails in the United States have experienced the impact of the national opioid epidemic, with a significant increase in deaths due to overdose. Between 2010 and 2019 (when the most recent data is available from the Department of Justice), jails experienced nearly 3 times the rate of death due to drug/alcohol intoxication (Carson, 2021a), and state prison systems experienced over 6 times the number of deaths due to drug/alcohol intoxication (Carson, 2021b).

To address this issue, many jurisdictions are implementing medication for opioid use disorder. The most recent data from the Bureau of Justice Statistics (Maruschak et al., 2023), which was from the midyear point of 2019, reports the following prevalence rates for local jails providing resources to address opioid use disorder:

- 63% conducted opioid use disorder screenings at intake;
- 54% provided medications to treat opioid withdrawal;
- 24% continued medication for opioid use disorder for individuals who had an active prescription from a methadone clinic at the time of their arrest;
- 19% initiated medication for opioid use disorder; and
- 25% provided overdose reversal medications upon release to persons with opioid use disorder.

The importance of treatment for substance use, particularly immediately upon release, is evidenced by the rate of overdose for those reentering the community. A recent study (Hartung et al., 2023) found that, of the over 18,000 individuals released from prison, 67% had a documented substance use disorder treatment need. The rate of opioid overdose within the first 2 weeks of release was high: 2,286.6 per 100,000 person years.

Enhanced reentry planning and supports

Another area where recovery principles are critical is at the interface between the correctional environment and the community (see Chapters 23 and 50). New federal funding opportunities are changing and will further change the face of reentry work, with the potential to fund some services prior to release via Medicaid. Under the Medicaid Inmate Exclusion Policy, Medicaid coverage has historically been deactivated during detention and incarceration. One strategy to address this issue has involved the Centers for Medicare and Medicaid Services (CMS) authorizing certain services that can be covered prior to release. To that end, CMS released a letter encouraging states to apply for the *Medicaid Reentry Section 1115 Demonstration Waiver Opportunity* (CMS, 2023). The waiver allows states the opportunity to apply to activate Medicaid coverage for IPs within 90 days of release. Each interested state is required to submit a proposal as to how the program would be administered in their state. States can individualize their plan for providing coverage, but three service areas are required: (a) case management, (b) medication-assisted treatment and counseling, and (c) at least a 30-day supply of all prescription medication. Although these are newly emerging opportunities, they demonstrate a recognition of the critical importance of whole-person and cross-system collaboration to prioritize long-term recovery strategies for individuals returning to communities from carceral settings.

Initial steps for implementing a recovery-based model in a correctional setting

Training for institutional leaders

For correctional systems to fully benefit from recovery model concepts, the leadership throughout the system must embrace the basic tenets of this model. Initial training must be provided to all leaders in the institution to gain initial buy-in and long-term adherence to recovery-based principles. After such training, the leadership group, composed of correctional and mental health professionals, can work collaboratively to implement the aspects of the model that seem to fit best, while considering all safety and security concerns.

Planning

Without a well-defined and structured approach supported by all key stakeholders, recovery-focused programming will not succeed. A small preplanning committee should include key stakeholders from the correctional system and mental health administration (including high-ranking individuals with decision-making power). This group will identify how the recovery-based model can be supported and implemented in their system. This group should hold regular meetings to review the literature on recovery, attend training, and visit recovery-based programs. Individuals with experience designing mental health units in correctional settings will be particularly helpful in leadership roles, especially if additional mental health units are contemplated.

Implementation

Once the vision for the systemic implementation has been determined, an oversight committee should be established to work out the details. The participants may include general planning committee members and a larger group of professionals with experience providing mental health services to IPs. It would be helpful, when feasible, to include "consumers" in the planning process. A group of IPs with mental health needs should be recruited from the general population for membership in the workgroup. To maintain the integrity and security of the system, the process for selecting this group of IPs must be thorough. Also, the IP participants should not be privy to information that would pose a security risk (e.g., detailed plans, descriptions of facility design, schedules for transferring IPs between facilities). IP members provide consumer-based input into the planning of the treatment program (e.g., identify needs and incentives for active participation).

Leadership and infrastructure with services to focus on recovery

Use of a system where officers and treatment staff are trained to deliver services respectfully can help make an institution more recovery oriented. Programs and services that focus on an individual's strengths, instead of on barriers to success, comport with a recovery orientation and can help individuals take responsibility for their actions. This might require major institutional adjustments. However, in the authors' experience, this can best occur when the leadership embraces these approaches and demonstrates them through role modeling while training and supporting staff with this new way of thinking. This is best done when leadership emphasizes how these approaches will improve safety and security. The leaders should emphasize that these philosophical shifts do not equate to ignoring the critical need for caution and vigilance and that policies and protocols on safety and security will be enforced.

Summary

The recovery model provides correctional systems with unique opportunities to engage individuals with serious mental illness and other mental health needs more fully. Application in correctional settings requires adjustments and flexibility related to recovery frameworks used in the community, but the underlying philosophy can still be used. To provide a comprehensive program, the basic tenets of recovery should be combined with evidence-based practice in correctional settings. This will benefit the entire IP population and correctional staff by increasing safety and security. Promoting recovery is also in the interest of public safety, as the vast majority of IPs will be released to the community. By providing programs based on evidence, including criminogenic risk factors, coupled with individual-focused recovery-based initiatives for IPs with mental illness, the chance of successful reintegration into society improves.

REFERENCES

Alcoholics Anonymous. (2014). *Historical data: The birth of A.A. and its growth in U.S./Canada.* http://www.aa.org/lang/en/subpage.cfm?page=288

Andrews, D. A., & Bonta, J. (2010). *The psychology of criminal conduct.* Matthew Bender & Company, a member of the LexisNexis Group.

Andrews, D. A., Bonta, J., & Wormith, S. J. (2006). The recent past and near future of risk and/or need assessment. *Crime and Delinquency, 52*, 7–27.

Andrews, D. A., Zinger, I., Hoge, R. D., Bonta, J., Gendreau, P., & Cullen, F. T. (1990). Does correctional treatment work? A psychologically informed meta-analysis. *Criminology, 28*, 369–404.

Anthony, W. A. (1993). Recovery from mental illness: The guiding vision of the mental health service system in the 1990s. *Psychosocial Rehabilitation Journal, 16*(4), 11–23.

Anthony, W. A. (2000). A recovery-oriented system: Setting some system level standards. *Psychiatric Rehabilitation Journal, 24*(2), 159–168.

Appelbaum, K. L., & Zaitchik, M. C. (1995). Mental health professionals play critical role in presentencing evaluations. *Mental & Physical Disability Law Reporter, 19*(5), 677–684.

Blair-Lawton, D., Mordoch, E., & Chernomas, W. (2020). Putting on the same shoes: Lived experiences of women who are reincarcerated. *Journal of Forensic Nursing, 16*(2), 99–107.

Bosworth, M. (2010). *Explaining U.S. imprisonment.* Sage Publications.

Bureau of Justice Administration. (2022). *Peer recovery support services in correctional settings.* https://bja.ojp.gov/library/publications/peer-recovery-support-services-correctional-settings

Carson, E. A. (2021a). *Mortality in local jails, 2000–2019—Statistical tables.* Department of Justice, Bureau of Justice Statistics.

Carson, E. A. (2021b). *Mortality in state and federal prisons, 2001–2019—Statistical tables.* Department of Justice, Bureau of Justice Statistics.

Center for Health Care Strategies. (2024). *Trauma Informed Care Implementation Resource Center.* https://www.traumainformedcare.chcs.org/resource/samhsas-national-center-for-trauma-informed-care/

Centers for Medicare and Medicaid Services. (2023, April 17). *HHS letter.* https://www.cms.gov/newsroom/press-releases/hhs-releases-new-guidance-encourage-states-apply-new-medicaid-reentry-section-1115-demonstration

Clossey, L., & Rheinheimer, D. (2013). Exploring the effect of organizational culture on consumer perceptions of agency support for mental health recovery. *Community Mental Health Journal, 50*(4), 427–434.

Côté, G., & Hodgnis, S. (1990). Co-occurring mental disorders among criminal offenders. *Bulletin of the American Academy of Psychiatry & the Law, 18*(3), 271–281.

Davidson, L., & Rowe, M. (2008). *Peer support within criminal justice settings: The role of forensic peer specialists.* CMHS National GAINS Center.

Deegan, P. E. (1988). Recovery: The lived experience of rehabilitation. *Psychosocial Rehabilitation Journal, 11*(4), 11–19.

Dekhtyar, M., Beasley, C. R., Jason, L. A., & Ferrari, J. R. (2012). Hope as a predictor of reincarceration among mutual-help recovery residents. *Journal of Offender Rehabilitation, 51*, 474–483.

Fallot, R. D., & Harris, M. (2002). The Trauma Recovery and Empowerment Model (TREM): Conceptual and practical issues in a group intervention for women. *Community Mental Health Journal, 38*, 475–485.

Hare, R. D. (2003). *The Hare Psychopathy Checklist–Revised* (2nd ed.). Multi-Health Systems. (Original work published 1991)

Harris, M. (2014). *Trauma Recovery and Empowerment (TREM) and Men's Trauma Recovery and Empowerment (M-TREM).* http://www.communityconnectionsdc.org/web/page/657/interior.html

Hartung, D. M., McCracken, C. M., Nguyen, T., Kempany, K., & Waddell, E. N. (2023). Fatal and nonfatal opioid overdose risk following release from prison: A retrospective cohort study using linked administrative data. *Journal of Substance Use and Addiction Treatment, 147*, 208971.

Heilbrun, K., Hart, S. D., Hare, R. D., Gustafson, D., Nunez, C., & White, A. (1998). Inpatient and post-discharge aggression in mentally disordered offenders: The role of psychopathy. *Journal of Interpersonal Violence, 13*, 514–527.

Hill, C. D., Rogers, R., & Bickford, M. E. (1996). Predicting aggressive and socially disruptive behavior in a maximum security forensic psychiatric hospital. *Journal of Forensic Sciences, 41*(1), 56–59.

Interagency Task Force on Trauma Informed Care. (2018). *National Strategy for Trauma Informed Care Operating Plan.* https://www.samhsa.gov/sites/default/files/trauma-informed-care-operating-plan.pdf

Loeb, S. J., Hollenbeak, C. S., Penrod, J., Smith, C. A., Kitt-Lewis, E., & Crouse, S. B. (2013). Care and companionship in an isolating environment: Inmates attending to dying peers. *Journal of Forensic Nursing, 9*(1), 35–44.

Lynch, S. M., Health, N. M., Mathews, K. C., & Cepeda, G. J. (2012). Seeking Safety: An intervention for trauma-exposed incarcerated women? *Journal of Trauma and Dissociation, 13*(1), 88–101.

Maruschak, L. M., Minton, T. D., & Zeng, Z. (2023). *Opioid use disorder screening and treatment in local jails, 2019.* U.S. Department of Justice, Office of Justice Programs, Bureau of Justice Statistics.

Miller, L. D., & Massaro, J. (2008). *Overcoming legal impediments to hiring forensic peer specialists.* CMHS National GAINS Center.

Miller, N. A., & Najavits, L. M. (2012). Creating trauma-informed correctional care: A balance of goals and environment. *European Journal of Psychotraumatology, 3*, 17246.

Morgan, R. D., Fisher, W. H., Duan, N., Mandracchia, J. T., & Murray, D. (2010). Prevalence of criminal thinking among state prison inmates with serious mental illness. *Law and Human Behavior, 34*, 324–336.

Najavits, L. M. (2002). *Seeking Safety: A treatment manual for PTSD and substance abuse*. Guilford Press.

Najavits, L. M. (2006). Managing trauma reactions in intensive addiction treatment environments. *Journal of Chemical Dependency Treatment*, *8*, 153–161.

Onken, S. J., Craig, C. M., Ridgway, P., Ralph, R. O., & Cook, J. A. (2007). An analysis of the definitions of recovery: A review of the literature. *Psychiatric Rehabilitation Journal*, *31*, 9–22.

Osher, F., D'Amora, D. A., Plotkin, M., et al. (2012). *Adults with behavioral health needs under correctional supervision: A shared framework for reducing recidivism and promoting recovery*. Council of State Governments Justice Center, Criminal Justice/Mental Health Consensus Project.

Owens, B., Wells, J., Pollock, J., Muscat, B., & Torres, S. (2008). *Gendered violence and safety: A contextual approach to improving security in women's facilities*. U.S. Department of Justice, Office of Justice Programs, National Institute of Justice.

Pouncey, C. L., & Lukens, J. M. (2010). Madness versus badness: The ethical tension between the recovery movement and forensic psychiatry. *Theoretical Medicine and Bioethics*, *31*, 93–105.

Pratt, C., Yanos, P. T., Kopelovich, S. L., Koerner, J., & Alexander, M. J. (2013). Predictors of criminal justice outcomes among mental health courts participants: The role of perceived coercion and subjective mental health recovery. *International Journal of Forensic Mental Health*, *12*(2), 116–125.

President's New Freedom Commission on Mental Health. (2002). *Transforming mental health care in America*. http://govinfo.library.unt.edu/mentalhealthcommission/reports/FinalReport/FullReport-1.htm

Prison Rape Elimination Act of 2003, Pub. L. 108–179 (2003).

Sarchiapone, M., Carli, V., Cuomo, C., Marchetti, M., & Roy, A. (2009). Association between childhood trauma and aggression in male prisoners. *Psychiatry Research*, *165*, 1–2, 187–192.

Smith, P., Gendreau, P., & Swartz, K. (2009). Validating the principles of effective intervention: A systematic review of the contributions of meta-analysis in the field of corrections. *Victims and Offenders*, *4*, 148–169.

Substance Abuse and Mental Health Services Administration. (2012). *SAMHSA's working definition of recovery*. U.S. Department of Health and Human Services.

Substance Abuse and Mental Health Services Administration. (2014). *SAMHSA announces a working definition of "recovery" from mental disorders and substance use disorders*. http://www.samhsa.gov/newsroom/advisories/1112223420.aspx

Washington v. Harper, 494 U.S. 2010 (1990).

Wolff, N., & Shi, J. (2012). Childhood and adult trauma experiences of incarcerated persons and their relationship to adult behavioral health problems and treatment. *International Journal of Environmental Research and Public Health*, *9*, 1908–1926.

42

Individual psychotherapy

James L. Knoll IV and Adam Bernstein

Introduction

The abandonment of the medical model in carceral settings about half a century ago left a scorched earth policy for rehabilitation and, in turn, for psychotherapeutic efforts with incarcerated persons (IPs; Martinson, 1974). Fortunately, much progress has been made since the 1970s (Simon, 2013). Along with the imperative of improving psychiatric treatment in carceral settings, mental health professionals have brought back the science of psychotherapeutic intervention, this time reinforced by a social science evidence base (Ameen et al., 2010; Andrews et al., 2011; Novalis et al., 2022; Sapp, 2023; Trestman et al., 2021).

This chapter discusses practical and theoretical aspects of individual psychotherapy with IPs, followed by an overview of evidence-based paradigms for psychotherapy in carceral settings. While much of the evidence base supports cognitive-behavioral approaches, the importance of maintaining competence in psychodynamically informed therapy is also discussed.

Practical considerations

Style

Therapeutic style is cultivated over time. In carceral settings, effective psychotherapy style includes at least three main ingredients: dignity preservation, genuineness, and meaning making. IPs have often had their dignity stripped away in the process of criminal adjudication and carceral conformity. Dignity-conserving approaches are highly recommended and may be helpful in establishing rapport and trust (Testoni et al., 2024). Being genuine is a way to respect an individual's dignity, and many IPs are quick to notice disingenuous attempts to connect therapeutically. Being genuine does not refer to relaxing one's style but rather to responding in a relatively undefended way and without making value judgments. A useful rule to keep in mind is: when in doubt, be human (Gabbard, 2010). Finally, meaning making is an important element of a therapist's approach in carceral settings; this is described in the next section.

Common themes

Carceral psychotherapy brings the therapist in contact with the harsh realities of IPs' difficult and traumatic life circumstances. Salient themes can be expected to arise repeatedly, such as nihilism and the need to find meaning. Clinical observations suggest that a significant portion of IPs struggle with a persecutory mindset (Hyatt-Williams, 1998) and develop a nihilistic attitude toward treatment and life (Knoll, 2009). Such cognitions reduce their ability to participate in and benefit from treatment efforts. Regardless of the type of individual therapy used, therapists will likely encounter IPs' sense of hopelessness and need to find meaning in their personal struggles. Psychiatrist Viktor Frankl's experience as a Nazi concentration camp prisoner led him to conclude that a primary motivation is a drive to find meaning and purpose in life (Frankl, 1959/1963). In contrast, a failure to find meaning may result in hopelessness, suicidality, and self-defeating actions (Edwards & Holden, 2001). Trauma literature and research suggest that meaning making can be a "central process in healing from trauma or loss" (Lemaire, 2011, p. 187). The path to reconstructing meaning will depend on the individual's background, culture, and spiritual beliefs. A common central theme to meaning making involves intolerable conditions causing one to reach one's limit—followed by acceptance, dissolution of defenses, and finally positive transformation (Andresen, 1991; Chodron, 2008). IPs have frequently experienced substantial loss and deep existential crises. In the past decade, renewed research interest in the importance of loss of meaning has suggested that for IPs, meaning modulates distress, hopelessness, and suicide risk (Marco et al., 2016; Vanhooren et al., 2017a).

Setting

The therapy setting depends on the security level of the IP, the security level of the facility, and overall institutional resources. The therapist should strive to see the IP in a private room; convenience does not justify acquiescing to cell-front therapy or similarly non-confidential arrangements. Attention should also be paid to the IP's comfort and freedom of movement in the therapeutic setting. Common correctional practices such as shackling IPs behind their backs during mental health assessments can deter individuals from engaging in therapy, so some settings offer programming modules as an alternative. The key is to secure a setting that conveys a sense of confidentiality and safety for both patient and therapist. Ultimately, carceral institution administrators have the responsibility to ensure that clinical staff have appropriate space and adequate resources for treatment efforts, and it is appropriate for carceral mental health leaders to advocate for confidential therapy space when it is lacking.

Informed consent

The patient's right to consent to treatment is a basic ethical principle in medicine (Appelbaum, 2007). To give legally and ethically appropriate consent, the patient must be competent, have adequate information about the proposed treatment, and be in a position to choose the treatment voluntarily. Strong arguments have been made in favor of psychiatrists obtaining informed consent for psychotherapy (Gutheil & Appelbaum, 2020; Traschel et al., 2015). Informed consent for psychotherapy supports patient autonomy, explains risks and benefits, and provides reasonable alternatives to treatment. It is recommended that the carceral therapist obtain and document the IP's informed consent for therapy in the initial meeting (Appelbaum, 1997).

Confidentiality

The therapist should explain the limits of confidentiality and, in particular, the limits that apply to the correctional setting. No clear consensus exists among correctional and forensic mental health staff about how to approach explaining limits to confidentiality (Bruggen et al., 2013), but standards of IP confidentiality should generally be the same as those in the community (Pinta, 2009). The usual exceptions to confidentiality continue to apply in carceral settings, such as risk of harm to self or others (American Academy of Psychiatry and the Law, 2018). Ideally, in the first session, the IP should be informed about circumstances that may require the therapist to breach confidentiality (Mossman, 2006; Pinta, 2010). There are some important exceptions to confidentiality specific to the carceral setting. These include when IPs inform the therapist that they are an escape risk, are involved in a prison riot, or are involved in some activity that could potentially cause turmoil or harm within the facility (American Psychiatric Association, 2016). The carceral therapist should be clear about any other exceptions to confidentiality that may be specified in the facility's policies and procedures. For example, clinicians may be required to disclose sexual activity between IPs under the Prison Rape Elimination Act (see Chapter 70) or episodes of child abuse under state-mandated reporting statutes.

Psychotherapeutic approaches

Engaging, cost-effective, and evidence-based approaches are preferred in today's budget-restricted, underresourced carceral settings. The number of therapeutic programming options delivered in group and manualized form has grown faster than evidence-based individual therapies. However, many of the newer evidence-based programs incorporate individual sessions within their overall paradigm. Cognitive-behavioral therapy has been the most widely studied therapy in carceral settings (Simpson et al., 2022). Preliminary evidence for the effectiveness of dialectical behavior therapy (DBT), acceptance and commitment therapy, compassion-focused therapy, and mindfulness-based approaches has been reported, particularly for reducing aggression and violent behavior (Cunha et al., 2024; McCann & Ball, 2021).

DBT has been shown to be an effective approach for both male and female IPs. DBT has been modified for a correctional setting (DBT-Corrections Modified) and used to help reduce impulsive–aggressive behaviors, particularly those resulting in disciplinary tickets (Shelton et al., 2009, 2011). This approach is often used in conjunction with group sessions and manuals.

START NOW, first developed in Connecticut's prisons, is a psychotherapy program integrating cognitive-behavioral therapy and motivational interviewing (MI) that is designed for impulsive–aggressive behavior in high-security settings (Shelton & Wakai, 2011). START NOW's materials are available online without cost, and it has been implemented in 21 states and seven countries (Carilion Clinic, 2024). The program has been shown to have high satisfaction rates among IPs, as well as decreased psychiatric hospitalizations (Kersten, 2016).

MI is an evidence-based therapy used to facilitate behavior change (Triana & Olson, 2013). In the carceral setting, MI is used to engage and build motivation for treatment. MI is now being utilized as a brief intervention to decrease jail recidivism in IPs with substance use disorders, as well as for suicidal patients (Cigrang et al., 2020; Zerler, 2009). Additionally, MI can be modified for use with individuals with intellectual disabilities (Frielink & Embregts, 2013). There are four main strategies in MI, which are easily taught to multidisciplinary therapists (Miller & Moyers, 2006; Miller & Rollnick, 2002, 2009). The first principle involves engaging patients by appropriately expressing empathy and acceptance of their unique issues. The second principle is to elicit dialogue about change. This is done by developing important areas of discrepancy, such as assisting IPs in describing differences in current personal efficacy versus how they would like things to be in the future. The third principle is called "rolling with resistance." This requires therapists to pay attention to defensiveness and recognize it as a signal that a modified approach to the issue is needed. The fourth principle is to support self-efficacy by reinforcing expressions of willingness to understand therapist input, acknowledge problems, and take steps toward positive change.

The mindfulness movement

The New York State Department of Corrections and Community Supervision, in collaboration with the New York State Office of Mental Health, has developed an intervention for IPs with serious mental illness and/or severe personality disorders who are difficult to engage, behaviorally challenging, and frequently sentenced to punitive isolation. The program is held in a facility called the residential mental health unit. The residential mental health unit places heavy emphasis on programming, psychotherapy, and behavioral analysis and helps engage patients by expunging their punitive isolation time after successful program participation. The program uses daily multidisciplinary ratings for behavioral analysis, symptom checklists, and measures of improvement. The psychotherapy approach of mindfulness is strongly emphasized (Pankovics & Martinovic, 2024; Spina, 2023). Mindfulness training helps IPs learn to focus their attention on moment-by-moment experience and has become popular as a complementary therapeutic strategy for medical and psychiatric conditions (Marchand, 2012; Robins et al., 2012). Evidence suggests a role as an adjunct treatment for depression, anxiety, pain management, and general psychological health.

Special considerations for incarcerated persons with long sentences

IPs who have received long sentences of incarceration, such as life without the possibility of parole, must be viewed with a sharper lens. Ernest Becker postulated that the mere thought of death is too overwhelming, and thus people must do everything in their power to deny the fact (Becker, 1973). Individuals with life sentences are perhaps the most intimately aware of the passage of time and their mortality. Building on Becker and others like Yalom (1980), existential isolation has received increasing attention. Although research is limited on this topic in the carceral setting, Sease et al. (2022) propose authentic therapeutic alliance building as a strategy to overcome existential isolation. In a direct response to the loneliness aspect of prolonged incarceration, both existential therapy and acceptance and commitment therapy showed significant decreases in such emotions, without a significant difference between the two therapies (Ziaee, 2022).

Returning to the importance of meaning in the lives of long-term IPs, meaning making and existential therapies aimed at enhancing posttraumatic growth help regulate distress and reduce hopelessness (Reading & Bowen, 2014; Vanhooren et al., 2017b). As adjuncts to these efforts, bibliotherapy and therapeutic journaling can serve as a collaborative therapeutic process that is inexpensive and may help patients organize and clarify their thoughts (Pardini et al., 2014; Wong et al., 2018).

Psychodynamic knowledge in carceral psychotherapy

There are many reasons to maintain a broad psychodynamic viewpoint of IPs and carceral systems of care, even when psychodynamic psychotherapy is not used. Psychodynamically oriented therapists have subjected their approach to the scientific method in recent years (Gabbard, 2010; Gerber et al., 2011; Perry & Bond, 2012), and important lessons have been learned. For example, nonpsychodynamic therapies may be effective, in part, because more skilled practitioners use techniques that have long been central to psychodynamic theory and practice (Shedler, 2010). Therapists find themselves employing a mix of evidence-based treatments with other empirically supported approaches and a good measure of creativity (Douglas, 2011; Vaillant, 2012).

In addition to its instructive focus on the therapeutic relationship and countertransference, psychodynamic theory involves other distinctive features that are of particular concern to carceral therapists. These features include identification of recurring behavior or thought patterns, understanding of interpersonal relations, and recognizing styles of emotional expression (Gabbard, 2010). An understanding of the patient's childhood development is critical to the therapeutic relationship, approach, and goal setting.

Regardless of the psychotherapy approach used, there remains a need to understand transference and countertransference themes. Countertransference of a therapist to an IP may provide valuable data about emotions and cognitions induced in others, which will inform future therapy directions. Specific personality disorders and styles are associated with fairly consistent emotional responses in therapists, allowing the therapist to make diagnostic and therapeutic use of these responses (Colli et al., 2013). For example, therapist countertransference involving feeling devalued, criticized, or mistreated has been associated with patient diagnoses of antisocial personality disorder, paranoid personality disorder, and narcissistic personality disorder (Perry et al., 2013).

Forensic psychotherapists place importance on understanding the meaning of a violent act for the individual and believe that a "psychodynamic approach can … inform effective therapeutic interventions in hard-to-treat patients" (Yakely & Adshead, 2013, p. 38; see also Keogh, 2022; Papapietro & Adshead, 2016). Forensic psychotherapists are particularly interested in how an individual's criminogenic needs and behavior may represent a repetition of early experience. For individuals serving long sentences, psychodynamic therapy can help them to make connections between traumatic childhood experiences and their adult functioning (Mulay et al., 2017).

The use of psychodynamic thinking also helps in understanding treatment team dynamics and managing multidisciplinary staff's responses to IPs. Unexplored countertransference in staff may result in a host of adverse outcomes such as staff division, boundary violations, breaches of security, and a toxic team milieu. Encouraging staff to recognize and manage these emotions, as well as discussing them in supervision and designated team meetings, can help mitigate these outcomes.

Understanding early development

IPs often share similar developmental histories that profoundly affect and challenge psychotherapeutic efforts (Farrington, 2020; Tärnhäll et al., 2023). It helps to have a good understanding of a patient's developmental history prior to treatment. Histories of neglect and trauma are common in IPs (see Chapter 36), and they forewarn about difficulties with treatment readiness, trust in the therapeutic alliance, and realistic treatment goal setting. Childhood abuse and neglect are associated with an increased risk of personality disorders (Johnson et al., 1999), as well as adult criminal behavior (Lykken, 1998). Object relations theory suggests that children who experience developmentally adverse events develop distorted internal models of interpersonal relationships and self-regulation (Craissati & Beech, 2006; Maia et al., 2025). Early maltreatment and adverse conditions are theorized to play a role in creating structural changes in the brain, as evidenced by preliminary neuroimaging findings (McCollum, 2006). Childhood exposure to violence and abuse may adversely affect infant neurocircuitry, leading to underdevelopment in the frontal and prefrontal cortex (Keeshin et al., 2012). Childhood abuse and stress can result in chronically increased cortisol levels, leading to hippocampal volume loss and associated learning problems (Bair-Merritt et al., 2013). Such neuropsychiatric deficits may produce problems in behavioral self-regulation, emotional regulation, and executive function that may significantly affect the IP's treatment readiness (Fishbein et al., 2009).

Common countertransference themes

Regardless of theoretical orientation, the carceral therapist will need to manage internal reactions flowing from their work with IPs (Mulay & Cain, 2018). Recognizing and making use of countertransference with IPs, particularly those with antisocial traits, is critical to therapy success, cohesive staff functioning, and safety. The term "countertransference" is used here in its broadest sense to mean the emotional reaction of the therapist to the patient (Ursano et al., 1991). Regardless of style, therapists working with IPs invariably come to realize that treatment cannot be a dispassionate, technical endeavor (Freidrich, 2006). The therapist must recognize, tolerate, and "hold" the IP's feelings in a safe way (Slochower, 1991). Lack of attention to countertransference may cause the therapist to avoid internal discomfort reflexively by responding in an attacking or rejecting manner. IPs with strong psychopathic traits may engender particularly corrosive countertransference emotions, causing the therapist to feel controlled or deceived.

Carceral therapists may find themselves using psychological defenses such as isolation of affect to deal with unpleasant or difficult emotional reactions to some patients. An absence or lack of feelings about the patient will be the hallmark of this reaction. This type of reaction can create excessive distance from the IP or cause the therapist to overlook important clinical warning signs.

Although common, countertransference should not be confused with compassion fatigue. Compassion fatigue is the provider's emotional reactions that result from overexposure to a patient's suffering (Figley, 1995). Such overexposure is cumulative, and the therapist slowly absorbs the emotional weight, which has negative professional and personal effects. Distinct from countertransference, compassion fatigue is not necessary to the therapeutic process (Berzoff & Kita, 2010), and clinicians delivering psychotherapy in a carceral setting should be mindful of this difference.

Therapeutic nihilism is a countertransference reaction experienced with difficult-to-treat or help-rejecting IPs and with those with strong psychopathic traits (Knoll, 2009; Meloy, 1988). Many therapists assume that all such individuals are similar in their lack of response and that, therefore, treatment is pointless. This reaction should be tempered by the fact that IPs comprise a heterogeneous group with unique personal characteristics. There is no evidence that all IPs are immune to treatment efforts (Barbaree, 2005; Salekin, 2002). The therapist must carefully navigate between the Scylla and Charybdis of therapeutic nihilism and therapeutic naiveté (Knoll, 2009). This is a challenge requiring efforts to prohibit moral judgment from impinging upon an objective, professional approach.

Malignant pseudo-identification is a potentially hazardous reaction described in the treatment of highly antisocial patients (Knoll, 2009; Meloy, 1988). It involves the process by which the IP consciously imitates (or unconsciously simulates) the narcissistic characteristics of the therapist. This results in a strengthening of the therapist's identification with the IP, which may cause the therapist to become vulnerable to manipulation. The process may involve the IP simulating the values, beliefs, or even mannerisms of the therapist. The pseudo-flattery may be taken as a positive sign of improvement by the therapist, who then assumes a therapeutic alliance and healthy identification.

Some IPs may realistically carry a poor long-term prognosis. Such cases have the potential to induce subtle feelings of worthlessness and self-devaluation in the therapist. Similar self-devaluing reactions include excessive questioning of one's abilities, as well as feelings that one's work with IPs is insignificant. Some IPs may demonstrate attitudes that the therapist will find disgusting or off-putting. Such countertransferential feelings should receive close attention by the therapist, as they may signal a critical theme for the patient at best and at worst may subtly signify the phenomenon of malignant alienation in both therapist and carceral staff. Malignant alienation describes a process of deterioration in relationships with staff that precedes suicide (Whittle, 1997). Clearly, this a critical concept in terms of individual therapy, as well as potentially life-saving. Fortunately, psychodynamic theory provides some understanding and guidance about malignant alienation (Gordon, 2002; Watts & Morgan, 1994). Feelings of hatred may be acted upon by the therapist in the form of inappropriate criticisms, hostile remarks, or premature withdrawal of care. In all such cases, supervision and case consultation are highly recommended. The therapist must be particularly thoughtful if the patient's crime touches on a specific area of sensitivity for the therapist (Hyatt-Williams, 1998). A reflective processing of such countertransference may be required on a treatment team level. This is especially important when other staff also have conscious or unconscious wishes to destroy or punish the IP.

Summary

Individual psychotherapy with IPs can be as gratifying as it is challenging. The evidence base for correctional psychotherapy approaches is advancing, with an emphasis on cognitive-behavioral methods and mindfulness training. However, there remains an important place for psychodynamic competence, particularly in the areas of biopsychosocial formulations and effective management of countertransference. The carceral therapist's effectiveness will be enhanced by regular use of consultation and supervision.

REFERENCES

Ameen, C. A., Loeffler-Cobia, J., Clawon, E., & Guevara, M. (2010). *Evidence-based practice skills assessment for criminal justice organizations, Version 1.0*. National Institute of Corrections.

American Academy of Psychiatry and the Law. (2018). Practice resource for prescribing in corrections *Journal of the American Academy of Psychiatry and the Law*, *46*(2 Suppl.), S2–50.

American Psychiatric Association. (1997). American Psychiatric Association resource document on principles of informed consent in psychiatry. *Journal of American Academy of Psychiatry Law*, *25*(1), 121.

American Psychiatric Association. (2016). *Psychiatric services in jails and prisons* (3rd ed.). American Psychiatric Publishing.

Andresen, J. J. (1991). Biblical job: Changing the helper's mind. *Contemporary Psychoanalysis*, *27*(3), 454–481.

Andrews, D. A., Bonta, J., & Wormith, J. S. (2011). The Risk-Need-Responsivity (RNR) Model: Does adding the good lives model contribute to effective crime prevention? *Criminal Justice and Behavior*, *38*(7), 735–755.

Appelbaum, P. (1997). Informed consent to psychotherapy: Recent developments. *Psychiatric Services*, *48*(4), 445.

Appelbaum, P. (2007). Assessment of patients' competence to consent to treatment. *New England Journal of Medicine*, *357*(18), 1834–1840.

Bair-Merritt, M., Zuckerman, B., Augustyn, M., & Cronholm, P. F. (2013). Silent victims—An epidemic of childhood exposure to domestic violence. *New England Journal of Medicine*, *369*(18), 1673–1675.

Barbaree, H. (2005). Psychopathy, treatment behavior, and recidivism: An extended follow-up of Seto and Barbaree. *Journal of Interpersonal Violence*, *20*(9), 1115–1131.

Becker, E. (1973). *The denial of death*. Free Press.

Berzoff, J., & Kita, E. (2010). Compassion fatigue and countertransference: Two different concepts. *Clinical Social Work Journal*, *38*(3), 341–349.

Bruggen, M. C., Eytan, A., Gravier, B., & Elger, B. S. (2013). Medical and legal professionals' attitudes towards confidentiality and disclosure of clinical information in forensic settings: A survey using case vignettes. *Medical Science Law*, *53*(3), 132–148.

Carilion Clinic. (2024). *START NOW*. https://www.carilionclinic.org/start_now#about

Chodron, P. (2008). *Comfortable with uncertainty: 108 teachings on cultivating fearlessness and compassion*. Shambhala Publications.

Cigrang, J. A., Fedynich, A. L., Nichting, E., Frederick, S. A., Schumm, J. A., & Auguste, C. B. (2020). Brief motivational interview–based intervention for women in jail with history of drug addiction and sex-trading. *Professional Psychology: Research and Practice, 51*(1), 25.

Colli, A., Tanzilli, A., Dimaggio, G., & Lingiardi, V. (2013). Patient personality and therapist response: An empirical investigation. *American Journal of Psychiatry, 171*(1), 102–108.

Craissati, J., & Beech, A. (2006). The role of key developmental variables in identifying sex offenders likely to fail in the community: An enhanced risk prediction model. *Child Abuse & Neglect, 30*(4), 327–339.

Cunha, O., Pereira, B., Sousa, M., & Rodrigues, A. C. (2024). Cognitive behavioural "thirdwave" therapies in the treatment of justice-involved individuals: A systematic review. *Aggression and Violent Behavior, 76*, 101923.

Douglas, C. (2011). Studying the efficacy of psychodynamic psychotherapy. Letters to the editor. *American Journal of Psychiatry, 168*, 649.

Edwards, M., & Holden, R. (2001). Coping, meaning in life, and suicidal manifestations: Examining gender differences. *Journal of Clinical Psychology, 57*(12), 1517–1534.

Farrington, D. P. (2020). Human development and criminal careers. In M. Vogel (Ed.), *Crime, inequality and the state* (pp. 223–244). Routledge.

Figley, C. R. (Ed.). (1995). *Compassion fatigue: Coping with secondary traumatic stress disorder in those who treat the traumatised.* Brunner/Mazel.

Fishbein, D., Sheppard, M., Hyde, C., et al. (2009). Deficits in behavioral inhibition predict treatment engagement in prison inmates. *Law and Human Behavior, 33*(5), 419–435.

Frankl, V. E. (1963). *Man's search for meaning.* Simon and Schuster. (Original work published 1959)

Friedrich, M. & Leiper, R. (2006). Countertransference reactions in therapeutic work with incestuous sexual abusers. *Journal of Child Sex Abuse, 15*(1), 51–68.

Frielink, N., & Embregts, P. (2013). Modification of motivational interviewing for use with people with mild intellectual disability and challenging behaviour. *Journal of Intellectual and Developmental Disability, 38*(4), 279–291.

Gabbard, G. (2010). *Long-term psychodynamic psychotherapy: A basic text.* American Psychiatric Association Publishing.

Gerber, A. J., Kocsis, J. H., Milrod, B. L., et al. (2011). A quality-based review of randomized controlled trials of psychodynamic psychotherapy. *American Journal of Psychiatry, 168*(1), 19–28.

Gordon, H. (2002). Suicide in secure psychiatric facilities. *Advances in Psychiatric Treatment, 88*(6), 408–417.

Gutheil, T. G., & Appelbaum, P. S. (2020). *Clinical handbook of psychiatry and the law.* Wolters Kluwer.

Hyatt-Williams, A. (1998). *Cruelty, violence and murder: Understanding the criminal mind.* Jason Aronson.

Johnson, J., Cohen, P., Brown, J., et al. (1999). Childhood maltreatment increases risk for personality disorders during early adulthood. *Archives of General Psychiatry, 56*(7), 600–606.

Keeshin, B. R., Cronholm, P. F., & Strawn, J. R. (2012). Physiologic changes associated with violence and abuse exposure an examination of related medical conditions. *Trauma, Violence, & Abuse, 13*(1), 41–56.

Keogh, T. (2022). Bringing our light out from under the bushel: The unrealised potential of forensic psychotherapy. *International Journal of Forensic Psychotherapy, 4*(2), 131–143.

Kersten, L., Cislo, A. M., Lynch, M., Shea, K., & Trestman, R. L. (2016). Evaluating START NOW: A skills-based psychotherapy for inmates of correctional systems. *Psychiatric Services, 67*(1), 37–42.

Knoll, J. (2009). Treating the morally objectionable. In J. Andrade (Ed.), *Handbook of violence risk assessment and treatment: New approaches for mental health professionals* (pp. 311–345). Springer Publishing Company.

Lemaire, C. (2011). Grief and resilience. In F. Stoddard, A. Pandya, & C. Katz (Eds.), *Disaster psychiatry: Readiness, evaluation, and treatment* (pp. 179–199). American Psychiatric Publishing.

Lykken, D. T. (1998). The case for parental licensure. In T. Milton, E. Simonsen, M. Birket-Smith, & R. D. Davis (Eds.), *Psychopathy: Antisocial, criminal, and violent behavior* (pp. 122–143). Guilford Publications.

Maia, B., Cruz, A. R., & Cunha, O. (2025). Adverse and positive childhood experiences and emotional regulation difficulties in a sample of incarcerated men. *Behavioral Sciences, 15*(6), 828.

Marchand, W. R. (2012). Mindfulness-based stress reduction, mindfulness-based cognitive therapy, and zen meditation for depression, anxiety, pain, and psychological distress. *Journal of Psychiatric Practice, 18*(4), 233–252.

Marco, J., Pérez, S., & García-Alandete, J. (2016). Meaning in life buffers the association between risk factors for suicide and hopelessness in participants with mental disorders. *Journal of Clinical Psychology, 72*(7), 689–700.

Martinson, R. (1974). What works? Questions and answers about prison reform. *Public Interest, 35*, 22.

McCann, R., & Ball, E. M. (2021). Comprehensive DBT forensic and correctional programs: Orchids, not dandelions. In L. A. Dimeff, S. L. Rizvi, & K. Koerner (Eds.), *Dialectical behavior therapy in clinical practice: Applications across disorders and settings* (2nd ed., pp. 182–203). Guilford Press.

McCollum, D. (2006). Child maltreatment and brain development. *Minnesota Medicine, 89*(3), 48–50.

Meloy, J. (1988). *The psychopathic mind: Origins, dynamics, and treatment.* Jason Aronson.

Miller, W. R., & Moyers, T. B. (2006). Eight stages in learning motivational interviewing. *Journal of Teaching in the Addictions, 5*(1), 3–17.

Miller, W. R., & Rollnick, S. (2002). *Motivational interviewing: Preparing people for change.* Guilford Press.

Miller, W. R., & Rollnick, S. (2009). Ten things that motivational interviewing is not. *Behavioural and Cognitive Psychotherapy, 37*(2), 129.

Mossman, D. (2006). Critique of pure risk assessment or, Kant meets Tarasoff. *University of Cincinnati Law Review, 75*, 523.

Mulay, A. L., & Cain, N. M. (2018). Managing countertransference in correctional treatment settings: An updated perspective. *Journal of Forensic Psychology Research and Practice, 18*(1), 1–18.

Mulay, A. L., Kelly, E., & Cain, N. M. (2017). Psychodynamic treatment of the criminal offender: Making the case for longer-term treatment in a longer-term setting. *Psychodynamic Psychiatry, 45*(2), 143–173.

Novalis, P. N., Virginia Singer, D. N. P., & Novalis, C. M. (2022). *Psychotherapy in corrections: A supportive approach.* American Psychiatric Association Publishing.

Pankovics, N., & Martinovic, M. (2024). Freedom from within: A meta-analytic review of mindfulness meditation-based interventions in prisons. *European Journal of Behavioral Sciences, 7*(2), 1–22.

Papapietro, D., & Adshead, G. (2016). Forensic psychotherapy: Psychodynamic therapy with offenders. In E. Griffith, M. A. Norko, A. Buchanan, M. V. Baranoski, & H. Zonana (Eds.), *Bearing witness to change* (pp. 253–266). CRC Press.

Pardini, J., Scogin, F., Schriver, J., Domino, M., Wilson, D., & LaRocca, M. (2014). Efficacy and process of cognitive bibliotherapy for the treatment of depression in jail and prison inmates. *Psychological Services, 11*(2), 141–152.

Perry, J. C., & Bond, M. (2012). Change in defense mechanisms during long-term dynamic psychotherapy and five-year outcome. *American Journal of Psychiatry, 169*(9), 916–925.

Perry, J. C., Presniak, M. D., & Olson, T. R. (2013). Defense mechanisms in schizotypal, borderline, antisocial, and narcissistic personality disorders. *Psychiatry: Interpersonal & Biological Processes, 76*(1), 32–52.

Pinta, E. R. (2009). Decisions to breach confidentiality when prisoners report violations of institutional rules. *Journal of the American Academy of Psychiatry and the Law, 37*(2), 150–154.

Pinta, E. R. (2010). Tarasoff duties in prisons: Community standards with certain twists. *Psychiatric Quarterly, 81*(2), 177–182.

Reading, L., & Bowen, E. (2014). A thematic analysis of how prisoners overcome suicidality. *International Journal of Prisoner Health, 10*(4), 212–227.

Robins, C. J., Keng, S., Ekblad, A. G., & Brantley, J. G. (2012). Effects of mindfulness-based stress reduction on emotional experience and expression: A randomized controlled trial. *Journal of Clinical Psychology, 68*(1), 117–131.

Salekin, R. (2002). Psychopathy and therapeutic pessimism: Clinical lore or clinical reality? *Clinical Psychology Review, 22*, 79–112.

Sapp, K. (2023). *Understanding offending populations and the power of correctional psychotherapy: Unlocking insights.* Springer International Publishing.

Sease, T. B., Cox, C. R., & Knight, K. (2022). Existential isolation and well-being in justice-involved populations. *Frontiers in Psychology, 13*, 1092313.

Shedler, J. (2010). The efficacy of psychodynamic psychotherapy. *American Psychologist, 65*(2), 98.

Shelton, D., Kesten, K., Zhang, W., & Trestman, R. (2011). Impact of a Dialectic Behavior Therapy—Corrections Modified (DBT-CM) upon behaviorally challenged incarcerated male adolescents. *Journal of Child and Adolescent Psychiatric Nursing, 24*(2), 105–113.

Shelton, D., Sampl, S., Kesten, K. L., Zhang, W., & Trestman, R. L. (2009). Treatment of impulsive aggression in correctional settings. *Behavioral Sciences & the Law, 27*(5), 787–800.

Shelton, D., & Wakai, S. (2011). A process evaluation of START NOW Skills Training for inmates with impulsive and aggressive behaviors. *Journal of the American Psychiatric Nurses Association, 17*(2), 148–157.

Simon, J. (2013). The return of the medical model: Disease and the meaning of imprisonment from John Howard to Brown v. Plata. *Harvard Civil Rights-Civil Liberty Law Review, 48*, 217–325.

Simpson, A. I., Gerritsen, C., Maheandiran, M., Adamo, V., Vogel, T., & Jones, R. M. (2022). A systematic review of reviews of correctional mental health services using the STAIR Framework. *Frontiers in Psychiatry, 12*, 1–15.

Slochower, J. (1991). Variations in the analytic holding environment. *International Journal of Psycho-Analysis, 72*(4), 709.

Spina, F. (2023). The importance of mindfulness meditation in correctional settings. *Journal of Correctional Education (1974–), 74*(2), 56–71.

Tärnhäll, A., Björk, J., Wallinius, M., Gustafsson, P., & Hofvander, B. (2023). Offending trajectories in violent offenders: criminal history and early life risk factors. *International Journal of Offender Therapy and Comparative Criminology, 67*(2–3), 270–290.

Testoni, I., Scardigli, F., Toniolo, A., & Gabriele Gionti, S. J. (Eds.). (2024). *Eternity between space and time: From consciousness to the cosmos.* Walter de Gruyter GmbH.

Trachsel, M., Holtforth, M. G., Biller-Andorno, N., et al. (2015). Informed consent for psychotherapy: Still not routine. *Lancet Psychiatry, 2*, 775–777.

Trestman, R. L., Truong, A. Y., Kablinger, A. S., Hartman, D. W., McNamara, R. S., Seidel, R. W., Hartman, C. W., & Sylvester-Johnson, A. (2021). *START NOW: An effective mental health intervention.* https://vtechworks.lib.vt.edu/server/api/core/bitstreams/9e4e3e20-ac9d-4334-ba66-ac2f5941190e/content

Triana, A. C., & Olson, M. (2013). Motivational interviewing as a pedagogical approach in behavioral science education: "Walking the talk." *International Journal of Psychiatry Medicine, 45*(4), 389.

Ursano, R., Sonnenberg, S., & Lazar, S. (1991). *Concise guide to psychodynamic psychotherapy.* American Psychiatric Press.

Vaillant, G. (2012). Lifting the field's "repression" of defenses. *American Journal of Psychiatry, 169*(9), 885–887.

Vanhooren, S., Leijssen, M., & Dezutter, J. (2017a). Loss of meaning as a predictor of distress in prison. *International Journal of Offender Therapy and Comparative Criminology, 61*(13), 1411–1432.

Vanhooren, S., Leijssen, M., & Dezutter, J. (2017b). Ten prisoners on a search for meaning: A qualitative study of loss and growth during incarceration. *Humanistic Psychologist, 45*(2), 162–178.

Watts, D., & Morgan, G. (1994). Malignant alienation: Dangers for patients who are hard to like. *British Journal of Psychiatry, 164*(1), 11–15.

Whittle, M. (1997). Malignant alienation. *Journal of Forensic Psychiatry, 8*(1), 5–10.

Wong, Y. J., Owen, J., Gabana, N. T., Brown, J. W., Mcinnis, S., Toth, P., & Gilman, L. (2018). Does gratitude writing improve the mental health of psychotherapy clients? Evidence from a randomized controlled trial. *Psychotherapy Research, 28*(2), 192–202.

Yakeley, J., & Adshead, G. (2013). Locks, keys, and security of mind: Psychodynamic approaches to forensic psychiatry. *Journal of the American Academy of Psychiatry and the Law, 41*(1), 38–45.

Yalom, I. D. (1980). *Existential psychotherapy.* Basic Books.

Zerler, H. (2009). Motivational interviewing in the assessment and management of suicidality. *Journal of Clinical Psychology, 65*(11), 1207–1217.

Ziaee, A., Nejat, H., Amarghan, H. A., & Fariborzi, E. (2022). Existential therapy versus acceptance and commitment therapy for feelings of loneliness and irrational beliefs in male prisoners. *European Journal of Translational Myology, 32*(1), 102171.

43

Group psychotherapy

Brittany Brizendine and Ruben Valencia[1]

Introduction

In the evolving landscape of correctional psychiatry, group psychotherapy emerges as a vital therapeutic modality. It serves as both a stand-alone treatment and an adjunctive treatment to a variety of subpopulations within the correctional milieu. This chapter draws from a robust body of literature, outlining the efficacy of group psychotherapy across diagnostic categories and settings, emphasizing attention to gender-responsive and trauma-informed care, as well as cultural competence. While examining evidence-based approaches, this chapter serves as a guide to the application of group psychotherapy and nuanced understanding of operational logistics in the field of correctional psychiatry using a thoughtful, informed, and empathetic approach to incarcerated persons (IPs).

Overview

A growing body of research offers strong empirical support for the efficacy of group treatment across diverse diagnoses and settings (Barlow et al., 2015). Additionally, many outcome studies have demonstrated similar efficacy of group treatment as compared to individual treatment (Morgan & Flora, 2002; Yoon et al., 2017). Research highlights the efficacy of group treatment for IPs, examining a variety of outcome measures such as recidivism, disciplinary behavior, and substance misuse (Allen et al., 2001; Little et al., 2000; Sandahl et al., 1998). Several key elements have been identified as contributing to successful group outcomes within and outside of the correctional setting. Outcomes of group therapy are most positive when participants are appropriately selected, goals of treatment are carefully defined, and the group facilitator is adequately trained and skilled (Barlow, 2004). Further, literature supports the concept of conditions, processes, and mediators as "therapeutic factors" that drive therapeutic change (Yalom, 2005). According to Barlow (2013), ability of the leader to promote appropriate therapeutic factors effectively is a core competency. Yalom identified the following 11 therapeutic factors of group therapy:

1. Installation of hope
2. Universality
3. Imparting information
4. Altruism
5. Corrective recapitulation of the primary family group
6. Development of socializing techniques
7. Imitative behavior
8. Interpersonal learning
9. Group cohesiveness
10. Catharsis
11. Existential factors

While many studies have attempted to rank the importance of Yalom's therapeutic factors, no universal hierarchy has been identified (Greene et al., 2020). However, group cohesion has consistently been a strong predictor of positive therapeutic outcome (Burlingame et al., 2011). Group leaders can support group cohesion through use of structure, modeling appropriate delivery of feedback, and intentionally maintaining a therapeutic emotional climate (Burlingame et al., 2002). For IPs, the theoretical orientation of the facilitator can contribute to positive outcomes. According to Andrews and colleagues (1990), directive approaches that target criminogenic needs such as cognitive-behavioral therapy (CBT) should be utilized with incarcerated populations. Most empirically supported interventions for offender populations use a CBT framework (Andrews et al., 1990). While the body of research regarding the efficacy of group treatment with IPs continues to grow, there are several considerations related to the structure and logistics of group development that can influence positive outcomes. Many of these considerations can pose obstacles in correctional settings, and thoughtful adjustments are often necessary.

Logistics of supporting quality group therapy

Group structure

Several decisions regarding the group's structure, including the size of the group, composition, length, and entry and exit points, must be determined through a needs assessment prior to pregroup interviews and member selection. When a group is in high demand, there may be little opportunity to limit size or close the group to rolling

1. The authors acknowledge the contributions of Shama Chaiken, who was a coauthor of this chapter in the textbook's first edition.

entrance. Fortunately, cognitive-behavioral group therapy (CBGT) and psychoeducation groups support larger group membership (Rutan et al., 2020a). Although closed groups, where a consistent cohort moves through the group together, are preferred by many clinicians, they are often difficult to develop in correctional settings because group attrition inhibits efficiency of providing care to a high volume of IPs. However, open groups that allow new members after the start of the group lend themselves to several benefits that can be explored by a skilled leader. Rutan et al. (2020a) note the opportunity to observe and facilitate appropriate group accommodation to new members, as well member assimilation into the group. Further, open groups provide an opportunity to revisit group boundaries, structure, and core learnings.

In addition to utilizing CBGT as a directive treatment modality, the use of homework in the correctional setting is a critical element of group structure. Morgan and Flora (2002) suggest that correctional environments inhibit externalization of gains made in therapeutic sessions, but the use of homework significantly improves positive outcomes. Empirical data supports that use of homework facilitates generalization of therapeutic gains to the external world (Cormier & Cormier, 1991).

Group length and duration

Similar to the general population, the length and duration of treatment in a correctional setting depend on treatment goals and member acuity. Inpatient group therapy is frequently conducted several times a week for brief periods, while outpatient sessions are usually weekly or biweekly over several months. To support structure and cohesion, active planning and discussion of termination should begin in the first session and continue throughout treatment to prepare the IP and allow for appropriate emotional closure (Linehan, 1993). In the correctional setting, it is critical for the facilitator to predict sudden membership loss throughout treatment and appropriately prepare members for how member entry and attrition will be handled.

Group type and facilitator

While CBGT is the group treatment of choice, several other group modalities are utilized in the correctional setting and can contribute to a well-rounded treatment approach. Process groups, focused on the "here and now," facilitated by master's- and doctorate-level clinicians, can be particularly effective with motivated, homogenous groups. Contemporary process groups have focused on increasing structure and gaining empirical support, and they have been shown to be particularly beneficial for grief, anxiety, and depression (Burlingame et al., 2013). In correctional settings where group demand is high and there are varying levels of member acuity, it can be common to find a variety of therapeutic, psychoeducational, skill-building, and recreational group offerings. Recreational therapists have a diverse skillset and can lead groups focused on sports, games, art, music, drama, and reading, which are used to encourage improvement in social skills, exploration of relationships, and the reduction of isolation. Medical staff such as nurses, medical assistants, and licensed psychiatric technicians are often utilized to facilitate structured psychoeducational groups focused on medication management and skill building.

Pregroup interviews

As a contributor to group cohesion and a critical component of CBGT, group structure plays a critical role in positive therapeutic change. Pregroup interviews can be utilized to prepare IPs for their role in the group, other group members' roles, treatment expectations, appropriate boundaries, expected outcomes, and effective approaches to communication (Greene et al., 2020). Expectation setting in corrections should also give special consideration to factors unique to the setting, such as safety precautions, group disruption, limits to confidentiality, and sudden departure of members.

Group therapy facilitator skills

A central role of the facilitator in the correctional setting is to support participants to interact without aggressive, violent, destructive, or other inappropriate behavior during the session (Chaiken et al., 2005). Additionally, an effective facilitator will strategically focus on a given therapeutic factor, consistently identify where the group is developmentally, relate consistently to treatment goals, maintain safety within the group, and consistently reinforce boundaries (Rutan et al., 2020b). Effective facilitation of group therapy requires an artful balance of empathic support and confrontation (Kominars & Dornheim, 2004). Wherever possible, a group facilitator should reinforce group norms and behavioral expectations that support therapeutic work (Rutan et al., 2020b). In correctional settings, there may be added challenges to maintaining boundaries such as timekeeping due to the unpredictable nature of the setting. However, boundary violations, controllable or not, offer an opportunity for the skilled leader to process the violation, discuss impact to the group, identify aspects where there may be agency to avoid the same situation in the future, and engage in problem solving. Research has found that facilitators who draw on specific examples from the group create a more meaningful learning experience (Morgan et al., 2006).

Due to the challenging setting in corrections, risk of burnout, and potential for trauma, a skilled facilitator will prioritize self-care. Strategies to prevent burnout and foster a psychologically healthy workplace for facilitators providing group therapy include the following:

- Circumscribed time frames for groups with clear start and stop dates;
- Regular and predicable rotation of settings and member population;
- Clinical supervision and consultation;
- Inclusion and influence regarding patient selection, treatment planning, and program development;
- Positive and collaborative custody and clinical relationships;
- Maintenance of appropriate boundaries; and
- Robust personal wellness and self-care practices outside of the work setting.

Supervisors should meet regularly with facilitators to provide supervision and consultation. These meetings should have clear goals and objectives, including review of group syllabi, countertransference and transference, and decisions about self-disclosure.

Learning and intellectual disabilities

People with intellectual disabilities (IDs) face significant obstacles. Apart from cognitive impairments, they may also contend with comorbid mental health diagnoses, inadequate adaptive coping abilities, and a prevalence of maladaptive behaviors (Brown et al., 2013; see Chapter 57). Nearly a third of adults with intellectual and developmental disabilities display emotion dysregulation and challenging behaviors (Brown et al., 2013). While the effectiveness of current treatments is uncertain, dialectical behavior therapy (DBT), especially when combined with a modified skills curriculum (DBT-SS), has shown promise; in one study, substantial behavior improvements were observed over a 4-year period (Brown et al., 2013).

Accommodation and adaptation of materials for individuals with IDs present a considerable challenge across a variety of contexts but are critical to efficacy of treatment. A requirement for success with this population is concrete, repetitious training using simple terms (Shively, 2004). Those exhibiting memory processing deficits or who encounter challenges in assimilating new information may not be suitably placed within psychoeducational or psychotherapy groups alongside patients possessing more advanced cognitive functioning. Effective care in correctional settings includes adhering to best practice treatment principles of risk, need, and responsivity (see Chapter 41). Responsivity involves tailoring the treatment to the learning styles of the patients (Chapman & Ivanoff, 2018). By aligning the treatment approach with the intellectual capabilities of group participants, one can ensure that the treatment provided is the most beneficial for all involved.

Restrictive housing units

Placing IPs with severe mental illness in restrictive housing should be minimized or avoided due to the deleterious effects, but when necessary, group therapy in these units can be conducted in an environment that is safe for both IPs and staff. This usually involves providing a barrier between each IP and staff such as a programming module; the module is designed with protective measures that ensure a secure environment, preventing unauthorized access by other individuals while not requiring the IP to be in mechanical restraints. If the IP does not feel safe or the group facilitator fears for anyone's safety, the clinical environment cannot effectively foster therapeutic change, as physical and psychological safety are necessary conditions for supporting therapeutic factors (Greene et al., 2020).

Confidentiality issues

Group therapy necessitates comprehensive informed consent procedures; ethics codes specify that the facilitator must clarify everyone's roles, responsibilities, and confidentiality boundaries and limits at the group's inception. The facilitator has a duty to keep group discussions confidential, barring any legally mandated reporting obligations. While group participants are urged to respect confidentiality, their adherence isn't governed by professional ethics standards, meaning that group facilitators cannot assure complete confidentiality of disclosures made within the group. As such, informed consent requires that participants understand that the facilitator does not have the ability to protect the confidentiality of information disclosed during group therapy (Chaiken et al., 2005). Disclosures outside the group by members can breach trust, diminish intervention effectiveness, and expose individuals to potential hostility, leading others to withhold engagement.

Providers who treat IPs often are required to make decisions about disclosure of information, especially when patients reveal violent thoughts. Facilitating group therapy in a correctional environment is full of ethical dilemmas, which can be stressful to the facilitator, who often has to weigh the balance of the ethical and legal obligation to report, taking away from the therapeutic process. This underscores the necessity of the facilitators having comprehensive training in limits to confidentiality and mandated reporting, especially as it relates to the correctional environment.

Cultural competence and gang culture

Heterogeneity of group participants can either facilitate the group process or hinder communication and trust (Yalom, 2005). It is the facilitator's responsibility to match appropriate therapeutic interventions to specific cultural groups. For example, some groups experienced more positive outcomes with a direct confrontational approach to substance use, while the same approach led to higher dropout rates in other groups (Pérez-Arce et al., 1993). Facilitators must consistently identify and assess their cultural competency to work within their scope and seek additional information when working with individuals from a cultural group with which they are less familiar. Cultural competency with respect to gang affiliation is foundational for creating physical and psychological safety in the correctional group setting. It is the facilitator's responsibility to work closely with custodial, educational, and clinical staff to understand the risk of heterogenous gang affiliation of group members (see Chapter 64). A skilled facilitator will manage risk through group inclusionary criteria, expectation setting and behavioral agreements in the pregroup interview, and management of boundaries during group treatment.

In addition to inter-subgroup dynamics, an astute facilitator will be educated on the general social norms and "politics" surrounding gang culture that may impact the safety of the facilitator, members, or therapeutic process. For example, some gang cultures discourage mental health treatment, and there may be a safety risk to individuals who are known to participate. Additionally, gang cultures tend to place high value on the idea of respect and will have varying degrees of comfort regarding confrontation by the facilitator and other members during the therapeutic process. It is expected that identifying and facilitating member vulnerability can pose a risk in the correctional setting, particularly in heterogeneous groups.

While subculture social norms and expectations can often be limiting, it is critical to understand the differences between groups, as many gang cultures understand the need for mental health services. Fortunately, for many mental health diagnoses, the similarity and intensity of the disorder outweigh the heterogeneity of other subgroup membership, and group treatment is effective for achieving positive outcomes (Yalom & Leszcz, 2020).

Women: trauma-informed care

Compared to their male counterparts, incarcerated women exhibit distinct risk factors for offending, including high rates of interpersonal victimization; physical, emotional, and sexual abuse; and exposure to family and community violence (Green et al., 2016). Incarcerated women are often survivors of complex psychological trauma, which is characterized as stemming from exposure to repeated, severe stressors early in life, often by caregivers or responsible adults (Ford & Courtois, 2009). Consequently, complex posttraumatic outcomes arise, encompassing alterations in cognition, emotions, physiological responses, and interpersonal relationships during critical socioemotional and psychobiological development. Estimated prevalence rates of posttraumatic stress disorder (PTSD) in incarcerated women vary from 21.1% (Baranyi et al., 2018) to 44% (Harner et al., 2015). As such, treatment for incarcerated women must be gender responsive and trauma informed (see Chapters 36 and 55). In fact, many correctional systems recognize this and are becoming trauma-informed organizations, whereby they are changing policies and practices of the department to foster a culture that is resistant to retraumatization.

There are a number of group-based programs to be considered for this population, including Seeking Safety, an evidence-based treatment for PTSD, substance misuse, and emotion dysregulation; Helping Women Recover and Beyond Trauma, a treatment for women who have substance use disorders (SUDs) and are likely to have co-occurring trauma histories such as sexual or physical abuse; and the Trauma Recovery and Empowerment Model, a group therapy designed for women trauma survivors with comorbid SUDs and/or mental health conditions. Regardless of the theoretical framework utilized, treatment providers must familiarize themselves with the trauma-informed care approach when working with incarcerated women.

Structured approaches to group therapy

Cognitive-behavioral therapies

CBGT has been shown to be as effective as individual therapy (Sochting, 2014) and is often utilized in the correctional setting because of its directive, highly structured, and time-limited model that allows for higher membership. A meta-analysis by Morgan and Flora (2002) found that CBT or general behavioral approaches yielded the most positive outcomes in correctional settings. Further, there is moderate evidence to suggest improvement of anxiety and depression in correctional settings with the use of CBT (Yoon et al., 2017). The approach of CBGT lends well to structure and predictability, which supports group cohesion and safety. CBGT can also increase engagement through the use of homework and encouragement for members to share their experience of assignments and activities (Rutan et al., 2020b). Increasing engagement is an excellent way to safeguard against member attrition and lack of participation, which are more prevalent in correctional settings.

Dialectical behavior therapy

DBT is an evidence-based treatment that addresses the therapeutic needs of patients exhibiting chronic suicidal ideation and diagnosed with borderline personality disorder (BPD; Linehan, 1993). DBT has been shown through randomized clinical trials to reduce suicide attempts and nonsuicidal self-injurious behavior (Linehan et al., 2015). DBT blends cognitive-behavioral techniques with mindfulness interventions and is composed of a weekly skills training group, DBT individual treatment, DBT phone coaching, and a DBT consultation team for the therapist. Chapman and Ivanoff (2018) noted BPD prevalence rates in forensic settings between 35% and 57% of the population, compared to the general population rate of approximately 1% to 2%.

Although DBT was originally validated as an evidence-based approach for patients diagnosed with BPD, empirical studies have demonstrated its efficacy in addressing a broad spectrum of additional psychological disorders (Linehan et al., 1999), including SUDs (estimated to be approximately 65% of the correctional population and another 20% who were under the influence at the time of their crime [National Institute on Drug Abuse, 2020]), depression (pooled prevalence rate is estimated to be 36.9% of the correctional population [Bedaso et al., 2020]), and PTSD (pooled prevalence rate ranged from 6.2% in men to 21.1% to 44% in women in the correctional population [Baranyi et al., 2018, Harner et al., 2015]).

Comprehensive DBT programs in correctional settings are difficult to implement for multiple reasons, including the need for all staff working in the unit to be DBT trained appropriately and relative to their classification. A significant distinction between implementing DBT in community settings versus correctional environments is the pronounced presence of antisocial traits, criminal involvement, and substance misuse among individuals in the latter, which has been found to have increased risk of violence to others (Chapman & Ivanoff, 2018). As discussed above, correctional settings have a disproportionately high prevalence of BPD, depression, and PTSD; this is juxtaposed with personality disorder treatment in correctional settings being scarce (McCann & Ball, 2021). These findings represent an opportunity to implement DBT in correctional settings and overcome obstacles for the betterment of IPs.

Peer mentorship

Peer mentorship programs in correctional settings can serve as a critical component of rehabilitation by leveraging the unique position of mentors who have direct experience with the criminal justice system (see Chapter 44). Peer mentors can provide mental health support, aid in recovery from SUDs, and encourage educational attainment and vocational training by leading peer support groups and connecting the IP with services and resources. Matthews (2021) explored peer mentorship in correctional settings, noting its growth as a rehabilitation method and the essential role of mentors' credibility and lived experience of incarceration and successful reintegration into society. Peer mentorship benefits an underserved IP population and bolsters the broader health care system's support for SUDs and beyond.

Integrated treatment for substance use disorders

Up to 85% of IPs either have a diagnosed SUD or were intoxicated at the time of their crime (National Institute on Drug Abuse, 2020). Corrections is uniquely positioned to treat and positively impact IPs with SUDs, including preventing intoxication and withdrawal, reducing overdose deaths both during confinement and upon reentry into the community, and helping people break their cycle of repeated imprisonment (Waller et al., 2024). IPs' psychosocial needs should be assessed, and they should be offered psychosocial treatment based on individual needs alongside pharmacotherapy for opioid use disorder (American Society of Addiction Medicine [ASAM], 2020). However, refusal of psychosocial treatment or lack of availability should not prevent or delay pharmacological treatment for opioid use disorder. Motivational interviewing techniques are standard in treatment of SUDs and should be utilized as necessary to encourage IPs to engage in treatment. Corrections-based treatment programs should tailor their psychosocial services with the awareness that many patients will also have concurrent mental health conditions (Waller et al., 2024). The ASAM recommends that individuals with SUDs incarcerated for more than 2 weeks should receive at least 4 hours of psychosocial services weekly, including individual or group therapy or psychoeducation, aiming eventually for jails to provide 9 or more hours weekly, comparable to community-based intensive outpatient programs.

Community reentry

IPs face significant challenges reentering into the community, such as securing housing, employment, and health care (see Chapter 23). Failure of adequate reentry into society can lead to recidivism, health complications, and increased mortality. These adversities are further exacerbated for those with mental health conditions (Galletta et al., 2021). IPs should receive assessment and planning prior to release, with prerelease groups serving as an efficient approach to fostering readiness for return to their community. Programs aimed at assisting IPs with mental illness in transitioning from jail or prison to community living can improve their access to health insurance, mental health care, and other health services (Hopkin et al., 2018).

Summary

Group psychotherapy in correctional settings has been shown to be an efficacious and economically viable treatment modality for a variety of mental health conditions, SUDs, and maladaptive characterological structures. Effective group psychotherapy requires evidence-based treatment, emphasizing the importance of facilitator training and appropriate patient selection. Significant nuances and precautions must be recognized when doing group psychotherapy in restrictive housing units. Given the demonstrated efficacy of the group treatment modality, correctional administrators are encouraged to consider integrating group psychotherapy as a comprehensive approach to the treatment of IPs, as this approach aligns with best practices and supports rehabilitation and reintegration into the community.

REFERENCES

Allen, L. C., MacKenzie, D. L., & Hickman, L. J. (2001). The effectiveness of cognitive behavioral treatment for adult offenders: A methodological, quality-based review. *International Journal of Offender Therapy and Comparative Criminology, 45*, 498–514.

American Society of Addiction Medicine. (2020). The ASAM national practice guideline for the treatment of opioid use disorder: 2020 focused update. *Journal of Addiction Medicine, 14*(2S Suppl. 1), 1–91.

Andrews, D. A., Zinger, I., Hoge, R. D., Bonta, J., Gendreau, P., & Cullen, F. T. (1990). Does correctional treatment work? A clinically relevant and psychologically informed meta-analysis. *Criminology, 28*, 369–404.

Baranyi, G., Cassidy, M., Fazel, S., Priebe, S., & Mundt, A. P. (2018). Prevalence of posttraumatic stress disorder in prisoners. *Epidemiologic Reviews, 40*(1), 166.

Barlow, S. (2004). A strategic three-year plan to teach group competencies. *Journal of the Specialists in Group Work, 29*, 113–126.

Barlow, S. H. (2013). *Specialty competencies in group psychology*. Oxford University Press.

Barlow, S., Burlingame, G. M., Greene, L. R., Joyce, A., Kalkauskas, F., Kinley, J., Klein, R. H., Kobos, J. C., Leszcz, M., MacNair-Semands, R., Paquin, J. D., Tasca, G. A., Whittingham, M., & Feirman, D. (2015). *Evidence-based practice in group psychotherapy* [American Group Psychotherapy Association Science to Service Task Force web document]. https://www.agpa.org/home/practice-resources/evidence-based-practice-in-group-psychotherapy

Bedaso, A., Ayalew, M., Mekonnen, N., & Duko, B. (2020). Global estimates of the prevalence of depression among prisoners: A systematic review and meta-analysis. *Depression Research and Treatment, 2020*, 3695209.

Brown, J. F., Brown, M. Z., & Dibiasio, P. (2013). Treating individuals with intellectual disabilities and challenging behaviors with adapted dialectical behavior therapy. *Journal of Mental Health Research in Intellectual Disabilities, 6*(4), 280–303.

Burlingame, G. M., Fuhriman, A., & Johnson, J. (2002). Cohesion in group psychotherapy. In J. Norcross (Ed.), *Psychotherapy relationships that work: Therapist contributions and responsiveness to patients* (pp. 71–87). Oxford University Press.

Burlingame, G. M., McClendon, D. T., & Alonso, J. (2011). Cohesion in group therapy. *Psychotherapy, 48*, 34–42.

Burlingame, G., Strauss, B., & Joyce, A. (2013). Change mechanisms and effectiveness of small group treatments. In M. J. Lambert (Ed.), *Bergin & Garfield's handbook of psychotherapy and behavior change* (6th ed., pp. 640–689). Wiley & Sons.

Chaiken, S., Thompson, C., & Shoemaker, W. (2005). Mental health interventions in correctional settings. In C. L. Scott & J. B. Gerbasi (Eds.), *Handbook of correctional mental health* (pp. 345–376). American Psychiatric Publishing.

Chapman, A. L., & Ivanoff, A. (2018). Forensic issues in borderline personality disorder. In B. Stanley & A. S. New (Eds.), *Borderline personality disorder* (pp. 403–419). Oxford University Press.

Cormier, W. H., & Cormier, L. S. (1991). *Interviewing strategies for helpers: Fundamental skills and cognitive behavioral interventions* (3rd ed.). Brooks/Cole.

Ford, J. D., & Courtois, C. A. (2009). Defining and understanding complex trauma and complex traumatic stress disorders. In C. A. Courtois & J. D. Ford (Eds.), *Treating complex traumatic stress disorders: An evidence-based guide* (pp. 13–30). Guilford Press.

Galletta, E., Fagan, T. J., Shapiro, D., & Walker, L. E. (2021). Societal reentry of prison inmates with mental illness: Obstacles, programs, and best practices. *Journal of Correctional Health Care, 27*(1), 58–65.

Green, B. L., Dass-Brailsford, P., Hurtado de Mendoza, A., Mete, M., Lynch, S. M., DeHart, D. D., & Belknap, J. (2016). Trauma experiences and mental health among incarcerated women. *Psychological Trauma: Theory, Research, Practice, and Policy, 8*(4), 455–463.

Greene, L. R., Barlow, S., & Kaklauskas, F. J. (2020). Therapeutic factors. In F. J. Kaklauskas & L. R. Greene (Eds.), *Core principles of group psychotherapy: An integrated theory, research, and practice training manual* (pp. 56–70). Routledge.

Harner, H. M., Budescu, M., Gillihan, S. J., Riley, S., & Foa, E. B. (2015). Posttraumatic stress disorder in incarcerated women: A call for evidence-based treatment. *Psychological Trauma: Theory, Research, Practice, and Policy, 7*(1), 58–66.

Hopkin, G., Evans-Lacko, S., Forrester, A., Shaw, J., & Thornicroft, G. (2018). Interventions at the transition from prison to the community for prisoners with mental illness: A systematic review. *Administration and Policy in Mental Health and Mental Health Services Research, 45*(4), 623–634.

Kominars, K., & Dornheim, L. (2004). *Group approaches in substance abuse treatment*. Sage Publications.

Linehan, M. M. (1993). *Cognitive behavioral treatment of borderline personality disorder*. Guilford Press.

Linehan, M. M., Korslund, K. E., Harned, M. S., et al. (2015). Dialectical behavior therapy for high suicide risk in individuals with borderline personality disorder: A randomized clinical trial and component analysis. *JAMA Psychiatry, 72*(5), 475–482.

Linehan, M. M., Schmidt, H., III, Dimeff, L. A., Craft, J. C., Kanter, J., & Comtois, K. A. (1999). Dialectical behavior therapy for patients with borderline personality disorder and drug-dependence. *American Journal on Addictions, 8*(4), 279–292.

Little, G., Robinson, K. D., Burnette, K. D., & Swan, S. (2000). Ten-year outcome data on MRT-treated DWI offenders. *Alternatives to Incarceration, 6*, 16–18.

Matthews, E. (2021). Peer-focused prison reentry programs: Which peer characteristics matter most? *Incarceration*, *2*(2), 1–19.

McCann, R., & Ball, E. (2021). Comprehensive DBT forensic and correctional programs: Orchids, not dandelions. In L. A. Dimeff, S. L. Rizvi, & K. Koerner (Eds.), *Dialectical behavior therapy in clinical practice: Applications across disorders and settings* (pp. 182–206). Guilford Press.

Morgan, R. D., & Flora, D. B. (2002). Group psychotherapy with incarcerated offenders: A research synthesis. *Group Dynamics: Theory, Research, and Practice*, *6*(3), 203–218.

Morgan, R. D., Kroner, D. G., & Mills, J. F. (2006). Group psychotherapy in prison: Facilitating change inside walls. *Journal of Contemporary Psychotherapy*, *36*, 137–144.

National Institute on Drug Abuse. (2020, June 1). *Criminal Justice DrugFacts*. Retrieved June 21, 2025, from https://nida.nih.gov/publications/drugfacts/criminal-justice

Pérez-Arce, P., Carr, K. D., & Sorensen, J. L. (1993). Cultural issues in an outpatient program for stimulant abusers. *Journal of Psychoactive Drugs*, *25*, 35–44.

Rutan, J. S., Greene, L. R., & Kaklauskas, F. J. (2020a). Preparing to begin a new group. In F. J. Kaklauskas & L.R. Greene (Eds.), *Core principles of group psychotherapy: An integrated theory, research, and practice training manual* (pp. 89–100). Routledge.

Rutan, J. S., Greene, L. R., & Kaklauskas, F. J. (2020b). Basic leadership tasks. In F. J. Kaklauskas & L. R. Greene (Eds.), *Core principles of group psychotherapy: An integrated theory, research, and practice training manual* (pp. 111–121). Routledge.

Sandahl, C., Herlitz, K., Ahlin, G., & Ronnberg, S. (1998). Time-limited group psychotherapy for moderately alcohol dependent patients: A randomized controlled clinical trial. *Psychotherapy Research*, *8*, 361.

Shively, R. (2004). Treating offenders with mental retardation and developmental disabilities. *Corrections Today*, *66*, 84–86, 141.

Sochting, I. (2014). *Cognitive behavioral group therapy: Challenges and opportunities*. Wiley.

Waller, R. C., Zaller, N. D., Baxter, L. E., et al. (2024). *Proposed framework for the ASAM criteria, 4th ed., Vol. 3: Correctional settings & community reentry*. ASAM Criminal Justice Expert Committee. The MedComms Group.

Yalom, I. D. (2005). *The theory and practice of group psychotherapy* (5th ed.). Basic Books.

Yalom, I. D., & Leszcz, M. (2020). *The theory and practice of group psychotherapy*. Basic Books.

Yoon, I. A., Slade, K. S., & Fazel, S. (2017). Outcomes of psychological therapies for prisoners with mental health problems: A systematic review and meta-analysis. *Journal of Consulting and Clinical Psychology*, *85*(8), 783–802.

44

Peer support programs

Melissa J. Lavoie and Charlotte M. Schwarz

Introduction

Structured peer support services have long played a role in promoting engagement with care among individuals with mental illness. While peer support services grew with the mental health service user movement of the 1970s and have become increasingly commonplace since, efforts to hire staff with a personal history of mental illness were made as early as the 18th century (Davidson et al., 2012). Through mutual understanding, social support, unconditional positive regard, and positive self-disclosure, peer specialists can support access to care and offer hope to individuals experiencing mental illness. This chapter outlines the development of peer support programs, their application to carceral environments, and their potential benefits and challenges.

Origins and definitions of peer support

The use of peer support draws from the recovery model, premised on the idea that a rehabilitative approach supports individuals with psychosocial challenges and psychiatric disorders to achieve their goals. Integral to this future-oriented paradigm is the use of peer support to promote social inclusion and a sense of belonging, as well as the expertise of lived experience (World Health Organization, 2013).

As such, the *peer* or *peer support worker* occupies a unique position in that they may "explicitly and intentionally instill hope and afford personal assistance" in the process of offering the trained skills that formalize their structured role (Zeng & Chung, 2018, p. 1). Peer support workers practice in a variety of settings such as drug courts, homeless shelters, and recovery community centers. In correctional settings, which are the focus of this chapter, a peer support worker is an individual with current or former criminal justice involvement in addition to the lived experience of recovery from substance use disorders (SUDs) and/or other mental health diagnoses. *Peer practice* encompasses aspects of the approach described here. A peer support worker receives specialized training, including possible certification, and may be a volunteer or paid employee of the correctional system. However, the peer support worker's distinct asset emerges from being "experientially credentialed" by their history navigating the health care and criminal justice systems (Davidson et al., 1999). In the literature and depending on the institutional setting, peer support workers may be referred to by other titles including peer specialists, peer recovery coaches, peer advocates, and peer recovery support specialists.

Peer support is an evidence-based model of care delivery between a peer support worker and the individual whose recovery and progress they are promoting. It includes a wide variety of interactions and activities that foster connectedness and resilience, ultimately striving for recovery and integration into the community. These services are supportive in nature rather than hierarchical and directive. They are characterized by a mutuality, also referred to as *peerness*, in the relationship between the peer support worker and the incarcerated person (IP). Other hallmarks include a nonjudgmental stance on the part of the peer support worker, a voluntariness on the part of the IP, and mutual respect and responsibility in this relationship-focused partnership (National Association of Peer Supporters, 2019). Given the pervasiveness of trauma experienced by IPs, trauma-informed peer support is a core principle of the interactions.

The Substance Abuse and Mental Health Services Administration (2023) has identified five core values to guide the training of peer specialists working in behavioral health services:

1. Recovery oriented: Peer workers hold out hope to those they serve, partnering with them to envision and achieve a meaningful and purposeful life. Peer workers help those they serve identify and build on strengths and empower them to choose for themselves, recognizing that there are multiple pathways to recovery.
2. Person centered: Peer recovery support services are always directed by the person participating in services. Peer recovery support is personalized to align with the specific hopes, goals, and preferences of the people served and to respond to specific needs the people have identified to the peer worker.
3. Voluntary: Peer specialists are partners or consultants to those they serve. They do not dictate the types of services provided or the elements of recovery plans that will guide their work with peers. Participation in peer recovery support services is always contingent on peer choice.
4. Relationship focused: The relationship between the peer worker and the peer is the foundation on which peer recovery support

services and support are provided. The relationship between the peer worker and peer is respectful, trusting, empathetic, collaborative, and mutual.

5. Trauma informed: Peer recovery support utilizes a strengths-based framework that emphasizes physical, psychological, and emotional safety and creates opportunities for survivors to rebuild a sense of control and empowerment.

Evidence base for peer support in justice-involved individuals

Much of the research relating to peer support draws from prior studies examining its benefits for individuals with SUDs and other psychiatric conditions. Furthermore, there is emerging interest in examining how peer support workers influence reentry outcomes for IPs.

In what Mowen and Boman (2018, p. 1) described as the "duality of the peer effect," formerly incarcerated individuals who are exposed to a relative's or friend's criminality face higher levels of recidivism; however, peer support workers can provide positive social support to promote resilience and reintegration through decreased substance use and recidivism. The evidence for the benefits of peer support encompasses several psychosocial factors. For one, peer support has been found to enhance self-esteem and confidence in interacting with others, which can increase an individual's sense of control and ability to bring about changes in their life (Davidson et al., 2012). Positive self-disclosure allows an individual to seize the narrative of their life's story, and peer support has been shown to increase a sense of hope and inspiration (Ratzlaff et al., 2006; Solomon, 2004). Accordingly, peer support programs have been shown to enhance personal well-being on measures of recovery orientation, confidence, and empowerment (Resnick & Rosenheck, 2008). Other demonstrated benefits include increased self-efficacy, perceived social support, positive relations with family and friends, improved quality of life, and decreased stress (Andreas et al., 2010). These findings likely extend to incarcerated men and women, though the evidence base is still developing. A study by Heidemann and colleagues (2014) explored the sources of support available to formerly incarcerated women and the influence of that support on life satisfaction; only support from "others" (a category that included peers, agency staff, and other professionals), but not friends or family, positively predicted life satisfaction.

Individuals being treated for a psychiatric illness on inpatient units have reported that peer support workers offer them encouragement and genuine support that allows them to envision a life beyond their current situation (Rooney et al., 2016). In correctional settings, peer practice harnesses empathy, often also allowing the peer's own success to set a positive expectation for the IP. An IP might not otherwise experience high expectations from a society in which they are marginalized. Another benefit of peer support programs has been to decrease participants' level of psychotic symptoms. Of note, individuals reported an increased amount of distress experienced due to these symptoms, possibly because they were challenged to do more than before, and their remaining symptoms were viewed as barriers (Davidson et al., 2012). Peer practice has also been shown to have benefits for the physical health of recently incarcerated individuals. In a randomized trial, Wang and colleagues (2012) demonstrated that people recently released from prison who were matched with a peer health worker had decreased rates of emergency department utilization compared to people who received expedited primary care.

The role of peer support in corrections

In correctional settings, peer specialists may assist clients through a wide range of services (Bureau of Justice Assistance, 2022; Davidson & Rowe, 2008; Razavi & Ayala, 2017). They augment, but do not duplicate, the roles of treatment providers, including psychotherapists, psychiatrists, and social workers. To promote effective interdisciplinary collaboration, it is crucial that organizations clearly delineate the separate responsibilities of peer specialists and other members of the health care team. While peer workers in correctional settings share the same core values as other peer specialists and offer many similar services, some supports they provide are specific to the needs of justice-involved individuals. Services peer specialists may be able to deliver include:

- Supporting individuals in engaging with drug courts and other pretrial supervision and diversion services;
- Facilitating support groups in correctional settings or among recently incarcerated persons in the community;
- Encouraging clients to engage in psychiatric and SUD treatment using motivational interviewing and positive self-disclosure;
- For clients not interested in treatment, supporting them in using harm reduction approaches to promote health and wellness;
- Offering psychoeducation and information about health and wellness;
- Supporting IPs in developing a personalized transition plan prior to release;
- Helping IPs identify and prepare for possible obstacles to recovery and successful reintegration into the community;
- Connecting clients to community-based mental health treatment and other services;
- Ensuring a warm hand-off between providers in corrections and in the community;
- Accompanying clients to treatment appointments and meetings with probation or parole;
- Supporting recently released individuals in overcoming barriers to housing and employment, such as by helping them obtain photo identification and enter wait lists for government-subsidized housing; and
- Offering crisis management and referral to a higher level of care when necessary
- Training colleagues on how to engage individuals with a history of criminal justice involvement.

Peer workers can play a crucial role in building and maintaining partnerships with community-based resources, including mental health clinics and SUD treatment programs. Peer supporters deliver services in the correctional setting and may also offer support to individuals after release. The lived experience of peer specialists uniquely enables them to provide trauma-informed and culturally relevant support both during and after incarceration. Peer support programs should encourage and support collaboration between peers and community resources such as Veterans Justice Outreach and community reentry coalitions (Razavi & Ayala,

2017). Involvement with these groups allows peer workers to understand the landscape of services offered in the community, provide more targeted referrals to resources, and facilitate a more effective and coordinated transition of care for individuals recently released from incarceration. In addition, the lived experience of peer workers enables them to offer valuable insights to community providers.

While the roles of peer support providers may remain largely the same in prisons and in jails, the duration and intensity of peer support services in each setting must necessarily be different. Given the shorter length of stay in jails, interventions may be briefer but more intense (Bureau of Justice Assistance, 2022). Considering the unpredictable length of stay in jails, peer specialists in those facilities must be flexible and able to adapt their schedule to best serve the highest need clients, often but not always individuals with an impending discharge. Prisons, on the other hand, may be better suited to the longer term interventions targeting a wider array of IPs. For instance, long-term establishment of support groups facilitated by peer specialists and with consistent groups of attendees who provide mutual accountability and social support would likely be more feasible in a prison than a jail.

Burden and Etwaroo (2020) have outlined five essential elements of comprehensive peer recovery support services in correctional settings, which are delineated below.

Trained peers

Recruiting a pool of prospective peer support workers begets questions as to the requirements for their employment, which will vary depending on whether they are paid or voluntary, and what state and institutional practice dictates. Although certification is not mandatory, it does have financial implications. The Centers for Medicare and Medicaid Services authorized states to bill Medicaid for peer provider services if a statewide training and certification process was in place and if peers received supervision by an appropriate mental health professional (Chapman et al., 2018). This led to the emergence of certifying bodies (e.g., the International Certification and Reciprocity Consortium or the Association for Addiction Professionals). Non–Centers for Medicare and Medicaid Services funding sources such as grants and drug court funds also exist to support peer programs. Regardless of funding or formalized certification, training to standardize knowledge and competencies is required to prepare peer support staff. This includes an understanding of the stages of change and recovery, as well as safety procedures in the correctional facility.

Choice and access

Self-direction and choice are core values of peer practice, and accordingly, they are essential elements of a peer support program. In the correctional setting, an IP's choices may be contingent on an interplay of factors such as their housing status, security level, and the staffing of the institution on a given day. However, elements of self-direction are supported even in these settings, such as whether or not to attend recreational activities or to participate actively in reentry planning. Thus, prisons and jails benefit from a strategy for making peer support accessible for IPs who choose to use it. For example, a correctional facility could deploy peer support workers onsite for "drop-in hours" or have them lead group discussions. Other corrections staff, such as officers and clinicians, should be educated about peer practice implementation as an available resource to coordinate promotion of this resource.

Recovery capital building

Recovery capital includes the internal and external factors that help someone initiate and sustain long-term recovery from addiction (Groshkova et al., 2012). Building this capital requires planning to articulate, outline, and develop an action plan for personal goals. It may involve practical aspects like finding housing, employment, or educational training, as well as more abstract skills for life and recovery. Frequent recovery check-ins allow an individual who is in recovery to reflect on challenges and seek guidance along the way.

Recovery peer support groups and activities

Comprehensive peer recovery support services incorporate elements of community building beyond one-on-one interactions. Groups or workshops, whether structured or semi-structured, educational or supportive, can foster social skills and a sense of purpose and belonging.

Reentry support

Reentry support links IPs to resources that will continue to support their goals in the community. With the implementation of Medicaid expansion in participating states under the Affordable Care Act, incarcerated adults released from prison or jail have increasing opportunities to seek health care, including peer support services.

Peer support for community reentry

Community reentry after incarceration represents a high-risk period for individuals with mental illness and SUDs. In the period following incarceration, individuals face an elevated risk of multiple adverse health outcomes, including hospitalization and drug-related death (Merrall et al., 2010; Wang et al., 2013). Individuals leaving incarceration must navigate multiple complex systems, including social service agencies, behavioral health clinics, and probation and parole services. They may experience barriers to obtaining employment, housing, insurance, and medical care. These challenges are compounded by the stigma faced by individuals with a history of incarceration.

Since reentry planning and transitioning into the community after release are especially fraught periods for an IP, the peer support worker's experience navigating this time can be an invaluable support. Peer specialists can augment existing psychiatric services in correctional facilities at the end of an IP's sentence and in the community to prepare for reentry, facilitate linkage to community services, and promote health and well-being upon release.

Peers can facilitate reentry by navigating logistical barriers such as transportation to parole or probation officers, securing stable housing, and ensuring adequate food and clothing. Their presence may serve to reduce stigma and bolster assertive advocacy, empowering formerly incarcerated individuals to seek out and use community resources that will further their integration. Peer support workers may encourage formerly incarcerated individuals to seek medical and psychiatric care, attend recovery groups, and prioritize positive engagement.

Challenges and drivers of success for peer support

Integrating peer support services into the correctional setting can be a challenge. In a setting where every aspect of the IP's daily life is monitored and controlled, the flexibility and customized nature of peer practice might seem at odds. In addition, security personnel in correctional settings may cite safety concerns as a reason to prohibit or stop peer support programs, thinking that peers will negatively influence each other or conspire in illegal activity. Even in systems that support the idea of peer recovery specialists, the risk of inappropriately using these trained peers to supplant staff functions, especially during periods of understaffing, may exist. Thus, the challenges in corrections include not just the risk of shutting down peer support programs prematurely but also of exploiting the incarcerated peer specialists.

Burden and Etwaroo (2020) enumerate certain drivers of success for integration of peer support services in the carceral setting. For one, the institution should have a defined vision of what successful peer practice implementation would look like in their facility. Setting a vision requires identifying the overall purpose of the program and evaluating the motivation for getting it off the ground. Identifying stakeholders is crucial for successful implementation to align the peer support program's values with the facility's organizational goals. This core team, including participants such as corrections leadership, security staff, and behavioral health staff, will ideally collaborate with the peer support program. Even at early stages of planning, the participation of peers with lived experience is critical for generating effective strategies and recommendations for future implementation.

Next, effective recruitment, hiring, and onboarding of peer support workers will set the program's course. A group interview format can be an effective means of assessing applicants' communication skills and suitability for teamwork (Repper & Watson, 2012). Fifteen to 20 peer specialists for every 1,500 IPs, with a minimum of 20 peers if the facility has a mental health disorder or co-occurring disorders program, is recommended by the Bureau of Justice Assistance (2022). A culture of ongoing training and support for peer specialists is another driver of success. Some peer support workers have experienced hurdles in terms of role confusion and limited opportunities for networking and support (Berry et al., 2011). Thus, they would benefit from supervision and a space to process ethical dilemmas that may arise in their role. The boundaries of clinical staff (such as psychiatrists, psychologists, and clinical social workers) as they relate to the boundaries of peer support staff should be clearly delineated and enforced. This minimizes splitting and empowers collaboration in the system.

It is crucial that peer supporters receive formal training, both before starting the role and as continuing education. Most states require peer specialists to obtain certification, and this certification may be necessary for reimbursement from Medicaid or private insurers (Stack et al., 2022). Peer specialist trainings vary in content but may include the following topics (Texas Institute for Excellence in Mental Health, 2016):

- The stages of change model of recovery;
- Motivational interviewing;
- Empathic communication skills;
- Conflict resolution;
- Signs and symptoms of mental illness;
- Overdose prevention;
- Group facilitation skills;
- Legal and ethical considerations, including confidentiality laws, mandatory reporting, and professional boundaries;
- Documentation; and
- Cultural competency and sensitivity.

Given the unique challenges faced by individuals with a history of criminal justice involvement, peer specialists working in correctional settings can also benefit from training specific to incarceration and reentry. This training might include information about the criminal justice system, services available to justice-involved individuals, and the ways in which incarceration contributes to trauma (Razavi & Ayala, 2017). It is also important that peer supporters understand any obligations they may have to inform correctional, probation, or parole authorities about certain issues, such as substance use, suspected rule infractions, or nonadherence to conditions of supervised release.

There is an intrinsic tension between peer support services and traditional correctional approaches. The voluntary, trauma-informed, and person-centered nature of peer support work may be difficult to foster in correctional settings, which have traditionally relied on authoritarian and punitive approaches to manage behavior. To successfully navigate these tensions and integrate peer support programs into correctional systems, organizations must engage diverse stakeholders, including wardens, correctional officers, and treatment providers.

In addition to cultural challenges, correctional facilities may also encounter logistical difficulties in implementing peer support programs. For instance, the inclusion of clients in restrictive housing units may present operational challenges. One successful program in Pennsylvania addressed these concerns by working closely with front-line correctional officers to ensure that peer services were in alignment with security priorities and that appropriate procedural enhancements were made prior to offering services on restrictive housing units (Bureau of Justice Assistance, 2022). The program has since been able to provide services in high-security areas of the facility, including psychiatric observation cells and diversionary treatment units. Preparing to launch the program on a small scale, with a target group for a set length of time, allows for an iterative approach. As the groundwork is laid with policies and procedures, it is natural that they will be refined and modified as unanticipated challenges and unexpected needs arise.

Programs that have used peer workers who are currently incarcerated may face resistance from staff. Staff may worry that giving IPs increased access to peers and to restricted areas of the facility may adversely impact security, for instance, by allowing the distribution of contraband (South et al., 2016). Close engagement with correctional officers in program development and frequent check-ins during program delivery are crucial in alleviating these concerns. Some studies have found that initial staff opposition to peer support services wanes over time as the value of those services becomes clear (Davies, 1994; Scott et al., 2004).

Examples of peer support programs

The following are aspects of peer support services implementation in various criminal justice settings around the United States, as described in the Bureau of Justice Assistance's 2022 manual on Peer Recovery Support Services in Correctional Settings and online resources accessed in April 2024:

- The West Tennessee State Penitentiary has a residential SUD program providing treatment while incarcerated and a continuum of support after release. This program uses therapeutic communities for IPs with SUDs. Residents progress through three phases lasting 3 to 4 months each. They are paired with a peer supporter who is another resident of the therapeutic community, modeling effective coping and self-help strategies.
- The Albany County Corrections and Rehabilitative Services center contracts with Catholic Charities' Project Safe Point to provide two certified recovery peer advocates who provide approximately 20 hours of in-jail support weekly.
- The Vermont Department of Corrections implemented the Open Ears Program, in which paid forensic peer recovery coaches facilitate one-on-one mentoring and groups with IPs. These forensic peer recovery coaches are themselves IPs who have been identified by corrections staff to undergo a week-long training. The coaching sessions occur in a private setting.
- The Multnomah County, Oregon, Sheriff's Office partners with the Mental Health Addiction Association of Oregon to provide peer specialists in county jails. A biweekly meeting among peer specialists, supervisors, and program directors has created a regular space for feedback and support.
- The Milwaukee County, Wisconsin, Behavioral Health Division partners with the Milwaukee County Jail and House of Corrections to provide resources for individuals with SUDs while incarcerated and after release. Peers are involved from the onset while developing programming.
- The Pennsylvania Department of Corrections identifies certified peer specialists, including a small percentage of individuals who have been sentenced to life in prison. The certified peer specialists receive the same training as their counterparts in the community, as well as additional training in evidence-based practices such as trauma-informed care, suicide prevention in the correctional setting, and Mental Health First Aid. The Pennsylvania Department of Corrections' Psychology Office assumed oversite of the peer practice program and has instituted regular staffing analysis and auditing processes.
- In Connecticut, the Department of Mental Health and Addiction Services partners with Advocacy Unlimited Inc.'s Recovery Support Specialist Training and Certification program to assist individuals in becoming Certified Recovery Support Specialists in Peer Delivered Services (covered by the Section 1115 Medicaid waiver). The training is free, though there are costs associated with the application.

Summary

Peer support programs harness the expertise of individuals with lived experience of mental illness, SUDs, and criminal justice involvement to support the recovery of IPs facing similar challenges. Effective peer support programs take an approach that is person centered, voluntary, recovery oriented, relationship focused, and trauma informed. In correctional settings, trained peer specialists can serve as role models in recovery, encourage and facilitate access to care for mental illness and SUDs, support harm reduction strategies for individuals uninterested in treatment, aid in community reentry planning, and educate staff about the experience of individuals with lived experience. Emerging evidence supports the efficacy of peer support programs in correctional settings despite the concerns about security that are sometimes cited in opposition, leading the Bureau of Justice Assistance and other national agencies to promote and fund the practice in recent years. Measures must be taken to ensure that peer support specialists are adequately trained and are not being asked inappropriately to replace staff functions, but when implemented properly, such programs can enhance individuals' recovery during incarceration.

REFERENCES

Andreas, D., Ja, D. Y., & Wilson, S. (2010). Peers Reach Out Supporting Peers to Embrace Recovery (PROSPER): A Center for Substance Abuse Treatment Recovery Community Services program. *Alcoholism Treatment Quarterly*, *28*(3), 326–338.

Berry, C., Hayward, M. I., & Chandler, R. (2011). Another rather than other: Experiences of peer support specialist workers and their managers working in mental health services. *Journal of Public Mental Health*, *10*(4), 238–249.

Burden, E., & Etwaroo, E. (2020). Peer recovery support services in New York opioid intervention courts: Essential elements and processes for effective integration. *Federal Probation Journal*, *84*, 50.

Bureau of Justice Assistance. (2022). *Peer recovery support services in correctional settings*. U.S. Department of Justice. https://bja.ojp.gov/library/publications/peer-recovery-support-services-correctional-settings

Chapman, S. A., Blash, L. K., Mayer, K., & Spetz, J. (2018). Emerging roles for peer providers in mental health and substance use disorders. *American Journal of Preventive Medicine*, *54*(6), S267–S274.

Davidson, L., Bellamy, C., Guy, K., & Miller, R. (2012). Peer support among persons with severe mental illnesses: A review of evidence and experience. *World Psychiatry*, *11*(2), 123–128.

Davidson, L., Chinman, M., Kloos, B., Weingarten, R., Stayner, D., & Tebes, J. K. (1999). Peer support among individuals with severe mental illness: A review of the evidence. *Clinical Psychology: Science and Practice*, *6*(2), 165–187.

Davidson, L., & Rowe, M. (2008). *Peer support within criminal justice settings: The role of forensic peer specialists*. CMHS National Gains Center. https://static1.squarespace.com/static/599ee1094c0dbff62a07fc13/t/59af1347dbe3974ceaa105ce/1376071906957/ForensicPeerGAINSCenter+1.pdf

Davies, B. (1994). The Swansea listener scheme: Views from the prison landings. *Howard Journal of Criminal Justice*, *33*(2), 125–135.

Groshkova, T., Best, D., & White, W. (2012). The assessment of recovery capital: Properties and psychometrics of a measure of addiction recovery strengths. *Drug and Alcohol Review*, *32*(2), 187–194.

Heidemann, G., Cederbaum, J. A., & Martinez, S. (2014). "We walk through it together": The importance of peer support for formerly incarcerated women's success. *Journal of Offender Rehabilitation*, *53*(7), 522–542.

Merrall, E. L., Kariminia, A., Binswanger, I. A., et al. (2010). Meta-analysis of drug-related deaths soon after release from prison. *Addiction*, *105*(9), 1545–1554.

Mowen, T. J., & Boman, J. H. (2018). The duality of the peer effect: The interplay between peer support and peer criminality on offending and substance use during reentry. *Crime & Delinquency*, *64*(8), 1094–1116.

National Association of Peer Supporters. (2019). *National practice guidelines for peer specialists and supervisors.*

Ratzlaff, S., McDiarmid, D., Marty, D., & Rapp, C. (2006). The Kansas Consumer as Provider program: Measuring the effects of a supported education initiative. *Psychiatric Rehabilitation Journal*, *29*(3), 174–182.

Razavi, M., & Ayala, J. (2017). *Substance use disorder forensic peer 10 best practices curriculum.* Regional Facilitation Center. https://static1.squarespace.com/static/5a0de0f94c0dbf779166a592/t/5ebf007355cc77112e7d4860/1589575797697/Substance+Use+Disorder+Forensic+Peer+Best+Practices.pdf

Repper, J., & Watson, E. (2012). A year of peer support in Nottingham: Lessons learned. *Journal of Mental Health Training, Education and Practice*, *7*(2), 70–78.

Resnick, S. G., & Rosenheck, R. A. (2008). Integrating peer-provided services: A quasi-experimental study of recovery orientation, confidence, and empowerment. *Psychiatric Services*, *59*(11), 1307–1314.

Rooney, J. M., Miles, N., & Barker, T. (2016). Patients' views: Peer support worker on inpatient wards. *Mental Health and Social Inclusion*, *20*(3), 160–166.

Scott, D., Harzke, A. J., Mizwa, M. B., et al. (2004). Evaluation of an HIV peer education program in Texas prisons. *Journal of Correctional Health Care*, *10*(2), 151–173.

Solomon, P. (2004). Peer support/peer provided services underlying processes, benefits, and critical ingredients. *Psychiatric Rehabilitation Journal*, *27*(4), 392–401.

South, J., Woodall, J., Kinsella, K., & Bagnall, A.-M. (2016). A qualitative synthesis of the positive and negative impacts related to delivery of peer-based health interventions in prison settings. *BMC Health Services Research*, *16*(1), 1–8.

Stack, E., et al. (2022). Peer recovery support services across the continuum: In community, hospital, corrections, and treatment and recovery agency settings—A narrative review. *Journal of Addiction Medicine*, *16*(1), 93–100.

Substance Abuse and Mental Health Services Administration. (2023). *Core competencies for peer workers.* https://www.samhsa.gov/brss-tacs/recovery-support-tools/peers/core-competencies-peer-workers

Texas Institute for Excellence in Mental Health. (2016). *Peer specialist training & certification programs: National overview 2016.* https://sites.utexas.edu/mental-health-institute/files/2017/01/Peer-Specialist-Training-and-Certification-Programs-A-National-Overview-2016-Update-1.5.17.pdf

Wang, E. A., Hong, C. S., Shavit, S., Sanders, R., Kessell, E., & Kushel, M. B. (2012). Engaging individuals recently released from prison into primary care: A randomized trial. *American Journal of Public Health*, *102*(9), e22–e29.

Wang, E., Wang, Y., & Krumholz, H. (2013). A high risk of hospitalization following release from correctional facilities in Medicare beneficiaries: A retrospective matched cohort study, 2002 to 2010. *JAMA Internal Medicine*, *173*(17), 1621–1628.

World Health Organization. (2013). *Mental health action plan 2013–2020.* http://apps.who.int/iris/bitstream/10665/89966/1/9789241506021_eng.pdf

Zeng, G., & Chung, D. (2018). The stepped model of peer provision practice: Capturing the dynamics of peer support work in action. *Journal of Mental Health Training, Education and Practice*, *14*(2), 106–118.

SECTION VIII

Substance use disorders

45

Substance use in facilities

Jason D. Ourada[*]

Introduction

Substance use by incarcerated persons (IPs) poses challenges for correctional psychiatrists. Substance use disorders (SUDs) are common among IPs, with higher prevalence usually found in those with other psychiatric conditions. Correctional psychiatrists assess and treat patients with SUDs and provide consultation for other staff regarding mental status changes, psychiatric emergencies, intoxication, medically supervised withdrawal, protracted abstinence syndromes, psychiatric medication management, motivational interviewing, assessment of stages of change, individualized interdisciplinary treatment, and discharge planning. Knowledge about substance use in correctional facilities fosters competent clinical intervention and enhances management at all levels.

Psychiatrists who work in jails and prisons have the challenging task of maintaining therapeutic alliances with patients who have co-occurring psychiatric conditions and SUDs and who also may be currently using substances. Patients might not spontaneously report substance use during incarceration because they fear retribution by correctional staff or not receiving needed treatment for medical and mental health problems. Psychiatrists need to remain aware of this and to screen for substance use and SUDs as part of comprehensive treatment planning. The clinical challenges in specific jails and prisons differ, and the substances found in these facilities vary geographically. This chapter highlights these differences, outlines clinical management, and describes an interdisciplinary approach to intervention.

Substances commonly found in correctional settings

Although psychiatrists may know the commonly used substances in their facilities, no formal systems exist for collecting this data (Rowell et al., 2012). Some studies have used interviews and self-report in gathering information, such as a Plourde and Brochu's (2002) study of use of cocaine, cannabis, and hallucinogens in Canadian prisons. Most studies have focused on classes of illicit substances such as opioids, stimulants, cannabis, and alcohol. Opioid use was shown to continue at higher rates than cocaine and methamphetamine in a study of persistent substance use in correctional facilities (Strang et al., 2006). External factors, such as economic forces, and the opioid withdrawal syndrome may contribute to ongoing opioid use in correctional facilities.

A 2010 Spanish study quantitatively examined substances in the wastewater of a Catalonian prison using liquid chromatography–tandem mass spectrometry. Methadone (prescribed by medical staff for treatment of opioid use disorder) was the most prevalent, followed by alprazolam, ephedrine, cannabis, heroin, cocaine, 3,4-methylenedioxy-methamphetamine (MDMA), methamphetamine, and amphetamine (Postigo et al., 2011). Brewer and colleagues' (2016) study in the Oregon Department of Corrections compared wastewater analysis with random urinalyses, as the latter is expected to be prone to bias because IPs may learn which days of the week random urinalyses are conducted. Methamphetamine was observed in each sample of prison wastewater, with no significant difference between random urinalysis testing and nontesting days, suggesting that knowledge of testing days did not change behavior in terms of methamphetamine use.

Most state prison systems ban indoor tobacco use, and many also prohibit tobacco use on outdoor grounds (Cork, 2012). Even in systems that have bans, however, tobacco products manage to enter facilities.

The illicit substances available in correctional facilities may closely resemble those in the local community; therefore, geographic trends are important. For example, methamphetamine use in the United States has been most prevalent in the West (1.1% of the general population), Midwest (0.8% of the general population), and South (0.7% of the general population; C. M. Jones et al., 2022). Psychiatrists who work in facilities in these regions may encounter methamphetamine use more frequently than psychiatrists elsewhere. In recent years, substance use in correctional facilities has come to include fentanyl and novel psychoactive substances (NPSs), especially synthetic cannabinoids.

[*] The author acknowledges the contributions of Kenneth L. Appelbaum, who was a coauthor of this chapter in the textbook's first edition.

Origins of substances in facilities

Substance use in correctional facilities may be associated with gang activity and the smuggling of substances and contraband such as mobile phones and drug paraphernalia by staff and IPs. Mobile phones can aid coordination of smuggling, and novel and creative methods for this activity continually challenge efforts to curb the flow of substances into facilities. Visitation provides a common means of entry (*Washington Times*, 2010).

One technique involves passing balloons filled with drugs from mouth to mouth when kissing (Ferranti, 2013; Malcolm, 1989). The recipient swallows the balloon and later recovers it by vomiting or collecting from feces. If suspected of such behavior, the IP may be housed in a cell with no running water (i.e., a dry cell) until the material passes. Another smuggling technique includes passing small packages during visits and concealment in oral, vaginal, or anal cavities to evade normal search procedures (Malcolm, 1989). A 2014 case report outlined an accidental death via intravaginal absorption of methamphetamine by a 23-year-old woman in custody in a county jail who was discovered in a holding cell unconscious and unresponsive. At autopsy, multiple small plastic packages were found in her vagina (P. Jones et al., 2014).

Media reports describe dissolving buprenorphine on papers and mailing them to IPs (Goodnough & Zezima, 2011) or hiding buprenorphine strips beneath stamps (Zoch, 2019). Attempts to drop drugs and tobacco into recreation yards from drones have occurred in correctional facilities in the United States and Canada, and paint guns and catapults have been used to launch drugs over perimeter fences (Doyle & Williams, 2013; Ernst, 2013; *Washington Times*, 2010).

In contrast to opioids and other illicit substances that must be brought into facilities from the outside, alcohol is typically manufactured inside correctional facilities. Alcohol brewed in prison, known as "pruno" or "hooch," is usually made from fruit, water, ketchup, and sugar mixed in a plastic bag and allowed to ferment over several days (Centers for Disease Control and Prevention, 2012, 2013). Hand sanitizers provide another source of alcohol (Doyon & Welsh, 2007).

Clinical presentation and assessment

About a third of IPs use substances during their incarceration, which is associated with adverse health and criminal justice outcomes (Austin et al., 2023). Key modifiable risk factors are psychiatric morbidity and poor prison conditions; nonmodifiable factors included previous substance use and criminal history linked to substance use. Favril (2023) found that, of those IPs who recently used substances in the community, half (52%) continued to do so while incarcerated. Factors independently associated with continuation (versus cessation) were young age, history of SUD treatment in the community, polysubstance use, and poor mental health. In a secondary analysis, initiation of substance use while in prison (defined as those who had not used substances for 12 months prior to incarceration) was related to young age, prior incarceration, low education, serving more than 36 months, and being prescribed psychotropic medication. Of note, having a drug-related index offense did not correlate with substance use during incarceration. In another study, Gillespie (2015) found drug use inside prison to be associated with young age, White race, greater number of years incarcerated, nonparticipation in religious services, drug-related activities in the community, negative attitudes toward correctional rules, and facility overcrowding.

A thorough intake history of substance use, including prior overdoses and complicated withdrawal syndromes such as delirium tremens, will inform treatment staff about the likelihood of continued use and associated risks during incarceration (see Chapter 16). Patients, however, may underreport their history to bypass confinement to an infirmary for medical observation or to avoid housing in a setting focused on treatment of an SUD, like a therapeutic community. Some want to avoid detection of their problem by mitigating withdrawal symptoms in general population with smuggled substances. Other helpful components of the intake assessment include collateral information, findings on physical examination, toxicology screens, and general laboratory tests. In the absence of a knowledgeable and comprehensive diagnostic assessment, correctional psychiatrists may fail to detect an IP's SUD (Fazel et al., 2006).

Laboratory specimens used in drug testing include urine, blood, hair, saliva, sweat, and nails (toenails or fingernails). Different specimens provide different levels of specificity, sensitivity, and accuracy (Moeller et al., 2008). Drug screening by immunoassay requires confirmation of positive results with more sensitive methods such as gas or liquid chromatography coupled with mass spectrometry. Detection times for specific substances and means of collection differ. Urine and hair samples (especially head and body hair) have the advantages of long detection windows and ease of collection. Blood and saliva samples offer shorter and narrower windows of detection. Oral fluid samples may require longer collection times and yield lower volumes, which can necessitate collection of a different type of sample (Drummer, 2006). Many psychiatric and nonpsychiatric medications can cause false-positive immunoassay results: bupropion, trazodone, and chlorpromazine on amphetamine screens; lamotrigine and venlafaxine on phencyclidine screens; bupropion, buspirone, doxepin, fluoxetine, haloperidol, risperidone, sertraline, and trazodone on lysergic acid diethylamide (LSD) screens; diphenhydramine, clomipramine, chlorpromazine, quetiapine, and thioridazine on methadone screens; and sertraline on benzodiazepine screens (Brahm et al., 2010; Saitman et al., 2014).

An IP's substances of choice in the community may shift to those that are more readily available during incarceration. Therefore, a prior diagnosis of a particular SUD should not deter consideration of current use of other, or multiple, substances. Substance use by injection may continue or commence during incarceration. In a study in Irish prisons, 70.5% of injection drug–using individuals reported sharing needles while incarcerated (Allwright et al., 2000). Psychiatric emergencies, bloodborne pathogen exposure, overdose, self-injury, and suicide are potential consequences of substance use in correctional facilities.

Because of the many substances found in correctional facilities, psychiatrists should consider a broad differential diagnosis when evaluating altered mental status. Intoxication or withdrawal can present with acute anxiety, perceptual changes, delusions, suicidal or homicidal thinking, and other signs and symptoms associated with mental and medical illnesses. For example, the underground market for tobacco in facilities with bans warrants consideration of nicotine withdrawal in IPs who present with irritability, difficulty concentrating, anxiety, depression, restlessness, or insomnia (Hughes, 2007).

General psychiatric disorders often accompany SUDs, and the transition into correctional facilities can affect the expression of both conditions. When thrust into an environment with restricted access to substances and, in some cases, restrictive formularies (Morris et al., 2020), symptoms of psychiatric disorders and of SUDs (including withdrawal and craving) may appear. Understanding how this transition period affects an IP's mental health helps guide treatment planning.

Commonly used substances

The following review of intoxication and withdrawal syndromes focuses on commonly used substances in correctional settings: cannabis, stimulants, alcohol, opioids, and NPSs. More extensive discussions of withdrawal management, addiction programming, pharmacotherapy, and community reentry can be found in Chapters 46, 47, 49, and 50, respectively.

Cannabis

Cannabis was the drug most used by IPs in one Canadian study (Plourde & Brochu 2002). Initial effects of cannabis intoxication include relaxation, euphoria, slowed time perception, altered sensory perception, increased awareness of the environment, and increased appetite. Higher doses, repeated use, or a stressful setting is associated with adverse effects such as hypervigilance, anxiety, suspicion, derealization and depersonalization (commonly associated with altered time sense), acute panic, illusions or hallucinations (usually auditory or visual), psychosis, and delirium (Wilkins et al., 2019). Management of cannabis intoxication occasionally requires benzodiazepines or antipsychotic medications (Wilkins et al., 2019) and, more rarely, infirmary observation. Cannabis withdrawal presents with irritability, nervousness, sleep difficulty, decreased appetite, restlessness, depressed mood, and physical discomfort (American Psychiatric Association, 2022). Rare case reports exist of brief psychotic episodes occurring after withdrawal from heavy cannabis use (Marín et al., 2021; Ramos et al., 2022). When compared with the severity of other withdrawal syndromes, correctional staff might not view cannabis intoxication and withdrawal as requiring treatment. Therefore, correctional psychiatrists can offer education about these risks.

Stimulants

Stimulants, including cocaine, amphetamine, and methamphetamine, may be used by ingestion, nasal insufflation, inhalation, injection, or rectal insertion. Stimulants increase catecholamine neurotransmitter and sympathetic nervous system activity and may cause physiologic changes, including mydriasis, tachycardia, palpitations, tremor, hyperreflexia, and mild fever (Wilkins et al., 2019). Intoxication is associated with increased energy, alertness, and euphoria, as well as decreased fatigue, need for sleep, and appetite. With chronic use, stimulant intoxication can cause anxiety, panic, irritability, hypervigilance, grandiosity, impaired judgment, stereotyped behavior, persecutory delusions, and hallucinations (including tactile hallucinations, i.e., formication). Severe intoxication may produce a potentially fatal delirium with agitation. Cocaine intoxication sometimes requires hospitalization because of asthma exacerbation, arrhythmia, myocardial or cerebral infarction, rhabdomyolysis, acute renal failure, or seizures. Other adverse effects include agitation and psychosis that require treatment with benzodiazepines, antipsychotic medications, or both. Care should be taken if using antipsychotics, however, as they may exacerbate cardiovascular effects, lower the seizure threshold, and increase the risk of hyperthermia.

Alcohol

Psychiatric evaluation may be crucial to the detection of alcohol intoxication and withdrawal, especially when perceptual disturbances and delusional thinking are prominent. Autonomic instability, diaphoresis, and tremor provide clues to alcohol withdrawal as the etiology of mental status changes (Gottlieb et al., 2024). Complicated withdrawal syndromes can cause acute mental status changes among patients who have been in the general population for extended periods but have developed physiological dependence on alcohol manufactured within the facility. Particularly in prisons where IPs serve long sentences and alcohol production may be sophisticated, psychiatrists should consider the possibility of regular drinking, intoxication, and physiological dependence. Doyon and Welsh (2017) reported an IP's intoxication and agitation stemming from ethyl alcohol from hand sanitizer that required haloperidol and fluid repletion in an emergency department. Rhabdomyolysis cases in the corrections system are often attributed to overexertion during exercise. However, given a case report of rhabdomyolysis associated with consumption of prison-made alcohol, this potential cause should also be considered in the differential (Soares et al., 2022).

Cases of botulism from the use of raw potatoes in the production of pruno have been reported (Centers for Disease Control and Prevention, 2012; Vugia et al., 2009). The second and third largest botulism outbreaks in the United States since 2006 occurred in a Utah prison in 2011 and an Arizona prison in 2012 consequent to the use of raw potatoes in manufacturing pruno. The Utah outbreak cost an estimated $500,000 and resulted in the hospitalization of eight people (Centers for Disease Control and Prevention, 2012). In the Arizona outbreak, seven of the eight affected IPs were intubated for 11 to 14 days before receiving tracheostomies (Centers for Disease Control and Prevention, 2013). The patients in these cases presented with common signs and symptoms of botulism, including blurry vision, dysarthria, dysphagia, shortness of breath, and generalized muscle weakness. Complicating diagnostic assessment, the onset of botulism occurs 12 to 36 hours after the consumption of pruno, when the IP no longer has the slurred speech, motor incoordination, and mental status changes associated with alcohol intoxication (Vugia et al., 2009).

Opioids

Opioid use by IPs presents medical and mental health staff with significant challenges. With injection substance use, the potential exists for the transmission of infectious disease and greater risk for overdose (intended and unintended). Buprenorphine suppresses opioid withdrawal symptoms in opioid-tolerant individuals, and IPs not tolerant to opioids can experience euphoria by taking buprenorphine sublingually, intranasally, or intravenously. In a case report by George and colleagues (2009), an outpatient in a British clinic for substance treatment admitted he was smuggling opioids into a correctional facility when his routine methadone dose of 110 mg was abruptly reduced to 40 mg while incarcerated, which predictably led to intense opioid withdrawal symptoms. Abrupt cessation of opioids, as commonly occurs at the time of incarceration, can cause sleep disturbance that can last for weeks to months (Chakravorty et al., 2018). A literature review found numerous cases of psychosis occurring days following opioid withdrawal that remitted when opioids were restarted (Lozano-López et al., 2021).

Fentanyl has led to unprecedented rates of fatal overdose in the United States, and IPs are particularly vulnerable because tolerance generally decreases during incarceration. Kaplowitz and colleagues' (2021) literature search found that between January 2013 and March 2021, 179 fentanyl overdoses in correctional facilities (76 fatal) were reported by the lay press, with 77% occurring in jails and the remainder in prisons. The authors endorsed staff and IP education on fentanyl, the availability of naloxone, and the expansion of medications for opioid use disorder in these settings.

The risk of overdose and death from opioid use makes detection, rapid triage, and medical intervention crucial. Opioid overdose is characterized by the classic signs of depressed mental status, decreased respiratory rate, decreased bowel sounds, and miotic pupils (Tetrault & O'Connor, 2019). The National Commission on Correctional Health Care's position statement, reaffirmed in 2021, called for naloxone kits to be available to health care staff, custody staff, and even IPs directly, in accordance with state laws (National Commission on Correctional Health Care, 2021).

Novel psychoactive substances

In recent years, the use of NPSs in carceral settings has become a cause of concern internationally (Vaccaro et al., 2016). The use of NPSs in prisons has led to increased levels of violence, organized crime, bullying, aggression, and debt. NPSs have also been shown to induce unpredictable health risks. Due to the structural diversity of NPSs, they are largely classified according to their substance groups, for example, aminoindanes, phencyclidine-type substances, phenethylamines, piperazines, plant-based substances, synthetic cannabinoids, synthetic cathinones (i.e., bath salts), tryptamines, and "other" substances such as designer opioids and benzodiazepines. Synthetic cannabinoids were by far the dominant NPS group reported, followed to a lesser extent by synthetic cathinones, synthetic opioids, new benzodiazepines, and stimulants. "Wasp dope" is created from pyrethroid-containing insecticides, produces a methamphetamine-like high, and has been reported by media sources as having infiltrated correctional facilities (White, 2020; Young et al., 2021). The literature suggests that most NPSs, in particular synthetic cannabinoids, are smuggled via paper and herbal matrices into prison, predominantly using postal services. Corraza et al. (2020) reported on psychiatric manifestations of NPS in IPs, including slurred speech, hallucinations, depression, suicidal ideation, fear, mistrust, anger outbursts, self-harm, and other risky behaviors.

Consultative role of the correctional psychiatrist

Correctional psychiatrists play important roles in staff education about SUDs, consulting in clinical situations, and crafting policies. All correctional, medical, and mental health staff need a basic understanding of SUDs. Psychiatrists can provide education through formal presentations and day-to-day interactions with other staff about the nature of SUDs, especially signs of intoxication and overdose, and factors that contribute to substance use by IPs.

As clinical consultants, psychiatrists help with diagnosis, including assessing for the presence and contribution of coexisting medical or mental disorders, general treatment planning, and the interpretation of toxicology screens. Consultations can involve direct clinical evaluation of IPs with mental status changes. Delirium tremens from alcohol or benzodiazepine withdrawal, for example, may resemble psychosis or acute intoxication with substances other than alcohol. In these cases, consultation with medical staff is important to coordinate care and inform decisions about transfer to an emergency department.

All facilities need policies regarding screening for, detecting, and treating SUDs. By playing an active role in developing these policies, psychiatrists will enhance the provision of appropriate services and care.

Discipline related to substance use

Many custody and administrative staff view substance use differently from psychiatrists and other health providers. According to a U.S. Department of Justice report (Wilson, 2000), potential sanctions for IPs found using substances include new charges (39.3% of jurisdictions) and time added to the current sentence (20.3% of jurisdictions). Administrative sanctions, by the percentage of jurisdictions that impose them, include loss of privileges (69.9%), loss of time credited for early release (i.e., "good time," 52.2%), reclassified security level (48.9%), increased testing (25.4%), and mandatory treatment (8.0%). Widra (2024) commented on an ongoing and ineffective punitive approach to drug use inside correctional facilities, including sanctions like restrictive housing, loss of visitation, and financial penalties. Custody staff have understandable concerns about the presence of controlled substances or other contraband, especially because of the increased risk of violence or disruptive behaviors associated with IPs who possess them (Friedmann et al., 2008).

The relatively low utilization of treatment-focused approaches by correctional facilities suggests an opportunity for enhanced education of correctional administrators on the nature of SUD as a disease and treatments that may promote positive health outcomes. Punitive administrative sanctions do not address the clinical symptoms (e.g., craving, anxiety, and mood instability) that are associated with continued substance use. Medication for alcohol or opioid use disorders, when available and appropriate, may decrease demand for illicit substances in correctional facilities. Correctional psychiatrists can inform their custody counterparts about the advantages of a clinical approach that might, for example, include contingency management strategies (e.g., re-earning "good time" and privileges).

Security staff monitor for illicit substances and other contraband with pat-downs, drug-sniffing dogs, radiography, metal detectors, mail scanning, and similar methods. They also collect blood, urine, or other specimens to test for recent substance use by IPs. Medical and mental health providers, however, do not participate in drug analyses done for nonclinical reasons. Nevertheless, custody staff might seek psychiatric input to help them understand the general use and interpretation of toxicology screening. Psychiatrists provide a service to the system and IPs by ensuring that custody staff understand the accuracy and limitations of testing and by avoiding sanctions for false-positive drug test results caused by legitimately prescribed medications.

In other cases, IPs have received undeserved punishment for an inability to provide urine samples. Paruresis, sometimes referred to as shy bladder or psychogenic urinary retention, involves difficulty initiating or sustaining urination while being observed or potentially observed by others (see Chapter 35). Symptoms range in severity and can vary for individuals at different times and under different circumstances (Boschen, 2008; Vythilingum et al., 2002; Zgourides, 1987). Sometimes it is impossible for affected individuals to provide a witnessed urine sample or an unwitnessed sample under time pressure. The recognizably situational and psychogenic nature of the condition makes physiological evaluation fruitless and unnecessary. Instead, IPs who claim to have this difficulty need accommodation by allowing them to void unobserved in a dry cell or, when necessary, to provide alternative samples such as blood or saliva. Attempts at fluid loading or prolonged observation until an IP voids risks bladder damage and water intoxication (Klonoff & Jurow, 1991). In addition, courts in the United States have recognized paruresis as a condition covered by the Americans With Disabilities Act (1990). Correctional systems risk successful litigation if they sanction IPs who cannot provide urine samples instead of offering them reasonable accommodations (*Dwyer v. Dubois*, 1998).

Summary

Substance use by IPs presents clinical and systemic challenges for correctional psychiatrists. The interplay among mental health, medical, and custody staff regarding screening, detection, triage, management, and treatment lies at the heart of these challenges. Correctional psychiatrists make important contributions by providing direct assessment and treatment to IPs and by offering educational, clinical, and policy consultations to other staff. These contributions help prevent potentially life-threatening complications of intoxication and withdrawal, ensure integrated and evidence-based care, and avoid misguided or ill-informed disciplinary or other institutional practices.

REFERENCES

Allwright, S., Bradley, F., Long, J., Barry, J., Thornton, L., & Parry, J. V. (2000). Prevalence of antibodies to hepatitis B, hepatitis C, and HIV and risk factors in Irish prisoners: Results of a national cross sectional survey. *BMJ, 321*(7253), 78–82.

American Psychiatric Association. (2022). *Diagnostic and statistical manual of mental disorders* (5th ed., text rev.).

Americans with Disabilities Act of 1989, 42 U.S.C. sec. 12132 (1990).

Austin, A., Favril, L., Craft, S., Thliveri, P., & Freeman, T. P. (2023). Factors associated with drug use in prison: A systematic review of quantitative and qualitative evidence. *International Journal on Drug Policy, 122*, 104248.

Boschen, M. J. (2008). Paruresis (psychogenic inhibition of micturition): Cognitive behavioral formulation and treatment. *Depression and Anxiety, 25*, 903–912.

Brahm, N. C., Yeager, L. L., Fox, M. D., et al. (2010). Commonly prescribed medications and potential false-positive urine drug screens. *American Journal of Health System Pharmacy, 67*, 1344–1350.

Brewer, A. J., Banta-Green, C. J., Ort, C., Robel, A. E., & Field, J. (2016). Wastewater testing compared with random urinalyses for the surveillance of illicit drug use in prisons. *Drug and Alcohol Review, 35*(2), 133–137.

Centers for Disease Control and Prevention. (2012). Botulism from drinking prison-made illicit alcohol—Utah 2011. *Morbidity and Mortality Weekly Report, 61*, 782–784.

Centers for Disease Control and Prevention. (2013). Notes from the field: Botulism from drinking prison-made illicit alcohol—Arizona, 2012. *Morbidity and Mortality Weekly Report, 62*, 88–88.

Chakravorty, S., Vandrey, R. G., He, S., & Stein, M. D. (2018). Sleep management among patients with substance use disorders. *Medical Clinics of North America, 102*(4), 733–743.

Corazza, O., Coloccini, S., Marrinan, S., et al. (2020). Novel psychoactive substances in custodial settings: A mixed method investigation on the experiences of people in prison and professionals working with them. *Frontiers in Psychiatry, 11*, 460.

Cork, K. (2012). *Tobacco behind bars: Policy options for the adult correctional population*. Public Health Law Center at William Mitchell College of Law. http://publichealthlawcenter.org/sites/default/files/resources/phlc-policybrief-tobaccobehindbars-adultcorrections-2012.pdf

Doyle, J., & Williams, D. (2013). *Gang foiled as they fling drugs and mobiles to inmates over prison wall with 8ft catapult*. http://www.dailymail.co.uk/news/article-2389469/Gang-foiled-fling-drugs-mobiles-inmates-Midlands-prison-wall-8ft-CATAPULT.html

Doyon, S., & Welsh, C. (2007). Intoxication of a prison inmate with an ethyl alcohol-based hand sanitizer. *New England Journal of Medicine, 356*(5), 529–530.

Drummer, O. H. (2006). Drug testing in oral fluid. *Clinical Biochemist Reviews, 27*(3), 147–159.

Dwyer v. Dubois, Massachusetts Superior Court Civil Action No. 95-05162-G (1998).

Ernst, D. (2013). *Special delivery: Drone drops contraband into Georgia prison yard*. http://www.washingtontimes.com/news/2013/nov/27/drone-drops-contraband-georgia-prison-yard/

Favril, L. (2023). Drug use before and during imprisonment: Drivers of continuation. *International Journal on Drug Policy, 115*, 104027.

Fazel, S., Bains, P., & Doll, H. (2006). Substance abuse and dependence in prisoners: A systematic review. *Addiction, 101*(2), 181–191.

Ferranti, S. (2013). *Inside the Aryan Brotherhood's prison heroin empire*. http://www.salon.com/2013/03/19/inside_the_aryan_brotherhoods_prison_heroin_empire_partner/

Friedmann, P. D., Melnick, G., Jiang, L., et al. (2008). Violent and disruptive behavior among drug-involved prisoners: Relationship with psychiatric symptoms. *Behavioral Sciences and the Law, 26*(4), 389–401.

George, S., Clayton, S., Namboodiri, V., et al. (2009). "Up yours": Smuggling illicit drugs into prison. *BMJ Case Reports, 2009*, bcr06.2009.1935.

Gillespie, W. (2005). A multilevel model of drug abuse inside prison. *Prison Journal, 85*(2), 223–246.

Goodnough, A., & Zezima, K. (2011). *When children's scribbles hide a prison drug*. http://www.nytimes.com/2011/05/27/us/27smuggle.html?pagewanted=all&_r=0

Gottlieb, M., Chien, N., & Long, B. (2024). Managing alcohol withdrawal syndrome. *Annals of Emergency Medicine, 84*(1), 29–39.

Hughes, J. R. (2007). Effects of abstinence from tobacco: Valid symptoms and time course. *Nicotine and Tobacco Research, 9*(3), 315–327.

Jones, C. M., Houry, D., Han, B., Baldwin, G., Vivolo-Kantor, A., & Compton, W. M. (2022). Methamphetamine use in the United States: Epidemiological update and implications for prevention, treatment, and harm reduction. *Annals of the New York Academy of Sciences, 1508*(1), 3–22.

Jones, P., Mutsvunguma, R., & Prahlow, J. A. (2014). Accidental death via intravaginal absorption of methamphetamine. *Forensic Science, Medicine, and Pathology*, *10*(2), 234–238.

Kaplowitz, E., Truong, A. Q., Macmadu, A., et al. (2021). Fentanyl-related overdose during incarceration: A comprehensive review. *Health & Justice*, *9*(1), 13.

Klonoff, D. C., & Jurow, A. H. (1991). Acute water intoxication as a complication of urine drug testing in the workplace. *Journal of the American Medical Association*, *265*(1), 84–85.

Lozano-López, M. T., Gamonal-Limcaoco, S., Casado-Espada, N., Aguilar, L., Vicente-Hernández, B., Grau-López, L., et al. (2021). Psychosis after buprenorphine, heroin, methadone, morphine, oxycodone, and tramadol withdrawal: A systematic review. *European Review for Medical and Pharmacological Sciences*, *25*(13), 4554–4562.

Malcolm, A. H. (1989). *Explosive drug use creating new underworld prisons.* http://www.nytimes.com/1989/12/30/us/explosive-drug-use-creating-new-underworld-prisons.html?pagewanted=print&src=pm

Marín, J., Pérez de Mendiola, X., Fernández, S., & Chart, J. P. (2021). Cannabis withdrawal induced brief psychotic disorder: A case study during the national lockdown secondary to the COVID-19 pandemic. *Journal of Addictive Diseases*, *39*(4), 579–584.

Moeller, K. E., Lee, K. C., & Kissack, J. C. (2008). Urine drug screening: Practical guide for clinicians. *Mayo Clinic Proceedings*, *83*(1), 66–76.

Morris, N. P., Hirschtritt, M. E., & Tamburello, A. C. (2020). Drug formularies in correctional settings. *Journal of the American Academy of Psychiatry and the Law*, *48*(1), 2–6.

National Commission on Correctional Health Care. (2021). *Position statement on naloxone in correctional facilities for the prevention of opioid overdose deaths.* https://www.ncchc.org/wp-content/uploads/Naloxone-in-Correctional-Facilities-for-the-Prevention-of-Opioid-Overdose-Deaths-1.pdf

Plourde, C., & Brochu, S. (2002). Drugs in prison: A break in the pathway. *Substance Use and Misuse*, *37*(1), 47–63.

Postigo, C., de Alda, M. L., & Barcelo, D. (2011). Evaluation of drugs of abuse use and trends in a prison through wastewater analysis. *Environment International*, *37*(1), 49–55.

Ramos, B., Santos Martins, A. F., & Lima Osório, E. S. (2022). Psychotic cannabis withdrawal: A clinical case. *Cureus*, *14*(11), e31465.

Rowell, T. L., Wu, E., Hart, C. L., et al. (2012). Predictors of drug use in prison among incarcerated Black men. *American Journal of Drug and Alcohol*, *38*(6), 593–597.

Saitman, A., Park, H. D., & Fitzgerald, R. L. (2014). False-positive interferences of common urine drug screen immunoassays: A review. *Journal of Analytical Toxicology*, *38*(7), 387–396.

Soares, M. H., Izquierdo-Pretel, G., & Ramesar, L. A. (2022). Rhabdomyolysis associated with "pruno" prison-made alcohol intake in corrections facility: A case report. *Cureus*, *14*(10), e30933.

Stallwitz, A., & Stover, H. (2007). The impact of substitution treatment in prisons—A literature review. *International Journal of Drug Policy*, *18*(6), 464–474.

Strang, J., Gossop, M., Heuston, J., et al. (2006). Persistence of drug use during imprisonment: Relationship of drug type, recency of use and severity of dependence to use of heroin, cocaine and amphetamine in prison. *Addiction*, *101*(8), 1125–1132.

Tetrault, J. M., & O'Connor, P. G. (2019). Management of opioid intoxication and withdrawal. In S. C. Miller (Ed.), *The ASAM principles of addiction medicine* (6th ed., pp. 741–756). Wolters Kluwer.

Vaccaro, G., Massariol, A., Guirguis, A., Kirton, S. B., & Stair, J. L. (2022). NPS detection in prison: A systematic literature review of use, drug form, and analytical approaches. *Drug Testing and Analysis*, *14*(8), 1350–1367.

Vugia, D. J., Mase, S. R., Cole, B., et al. (2009). Botulism from drinking pruno. *Emerging Infectious Diseases*, *15*(1), 69–71.

Vythilingum, B., Stein, D. J., & Soifer, S. (2002). Is "shy bladder syndrome" a subtype of social anxiety disorder? A survey of people with paruresis. *Depression and Anxiety*, *16*(2), 84–87.

Washington Times. (2010, January 27). *Drugs inside prison walls.* http://www.washingtontimes.com/news/2010/jan/27/drugs-inside-prison-walls/print/

White, D. (2020, October 14). *Florida law enforcement reports inmates getting high with wasp spray in disturbing "wasping" trend.* https://www.firstcoastnews.com/article/news/local/florida-law-enforcement-reports-inmates-getting-high-with-wasp-spray-in-disturbing-wasping-trend/77-3e7d9cb4-0abf-4bcf-8175-1a360aaaa9d

Widra, E. (2024). *Addicted to punishment: Jails and prisons punish drug use far more than they treat it.* https://www.prisonpolicy.org/blog/2024/01/30/punishing-drug-use/

Wilkins, J. N., Danovitch, I., & Gorelick, D. A. (2019). Management of stimulant, hallucinogen, marijuana, phencyclidine, and club drug intoxication and withdrawal. In S. C. Miller (Ed.), *The ASAM principles of addiction medicine* (6th ed., pp. 757–780). Wolters Kluwer.

Wilson, D. J. (2000). *Drug use, testing, and treatment in jails.* U.S. Department of Justice, Bureau of Justice Statistics. https://bjs.ojp.gov/content/pub/pdf/duttj.pdf

Young, A. M., Livingston, M., Vickers-Smith, R., & Cooper, H. L. F. (2021). Emergence of wasp dope in rural Appalachian Kentucky. *Addiction (Abingdon, England)*, *116*(7), 1901–1907.

Zgourides, G. D. (1987). Paruresis: Overview and implications for treatment. *Psychological Reports*, *60*(3 Pt. 2), 1171–1176.

Zoch, R. (2019). *Suboxone and spice: 7 things COs need to know.* https://www.corrections1.com/products/facility-products/body-scanners/articles/suboxone-and-spice-7-things-cos-need-to-know-dXEYM4DDnTD5PWpm/

46

Detoxification or supervised withdrawal

Rebecca A. Ballard

Introduction

Intoxication and withdrawal can mimic signs and symptoms of an acute mental health episode or the exacerbation of an underlying medical illness like hypoglycemia or encephalopathy. One of the most difficult challenges a receiving clinician may face is determining whether the altered mental status presentation is due to a medical condition, a psychiatric illness, intoxication or withdrawal from a substance, or a combination of these. Using substances while taking psychiatric medications can alter pharmacology and exacerbate the side effects of prescribed medications, potentially causing a lack of clinical response, nonadherence, or dangerous physical effects. Substance use also puts the patient at risk for trauma (e.g., via motor vehicle accidents or physical altercations) and exposure to infections from high-risk behaviors while intoxicated.

Detoxification, or medically supervised withdrawal (MSW), is not considered a treatment for a substance use disorder but rather a means to stabilize a patient so mental health needs can be assessed and indications for treatment can be identified. Medication for opioid use disorders is addressed in more detail in Chapter 49. When indicated and available, agonist medication for opioid use disorder (MOUD, e.g., buprenorphine, methadone) may be an appropriate strategy both to avoid or mitigate withdrawal symptoms and for maintenance treatment. If MOUD is not to be initiated, either because the receiving facility does not yet offer it, the staff are not yet trained, it is not indicated, or the patient does not want it, standardized medical management approaches during supervised withdrawal should be used, as presented here. Once a patient's physical and mental conditions are stabilized, either with maintenance medications or supervised withdrawal, the clinician can more accurately assess the patient's diagnosis and long-term treatment needs.

Alcohol

Alcohol intoxication

Many people assert that using alcohol helps them feel better and improves their thinking or mood. This may be due to alcohol's inherent sedating, euphoric, and amnesic effects that provide a temporary escape from unpleasant feelings for those with depression, posttraumatic stress disorder, and similar conditions. Some with poor coping skills may have learned from family or peers that alcohol can make problems better when, in fact, the exact opposite is usually the case (Shivani et al., 2002).

Signs and symptoms of alcohol intoxication vary considerably. Emotions are often intensified during acute intoxication while judgment becomes poor. Underlying mental health conditions may come to the forefront and intoxicated individuals may demonstrate unpredictable behaviors. In general, disinhibition and euphoria are transitory, with continued alcohol use culminating in ataxia, nausea or vomiting, and heavy sedation (Victor & Adams, 1953). Patients who drink habitually often require more alcohol to have the same effect. With tolerance comes dependence and with dependence comes the risk for withdrawal. The disinhibition that occurs with intoxication all too often leads to criminal behavior, ranging from disturbance of the peace to driving violations to homicide. In vulnerable persons, the subsequent lack of access to alcohol during the process of arrest predictably leads to withdrawal.

Alcohol withdrawal and management

Incarcerated persons (IPs) who were recently in the community (either after an arrest or otherwise returning to custody) are at high risk of withdrawal from various substances, alcohol being one of the most common and perhaps the most dangerous (Stuart & Rich, 2018). Alcohol dampens the body's adrenergic system, causing it to be depressed during chronic use. Discontinuing alcohol suddenly ("going cold turkey") puts the patient at risk for a storm of norepinephrine and its metabolites, which may lead to anxiety, tremors, tachycardia, hypertension, hallucinations, confusion, and seizures. When severe, alcohol withdrawal culminates in the syndrome of delirium tremens (DTs). Patients with DTs require intensive hospitalization as its mortality rate is about 5% (Hasin et al., 2007). Alcohol withdrawal is dangerous not only in its severity but also in its timing. While early symptoms of withdrawal may begin within 8 hours of a substantial reduction in alcohol use, the greatest risk of seizures and DTs peaks at 48 to 72 hours after cessation (Day & Daly, 2022). This is the time frame when many IPs arrive at intake centers. An even more dangerous situation is when intake screening is performed prior to the at-risk period and the patient is "cleared" to be housed in a unit with no perceived need for monitoring.

A medical evaluation is essential to look for conditions that may be comorbid or may mimic alcohol withdrawal. The greatest risk of missing another potentially serious medical condition is during the first 48 hours upon arrival. Head trauma, with or without subdural hematomas, metabolic derangements like hypoglycemia, infections such as meningitis, pancreatitis, end-stage liver disease, gastrointestinal bleeding, and other drug intoxications can present similarly to alcohol withdrawal (Mayo-Smith et al., 2004). An accurate diagnosis of another medical condition is imperative and may avoid inappropriate administration of sedatives for alcohol withdrawal, which can complicate medical assessment (Hecksel et al., 2008).

There is a great deal of literature on the methods for safely managing a patient's withdrawal from alcohol. Intake facility "alcohol detox" protocols are primarily based on available resources, particularly nursing care and scope of service. The frequency of nursing assessments and whether the medical unit can offer intravenous fluids, for example, will dictate how severe the withdrawal symptoms can become before transfer to a higher level of medical care is necessary. The revised Clinical Institute Withdrawal Assessment for Alcohol Scale (CIWA-Ar) is the most widely used and researched monitoring tool (American Society of Addiction Medicine, 2001; Sullivan et al., 1989). The CIWA-Ar is freely available and evaluates a patient's symptoms (nausea, anxiousness, tactile/auditory/visual disturbances, and headache) and signs (pulse, blood pressure, tremor, sweats, agitation, and orientation) to create the score used to guide dosing (American Society of Addiction Medicine, 2001; Sullivan et al., 1989). The CIWA-Ar is often administered by a nurse who records the absence or severity of specific signs and symptoms of withdrawal. All patients in withdrawal from alcohol need to be treated using a benzodiazepine (BZD) taper to decrease the risk of significant morbidity and mortality. BZDs are the mainstay of MSW from alcohol as they bind the same receptors, mitigating the adrenergic response, though BZDs are rarely needed if the CIWA-Ar score is less than 10 (Sullivan et al., 1989). Patients at risk for alcohol withdrawal should have CIWA-Ar scores reassessed every 1 to 2 hours. While a symptom-triggered protocol is often used, whereby a CIWA-Ar score determines BZD dosing, a single preset BZD taper is another strategy. A standardized taper offers every patient the same dosages of lowering-strength BZDs over a certain period. For either method any BZD can be used, but those with a longer half-life are preferred, such as chlordiazepoxide and diazepam. These medications are dosed less frequently which may simplify management. However, this long half-life is not optimal for patients who have cirrhosis and could become overly sedated as their livers metabolize BZDs more slowly. In these patients, a shorter acting BZD without active metabolites such as oxazepam or lorazepam may be preferred (Day & Daly, 2022).

Since many patients who chronically use alcohol do not eat a well-balanced diet, nutritional deficiencies often exist. Any protocol for MSW from alcohol must include vitamin supplementation with thiamine. Thiamine deficiency may precipitate Wernicke's encephalopathy (ataxia, ocular weakness, nystagmus, and cognitive dysfunction). Adequate thiamine levels must be present, especially if the patient is to receive glucose. Glucose administration in the setting of thiamine deficiency increases the risk and severity of Wernicke's encephalopathy (Mayo-Smith & Krishnamurthy, 2011). Korsakoff psychosis (also known as Korsakoff's syndrome), a permanent amnesic dementia, may remain, especially when treatment with thiamine is delayed (Westermeyer et al., 2021). Magnesium deficiency is also common in patients with alcohol use disorder, but there is no current literature suggesting that repletion of this nutrient improves the patient's clinical status. However, most protocols include a multivitamin (Carlson & Kennedy, 2006). Even though withdrawal seizures can occur in the absence of DTs, studies do not support the use of prophylactic antiepileptic medications (Minozzi et al., 2010).

As MSW progresses, underlying mental disorders may be uncovered. The patient thus becomes increasingly uncomfortable from both the managed symptoms of withdrawal and the now-untreated mental illness. Except when these mental status changes are better assessed as delirium (which, in the absence of another medical explanation, may suggest undertreatment of the withdrawal syndrome), the clinician should not wait until MSW is complete to initiate psychiatric and substance use treatment as indicated. Mental health assessments on patients should begin at entry into the correctional facility and continue through the MSW process as needed, with follow-up performed once the patient is medically cleared to determine what further psychiatric care, if any, is appropriate (Peters & Bekman, 2007).

Opioids

Opioid intoxication

As with alcohol, patients with mental illness may turn to opioids for various reasons. Although the "high" obtained from these substances can be the driving factor behind their use, patients may use them to manage symptoms of their underlying psychiatric disorder. Opioids, including heroin, fentanyl, and narcotic pain medications, give the user a dissociative feeling or "numbing" sensation. Patients with depression, posttraumatic stress disorder, or other disorders may use opioids to avoid memories, thoughts, feelings, or emotions that are too painful for them to experience. Overdoses of opioids, either alone or combined with alcohol, BZDs, gabapentinoids, or other sedatives, cause respiratory depression that can be fatal (Hahn et al., 2022). With habitual use of opioids, the body quickly develops tolerance and craves the drug, both physically and mentally. The patient is forced to seek frequent "hits" throughout the day to avoid unpleasant withdrawal effects; this often interferes with work and relationships (National Institute on Drug Abuse, 2013a). Patients may become incarcerated due to use, sale, or possession of the substance, as well as for the crimes committed while intoxicated or during periods of relative sobriety to support the expense of the habit.

Opioid use can put patients at risk for medical problems that differ from those seen with alcohol. The stigma associated with intravenous use, including the danger of contracting bloodborne pathogens like HIV, hepatitis B, or hepatitis C, may reduce a patient's motivation to seek treatment for an opioid use disorder. It is often during a period of incarceration that a patient discovers their HIV or hepatitis infection. The clinician should take this opportunity to educate the patient about the disease and offer advice on self-care and prevention of spread, including treatment of the opioid use disorder (Carlson & Kennedy, 2006).

Methadone (a long-acting, full-agonist opioid) and buprenorphine (a long-acting partial opioid agonist/antagonist) are among the U.S. Food and Drug Administration (FDA)–approved medications used to treat opioid use disorder. If patients with opioid use disorder do not continue their maintenance medications prescribed in the community, or if they are opioid tolerant and not offered MOUD, then they will likely experience an opioid withdrawal syndrome.

Opioid withdrawal and management

An adage regarding opioid withdrawal is "you won't die, but you feel like you're going to die." This is a fairly accurate description; however, deaths do occur from complications of opioid withdrawal. Opioid withdrawal is a miserable process that patients try to avoid by continuing to use opiates. Signs and symptoms include generalized deep body aches ("bones hurt"), nausea, vomiting, diarrhea, leg cramps ("kicking"), piloerection ("skin crawling"), sneezing, yawning, watery eyes, and insomnia. Most patients will experience some adverse effects of opioid withdrawal. Although alcohol withdrawal carries a much higher mortality risk, opioid withdrawal can be severe, even fatal, if dehydration and electrolyte imbalances are left untreated. If nausea prevents the patient from holding down fluids, intravenous replacement may be required. Low potassium levels and other electrolyte imbalances from vomiting and diarrhea can lead to arrhythmias or sudden cardiac death. Dehydration can precipitate rhabdomyolysis and acute renal failure (Fudala & Johnson, 2011). Pierce (1967) described suicides among IPs in opioid withdrawal. This syndrome lasts 2 to 4 days and can last up to 2 weeks if the patient was using a long-acting opioid such as methadone (Tetrault et al., 2011).

As with alcohol withdrawal, a medical assessment should be performed to identify any condition that may mimic or coexist with opioid withdrawal. In a correctional setting where MOUD is not offered or is not wanted by the patient, the patient should be monitored for the need for MSW.

The Clinical Opiate Withdrawal Scale (COWS) assessment tool can be used to evaluate and medicate patients to help them feel less uncomfortable (California Society of Addiction Medicine, 2011; Wessen & Ling, 2003). Unlike alcohol detoxification, there is not a standard medication taper or protocol so correctional facilities have various strategies for symptom relief, ranging from prescribing nothing to offering several pharmaceutical agents. If MOUD is not employed, withdrawal treatment is symptomatic. Symptom-based protocols usually include an antiemetic for nausea, an antidiarrheal agent, analgesics for aches and pains, and clonidine to mitigate some of the most uncomfortable sensations (Tetrault et al., 2011). Muscle relaxants are controversial in their medical necessity and are not ubiquitous in protocols. Sleep agents are also not standard but may be used in some protocols. When short-term and non-BZD medications are used for such concerns, this should mitigate the risk of iatrogenic substance use disorders.

Pregnant patients who use opiates or are on MOUD should continue to receive this treatment as any withdrawal syndrome poses the risk of miscarriage. Methadone and buprenorphine are effective medications in mitigating the withdrawal effects of opioids and decreasing the risk to the fetus (Krans et al., 2021). The COWS score is often used to help dose the methadone for maintenance during pregnancy. Incarcerated pregnant patients should be referred to a high-risk obstetrician with relevant experience.

Other sedatives

Sedative intoxication

BZD intoxication is primarily manifested by varying degrees of somnolence and stupor, especially if combined with alcohol. Short-acting BZDs have the highest risk of physical and mental dependence due to their quick onset and offset. As an anxiolytic, patients sometimes may use more than prescribed (Weaver, 2015). Patients who find their prescribed dosage inadequate to manage their symptoms may use their medication more frequently or purchase more from the street market. Street BZDs are popular among those with and without a diagnosed mental illness. Unfortunately, overuse for perceived uncomfortable emotions like sadness and regret can lead to inappropriate usage, tolerance, and physical dependency (National Institute on Drug Abuse, 2011). Because BZDs are prescribed medications that are often not readily available for long-term use in correctional facilities, withdrawal may be a consequence of arrest (Tamburello et al, 2022).

Sedative withdrawal and management

Since BZDs stimulate the same receptors as alcohol, the withdrawal syndrome and the health risks are similar, though the onset of BZD withdrawal symptoms is typically delayed (up to 7 to 10 days after last use) by comparison (Weaver, 2015). Patients should be tapered off BZDs as abrupt discontinuation can lead to dangerous physical effects such as elevated blood pressure, tachycardia, and seizures. As with alcohol, any BZD can be used for the tapering process. Many facilities use chlordiazepoxide as it is long acting and staff are often familiar with it from MSW for alcohol use disorder. For those who use BZDs and alcohol concomitantly, chlordiazepoxide is preferred since it will treat both withdrawal syndromes (Carlson & Kennedy, 2006). Short-acting BZD tapers, such as clonazepam or lorazepam, can be used if no alcohol use is suspected. These tapers are usually done over a 7- to 10-day period. Patients may experience more emotional difficulty as they notice the effects of their prescribed medication dwindle; therefore, long-acting medication whose dosage is unfamiliar to them may help reduce anxiety about the process. Though less urgent than for alcohol use disorder, some facilities use vitamins in standard protocols as they are inexpensive and have no adverse effects.

Gabapentin and pregabalin have withdrawal syndromes like those for BZDs and should be tapered if they are to be discontinued (Naveed et al., 2018; Tran et al., 2005). Although now rarely prescribed or misused, barbiturates can induce a serious withdrawal syndrome like alcohol with delirium and seizures; these medications should also be tapered (Ciraulo & Knapp, 2011). Tapering doses of phenobarbital, a very long-acting (up to 100-hour half-life) barbiturate available as an elixir, is an alternative strategy for the management of short-acting BZD withdrawal (Weaver, 2015).

Cannabinoids and synthetic cannabinoids

With the recent wave of reforms decriminalizing marijuana, use of cannabinoids may increase in the community. Synthetic compounds with cannabinoid-like properties are either illicit (such as "spice" or "K2") or are FDA-approved medications (such as dronabinol). Natural cannabis induces sedative, analgesic, and euphoric effects. Severe intoxication is rare, presenting as dysphoria or agitation and hyperemesis. Physical signs include slurred speech, ataxia, increased appetite, red eyes, tachycardia, hyper- or hypotension, tachypnea, and nystagmus (Ashton, 2001). The patient may also develop panic attacks, delirium, myoclonic jerking (Dow et al., 1984), and acute psychosis (Barkus, 2016). Management of the severely intoxicated individual is supportive with limited exposure to excess external stimuli.

Low-dose, short-acting BZDs may help with mild to moderate agitation. Marked agitation may be due to concomitantly used substances. Myocardial infarction, pneumothorax, and bronchospasm have been reported in rare cases (Ashton, 2001, Khoj et al., 2024).

Cannabis withdrawal may occur in individuals who habitually use 3 times a week or more and abruptly stop. Symptoms include sleep disturbances, irritability, headache, and transient depression (Livne et al., 2019); they begin within 24 to 72 hours and resolve after 1 to 2 weeks (Budney et al., 2003). There is no specific management for cannabis withdrawal.

The illicit forms of synthetic cannabinoids have similar effects as the natural source but they may last longer (possibly for days), are more intense, and have greater potential for life-threatening toxicity (Darke et al., 2020; Grigg et al., 2019). Seizures, hallucinations, and coma are common, as well as respiratory depression, rhabdomyolysis, hyperthermia, and kidney injury (Riederer et al., 2016). Monitoring in an emergency room setting is recommended for intoxication beyond mild severity due to the potential for severe agitation, violent and unpredictable behavior, and life-threatening complications.

Withdrawal from synthetic cannabinoids can cause serious deleterious effects. Individuals may experience psychosis, delirium, hypertension, tachycardia, and diaphoresis. The risk of seizures, cardiac arrhythmias, and acute kidney injury is significant (Grigg et al., 2019), and the individual may need inpatient care, including treatment with the FDA-approved synthetic cannabinoid dronabinol (Levin et al., 2011).

Stimulants

Recently incarcerated persons infrequently present with an acute high from stimulants as the effects are short-lived, lasting only a few hours. However, patients can present acutely intoxicated by ingesting or inhaling substances on their person at the time of arrest to dispose of evidence of illegal substances. People intoxicated on stimulants typically are in a hyperactive state—physically and mentally—characterized by tachycardia, high blood pressure, sweating, inability to focus, and, in severe cases, rhabdomyolysis or seizures. Patients may develop chest discomfort, either from cardiac or noncardiac sources. Increased cardiac demand or cocaine-induced coronary arterial spasms put patients at risk for cardiac damage (Wilkins et al., 2011). Complaints of chest discomfort should be evaluated in an emergency medical facility.

Serotonin syndrome is a serious, potentially life-threatening complication of amphetamine use and overdose. Excess serotonin produces autonomic (hyperthermia, tachycardia), cognitive (agitation, hallucinations, coma), and somatic effects (clonus, myoclonus) (Boyer and Shannon, 2005). Long-term, chronic methamphetamine (i.e., "meth") use has been associated with severe dental decay, mood changes, violent behavior, weight loss, anxiety, paranoia, and delusions (National Institute on Drug Abuse, 2010).

Intoxication with any stimulant can resemble an acute manic episode, making it difficult to exclude mental illness as a cause of the behavior. Urine drug testing in the acute setting may be helpful in guiding management, especially if the diagnosis of intoxication (or the specific substance used) is in question. Police lockups might regularly hold individuals who are acutely intoxicated with stimulants even though they are rarely prepared to manage them medically. In these situations, transfer of the IP to an emergency medical facility for appropriate management is recommended.

There are no medications either FDA approved or otherwise indicated to address stimulant withdrawal. Related symptoms are rarely life-threatening, but they are uncomfortable. Patients may experience fatigue, agitation, changes in appetite, or bad dreams. The psychological effects of dysphoria, insomnia or hypersomnia, and intense cravings are more concerning for the risk of relapse (Hill & Weiss, 2011; Paczynski & Gold, 2011). There are no specific protocols for MSW for stimulants and care is supportive. Increased suicide monitoring is recommended as the risk of suicidal ideation is high during withdrawal. Stimulant-induced psychosis is not a typical withdrawal symptom but may be present with intoxication and may continue even after the acute effects of the substance have worn off. These patients should be monitored closely. If their psychosis persists after the physiological effects of the stimulant have passed, use of antipsychotic medication may be considered (Carlson & Kennedy, 2006).

3,4-Methylenedioxy-methamphetamine

The substance 3,4-methylenedioxy-methamphetamine (MDMA) is a popular club drug, also referred to as "ecstasy" or "molly." Because it is both a stimulant and a hallucinogen, the patient may experience sensations of euphoria, increased energy, emotional empathy, and warmth, while sensory perceptions are dulled. MDMA has the same cardiac risks as stimulants and in high dosages can interfere with temperature regulation. Teeth clenching, vision changes, and sleep or appetite disturbances are commonly seen with intoxication (National Institute on Drug Abuse, 2013b). Intoxication can be associated with serotonin syndrome as well as rhabdomyolysis and liver and kidney damage (Wilkins et al., 2011). Patients may commit criminal acts while under the influence. The acute effects usually will have resolved by the time the patient is seen for initial evaluation unless hidden portions are ingested during the postarrest period.

There are no protocols for MSW from MDMA as the symptoms of withdrawal (anxiety, depression, fatigue) are usually transient and there are no specific treatments available (Carlson & Kennedy, 2006). Clinicians of patients recently admitted to correctional facilities from the community should know that young persons who use MDMA have higher rates of suicidal behaviors in general and a drop in serotonin levels in the early days after last use of MDMA may increase risk (Kim et al., 2011).

Other substances

Hallucinogens, phencyclidine (PCP), and ketamine are psychoactive substances that have few effects of intoxication beyond altered mental status. These include psychosis induced by PCP, which can last for months, as well as persistent hallucinosis from hallucinogens (American Psychiatric Association, 2022). Inhalants can be damaging to the central nervous system and can cause cardiac, kidney, and liver damage (National Institute on Drug Abuse, 2012). These substances have a low risk of dependence as they do not cause neurologic changes in the brain that produce physical dependence. However, patients may want to continue to use these agents for the effect and may become psychologically dependent (Wilkins et al., 2011).

There are no specific withdrawal syndromes, no specific medications, and no MSW protocols associated with these families of substances. The patient may experience some anhedonia, fatigue, or insomnia in the context of cessation, though rarely is medical intervention necessary. Baseline psychological health should be assessed after the acute intoxication phase has resolved (Carlson & Kennedy, 2006).

Combined substances

Patients often combine illicit substances, prescribed controlled substances, and alcohol. Depending on which substances are combined, the effects will vary. Alcohol and BZDs will potentiate each other's sedative and respiratory depressive effects, as is true if combined with opioids. Combinations of stimulants (e.g., methamphetamine or MDMA) and depressants (e.g., alcohol, opioids, or cannabinoids) are often used to mitigate each other's adverse effects. Combinations (e.g., opioids and gabapentinoids) may give a faster, more intense high. Combining drugs puts the patient at risk for more physical injury and adverse psychological effects, thus complicating the clinician's attempts at treatment. If multiple substances have been identified in a withdrawal syndrome, MSW for each identified substance should be followed.

Summary

Persons with mental illness and substance use have a higher risk of arrest and incarceration (Peters & Bekmen, 2007). For those actively or recently using drugs, MSW protocols used in the community are effective in correctional settings with few modifications, depending on available medication, scope of service, and staff resources (Wright et al., 2011). As acceptance of and access to MOUD grow, continuity with community treatment will lessen the need for MSW for those with opioid dependance. The psychiatrist should follow the patient from intake screening through completion of MSW to determine the patient's needs for mental health treatment and psychotropic medications, if any. Early recognition and differentiation between the physiological and withdrawal effects of substances and other mental health disorders will help the clinician provide the most efficacious treatment.

REFERENCES

American Psychiatric Association. (2022). *Diagnostic and statistical manual of mental disorders* (5th ed., text rev.).

American Society of Addiction Medicine. (2001). *Addiction medicine essentials—Clinical Institute Withdrawal Assessment of Alcohol Scale, Revised (CIWA-Ar)*. http://www.chce.research.va.gov/apps/PAWS/pdfs/ciwa-ar.pdf.

Ashton, C. H. (2001). Pharmacology and effects of cannabis: A brief review. *British Journal of Psychiatry, 178*, 101.

Barkus, E. (2016). High-potency cannabis increases the risk of psychosis. *Evidence-Based Mental Health, 19*(2), 54.

Boyer, E. W., & Shannon, M. (2005). The serotonin syndrome. *New England Journal of Medicine, 352*(11), 1112–1120.

Budney, A. J., Moore, B. A., Vandrey, R. G., & Hughes, J. R. (2003). The time course and significance of cannabis withdrawal. *Journal of Abnormal Psychology, 112*(3), 393.

California Society of Addiction Medicine. (2011). *Clinical Opiate Withdrawal Scale*. http://www.csam-asam.org/buprenorphine-info

Carlson, H. B., & Kennedy, J. A. (2006). The treatment of alcohol and other drug withdrawal syndromes in persons taken into custody. In M. Puisis (Ed.), *Clinical practice in correctional medicine* (2nd ed., pp. 387–399). Mosby Elsevier.

Ciraulo, D. A., & Knapp, C. (2011). Sedative–hypnotics. In P. Ruiz & E. Strain (Eds.), *Lowinson and Ruiz's substance abuse: A comprehensive textbook* (5th ed., pp. 255–266). Lippincott Williams & Wilkins.

Darke, S., Duflou, J., Farrell, M., Peacock, A., & Lappin, J. (2020). Characteristics and circumstances of synthetic cannabinoid-related death. *Clinical Toxicology, 58*(5), 368.

Day, E., & Daly, C. (2022). Clinical management of the alcohol withdrawal syndrome. *Addiction (Abingdon, England), 117*(3), 804–814.

Dow, G. J., Meyers, F. H., Stanton, W., & Devine, M. L. (1984). Serious reactions to oral delta-9-tetrahydrocannabinol in cancer chemotherapy patients. *Clinical Pharmacology, 3*(1), 14.

Fudala, P. J., & Johnson, R. E. (2011). Alternative pharmacotherapies for opioid addiction. In P. Ruiz & E. Strain (Eds.), *Lowinson and Ruiz's substance abuse: A comprehensive textbook* (5th ed., pp. 494–500). Lippincott Williams & Wilkins.

Grigg, J., Manning, V., Arunogiri, S., & Lubman, D. I. (2019). Synthetic cannabinoid use disorder: An update for general psychiatrists. *Australasian Psychiatry, 27*(3), 279.

Hahn, J., Jo, Y., Yoo, S. H., Shin, J., Yu, Y. M., & Ah, Y. M. (2022). Risk of major adverse events associated with gabapentinoid and opioid combination therapy: A systematic review and meta-analysis. *Frontiers in Pharmacology, 13*, 1009950.

Hasin, D. S., Stinson, F. S., Ogburn, E., & Grant, B. F. (2007). Prevalence, correlates, disability, and comorbidity of DSM-IV alcohol abuse and dependence in the United States: Results from the National Epidemiologic Survey on Alcohol and Related Conditions. *Archives of General Psychiatry, 64*(7), 830–842.

Hecksel, K. A., Bostwick, J. M., Jaeger, T. M., & Cha, S. S. (2008). Inappropriate use of symptom-triggered therapy for alcohol withdrawal in the general hospital. *Mayo Clinic Proceedings, 83*(3), 274–279.

Hill, K. P., & Weiss, R. D. (2011). Amphetamines and other stimulants. In P. Ruiz & E. Strain (Eds.), *Lowinson and Ruiz's substance abuse: A comprehensive textbook* (5th ed., pp. 238–254). Lippincott Williams & Wilkins.

Khoj, L., Zagà, V., Amram, D. L., Hosein, K., Pistone, G., Bisconti, M., Serafini, A., Cammarata, L. M., Cattaruzza, M. S., & Mura, M. (2024). Effects of cannabis smoking on the respiratory system: A state-of-the-art review. *Respiratory Medicine*, 221:107494.

Kim, J., Fan, B., Liu, X., Kerner, N., & Wu, P. (2011). Ecstasy use and suicidal behavior among adolescents: Findings from a national survey. *Suicide & Life-Threatening Behavior, 41*(4), 435–444.

Kinner, S., & Rich, J. (Eds.) (2018). *Drug use in prisoners: Epidemiology, implications, and policy responses*. (pp: 57–70). Oxford University Press.

Krans, E. E., Kim, J. Y., Chen, Q., et al. (2021). Outcomes associated with the use of medications for opioid use disorder during pregnancy. *Addiction, 116*, 3504–3514.

Levin, F. R., Mariani, J. J., Brooks, D. J., Pavlicova, M., Cheng, W., & Nunes, E. V. (2011). Dronabinol for the treatment of cannabis dependence: A randomized, double-blind, placebo-controlled trial. *Drug and Alcohol Dependence, 116*(1–3), 142.

Livne, O., Shmulewitz, D., Lev-Ran, S., & Hasin, D. S. (2019). DSM-5 cannabis withdrawal syndrome: Demographic and clinical correlates in U.S. adults. *Drug and Alcohol Dependence, 195*, 170.

Mayo-Smith, M. F., Beecher, L. H., Fischer, T. L., et al. (2004). Working Group on the Management of Alcohol Withdrawal Delirium, Practice Guidelines Committee, American Society of Addiction Medicine. Management of alcohol withdrawal delirium. An evidence-based practice guideline. *Archives of Internal Medicine, 164*(13), 1405–1412.

Mayo-Smith, M. F., & Krishnamurthy, A. (2011). Management of alcohol intoxication and withdrawal. In C. A. Cavacuiti (Ed.), *Principles of addiction medicine—The essentials* (pp. 204–211). Lippincott Williams & Wilkins.

Minozzi, S., Amato, L., Vecch, S., & Davoli, M. (2010). Anticonvulsants for alcohol withdrawal. *Cochrane Database for Systemic Review, 17*(3), CD005064.

National Institute on Drug Abuse. (2010). *InfoFacts: Methamphetamine.* http://www.drugabuse.gov/publications/drugfacts/methamphetamine

National Institute on Drug Abuse. (2011). *InfoFacts: Commonly abused prescription drugs chart.* http://www.drugabuse.gov/drugs-abuse/commonly-abused-drugs/commonly-abused-prescription-drugs-chart

National Institute on Drug Abuse. (2012). *InfoFacts: Inhalants.* http://www.drugabuse.gov/publications/drugfacts/inhalants

National Institute on Drug Abuse. (2013a). *InfoFacts: Heroin.* http://www.drugabuse.gov/publications/drugfacts/heroin

National Institute on Drug Abuse. (2013b). *InfoFacts: MDMA (ecstasy or molly).* http://www.drugabuse.gov/publications/drugfacts/mdma-ecstasy-or-molly

Naveed, S., Faquih, A. E., & Chaudhary, A. M. D. (2018). Pregabalin-associated discontinuation symptoms: A case report. *Cureus, 10*(10), e3425.

Paczynski, R. P., & Gold, M. S. (2011). Cocaine and crack. In P. Ruiz & E. Strain (Eds.), *Lowinson and Ruiz's substance abuse: A comprehensive textbook* (5th ed., pp. 191–213). Lippincott Williams & Wilkins.

Peters, R. H., & Bekman, N. M. (2007). Treatment reentry approaches for offenders with co-occurring disorders. In R. Greifinger (Ed.), *Public health behind bars—From prisons to communities* (pp. 368–384). Springer.

Pierce, J. I. (1967). Suicide and mortality amongst heroin addicts in Britain. *British Journal of Addiction to Alcohol and Other Drugs, 62*(3), 391–398.

Riederer, A. M., Campleman, S. L., Carlson, R. G., et al. (2016). Acute poisonings from synthetic cannabinoids—50 U.S. toxicology investigators consortium registry sites, 2010–2015. *Toxicology Investigators Consortium (ToxIC), 65*(27), 692.

Shivani, R., Goldsmith, R. J., & Anthenelli, R. M. (2002). *Alcoholism and psychiatric disorders—Diagnostic challenges.* National Institute on Alcohol Abuse and Alcoholism. http://pubs.niaaa.nih.gov/publications/arh26-2/90-98.htm

Sullivan, J. T., Sykora, K., Schneiderman, J., Naranjo, C. A., & Sellers, E. M. (1989). Assessment of alcohol withdrawal: The revised Clinical Institute Withdrawal Assessment for Alcohol Scale (CIWA-Ar). *British Journal of Addiction, 84*(11), 1353–1357.

Tamburello, A., Penn, J., Ford, E., et al. (2022). The American Academy of Psychiatry and the Law practice resource for prescribing in corrections. *Journal of the American Academy of Psychiatry and the Law, 50*(4 Suppl.), S1–S62.

Tetrault, J. M., O'Connor, P. G., & Krishnamurthy, A. (2011). Management of opioid intoxication and withdrawal. In C. A. Cavacuiti (Ed.), *Principles of addiction medicine—The essentials* (pp. 223–228). Lippincott Williams & Wilkins.

Tran, K. T., Hranicky, D., Lark, T., & Jacob, N. J. (2005). Gabapentin withdrawal syndrome in the presence of a taper. *Bipolar Disorders, 7*(3), 302–304.

Victor, M., & Adams, R. D. (1953). The effect of alcohol on the nervous system. *Research Publications—Association for Research in Nervous and Mental Disease, 32*, 523–526.

Weaver, M. F. (2015). Prescription sedative misuse and abuse. *Yale Journal of Biology and Medicine, 88*(3), 247–256.

Wessen, D. R., & Ling, W. (2003). The Clinical Opiate Withdrawal Scale (COWS). *Journal of Psychoactive Drugs, 35*(2), 253–259.

Westermeyer, J. J., Soukup, B., Mayer, J., & Lee, K. (2021). Identifying, assessing, and treating Korsakoff syndrome patients: Updated perspectives. *Journal of Nervous and Mental Disease, 209*(8), 592–599.

Wilkins, J. N., Danovitch, I., Gorelick, D. A., & Krishnamurthy, A. (2011). Management of stimulant, hallucinogen, marijuana, phencyclidine, and club drug intoxication and withdrawal. In C. A. Cavacuiti (Ed.), *Principles of addiction medicine—The essentials* (pp. 229–244). Lippincott Williams & Wilkins.

Wright, T. M., Cluver, J. S., Myrick, H., & Krishnamurthy, A. (2011). Management of intoxication and withdrawal: General principles. In C. A. Cavacuiti (Ed.), *Principles of addiction medicine—The essentials* (pp. 199–203). Lippincott Williams & Wilkins.

47

Treatment models for substance use disorders

Ingrid A. Binswanger and Jennifer M. Tippett[1]

Introduction

Substance use and substance use disorders (SUDs) are prevalent among individuals involved with criminal legal systems. In the United States, approximately 21% of persons in state prisons met criteria for an alcohol use disorder (Maruschak et al., 2021), and 40% of persons in state prisons met criteria for another SUD before being incarcerated. Across studies in 10 countries, a higher proportion of incarcerated women had drug use disorders than men (51% versus 30%; Fazel et al., 2017). Drugs and alcohol may be a factor leading to or involved in the event leading to incarceration (Maruschak et al., 2021). In 2022, 46% of incarcerated persons (IPs) in U.S. federal prisons were incarcerated for drug-related convictions, with fentanyl exceeding heroin as a cause for Drug Enforcement Administration arrests (Motivans, 2024). Tobacco use disorders are more common in IPs than in the community (Binswanger et al., 2009; Spaulding et al., 2018). Problems with gambling are also a concern, with approximately 31% of IPs affected (Tørdal et al., 2024). Thus, it is critical to provide a wide range of evidence-based SUD treatments to IPs.

This chapter describes the evolution of SUD treatment within jails and prisons from the mutual aid societies of the late 1700s to contemporary practices such as cognitive-behavioral approaches, therapeutic communities (TCs), and pharmacotherapy. While not treatment per se, drug courts, which seek to divert people with SUDs from incarceration, and harm reduction are addressed. Throughout the chapter, it is important to note that drug policies have led to exceedingly large numbers of IPs, that mandated or coercive treatment is highly controversial, that noncorrectional and voluntary settings are the preferred settings in which to provide treatment for SUDs, and that the evidence base supporting the positive effects of correctional-based treatments on meaningful outcomes for affected individuals is lacking. Furthermore, recidivism outcomes, which are legal rather than clinical, and outcome measures exclusively focused on substance use are not equivalent to person-centered treatment outcomes and recovery domains.

Screening, diagnosis, and assessment

Changes to psychiatry's conceptualization of SUDs, often operationalized in diagnostic criteria, have affected prevalence estimates for SUDs in IPs over time. Released in 2013, the *Diagnostic and Statistical Manual of Mental Disorders*, fifth edition (DSM-5) included changes to the psychiatric diagnostic system. Most notably, it combined substance dependence and abuse into a single category of substance use disorder. Historically, the distinction between substance abuse and dependence was based on the concept that abuse represented a milder form of behavior, with dependence as the more severe manifestation (American Psychiatric Association [APA], 2013, pp. 481–485). Individuals who met the criteria for substance abuse could present with severe symptomatology but no symptoms of dependence. A unitary diagnostic category was created, and individuals are now assessed on a continuum from mild to severe. In the DSM-5, two or three symptoms are needed for a diagnosis of mild SUD, each substance is addressed separately (e.g., alcohol use disorder), and craving was added to the list of criteria. Additionally, the "problems with law enforcement" criterion was eliminated (APA, 2013, p. 815); this makes the diagnosis internationally more applicable, given that national policies regarding the legality of substance use vary. Gambling disorder was also added to the DSM-5 (APA, 2013). The diagnostic criteria for substance-related disorders were not substantially changed in the DSM, fifth edition, text revision (DSM-5-TR; APA, 2022).

Systematic screening and diagnostic assessment in jails, prisons, and community criminal legal settings are critical to ensuring that the appropriate individuals are offered evidence-based behavioral and medication treatments, recovery supports, and harm reduction services. Individuals need treatment recommendations matched to their needs, functioning, and preferences (Taxman et al., 2013). Accurate assessment and diagnosis should therefore guide tailored treatment recommendations, when available. Available screeners include the Alcohol, Smoking, and Substance Involvement Screening Test, the Alcohol Use Disorders Identification Test, and the Texas

1. The authors acknowledge the contributions of Patrece Hairston, who was a coauthor of this chapter in the first edition of this textbook.

Christian University Drug Screen 5, among others (Bureau of Justice Assistance, 2022).

Early treatment modalities

In the late 1700s, the physician Benjamin Rush began an educational campaign to warn against the potential dangers of consuming distilled alcoholic beverages. Regarded as the "father of American psychiatry," Rush advocated for the understanding of "alcoholism" as a medical disease in need of ongoing treatment. Based primarily on physical observation, Rush described medical conditions that he believed were caused by consuming large amounts of distilled alcoholic spirits (Katcher, 1993; White, 1998). He identified symptoms such as stomach discomfort, vomiting, liver damage, "madness," and tremors (after abstaining). Although he was astute in his clinical observations, treatment recommendations included whippings, sticking a feather down the throat to force vomiting, dunking patients in cold water, and inducing sweats. Despite the promotion of these early punitive remedies, Rush also advocated for "sober houses," medical communities that focused on treating individuals with alcohol problems (White, 1998). Decades later, this idea would lay the foundation for inpatient treatment modalities.

Throughout the 1800s, the temperance movement gained momentum; abstinence from alcoholic beverages was permeating the broader culture. During this century, the idea of developing "inebriate asylums" was born and propagated by Samuel Woodward, a physician who championed "moral therapy" and supported a warm, compassionate approach to care (Blocker et al., 2003). Before the establishment of these institutions, many with SUDs were housed primarily in prisons and housing facilities serving individuals with low income (Dadoly et al., 2005). Using a "patient-centered" approach to care, Woodward recommended occupational therapy, games, and spiritual treatments. He advocated against the use of physical violence and restraints. In addition to the creation of early inpatient psychiatric facilities for individuals with SUDs and mental health conditions, he focused on treatment rather than punishment. The late 1800s spawned the continued development of alcohol-focused mutual aid societies (White, 1998).

In the early 1900s, most "inebriate asylums" and private treatment facilities closed for a brief period (White, 1998). Sadly, state laws in the United States called for mandatory sterilization of "defective" citizens, including individuals with SUDs (Blocker et al., 2003). In 1935, chemical aversive conditioning was introduced in inpatient settings for alcohol use disorder (Lemere & Voegtlin, 1950; White, 1998; G. Wilson, 1987). Individuals were given nausea-inducing drugs as a means of conditioning an aversion to the smell and taste of alcoholic beverages. Early research studies touted success but were later criticized for being methodologically flawed (G. Wilson, 1987).

During the mid-1900s, Alcoholics Anonymous (AA) was founded on the concept that the company and encouragement of peers could be effective. Similar to mutual aid societies, AA focused on abstinence, although it developed the 12-step model (Kurtz, 1979; White, 1998). A protocol was developed in 1966 specifically for IPs, which has been periodically updated and supplemented with resources for staff (Alcoholics Anonymous World Services, 2017). Narcotics Anonymous was founded in 1953 to address the use of drugs. AA and similar mutual aid models remain common in jails, prisons, probation, and post-release settings, despite mixed findings on their long-term effectiveness (Bahr et al., 2012).

Throughout the 1700s and 1800s, treatment options were scarce and dependent on citizen-led social organizations. In the 1900s, these expanded to include inpatient and outpatient programs, and the medical and psychiatric community began to conceptualize SUDs as brain and behavioral disorders. The concept of levels of care emerged to guide decision-making around treatment setting and intensity; this concept has persisted as the American Society of Addiction Medicine's criteria for adult addiction treatment (American Society of Addiction Medicine, 2023).

In the early 2000s, more than half of IPs in U.S. state prisons met criteria for an SUD, but only less than half of those reported participating in treatment in prison; most of that was alcohol and drug use education and self-help groups (Taxman et al., 2007). Of those IPs who received treatment, many received programming that was not appropriate to their needs. Less than 1% received medications for maintenance (Mumola & Karberg, 2006). Additionally, tobacco bans became increasingly prevalent, and access to alcohol and drugs was limited via enforcement mechanisms, leading to withdrawal for individuals with SUDs entering facilities from the community. Among people entering jails and prisons, treatment of withdrawal has historically been limited (Mumola & Karberg 2006; see Chapter 46), despite its significant discomfort and medical risks.

Contemporary interventions

Treatment of IPs for SUD has been increasingly recognized as ethical and essential to improve outcomes during and after incarceration and consistent with international standards (e.g., Council of Europe International Co-operation Group on Drugs and Addictions, 2022). Treatment has evolved to account for empirical research and cultural and sociopolitical shifts in attitudes toward SUDs, treatment, and harm reduction. Contemporary programming is increasingly aimed at being integrative, including behavioral and pharmacotherapeutic modalities as well as holistic programming that accounts for social determinants of health and multilevel (i.e., individual, family, and community) influences on outcomes (Brinkley-Rubenstein, 2013; Howell et al., 2021).

Contemporary approaches also consider the continuum of involvement in the criminal legal system, the importance of early prerelease planning, and overdose prevention. The increased risk of drug-related death (i.e., overdose) after release from prison has been documented in international studies (Binswanger et al., 2007; Borschmann et al., 2024). As a result, overdose education and naloxone provision should be integrated into programming. Community-based treatment may be interrupted during incarceration, leading to withdrawal and difficulty reinitiating treatment after release (Binswanger, 2019).

Formerly incarcerated individuals face challenges when they return to community settings, as they rapidly and sometimes unexpectedly move from enforced abstinence and limited independence to routine exposure to drugs and alcohol while trying to meet basic needs for housing and income (Binswanger et al., 2011). Nicotine and tobacco products are frequently banned in U.S. prisons and jails, and a return to these substances is common after release (Martin et al., 2022). Thus, there is an ongoing need for programming that supports continuity of care to improved postrelease outcomes. Such strategies include in-reach, peer support, patient navigation, and case management (Substance Abuse and Mental Health Services Administration, 2023; see Chapter 50). Peer navigators with lived experience can play an important role in bridging treatment between correctional and community settings, particularly for subgroups of IPs such as women (Tillson et al., 2022).

Finally, the COVID-19 pandemic made remote or telehealth-assisted treatment modalities for IPs essential, leading to the development of new and adapted programming (see Chapter 21). For instance, some telehealth programs have integrated group-based counseling to support tobacco cessation (Valera et al., 2024).

Cognitive-behavioral models

Behavioral and cognitive-behavioral therapeutic models are the most common approaches for SUDs in correctional settings. This is largely due to the effectiveness of these modalities in treating a range of behavioral disorders (Hofmann et al., 2012). Cognitive-behavioral therapy (CBT) for SUDs has shown effectiveness in IPs compared to drug and alcohol education or no treatment at all (Landenberger & Lipsey, 2005; Pearson et al., 2002; D. B. Wilson et al., 2005). Program goals have often focused on "criminal recidivism," but evaluating effectiveness should account for the complex relationships between substance use and crime and legal involvement, which are highly dependent on legal and structural factors.

The underlying tenets of CBT include identifying thinking patterns, modifying beliefs and attitudes, and changing behaviors (Beck, 1995). As a therapeutic approach, CBT is effective for a range of addictive, behavioral, and psychiatric conditions. Programs have been adapted to the needs of IPs, often using cognitive-behavioral frameworks with added features. Implementation fidelity and participant adherence have been major concerns in the delivery of treatment services. Table 47.1 lists several key programs, and below we highlight several of these.

Strategies for Self-Improvement and Change

Strategies for Self-Improvement and Change is a long-term, multiphasic cognitive-behavioral intervention developed for adults in the criminal legal system intended to develop skills and understanding of the internal processes (thoughts, emotions, beliefs, attitudes) and external events or circumstances that lead to substance use (Wanberg & Milkman, 2008). The curriculum consists of 12 treatment modules with three phases: Phase I is focused on relationships, self-disclosure, self-awareness, and a relapse/recidivism prevention plan; phase II involves active practice and change implementation (Wanberg & Milkman, 2008), including managing cravings, regulating emotions, and developing more effective interpersonal relationships; and phase III is a maintenance phase focused on healthy living skills.

Table 47.1 CBT-based modalities adapted for correctional use

Name	Reference
Strategies for Self-Improvement and Change	Wanberg and Milkman (2008)
Moral Reconation Therapy	Little and Robinson (1988)
Reasoning and Rehabilitation	Ross and Fabiano (1985)
Reasoning and Rehabilitation-2	Ross et al. (n.d.)
Thinking for a Change	Bush et al. (1997)
Relapse Prevention Therapy	Marlatt et al. (2002)
START NOW	Sampl et al. (2018)

Moral Reconation Therapy

Originally developed for prison-based TCs, Moral Reconation Therapy (MRT) is focused on moral reasoning and factors that contribute to crime (Little & Robinson, 1988). Within a cognitive-behaviorist framework, MRT was influenced by Lawrence Kohlberg's theory of moral development, which asserts that moral development progresses through six stages, with few adults reaching the final stage (Kohlberg, 1969; Milkman & Wanberg, 2007). Advocates of MRT assert that character and personality traits are a significant but underaddressed reason for crime after release (Milkman & Wanberg, 2007). Participants progress through MRT's 16 steps, focused on setting goals and building skills. This curriculum is conducted in open groups and has been adapted for correctional- and community-based settings. A 2012 meta-analysis of MRT indicated effectiveness in reducing rearrest (Ferguson & Wormith, 2012). However, a more recent randomized trial of MRT among justice-involved veterans treated in a noncorrectional setting suggests limited effectiveness compared with usual care across a range of outcomes, including substance use (Blonigen et al., 2022).

Reasoning and Rehabilitation

Reasoning and Rehabilitation (R&R) is a 35-session CBT program that focuses on attitudes and perspectives, emotion regulation and self-control, and interpersonal problem solving (Ross & Fabiano, 1985). Developed for institutional, community corrections, and reentry programs, participants learn problem-solving skills, coping with provocation, empathy, and assertive communication. Focused on participant engagement, R&R includes activities, games, role playing, and modeling to encourage skill development. This program was developed to be run by health professionals with various levels of education (Milkman & Wanberg, 2007). However, certain skills among facilitators are necessary for its successful implementation (Ross & Fabiano, 1985; Ross et al., 1986). R&R-2 is a shorter version tailored to subpopulations of IPs (Ross & Hilborn, 2008; Ross et al., n.d.). Joy Tong and Farrington's (2006) meta-analysis found R&R to be effective across various international community and institutional studies.

START NOW

Many modern programs in correctional settings incorporate trauma-informed and strengths-based interventions (Miller & Najavits, 2012; Wolff et al., 2015). START NOW is a manualized, skills-based program that does not specifically focus on substance use but incorporates content related to it (Trestman et al., 2021). The program utilizes group therapy to present 32 sessions broken down into four units (foundational, emotion management, interpersonal, and future-focused skills) in a CBT framework (Kersten et al., 2016). Units focus on promoting self-control in the context of emotions and stressors, understanding and coping with emotions, building relationships, and creating personal goals and future-forward thinking. START NOW includes functional analysis, role play, exercises, and group discussions (Sampl et al., 2018; Trestman et al., 2021). The evolution of programming highlights the individual's history with increasing emphasis on personal accountability, control, and skills.

Motivational interviewing

Motivational interviewing (MI) evolved from the person-centered teachings of Carl Rogers and bridges the gap between evidence-based practice and the therapeutic relationship (Miller & Moyers, 2017). The National Institute of Corrections and the U.S. Department of Education have encouraged MI in correctional settings (Iarussi et al., 2016). MI recognizes the importance of personal motivation in treatment engagement and outcomes and seeks to resolve ambivalence by evoking intrinsic motivation for changed behavior. MI has eight stages: openness to collaboration with clients' own expertise, proficiency in client-centered counseling including accurate empathy, recognition of key aspects of client speech that guide the practice of MI, eliciting and strengthening client change talk, rolling with resistance, negotiating change plans, consolidating client commitment, and switching flexibly between MI and other intervention styles. Pederson and colleagues' (2021) review of available studies of MI in justice-involved individuals found no evidence of benefit in terms of reducing substance use and suggested a need for more research.

Therapeutic communities

TCs are intensive facility-based residential treatment models with 6 to 12 months of participation (Kooyman, 1993; Mitchell et al., 2007). Specific programming varies, but most share some elements, such as separation from the general population and immersive recovery-related interventions. The TC builds a social climate to support change and involves resident peers in service delivery (Kooyman, 1993; see Chapter 44). A meta-analysis suggests that participation in TCs reduces postrelease drug use, though prison-based TCs followed by aftercare in the community are more effective (Mitchell et al., 2007).

Drug courts

Drug courts are a system-level intervention to address SUDs and promote diversion from incarceration to treatment (National Treatment Court Resource Center, 2024; U.S. Department of Justice Office of Justice Programs, 2004). The most effective drug courts provide high-intensity programming, emphasize recovery, and predictably apply rewards and sanctions (Longshore et al., 2001; Mitchell et al., 2012). The implementation of drug courts may decrease recidivism among adults, with uncertain benefits for individuals with severe SUDs (Mitchell et al., 2012). A 15-year study in Baltimore found no difference in terms of mortality with drug court involvement, though the authors noted only that only 7% of participants received pharmacotherapy for SUDs (Kearley et al., 2019).

Pharmacotherapy and naloxone

Traditionally, evidence-based pharmacological treatments, such as methadone and buprenorphine, were largely unavailable to IPs (Rich et al., 2005). However, pharmacological treatments can effectively be provided in jails and prisons, are guideline concordant, and are increasingly legally mandated in the United States (see Chapter 49). Models for justice-involved persons include in-facility care, telehealth, peer recovery support services, mobile vans, and Transitions Clinics (Ford et al., n.d.; Tilson et al., 2022). Many of these approaches integrate the provision of naloxone (an opioid antidote that reverses respiratory depression in opioid overdose) for IPs in jails and prisons and those being released (Wenger et al., 2019). Given the high risk of overdose death during the transitional period (Binswanger et al., 2007; Wakeman et al., 2009), holistic programming that integrates psychosocial approaches, pharmacotherapy, and overdose prevention is critical.

Summary

The development of treatment for SUDs in corrections was influenced by mutual aid societies, the temperance movement, and AA. Contemporary behavioral approaches are highly influenced by CBT, integrate pharmacotherapy, and address overdose risk after release. While many programs to address SUDs among IPs exist, many do not receive adequate care and continue to experience overdoses. Clinicians, staff, researchers, and people with lived experience need to continue to advocate for improved and enhanced dissemination of integrated, holistic, noncoercive, evidence-based behavioral and pharmacological treatment for SUDs across the continuum of criminal legal involvement.

REFERENCES

Alcoholics Anonymous World Services. (2017). *AA in correctional facilities*. http://www.aa.org/pdf/products/p-26_AAinCF.pdf

American Psychiatric Association. (2013). *Diagnostic and statistical manual of mental disorders* (5th ed.).

American Psychiatric Association. (2022). *Diagnostic and statistical manual of mental disorders* (5th ed., text rev.).

American Society of Addiction Medicine. (2023). *The ASAM Criteria. Treatment criteria for addictive, substance-related, and co-occurring conditions* (Vol. 1).

Bahr, S., Masters, A., & Taylor, B. (2012). What works in substance abuse treatment programs for offenders? *Prison Journal*, *92*(2), 155–174.

Beck, J. (1995). *Cognitive therapy: Basics and beyond*. Guilford Publications.

Binswanger, I. A. (2019). Opioid use disorder and incarceration—Hope for ensuring the continuity of treatment. *New England Journal of Medicine*, *380*(13), 1193–1195.

Binswanger, I. A., Krueger, P. M., & Steiner, J. F. (2009). Prevalence of chronic medical conditions among jail and prison inmates in the USA compared with the general population. *Journal of Epidemiology and Community Health*, *63*(11), 912–919.

Binswanger, I. A., Nowels, C., Corsi, K. F., et al. (2011). Return to drug use and overdose after release from prison: A qualitative study. *Substance Abuse*, *32*(1), 57–58.

Binswanger, I., Stern, M., Deyo, R., Heagerty, P., Cheadle, A., & Elmore, J. (2007). Release from prison: A high risk of death for former inmates. *New England Journal of Medicine*, *356*(2), 157–165.

Blocker, J., Fahey, D., & Tyrell, I. (2003). *Alcohol and temperance in modern history: An international encyclopedia*. ABC-CLIO.

Blonigen, D. M., Cucciare, M. A., Byrne, T., et al. (2022). A randomized controlled trial of moral reconation therapy to reduce risk for criminal recidivism among justice-involved adults in mental health residential treatment. *Journal of Consulting and Clinical Psychology*, *90*(5), 413–426.

Borschmann, R., The Mortality After Release from Incarceration Consortium (MARIC) Collaborators, & Kinner, S. (2024). Rates and causes of death after release from incarceration among 1 471 526 people in eight high-income and middle-income countries: An individual participant data meta-analysis. *Lancet (London, England), 403*(10438), 1779–1788.

Brinkley-Rubenstein, L. (2013). Incarceration as a catalyst for worsening health. *Health & Justice, 1*(1), 3.

Bureau of Justice Assistance. (2022). *Screening for substance use disorders in jails.* https://www.cossup.org/Content/Documents/Articles/AHP_Screening_for_Substance_Use_Disorders_in_Jails.pdf

Bush, J., Glick, B., & Taymans, J. (1997). *Thinking for a change.* National Institute of Corrections, U.S. Department of Justice.

Council of Europe International Co-operation Group on Drugs and Addictions. (2022). *Standards for treatment of people with drug use disorders in custodial settings.* https://rm.coe.int/stantards-for-treatment-of-people-with-drug-use-disorders-in-custodial/1680a9b0cd

Dadoly, J., Levin, L., & Palmer, L. (2005). *Dr. Samuel B. Woodward: A 19th-century pioneer in American psychiatric care.* Presented at Medical Library Association Annual Meeting, San Antonio, TX.

Fazel, S., Yoon, I. A., & Hayes, A. J. (2017). Substance use disorders in prisoners: An updated systematic review and meta-regression analysis in recently incarcerated men and women. *Addiction, 112*(10), 1725–1739.

Ferguson, L. M., & Wormith, J. S. (2012). Meta-analysis of Moral Reconation Therapy. *International Journal of Offender Therapy and Comparative Criminology, 57*(9), 1076–1106.

Ford, B. R., Ho, S. J., Puglisi, L. B., et al. (n.d.). *A roadmap to evaluating 1115 reentry waiver outcomes: Ensuring a safe and health reentry from incarceration to communities.* https://transitionsclinic.org/wp-content/uploads/2024/01/A-Roadmap-to-Evaluating-1115-Reentry-Waiver-Outcomes.pdf

Hofmann, S. G., Asnaani, A., Vonk, I. J., Sawyer, A. T., & Fang, A. (2012). The efficacy of cognitive behavioral therapy: A review of meta-analyses. *Cognitive Therapy and Research, 36*, 427–440.

Howell, B., Puglisi, L., Clark, K., et al. (2021). The Transitions Clinic Network: Post Incarceration Addiction Treatment, Healthcare, and Social Support (TCN-PATHS): A hybrid type-1 effectiveness trial of enhanced primary care to improve opioid use disorder treatment outcomes following release from jail. *Journal of Substance Abuse Treatment, 128*, 108315.

Iarussi, M. M., Vest, R., Booker, A. T., & Powers, D. F. (2016). Motivational interviewing training in correctional education. *Journal of Correctional Education, 67*(1), 39–57.

Joy Tong, L. S., & Farrington, D. P. (2006). How effective is the "Reasoning and Rehabilitation" programme in reducing re-offending? A meta-analysis of evaluations in four countries. *Psychology, Crime & Law, 12*(1), 3–24.

Katcher, B. (1993). Benjamin Rush's educational campaign against hard drinking. *American Journal of Public Health, 83*(2), 273–281.

Kearley, B. W., Cosgrove, J. A., Wimberly, A. S., & Gottfredson, D. C. (2019). The impact of drug court participation on mortality: 15-year outcomes from a randomized controlled trial. *Journal of Substance Abuse Treatment, 105*, 12–18.

Kersten, L., Cislo, A. M., Lynch, M., et al. (2016). Evaluating START NOW: A skills-based psychotherapy for inmates of correctional systems. *Psychiatric Services, 67*(1), 37–42.

Kohlberg, L. (1969). Stage and sequence: The cognitive-development approach to socialization. In D. Goslin (Ed.), *Handbook of socialization theory and research* (pp. 347–480). Rand McNally.

Kooyman, M. (1993) *The therapeutic community for addicts: Intimacy, parent involvement, and treatment success.* Swets and Zeitlinger Publishers.

Kurtz, E. (1979). *Not God: A history of Alcoholics Anonymous.* Harper and Row Publishers.

Landenberger, N. A., & Lipsey, M. W. (2005). The positive effects of cognitive–behavioral programs for offenders: A meta-analysis of factors associated with effective treatment. *Journal of Experimental Criminology, 1*(4), 451–476.

Lemere, F., & Voegtlin, W. (1950). An evaluation of aversion treatment. *Quarterly Journal of Studies on Alcohol, 11*, 199–204.

Little, G., & Robinson, K. (1988). Moral Reconation Therapy: A systematic, step-by-step treatment system for treatment resistant clients. *Psychological Reports, 62*, 135–151.

Longshore, D., Turner, S., Morral, A., et al. (2001). Drug courts: A conceptual framework. *Journal of Drug Issues, 31*, 7–26.

Marlatt, G., Parks, G., & Witkiewitz, K. (2002). *Clinical guidelines for implementing Relapse Prevention Therapy: A guideline developed for the Behavioral Recovery Management Project.* https://www.drugsandalcohol.ie/13620/1/NTA_RPT.pdf

Martin, R. A., Stein, L. A. R., Kang, A., et al. (2022). Circumstances around cigarette use after enforced abstinence from smoking in an American prison. *Journal of Addiction Medicine, 16*(6), e405–e411.

Maruschak, L. M., Bronson, J., & Alper, M. (2021). *Alcohol and drug use and treatment reported by prisoners.* https://bjs.ojp.gov/sites/g/files/xyckuh236/files/media/document/adutrpspi16st.pdf

Milkman, H., & Wanberg, K. (2007). *Cognitive-behavioral treatment: A review and discussion for corrections professionals.* https://s3.amazonaws.com/static.nicic.gov/Library/021657.pdf

Miller, W. R., & Moyers, T. B. (2006). Eight stages in learning motivational interviewing. *Journal of Teaching in the Addictions, 5*(1), 3–17.

Miller, W. R., & Moyers, T. B. (2017). Motivational interviewing and the clinical science of Carl Rogers. *Journal of Consulting and Clinical Psychology, 85*(8), 757–766.

Miller, N. A., & Najavits, L. M. (2012). Creating trauma-informed correctional care: A balance of goals and environment. *European Journal of Psychotraumatology, 3.* https://doi.org/10.3402/ejpt.v3i0.17246

Mitchell, O., Wilson, D., Eggers, A., & MacKenzie, D. (2012). Assessing the effectiveness of drug courts on recidivism: A meta-analytic review of traditional and non-traditional drug courts. *Journal of Criminal Justice, 40*, 60–71.

Mitchell, O., Wilson, D., & MacKenzie, D. (2007). Does incarceration-based drug treatment reduce recidivism? A meta-analytic synthesis of research. *Journal of Experimental Criminology, 3*(4), 353–375.

Motivans, M. (2024). *Federal justice statistics, 2022.* https://bjs.ojp.gov/document/fjs22.pdf

Mumola, C. J., & Karberg, J. C. (2006). *Drug use and dependence, state and federal prisoners, 2004* (NCJ 213530). U.S. Department of Justice, Office of Justice Programs, Bureau of Justice Statistics.

National Treatment Court Resource Center. (2024). *Program evaluation tools.* https://ntcrc.org/program-evaluation-tools

Pearson, F. S., Lipton, D. S., Cleland, C. M., & Yee, D. S. (2002). The effects of behavioral/cognitive-behavioral programs on recidivism. *Crime and Delinquency, 48*, 476–496.

Pederson, S. D., Curley, E. J., & Collins, C. J. (2021). A systematic review of motivational interviewing to address substance use with justice-involved adults. *Substance Use & Misuse, 56*(5), 639–649.

Rich, J. D., Boutwell, A. E., Shield, D. C., et al. (2005). Attitudes and practices regarding the use of methadone in US state and federal prisons. *Journal of Urban Health, 82*, 411–419.

Ross, R., & Fabiano, E. (1985). *Time to Think: A cognitive model of delinquency prevention and offender rehabilitation*. Institute of Social Sciences and Arts.

Ross, R., Fabiano, E., & Ross, R. (1986). *Reasoning and rehabilitation: A handbook for teaching cognitive skills* (Vols. 1 & 2). T3 Associates.

Ross, R., & Hilborn, J. (2008). *Rehabilitating rehabilitation: Neurocriminology for treatment of antisocial behavior*. Cognitive Centre of Canada.

Ross, R., Hillborn, J., & Little, P. (n.d.). *Reasoning & Rehabilitation 2 Short Version for Adults. Program overview.*

Sampl, S., Trestman, R. L., Krauss, W. J., & Guiher, J. (2018). *START NOW facilitator manual* published by Carilion Clinic. https://www.carilionclinic.org/sites/default/files/2019-07/START_NOW_facilitator_manual_v3.0_05242018.pdf

Spaulding, A. C., Eldridge, G. D., Chico, C. E., et al. (2018). Smoking in correctional settings worldwide: Prevalence, bans and interventions. *Epidemiologic Reviews, 40*(1), 82–95.

Substance Abuse and Mental Health Services Administration. (2023). *Best practices for successful reentry from criminal justice settings for people living with mental health conditions and/or substance use disorders*. https://store.samhsa.gov/sites/default/files/pep23-06-06-001.pdf

Taxman, F. S., Perdoni, M., & Caudy, M. (2013). The plight of providing appropriate substance abuse treatment services to offenders: Modeling the gaps in service delivery. *Victims & Offenders, 8*(1), 70–93.

Taxman, F. S., Perdoni, M. L., & Harrison, L. D. (2007). Drug treatment services for adult offenders: The state of the state. *Journal of Substance Abuse Treatment, 32*(3), 239–254.

Tillson, M., Fallin-Bennett, A., & Staton, M. (2022). Providing peer navigation services to women with a history of opioid misuse pre- and post-release from jail: A program description. *Journal of Clinical and Translational Science, 6*(1), e106.

Tørdal, E. V., Pallesen, S., Sagoe, D., Jones, L. Ø., & Mahjabeen, F. (2024). The prevalence of gambling problems in prison populations: A systematic review and meta-analysis. *Journal of Behavioral Addictions, 13*(1), 25–35.

Trestman, R. L., Kalinger, A., Truong, A., et al. (2021). *Start Now: An effective mental health intervention*. https://www.scientia.global/wp-content/uploads/Robert_Trestman/Robert_Trestman.pdf

U.S. Department of Justice Office of Justice Programs. (2004). *Defining drug courts: The key components*. https://www.ojp.gov/pdffiles1/bja/205621.pdf

Valera, P., Malarkey, S., Smith, N., & McLaughlin, C. (2024). Exploring the role of telehealth: A novel approach to group-based smoking cessation treatment for men incarcerated in a rural state prison. *Journal of Telemedicine and Telecare, 30*(1), 142–150.

Wakeman, S. E., Bowman, S. E., McKenzie, M., Jeronimo, A., & Rich, J. D. (2009). Preventing death among the recently incarcerated: An argument for naloxone prescription before release. *Journal of Addictive Diseases, 28*, 124–129.

Wanberg, K., & Milkman, H. (2008). *Criminal conduct and substance abuse treatment: Strategies for self-improvement and change, pathways to responsible living, providers' guide*. Sage Publications.

Wenger, L. D., Showalter, D., Wheeler, E., et al. (2019). *A primer for implementation of overdose education and naloxone distribution in jails and prisons*. RTI International. https://harmreduction.org/wp-content/uploads/2020/09/A-primer-for-implementation-of-OEND-in-jails-and-prisons-Wenger-2019-RTI.pdf

White, W. (1998). *Slaying the dragon: The history of addiction treatment and recovery in America*. Chestnut Health Systems.

Wilson, D. B., Bouffard, L. A., & MacKenzie, D. L. (2005). A quantitative review of structured, group-oriented, cognitive-behavioral programs for offenders. *Journal of Criminal Justice and Behavior, 32*(2), 172–204.

Wilson, G. (1987). Chemical aversion conditioning as a treatment for alcoholism: A re-analysis. *Behaviour Research and Therapy, 25*(6), 503–516.

Wolff, N., Huening, J., Shi, J., Frueh, C., Hoover, D. R., & McHugo, G. (2015). Implementation and effectiveness of integrated trauma and addiction treatment for incarcerated men. *Journal of Anxiety Disorders, 30*, 66–80.

48

Dual diagnosis

CJ Appleton and Faye S. Taxman

Introduction

The World Health Organization (WHO) defines dual diagnosis as the co-occurrence of a psychoactive substance use disorder (SUD) and another psychiatric disorder within the same individual (Vitali et al., 2018). The presence of both SUD and mental illness is high in the criminal justice population. So, it comes as no surprise that the prevalence of comorbid disorders within the justice population is much higher than that of the general population (Peters et al., 2017). What we know about effective dual diagnosis treatment comes from the general treatment literature, which lacks an integrated understanding of the unique needs of the justice population (Taxman & Belenko, 2012). What is needed is a merging of the dual diagnosis and criminal justice literature to highlight important gaps in our understanding, identify promising intervention strategies, and inspire new approaches to researching justice-involved individuals with dual diagnosis.

This chapter first defines dual diagnosis, discusses the complex relationship between the disorders, and highlights the implications of the high prevalence of dual diagnosis individuals within the justice population. Next, it describes general treatment philosophies and guidelines regarding dual diagnosis treatment while describing the unique criminogenic needs of the justice population that must be considered. Finally, this chapter reviews current interventions that show promising results and discusses important implementation challenges that prevent effective treatment for justice-involved individuals with dual diagnosis.

What is dual diagnosis?

To be categorized as dual diagnosis, an individual must meet the *Diagnostic and Statistical Manual of Mental Disorders*, fifth edition, text revision (DSM-5-TR) criteria for both a mental disorder and an SUD (American Psychiatric Association, 2022). The DSM-5-TR defines a mental disorder as "a syndrome characterized by a clinically significant disturbance in an individual's cognition, emotion regulation, or behavior that reflects a dysfunction in the psychological, biological, or development processes underlying mental functioning" (Stein et al., 2021, p. 895). On the other hand, an SUD involves patterns of symptoms caused by using a substance that an individual continues taking despite its adverse effects. These negative effects can be grouped into four categories: impaired control, physical dependence, social problems, and risky use.

For those with dual diagnosis, both substance use and psychiatric disorders have an independent developmental course but influence the other. For instance, having one disorder increases the likelihood of developing the other. The lifetime prevalence of SUDs for individuals with a serious mental illness like bipolar disorder, schizophrenia, major depression, or anxiety disorder is approximately 50%, compared to 15% in the general population (Cohn & Mueser, 2012). Similarly, within the United States, about half of the people seeking treatment for SUDs are diagnosed as having a co-occurring mental health disorder (Subodh et al., 2018). Furthermore, the relationship between the two disorders is dynamic, resulting in a diverse spectrum of case types. Examples of this complex relationship include (a) a primary mental disorder that causes the increased substance intake and the possible development of an addiction; (b) substance use and/or withdrawal from it leading to a psychiatric symptomatology or established disorder; (c) the reversible/temporary worsening of a psychiatric condition due to the substance intake; and (d) the coexistence, independently developed, of substance use and mental disorder (Vitali et al., 2018). Taken together, having not one but two co-occurring disorders that increase the prevalence and exacerbate the symptoms of the other makes the challenges of the dual diagnosis population intricate and difficult to manage.

Individuals with dual diagnosis are an especially vulnerable population with a unique and complex set of needs. Compared to mental illness alone, dual diagnosis is associated with a range of negative outcomes, including high levels of service use and problems handling social, legal, and lifestyle matters (Pinderup, 2018; Rassool, 2006). Major problems associated with dual diagnosis are an increased likelihood of self-harm, increased risk of HIV infection, increased use of institutional services, poor compliance with medication/treatment, homelessness, risk of violence, risk of victimization, higher recidivism, contact with the criminal justice system, and poor social outcomes (e.g., family, peers; Pinderup, 2018; Rassool, 2006). Additionally, Black, Indigenous, and other people of color with dual diagnosis face additional challenges that stem from additive stigma, prejudice, institutional racism, and ethnocentric intervention strategies (Rassool, 2006; see Chapter 22).

Dual diagnosis within the justice-involved population

The prevalence of both serious mental illness (17% to 34%) and lifetime SUD (70% to 86%) is much higher in justice-involved populations than in the general population (Cohn & Mueser, 2012). Consequently, we also see increased numbers of justice-involved people with dual diagnosis. An estimated 24% to 34% of women and 12% to 15% of men in the criminal justice system have dual diagnosis, compared to approximately 1.3% of the general population (Peters et al., 2017). Justice-involved people with dual diagnosis suffer from worse outcomes throughout the different components of the criminal justice system. For instance, they are more likely to be arrested, and law enforcement is more likely to use force when they are arrested. They are less likely to post bond and more likely to be sentenced to jail or prison and experience longer sentences. While incarcerated, they are more likely to have behavioral problems, which leads to punishments that can exacerbate mental health symptoms (i.e., restrictive housing). Finally, upon reentry to the community, individuals with dual diagnosis often do not have enough psychiatric medication, experience delays in seeing their psychiatrist, lack basic needs (clothes, housing, transportation), and experience employment difficulties (Peters et al., 2017). These difficulties combine to put dually diagnosed people at greater risk for criminal outcomes upon release, such as rearrest or technical violation of probation/parole (Cohn & Mueser, 2012).

Justice-involved people with dual diagnosis have been found to cluster into several types. Individuals with mood or anxiety disorders combined with SUD represent one cluster. The prevalence of mood disorders, anxiety disorders, and SUD in justice-involved populations is high (Steadman et al., 2009). This population suffers from impaired social functioning, is at greater risk for substance use relapse, and has more difficulty with SUD treatment when compared to individuals who do not have a co-occurring mental health disorder (Cohn & Mueser, 2012). Another cluster represents those with a schizophrenia spectrum disorder combined with SUD. Between 33% and 66% of individuals diagnosed with schizophrenia meet the criteria for an SUD at some point in their life (Cohn & Mueser, 2012; Swartz et al., 2006). When compared to those with only schizophrenia, this population is more likely to be male, have greater mood problems, suffer higher rates of suicide, maintain worse medication adherence, experience a higher rate of relapse, and have high criminal justice involvement (Constantine et al., 2010; Tiet & Mausbach, 2007). The final cluster is those who have antisocial personality disorder (ASPD), schizophrenia, and SUD. This group is especially important to focus on regarding violence risk assessment and management. For instance, while many believe that substance use drives the majority of violence perpetration among dual diagnosis individuals (Elbogen et al., 2006), others have noted that the presence of ASPD may better explain the prevalence of violent behavior in the dual diagnosis population. ASPD is characterized by a long-standing pattern of aggression and violence dating back to childhood and is the single greatest risk factor for the development of an SUD for both those in the general population and those with serious mental illness (Cohn & Mueser, 2012).

Ultimately, the higher prevalence of comorbid disorders, increased risk of justice involvement, worse outcomes within the justice system, and complications for successful reentry all identify justice-involved individuals with dual diagnosis as prime candidates for treatment. The following section will review various treatment/intervention approaches for dual diagnosis individuals and discuss what special considerations should be given to the justice-involved population.

Treatment approaches for individuals with dual diagnosis

To intervene appropriately with dual diagnosis individuals, it is essential to consider the unique characteristics of the population. Fantuzzi and Mezzina (2020) suggest that proper treatment for dual diagnosis individuals should be multidimensional to reflect the population's dynamic nature and complex needs. Effective treatment approaches consider the type and level of severity for both mental health and SUD and employ a combination of pharmacological and psychosocial treatments to address them (Hughes, 2006). When directed at mental health symptoms, pharmacological treatments such as mood stabilizers, antipsychotics, and antidepressants are used to affect the neurobiological changes associated with mood, anxiety, and psychotic disorders. When directed at substance use, pharmacological treatments include medications for reducing the symptoms of withdrawal, maintenance medications, and agents for managing cravings (Subodh et al., 2018; see Chapter 49). On the other hand, psychosocial interventions such as family interventions, motivational interviewing (MI), motivation enhancement therapy, relapse prevention counseling, contingency management, cognitive-behavioral therapy (CBT), and other behavior therapies are used in conjunction with pharmacological treatments to assist individuals in altering their lifestyle and thinking patterns as they learn to manage their disease(s) (Subodh et al., 2018; see Chapter 47).

Over the years, research has developed various guidelines for effective intervention with dual diagnosis populations. For instance, Osher and Kofoed (1989) identified a four-stage framework (engagement, motivation to change, treatment, and relapse prevention) for therapeutic interventions with individuals with dual diagnosis. Engagement focuses on developing and maintaining a therapeutic alliance between clinical staff and the dual diagnosis client. Guidelines for developing this engagement include motivating clients to see the benefits of treatment and taking a nonconfrontational, empathetic, and committed approach. Other approaches include offering to help meet basic needs (food, clothing, shelter), providing assistance with legal matters, involving family, and meeting clients in settings where they feel safe (Rethink & Turning Point, 2004). The motivation stage draws on the principles of MI and is contingent on the strength of the working relationship between staff and client. The motivation stage aims to create a collaborative environment that empowers clients to gain insight into their problems and develop solutions. Active treatment involves the client's persuasion of the treatment's value and benefits. To this end, staff and client need to agree upon the goals of treatment and for the treatment of both disorders to be integrated. Relapse prevention acknowledges the reality that both mental health and SUDs are chronic relapsing conditions. Given this context, relapse is approached as a learning opportunity and not a failure of the client (Rassool, 2006).

Models of intervention for the dual diagnosis population are based on whether the services provided are identified as serial, parallel, integrated, or shared care. In the serial or sequential model, one treatment follows the other, but they are not offered simultaneously.

Parallel models are based on treatment being delivered by both SUD and mental health providers concurrently. The weaknesses of the sequential and parallel models stem from the need for more effective collaboration between service providers. Poor coordination and communication between parties leads to difficulty engaging patients in treatment (Edeh, 2002). The integrated model is based on a single treatment system where an individual's SUD and mental health problems are treated simultaneously by the same practitioner. The shared care model involves delivering parallel treatment with close collaboration and communication between teams and carefully timing interventions (Rassool, 2006). While no solid empirical evidence supports one treatment model over the rest, integrated treatment has become the gold standard for dual diagnosis management (Subodh et al., 2018).

Treating justice-involved people with a dual diagnosis

Dual diagnosis individuals involved in the justice system must contend with a significant number of mental health (e.g., psychiatric symptoms, increased risk of self-harm, impaired functioning) and substance use (e.g., withdrawal, self-medicating for psychiatric symptoms, peer pressure to use) risks and needs when attempting to change their behavior. However, dual diagnosis individuals with justice involvement have unique criminogenic needs that must also be addressed. Criminogenic needs are dynamic, changeable risk factors empirically connected to offending behavior (Andrews & Bonta, 2010). Within the risk–need–responsivity model, criminogenic needs are assessed and targeted with intervention efforts. Criminogenic needs include antisocial cognition, antisocial personality patterns, antisocial peers, dysfunctional family relationships, dysfunctional relationships with school/work, too much unstructured leisure time, and substance misuse (Ziv, 2017). The risk–need–responsivity model calls for the limited resources of the justice system to be focused on those with the greatest severity and number of criminogenic needs. Justice-involved persons with dual diagnosis are at a higher risk of recidivism and report higher levels of risk factors compared to other justice-involved populations (Peters et al., 2017). As such, the justice-involved dual diagnosis populations should be a primary focus of carceral intervention.

Having discussed the unique needs/risks of dual diagnosis inside and outside of the justice context, we next review treatment interventions that have been used to address both SUD and mental health disorders and discuss adaptations that have been made to them to treat those with dual diagnosis specifically. Within these, we will review integrated dual disorder treatment (IDDT), MI, CBT, and therapeutic communities (TCs).

Integrated Dual Disorder Treatment

IDDT is a manualized, evidence-based intervention for the integrated; Kikkert et al., 2018 treatment of individuals with dual diagnosis (Mueser et al., 2003). The core philosophy of IDDT embraces the principles of proactive and empathic outreach, continuity of care, stage-specific treatment, and education and engagement of family members (Osher & Kofoed, 1989; Young et al., 2014). The IDDT model includes a multidisciplinary team that has been trained in the treatment of both substance use and psychiatric disorders. These teams focus on psychological, pharmacological, educational, and social interventions, which teams employ in a stage-matched fashion based on the trans-theoretical stages of the change model: precontemplation, contemplation, preparation, action, and maintenance (Fantuzzi & Mezzina, 2020). A key feature of IDDT is providing integration of mental health and SUDs within the same program setting and by the same staff who have expertise in both disorders (Peters et al., 2017). IDDT has been successfully adapted for use with criminal justice populations. In fact, most comprehensive dual diagnosis programs in justice settings (jails/prisons) provide an IDDT approach (Fletcher & Chandler, 2014). The intensive and highly structured nature of IDDT works especially well to address the needs of justice-involved dual diagnosis individuals. Effective adaptations of IDDT for justice-involved populations include an additional focus on criminal thinking and other criminogenic need areas (Peters et al., 2017).

Motivational interviewing

MI was developed for use with those struggling with SUDs. MI is designed to work constructively through many challenges associated with making cognitive and behavioral changes. At its core, MI begins with developing a collaborative relationship between practitioner and client. MI encourages practitioners to move from being overly directive of their clients to taking more of a guiding role. The guiding role must follow four processes: engaging, focusing, evoking, and planning. Engaging involves the development of a therapeutic alliance between the two parties and is considered a prerequisite for any further work. Focusing is the process through which the helper maintains a particular direction in the change conversation. Evoking involves eliciting from the client their motivations for change. Planning happens when the client displays a readiness for change, at which point the helper assists with goals and activities that the client agrees with (Miller & Rollnick, 1991). MI is considered an evidence-based practice and is promoted for use within the risk–need–responsivity model, the predominant rehabilitative framework used in corrections. However, despite its pervasive use, few studies have assessed the various uses of MI with justice populations and its impact on criminal justice outcomes (McMurran, 2009).

Martino and colleagues (2002) adapted MI for dual diagnosis patients, creating dual diagnosis motivational interviewing (DDMI). DDMI includes four considerations for assisting those with dual diagnosis: adopting an integrated approach that equally emphasizes SUD and mental illness; accommodating the cognitive impairments that patients with psychotic disorders present; modifying the core skills of MI (i.e., asking open-ended questions, active listening, reflecting, and affirming) to accommodate the challenges of dual disorder patients; and modifying MI strategies to integrate personalized and engaged feedback, use of decisional balance matrices, and other clinical tools. The adaptations made within the DDMI are aimed at accommodating the interplay between SUD and psychotic functioning. Most of the adaptations use MI and other clinical tools to address ambivalence toward treatment for psychiatric disorders and medication adherence. DDMI has not yet been tested with a justice-involved population, but its emphasis on incorporating psychiatric conditions and its functionality make it potentially useful for this population.

Cognitive-behavioral therapy

The CBT model is one of the most effective psychotherapies for individuals with SUD, as well as those within the criminal justice system (Andrews & Bonta, 2010; Lipsey & Landengerger, 2006). Specifically, the CBT approach aims to alter maladaptive thinking styles like poor moral reasoning, deficient empathy, a strong need for dominance and superiority, and a sense of entitlement that influence criminal and antisocial behavior (Cohn & Mueser, 2012). CBT focuses on teaching participants new skills to increase awareness of problematic thinking patterns, increase control over certain emotions (i.e., anger), and prevent substance use relapse (Taxman, 2015). Many CBT modules include behavioral techniques, social skills training, contingency management strategies, self-monitoring, and the use of token economies (Cohn & Mueser, 2012).

CBT programs, including ones that include anger management and interpersonal problem-solving components, seem to be more effective in targeting criminal outcomes compared to behavioral-only interventions (Lipsey & Landengerger, 2006; McMurran et al., 2008). Moreover, there are several CBT curricula that have integrated aspects of criminal thinking or antisocial cognitions. Some of these include Aggression Replacement Training, Criminal Conduct and Substance Abuse, Moral Reconation Therapy, Thinking for Change, and Reasoning and Rehabilitation (Taxman, 2015; see Chapter 47). Integrating CBT to address the unique criminogenic needs is important to treat the justice-involved population effectively. Still, there is no research evidence that these programs are able to address the comorbid substance use, mental health, and criminogenic needs of the justice-involved dual diagnosis population.

Less is known about how best to adapt CBT curricula to address the needs of dual diagnosis individuals. However, suggested modifications to CBT include the following: using a slower pace when going through therapy and group sessions; adding practice sessions; focusing attention on both symptoms of mental illness and relapse for substances; emphasizing medication adherence strategies; and integrating behavioral therapy with skills to advance stability in the community regarding housing, social supports, and transition across justice settings (Taxman, 2015).

Therapeutic communities

The TC model was originally developed for the treatment of disenfranchised, socially isolated individuals with SUD. The TC model has been recognized as an evidence-based practice that has shown positive effects on abstinence, employment, interpersonal functioning, and reduced criminal involvement (Cohn & Mueser, 2012; Mitchell et al., 2007). The TC approach includes a focus on the whole individual, including a daily regimen that is structured to resocialize the individual, develop personal responsibility, engage in self-help in managing life difficulties, use peer social networks as a healing agent, and pursue change as a gradual developmental process (Taxman, 2015). To be successful, a TC must take place over an extended period (generally 6 to 12 months), and individuals must live within a 24-hour residential setting. This way, life skills and prosocial thinking (e.g., work, self-reliance, prosocial values) can be learned and integrated without outside distraction.

TCs have been shown to be effective with dual diagnosis populations. Because of this, TCs have been adapted to treat individuals with dual diagnosis within the justice system (De Leon, 2000; Sacks et al., 2004; Van Stelle et al., 2004; Zhang et al., 2011). The modified TC for dual diagnosis patients addresses psychiatric symptoms, cognitive impairments, and functionality. Within the prison setting, adaptations include segregating TC participants from the general population, group and community meetings, reinforcement/reward systems, using program graduates as aids for current enrollees, and incorporating a team treatment approach (Cohn & Mueser, 2012). The modified TC for dual diagnosis also features a less intense treatment schedule, addressing criminal thinking and behavior by providing psychosocial education to help participants understand the connection between substance use, mental illness, and criminality.

Implementation challenges for treating dual diagnosis

There are several challenges to treating justice-involved people with dual diagnosis effectively. One of the most fundamental components of developing and directing effective intervention is a comprehensive understanding of the target population for the intervention. Unfortunately, the heterogeneity of the dual diagnosis population makes delivering effective interventions challenging. Some work has attempted to document the typical ways that mental health disorders and SUDs cluster, but the research base is not yet close to a comprehensive understanding of the many ways the two disorders can coexist and the implications of this for intervention. While a broad group of the dual diagnosis population may have overlapping needs, the lack of specificity regarding the nature and severity of alcohol and/or drug use disorders within the spectrum of serious mental illnesses makes generalizing study outcomes difficult (Cohn & Mueser, 2012).

Moreover, although the literature notes that the integrated treatment model is the gold standard for treating dual diagnosis, from a pragmatic standpoint, these services are rare and difficult to access. For instance, in the United States, 18% of addiction programs and 9% of mental health programs offer integrated services, and people with dual diagnosis report receiving integrated services between 7% and 9% of the time (Fantuzzi & Mezzina, 2020). Instead of an integrated approach, often dual diagnosis clients receive treatment for each of their mental health disorders and SUDs separately in a sequential or parallel approach. However, too often, the two sets of experts evaluate the client individually and are not in communication, which limits the efficiency and effectiveness of the treatment (Murthy & Chand, 2012). Furthermore, among the services that exist in the community, many lack a specific focus for the dual diagnosis population. As noted in this chapter, individuals with dual diagnosis present unique needs and risks for which organizations should have guidelines and policies to address. In the absence of these policies and guidelines, therapeutic decisions are often left to the discretion of practitioners, which limits positive outcomes. Add to this the resource limitations and interagency communication limitations of the justice system, and one can imagine the precarious structural landscape that those with dual diagnosis must navigate to receive treatment.

A major barrier to treating dual diagnosis is the need for more organizational support for treatment staff to treat the dual diagnosis population differently from those with a single disorder. Pinderup (2018) notes a number of difficulties that staff have when treating those with dual diagnosis. First, practitioners report an insufficient knowledge of treating mental health patients with comorbid SUD. Consequently, the insufficient knowledge of dual diagnosis treatment, combined with the lack of specialized clinical skills, can lead to negative attitudes toward the dual diagnosis clients (Adams, 2008; Richmond & Foster, 2003). Next, the standardization of treatment approaches often utilizes predefined treatment packages that do not consider the unique needs of dual diagnosis. Finally, a division between service providers impacts treating dual diagnosis clients. Poor communication between parties and unclear policies may confuse practitioners about who has the responsibility to address specific factors with a patient.

Summary

Research has noted an increased prevalence of comorbid SUD and mental illness within the general population, and a growing body of research has begun to identify guidelines and best practices to treat these dual diagnosis individuals. Despite this, we do not fully understand the effects of dual diagnosis in diverse populations, the various ways the two disorders are interrelated, and what external characteristics potentially complicate treatment efforts. Justice-involved dual diagnosis individuals exist within this gap in our knowledge. The prevalence of dual diagnosis is far greater among those with justice involvement than it is in the general population. Additionally, justice involvement carries with it unique treatment needs (e.g., criminogenic needs) and limitations (e.g., justice system organization, resource limitation, coerced treatment) that have yet to be understood from a research standpoint. Moreover, even our most promising dual diagnosis treatments, IDDT, MI, CBT, and TC, have not been properly evaluated for their impact on substance use, mental health, and criminal legal outcomes. More research is needed to address these limitations and provide evidence-based guidance on how to best treat justice-involved individuals with dual diagnosis.

REFERENCES

Adams, M. W. (2008). Comorbidity of mental health and substance misuse problems: A review of workers' reported attitudes and perceptions. *Journal of Psychiatric and Mental Health Nursing, 15*(2), 101–108.

American Psychiatric Association. (2022). *Diagnostic and statistical manual of mental disorders* (5th ed., text rev.).

Andrews, D. A., & Bonta, J. (2010). *The psychology of criminal conduct.* Routledge.

Cohn, A., & Mueser, K. T. (2012). Treatments for offenders with dual diagnosis. In *Alcohol-related violence: Prevention and treatment* (pp. 249–283).

Constantine, R., Andel, R., Petrila, J., et al. (2010a). Characteristics and experiences of adults with a serious mental illness who were involved in the criminal justice system. *Psychiatric Services, 61*(5), 451–457.

De Leon, G. (2000). *The therapeutic community: Theory, model, and method.* Springer Publishing Company.

Edeh, J. (2002). Dual or separate services? In Dual diagnosis: Substance misuse and psychiatric disorders (Rasool G.H., ed). p. 204–216. Blackwell, Oxford.

Elbogen, E. B., Van Dorn, R. A., Swanson, J. W., Swartz, M. S., & Monahan, J. (2006). Treatment engagement and violence risk in mental disorders. *British Journal of Psychiatry, 189*(4), 354–360.

Fantuzzi, C., & Mezzina, R. (2020). Dual diagnosis: A systematic review of the organization of community health services. *International Journal of Social Psychiatry, 66*(3), 300–310.

Fletcher, B. W., & Chandler, R. K. (2014). *Principles of drug abuse treatment for criminal justice populations: A research-based guide* (Publication No. NIH 06-5316). National Institute on Drug Abuse. https://nida.nih.gov/sites/default/files/txcriminaljustice_0.pdf

Hughes, L. (2006). *Closing the gap: A capability framework for working effectively with people with combined mental health and substance use problems (dual diagnosis).* Center for Clinical and Academic Workforce Innovation, University of Lincoln.

Kikkert, M., Goudriaan, A., De Waal, M., Peen, J., & Dekker, J. (2018). Effectiveness of Integrated Dual Diagnosis Treatment (IDDT) in severe mental illness outpatients with a co-occurring substance use disorder. *Journal of Substance Abuse Treatment, 95*, 35–42.

Lipsey, M. W., & Landenberger, N. A. (2006). Cognitive-behavioral interventions. In Brandon C. Welsh & David P. Farrington (Eds.), *Preventing crime: What works for children, offenders, victims and places* (pp. 57–71). Springer.

Martino, S., Carroll, K., Kostas, D., Perkins, J., & Rounsaville, B. (2002). Dual diagnosis motivation interviewing: A modification of motivational interviewing for substance-abusing patients with psychotic disorders. *Journal of Substance Abuse Treatment, 23*(40), 297–308.

McMurran, M. (2009). Motivational interviewing with offenders: A systematic review. *Legal and Criminological Psychology, 14*(1), 83–100.

McMurran, M., Theodosi, E., Sweeney, A., & Sellen, J. (2008). What do prisoners want? Current concerns of adult male prisoners. *Psychology, Crime & Law, 14*(3), 267–274.

Miller, W. R., & Rollnick, S. (1991). *Motivational interviewing: Preparing people to change addictive behavior.* Guilford Press.

Mitchell, O. J., Wilson, D. B., & MacKenzie, D. L. (2007). Does incarceration-based treatment reduce recidivism? A meta-analytic synthesis of the research. *Journal of Experimental Criminology, 3*(4), 353–375.

Mueser, K., Noordsy, D., Drake, R., & Fox, L. (2003). *Integrated treatment for dual disorders: A guide to effective practice.* Guilford Press.

Murthy, P., & Chand, P. (2012). Treatment of dual diagnosis disorders. *Current Opinion in Psychiatry, 25*(3), 194–200.

Osher, F. C., & Kofoed, L. L. (1989). Treatment of patients with psychiatric and psychoactive substance abuse disorders. *Hospital and Community Psychiatry, 40*, 1025–1030.

Peters, R. H., Young, M. S., Rojas, E. C., & Gorey, C. M. (2017). Evidence-based treatment and supervision practices for co-occurring mental and substance use disorders in the criminal justice system. *American Journal of Drug and Alcohol Abuse, 43*(4), 475–488.

Pinderup, P. (2018). Challenges in working with patients with dual diagnosis. *Advances in Dual Diagnosis, 11*(2), 60–75.

Rassool, G. H. (Ed.). (2007). Dual diagnosis nursing. John Wiley & Sons, Incorporated.

Rethink & Turning Point. (2004). *Dual diagnosis toolkit mental health and substance misuse. A practical guide for professionals and practitioners.*

Richmond, I., & Foster, J. (2003). Negative attitudes towards people with co-morbid mental health and substance misuse problems: An investigation of mental health professionals. *Journal of Mental Health, 12*(4), 393–403.

Sacks, S., Sacks, J. Y., McKendrick, K., Banks, S., & Stommel, J. (2004). Modified TC for MICA offenders: Crime outcomes. *Behavioral Sciences & the Law, 22*(4), 477–501.

Steadman, H., Osher, F., Robbins, P. C., Case, B., & Samuels, S. (2009). Prevalence of serious mental illness among jail inmates. *Psychiatric Services, 60*(6), 761–765.

Stein, D. J., Palk, A. C., & Kendler, K. S. (2021). What is a mental disorder? An exemplar-focused approach. *Psychological Medicine, 51*(6), 894–901.
Subodh, B. N., Sharma, N., & Shah, R. (2018). Psychosocial interventions in patients with dual diagnosis. *Indian Journal of Psychiatry, 60*(Suppl. 4), S494–S500.
Swartz, M. S., Wagner, H. R., Swanson, J. W., Stroup, T. S., McEvoy, J. P., Canive, J. M., & Khan, A. (2006). Substance use in persons with schizophrenia: Baseline prevalence and correlates from the NIMH CATIE study. *Journal of Nervous and Mental Disease, 194*(3), 164–172.
Taxman, F. S. (2015). Dual diagnosis. In R. L. Trestman, K. Appelbaum, & J. Metzner (Eds.), *Oxford textbook of correctional psychiatry* (p. 254). Oxford University Press.
Taxman, F. S., & Belenko, S. (2012). *Implementing evidence-based practices in community corrections and addiction treatment.* Springer.
Tiet, Q. Q., & Mausbach, B. (2007). Treatments for patients with dual diagnosis: A review. *Alcoholism: Clinical and Experimental Research, 31*(4), 513–536.
Van Stelle, K. R., Blumer, C., & Moberg, D. P. (2004). Treatment retention of dually diagnosed offenders in an institutional therapeutic community. *Behavioral Sciences & the Law, 22*(4), 585–597.
Vitali, M., Sorbo, F., Mistretta, M., Coriale, G., Messina, M. P., Alessandrini, G., … Ceccanti, M. (2018). Drafting a dual diagnosis program: A tailored intervention for patients with complex clinical needs. *Rivista di psichiatria, 53*(3), 149–153.
Young, M., Barrett, B., Engelhardt, M., & Moore, K. (2014). Six month outcomes of an integrated assertive community treatment team serving adults with complex behavioral health and housing needs. *Community Mental Health Journal, 50*(4), 474–479.
Zhang, S. X., Roberts, R. E. L., & McCollister, K. E. (2011). Therapeutic community in a California prison: Treatment outcomes after 5 years. *Crime & Delinquency, 57*(1), 82–101
Ziv, R. (2017). *The future of correctional rehabilitation: Moving beyond the RNR model and good lives model debate.* Routledge.

49

Pharmacotherapy for substance use disorders

James Q. Zhou and Sarah E. Wakeman[1]

Introduction

According to the Substance Abuse and Mental Health Services Administration (SAMHSA; 2023), over 17% of people in the United States have a substance use disorder (SUD). Opioids are the largest contributor to the global burden of disease from substance use, resulting in 55% of drug-related deaths in 2010 and an estimated cost of 9.2 million disability-adjusted life years (Degenhardt et al., 2013). Injecting substance users, the majority of whom use opioids, are at especially high risk for bloodborne pathogens, homelessness, and incarceration (Degenhardt et al., 2017). One in five incarcerated persons (IPs) is admitted to correctional facilities in the United States for drug-related offenses, with the prevalence of active SUD there ranging from 60% to 84% (SAMHSA, 2023; Toyoshima et al., 2021). Opioid overdose is the leading cause of postrelease deaths (Binswanger et al., 2013), with rates occurring 40 to 120 times higher than the general population (Toyoshima et al., 2021). Specifically for alcohol use disorder (AUD), 20% to 23% of IPs in the United States are thought to meet diagnostic criteria (Fazel et al., 2017), compared to just over 10% in the community (SAMHSA, 2023). This chapter presents the background, best practices, and evidence base for the use of pharmacotherapy for SUD treatment within correctional settings.

Despite the high prevalence of SUDs and the potential consequences of undertreatment, few IPs receive any form of treatment for these while incarcerated. Mumola and Karberg (2006) noted that only 15% to 17% of IPs in the United States received SUD treatment from a trained professional. Most often, SUD treatment consists of psychosocial therapies, group counseling, and sometimes therapeutic communities (TCs). Traditional TCs are residential drug-free programs that focus on behavioral modification and psychosocial skill building, often actively discouraging pharmacological treatment (Bruce et al., 2007). Wakeman and colleagues (2020), in a large real-world study of persons in various treatment modalities for opioid use disorder (OUD) in the community, found that, among the 12.5% who were treated with methadone or buprenorphine, this was the only group with a reduced risk of overdose at 3- and 12-month follow-ups. Rarely are these more efficacious pharmacotherapies offered in jails and prisons.

Only modest gains have been made in recent years in access to SUD pharmacotherapy. A 2019 Bureau of Justice Statistics report found that 24% of jail jurisdictions continued pharmacotherapy for IPs already engaged in treatment preincarceration, while 19% of jurisdictions initiated de novo pharmacotherapy (Maruschak et al., 2023). A survey by Scott and colleagues (2021) of 21 U.S. prison systems found that only 7% of facilities offered comprehensive medications for opioid use disorder (MOUD).

Medically supervised withdrawal

Medically supervised withdrawal (MSW, previously called "detoxification") refers to the use of pharmacological treatments to minimize the symptoms of substance withdrawal in the period immediately following cessation of use (Mattick & Hall, 1996). MSW alone is not treatment and by itself does not lead to any reduction in long-term substance use, though, if needed, it will signal a serious SUD that requires further attention. The worthy aim of MSW is to achieve a safe and humane withdrawal from alcohol or drugs (American Society of Addiction Medicine, 2020; Mattick & Hall, 1996; see Chapter 46).

Opioid withdrawal syndrome, while classically not considered life-threatening, has been associated with deaths in IPs via dehydration, hypovolemia, or suicide (Larney et al., 2014). In the absence of appropriate MSW for opioids, IPs may attempt to seek relief through other means, such as feigning withdrawal from different substances (like alcohol) or psychiatric symptoms, intentionally injuring themselves, or obtaining medications from other IPs (Mitchell et al., 2009). Such behaviors are unsafe for the patient and do not address the underlying problem. Continuation of MOUD from the community or initiation of MOUD, if clinically indicated, will prevent the development of opioid withdrawal and the need for MSW.

1. The authors acknowledge the contributions of Josiah D. Rich, who was a coauthor of this chapter in the first edition of this textbook.

Pharmacological treatments for opioid use disorder

Decades of evidence have demonstrated that strategies involving MSW alone, regardless of duration or the type of medication used, result in the dismal outcome of 65% to 90% of people returning to drug use within months (Broers et al., 2000; Weiss et al., 2011). In contrast, both methadone and buprenorphine have been shown to be clinically effective and cost-effective (Connock et al., 2007), with a 34% to 38% relative risk reduction for fatal opioid overdoses compared to nonpharmacological strategies (Heimer et al., 2024). Adequately dosed opioid agonist therapy results in treatment retention rates of 60% to 80%, with only 20% of those treated using any opioids at 1 year (Mattick et al, 2014). MOUD has been shown to reduce behaviors that are risk factors for transmission of hepatitis C and HIV, as well as improve adherence to their treatments (Taweh et al., 2021). A second-line pharmacological treatment for individuals who decline opioid agonist therapy is the opioid antagonist naltrexone.

Professional organizations, including the American Psychiatric Association and the National Commission for Correctional Health Care, support the use of MOUD in correctional settings (American Psychiatric Association, 2020; National Commission for Correctional Health Care, 2021). In a 2020 position statement, the American Society of Addiction Medicine wrote that access to all U.S. Food and Drug Administration (FDA)–approved MOUD is standard of care for all IPs (American Society of Addiction Medicine, 2020). Recent studies conducted within correctional facilities suggest that the benefits of pharmacotherapy extend to justice-involved populations (Malta et al., 2019; McKenzie et al., 2012).

Despite the evidence base and support of professional organizations, many barriers within correctional systems exist to limit MOUD's widespread adoption. These include institutional factors (such as lack of capacity or specialized providers), programmatic factors (such as lack of evidence-based protocols), attitudinal factors (such as stigma and concerns about diversion), and systemic factors (such as inadequate coordination of postrelease care). These barriers are often interdependent and are difficult to break without simultaneous interventions aimed toward the full scope of the problem (Grella et al., 2020).

In recent years, IPs with OUD have filed legal challenges against correctional facilities citing the Eighth Amendment, Title II of the Americans With Disabilities Act, or the Rehabilitation Act of 1973. Judges have largely ruled in favor of the plaintiffs, dismissing arguments that antagonist therapy (naltrexone) or MSW alone is a sufficient form of treatment (Toyoshima et al., 2021). Rhode Island, in 2016, and Vermont, in 2018, were early adopters of comprehensive MOUD programs in statewide correctional systems. Rhode Island saw a 60.5% reduction in postrelease opioid overdose deaths in the year after the program was implemented (Green et al., 2018), while Vermont saw a one-third reduction in nonfatal overdoses and a greater than 60% reduction in fatal overdoses following release (Klemperer et al., 2023).

Methadone

Methadone, a full mu-opioid receptor agonist, was first demonstrated in 1965 to be effective in markedly reducing heroin use (Dole & Nyswander, 1965). Methadone's high oral bioavailability, long half-life, and slow onset of action allows for once-daily oral dosing and leads to less euphoria than other opioids. A Cochrane review found that when methadone is used for OUD, higher dosages (up to 100 mg daily) are associated with increased treatment retention, reduced opioid use, decreased withdrawal symptoms, and increased abstinence from cocaine (Faggiano et al., 2003).

Prerelease methadone treatment has been repeatedly shown to improve health-related outcomes during and after incarceration (Malta et al., 2019; see Chapter 50). Larney and colleagues (2014) demonstrated that MOUD, primarily methadone, led to a 74% reduction in all-cause mortality during the entire incarceration period compared to no MOUD among Australian IPs. This effect was particularly pronounced during the first 4 weeks of incarceration, where the all-cause mortality hazard was 94% lower in the MOUD group (Larney et al., 2014). Brinkley-Rubenstein and colleagues (2018) found that IPs in Rhode Island were more likely to continue engagement with a methadone treatment program compared to those who received only MSW. Furthermore, IPs in the Connecticut jail system who received methadone experienced an 18.8% absolute risk reduction of reincarceration after 1 year compared to those who received only MSW (Westerberg et al., 2016). Overall, initiation of methadone during incarceration and prior to release is significantly more effective for increasing treatment retention, reducing drug use, and reducing acquisitive crime than either counseling alone or referral to methadone treatment upon release (Gordon et al., 2008; McKenzie et al., 2012).

Buprenorphine

Buprenorphine is a partial mu-opioid receptor agonist first developed in the 1960s for analgesia and subsequently determined to be an effective MOUD (Bart, 2012). Like methadone, buprenorphine reduces cravings and other opioid use. Its partial agonism results in less euphoria and a ceiling effect for respiratory depression that, combined with its relatively long half-life, establishes its value for the management of OUD (Bruce et al., 2007).

The efficacy of buprenorphine is dose dependent. Most patients stabilize on 12 to 16 mg daily, although higher dosages of 16 to 32 mg likely improve treatment retention (Bart, 2012; Fareed et al., 2012). With flexible dosing, buprenorphine is as effective as methadone in reducing other opioid use and retaining individuals in treatment (Mattick et al., 2014).

Within correctional facilities, there is growing experience with buprenorphine. At the Riker's Island jail in New York City, buprenorphine was more acceptable than, and as effective as, methadone in reducing self-reported postrelease recurrence of opioid use, reincarceration, and criminal activity (Magura et al., 2009). In Rhode Island, prerelease buprenorphine demonstrated reasonable retention rates 6 months after release (Zaller et al., 2013). Buprenorphine has an advantage over methadone for prerelease populations who are not opioid tolerant, as it can be safely titrated to a dose that blocks the effects of other opioids within a week (Zaller et al., 2013), whereas methadone can take months (Gordon et al., 2008).

Concerns about diversion are a barrier to MOUD implementation in correctional settings. While costly, injectable extended-release buprenorphine (XR-BUP) carries a low risk of diversion and reduces administration time, given its once-monthly dosing (Martin et al., 2022). After the Rhode Island Department of Corrections implemented their statewide comprehensive MOUD program, no attempts at XR-BUP diversion were documented, and many IPs were able to successfully transition from preincarceration methadone to XR-BUP.

Upon release, 70% of XR-BUP recipients continued to engage in OUD-related care, though not necessarily continuing with XR-BUP because of financial and insurance barriers (Martin et al., 2022). A similar study by Lee and colleagues (2021) demonstrated a 69% XR-BUP postrelease continuation rate among IPs in New York City, compared to just 35% among sublingual buprenorphine recipients.

Naltrexone

Naltrexone, a semi-synthetic mu- and kappa-opioid receptor antagonist, was first synthesized in the 1960s and can be administered in oral or intramuscular formulations. As an antagonist, it blocks the effects of opioids for 24 to 48 hours following oral administration and for 28 days following an intramuscular extended-release naltrexone (XR-NTX) dose of 380 mg. As a treatment for OUD, naltrexone's ability to block the reinforcing effects of opioids seemed promising as a means of extinguishing the reward associated with ongoing opioid use (Bart, 2012). In practice, the results have been less impressive due to poor rates of treatment retention.

In Lee and colleagues' (2016) study of opioid-abstinent individuals with a history of criminal legal system involvement who were offered opioid agonist therapy and declined, XR-NTX resulted in an absolute relative reduction in OUD recurrence rate of 21% and a longer median time to recurrence, though there were no differences in recidivism or in overdoses compared to those who received psychosocial therapies alone. A subsequent head-to-head comparison of buprenorphine to XR-NTX in nonincarcerated patients demonstrated better outcomes for buprenorphine and highlighted the challenges in initiating XR-NTX, as 28% of those randomized to XR-NTX dropped out before their first dose, compared to 6% for the buprenorphine group (Lee et al., 2017). A small study by Friedmann et al. (2018) suggested that IPs who received their first XR-NTX dose prior to release were more likely to have better treatment retention and greater rates of abstinence compared to those who received their index injection after release. These findings support XR-NTX as a second-line therapy for OUD that is superior to no medication at all and should be considered among individuals who are offered opioid agonist therapy and decline. In a survey of IPs in Rhode Island eligible for their comprehensive MOUD program, only 2.5% preferred a naltrexone product over agonist options (Kaplowitz et al., 2022).

While indicated for the blockage of opioids, oral naltrexone is not approved by the FDA for treatment of OUD (FDA, 2024) and is generally not recommended by SUD experts. Research for oral naltrexone has demonstrated poor adherence and therefore no benefit over placebo (Coviello et al., 2010).

Despite being widely accepted as superior to naltrexone, many correctional administrators believe that providing agonist therapy is tantamount to rewarding bad behavior, whereas antagonist therapy, a blocking agent that does not provide euphoria, is more in line with a correctional mindset. Naltrexone continues to be the most widely offered MOUD in U.S. correctional systems despite an economic modeling study showing that naltrexone alone is both less cost-efficient and less effective at preventing deaths than offering a comprehensive MOUD program (Chatterjee et al., 2023). An American Psychiatric Association (2020) position statement explicitly opposes offering only a naltrexone product as MOUD in jails and prisons.

Naloxone

Naloxone is an opioid blocker that must be administered parenterally (most often intranasally or by intramuscular injection) and is intended as a rescue treatment for opioid overdose (National Institute on Drug Abuse, 2022). It is not for the maintenance treatment of any substance use disorders, but its availability to people with high-risk opioid use may save lives. Research supports take-home doses of naloxone for IPs as a low-cost and effective method for reducing deaths in the community (Bird et al., 2016; Leung et al., 2021).

Pharmacological treatments for alcohol use disorder

As with OUD, MSW from alcohol alone rarely results in long-term sobriety. Unlike for OUD, pharmacotherapy for AUD is less efficacious but still offers meaningful benefits and is widely underused. Three medications are approved by the FDA for the treatment of AUD: naltrexone, acamprosate, and disulfiram.

A meta-analysis found that naltrexone is generally well tolerated within correctional settings, and its benefits for AUD approximately mirror those seen among the general population. Compared to placebo, naltrexone reduces alcohol consumption, increases medication adherence for other medical conditions, and may reduce recidivism (Slavin-Stewart et al., 2021).

In the community, acamprosate demonstrates similar improvements to alcohol consumption as oral naltrexone. Acamprosate is usually taken 3 times a day, compared to once a day for oral naltrexone, which may complicate adherence (Jonas et al., 2014). A Swedish cohort did not show improvements in most justice-related outcomes when comparing before and after treatment with acamprosate (Molero et al., 2018). Due to the sparsity of evidence for justice-involved individuals and its high cost, the American Academy of Psychiatry and the Law concluded that the role of acamprosate in correctional settings is "unclear" (American Academy of Psychiatry and the Law, 2018).

Most studies of disulfiram within correctional settings are dated and lack sufficient methodical and statistical rigor. Some studies weakly suggest that disulfiram may reduce alcohol consumption and rearrest rates (Slavin-Stewart et al., 2021). However, adherence with disulfiram is a concern in any setting. In each of four studies between 1966 and 1983, release to the community for IPs with AUD was contingent upon clinic visits and observed ingestion of disulfiram, which is impractical to implement consistently (Slavin-Stewart et al., 2021).

Pharmacotherapy for stimulant use disorder

There are no FDA-approved medication options for other SUDs common in IPs, such as stimulant use disorders, which suggests an important need to be addressed. Numerous pharmacotherapies have been studied in the community, including psychostimulants, n-acetylcysteine, opioid agonist therapy, disulfiram, and antidepressants, with inadequate evidence to recommend their widespread use. Contingency management has thus far demonstrated the best outcome with respect to treatment of stimulant use disorders, but it is unclear if this finding is generalizable to justice-involved individuals (Ronsley et al., 2020). A study of a contingency-based program for parolees found it ineffective for those who preferred opioids or stimulants (Friedmann et al., 2012).

Aftercare services

Linkage of IPs who received MOUD or other pharmacotherapy in prison or jail to these services in the community is necessary (see Chapter 50). All state Medicaid programs support at least one form of MOUD, most often buprenorphine (SAMHSA, 2019). Hamilton and colleagues (2022) suggest a peer support specialist model for justice-involved persons with OUD, citing research supporting its value for improving adherence with treatment in the community (see Chapter 44).

Summary

SUD is highly prevalent among IPs, and the chronic, recurring nature of these disorders within the context of criminalized drug use results in high rates of recidivism, cost, spread of disease, and mortality. MSW by itself does not treat SUD. Pharmacotherapy for SUD, particularly for opioids, has a robust evidence base. Untreated OUD is associated with HIV, hepatitis C, acquisitive crime, death by overdose, and all-cause mortality. Substantial evidence argues that these risks are reduced through long-term treatment with agonist medications such as methadone and buprenorphine.

Despite convincing evidence from years of research that establishes the efficacy of buprenorphine and methadone for the treatment of OUD, most correctional facilities do not offer these life-saving medications. Lack of understanding about the disease model of OUD, persistent stigma that pharmacotherapy is simply a "substitute," the challenging logistics of administering controlled medications, fear of diversion, and the punitive culture common to many correctional facilities have limited the use of these treatments. Though there are differences in environment and drug use patterns between community and correctional settings, recent studies conducted specifically within the latter demonstrate that opioid agonist therapy significantly improves health-related outcomes. The evidence base, along with the statements of professional organizations, supports offering comprehensive MOUD as clinically appropriate throughout the period of incarceration. Direct linkage to community treatment programs for continuity of care is essential.

While the evidence base is modest, pharmacotherapy for AUD is an important and underused tool. Additional well-designed studies are needed to assess the impact of medications for AUD for IPs. The lack of recommended pharmacotherapies for other SUDs common in IPs like stimulant use disorder is a need to be addressed.

The time has come to reexamine SUD treatment practices within jails and prisons. Incarceration offers an opportunity to engage a highly marginalized population with a disproportionate burden of disease and mortality.

REFERENCES

American Academy of Psychiatry and the Law. (2018). Practice resource for prescribing in corrections. *Journal of the American Academy of Psychiatry and the Law, 46*(2 Suppl.), S2–S50.

American Psychiatric Association. (2020). *Position statement on pharmaceutical marketing to justice entities regarding medication treatment for substance use disorders.* https://psychiatry.org/getattachment/93e24bc4-ea89-4f29-aacf-71e093c88b6b/Position-Pharmaceutical-Marketing-Justice-Entities.pdf

American Society of Addiction Medicine. (2020). *Public policy statement on treatment of opioid use disorder.* https://www.asam.org/docs/default-source/public-policy-statements/2020-statement-on-treatment-of-oud-in-correctional-settings.pdf

Bart, G. (2012). Maintenance medication for opiate addiction: The foundation of recovery. *Journal of Addictive Diseases, 31*(3), 207–225.

Binswanger, I. A., Blatchford, P. J., Mueller, S. R., & Stern, M. F. (2013). Mortality after prison release: Opioid overdose and other causes of death, risk factors, and time trends from 1999 to 2009. *Annals of Internal Medicine, 159*(9), 592–600.

Bird, S. M., McAuley, A., Perry, S., & Hunter, C. (2016). Effectiveness of Scotland's National Naloxone Programme for reducing opioid-related deaths: A before (2006–10) versus after (2011–13) comparison. *Addiction (Abingdon, England), 111*(5), 883–891.

Brinkley-Rubinstein, L., McKenzie, M., Macmadu, A., et al. (2018). A randomized, open label trial of methadone continuation versus forced withdrawal in a combined US prison and jail: Findings at 12 months post-release. *Drug and Alcohol Dependence, 184*, 57–63.

Broers, B., Giner, F., Dumont, P., & Mino, A. (2000). Inpatient opiate detoxification in Geneva: Follow-up at 1 and 6 months. *Drug and Alcohol Dependence, 58*(1–2), 85–92.

Bruce, R. D., Smith-Rohrburg, D., & Altice, F. L. (2007). Pharmacological treatment of substance abuse in correctional facilities: Prospects and barriers to expanding access to evidence-based therapy. In R. Greifenger (Ed.), *Public health behind bars: From prisons to communities* (pp. 385–411). Springer.

Chatterjee, A., Weitz, M., Savinkina, A., et al. (2023). Estimated costs and outcomes associated with use and nonuse of medications for opioid use disorder during incarceration and at release in Massachusetts. *JAMA Network Open, 6*(4), e237036.

Connock, M., Juarez-Garcia, A., Jowett, S., et al. (2007). Methadone and buprenorphine for the management of opioid dependence: A systematic review and economic evaluation. *Health Technology Assessment, 11*, 9.

Coviello, D. M., Cornish, J. W., Lynch, K. G., et al. (2010). A randomized trial of oral naltrexone for treating opioid-dependent offenders. *American Journal on Addictions, 19*(5), 422–432.

Degenhardt, L., Peacock, A., Colledge, S., et al. (2017). Global prevalence of injecting drug use and sociodemographic characteristics and prevalence of HIV, HBC, and HCF in people who inject drugs: A multistage systematic review. *Lancet Global Health, 5*(12), e1192–e1207.

Degenhardt, L., Whiteford, H. A., Ferrari, A. J., et al. (2013). Global burden of disease attributable to illicit drug use and dependence: Findings from the Global Burden of Disease Study 2010. *Lancet, 382*(9904), 1564–1574.

Dole, V. P., & Nyswander, M. (1965). A medical treatment for diacetylmorphine (heroin) addiction: A clinical trial with methadone hydrochloride. *Journal of the American Medical Association, 193*(8), 646–650.

Faggiano, F., Vigna-Taglianti, F., Versino, E., & Lemma, P. (2003). Methadone maintenance at different dosages for opioid dependence. *Cochrane Database of Systematic Reviews, 3*, CD002208.

Fareed, A., Vayalapalli, S., Casarella, J., & Drexler, K. (2012). Effect of buprenorphine dose on treatment outcome. *Journal of Addictive Diseases, 31*(1), 8–18.

Fazel, S., Yoon, I. A., Hayes, & A. J. (2017). Substance use disorders in prisoners: An updated systematic review and meta-regression analysis in recently incarcerated men and women. Addiction, 112(10), 1725–1739.

Friedmann, P. D., Green, T. C., Taxman, F. S., et al. (2012). Collaborative behavioral management among parolees: Drug use, crime and re-arrest in the Step'n Out randomized trial. *Addiction (Abingdon, England)*, *107*(6), 1099–1108.

Friedmann, P. D., Wilson, D., Hoskinson, R., Poshkus, M., & Clarke, J. G. (2018). Initiation of extended release naltrexone (XR-NTX) for opioid use disorder prior to release from prison. *Journal of Substance Abuse Treatment*, *85*, 45–48.

Gordon, M. S., Kinlock, T. W., Schwartz, R. P., & O'Grady, K. E. (2008). A randomized clinical trial of methadone maintenance for prisoners: Findings at 6 months post-release. *Addiction*, *103*(8), 1333–1342.

Green, T. C., Clarke, J., Brinkley-Rubinstein, L., et al. (2018). Postincarceration fatal overdoses after implementing medications for addiction treatment in a statewide correctional system. *JAMA Psychiatry*, *75*(4), 405–407.

Grella, C. E., Ostile, E., Scott, C. K., Dennis, M., & Carnavale, J. (2020). A scoping review of barriers and facilitators to implementation of medications for treatment of opioid use disorder within the criminal justice system. *International Journal of Drug Policy*, *81*, 102768.

Hamilton, J., Ti, L., Korchinski, M., & Nolan, S. (2022). Peer support specialists: An underutilized resource in the criminal justice system for opioid use disorder management? *Journal of Addiction Medicine*, *16*(2), 132–134.

Heimer, R., Black, A. C., Lin, H., et al. (2024). Receipt of opioid use disorder treatments prior to fatal overdoses and comparison to no treatment in Connecticut, 2016–17. *Drug and Alcohol Dependence*, *254*, 111040.

Jonas, D. E., Amick, H. R., Feltner, C., et al. (2014). Pharmacotherapy for adults with alcohol use disorders in outpatient settings: A systematic review and meta-analysis. *JAMA*, *311*(18), 1889–1900.

Kaplowitz, E., Truong, A. Q., Berk, J., et al. (2022). Treatment preference for opioid use disorder among people who are incarcerated. *Journal of Substance Abuse Treatment*, *137*, 108690.

Klemperer, E. M., Wreschnig, L., Crocker, A., et al. (2023). The impact of the implementation of medication for opioid use disorder and COVID-19 in a statewide correctional system on treatment engagement, postrelease continuation of care, and overdose. *Journal of Substance Use and Addiction Treatment*, *152*, 209103.

Larney, S., Gisev, N., Farrell, M., et al. (2014). Opioid substitution therapy as a strategy to reduce deaths in prison: Retrospective cohort study. *BMJ Open*, *4*(4), e004666.

Lee, J. D., Malone, M., McDonald, R., et al. (2021). Comparison of treatment retention of adults with opioid addiction managed with extended-release buprenorphine vs daily sublingual buprenorphine-naloxone at time of release from jail. *JAMA Network Open*, *4*(9), e2123032.

Lee, J. D., Nunes, E. V., Novo, P., et al. (2017). Comparative effectiveness of extended-release naltrexone versus buprenorphine-naloxone for opioid relapse prevention (X:BOT): A multicentre, open-label, randomized controlled trial. *The Lancet*, *391*(10118), 309–318.

Leung, T. C., Colyer, S., & Zehireva, S. (2021). An outcome study on the naloxone education/dispensing program for departure patients at Cermak Health Services of Cook County. *Journal of Correctional Health Care: Official Journal of the National Commission on Correctional Health Care*, *27*(1), 11–13.

Magura, S., Lee, J. D., Hershberger, J., et al. (2009). Buprenorphine and methadone maintenance in jail and post-release: A randomized controlled clinical trial. *Drug and Alcohol Dependence*, *99*(1–3), 222–230.

Malta, M., Varatharajan, T., Russell, C., et al. (2019). Opioid-related treatment, interventions, and outcomes among incarcerated persons: A systematic review. *PLoS Medicine*, *16*(12), e1003002.

Martin, R. A., Berk, J., Rich, J. D., et al. (2022). Use of long-acting injectable buprenorphine in the correctional setting. *Journal of Substance Abuse Treatment*, *142*, 108851.

Maruschak, L. M., Minton, T. D., & Zeng, Z. (2023). *Opioid use disorder screening and treatment in local jails, 2019* (NCJ 305179). Bureau of Justice Statistics.

Mattick, R. P., Breen, C., Kimber, J., & Davoli, M. (2014). Buprenorphine maintenance versus placebo or methadone maintenance for opioid dependence. *Cochrane Database of Systematic Reviews*, *2*, CD002207.

Mattick, R. P., & Hall, W. (1996). Are detoxification programmes effective? *Lancet*, *347*(8994), 97–100.

McKenzie, M., Zaller, N., Dickman, S. L., et al. (2012). A randomized trial of methadone initiation prior to release from incarceration. *Substance Abuse*, *33*(1), 19–29.

Mitchell, S. G., Kelly, S. M., Brown, B. S., et al. (2009). Incarceration and opioid withdrawal: The experiences of methadone patients and out of treatment heroin users. *Journal of Psychoactive Drugs*, *41*(2), 145–152.

Molero, Y., Zetterqvist, J., Binswanger, I. A., et al. (2018). Medications for alcohol and opioid use disorders and risk of suicidal behavior, accidental overdoses, and crime. *American Journal of Psychiatry*, *175*(10), 970–978.

Mumola, C. J., & Karberg, J. C. (2006). *Drug use and dependence, State and federal prisoners, 2004* (NCJ 213530). Bureau of Justice Statistics.

National Commission on Correctional Health Care. (2021). *Position statement: Opioid use disorder in correctional settings*. https://www.ncchc.org/opioid-use-disorder-treatment-in-correctional-settings

National Institute on Drug Abuse. (2022). *Naloxone DrugFacts*. https://nida.nih.gov/publications/drugfacts/naloxone

Ronsley, C., Nolan, S., Knight, R., et al. (2020). Treatment of stimulant use disorder: A systematic review of reviews. *PLOS ONE*, *15*(6), e0234809.

Scott, C. K., Dennis, M. L., Grella, C. E., Mischel, A. F., & Carnevale, J. (2021). The impact of the opioid crisis on U.S. state prison systems. *Health & Justice*, *9*(1), 17.

Slavin-Stewart, C., Minhas, M., Turna, J., et al. (2021). Pharmacological interventions for alcohol misuse in correctional settings: A systematic review. *Alcoholism: Clinical and Experimental Research*, *46*(1), 13–24.

Substance Abuse and Mental Health Services Administration. (2019). *Use of medication-assisted treatment for opioid use disorder in criminal justice settings*. https://store.samhsa.gov/product/Use-of-Medication-Assisted-Treatment-for-Opioid-Use-Disorder-in-Criminal-Justice-Settings/PEP19-MATUSECJS

Substance Abuse and Mental Health Services Administration. (2023). *HHS, SAMHSA release 2022 National Survey on Drug Use and Health data*. https://www.samhsa.gov/newsroom/press-announcements/20231113/hhs-samhsa-release-2022-nsduh-data

Taweh, N., Schlossberg, E., Frank, C., et al. (2021). Linking criminal justice-involved individuals to HIV, hepatitis C, and opioid use disorder prevention and treatment services upon release to the community: Progress, gaps, and future directions. *International Journal of Drug Policy*, *96*, 103283.

Toyoshima, T., McNiel, D. E., Schonfeld, A., & Binder, R. (2021). The evolving medicolegal precedent for medications for opioid use disorder in U.S. jails and prisons. *Journal of the American Academy of Psychiatry and the Law*, *49*(4), 545–552.

U.S. Food and Drug Administration. (2024). *Revia (naltrexone) product information.* https://www.accessdata.fda.gov/drugsatfda_docs/label/2013/018932s017lbl.pdf

Wakeman, S. E., Larochelle, M. R., Ameli, O., et al. (2020). Comparative effectiveness of different treatment pathways for opioid use disorder. *JAMA Network Open*, *3*(2), e1920622.

Weiss, R. D., Potter, J. S., Fiellin, D. A., et al. (2011). Adjunctive counseling during brief and extended buprenorphine-naloxone treatment for prescription opioid dependence: A 2-phase randomized controlled trial. *Archives of General Psychiatry*, *68*(12), 1238–1246.

Westerberg, V. S., McCrady, B. S., Owens, M., & Guerin, P. (2016). Community-based methadone maintenance in a large detention center is associated with decreases in inmate recidivism. *Journal of Substance Abuse Treatment*, *70*, 1–6.

Zaller, N., McKenzie, M., Friedmann, P. D., et al. (2013). Initiation of buprenorphine during incarceration and retention in treatment upon release. *Journal of Substance Abuse Treatment*, *45*(2), 222–226.

50

Transition of substance use disorder treatment to the community

Nadeen Ibrahim and Jaimie P. Meyer

Introduction

People with substance use disorders (SUDs) are disproportionately impacted by the criminal legal system, and SUDs are often untreated or undertreated during incarceration. Relapse to substance use following incarceration is a major driver of morbidity and mortality and may result in people experiencing further criminal legal system involvement, generating a revolving door of cyclic incarceration and widening health disparities. Over the past several decades, some programs have provided support for people with SUDs as they transition from carceral settings to the community, but many programs do not deploy evidence-based practices. This chapter discusses best practices and evidence-based models for the management of SUDs to help people successfully transition from carceral settings to communities. We address a range of interventions that include treatment of SUDs during incarceration and prior to release, alternatives to incarceration, transitional case management, adherence support, and harm reduction.

Epidemiology of substance use disorders among incarcerated people

People with SUDs are disproportionately impacted by the criminal legal system because of criminalization of substance use that penalizes people with SUDs. Common social and structural determinants also drive both health and incarceration outcomes, including poverty, homelessness, and racism. An estimated 85% of people incarcerated in U.S. prisons have unhealthy substance use, including 65% who have an SUD and an additional 20% who do not meet criteria for an SUD but were under the influence of substances or intoxicated at the time an offense occurred (National Institute on Drug Abuse, 2020).

Opioid use disorder (OUD) is especially prevalent among incarcerated people, which parallels the high and rising prevalence of OUD in U.S. community settings. Opioid use increases the odds of any criminal legal system involvement, and the frequency of criminal legal system involvement also increases with the severity of opioid use (Substance Abuse and Mental Health Services Administration [SAMHSA], 2019). Current estimates suggest that 19% or more of people in jail report regular opioid use, and among people incarcerated in state prisons, as many as 17% regularly used opioids prior to incarceration (SAMHSA, 2019).

Opioid use and opioid-related overdoses resulted in the United States declaring the opioid crisis a public health emergency in 2017 (SAMHSA, 2019). The opioid crisis has been characterized by exorbitantly high rates of opioid overdose-related deaths, wherein poisoning became the leading cause of accidental deaths for the first time in U.S. history (Centers for Disease Control and Prevention, 2020), mostly related to high-potency synthetic opioids, including fentanyl (Centers for Disease Control and Prevention, 2023). Similarly, drug overdose (primarily due to opioids) is the leading cause of death for people returning to communities from jail or prison (Binswanger et al., 2013; Joudrey et al., 2019). In a large retrospective cohort of 33,811 people returning to communities from Washington State prisons between 2014 and 2018, the all-cause mortality rate was 747 per 100,000 person years, and drug overdose (related to psychostimulants and opioids) was the leading cause of death, which was highest during the first 2 weeks following return to communities (O'Connor et al., 2022). Nonfatal overdoses following prison release are even more common than fatal overdoses (Hartung et al., 2023). When incarceration cannot be avoided altogether, these facts confirm a pressing need for identifying and treating people's SUDs while they are incarcerated and before they return to communities.

Addressing substance use disorders in carceral settings

Given the high prevalence of SUDs among people impacted by the criminal legal system, evidence-based strategies are urgently needed to effectively address SUDs in this population and to curb postrelease drug-related morbidity and mortality.

Treatment for substance use disorders during incarceration

Evidence-based treatment for SUDs, which is addressed in more detail elsewhere (Chapters 47 to 49), includes a combination of behavioral and pharmacological interventions. We will focus here on management of OUD, which is highly prevalent among people in carceral settings and arguably has the greatest impact on postrelease morbidity and mortality. Medications for opioid use disorder (MOUD), when provided during incarceration, have been shown to reduce opioid use and opioid-related overdoses postrelease, decrease the risk of prison recidivism (Evans et al., 2022), promote treatment retention, and substantially reduce overdose-related mortality following release from jail or prison (Hoffman et al., 2019; SAMHSA, 2019). There are currently three MOUD options that are available and strongly evidence based, regardless of treatment setting: (a) methadone, an opioid receptor agonist; (b) buprenorphine, a partial agonist; and (c) naltrexone, an opioid antagonist. All three medications block opioid effects on the brain, reduce cravings, alleviate withdrawal symptoms, reduce the risk of opioid overdose, reduce the risk of HIV and hepatitis C, and reduce substance use (Hoffman et al., 2019). Each medication has varying formulations, advantages, and disadvantages, but all three can be used to treat people with OUD successfully while they are in carceral settings and help facilitate a successful transition to the community.

Despite demonstrated need, implementation of evidence-based SUD treatment programs during incarceration is relatively limited. In 2017, just 30 out of 5,100 prisons and jails in the United States offered methadone or buprenorphine to incarcerated people (SAMHSA, 2019). Until recently, most MOUD programs during incarceration were restricted to people who were pregnant, those who were receiving MOUD prior to incarceration, or those who had imminent release dates (Weizman et al., 2021). Instead of deploying evidence-based MOUD, many carceral facilities have relied solely on behavioral programs that promoted education, detoxification, and abstinence, which did not achieve the same level of benefit in terms of SUD outcomes compared to MOUD, including for people with or without HIV (Kinlock et al., 2009; Springer et al., 2010).

More recently, some states have begun to shift their policies to recognize SUD as a medical disorder that is chronic, relapsing, and remitting rather than a moral failing. Litigation victories and settlements in places like New York and Michigan, investigations led by the U.S. Department of Justice in places like Massachusetts and Kentucky, legislative efforts in New York and Colorado, and executive action in Ohio have all helped facilitate the expansion of MOUD programs in carceral settings (Longley et al., 2023). In 2016, Rhode Island implemented the first statewide, comprehensive MOUD program in the United States (Green et al., 2018). It is currently the only state that screens every person who comes into state prisons or jails for OUD and offers all three forms of MOUD in conjunction with counseling. The program also offers people who have undergone detoxification during incarceration the opportunity to start any of the three medications before release, with appointments arranged for continued treatment in the community. Data on MOUD in Rhode Island illustrate that the program has successfully reduced overdose deaths and supported long-term continuity of care (Green et al., 2018). Between January 2018 and October 2020, following the expansion of MOUD in Rhode Island prisons and jails, the availability of MOUD in jails and prisons across the United States increased by 471.3% (Dadiomov et al., 2022). As of August 2023, approximately 62.4% of 1,028 surveyed jails and 42.8% of 876 surveyed state prisons offered at least one form of MOUD (Jail and Prison Opioid Project, 2024; NORC at the University of Chicago, 2023).

Gender-responsive SUD treatment is particularly important for incarcerated women, who often experience comorbid trauma (see Chapter 55). Best practice for the management of SUDs in women experiencing transitions from carceral to community settings is for transitional programs that include gender-responsive programming and strengths-based individual case management for comorbid mental health conditions (Edwards et al., 2022). Recidivism to prison or jail is not a strong measure of program efficacy for people with SUDs because it is measured inconsistently and focuses on deficits rather than strengths, whereas strengths-based programming is an important component of gender responsiveness (Edwards et al., 2022). For both women and men, treatment retention and prevention of overdose are stronger markers of programmatic success.

Discharge planning

To ensure that people with SUDs successfully transition to communities, prerelease discharge planning is required, incorporating several key components (Figure 50.1): screening for SUDs, briefly intervening, and referring to or directly providing evidence-based treatment; MOUD as indicated in conjunction with counseling; adherence support; discharge planning and transitional case management that includes accessing medical and social programs; and harm reduction with naloxone for overdose prevention and HIV pre-exposure prophylaxis (PrEP) for HIV prevention. Comprehensive transitional programs for incarcerated people with SUDs should also incorporate diagnosis and treatment of comorbid psychiatric disorders during incarceration (see Chapter 48) with transition to

Intervention	During incarceration	Prior to release	Post-release	Comorbid conditions addressed
SBIRT	X	X	X	SUDs
Medications for opioid use disorders	X	X	X	SUDs
Counseling	X	X	X	SUDs
Adherence support	X	X	X	SUDs, HIV, psychiatric disorders
Discharge planning		X	X	SUDs, HIV, psychiatric disorders
Case management Navigation		X	X	SUDs, HIV, psychiatric disorders, SDOH
Naloxone		X	X	Overdose prevention
PrEP		X	X	HIV prevention

Figure 50.1 Key Elements of Pre-Release Discharge Planning for People with Substance Use Disorders

SUDs = substance use disorders; SDOH = social determinants of health; SBIRT = screening, brief intervention, (referral to) treatment; PrEP = HIV pre-exposure prophylaxis.

integrated community mental health treatment programs (Lincoln et al., 2006).

Alternatives to incarceration

One important approach to mitigate the risk of postrelease overdose and enabling continuity of care of SUDs is to implement alternatives to incarceration (see Chapter 6). Drug courts, for instance, offer individuals with SUDs or those with drug-related charges the opportunity to enroll in long-term drug treatment with regular court supervision (U.S. Department of Justice, 2020). The main components of drug courts include (a) participation over a series of months or years to establish and maintain long-term recovery strategies; (b) frequent and random urine toxicology to monitor substance use; (c) clinical treatment for SUDs; (d) individualized case management services, connecting participants to employment opportunities, community service, prosocial activities, and education; (e) required frequent appearances in court; (f) rewards for maintaining treatment plans and sanctions for failure to meet obligations; and (g) support and encouragement from the drug court team (National Treatment Court Resource Center, 2019). Some drug courts are adapted for target populations such as youths and families or veterans (U.S. Department of Justice, 2020). For young adults who have SUDs, juvenile drug treatment courts serve as comprehensive alternatives to incarceration that include individual and family counseling, education, and other holistic intervention and treatment services (U.S. Department of Justice, 2020). Similarly, family treatment courts provide SUD treatment and social services to parents and children involved in the child welfare system. Program goals are to ensure that "children have safe, nurturing, and permanent homes; parents achieve stable recovery; and family members receive needed support and services to improve family functioning" (U.S. Department of Justice, 2020, para. 5). Ultimately, drug courts present an important alternative to incarceration for people with SUDs who need treatment and support. They are evidence based, effective, and cost-effective, and they support community-based continuity of care.

Services to facilitate community transition

Transitional case management

As jails and prisons begin to implement comprehensive MOUD programs, people need linkages to continuous care in communities, where they can seek care following release. In addition to treatment for SUDs, people with SUDs need treatment for comorbid conditions and social support to sustain positive health outcomes as they transition from carceral to community settings. Recent research has considered the influence of social determinants of health in treatment outcomes after incarceration (Sugarman et al., 2020). The World Health Organization defines social determinants of health as the social, physical, and economic conditions in society that impact health, including socioeconomic status, education, employment, housing, food security, and structural oppression (World Health Organization, 2024). Prior research has identified social determinants of health as important barriers to receiving care postrelease, specifically in terms of medication adherence (Sugarman et al., 2020).

Transitional case management, which involves the coordination of medical and psychosocial care for individuals with complex medical needs like people with SUDs (Springer et al., 2011), is one method of addressing social determinants of health and ensuring individuals can continue to access and engage in health care services postrelease (Loeliger et al., 2018). Transitional case management can play a key role in assisting people with accessing medical and social entitlement programs. People living with HIV and SUDs are an important subpopulation to target for transitional case management because continuity of care (for both HIV and SUDs) is critical to achieve and sustain positive health outcomes. For example, a study of people with HIV from jails and prisons found a significant positive association between receiving transitional case management and successfully linking to community-based HIV care, demonstrating the effectiveness of transitional case management in improving HIV treatment outcomes (Loeliger et al., 2018). When paired with evidence-based HIV and SUD treatment, case management services can provide a seamless system of care to reduce recidivism, maintain overall health, and reduce the potential harms of drug use.

Transitional case management is particularly important for the effective management of comorbid HIV among people with SUDs. For people with HIV, for example, social determinants of health can compromise antiretroviral therapy adherence. Lower education, poverty, unemployment, and experiences of sexism, racism, and homophobia have all been associated with reduced antiretroviral therapy adherence (Benson et al., 2020). Health disparities are exacerbated for people who have experienced incarceration, which significantly disrupts continuity of care for SUDs and HIV. A study of health care access for women with HIV living in Canada identified recent incarceration as a primary factor contributing to disengagement from HIV care, reporting a care attrition rate of 30% following prison release (Kerkerian et al., 2018). A growing body of research suggests that social determinants of health present barriers to SUD and HIV care postrelease, but few interventions have included a component that specifically addresses social determinants of health (Sugarman et al., 2020). Further research is needed on how best to optimize social determinants of health and integrate case management into HIV and SUD comprehensive care (Sugarman et al., 2020).

Patient and peer navigation

Beyond transitional case management, recent research suggests other promising interventions for the continuous management of SUDs and HIV to support people transitioning from carceral to community settings. A 2022 review by Dauria et al. highlighted the efficacy of interventions including patient navigation alongside SUD treatment (Dauria et al., 2022).

Patient navigation typically involves professionals who guide patients through the treatment process, whereas peer navigation typically involves people with shared experiences with those receiving the intervention to destigmatize treatment and foster a trusting environment (Cunningham et al., 2018). Both forms of navigation may improve outcomes by educating patients, addressing barriers to care, providing psychosocial support, conducting outreach, disseminating community resources, and engaging in patient advocacy (Rohan et al., 2018). A 2021 review examined the impact of peer and patient navigation on people's engagement in HIV, hepatitis C, and OUD prevention and treatment services during the transition from carceral settings to the community. They found that both patient and peer navigation programs successfully increased linkage to care, reduced time to medication initiation, and increased the likelihood of medication initiation and adherence across multiple studies (Taweh et al., 2021). One study directly compared a peer navigation intervention to standard transitional case management on HIV viral suppression among men and transgender women with HIV who were released from jail (Dauria et al., 2022). The peer navigation intervention entailed regular counseling on goal setting and problem solving around barriers to HIV care and adherence, starting while participants were still in jail and continuing postrelease. Navigators accompanied participants to two HIV care visits, then facilitated communication with clinicians during visits (Cunningham et al., 2018). Compared to standard case management, the peer navigation intervention was significantly more successful at sustaining HIV viral suppression. The adjusted probability of viral suppression among controls declined from 52% at baseline to 30%, while the intervention group sustained viral suppression at 49% from baseline to 12 months, for a significant difference-in-difference of 22% (Cunningham et al., 2018).

Similar navigation models could help people with SUDs engage in treatment following return to their communities. Many peer navigation interventions begin during incarceration and extend into community transition. Peer recovery support services are an evidence-based model of care that offer a qualified peer support practitioner who assists individuals with their recovery from substance use and mental health conditions (Bureau of Justice Assistance, 2022). In addition to one-on-one recovery check-ins, comprehensive peer recovery support service programs include peer support groups, health education, stress and emotional management, crisis prevention, and community-building activities. Peer recovery support service programs link individuals to treatment and recovery supports in the community, including treatment for SUDs.

Adherence support

Transitional programs can incorporate effective ways to overcome problematic medication adherence common among people with SUDs, particularly when they address social determinants of health that can present major barriers to medication adherence (Anand et al., 2010; Springer et al., 2011). Homelessness (or housing instability) and unemployment, for example, can significantly impair one's ability to adhere to therapy, including MOUD. Among people living with HIV who were formerly incarcerated, factors such as medication burden, forgetfulness, mental health and emotional difficulties, and perceived conflict between substance use and medication adherence are also barriers to medication adherence (Rowell-Cunsolo & Hu, 2020). Further research is needed on barriers to adherence to MOUD during the postincarceration period, when people are most vulnerable to relapse to substance use and fatal overdose (Lim et al., 2023).

Some examples of adherence support that have been demonstrated to be effective in community settings include the use of reminders, adherence counseling support, and directly administered therapy (Springer et al., 2011). While directly administered therapy (either for HIV, known as directly administered antiretroviral therapy, or for MOUD, like methadone) can support adherence and reduce diversion, it is not feasible or cost-effective to implement in all settings. Moreover, directly observed therapy may mimic the lack of autonomy people experience in carceral settings instead of building self-efficacy.

Cues and reminders may be useful for patients for whom a major reason for missed doses is "forgetting" because of chaotic living conditions comorbid psychiatric disorders, or HIV- or SUD-associated cognitive impairment (Springer et al., 2011). Mobile health (mHealth) interventions have demonstrated efficacy at reducing potential gaps in care. Drawing from another HIV-specific example, a 2020 randomized controlled trial recruited people with HIV currently or recently incarcerated within the DC Department of Corrections and randomized them to a control group or one that received an mHealth intervention involving adherence support delivery through text messaging (Uhrig Castonguay et al., 2020). Text message content included HIV appointment reminders, medication adherence, prevention reminders, and barriers to care following release from jail; participants could customize the timing, frequency, and message content throughout the study period. The most preferred appointment reminder message was "Hey how you feeling? Don't forget to give a call and make your appointment" (19/57, 33%). The most preferred message about medication adherence was "Don't forget your skittles!" (31/57, 54%). Sixty-three percent (36/57) of participants chose to receive daily (versus weekly) messages from this category at baseline (Uhrig Castonguay et al., 2020). Adherence reminder systems have been implemented both nationally and globally in high-HIV-burden countries like South Africa, where several adherence monitoring and support interventions among people initiating antiretroviral therapy are currently being evaluated (Jennings et al., 2023).

Adherence counseling strategies have been shown to change patients' knowledge, attitudes, and beliefs about medical treatment and to improve their adherence to complex medication regimens (Leeman et al., 2010). Peer navigation and patient navigation are emerging adherence support strategies, as described above. A recent review demonstrated the effectiveness of mobile health units to support medication adherence, wherein individuals are linked to a mobile health unit within their community that provides integrated infectious disease and SUD prevention and treatment services (Taweh et al., 2021). In one study that reviewed the efficacy of mobile health units in people transitioning from jail, researchers found that a mobile van located directly outside of the Baltimore City jail significantly increased buprenorphine and naltrexone initiation and improved adherence, compared to linkage to care as usual (Krawczyk et al., 2019).

Medication adherence may also be supported by using long-acting injectable MOUD, obviating the need for daily oral medications that require more frequent adherence. Extended-release buprenorphine (XR-BUP) and extended-release naltrexone (XR-NTX), both monthly injectable long-acting MOUDs, have gained traction as effective forms of adherence support for people transitioning from jail or prison. When compared with daily sublingual buprenorphine, XR-BUP offered prior to release from jail led to increased buprenorphine treatment retention postrelease, wherein 69% of XR-BUP participants versus 35% of sublingual buprenorphine participants adhered to treatment at 8 weeks postrelease (Lee et al., 2021). Both XR-BUP and XR-NTX have been found to be highly acceptable across multiple studies. People using XR-NTX have consistently confirmed that the medication effectively blocked euphoric effects of opioids, noted low potential for misuse, reported no overdoses, and experienced fewer cravings and improved treatment adherence

(Velasquez et al., 2019). Extended-Release Injectable Treatments in the Criminal Justice System (EXIT-CJS), a multisite open-label randomized controlled trial comparing the effectiveness of XR-BUP and XR-NTX in people involved in the criminal legal system, is currently in progress (Waddell et al., 2021).

Harm reduction

In addition to treating SUDs and supporting treatment adherence, harm reduction is an important approach to reducing morbidity and mortality among people with SUDs transitioning from carceral to community settings. Given the extraordinarily high rates of opioid overdose mortality following prison and jail release, the National Commission on Correctional Health Care recommends provision of take-home naloxone and education on overdose and naloxone use prior to release (Horton et al., 2017; National Commission on Correctional Health Care, 2020). The largest study on take-home naloxone to date, known as NALoxone InVEstigation (N-ALIVE), randomized 1,685 people leaving 16 prisons in the United Kingdom to receive take-home naloxone or control. Although naloxone was used frequently to successfully prevent fatal overdose, randomization was stopped early because, two-thirds of the time, naloxone was administered to people other than study participants, which made outcomes more difficult to measure (Meade et al., 2018; Parmar et al., 2017). Even without naloxone provision to people prior to release, which might not be feasible in all settings, overdose awareness and prevention are important. For example, a study conducted in New York City's Rikers Island jail trained jail visitors on naloxone use, finding that it was effective in reaching people with OUD prior to incarceration and following release from jail (Huxley-Reicher et al., 2018).

HIV prevention is another important component of harm reduction among people with SUDs transitioning from prisons and jails. PrEP, including long-acting injectable formulations, is a promising intervention for people with SUDs at high risk for HIV upon transitioning from carceral settings. In one pilot demonstration project, women who were recently released from incarceration or on community supervision successfully initiated PrEP in a low-barrier-to-access setting using telehealth (Meyer et al., 2022). To date, PrEP implementation behind bars is limited (Murphy et al., 2022). One study examining the awareness, acceptability, and adoption of long-acting injectable PrEP among Black sexual minority men and transgender women in jail identified several major barriers to PrEP adoption during incarceration, including stigma, potential misuse, needle aversion (in relation to long-acting injectable PrEP), and need for additional clinic time (Jones et al., 2023). Participants indicated that PrEP e-prescription could help support continuity of care postrelease and highlighted reduced stigma, convenience, and longer term HIV protection as benefits for long-acting injectable PrEP (Jones et al., 2023). Study findings provided context-specific information to inform the implementation of future PrEP interventions in jail settings for people at high risk of HIV during incarceration or following release (Jones et al., 2023).

Summary

Management of SUDs for incarcerated people includes evidence-based treatment such as MOUD during incarceration, alternative-to-incarceration programs, transitional case management, adherence support, and provision of long-acting injectable MOUD to help people successfully transition from carceral to community settings. These approaches are important for sustaining continuity of care for SUDs and comorbid conditions (including HIV and psychiatric disorders) and reducing SUD-related morbidity and mortality for people impacted by the criminal legal system. To overcome logistical constraints and provide evidence-based care for SUDs in carceral settings, innovative solutions are urgently needed that involve partnerships between all existing stakeholders, including individual patients with SUDs and lived experiences of incarceration, practitioners within the criminal legal system, and communities.

REFERENCES

Anand, P., Springer, S. A., Copenhaver, M. M., & Altice, F. L. (2010). Neurocognitive impairment and HIV risk factors: a reciprocal relationship. *AIDS and Behavior*, *14*(6), 1213–1226.

Benson, C., Wang, X., Dunn, K. J., Li, N., Mesana, L., Lai, J., Wong, E. Y., Chow, W., Hardy, H., Song, J., & Brown, K. (2020). Antiretroviral adherence, drug resistance, and the impact of social determinants of health in HIV-1 patients in the US. *AIDS and Behavior*, *24*(12), 3562–3573.

Binswanger, I. A., Blatchford, P. J., Mueller, S. R., & Stern, M. F. (2013). Mortality after prison release: Opioid overdose and other causes of death, risk factors, and time trends from 1999 to 2009. *Annals of Internal Medicine*, *159*(9), 592–600.

Bureau of Justice Assistance. (2022). *Peer recovery support services in correctional settings* (NCJ 304806). https://bja.ojp.gov/library/publications/peer-recovery-support-services-correctional-settings

Centers for Disease Control and Prevention. (2020). *Leading causes of death*. https://www.cdc.gov/injury/wisqars/LeadingCauses.html

Centers for Disease Control and Prevention. (2023). *CDC WONDER online database: National drug involved overdose deaths 1999–2021.* https://nida.nih.gov/research-topics/trends-statistics/overdose-death-rates

Cunningham, W. E., Weiss, R. E., Nakazono, T., Malek, M. A., Shoptaw, S. J., Ettner, S. L., & Harawa, N. T. (2018). Effectiveness of a peer navigation intervention to sustain viral suppression among HIV-positive men and transgender women released from jail: The LINK LA randomized clinical trial. *JAMA Internal Medicine*, *178*(4), 542–553.

Dadiomov, D., Trotzky-Sirr, R., Shooshtari, A., & Qato, D. M. (2022). Changes in the availability of medications for opioid use disorder in prisons and jails in the United States during the COVID-19 pandemic. *Drug and Alcohol Dependence*, *232*, 109291.

Dauria, E. F., Kulkarni, P., Clemenzi-Allen, A., Brinkley-Rubinstein, L., & Beckwith, C. G. (2022). Interventions designed to improve HIV continuum of care outcomes for persons with HIV in contact with the carceral system in the USA. *Current HIV/AIDS Reports*, *19*(4), 281–291.

Edwards, L., Jamieson, S. K., Bowman, J., Chang, S., Newton, J., & Sullivan, E. (2022). A systematic review of post-release programs for women exiting prison with substance-use disorders: Assessing current programs and weighing the evidence. *Health Justice*, *10*(1), 1.

Evans, E. A., Wilson, D., & Friedmann, P. D. (2022). Recidivism and mortality after in-jail buprenorphine treatment for opioid use disorder. *Drug and Alcohol Dependence*, *231*, 109254.

Green, T. C., Clarke, J., Brinkley-Rubinstein, L., Marshall, B. D. L., Alexander-Scott, N., Boss, R., & Rich, J. D. (2018).

Postincarceration fatal overdoses after implementing medications for addiction treatment in a statewide correctional system. *JAMA Psychiatry*, *75*(4), 405–407.

Hartung, D. M., McCracken, C. M., Nguyen, T., Kempany, K., & Waddell, E. N. (2023). Fatal and nonfatal opioid overdose risk following release from prison: A retrospective cohort study using linked administrative data. *Journal of Substance Use and Addiction Treatment*, *147*, 208971.

Hoffman, K. A., Ponce Terashima, J., & McCarty, D. (2019). Opioid use disorder and treatment: Challenges and opportunities. *BMC Health Services Research*, *19*(1), 884.

Horton, M., McDonald, R., Green, T. C., Nielsen, S., Strang, J., Degenhardt, L., & Larney, S. (2017). A mapping review of take-home naloxone for people released from correctional settings. *International Journal on Drug Policy*, *46*, 7–16.

Huxley-Reicher, Z., Maldjian, L., Winkelstein, E., Siegler, A., Paone, D., Tuazon, E., Nolan, M. L., Jordan, A., MacDonald, R., & Kunins, H. V. (2018). Witnessed overdoses and naloxone use among visitors to Rikers Island jails trained in overdose rescue. *Addictive Behaviors*, *86*, 73–78.

Jail and Prison Opioid Project. (2024). *Who has access to medication for opioid use disorder (MOUD) in correctional settings?* https://prisonopioidproject.org/#fn2

Jennings, L., West, R. L., Halim, N., Kaiser, J. L., Gwadz, M., MacLeod, W. B., Gifford, A. L., Haberer, J. E., Orrell, C., & Sabin, L. L. (2023). Protocol for an evaluation of adherence monitoring and support interventions among people initiating antiretroviral therapy in Cape Town, South Africa—A multiphase optimization strategy (MOST) approach using a fractional factorial design. *Trials*, *24*(1), 310.

Jones, M. D., Jones, K., Almirol, E., et al. (2023). Examining the awareness, acceptability, and adoption of conventional and non-conventional forms of pre-exposure prophylaxis (PrEP) for HIV prevention among jail-involved Black sexual minority men (BSMM) and Black transgender women (BTW) in two diverse US cities. *AIDS and Behavior*, *27*(4), 1304–1313.

Joudrey, P. J., Khan, M. R., Wang, E. A., Scheidell, J. D., Edelman, E. J., McInnes, D. K., & Fox, A. D. (2019). A conceptual model for understanding post-release opioid-related overdose risk. *Addiction Science & Clinical Practice*, *14*(1), 17.

Kerkerian, G., Kestler, M., Carter, A., Wang, L., Kronfli, N., Sereda, P., Roth, E., Milloy, M. J., Pick, N., Money, D., Webster, K., Hogg, R. S., de Pokomandy, A., Loutfy, M., Kaida, A., on behalf of the Canadian HIV Women's Sexual and Reproductive Health Cohort Study (CHIWOS) Research Team. (2018). Attrition across the HIV cascade of care among a diverse cohort of women living with HIV in Canada. *JAIDS Journal of Acquired Immune Deficiency Syndromes*, *79*(2), 226–236.

Kinlock, T. W., Gordon, M. S., Schwartz, R. P., Fitzgerald, T. T., & O'Grady, K. E. (2009). A randomized clinical trial of methadone maintenance for prisoners: Results at 12 months postrelease. *Journal of Substance Abuse Treatment*, 37(3), 277–85.

Krawczyk, N., Buresh, M., Gordon, M. S., Blue, T. R., Fingerhood, M. I., & Agus, D. (2019). Expanding low-threshold buprenorphine to justice-involved individuals through mobile treatment: Addressing a critical care gap. *Journal of Substance Abuse Treatment*, *103*, 1–8.

Lee, J. D., Malone, M., McDonald, R., Cheng, A., Vasudevan, K., Tofighi, B., Garment, A., Porter, B., Goldfeld, K. S., Matteo, M., Mangat, J., Katyal, M., Giftos, J., & MacDonald, R. (2021). Comparison of treatment retention of adults with opioid addiction managed with extended-release buprenorphine vs daily sublingual buprenorphine-naloxone at time of release from jail. *JAMA Network Open*, *4*(9), e2123032.

Leeman, J., Chang, Y. K., Lee, E. J., Voils, C. I., Crandell, J., & Sandelowski, M. (2010). Implementation of antiretroviral therapy adherence interventions: A realist synthesis of evidence. *Journal of Advanced Nursing*, *66*(9), 1915–1930.

Lim, S., Cherian, T., Katyal, M., Goldfeld, K. S., McDonald, R., Wiewel, E., Khan, M., Krawczyk, N., Braunstein, S., Murphy, S. M., Jalali, A., Jeng, P. J., MacDonald, R., and Lee, J. D. (2023). Association between jail-based methadone or buprenorphine treatment for opioid use disorder and overdose mortality after release from New York City jails 2011–17. *Addiction*, *118*(3), 459–467.

Lincoln, T., Kennedy, S., Tuthill, R., Roberts, C., Conklin, T. J., & Hammett, T. M. (2006). Facilitators and barriers to continuing healthcare after jail: A community-integrated program. *Journal of Ambulatory Care Management*, *29*(1), 2–16.

Loeliger, K. B., Altice, F. L., Desai, M. M., Ciarleglio, M. M., Gallagher, C., & Meyer, J. P. (2018). Predictors of linkage to HIV care and viral suppression after release from jails and prisons: A retrospective cohort study. *Lancet HIV*, *5*(2), e96–e106.

Longley, J., Weizman, S., Brown, S., & LaBelle, R. (2023). *A national snapshot update: Access to medications for opioid use disorder in U.S. jails and prisons.* O'Neill Institute for National and Global Health Law at Georgetown Law Center. https://oneill.law.georgetown.edu/wp-content/uploads/2023/02/ONL_Revised_50_State_P5.pdf

Meade, A. M., Bird, S. M., Strang, J., Pepple, T., Nichols, L. L., Mascarenhas, M., Choo, L., & Parmar, M. K. B. (2018). Methods for delivering the UK's multi-centre prison-based naloxone-on-release pilot randomised trial (N-ALIVE): Europe's largest prison-based randomised controlled trial. *Drug and Alcohol Review*, *37*(4), 487–498.

Meyer, J. P., Price, C. R., Ye, Y., Qin, Y., Tracey, D., Demidont, A. C., Melbourne, K., & Altice, F. L. (2022). A PrEP demonstration project using eHealth and community outreach to justice-involved cisgender women and their risk networks. *AIDS and Behavior*, *26*(12), 3807–3817. https://doi.org/10.1007/s10461-022-03709-2

Murphy, M., Sosnowy, C., Rogers, B., Napoleon, S., Galipeau, D., Scott, T., Tao, J., Berk, J., Clarke, J., Nunn, A., & Chan, P. A. (2022). Defining the pre-exposure prophylaxis care continuum among recently incarcerated men at high risk for HIV infection: Protocol for a prospective cohort study. *JMIR Research Protocol*, *11*(2), e31928.

National Commission on Correctional Health Care. (2020). *Naloxone in correctional facilities for the prevention of opioid overdose deaths.* https://www.ncchc.org/position-statements/naloxone-in-correctional-facilities-for-the-prevention-of-opioid-overdose-deaths-2020/

National Institute on Drug Abuse. (2020). *Criminal justice DrugFacts.* https://nida.nih.gov/publications/drugfacts/criminal-justice

National Treatment Court Resource Center. (2019). *What are drug courts?* https://ntcrc.org/what-are-drug-courts/

NORC at the University of Chicago. (2023). *JCOIN's national survey of substance use services in jails: Describing U.S. jails and their screening, treatment, recovery, and re-entry practices.* https://jcoinctc.org/MAT-results-from-JCOIN-national-jail-survey/

O'Connor, A. W., Sears, J. M., & Fulton-Kehoe, D. (2022). Overdose and substance-related mortality after release from prison in Washington State: 2014–2019. *Drug and Alcohol Dependence*, *241*, 109655.

Parmar, M. K. B., Strang, J., Choo, L., Meade, A. M., & Bird, S. M. (2017). Randomized controlled pilot trial of naloxone-on-release to prevent post-prison opioid overdose deaths. *Addiction*, *112*(3), 502–515.

Rohan, E. A., McDougall, R., & Townsend, J. S. (2018). An exploration of patient navigation and community health worker activities across national comprehensive cancer control programs. *Health Equity*, *2*(1), 366–374.

Rowell-Cunsolo, T. L., & Hu, G. (2020). Barriers to optimal antiretroviral therapy adherence among HIV-infected formerly incarcerated individuals in New York City. *PLoS One*, *15*(6), e0233842.

Springer, S., Chen, S., & Altice, F. (2010). Improved HIV and substance abuse treatment outcomes for released HIV-infected prisoners: The impact of buprenorphine treatment. *Journal of Urban Health*, *87*(4), 592–602.

Springer, S. A., Spaulding, A. C., Meyer, J. P., & Altice, F. L. (2011). Public health implications of adequate transitional care for HIV-infected prisoners: Five essential components. *Clinical Infectious Diseases: An Official Publication of the Infectious Diseases Society of America*, *53*(5), 469–479.

Substance Abuse and Mental Health Services Administration. (2019). *Use of medication-assisted treatment for opioid use disorder in criminal justice settings* (HHS Publication No. PEP19-MATUSECJS). National Mental Health and Substance Use Policy Laboratory.

Sugarman, O. K., Bachhuber, M. A., Wennerstrom, A., Bruno, T., & Springgate, B. F. (2020). Interventions for incarcerated adults with opioid use disorder in the United States: A systematic review with a focus on social determinants of health. *PLoS One*, *15*(1), e0227968.

Taweh, N., Schlossberg, E., Frank, C., Nijhawan, A., Kuo, I., Knight, K., & Springer, S. A. (2021). Linking criminal justice-involved individuals to HIV, hepatitis C, and opioid use disorder prevention and treatment services upon release to the community: Progress, gaps, and future directions. *International Journal on Drug Policy*, *96*, 103283.

Uhrig Castonguay, B. J., Cressman, A. E., Kuo, I., Patrick, R., Trezza, C., Cates, A., Olsen, H., Peterson, J., Kurth, A., Bazerman, L. B., & Beckwith, C. G. (2020). The implementation of a text messaging intervention to improve HIV continuum of care outcomes among persons recently released from correctional facilities: Randomized controlled trial. *JMIR Mhealth Uhealth*, *8*(2), e16220.

U.S. Department of Justice. (2020). *Drug courts, special feature, overview*. https://www.ojp.gov/feature/drug-courts/overview

Velasquez, M., Flannery, M., Badolato, R., Vittitow, A., McDonald, R. D., Tofighi, B., Garment, A. R., Giftos, J., & Lee, J. D. (2019). Perceptions of extended-release naltrexone, methadone, and buprenorphine treatments following release from jail. *Addiction Science & Clinical Practice*, *14*(1), 37.

Waddell, E.N., Springer, S.A., Marsch, L.A., Farabee, D., Schwartz, R.P., Nyaku, A., Reeves, R., Goldfeld, K., McDonald, R.D., Malone, M., Cheng, A., Saunders, E.C., Monico, L., Gryczynski, J., Bell, K., Harding, K., Violette, S., Groblewski, T., Martin, W., ... Lee, J. D. (2021). Long-acting buprenorphine vs. naltrexone opioid treatments in CJS-involved adults (EXIT-CJS). *Journal of Substance Abuse Treatment, 128*, 108389.

Weizman, S., Perez, J. E., Manoff, I., Baney, M., & El-Sabawi, T. (2021). *National snapshot: Access to medications for opioid use disorder in U.S. jails and prisons.* O'Neill Institute for National and Global Health Law at Georgetown Law Center. https://oneill.law.georgetown.edu/wp-content/uploads/2021/07/National-Snapshot-Access-to-Medications-for-Opioid-Use-Disorder-in-U.S.-Jails-and-Prisons.pdf

World Health Organization. (2024). *Social determinants of health.* https://www.who.int/health-topics/social-determinants-of-health#tab=tab_1

SECTION IX

Self-injury, aggression, and misconduct

51

Suicide risk reduction

Lindsay M. Hayes and Jeffrey L. Metzner

Introduction

The risk of suicide is a significant concern for both incarcerated persons (IPs) and those responsible for their care. This chapter reviews issues relevant to prevalence, identification of risk despite denial, intake screening and assessment, safe and humane housing, stability, continuous quality improvement, and other risk reduction strategies. Understanding the causes of why a suicidal individual would deny ideation when asked and formulating an effective systemic response are highlighted.

Prevalence of suicide in jails and prisons

Suicide continues to be the leading single cause of death in local jails and a leading cause of death in state prisons throughout the country. Local jails had 289 deaths by suicide in 2000, whereas there were 355 such deaths in 2019 (Carson, 2021). The suicide rate within local jails was 48 deaths per 100,000 IPs in 2000, with a similar rate of 49 per 100,000 in 2019. The percentage of jail suicides that occurred in the first 24 hours of confinement decreased between the 5-year periods of 2000–2004 (22%) and 2015–2019 (12%; Carson, 2021). The largest percentage of jail suicides occur between 2 and 7 days (Carson, 2021; Hayes, 2012). In addition, some jail suicides occur within close proximity to a court hearing, telephone call, or visit (Hayes, 2012).

From 2001 to 2019, the number of suicides in state prisons increased annually by 85%, from 168 to 311 (Carson, 2021). The suicide rate within state prisons grew significantly from 14 deaths per 100,000 IPs in 2001 to 27 per 100,000 in 2019 (Carson, 2021). The largest percentage of prison suicides occur between 1 and 5 years of confinement. In one study, almost half of the individuals committed suicide within 4 months of transferring between prisons (Daniel & Fleming, 2006). Most individuals who die by suicide had documented histories of both serious mental illness and suicidal behavior (Daniel & Fleming, 2006; He et al., 2001; Patterson & Hughes, 2008). One study analyzed mortality reviews of prison suicides and found that almost two thirds of individuals had recently received "adverse information" such as denial of parole or bad news from home, almost half had recent person-to-person conflict and/or received disciplinary action, and most evidenced some degree of psychological distress, manifested by anxiety or agitation in the period immediately preceding suicide (Kovasznay et al., 2004).

The vast majority of suicides in both local jails and state prisons are from asphyxiation by hanging or strangulation (Carson, 2021; Hayes, 2012). Most occur in single-occupancy cells (Daniel & Fleming, 2006; Hayes, 2012; Patterson & Hughes, 2008; Reeves & Tamburello, 2014; Way et al., 2007).

A disproportionate number of suicides take place in restrictive housing units (RHUs, i.e., segregation). For example, in California, segregated individuals represented 3% of the prison population but 37% of the suicides during 2022 (California Department of Corrections and Rehabilitation, 2023); in Texas, segregated individuals represented 30% of the prison population but 54% of the suicides during 2020–2022 (Texas Civil Rights Project & the University of Texas School of Law Civil Rights Clinic, 2023). In the federal prison system, segregated individuals represented 8% of the prison population but 46% of the suicides during 2014–2017 (U.S. Department of Justice, Office of the Inspector General, 2024). For purposes of comparison, an estimated 3.4% of IPs in state prisons throughout the country are housed in RHUs (Resnik et al., 2022). The majority of suicides in RHUs take place relatively soon after placement, often within the first 21 days (Patterson & Hughes, 2008) or 60 days (Way et al., 2007).

Although the rates of suicide in both jails and prisons greatly exceed that of the general population (Fazel et al., 2017; Garrett et al., 2022; Hayes, 2012), the current suicide rate in local jails (49 in 2019) is significantly less than it was in 1986, when that rate was 107 deaths per 100,000 IPs (Hayes, 1989). There are several probable reasons for the decrease, including national studies of jail suicide that gave a face to this long-standing and often ignored public health issue; increased awareness of suicide reflected in national correctional standards, focused training curricula, and more in-depth suicide risk inquiry during the intake process; litigation persuading (or sometimes forcing) counties and facility administrators to take corrective actions; and increased awareness and more positive attitudes that bad outcomes can be reduced (Hayes, 2016). Although suicide rates in local jails have decreased over the years, they remain too high, while rates in state prison systems have grown. Access to national data on jail and prison suicide is in jeopardy of ending, negatively impacting efforts to reduce deaths in custody (Goodwin, 2022). These data have recently been criticized as both inaccurate and underestimating deaths in custody (James, 2023). In light of the COVID-19 pandemic, staffing and other resources are being increasingly strained. Consistent efforts on the part of both custody and health care administrators and their respective staff are required to maintain and advance a suicide risk reduction strategy. This chapter details the critical components of this strategy.

Root of the problem: identifying suicide risk despite denial

A fundamental component of an agency's risk reduction strategy must be the ability to identify suicide risk despite the IP's denial and/or recanting of such risk. In other words, we must be able to identify and address why an otherwise suicidal individual would deny they were suicidal. Possible reasons could be:

- *They want to end their life and not be stopped*—This is the most challenging response, but as Shneidman (1987, p. 56) has offered, "Suicidal people use a particular logic, a style of thinking that brings them to the conclusion that death is the only solution to their problems. This style can be readily seen, and there are steps we can take to prevent suicide, if we know where to look."
- *They are unable or unwilling to articulate their thoughts*—As Jamison (1999, p. 150) has offered: "Were suicidal patients able or willing to articulate the severity of their suicidal thoughts and plans, little risk would exist."
- *They do not want to be ridiculed and/or ostracized by other IPs*—A correctional system's best prevention efforts are sometimes thwarted by peer, gang, cultural, or other pressures not to seek help.
- *Lack of privacy and confidentiality when conducting suicide risk inquiry*—The best phrased question is virtually meaningless when asked at the cell front or in an open and chaotic intake/reception area of the facility.
- *Manner in which the questions are asked or the weighted scale of inquiry*—The common intake screening question of "Are you thinking of hurting and/or killing yourself?" might be circumvented by a nurse as "You're not suicidal, right?" Suicide precautions are only initiated if the IP expresses suicidal ideation with the intent and plan to die.
- *The real and perceived punitive aspects of suicide precautions*—In the name of safety, we often create an environment that is so sterile and bleak that the suicidal person will recant their suicidal ideation at the first opportunity.

A sound risk reduction strategy acknowledges that a suicidal individual's denial of suicidal intent does not end inquiry; it increases the inquiry and builds a suicide prevention program to lessen the need for denial. A comprehensive suicide prevention program, based on national standards (National Commission on Correctional Health Care [NCCHC], 2019), should include at least eight essential components: staff training, intake screening/assessment, communication, safe housing, levels of observation/management, intervention, reporting, and mortality review. These components have been discussed previously by the authors (Hayes, 2016; Metzner & Hayes, 2020), but several are discussed here in the context of identifying risk despite denial.

Identification/assessment

Intake screening and assessment are critical to any correctional system's suicide prevention efforts. An IP can attempt suicide at any point during incarceration, beginning immediately following intake or reception and continuing through a stressful aspect of confinement. Although no single set of risk factors can be used to predict suicide, there is little disagreement about the value of screening and assessment in preventing suicide (American Psychiatric Association [APA], 2016; Spiers et al., 2006). In fact, identifying unique stressors, through the stress–vulnerability model, which encompasses biological vulnerability, stress, and protective factors (or lack thereof), has been utilized in the prison environment to better explain why IPs sometimes have a higher proclivity to suicide upon entrance to prison and restrictive housing (Bonner, 2006; Scott et al., 2023). Although IPs who become suicidal are often reluctant to express it to others upon demand, prior research has consistently reported that at least two thirds of all suicide victims communicate their intent prior to death and that any individual with a history of one or more suicide attempts is at a much greater risk for suicide than those who have never attempted (Pompili et al., 2016). In addition, research has consistently reported that both jail and prison suicide victims had high rates of mental illness and prior suicidal behavior (Daniel & Fleming, 2006; Hayes, 2012; He et al., 2001; Zhong et al., 2021). The key to identifying potentially suicidal behavior in IPs is through reasonably comprehensive inquiry during the intake/reception screening and assessment phases, as well as other high-risk periods of incarceration.

It would be reasonable to assume that a suicidal person might deny suicidal ideation when questioned in a physical environment that lacks both privacy and confidentiality. The booking area of any jail and reception area of a prison are commonly chaotic and noisy, an environment where staff feel pressure to process a high number of IPs in a short period of time. Two key ingredients for identifying suicidal behavior, time and privacy, are at a minimum. The ability to assess the potential for suicide by asking the IP a series of carefully worded questions, interpreting their response (including gauging the truthfulness of their denial of suicide risk), and observing their behavior is grossly compromised by an impersonal environment that lends itself to something quite the opposite. As a result, the clearly suicidal behavior of many individuals, as well as circumstances that may lend themselves to potential self-injury, is lost (Hayes, 2013).

Suicide risk inquiry during the intake screening process should be multilayered, including independent information from external sources regarding prior and current risk and specific inquiry of the IP. Through an automated electronic medical record or management system review, a determination as to whether the IP was a suicide risk during prior confinement in the facility and whether the arresting and/or transporting officer had any information that the IP was a suicide risk are of critical importance (Hayes, 2016; Metzner & Hayes, 2020). Specific inquiry of the IP should include, at a minimum, the following questions:

- Have you ever attempted suicide?
- Have you ever considered suicide?
- Are you now or have you ever been treated for mental health or emotional problems?
- Have you recently experienced a significant loss (relationship, death of family member/close friend, job, etc.)?
- Has a family member or close friend ever attempted or committed suicide?
- Do you feel there is nothing to look forward to in the immediate future (expressing helplessness and/or hopelessness)?
- Are you thinking of hurting and/or killing yourself?

Various correctional agencies utilize a numerical scale to rate signs and symptoms of potential suicidal behavior. The total number of points are placed in a risk level (e.g., "Low, Medium, or High"; "Caution or Warning"; etc.), and the IP is either placed on suicide precautions or not based on this numerical scoring. We should be suspicious of exclusive reliance on this approach because there are no known rating scales that are skillful enough to determine levels of potential lethality precisely, nor are there any available risk scales sensitive to the unique risk factors facing IPs. Further, there are no known suicide risk screening or assessment forms validated for the correctional environment (Berman & Canning, 2022). It is generally recommended that correctional facilities allow their staff wide discretion to place, at a minimum, IPs with active suicidal ideation on suicide precautions and refer all other potentially suicidal individuals (and not just those meeting rating scale criteria) to a qualified mental health professional for a comprehensive suicide risk assessment (NCCHC, 2019).

Within a reasonable period (and no greater than 14 days following admission), all individuals should receive postadmission mental health screening by mental health and/or trained medical staff (see Chapter 15). The screening should include inquiry into history of psychiatric treatment, violent and suicidal behavior, victimization, learning disabilities, cerebral trauma or seizures, and sex offenses; current mental status, psychotropic medication, suicidal ideation, drug and alcohol use, and orientation to person, place, and time; and emotional response to incarceration. Individuals with a positive screening for mental health issues should be referred to a qualified mental health professional for a full mental health evaluation (NCCHC, 2018a, 2018b).

Finally, given the strong association between suicide and restrictive housing placement (e.g., disciplinary and/or administrative segregation), any IP assigned to an RHU should receive a medical chart review and brief screening for suicide risk by health care staff prior to admission to ensure the placement is not contraindicated (NCCHC, 2019; see Chapter 10).

When an individual with no known predisposition for suicide enters a correctional facility, routine suicide risk inquiry through an intake or reception process will suffice. But when that same individual expresses suicidal ideation or is otherwise identified as a danger to themselves, completion of a comprehensive suicide risk assessment is required. Several quick screeners, such as the Columbia-Suicide Severity Rating Scale and its various iterations, have become somewhat in vogue within corrections during the past several years, but they are wrongly utilized as both a quick screening and assessment tool to assess suicide risk.

An adequate suicide risk assessment does not rely solely on the individual's affirmation or denial of suicidal intent (Knoll, 2010). If an individual's simple denial that they were suicidal was the only criterion utilized to assess suicide risk, then it would be unnecessary to ask any other questions during the intake screening or assessment process. It would also be unnecessary to involve clinicians because any nonclinician could listen to an individual deny they were suicidal and proceed accordingly (Hayes, 2016). Rather, the standard of care requires that a comprehensive assessment of suicide risk includes thorough questioning and observation by a qualified mental health professional, as well as timely review of collateral information (APA, 2003). An empathic interview with open-ended questions is critical for individuals who feel overwhelmed or have trouble putting their feelings into words (Powsner et al., 2023). As previously discussed by the authors (Metzner & Hayes, 2020), the suicide risk assessment should include a brief mental status examination, listing of chronic and acute risk factors (including prior history of suicidal behavior), listing of any protective factors, level of suicide risk (e.g., low, medium, or high), and a treatment plan.

Specifically, the clinician's thought process and documentation should include the information included in Table 51.1.

Table 51.1 Suicide risk assessment

- History of suicidal intent or suicide attempts:
- Is there a history of admitted suicidal intent or suicide attempt?
- Severity of ideation or attempt?
- Most recent?
- Family history of suicide?
- Degree of current suicidal ideation:
- Has the person thought about how they might end their life?
- Did or does the person have a plan?
- Does the person have the means to carry out the plan?
- Was or is the plan reasonable?
- Does the person express feelings of peace/resolution?
- Is the person attending to personal effects?
- Did the person write good-bye letters?
- Systematic inquiry into:
- Current mood
- Known risk factors—individual and group
- Known protective factors
- Stated intentions about suicide
- What has changed since attempt and/or last assessment?
- Evidence or absence of futuristic thinking
- Evidence of connectedness
- Effect of suicide precautions on denial of suicidal ideation:
- Is the person's current denial of suicidal ideation being influenced by the restrictive nature of the suicide precautions (e.g., restrictive clothing, shower, food, possessions, out-of-cell time)?
- If the person is removed from suicide precautions, what is the treatment plan?

Note. Reprinted with permission from Gold, L. H., & Frierson, R. L. (2020). *The American Psychiatric Association Publishing textbook of suicide risk assessment and management* (3rd ed., Table 21-5, p. 273). American Psychiatric Association. All Rights Reserved.

Reasonable efforts should be made to assess suicide risk in a private and confidential setting (Patterson & Hughes, 2008). Unless contraindicated by security concerns, custody personnel should always accommodate these clinical requests. Cell-front encounters should never be utilized for decisions that result in discharge from suicide precautions.

Safe and humane housing

In determining the most appropriate location to house a suicidal individual, there is often the tendency for correctional officials to physically isolate the IP. Such housing may occur in a "safety cell" or holding cell of a local jail or in an RHU of a prison. In one state, dry safety cells (i.e., without sink/toilet) utilized for housing suicidal individuals are approximately 6 by 7 feet in diameter and contain a flushing ring toilet that is mounted flush with the floor, padded walls, and viewing windows that are 4 inches wide and 24 inches long (California Building Code, 2022). This response may be more convenient for staff and provide a sense of risk reduction, but it is extremely detrimental to a suicidal individual. As previously indicated, isolation is directly related to suicidal behavior, and placement in sequestered housing not only exacerbates the individual's sense of alienation but also further serves to remove the individual from proper staff supervision (Morris & Izenberg, 2023). In addition, many cells designated to house suicidal individuals are not equipped with beds, forcing IPs to sleep on the cold cement floor with nothing other than a safety smock and plastic mat. These individuals are locked down in their cells 24 hours a day, with little or no opportunity to shower. They are prohibited visits, telephone calls, or recreation (U.S. Department of Justice, 2022). Further, safety smocks can be harmful because the suicidal individual may feel further humiliated, as well as ridiculed and ostracized by other IPs (Way et al., 2013). Even if out-of-cell activities were recommended by clinical staff, an individual clothed in a safety smock may decline the opportunity to leave their cell. Safety smocks, sometimes misused by staff as a punitive sanction, are frequently unnecessary if the suicidal individual is housed in a suicide-resistant cell (Hayes, 2016; NCCHC, 2019) and receives appropriate clinical interventions.

Housing that appears punitive to the IP creates unnecessary obstacles for the clinician attempting to assess the origins of risk. Take, for example, the scenario of a clinician assessing an individual on suicide precautions. The individual has been confined in their cell for a day or two, clothed only in a safety smock and lying on a plastic mat. The clinician approaches the individual at the cell front, within easy hearing distance of both other IPs and custody staff, and asks through the closed door, "Are you suicidal?" Given the circumstances they find themselves in, the likelihood of a suicidal individual answering affirmatively to that question, the result of which will be their continued placement under these harsh conditions, is highly questionable. As such, clinicians should be very concerned about these external factors negatively impacting their ability to assess the suicidality of their patients.

Recent research in the community has cited various reasons that suicidal ideation is not disclosed to providers, including shame, embarrassment, and fear of hospitalization (Blanchard & Farber, 2018; Fulginiti & Frey, 2019). In the correctional environment, research suggests that suicidal individuals are often reluctant to discuss their suicidal thoughts because of the likelihood of being exposed to the harsh conditions of suicide precautions, with the vast majority reporting that they did not want to be transferred to an observation cell (Way et al., 2013).

Correctional officials have previously argued that the conditions of suicide precautions were not intended to be punitive but rather driven by concern for the safety of the individual. A correctional agency's commitment to safety is not being challenged here. The safety of the suicidal individual is of inherent concern when developing a suicide prevention program, but the number and types of restrictions imposed in the name of safety must be reasonable and commensurate with the individual's level of suicide risk. These officials, as well as their health care staff, also argue that suicidal individuals are unpredictable and that bad news received during a family visit, telephone call, or court hearing might trigger suicidal ideation and/or a suicide attempt. This rationale, however, ignores the obvious: What better opportunity is there to observe an individual's reaction to potentially negative news than when they are on suicide precautions? It also ignores the possibility that interaction with the outside world can be therapeutic and reduce isolation.

Clinicians often also argue that these highly restrictive measures are effective in managing individuals suspected of being manipulative or malingering. Although distinguishable, perceived manipulative behavior and suicidal behavior are not mutually exclusive. Both types of behavior could occur (or overlap) in the same individual and cause serious injury and death. Several studies of self-harm and suicide in the correctional environment have found substantial coexistence of manipulative motive with both suicidal intent and potentially high lethality of self-harming behavior (Cummings & Thompson, 2009; Dear et al., 2000; Haycock, 1989). Others have observed that there were no reliable bases upon which to differentiate low-lethality suicide attempts perceived as manipulative from those attempts that ended in death but that reviewers concluded were not the act of manipulation (Haycock, 1989). Simply stated, IPs labeled as manipulative still commit suicide.

A recommended strategy to identify suicidal individuals and encourage them not to recant their ideation when they remain suicidal is not to house them in a sterile safety or segregated cell but rather in a general population setting such as a mental health unit or medical infirmary, located in close proximity to staff (Metzner & Hayes, 2020; NCCHC, 2018a, 2018b). Of course, housing a suicidal individual in a general population unit when their security level prohibits such assignment raises a challenging issue. The result, of course, will be the assignment of the suicidal individual to a housing unit commensurate with their security level. Within a correctional system, this assignment might be an RHU. However, housing assignments should not be based on decisions that heighten the depersonalizing aspects of incarceration; they should be based on the ability to maximize staff interaction with IPs. With that said, the most important consideration is that suicidal individuals must be housed in suicide-resistant, protrusion-free cells (Hayes, 2007a; NCCHC, 2019). Further, cancellation of routine out-of-cell activities (showers, visits, telephone calls, recreation, etc.), removal of clothing (excluding belts and shoelaces), and issuance of safety smocks, as well as the use of physical restraints (restraint chairs/boards, wraps, leather straps, etc.) should be avoided whenever possible and only utilized as a last resort for periods in which the suicidal individual is physically engaging in self-destructive behavior. Finally, unless exigent circumstances exist, court hearings should not be postponed for individuals on suicide precautions.

Stability

Documentation within the suicide risk assessment should not only include a sufficient description of the current behavior but also justification for either placement on or discharge from suicide precautions. The decision to discharge an IP from suicide precautions should always be made by a qualified mental health professional (APA, 2016; NCCHC, 2019). Following placement on suicide precautions, daily assessment should focus on current behavior, as well as changes in thoughts and behavior during the previous 24 hours. For example, if suicidal ideation is denied, the evaluator should ask, "How have your feelings and thoughts changed over the past 24 hours? What are some of the things you have done or can do to change these thoughts and feelings? What has changed that makes you no longer suicidal?" Following discharge from suicide precautions, periodic follow-up assessments based on an individualized safety plan are highly recommended. The safety plan should include a specific strategy that describes signs, symptoms, and the circumstances in which the risk for suicide is likely to recur, how recurrence of suicidal thoughts can be avoided, and actions the patient and clinician can take if suicidal thoughts do occur.

Continuous quality improvement

Continuous quality improvement not only allows the insight to confirm what goes well in the delivery of health care services to IPs but also provides the tools to identify and correct deficiencies and to sustain corrective actions (Schiff & Shansky, 2006). Sustainability of a comprehensive suicide prevention program can only be achieved through a continuous quality improvement process spearheaded by a multidisciplinary suicide prevention committee (Canning & Dvoskin, 2016; see Chapter 74). The committee meets regularly (monthly or quarterly) and oversees implementation of the agency's suicide prevention program, as well as corrective actions arising from mortality reviews of suicides. When sustainability of suicide prevention efforts begins to slip, the suicide prevention committee intercedes and restores program components to previously acceptable levels. With appropriate commitment and resources, the overall suicide prevention program can measure implementation and intermediate outcomes to better understand what metrics are best working to reduce the risk of suicide in the correctional environment (Obegi, 2024).

Unless the death was comprehensively examined, conclusions should never be made that an individual's suicide was not preventable (Hayes, 2013). The mortality review process is a critical ingredient to a correctional facility's suicide prevention program. The process can be instrumental in identifying systemic deficiencies (Patterson & Hughes, 2008). A thorough examination of an IP's death, encompassing both a mortality review and a psychological autopsy, is cited in most national standards (NCCHC, 2018a, 2018b) but often not done correctly. In many cases, a mortality review is not completed or is limited to a cursory review of the decedent's medical record by a health care professional, as well as a review of incident reports that summarize the emergency response to the incident. Although there are various references to psychological autopsies for custodial suicide in the literature (Aufderheide, 2000; Kovasznay et al., 2004), the process is often misunderstood and misused within the correctional environment. Rather than encompassing a thorough review of the medical record, an examination of the decedent's cell and belongings, and interviews with staff and IPs familiar with the decedent, as well as family members when appropriate, many of these critical components are ignored, with only medical record reviews completed and mislabeled as psychological autopsies (Hayes, 2022).

The primary purpose of a mortality review is to determine what happened in the case under review and what can be learned to help prevent future incidents. The multidisciplinary review should include (a) critical review of the circumstances surrounding the incident; (b) critical review of facility procedures relevant to the incident; (c) synopsis of all relevant training received by involved staff; (d) review of pertinent medical and mental health services/reports involving the decedent; (e) review of possible precipitating factors (i.e., circumstances that may have caused the decedent to engage in self-injury/suicide); and (f) recommendations, if any, for change in policy, training, physical plant, medical or mental health services, and operational procedures (Hayes, 2007b, 2022). Such recommendations should result in a corrective action plan that identifies specific deficiencies, responsible parties to address deficiencies, deadlines for completion, and methods for continuous quality improvement by the suicide prevention committee to ensure that corrective action is maintained.

Other risk reduction strategies

All correctional, medical, and mental health personnel and other staff who have regular contact with IPs should receive 8 hours of initial suicide prevention training, followed by 2 hours of refresher training each year (Hayes, 2016). The initial training should include instruction regarding administrator and staff attitudes about suicide and how negative attitudes impede suicide prevention efforts, why correctional environments are conducive to suicidal behavior, potential predisposing factors to suicide, high-risk suicide periods, warning signs and symptoms, how to identify suicidal individuals despite a denial of risk, components of the facility's suicide prevention policy, and liability issues. The 2-hour refresher training reviews selective topics discussed during the initial training and describes any changes to the facility's suicide prevention plan. The annual training should also include a general discussion of recent suicides and/or serious suicide attempts in the facility. In addition, all correctional and medical staff should receive recurrent training in standard first aid, cardiopulmonary resuscitation, and the use of emergency equipment located in each housing unit, with incorporation of mock drills into initial and refresher training (Hayes, 2016).

Furthermore, there are only two levels of supervision recommended for IPs identified as suicidal: close observation and constant observation (APA, 2016; NCCHC, 2019). Close observation is reserved for the individual who is not acutely suicidal but expresses suicidal ideation (e.g., expressing a wish to die without a specific threat or plan) and/or has a recent prior history of self-destructive behavior that places them at higher risk. Staff should observe such an individual at staggered intervals not to exceed 10 to 15 minutes (e.g., 5, 10, 7 minutes). In addition, an individual who denies suicidal ideation or does not threaten suicide but demonstrates other concerning behavior (through actions, current circumstances, or recent history) indicating the potential for self-injury should be placed on close observation. Close observation is often utilized as a step-down from constant observation status when a period of demonstrated stability is needed. Constant observation is reserved for the individual who is acutely suicidal, either threatening suicide with a specific plan or engaging in self-injurious behavior or a suicide attempt. Such an individual should be observed on a continuous, uninterrupted basis by assigned staff. Closed-circuit television monitoring may be used as a supplement to, but never as a replacement for, close or constant observation. Suicide prevention aides/companions, pulse oximetry, and other antisuicide technology products that separate staff from the suicidal individual are not recommended (Hayes, 2013).

Summary

Components of a basic suicide prevention program are well established and reflected in national standards, but these components often have the unintended consequence of deterring suicidal individuals from expressing their ideation and/or encouraging them to recant it. Creating a therapeutic environment that encourages suicidal individuals to express themselves, as well as developing effective strategies to identify those who do not, is critical to future suicide prevention efforts within correctional facilities. As suicide risk fluctuates based on changes in environment and circumstances, the assessment of suicide risk must not be seen as static; rather, it is an ongoing process throughout the individual's incarceration. In light of a changing correctional environment that includes more vulnerable individuals and fewer inpatient beds, there is a need for greater attention to proactive and creative measures that will reduce the risk of suicide in jails and prisons. As a prominent clinician once stated, "Most suicides, although by no means all, can be prevented. The breach between what we know and do is lethal" (Jamison, 1999, p. 25).

REFERENCES

American Psychiatric Association. (2003). Practice guideline for the assessment and treatment of patients with suicidal behaviors. *American Journal of Psychiatry, 160*(Suppl.), 1–60.

American Psychiatric Association. (2016). *Psychiatric services in correctional facilities* (3rd ed.).

Aufderheide, D. (2000). Conducting the psychological autopsy in correctional settings. *Journal of Correctional Health Care, 7*, 5–36.

Berman, A. L., & Canning, R. D. (2022). Proximal risk for suicide in correctional settings: A call for priority research. *Psychological Services, 19*, 407–412.

Blanchard, M., & Farber, B. A. (2018). It is never okay to talk about suicide: Patients' reasons for concealing suicidal ideation in psychotherapy. *Psychotherapy Research, 30*, 1–13.

Bonner, R. L. (2006). Stressful segregation housing and psychosocial vulnerability in prison suicide ideators. *Suicide & Life-Threatening Behavior, 36*, 250–254.

California Building Code, Title 24, Part 2, § 1231.2.5, Safety Cell (2022).

California Department of Corrections and Rehabilitation. (2023). *2022 annual report on suicides and suicide prevention efforts in the CDCR*. https://cchcs.ca.gov/wp-content/uploads/sites/60/2022-Annual-Report.pdf

Canning, R. D., & Dvoskin, J. A. (2016). Preventing suicide in detention and correctional facilities. In J. Wooldredge & P. Smith (Eds.), *The Oxford handbook of prisons and imprisonment* (pp. 1–31). Oxford University Press.

Carson, E. A. (2021). *Suicide in local jails and state and federal prisons, 2000–2019—Statistical tables*. Bureau of Justice Statistics Special Report. U.S. Department of Justice.

Cummings, D. L., & Thompson, M. N. (2009). Suicidal or manipulative? The role of mental health counselors in overcoming a false dichotomy in identifying and treating self-harming inmates. *Journal of Mental Health Counseling, 31*, 201–212.

Dear, G. E., Thomson, D. M., & Hills, A. M. (2000). Self-harm in prison: Manipulators can also be suicide attempters. *27*(2).

Daniel, A., & Fleming, J. (2006). Suicides in a state correctional system, 1992–2002: A review. *Journal of Correctional Health Care, 12*, 24–35.

Fazel, S., Ramesh, T., & Hawton, K. (2017). Suicide in prisons: An international study of prevalence and contributory factors. *Lancet Psychiatry, 4*, 946–952.

Fulginiti, A., & Frey, L. M. (2019). Exploring suicide-related disclosure motivation and the impact on mechanisms linked to suicide. *Death Studies, 43*, 562–569.

Garnett, M. F., Curtin, S. C., & Stone, D. M. (2022). *Suicide mortality in the United States, 2000–2020* (NCHS Data Brief, No. *433)*. National Center for Health Statistics.

Goodwin, G. (2022). *Deaths in custody: Additional action needed to help ensure data collected by DOJ are utilized* (GAO-22-106033). Government Accountability Office. https://www.hsgac.senate.gov/imo/media/doc/ Goodwin%20Testimony.pdf

Haycock, J. (1989). Manipulation and suicide attempts in jails and prisons. *Psychiatric Quarterly, 60*, 85–98.

Hayes, L. M. (1989). National study of jail suicide: Seven years later. *Psychiatric Quarterly, 60*, 7–29.

Hayes, L. M. (2007a). Suicide prevention and designing safer prison cells. In G. Dear (Ed.), *Preventing suicide and other self-harm in prison* (pp. 167–174). Palgrave MacMillan.

Hayes, L. M. (2007b). Responding to suicides in custody: Review processes. In G. Dear (Ed.), *Preventing suicide and other self-harm in prison* (pp. 206–214). Palgrave MacMillan.

Hayes, L. M. (2012). National study of jail suicide: 20 years later. *Journal of Correctional Health Care, 18*, 233–245.

Hayes, L. M. (2013). Suicide prevention in correctional facilities: Reflections and next steps. *International Journal of Law and Psychiatry, 36*, 188–194.

Hayes, L. M. (2016). *Training curriculum and program guide on suicide detection and prevention in jail and prison facilities*. National Center on Institutions and Alternatives.

Hayes, L. M. (2022). Reducing inmate suicides through the mortality review process. In R. Greifinger (Ed.), *Public health behind bars: From prisons to communities* (2nded., pp. 303–312). Springer Science and Business Media.

He, X. Y., Felthous, A. R., Holzer, C. E., Nathan, P., & Veasey, S. (2001). Factors in prison suicide: One-year study in Texas. *Journal of Forensic Sciences, 46*, 896–901.

James, N. (2023). *Death in custody reporting act: Background and legislative considerations* (CSR R47559). Congressional Research Service. https://crsreports.congress.gov/product/pdf/R/R47559/

Jamison, K. (1999). *Night falls fast—Understanding suicide*. Knopf.

Knoll, J. L. (2010). Suicide in correctional settings: Assessment, prevention, and professional liability. *Journal of Correctional Health Care, 16*, 188–204.

Kovasznay, B., Miraglia, R., Beer, R., & Way, B. (2004). Reducing suicides in New York state correctional facilities. *Psychiatric Quarterly, 75*, 61–70.

Metzner, J. L., & Hayes, L. M. (2020). Suicide prevention in jails and prisons. In L. Gold & R. Frierson (Eds.), *Textbook of suicide assessment and management* (3rd ed., pp. 265–277). American Psychiatric Publishing.

Morris, N. P., & Izenberg, J. M. (2023). Nowhere else to go-solitary confinement as mental health care. *JAMA, 330*, 17–18.

National Commission on Correctional Health Care. (2018a). *Standards for health services in jails*.

National Commission on Correctional Health Care. (2018b). *Standards for health services in prisons*.

National Commission on Correctional Health Care. (2019). *Suicide prevention resource guide*. https://www.ncchc.org/new-suicide-prevention-resource-guide-for-corrections/

Obegi, J. H. (2024). Monitoring a correctional suicide prevention program: The roles of implementation and intermediate outcomes. *Psychology, Public Policy, and Law, 30*, 59–65.

Patterson, R., & Hughes, K. (2008). Review of completed suicides in the California department of corrections and rehabilitation, 1999 to 2004. *Psychiatric Services, 59*, 676–682.

Pompili, M., Murri, B., Patti, S., et al. (2016). The communication of suicidal intentions: A meta-analysis. *Psychological Medicine, 46*, 2239–2253.

Powsner, S., Goebert, D., Richmond, J. S., & Takeshita, J. (2023). Suicide risk assessment, management, and mitigation in the emergency setting. *Focus: Journal of Lifelong Learning in Psychiatry, 21*, 8–17.

Reeves, R., & Tamburello, A. (2014). Single cells, segregated housing, and suicide in the New Jersey department of corrections. *Journal of the American Academy of Psychiatry and the Law, 42*, 484–488.

Resnik, J., Albertson, S., Li, G., & Taylor, J. (2022). *Time-in-cell: A 2021 snapshot of restrictive housing based on a nationwide survey of U.S. prison systems*. https://ssrn.com/abstract=4206981

Schiff, G. D., & Shansky, R. (2006). Challenges of improving quality in the correctional setting. In M. Puisis (Ed.), *Clinical practice in correctional medicine* (2nd ed., pp. 491–502). Mosby Elsevier.

Scott, R., Aboud, A., & Smith, T. (2023). Using the stress–vulnerability model to better understand suicide in prison populations. *Psychiatry, Psychology and Law, 30*, 299–333.

Shneidman, E. (1987, March). At the point of no return. *Psychology Today*.

Spiers, E. M., Pitt, S. E., & Dvoskin, J. A. (2006). Psychiatric intake screening. In M. Puisis (Ed.), *Clinical practice in correctional medicine* (pp. 285–291). Mosby Elsevier.

Texas Civil Rights Project & The University of Texas School of Law Civil Rights Clinic. (2023). *Solitary confinement in Texas: A crisis with no end*. Texas Civil Rights Project. https://aab91155-966e-43a7-af87-a209b39e1f8b.usrfiles.com/ugd/a4ea0d_7738c8c3097148ef814e8c157936335e.pdf

U.S. Department of Justice, Civil Rights Division. (2022). *Investigation of the Mississippi state penitentiary (Parchman)*. www.justice.gov/d9/press-releases/attachments/2022/04/20/mdoc_parchman_findings_report_0.pdf

U.S. Department of Justice, Office of the Inspector General. (2024). *Evaluation of issues surrounding inmate deaths in Federal Bureau of Prisons institutions*. https://oig.justice.gov/sites/default/files/reports/24-041.pdf

Way, B., Kaufman, A. R., Knoll, J. L., & Chlebowski, S.M. (2013). Suicidal ideation among inmate-patients in state prison: Prevalence, reluctance to report, and treatment preferences. *Behavioral Sciences & the Law, 31*, 230–238.

Way, B., Sawyer, D., Barboza, S., & Nash, R. (2007). Inmate suicide and time spent in special disciplinary housing in New York state prison. *Psychiatric Services, 58*, 558–560.

Zhong, S., Senior, M., Yu, R., Perry, A., Hawton, K., Shaw, J., & Fazel, S. (2021). Risk factors for suicide in prisons: A systematic review and meta-analysis. *Lancet Public Health, 6*, 164–174.

52

Self-injurious behaviors

Sharen Barboza[1]

Introduction

Self-injurious behavior (SIB) in correctional facilities has similarities and differences with occurrences in community settings. Along with some common precipitants, associated diagnoses, and effective interventions, the behavior in jails and prisons has unique aspects compared to other environments. This chapter provides an overview of SIB, with special focus on correctional considerations and challenges.

Definition

Diverse terminology and definitions have been used to describe SIB. In addition to "self-injury," commonly used terms have included "nonsuicidal self-injury," "self-harm," "self-mutilation," "suicide spectrum behavior," and "parasuicide." The terms "self-injury" and "SIB" in this chapter refer to acts intended to cause bodily harm but not death. These acts typically involve cutting, burning, self-hitting, self-biting, head banging, and ingesting or inserting foreign objects. SIB does not include damaging or risky behavior that does not have the primary goal of causing harm, such as tattooing, body piercing, substance misuse, or autoerotic acts.

Although the distinction between SIB and suicidal behaviors has important conceptual and treatment implications, the boundary is not always clear (O'Carroll et al., 1996). Determinations of intent rely primarily on self-reports, which have limited reliability, especially among incarcerated populations. Some individuals have ambivalence about the possibility of dying, have limited self-awareness or insight, and/or deliberately provide misleading self-reports regarding intent. Even a true absence of suicidal intent does not eliminate potential lethality. Therefore, awareness and treatment of incarcerated persons (IPs) who engage in SIB, regardless of intent, is important in reducing risk of injury and death (Yasmeen et al., 2023).

Reasons for self-injurious behaviors

In the broadest terms, SIB may be viewed as a response to an internal state or external circumstances. The behavior provides relief or escape from unpleasant emotions or cognitions in the former and adverse environments or interpersonal interactions in the latter. Regulation of negative affect such as anxiety and anger typically serves as the most prevalent function of SIB (Dixon-Gordon et al., 2012; Klonsky, 2007). Environmental and interpersonal factors play a role as well (Gardner et al., 2016), and they likely have greater significance in correctional settings than in the community for reasons described later in this chapter. Understanding the factors that trigger and support SIB has important implications for treatment and management.

Epidemiology

In community samples, 4% to 6% of adults report a history of SIB, with no significant gender differences in rate (Klonsky, 2011). Surveys of state and federal prisons in the United States found that 2% to 2.4% of IPs per year self-injure (Appelbaum et al., 2011; H. P. Smith & Kaminski, 2011). An international review of SIB in correctional settings revealed that, overall, 3.8% of IPs engage in SIB during incarceration (Favril et al., 2020). Rates in the other countries range from 0.7% in Israel (Vinokur & Levine, 2019) to 6.6% in the United Kingdom (Knight et al., 2017). Although relatively few IPs engage in this behavior, they do so often enough that almost all systems responding to the survey by Appelbaum and colleagues (2011) reported at least weekly incidents. More than 70% of systems in the United States reported episodes occurring several times per week to more than once per day. Almost half of the prison systems reported that they maintain no data related to SIB, and the remainder track only limited information. H. P. Smith and Kaminski (2011) found that 98% of U.S. facilities reported housing at least one individual who engaged in SIB.

1. The author acknowledges the contribution of Kenneth Applebaum, MD, who was the author of this chapter in the first edition of this textbook.

Diagnosis and assessment

SIB can occur in the context of several diagnoses or in the absence of an underlying psychiatric disorder. The *Diagnostic and Statistical Manual of Mental Disorders*, 5th edition, text revision (American Psychiatric Association, 2022) does not recognize SIB as a diagnostic category but includes "nonsuicidal self-injury" as a condition for further study and research. The same diagnostic considerations apply to IPs as to people in community settings; however, jail and prison environments often play a disproportionate role in supporting these behaviors.

Any psychiatric diagnosis elevates the risk for engaging in SIB while incarcerated, but the most common disorders are major depressive disorder, borderline personality disorder, anxiety disorders, and substance use disorders (Favril et al., 2020; Hakansson et al., 2011; Verdolini et al., 2017). Emerging research has also found SIB among individuals diagnosed with antisocial personality disorder (Yang et al., 2022). Unlike the routine treatment of these conditions in correctional settings, which are discussed elsewhere in this book, self-injury that occurs in the context of these disorders often has distinguishing characteristics. Additionally, studies have shown that large percentages of individuals who engage in SIB while incarcerated have past experiences of trauma (Knight et al., 2017; Walker et al., 2021).

Extreme acts of self-injury that result in significant tissue damage or permanent loss of functioning of a body organ occur most commonly in association with psychosis (Large et al., 2009). These acts include damage to or enucleation of the eye, amputation of a digit or limb, and genital mutilation unrelated to gender dysphoria. The psychiatrist should respond to such behaviors as psychiatric emergencies due to a psychotic disorder until proven otherwise.

Borderline personality disorder is the diagnosis most commonly associated with self-injury. SIB often serves to relieve overwhelming affective experiences of individuals with borderline personality disorder, and for some, the pain or the sight of blood counteracts dissociative states.

Self-injury among individuals with developmental and neurocognitive conditions typically presents as repeated, stereotypic self-injurious behaviors such as scratching, head banging and hitting, and hand biting (Furniss & Biswas, 2020).

IPs, however, often have motives for self-harm that have little to do with symptoms of a primary psychiatric disorder. Thus, the psychiatric assessment must focus on more than diagnosis. Without an understanding of the factors driving and supporting SIB, medical, mental health, and custody staff cannot formulate effective interventions or management plans. Adequate assessment requires sensitive but frank and direct history-taking.

Several self-report scales and structured interviews exist for assessment of self-injury (e.g., Faura-Garcia et al., 2020; Sansone & Sansone, 2010; Timberlake et al., 2020; Whitlock et al., 2014). Systematic reviews of risk assessment tools within correctional settings have focused primarily on suicide risk screening and have found limited predictive validity (Gould et al., 2018; Perry et al., 2010). There is initial evidence for the utility of self-harm risk screenings in correctional settings (Browne et al., 2023; Ryland et al., 2020). Although the instruments have high face validity, they need validation beyond the original sample. Whether through questionnaires or structured or unstructured interviews, the correctional psychiatrist needs to understand the history of the behavior and the function that it serves for the individual. Basic elements to explore include age of onset, known triggers, frequency, methods used, environmental and social context, severity, and outcomes. Working collaboratively with a psychologist or behaviorist to develop a functional analysis of the SIB will prove beneficial in understanding and providing effective interventions to reduce the behavior over time.

Precipitants for self-harm in correctional settings

Environmental factors (behavioral triggers and responses) play a key role in SIB, especially in jails and prisons. Self-injury can return a degree of control and autonomy to IPs who otherwise have limited means to affect their environment, cope with stress, communicate their needs/wants, or have those needs/wants addressed. Environmental triggers include interpersonal conflict, social isolation, relationship problems, and perceived injustice. Environmental responses that reinforce the behaviors can include positive and negative attention, change in housing, access to desired items or staff, temporary diversion (e.g., infirmary or hospital), desired medications, and disruption to the environment.

The highest rate of SIB occurs in restrictive housing and other segregated or punitive isolation units (Appelbaum et al., 2011; Favril et al., 2020; Kaba et al., 2014). As a group, IPs placed in restrictive settings may have a predisposition toward these behaviors, including an increased prevalence of serious psychiatric disorders (Lovell, 2008; O'Keefe & Schnell, 2007), increased levels of impulsivity, and a propensity toward violence. Nevertheless, the extreme conditions of confinement, including limited time out of cell, restricted privileges, isolation, and sensory overload or deprivation, can result in significant psychological distress (Grassian, 1983; P. S. Smith, 2006; see Chapter 10). For some individuals, physical pain provides a distraction and relief from mounting and intolerable psychological pain. The response by custody, medical, and mental health staff provides human contact, lessens the boredom and monotony of isolation, and can result in a temporary move to a less harsh setting. Additional reinforcement occurs if IPs obtain access to sought-after medications.

The most vexing situations for correctional staff arise when IPs use self-injury in response to interpersonal conflicts and anger, with a goal of retaliation for perceived insults or unjust sanctions (Doty et al., 2012). SIB impedes normal operations and diverts staff from other activities. IPs can exert control over the timing and severity of SIB, which can result in maximum disruption for the facility, effectively communicating the IP's anger and restoring a sense of empowerment.

Treatment and management of self-harm in correctional settings

Staff partnership

Effective management of self-injurious behaviors in correctional settings almost always requires cooperation among health care and custody staff. Disputes over who bears responsibility to address the problem serve little purpose, create discord, and impede progress. Whether these behaviors are driven by the presence of a psychotic disorder or are willful and deliberate acts of an individual who wants a change in housing, they are not signs of a mentally healthy person, and correctional psychiatrists need to participate actively in assessment and management of IPs who act this way. At the same time, however, custody staff evade their own responsibility if they expect mental health professionals to address the situation on their own. The demonstrably disturbed nature of the behavior, no matter how extreme or bizarre, does not make the matter a problem for mental health staff alone to solve. Effective interventions sometimes require creative use of privileges, property, or placement, none of which psychiatrists can order with a prescription. Structured, phase-based behavioral interventions, built in collaboration with the IP and custody staff, are effective in reducing the frequency and severity of self-injury (Andrade et al., 2014; Barboza & Wilson, 2011).

Treatment interventions

When psychiatric disorders contribute to self-injurious behavior, IPs should receive appropriate psychiatric treatment. Those who appear to have underlying depression may benefit from antidepressant medications. When command auditory hallucinations prompt self-injury, antipsychotic medication is likely indicated. Purely behavioral interventions may succeed for individuals with neurodevelopmental disabilities, although medication can sometimes play a role. Dialectical behavior therapy and cognitive-behavioral therapy, the most widely studied psychotherapeutic interventions for patients with borderline personality disorder and others who self-injure, have shown efficacy in reducing self-harm and improving functioning (Winicov, 2019), including in correctional settings (Shelton et al., 2009).

When a primary psychiatric disorder does not contribute to self-injury, pharmacotherapy has a limited role in reducing the behavior (Timberlake et al., 2020). Choice of agent relies on careful assessment of the underlying causes of self-injury, which are not always clear. In addition, medication rarely resolves the SIB and, at best, serves as an adjunct to environmental, interpersonal, and behavioral interventions described elsewhere in this chapter. The more challenging task for the correctional psychiatrist may entail tempering expectations for a simple pharmacological answer and resisting pressures to medicate inappropriately. Polypharmacy without compelling justification poses a particular problem. Discontinuation of medications after unsuccessful trials usually makes the most sense.

The absence of a serious psychiatric disorder as the primary cause of self-injury does not mean that mental health professionals have no role to play, even when the root cause involves conflict between the IP and custody staff. Dismissing the behavior as manipulative accomplishes nothing. It should come as no surprise that some IPs will resort to self-harm to achieve their goals when they have few other persuasive tools at their disposal. Identifying those goals actually provides the basis for formulating a predictable custody response and structuring effective behavioral interventions. All staff should view understanding the function of SIB as the first step in management.

Behavioral interventions are key. Behavior therapy may be part of individualized treatment plans or group programming in specialized residential treatment units. Extinction of SIB, however, is not a realistic goal for most individuals. Staff and the IP need to view a lessening of the frequency and/or severity of events as a successful outcome. Achieving this requires patience. Behaviors can actually worsen during initial phases of intervention. Progress takes months, even years, not days or weeks. The greatest likelihood of successful behavioral therapy occurs with the use of dialectical behavior therapy and cognitive-behavioral therapy principles, including patient agreement with specific goals and structured treatment strategies; close monitoring; skill enhancement; and a nonconfrontational, present-oriented approach (Lynch & Cozza, 2009; Winicov, 2019). Treatment providers who work with this population need ready access to support, consultation, and supervision.

Concerns sometimes arise about using behavioral rewards that gratify IPs' desires. Both custody and health care staff may fear outbreaks of contagion in which other IPs engage in SIB to achieve their own goals. Clinicians and administrators might also want to avoid appearing weak in the eyes of colleagues or IPs by giving in to a self-injurer's demands. Clinical experience, however, does not warrant excessive fear of contagion (Fagan et al., 2010). Very few individuals have the desire or the resolve to imitate serious self-harm to achieve their ends, and most IPs will acknowledge this if asked. As for concerns about the appearance of weakness, rejection of effective interventions merely because others will perceive it as a weakness is countertherapeutic and naïve. A more effective and professional strategy focuses on the use of evidence-based interventions that lead to real behavior change, not fears of others' perceptions. Managing self-injury is not a zero-sum game; both sides can achieve their desired goals. Getting there, however, requires motivation and remembering that rewards work better than punishments in shaping behaviors.

Staff reactions

Clinical and custody staff may face other personal and professional challenges when dealing with self-injurious IPs. Bizarre behaviors commonly encountered in correctional settings, such as foreign body insertion or ingestion, occur relatively infrequently in other settings and may unsettle some clinicians. Staff may be unwilling to admit these impacts (H. P. Smith et al., 2019), but if not acknowledged and addressed, feelings of distress or powerlessness can contribute to a loss of professional perspective, including use of pejorative language about self-injuring IPs. Along with the word "manipulative," dismissive terms such as "attention seeking" or "acting out" may arise. As a dangerous subtext, such terms minimize potential lethality. Published studies, as well as professional anecdotes, indicate that many self-inflicted fatalities occur in the apparent absence of suicidal intent among IPs deemed "manipulative" or "too antisocial" to kill themselves (Dear et al., 2000; H. P. Smith & Kaminski, 2010). Research has also shown that negative attitudes toward IPs who self-injure have been associated with increased hostility and lower quality of care (Hewson et al., 2022). With an awareness of personal distress and language use, the correctional psychiatrist can model appropriate responses and terminology for other staff.

Safety planning

The first edition of this chapter included a discussion about safety contracts. The limited utility of these "contracts" is now well understood by clinicians, especially in the absence of a well-established, therapeutic relationship. Instead, the use of safety planning interventions, as originally set forth by Stanley and Brown (2011), has proven to be a viable means of supporting individuals in collaboratively developing a list of warning signs, coping strategies, and resources that individuals can use instead of engaging in self-injury (Ferguson et al., 2021; Marshall et al., 2023).

Physical restraints

During an acute, ongoing episode of self-injury, an IP may need to be physically restrained when other reasonable interventions have failed to provide sufficient safety (see Chapter 25). Custody staff can apply restraints for security reasons; in some systems, medical staff can order them as a mental health intervention. Mental health restraints require clinical justifications and procedures. The American Psychiatric Association issued a resource document to help guide the use of mental health restraints in jails and prisons (Metzner et al., 2007). In recognition of the nontherapeutic aspects of the correctional environment, Appelbaum (2007) recommended that restraints only be used in response to SIB while arranging for transfer to an acute, inpatient setting. For similar reasons, standards in the United Kingdom limit the application of restraints to nonclinical prison correctional staff with security and custody responsibilities (O'Grady, 2007). Clearly, the use of physical restraints in carceral settings remains an unsettled topic, requiring careful consideration.

Suicide watch

Suicide watch, or the placement of an IP in isolation in a suicide-resistant room, with a tear-resistant smock, limited to no property, under the observation of staff, is often used in response to SIB (see Chapter 51). While the rationale for such placement is safety, far too often it is used as punishment, long after the acute risk of self-harm has passed. Suicide watch is not a treatment intervention. The placement of an individual on suicide watch is isolating, negatively affects therapeutic alliances, and fosters feelings of abandonment and shame. Placement on suicide watch should only occur when the individual demonstrates an imminent risk for ongoing SIB despite less restrictive interventions. Out-of-cell treatment should be provided daily, if not multiple times per day, with clear goals to be achieved, and removal from suicide watch should occur as soon as the goals have been met.

Hospitalization

When an IP engages in serious and ongoing SIB, transfer to a hospital may be considered. Psychiatric hospitalization runs the risk of reinforcing the behaviors, especially for IPs who seek respite from restrictive housing units. One recommended strategy involves providing IPs with infirmary placements as rewards for set amounts of time without SIB and avoiding such placements in response to SIB (Fagan et al., 2010). While symptoms often rapidly dissipate after hospitalization, this temporary intervention does not address the root cause of the problem when the harsh conditions of isolation contribute to psychological decompensation. A longer term solution involves the availability of housing units with less extreme isolation for IPs who need high security and treatment for SIB. Such units require creative collaboration among custody, medical, and mental health staff.

Trauma

In addition to discussing the prevalence, management, and treatment of IPs who engage in SIB, it is important to acknowledge and address trauma in the histories of these individuals. Research has shown that the majority of IPs who engage in self-injury have histories of interpersonal trauma, often early in life (Dixon-Gordon et al., 2012; Walker et al., 2021). Traumatic experiences can result in memories, emotions, and thoughts that serve as triggers for SIB. Further, challenges with trust and attachment often thwart the ability to form therapeutic alliances, which are required to facilitate effective treatment outcomes. Correctional psychiatrists should familiarize themselves with trauma-informed approaches (Substance Abuse and Mental Health Services Administration, 2023) and support their wider implementation within correctional settings.

Summary

SIB poses significant challenges for correctional facilities and significant risks to those who engage in the behavior. Although relatively few IPs engage in these acts, their impact is broad. The etiology and treatment of self-injury in jails and prisons have both similarities and differences with community settings. Effective management requires collaboration and a coordinated, planned response by clinical and custody staff. Treatment requires the use of evidence-based strategies. In most instances, this calls for a flexible approach to the environmental factors that contribute to the behavior. Maintaining a professional perspective and an openness to creative use of behavioral interventions increases the likelihood of success in lessening the frequency and severity of SIB.

REFERENCES

American Psychiatric Association. (2022). *Diagnostic and statistical manual of mental disorders* (5th ed., text rev.).

Andrade, J. T., Wilson, J. S., Franko, E., Deitsch, J., & Barboza, S. (2014). Developing the evidence base for reducing chronic inmate self-injury: Outcome measures for behavior management. *Corrections Today, 76*(6), 30–35.

Appelbaum, K. L. (2007). Commentary: The use of restraint and seclusion in correctional mental health. *Journal of the American Academy of Psychiatry & the Law, 35*, 431–435.

Appelbaum, K. L., Savageau, J. A., Trestman, R. L., Metzner, J. L., & Baillargeon, J. (2011). A national survey of self-injurious behavior in American prisons. *Psychiatric Services, 62*, 285–290.

Barboza, S., & Wilson, J. S. (2011). Behavior management plans decrease inmate self-injury. *Corrections Today, 73*(5), 34–37.

Browne, C., Chemjong, P., Korobanova, D., et al. (2023). Self-harm screening on prison entry: Assessing the predictive validity of self-harm history and recent ideation in men and women. *International Journal of Prisoner Health, 19*(3), 414–426.

Dear, G. E., Thomson, D. M., & Hills, A. M. (2000). Self-harm in prison: Manipulators can also be suicide attempters. *Criminal Justice and Behavior, 27*, 160–175.

Dixon-Gordon, K., Harrison, N., & Roesch, R. (2012). Non-suicidal self-injury within offender populations: A systematic review. *International Journal of Forensic Mental Health, 11*, 33–50.

Doty, S., Smith, H. P., & Rojek, J. (2012). Self-injurious behaviors in corrections: Informal social control and institutional responses in a state prison system. *Victims & Offenders: An International Journal of Evidence-Based Research, Policy, and Practice, 7*, 30–52.

Fagan, T. J., Cox, J., Helfand, S. J., & Aufderheide, D. (2010). Self-injurious behavior in correctional settings. *Journal of Correctional Health Care, 16*, 48–66.

Faura-Garcia, J., Orue, I., & Calvete, E. (2021). Clinical assessment of non-suicidal self-injury: A systematic review of instruments. *Clinical Psychology & Psychotherapy, 28*, 739–765.

Favril, L., Yu, R., Hawton, K., & Fazel, S. (2020). Risk factors for self-harm in prison: A systematic review and meta-analysis. *Lancet Psychiatry*, *7*, 682–691.

Ferguson, M., Rhodes, K., Loughhead, M., McIntyre, H., & Procter, N. (2022). The effectiveness of the safety planning intervention for adults experiencing suicide-related distress: A systematic review. *Archives of Suicide Research*, *26*(3), 1022–1045.

Furniss, F., & Biswas, A. B. (2020). Conceptualization and taxonomy of self-injurious behavior. In F. Furniss & A. B. Biswas (Eds.), *Self-injurious behavior in individuals with neurodevelopmental conditions* (pp. 1–18). Springer.

Gardner, K. J., Dodsworth, J., & Klonsky, E. D. (2016). Reasons for non-suicidal self-harm in adult male offenders with and without borderline traits. *Archives of Suicide Research*, *20*, 614–634.

Gould, C., McGeorge, T., & Slade, K. (2018). Suicide screening tools for use in incarcerated offenders: A systematic review. *Archives of Suicide Research*, *22*(3), 345–364.

Grassian, S. (1983). Psychopathological effects of solitary confinement. *American Journal of Psychiatry*, *140*, 1450–1454.

Hakansson, A., Bradvik, L., Schlyter, F., & Berglund, M. (2011). Variables associated with repeated suicide attempt in a criminal justice population. *Suicide and Life-Threatening Behavior*, *41*(5), 517–531.

Hewson, T., Gutridge, K., Bernard, Z., Kay, K., & Robinson, L. (2022). A systematic review and mixed-methods synthesis of the experiences, perceptions, and attitudes of prison staff regarding adult prisoners who self-harm. *BJPsych Open*, *8*, e102.

Kaba, F., Lewis, A., Glowa-Kollisch, S., et al. (2014). Solitary confinement and risk of self-harm among jail inmates. *American Journal of Public Health*, *104*(3), 442–447.

Klonsky, E. D. (2007). The functions of deliberate self-injury: A review of the evidence. *Clinical Psychology Review*, *27*, 226–239.

Klonsky, E. D. (2011). Non-suicidal self-injury in United States adults: Prevalence, sociodemographics, topography and functions. *Psychological Medicine*, *41*(9), 1981–1986.

Knight, B., Coid, J., & Ullrich, S. (2017). Non-suicidal self-injury in UK prisoners. *International Journal of Forensic Mental Health*, *16*(2), 172–182.

Large, M., Babidge, N., Andrews, D., et al. (2009). Major self-mutilation in the first episode of psychosis. *Schizophrenia Bulletin*, *35*, 1012–1021.

Lovell, D. (2008). Patterns of disturbed behavior in a supermax population. *Criminal Justice and Behavior*, *35*, 985–1004.

Lynch, T. R., & Cozza, C. (2009). Behavior therapy for nonsuicidal self-injury. In M. K. Nock (Ed.), *Understanding nonsuicidal self-injury: Origins, assessment, and treatment* (pp. 211–250). American Psychological Association.

Marshall, C. A., Crowley, P., Carmichael, D., et al. (2023). Effectiveness of suicide safety planning interventions: A systematic review informing occupational therapy. *Canadian Journal of Occupational Therapy*, *90*(2), 208–236.

Metzner, J. L., Tardiff, K., Lion, J., et al. (2007). Resource document on the use of restraint and seclusion in correctional mental health care. *Journal of the American Academy of Psychiatry & the Law*, *35*, 417–425.

O'Carroll, P. W., Berman, A., Maris, R. W., Moscicki, E. K., Tanney, B. L., & Silverman, M. M. (1996). Beyond the tower of Babel: A nomenclature for suicidology. *Suicide and Life-Threatening Behavior*, *26*(3), 237–252.

O'Grady, J. C. (2007). Commentary: A British perspective on the use of restraint and seclusion in correctional mental health care. *Journal of the American Academy of Psychiatry & the Law*, *35*, 439–443.

O'Keefe, M., & Schnell, M. (2007). Offenders with mental illness in the correctional system. *Journal of Offender Rehabilitation*, *45*, 81–104.

Perry, A. E., Marandos, R., Coulton, S., & Johnson, M. (2010). Screening tools assessing risk of suicide and self-harm in adult offenders: A systematic review. *International Journal of Offender Therapy and Comparative Criminology*, *54*(5), 803–828.

Ryland, H., Gould, C., McGeorge, T., Hawton, K., & Fazel, S. (2020). Predicting self-harm in prisoners: Risk factors and a prognostic model in a cohort of 542 prison entrants. *European Psychiatry*, *63*(1), e42.

Sansone, R. A., & Sansone, L. A. (2010). Measuring self-harm behavior with the self-harm inventory. *Psychiatry*, *7*(4), 16–20.

Shelton, D., Sampl, S., Kesten, K. L., Zhang, W., & Trestman, R. L. (2009). Treatment of impulsive aggression in correctional settings. *Behavioral Sciences & the Law*, *27*, 787–800.

Smith, H. P., & Kaminski, R. J. (2010). Incarcerated person self-injurious behaviors: Distinguishing characteristics within a retrospective study. *Criminal Justice and Behavior*, *37*, 81–96.

Smith, H. P., & Kaminski, R. J. (2011). Self-injurious behaviors in state prisons: Findings from a national survey. *Criminal Justice and Behavior*, *38*, 26–41.

Smith, H. P., Power, J., Usher, A. M., Sitren, A. H., & Slade, K. (2019). Working with prisoners who self-harm: A qualitative study on stress, denial of weakness, and encouraging resilience in a sample of correctional staff. *Criminal Behavior & Mental Health*, *29*, 7–17.

Smith, P. S. (2006). The effects of solitary confinement on prison incarcerated persons: A brief history and review of the literature. *Crime and Justice*, *34*, 441–528.

Stanley, B., & Brown, G. K. (2011). Safety planning intervention: A brief intervention to mitigate suicide risk. *Cognitive and Behavioral Practice*, *19*(2012), 256–264.

Substance Abuse and Mental Health Services Administration. (2023). *Practical guide for implementing a trauma-informed approach* (Publication No. PEP23-06-05-005). National Mental Health and Substance Use Policy Laboratory. https://store.samhsa.gov/sites/default/files/pep23-06-05-005.pdf

Timberlake, L. M., Beeber, L. S., & Hubbard, G. (2020). Non-suicidal self-injury: Management on the inpatient psychiatric unit. *Journal of the American Psychiatric Nurses Association*, *26*(1), 10–26.

Verdolini, N., Murru, A., Attademo, L., et al. (2017). The aggressor at the mirror: Psychiatric correlates of deliberate self-harm in male prison inmates. *European Psychiatry*, *44*, 153–160.

Vinokur, D., & Levine, S. Z. (2019). Non-suicidal self-harm in prison: A national population-based study. *Psychiatry Research*, *272*, 216–221.

Walker, T., Shaw, J., Gibb, J., et al. (2021). Lessons learnt from the narratives of women who self-harm in prison. *Crisis*, *42*(2), 255–262.

Whitlock, J. L., Exner-Cortens, D., & Purington, A. (2014). Validity and reliability of the non-suicidal self-injury assessment test (NSSI-AT). *Psychological Assessment*, *26*(3), 935–946.

Winicov, N. (2019). A systematic review of behavioral health interventions for suicidal and self-harming individuals in prisons and jails. *Heliyon*, *5*, e02379.

Yang, C., Wang, J., Shao, Y., Liu, M., & Geng, F., (2022). Antisocial and borderline personality traits and childhood trauma in male prisoners: Mediating effects of difficulties in emotional regulation. *Child Abuse & Neglect*, *132*, 105822.

Yasmeen, S. E., Stuewig, J. B., Wilson, J. S., et al. (2023). Escalation of suicidal spectrum behaviors during incarceration. *Criminal Justice and Behavior*, *50*(5), 766–782.

53

Aggression

Robert L. Trestman

Introduction

Managing aggression is a challenge for psychiatry in all settings. Recognizing opportunities for appropriate assessment and intervention in correctional settings is an important component of correctional psychiatry. Studies reflect significant risks of violence for both correctional officers and incarcerated persons (IPs). Prison homicide rates (eight per 100,000 IPs; Carson & Cowhig, 2020) are higher than estimated community homicide rates (5.9 per 100,000 persons; Centers for Disease Control and Prevention, 2019), and the rate of nonlethal violence is substantial. The data for assault are less clear, as definitions of what constitutes assault vary. One recent study of correctional officers found that 170 per 1,000 had experienced a serious assault (Lerman, 2017). For context, similar methodology estimates the rate of assault on police officers (the highest risk occupation) at 261 per 1,000 officers and community-based mental health clinicians at 68 per 1,000 clinicians. IP-on-IP physical assault has been estimated to occur in 20.3% of female and 18.1% of male IPs, and sexual assault is estimated to occur in 15.4% of female and 9.7% of male IPs (Caravaca-Sánchez et al., 2023). However assault is defined, correctional officers who have been the target of violence by IPs have an elevated risk of emotional exhaustion and burnout (Vaswani & Paul, 2019; see Chapter 65). This chapter reviews the factors that contribute to the broad range of assaultive behaviors observed in correctional settings and some of the pragmatic issues and opportunities for assessment, diagnosis, and treatment of aggressive behaviors, both impulsive and predatory.

Definitions

Aggression is an integral part of the human experience. Understanding the motivations and types of aggressive behavior underpins the ability to prevent, manage, or mitigate it. In broad terms, aggression is typically defined as either predatory/instrumental or impulsive acts of violence. Predatory aggression most often consists of premeditated behavior with a specific goal. Such goals might include robbery, intimidation, or revenge. In contrast, impulsive aggression is usually reactive in nature, responsive to an immediate stress or provocation. This simple dichotomy between predatory and impulsive aggression reasonably categorizes about 79% of aggressive behavior in violent individuals (Tapscott et al., 2012).

Making such a categorization has important value. It helps in determining how to manage the sequelae of the violence. In practice, though, the overlap of behaviors and motivations often seems to blur these descriptive boundaries. Some characteristics to consider in making this determination include the proximity of the triggering event (was there a planned delay between the triggering event and the assault, or was it immediately before the assault?), the activities immediately prior to the assault (was it a calm, controlled attack, or was there agitation and yelling?), an assessment of the motivation behind the assault (was there a motive such as revenge or dominance, or was it a reaction with no secondary gain?), and the level of insight into the consequences of the assaultive behavior (was there an absence or superficial expression of remorse, or was there meaningful remorse/recognition of overreaction?; Scott et al., 2008).

Within this dichotomy, subtypes exist. For example, aggression that stems from intoxication or during detoxification is usually considered impulsive. Aggression due to psychotic paranoia or in response to command auditory hallucinations would be considered planned or instrumental, but it logically would be managed very differently from predatory aggression intended to exact revenge.

Assessment

Many approaches have been devised to measure the nature of aggressive behaviors and their types, severity, frequency, and future risks. These include self-report questionnaires and structured interviews that fall into descriptive and predictive groupings. Relevant descriptive instruments include measures of impulsivity, aggression, and personality. One broadly used and well-validated assessment instrument for impulsivity is the Barratt Impulsiveness Scale, Version 11 (Barratt, 2000), which includes subscales for attention, lack of planning, and motor impulsivity. Measures of aggression per se typically target either a lifetime history of aggression or current levels of aggression. Lifetime measures are useful for baseline assessment but less sensitive to change (e.g., the Life History of Aggression; Timmins et al., 2022). Such instruments may be useful for making initial therapeutic recommendations. Other instruments that are sensitive to change over time include the well-researched Buss–Perry Aggression Questionnaire (BPAQ; Buss & Perry, 1992), with subscales measuring physical aggression, verbal aggression, hostility, and anger. The BPAQ is well suited to measuring the effectiveness of clinical treatment over time, with repeated measurements before, during, and after the intervention. A short form of the BPAQ has also been validated on IPs (Diamond & Magaletta, 2006).

Instruments widely used to predict relative risks of future aggression include actuarial assessments such as the Level of Service Inventory-Revised (LSI-R; Labrecque et al., 2014) and the Psychopathy Checklist-Revised (PCL-R; Hare, 2020) and structured clinical interviews such as the Historical Clinical Risk Management-20, Version 3 (HCR-20 V3; Challinor et al, 2021). A recent systematic review suggests that the predictive utility of almost all instruments (including the LSI-R, PCL-R, and HCR-20) is strongest for low-risk individuals and, at best, moderate for high-risk offenders (Ramesh et al., 2018). The rapid expansion of this area of study includes initiatives to define standards for risk assessment tools, allowing for a more meaningful evaluation of the validity and reliability of legacy and proposed instruments and interviews (Singh et al., 2013).

Demographic risk factors for violence in correctional settings

Several demographic variables have been associated with a risk of violent behavior in correctional settings. By far the strongest predictor of violence is age; younger IPs are more likely to demonstrate aggression. Compared to IPs who are 31 to 35 years old, the likelihood of violent behavior is 350% greater for those younger than 21 and 63% greater for those 21 to 25 years old (Cunningham & Sorensen, 2007). Level of education also predicts aggression during incarceration, with less education associated with greater risk (Berg & DeLisi, 2006). Gang membership also increases the risk of violence (Gaes et al., 2002). Based on demographic factors alone, the individuals at highest risk of violent behavior are younger than 21, without high school diplomas or equivalents, and gang members. While minority status has been associated with an increased risk of violent behavior in jail or prison, the relationship is complex (Schenk & Fremouw, 2012).

Differential diagnosis

Not every act of aggression is due to a diagnosable mental illness. The likelihood of a contributing diagnosis increases with the frequency of aggressive behavior and with the consistency of the nature of the aggression (Whiting et al., 2021).

The largest group of potential diagnoses includes disorders that have poor impulse control as one of their defining features. These disorders include borderline personality disorder, antisocial personality disorder, and intermittent explosive disorder (IED). While they share impulsivity as a characteristic, the manner of presentation varies dramatically among them. In general, aggressive behaviors found in borderline personality disorder tend to be emotionally reactive to perceived threats (see Chapter 37). Such threats may derive from misperceived behavior or motivation of those near them. Individuals with antisocial personality disorder, by definition, have a pattern of behavior that violates social norms and usually includes premeditated, impulsive, or mixed violence. Aggressive behaviors tend to serve an instrumental purpose of furthering the person's goals (monetary, status, or otherwise). Individuals with IED, again by definition, overreact to a situation with explosive violence. While they typically experience remorse subsequent to the event, that remorse does not prevent recurrence of overreactive aggression (American Psychiatric Association, 2022).

Schizophrenia has been associated with aggressive behavior, but the specifics have only recently been more clearly defined. The conditions under which individuals with schizophrenia are more likely to become aggressive include periods of no treatment, persecutory delusions, or active comorbid substance use (Keers et al., 2014; Silverstein et al., 2020).

Traumatic brain injury, a broad category associated with a host of potential injuries (Katzin et al., 2020), can cause impulsive aggression if the damage includes areas of the prefrontal cortex. Related impairments in executive function can result in disinhibition and serious violence (Fazel et al., 2011).

Traumatic life experiences may also play a role in aggression. One study of adult male violent individuals found a strong relationship between self-reported childhood trauma and subsequent violent behavior (Ternes et al., 2020). A separate, targeted meta-analysis also found strong relationships between childhood trauma and aggression perpetrated by women (Augsburger & Maercker, 2020).

Neurobiology

There has been a real interest in looking for neuropathological causes for serious aggression for decades. Recent work, much of it specifically with individuals convicted of violent offenses, has focused on functional and structural neuropathology in neuroimaging studies, neurotransmitter and neuroendocrine research, and the potential contribution of epigenetics (Felthous & Nassif, 2022; Klaus & Schutter, 2021; Richard et al., 2023). The collective findings suggest abnormalities but do not identify direct causative neuropathological lesions leading to violent behavior.

Differential therapeutics

Depending on the environment, resources, and diagnosis, differential therapeutics and management of the patient follow the assessment. In correctional settings, milieu management, psychotherapy, behavior management plans (see Chapter 54), and psychopharmacology each have a role to play.

Milieu management

Milieu management is not that different than what would occur on an inpatient psychiatric unit, with overall and individualized considerations made for the environment, potential stressors, and provocations related to aggression. Evidence suggests that effective milieu design and management are the most important factors in preventing aggression in correctional settings (Cooke, 2023). This is particularly an issue in units or environments with higher than expected overall levels of aggression. Such considerations include proper environment management (e.g., regular and random custody searches to eliminate weapons), appropriate grievance resolution protocols, humane conditions of confinement, and respectful treatment (Welsh et al., 2013). Perceptions of disrespectful treatment have a direct correlation with increased risk of violent thoughts (Butler & Maruna, 2009). After addressing unnecessary provocations and distressing situations, levels of aggressive behavior drop significantly (Cooke, 2023). Relevant concerns include staffing ratios, management of interpersonal grievances, fairness of the assignment of opportunities, and access to privileges, among other factors (Wortley, 2002). Treating the incarcerated population with dignity and respect and providing a safe environment substantially reduce the amount of violence on any correctional unit (Day et al., 2023). Of note, milieu management is an excellent approach for reducing both premeditated and impulsive aggression, while simultaneously improving staff morale (Cooke, 2023). A structured approach to reviewing the correctional milieu for violence risk factors has been developed and tested with positive results (Johnstone & Cooke, 2010). Another substantial concern in correctional settings, particularly prisons, is gang aggression. Chapter 64 reviews this specialized and challenging topic.

Psychotherapy

Psychotherapies have been developed or adapted for use in rehabilitation of IPs (see Chapters 42 and 43). While targeted psychotherapies in correctional settings have a limited evidence base, a range of cognitive-behavioral therapies (CBTs) have application to the reduction of violence and aggressive behavior. In a recent review of the literature, several randomized clinical trials and quasi-experimental studies supported the general effectiveness of CBT interventions in reducing violent behavior and reincarceration for violent offenses (Papalia et al., 2019). In this meta-analysis, 27 controlled studies involving 7,062 IPs with violent histories found small (10% to 20%) but clinically and statistically significant reductions in violent behavior and reincarceration. When the outcome measure is reduction in recidivism rather than violence per se, an extensive review of available interventions demonstrates clear support for CBT programs and argues against the effectiveness of sanctions and deterrence-based programs (Gannon et al., 2019). Substantial evidence supports the effectiveness in reducing recidivism of CBT that is implemented with fidelity to the model for IPs convicted of domestic and general violence, although uncertainty does exist with regard to the impact on sexual violence recidivism (Mews et al., 2017).

The commonalities among the interventions with positive findings include manual-based design with fidelity monitoring; skills-based training that includes emotion management, interpersonal relatedness, and impulse control; adequate duration to allow for skill acquisition through practice; and a reasonably supportive, reinforcing environment. Other CBT skills-based programs designed to meet these needs in correctional settings have been developed and are being evaluated (e.g., START NOW; Kersten et al., 2016). As a clear caveat for all such structured interventions, manual-guided treatment provides critical consistency in treatment programming; however, success requires therapeutic alliance and motivational engagement (Day et al., 2013). In parallel to CBT-based research findings, studies with mindfulness-based treatment paradigms have demonstrated positive but similarly modest benefits (Fix & Fix, 2013).

Psychopharmacology

In the 1980s, there was an attempt to develop a class of medications called serenics, medications targeted specifically at the reduction of aggressive behavior. While no new medication resulted from that attempt (Umukoro et al., 2013), a range of potential medications warrant consideration for the management of aggression. Based on the assessment and differential diagnosis, these medications include selective serotonin reuptake inhibitors, lithium, anticonvulsants, antipsychotics, and beta blockers.

Serotonin, a neurotransmitter with broad cortical distribution and complex inhibitory roles, has been proposed as having a key role in modulating impulsive aggression (Coccaro et al., 2015; da Cunha-Bang & Knudsen, 2021). Multiple studies have shown selective serotonin reuptake inhibitors to reduce impulsive aggression in patients with personality disorders (e.g., Rosell et al., 2023) and in those with traumatic brain injury (Fann et al., 2022). Fluoxetine has been the most studied agent in those with personality disorders, including double-blind randomized controlled studies, with effective doses ranging from 40 to 60 mg daily (Coccaro et al., 2015). Open-label studies using other selective serotonin reuptake inhibitors have generally found similar results.

Lithium has a very interesting history in the treatment of aggression, with clinical trials dating back as far as the 1970s. In two populations of aggressive prisoners, lithium was shown to reduce violent aggression (as measured by disciplinary infractions) over 3 months (Sheard et al., 1976) and 18 months (Tupin et al., 1973). A more recent review of the literature found substantial consistency supporting lithium's effectiveness in the treatment of aggression in multiple settings (Müller-Oerlinghausen & Lewitzka, 2010). Arguably, one reason that lithium has not been used more extensively is the need for therapeutic monitoring to avoid toxicity, particularly for renal function. However, with patients who allow appropriate monitoring, a therapeutic trial of lithium is an excellent consideration.

Anticonvulsants have also been used in the treatment of aggression for several decades. For individuals with impulsive aggression secondary to traumatic brain injury, valproate preparations have shown effectiveness in multiple case studies (Geracioti, 1994; Warden et al., 2006). One large, multisite, randomized clinical trial of divalproex studied patients with a history of impulsive aggression (46% with prior incarcerations) and *Diagnostic and Statistical Manual of Mental Disorders*, fourth edition, Cluster B personality disorders, IED, or posttraumatic stress disorder (Hollander et al., 2003). The patients with Cluster B personality disorders, but not those with posttraumatic stress disorder or IED, experienced substantial clinical and statistical improvement in impulsive aggression, irritability, and overall illness severity in a 12-week study. More limited data also exist supporting the use of carbamazepine (Warden et al., 2006), lamotrigine (Leiberich et al., 2008), and oxcarbazepine (Bellino et al., 2005). These studies used doses generally consistent with established therapeutic use in seizure or bipolar disorders.

Antipsychotics are commonly used in the management of acute aggression and agitation. Randomized clinical trials show inconsistent evidence that antipsychotic medications reduce violence in an unselected population (van Schalkwyk et al., 2018). Even within the schizophrenic spectrum of disorders, the heterogeneity of etiology may differentiate appropriateness of treatment with an antipsychotic, with some evidence supporting both positive psychotic symptom-driven aggression (e.g., persecutory delusions) and aggression secondary to cognition-impaired disinhibition. Among the antipsychotics, clozapine may be more effective in treating aggression in schizophrenia (and perhaps other psychiatric disorders) than other antipsychotics (Frogley et al., 2012). With the exception of clozapine, most other antipsychotics (whether first or second generation) appear similar and more modestly effective in the treatment of aggression. There is evidence that long-acting injectable antipsychotics may be superior to oral formulations in the reduction of violence risk, again with the exception of clozapine (Strassnig et al., 2020).

Beta blockers, most commonly propranolol, have demonstrated significant benefit in treating impulsive aggression in both case studies and randomized clinical trials (Scott et al., 2008). In doses ranging from 40 to 320 mg/day, positive results have been obtained in patients experiencing impulsive aggression secondary to traumatic brain injuries (Warden et al., 2006), psychotic disorders, and personality disorders (Scott et al., 2008; Silver et al., 1999). In one randomized study, two case examples are illustrative. Despite multiple previous clinical trials on other medications, these two individuals (one diagnosed with paranoid schizophrenia, the other with severe aggression associated with intellectual disability) were chronically aggressive in a forensic psychiatry unit, with seven and 21 aggressive episodes during the baseline assessment week, respectively. Following a month on propranolol, the frequency of aggressive outbursts dropped to an average of 1.5 and 1.75 per week, respectively (Silver et al., 1999).

Management of aggression

After assessment, differential diagnosis, and selection of therapeutic interventions, the real work may begin. Communicating the proposed interventions to all stakeholders, building support where needed (e.g., where milieu changes involve correctional staff), and gaining engagement of the patient are all required elements in this next phase. Sometimes it may be as simple as recommending participation in a therapy group or taking a new medication; often, it may require more extensive consensus building with a seriously challenging patient. Developing a methodology to measure improvement in targeted behaviors has equal importance to proposing interventions and engaging stakeholders. The time frame for measurement may range from weeks to months before significant improvement is seen in chronically disruptive or violent behavior. That time frame should be shared with the treatment team and the patient to avert expectations of unrealistically rapid responses and avoid disappointment.

Summary

Aggressive behavior is a common and challenging problem in correctional settings. To address aggression effectively, a thoughtful and comprehensive approach that may incorporate elements of environmental management, evaluation of potential motivating factors, differential diagnosis, and a coordinated intervention is needed. This always involves effective communication among stakeholders, including the patient. Recommended milieu changes and psychotherapeutic and/or pharmacological interventions need to be explicit. Consistent oversight and follow-up to measure the effects of each component of the intervention(s) are critical, as aggressive behavior may be both habitual and episodic.

REFERENCES

American Psychiatric Association. (2022). *Diagnostic and statistical manual of mental disorders* (5th ed., text rev.).

Augsburger, M., & Maercker, A. (2020). Associations between trauma exposure, posttraumatic stress disorder, and aggression perpetrated by women. A meta-analysis. *Clinical Psychology: Science and Practice*, *27*(1), e12322.

Barratt, E. S. (2000). Barratt Impulsiveness Scale, Version 11 (BIS 11). In A. J. Rush (Ed.), *Handbook of psychiatric measures*, Ed: Rush, A.J., (pp. 691–693). American Psychiatric Association.

Bellino, S., Paradiso, E., & Bogetto, F. (2005). Oxcarbazepine in the treatment of BPD: A pilot study. *Journal of Clinical Psychiatry*, *66*, 1111–1115.

Berg, M. T., & DeLisi, M. (2006). The correctional melting pot: Race, ethnicity, citizenship, and prison violence. *Journal of Criminal Justice*, *34*, 631–642.

Buss, A. H., & Perry, M. (1992). The Aggression Questionnaire. *Journal of Personality and Social Psychology*, *63*, 452–459.

Butler, M., & Maruna, S. (2009). The impact of disrespect on prisoners' aggression: Outcomes of experimentally inducing violence-supportive cognitions. *Psychology, Crime & Law*, *15*(2–3), 235–250.

Caravaca-Sánchez, F., Aizpurua, E., & Wolff, N. (2023). The prevalence of prison-based physical and sexual victimization in males and females: A systematic review and meta-analysis. *Trauma, Violence, & Abuse*, *24*(5), 3476–3492.

Carson, E. A., & Cowhig, M. P. (2020). *Mortality in state and federal prisons, 2001–2016—Statistical tables*. U.S. Department of Justice.

Centers for Disease Control and Prevention. (2019). *Age-adjusted death rates for selected causes of death, by sex, race, and Hispanic origin: United States, selected years 1950–2018*. https://www.cdc.gov/nchs/data/hus/2019/005-508.pdf

Challinor, A., Ogundalu, A., McIntyre, J. C., Bramwell, V., & Nathan, R. (2021). The empirical evidence base for the use of the HCR-20: A narrative review of study designs and transferability of results to clinical practice. *International Journal of Law and Psychiatry*, 78, 101729.

Coccaro, E. F., Fanning, J. R., Phan, K. L., & Lee, R. (2015). Serotonin and impulsive aggression. *CNS Spectrums*, *20*(3), 295–302.

Cooke, D. J. (2023). Exploring the wicked problem of violence in prison: Capturing the complexity of contexts. In A. J. Tamatea, A. J. Day, & D. J. Cooke (Eds.), *Preventing prison violence* (pp. 210–222). Routledge.

Cunningham, M. D., & Sorensen, J. R. (2007). Predictive factors for violent misconduct in close custody. *Prison Journal*, *87*(2), 241–253.

da Cunha-Bang, S., & Knudsen, G. M. (2021). The modulatory role of serotonin on human impulsive aggression. *Biological Psychiatry*, *90*(7), 447–457.

Day, A., Kozar, C., & Davey, L. (2013). Treatment approaches and offender behavior programs: Some critical issues. *Aggression and Violent Behavior*, *18*, 630–635.

Day, A., Malvaso, C. G., Galouzis, J. J., & Pilkington, R. (2023). An approach to preventing prison violence. In A. J. Tamatea, A. J. Day, & D. J. Cooke (Eds.), *Preventing prison violence* (pp. 199–209). Routledge.

Diamond, P. M., & Magaletta, P. R. (2006). The short-form Buss-Perry Aggression questionnaire (BPAQ-SF): A validation study with federal offenders. *Assessment*, *13*(3), 227–240.

Fann, J. R., Quinn, D. K., & Hart, T. (2022). Treatment of psychiatric problems after traumatic brain injury. *Biological Psychiatry*, *91*(5), 508–521.

Fazel, S., Lichtenstein, P., Grann, M., & Langstrom, N. (2011). Risk of violent crime in individuals with epilepsy and traumatic brain injury: A 35-year Swedish population study. *PLoS Medicine, 8*, e1001150.

Felthous, A. R., & Nassif, J. (2022). CNS glutamate in impulsive aggression. In Z. M. Pavlovic (Ed.), *Glutamate and neuropsychiatric disorders: Current and emerging treatments* (pp. 283–311). Springer International Publishing.

Fix, R. L., & Fix, S. T. (2013). The effects of mindfulness-based treatments for aggression: A critical review. *Aggression and Violent Behavior, 18*(2), 219–227.

Frogley, C., Taylor, D., Dickens, G., & Picchioni, M. (2012). A systematic review of the evidence of clozapine's anti-aggressive effects. *International Journal of Neuropsychopharmacology, 15*(9), 1351–1371.

Gaes, G. G., Wallace, S., Gilman, E., Klein-Saffran, J., & Suppa, S. (2002). The influence of prison gang affiliation on violence and other prison misconduct. *Prison Journal, 82*(3), 359–385.

Gannon, T. A., Olver, M. E., Mallion, J. S., & James, M. (2019). Does specialized psychological treatment for offending reduce recidivism? A meta-analysis examining staff and program variables as predictors of treatment effectiveness. *Clinical Psychology Review, 73*, 101752.

Geracioti, T. D. (1994). Valproic acid treatment of episodic explosiveness related to brain injury. *Journal of Clinical Psychiatry, 55*(9), 416–417.

Hare, R. D. (2020). The PCL-R assessment of psychopathy. In A. Felthous & H. Sass (Eds.), *The Wiley international handbook on psychopathic disorders and the law* (pp. 63–106). John Wiley and Sons.

Hollander, E., Tracey, K. A., Swann, A. C., et al. (2003). Divalproex in the treatment of impulsive aggression: Efficacy in Cluster B personality disorders. *Neuropsychopharmacology, 28*, 1186–1197.

Johnstone, L., & Cooke, D. (2010). PRISM: A promising paradigm for assessing and managing institutional violence: Findings from a multiple case study analysis of five Scottish prisons. *International Journal of Forensic Mental Health, 9*, 185–191.

Katzin, S., Andiné, P., Hofvander, B., Billstedt, E., & Wallinius, M. (2020). Exploring traumatic brain injuries and aggressive antisocial behaviors in young male violent offenders. *Frontiers in Psychiatry, 11*, 507196.

Keers, R., Ullrich, S., DeStavola, B. L., & Coid, J. W. (2014). Association of violence with emergence of persecutory delusions in untreated schizophrenia. *American Journal of Psychiatry, 171*(3), 332–339.

Kersten, L., Cislo, A. M., Lynch, M., Shea, K., & Trestman, R. L. (2016). Evaluating START NOW: A skills-based psychotherapy for inmates of correctional systems. *Psychiatric Services, 67*(1), 37–42.

Klaus, J., & Schutter, D. J. (2021). Functional topography of anger and aggression in the human cerebellum. *NeuroImage, 226*, 117582.

Labrecque, R. M., Smith, P., Lovins, B. K., & Latessa, E. J. (2014). The importance of reassessment: How changes in the LSI-R risk score can improve the prediction of recidivism. *Journal of Offender Rehabilitation, 53*(2), 116–128.

Leiberich, P., Nickel, M. K., Tritt, K., & Gil, F. P. (2008). Lamotrigine treatment of aggression in female borderline patients, Part II: An 18-month follow-up. *Journal of Psychopharmacology, 22*, 805–808.

Lerman, A. E. (2017). *Officer health and wellness: Results from the California correctional officer survey*. https://gspp.berkeley.edu/assets/uploads/research/pdf/executive_summary_08142018.pdf

Mews, A., Di Bella, L., & Purver, M. (2017). *Impact evaluation of the prison-based core sex offender treatment programme*. Ministry of Justice. https://www.gov.uk/government/publications/impact-evaluation-of-the-prison-based-core-sex-offender-treatment-programme

Müller-Oerlinghausen, B., & Lewitzka, U. (2010). Lithium reduces pathological aggression and suicidality: A mini-review. *Neuropsychobiology, 62*, 43–49.

Papalia, N., Spivak, B., Daffern, M., & Ogloff, J. R. (2019). A meta-analytic review of the efficacy of psychological treatments for violent offenders in correctional and forensic mental health settings. *Clinical Psychology: Science and Practice, 26*(2), e12282.

Ramesh, T., Igoumenou, A., Montes, M. V., & Fazel, S. (2018). Use of risk assessment instruments to predict violence in forensic psychiatric hospitals: A systematic review and meta-analysis. *European Psychiatry, 52*, 47–53.

Richard, Y., Tazi, N., Frydecka, D., Hamid, M. S., & Moustafa, A. A. (2023). A systematic review of neural, cognitive, and clinical studies of anger and aggression. *Current Psychology, 42*(20), 17174–17186.

Rosell, D. R., Slifstein, M., Thompson, J., et al. (2023). Serotonin transporter availability in physically aggressive personality disordered patients: Associations with trait and state aggression, and response to fluoxetine. *Psychopharmacology, 240*(2), 361–371.

Schenk, A. M., & Fremouw, W. J. (2012). Individual characteristics related to prison violence: A critical review of the literature. *Aggression and Violent Behavior, 17*, 430–442.

Scott, C. L., Quanbeck, C. D., & Resnick, P. J. (2008). Assessment of dangerousness. In R. E. Hales, S. C. Yudofsky, & G. Gabbard (Eds.), *The American Psychiatric Publishing textbook of psychiatry* (pp. 1655–1672). American Psychiatric Publishing.

Sheard, M. H., Marini, J. L., Bridges, C. I., & Wagner, E. (1976). The effect of lithium on impulsive aggressive behavior in man. *American Journal of Psychiatry, 133*(12), 1409–1413.

Silver, J. M., Yudovsky, S. C., Slater, J. A., et al. (1999). Propranolol treatment of chronically hospitalized aggressive patients. *Journal of Neuropsychiatry and Clinical Neurosciences, 11*, 328–335.

Silverstein, S. M., Del Pozzo, J., Roché, M., Boyle, D., & Miskimen, T. (2020). Schizophrenia and violence: Realities and recommendations. *Reviewing Crime Psychology, 17*, 181–202.

Singh, J. P., Yang, S., Bjorkly, S., et al. (2013). *Reporting standards for risk assessment predictive validity studies: The Risk Assessment Guidelines for the Evaluation of Efficacy (RAGEE) statement*. University of South Florida.

Strassnig, M. T., Nascimento, V., Deckler, E., & Harvey, P. D. (2020). Pharmacological treatment of violence in schizophrenia. *CNS Spectrums, 25*(2), 207–215.

Tapscott, J., Hancock, M., & Hoaken, P. (2012). Severity and frequency of reactive and instrumental violent offending: Divergent validity of subtypes of violence in an adult forensic sample. *Criminal Justice and Behavior, 39*, 202–219.

Ternes, M., Cooper, B. S., & Griesel, D. (2020). The perpetration of violence and the experience of trauma: Exploring predictors of PTSD symptoms in male violent offenders. *International Journal of Forensic Mental Health, 19*(1), 68–83.

Timmins, M. A., Berman, M. E., & Coccaro, E. F. (2022). Life history of experienced and witnessed aggression: Development of a new assessment instrument. *Journal of Psychiatric Research, 155*, 518–525.

Tupin, J. P., Smith, D. B., Clanon, T. L., et al. (1973). The long-term use of lithium in aggressive prisoners. *Comprehensive Psychiatry, 14*(4), 311–317.

Umukoro, S., Aladeokin, A., & Eduviere, A. T. (2013). Aggressive behavior: A comprehensive review of its neurochemical mechanisms and management. *Aggression and Violent Behavior, 18*(2), 195–203.

van Schalkwyk, G. I., Beyer, C., Johnson, J., Deal, M., & Bloch, M. H. (2018). Antipsychotics for aggression in adults: A meta-analysis. *Progress in Neuro-Psychopharmacology and Biological Psychiatry, 81*, 452–458.

Vaswani, N., & Paul, S. (2019). "It's knowing the right things to say and do": Challenges and opportunities for trauma-informed practice in the prison context. *Howard Journal of Crime and Justice*, *58*(4), 513–534.

Warden, D. L., Gordon, B., McAllister, T. W., et al. (2006). Guidelines for the pharmacologic treatment of neurobehavioral sequelae of traumatic brain injury. *Journal of Neurotrauma*, *23*(10), 1468–1501.

Welsh, E., Bader, S., & Evans, S. E. (2013). Situational variables related to aggression in institutional settings. *Aggression and Violent Behavior*, *18*, 792–796.

Whiting, D., Lichtenstein, P., & Fazel, S. (2021). Violence and mental disorders: A structured review of associations by individual diagnoses, risk factors, and risk assessment. *Lancet Psychiatry*, *8*(2), 150–161.

Wortley, R. (2002). *Situational prison control: Crime prevention in correctional institutions*. Cambridge University Press.

54

Behavior management plans

Henry Schmidt III, André Ivanoff, and William Kuo

Introduction

There are similarities and a connection between behavior management and treatment in definition and practice (Schmidt & Ivanoff, 2015). The principles of behaviorism and cognitive-behavioral therapies are all applicable to quality behavior management schemes, and they remain the best supported techniques for improving, maintaining, or decreasing specific behaviors. Managing the environment to promote the commitment of an incarcerated person (IP) to learn and employ skillful means toward prosocial behavior is also an important determinant in creating safe, secure environments within correctional settings.

Contingency management and new skill development are central to effective behavior management and form the backbone of the individual self-control discussion in this chapter. The shortest distance to effective behavior management in correctional settings is preventing functional behaviors already in the IP's repertoire from deteriorating. Behavior management programs should be intentionally structured to reward prosocial behaviors and provide reasonable punishment of behavior that undermines programming or personal and interpersonal stability. Ideally, the response to either functional or dysfunctional behavior would be reliable and quick to follow the target behaviors exhibited by the IP. Practically speaking, this requires that such responses fall within the responsibilities of the line staff working with IPs, who are always in proximity. This also implies that there are sufficient trained staff on the floor to be able to maintain an institution-determined rule structure and contingency schedule, which is often lacking from a staffing perspective.

IP behaviors are being reinforced or punished (i.e., behavior occurs, and then there is a response) every day in every unit. The only question is: Who is more effective and consistent in providing the response—the staff or the fellow IPs in the same institution? In all but a few settings, this competition or battle is waged daily, with some IPs forcefully attempting to sway the reinforcers for behavior in ways that will benefit themselves (or their group) and to align the punishments delivered in the unit to similarly benefit themselves or deprive others. For those individuals who have spent years in correctional settings (the majority in most adult settings), often across multiple incarcerations, learning the unwritten rules is a way of life, the first order of business, and critical to survival. Having a chance to influence or dictate these unwritten rules places one in a privileged place in the institution, and enforcers of the rules are typically well rewarded, as they maintain the rule makers at the top of the hierarchy and the benefits flow down to them. In units with insufficient staff, it is likely that the IPs are setting and enforcing their own rules.

The beginning of this chapter focuses on contingencies. *Contingencies* refer to any outcome consistently related to a given behavior. We press the button for the elevator because it consistently summons a car to pick us up and take us up or down in a building. While we may turn over rocks in a vacant lot and, to our surprise, find a gold coin, such behavior (rock turning) is unlikely to yield such a treasure consistently, and that single outcome is not likely to impact our behavior for long. Thus, consistent outcomes of a given behavior are one of the best predictors of its recurrence.

Contingencies

A discussion on contingencies should focus staff and administrators on the most salient aspect of an individual IP's behavior management within a correctional setting. Based on decades of experience in this field, the authors have concluded that it is almost impossible to prevent a behavior from occurring without resorting to illegal, unethical, and untenable practices. For instance, the only way to prevent someone from attacking another person is to maintain them in total isolation. Similarly, it is almost impossible to prevent someone who is intent on self-harming from doing so; even an IP in full restraints can bang their head against a wall or floor, and those with high intent can find or create the means to cut or scratch. Such IPs maintain a keen eye for anything on the floor or elsewhere that they can fashion to harm themselves, and they can easily hide such makeshift implements in their living spaces, on themselves, or with peers. However, establishing an appropriate structured milieu within a correctional housing unit and implementing individual behavior management plans, when clinically indicated, can decrease the frequency and severity of targeted behaviors in an ethical manner.

In correctional settings, staff may struggle to control the expression of a behavior by an IP but can have great opportunities to control outcomes. An important intervention is for staff to reduce IPs' access to the means to do significant harm to themselves or each other by blocking and removing contraband at every opportunity (environmental strategies). But fists, fingernails, feet, and so forth are all possible means of inflicting injury, and facilities are constructed of concrete and metal—immovable and potentially lethal materials when used for self-harm or violence. By focusing on outcomes (and protecting IPs from predation by others), the focus moves from staff control to IP self-control, which is the most stable and predictable form of behavior management (Chapman & Ivanoff, 2018; Papalia et al., 2019).

However, many programs cite prevention as their first, and often only, formal recourse to high-risk behavior. For individuals in low- or medium-security settings (who possess a natural aversion to pain, have reasons to abstain from infractions, and have enough skills to navigate the demanding social environments), prevention serves its purposes. Days or even weeks may pass without a fight or a self-injury. If this were true for all IPs in all correctional settings, there would be no need for the extensive training of staff and planning by teams to address egregious IP behavior.

Limitations

The absence of acute, visible, and extreme violence does not mean that all is well within facilities. Indebtedness via gambling or strong-arm methods, gang recruitment, and being deprived of meals, earned privileges, goods, personal belongings, or even the ability to take up space ("You aren't allowed to sit in a chair," "I get top bunk and your blanket") can create significant hardship for vulnerable individuals and lead to declines in physical and behavioral health. Such outcomes are often achieved via threats of direct physical violence or of harm to loved ones outside the walls, and actual violence may be infrequent. Programs and staff need to be structured to monitor behavioral deterioration and to investigate and eliminate its causes whenever possible. Since it is frequently not possible to prevent IPs from intimidating or threatening their peers, the focus should be on how staff respond to such behaviors. This demands well-trained staff who can identify threats to stability and behavioral health and intervene swiftly.

Formal and structured risk assessment for the population found in correctional settings is not very helpful in accurately predicting violent behaviors. Many individuals in correctional settings are likely to have a history of violence perpetration or being victims of interpersonal violence. Many have well-established, regularly reinforced habits of rule breaking, hiding behavior from authorities, and forming social networks with the intent to thwart rules or take advantage of others. Here, the very factors that are most likely to predict aggression and, similarly, self-harm or escape are likely to identify significant proportions of IPs as high risk upon entry. The fact that these are relatively low-frequency behaviors among all but a small minority of IPs makes prediction of specific times and places when an individual will act violently statistically improbable using population-based risk assessments. We will address below the use of an individualized, idiographic assessment process that enables us to improve our prediction of such behavior significantly when working with a cooperative IP or with attentive staff reports.

The responses most utilized in correctional settings to respond to high-risk or egregious behaviors are extremely limited and generally do little to address the risk of the individual who engaged in the behavior. The most typical response to a fight, self-harm, or effort to escape is to place the individual in a different setting. If two IPs do not get along and escalate that conflict to a physical fight, the belief is that separating those individuals will solve the problem. Similarly, for those who are self-harming, finding increasingly sterile environments will block access to most means, and for those who have tried to escape, placing them behind more barriers will impact the likely success of such behavior. None of these interventions, however, reduce the future likelihood of the individual engaging in such attempts. Individuals who perceive the benefits to outweigh the costs, or who are in a position where alternative problem-solving means are not accessible or successful, will continue to engage in the behaviors mentioned above. In some instances, they will escalate their attempts. Behavior management plans are essential for these IPs. When egregious behaviors occur, the response must be sure and swift to prevent behavioral contagion across the facility. Most who have worked in a correctional setting for a significant length of time have experienced this phenomenon. Extended contagion events are clear evidence that good behavior management is not being practiced and are always a wake-up call to review policy and practice, retrain staff, and engage the entire team of clinical and correctional staff in overt application of evidence-based responses.

Deterrence

As mentioned above, the element of deterrence has a role in behavior management (or, at least, event management). How the environment is structured, including clear and consistent contingencies mentioned above, can significantly impact the frequency of behavior expression before it has occurred. In the public sphere, deterrence tactics were found to be among the weakest predictors of crime rates across virtually all levels of the meta-analyses being reviewed (Pratt & Cullen, 2005) and vanish to near zero when multivariate effects are introduced (e.g., peer effects, self-control, criminogenic beliefs). On the other hand, the authors noted that "situational crime prevention" must go together with problem-solving policing to provide a complete theoretical and practical approach to crime reduction in communities. The same is true within correctional settings.

Place management

Place management theory synthesizes the dialectic between managing the environment (situational measures) within a correctional housing unit and supporting IPs to manage their own behavior. This theory is based on the empirically demonstrated proposition that "engaging the managers of high crime locations can reduce crime at these places" (Eck, 2015, p. 5; Madensen, 2007; St. John, 2023). As operationalized by Madensen (2007), place management includes four important elements: *organization of physical space*, *regulation of conduct* (where behavioral principles are emphasized), *control of access*, and *acquisition of resources*. Hoke's (2013) mixed-method design study tested the general applicability of these elements in selected housing units within a jail while incorporating social components to create a blended situational and social approach. This allows managers to manipulate both physical and social characteristics of the environment to regulate the occurrence of specific behavior effectively. There is limited research applying place management in correctional settings. This chapter will explain how these elements were operationalized in Hoke's (2013) study to illustrate how place management and a behavioral management plan (BMP) like the Egregious Behavior Protocol, discussed later in this chapter (Swenson et al., 2001), can be concurrently used to complement each other. It should be emphasized that such a model required significant training of correctional staff in the selected housing units.

Physical space involved assigning correctional officers responsibility for the organization, repair, and upkeep of the housing unit, as well as for decentralized unit decision- making. Officers were instructed that active supervision requires continual movement and interaction. They were also allowed to modify the layout of the furnishings to create spaces comfortable for them and to increase the amount of their interaction with the IPs (Hoke, 2013). Ideally, the decisions about space would be shared, considering IPs' concerns and preferences, as well as officers' comfort, without diminishing safety, security, or orderliness. Tolerable and safe living and working conditions are a prerequisite to effective behavior management.

Regulation of conduct included training officers to identify acceptable standards of conduct, communicating those standards to IPs individually and in groups, enforcing behavioral expectations, identifying and responding to unwanted behaviors as they arise, and informing IPs of any changes to the operation of the unit. Officers were taught how to identify aggressive and vulnerable IPs, manage behavior, and use the housing design to address IPs who had concerning behavior. Regular communication between officers and IPs was normalized and expected as part of institutional life. Officers were encouraged to model positive behavior and understand the value of reinforcement in maintaining positive behavior, allowed to create any reasonable reinforcers, and advised to act in a manner that promoted communication and built respect (Hoke, 2013). Ideally, officers used both positive and negative reinforcers to increase wanted behaviors and some combination of extinction and punishment to decrease or stop unwanted behaviors.

Control of access was operationalized by allowing housing unit officers to determine who should stay or be removed from a unit. Prior to the study, IPs were designated as minimum, medium, or maximum custody using a risk-based, objective classification system upon admission and housed separately based on their designation. Exceptions included the sole female housing unit and special populations (e.g., medical, suicide observation, and restrictive housing units). An IP's designation was limited and controlled by only a few members of the administrative team. After adequate training, officers were allowed to change an IP's cell assignment within the unit and decide whether someone would be removed from the unit (Hoke, 2013). This element allowed for a more dynamic system and accounted for the fact that risk levels change over time.

Acquisition of resources included decentralizing the control of resources (e.g., toilet paper, blankets, food trays, or directly requesting the repair of unit fixtures) from the administration to individual housing unit officers. Housing unit officers were given responsibility for making most decisions related to unit management (Hoke, 2013). It would be most effective for IPs to have some say in the choice of resources available in day-to-day programming and as reinforcers for improved behavior. Loss of access to those resources due to poor behavior can be a motivator to get back on course and make different behavioral choices.

There is significant overlap between the important components of BMPs and the *regulation of conduct* element, including fully orienting IPs to behavioral expectations, addressing behaviors as they arise, and using reinforcers and modeling to increase wanted behaviors. The complement between place management and BMPs lies in the transaction between the correctional environment and the IP. Decentralizing unit decision-making and control of resources from administration and generally providing officers with more autonomy increases the effective use of behavioral principles and, by extension, BMPs.

The individual elements of place management and changes in IP behaviors were correlational, and therefore it is difficult to establish causal links. Qualitative data indicated that *acquisition of resources* and *regulation of conduct* were especially important in managing IPs' behavior. Responsiveness to IP behavior, including the officers' ability to change housing units or directly acquire resources and meet IPs' basic needs in a more immediate manner, were also important. Being more responsive changed the dynamic of the relationship and was directly related to the quality of the interaction between officers and IPs. Officers who were more responsive to IPs and tried to manage the unit through better quality interactions received better compliance from IPs and were treated with greater respect. Officers were also seen as a legitimate resource since they made most of the housing unit decisions (Hoke, 2013).

Regulation of conduct seemed to be the most critical concept in place management. Increased officer involvement in the housing unit and the development of clear and consistent standards and rules were important to regulate behavior. Increased officer involvement improved levels of communication between officers and IPs, made officers appear more approachable, and increased IPs' willingness to comply with directions. The consistent enforcement of standards of conduct was essential (Hoke, 2013). Liebling (2004) suggested that IPs are more likely to comply with institutional rules when they view authority as legitimate, which has been linked to the perception of fairness and consistency (Sparks & Bottoms, 2008, Sparks et al., 1996). The perception of fairness is also related to the clarity and consistent reinforcement of rules. This consistent reinforcement and clarification of rules and procedures, along with strong officer–IP relationships, increases the IP's perception of fairness (Liebling, 2004).

Similarly, Sparks and Bottoms (2008) suggested that personal credibility is developed when IPs perceive officers to have a more consistent and fair approach. When personal credibility is developed, it enhances the IP's willingness to comply with organizational directives. Hoke's (2013) qualitative data suggests officers who developed higher levels of personal credibility found it easier to manage IP behavior than those with lower personal credibility.

Hoke (2013) identified and proposed *social legitimacy* as a fifth element of place management that particularly enhanced the *acquisition of resources* and *regulation of conduct* elements. Increasing the frequency of interactions between officers and IPs alone is not enough to develop social legitimacy, as the quality of interaction is crucial. This further highlights the importance of the bidirectional, transactional relationship between the correctional environment and IPs. Overall, Hoke (2013) found a significant decrease in the number of written misconduct reports in the place management housing units postintervention, with no significant changes in the control unit. At 4 months postintervention, there were continued reports of positive behavioral change.

An application of behavior management: the Egregious Behavior Protocol

The Egregious Behavior Protocol is an approach to behavioral management that combines the elements described above: contingency management for an IP's behavior and a staff-directed program. The

Egregious Behavior Protocol is a structured protocol for responding to IPs' high-risk behavior that has been taught for over 2 decades in correctional settings. The protocol was initially discussed in an article on the application of dialectical behavior therapy (DBT) in an inpatient setting (McCann et al., 2000; Swenson et al., 2001) and was elaborated by McCann et al. (2007). This protocol is designed to address high-risk behavior in correctional settings (e.g., threats to life, health, or program functioning) and lead to increasing self-control of behavior of the IP (Juvenile Rehabilitation Administration, 2002).

IPs are oriented to the protocol as part of the orientation to the institution. Behaviors that lead to the protocol are specified. Intake assessments should identify the occurrence of past behaviors that would merit the response, and staff should monitor all new IP behavior carefully for indicators of current behaviors of high concern: aggression, self-harm, efforts to escape, creation of weapons, or disruption of stable programming.

It is important to clarify during the orientation all actions that count as occurrences of the behavior. For example, an aggressive IP is told that verbal threats, threatening stares, closed fists, a fighting stance, and punching or other physical contact with other IPs or staff are all considered aggressive acts. Possessing or manufacturing a weapon and encouraging others to fight are behaviors that would lead to application of the protocol. Those with histories of self-injury or suicidal behavior are informed that statements, threats, notes, journal entries, and possession of contraband to use for self-harm are causes for placement on the protocol.

Once the IP is oriented to the protocol, normal programming begins. Privileges and rewards are earned based on the unit's merit level system or token economy, and the IP is informed of program expectations and may participate in education or work details. Staff provide regular feedback to IPs regarding their behavior while modeling skillful and prosocial interactions and speech. Staff resources are directed to coaching IPs on the unit when they demonstrate distress or low-level rule violations. Such coaching identifies the observed behavior calling for staff response (e.g., "You look upset right now"), states the staff's concerns ("Are you able to calm yourself down? Do you need some help?"), and provides concrete skills coaching ("Would it help if you sat over here and took some deep breaths or distracted yourself with this puzzle?"). IPs who follow the suggestions will hopefully be naturally reinforced (they feel calmer), and staff may provide additional verbal or arbitrary reinforcement (points or tokens) to strengthen the likelihood that the IP will engage in the same problem solving in future events. In many situations, once staff have established credibility as supportive and caring, these interventions head off a crisis. In instances where it is not effective and the IP engages in a serious rule violation behavior, the Egregious Behavior Protocol is implemented.

Egregious Behavior Protocol: step by step

Following the IP's egregious behavior, restoring safety and security is the first intervention. Fighting IPs are restrained, as necessary, and then separated. A self-injuring IP's actions are stopped, means to self-harm are removed, and the IP is placed in a setting with minimal means to self-harm. Medical attention is obtained, if needed. The IP is then informed that they are "off program" while the protocol is completed. Importantly, regular programming continues for all IPs not involved in the incident, and lockdowns are limited to the amount of time needed to secure the setting. It is important, therefore, that an engaging and active program for IPs is in place, including education, recreation, entertainment, social activities, and other appropriate privileges.

The protocol outlines a series of tasks for the IP to accomplish to restore full privileges and programming. The first is to make a commitment not to engage in egregious behavior(s). Conversations between staff and the IP initially focus on this issue, until commitment is obtained. Interactions between the IP and peers on the unit are restricted until this occurs. Staff need to be well trained to keep the focus on this topic or to end the conversation and return later. The protocol is not an opportunity for IPs to get unfettered one-on-one time with staff.

The next task is completion of a chain or behavioral analysis of the incident (Ivanoff & Schmidt, 2010). This analysis identifies the environmental cue that preceded the incident, thoughts/emotions/action urges that led to the behavior, and actual or expected outcomes that may have reinforced the behavior. Vulnerabilities (contextual variables that increase the likelihood of responding to the cue with egregious behavior) are also identified. This information should be documented in the IP's chart and is used in the development of an individualized treatment plan.

Staff then work with the IP to learn and practice skills that are identified as directly applicable to preventing the recurrence of egregious behavior. These may address vulnerabilities, tolerance of cues, or dysfunctional links (e.g., thoughts, problem solving) in the chain. A list of skills that IPs can practice when feeling distressed, angry, or anxious can be taught to officers and passed on to IPs. Implementation of the "toolbox" of DBT skills (Linehan, 2015a, 2015b), which provides methods for emotion regulation, distress tolerance, reality acceptance, interpersonal effectiveness, and mindfulness, should occur. Cognitive modification is also an important component of treatment with most egregious behaviors, to address beliefs that support the use of the behavior or the avoidance of more skillful means (Ivanoff & Schmidt, 2010; Ivanoff & Marotta, 2018; Tolisano et al., 2017).

IPs show their commitment to the BMP by demonstrating to staff and clinicians how they will use the skills, describing the steps, and then participating in structured role plays (or using the skills during their normal activities while on the protocol). Demonstration of proficiency—not perfection—in the skills, along with ongoing commitment to use skills when needed, is required for reinstatement of privileges.

Next, a "correction–overcorrection" is developed by the IP to address harm that may have been caused by the egregious behavior, as possible. This may begin with apologies to those affected but would also generally include a service project designed to improve the individual or unit experiences of others. This is not necessarily a grand project; the goal is to craft something meaningful to those receiving it. Most IPs will not be in a situation to pay for replacement of damaged items or medical bills for any injuries caused. If fighting is the target behavior, then problem solving with all parties involved is necessary, until agreement is reached that the issue is resolved and a shared commitment exists not to harm the other. Readers familiar with the principles of restorative justice (Pointer, 2021) will understand such practices.

As the IP works through the Egregious Behavior Protocol, rewards or small privileges may be extended to reinforce IP willingness and the steps they have taken. Full privileges are restored once IPs have completed the protocol and as they demonstrate their ability to successfully implement skills to avoid egregious behavior in the presence of future cues. For those who continue to engage in similar egregious behaviors, a return to full programming may require more time and demonstrated practice than for first-time offenders. Clinicians and staff together orchestrate the restrictions, practice opportunities, and ultimately determine when the IP earns a return to full programming. The relationships and trust built between staff and the IP are critical here, and staff follow-through in coaching, rewarding, and moving IPs through the protocol also assists in building a constructive relationship for future interactions. Staff commitment to safety in the milieu benefits all who live and work there.

It is important to balance the change demanded from the IP with staff interventions designed to maintain the IP's motivation to complete the task at hand. Burying IPs in sanctions or seemingly insurmountable lists of tasks may needlessly delay (or even prevent) them from applying themselves to the process. Further, the removal from basic daily programming is likely to be most salient when daily programming is meaningful and rewarding for IPs. To "climb the ladder" of the protocol, there needs to be something worth reaching at the top. Thus, a fully developed BMP will include elements that all IPs want to access, ensuring that removal from the program (response cost) will be meaningful and that rejoining the program will be a goal worth striving for. Staff who are present, know the IP well, are fair and consistent, and who can structure practice opportunities and model the behaviors expected are all aspects of place management, as described above. The goal is to transfer management of the IP's behavior from the staff to the IPs themselves by teaching new skills and providing incentives for using them.

The above discussion regarding an Egregious Behavior Protocol occurred in a housing unit where place management has been implemented. However, few correctional facilities have implemented such a model. BMPs are often effectively used in special housing units such as a special needs unit or mental health unit. Many of the principles previously described regarding the Egregious Behavior Protocol can be adapted to BMPs in such units.

Summary

BMPs such as the Egregious Behavior Protocol are built on the foundation of well-established behavioral principles and are most effective when incorporated and applied systematically by well-trained staff. This chapter explains the importance of bidirectional transactions between the environment and IPs in managing behaviors. There are many commonalities between BMPs and place management elements, and the two ideas can complement and enhance each other to enhance IP and staff safety in correctional settings.

REFERENCES

Chapman, A., & Ivanoff, A. (2018). Forensic issues in borderline personality disorder. In B. Stanley & A. New (Eds.), *Borderline personality disorder* (pp. 403–421). Oxford University Press.

Eck, J. E. (2015). Who should prevent crime at places? The advantages of regulating place managers and challenges to police services. *Policing*, *9*(3), 223–233.

Hoke, S. A. (2013). *Place management in a correctional setting*. https://scholarshare.temple.edu/handle/20.500.12613/1451

Ivanoff, A., & Marotta, P. (2018). DBT in forensic settings. In M. A. Swales (Ed.), *The Oxford handbook of dialectical behavior therapy* (pp. 617–644). Oxford University Press.

Ivanoff, A., & Schmidt, H. (2010). Functional assessment in forensic settings: A valuable tool for preventing and treating egregious behavior. *Journal of Cognitive Psychotherapy: An International Quarterly*, *24*(2), 81–91.

Juvenile Rehabilitation Administration. (2002). *The integrated treatment model report*. Washington State Department of Social and Health Services.

Liebling, A. (2004). *Prisons and their moral performance: A study of values, quality, and prison life*. Oxford University Press.

Linehan, M. M. (2015a). *DBT skills training manual: 2nd edition*. Guilford Press.

Linehan, M. M. (2015b). *Handouts and worksheets for DBT skills training*. Guilford Press.

Madensen, T. D. (2007). *Bar management and crime: Toward a dynamic theory of place management and crime hotspots*. University of Cincinnati, Cincinnati.

McCann, R., Ball, E., & Ivanoff, A. (2000). Creating a life worth living for those who don't think others deserve it: The CMHIP forensic DBT model. *Cognitive and Behavioral Practice*, *7*(4), 447–456.

McCann, R., Ivanoff, A., Schmidt, H., & Beach, B. (2007). DBT in residential forensic settings. In L. Dimeff, K. Koerner, & C. Sanderson (Eds.), *Dialectical behavior therapy in clinical practice* (pp. 112–144). Guilford Press.

Papalia, N., Spivak, B., Daffern, M., & Ogloff, J. R. P. (2019). A meta-analytic review of the efficacy of psychological treatments for violent offenders in correctional and forensic mental health settings. *Clinical Psychology Science and Practice*, *26*(2), e12282.

Pointer, L. (2021). *The restorative justice ritual*. Routledge Press.

Pratt, T. C., & Cullen, F. T. (2005). Assessing macro-level predictors and theories of crime: A meta analysis. In Michael Tonry (Ed.), *Crime and justice: A review of research* (Vol. 32, pp. 373–450). University of Chicago Press.

Schmidt, H., III, & Ivanoff, A. M. (2015). Behavior management plans. In R. L. Trestman, K. L. Applebaum, & J. L. Metzner (Eds.), *Oxford textbook of correctional psychiatry* (pp. 286–292). Oxford University Press.

Sparks, R., & Bottoms, A. (2008). Legitimacy and imprisonment: Some notes on the problem of order ten years after. In J. M. Byrne, D. Hummer, & F. S. Taxman (Eds.), *The culture of prison violence* (pp. 91–104). Pearson.

Sparks, R., Bottoms, A. E., & Hay, W. (1996). *Prisons and the problem of order*. Clarendon Press.

St. John, V. J. (2023). Blood on the walls: The influence of place management on jail and prison victimization. *Journal of Qualitative Criminal Justice and Criminology*, *12*(3), 362–403.

Swenson, C. R., Sanderson, C., Dulit, R. A., & Linehan, M. M. (2001). The application of dialectical behavior therapy for patients with borderline personality disorder on inpatient units. *Psychiatric Quarterly*, *72*(4), 307–324.

Tolisano, P., Sondik, T. M., & Dike, C. C. (2017). A positive behavioral approach for aggression in forensic psychiatric settings. *Journal of the American Academy of Psychiatry and the Law*, *45*(1), 31–39.

SECTION X
Distinct populations

55

Incarcerated women

Catherine F. Lewis

Introduction

Despite a roughly equal number of men and women in the general population, women consistently have lower rates of incarceration than their male peers (Carson & Kluckow, 2023). The difference is not trivial; there were more than 10 times as many men as women incarcerated in the United States in 2022 (Carson & Kluckow, 2023).

Issues specific to incarcerated women now confront the U.S. correctional system in part as a multigenerational product of the War on Drugs from the mid-1980s to the mid-1990s. During that period, the number of women incarcerated rose 888% (Mauer et al., 1999). Nonviolent drug-related charges accounted for the bulk of the rise. As the correctional system began to experience an influx of women, it became clear that they were different from their male peers. The differences included epidemiology of psychiatric disorders, intensity of health service use, social stressors, and patterns of offending. The logical question arose as to whether women needed a different treatment approach in the correctional system than men. The term "gender-responsive programming" emerged and represented the idea that women have specific needs distinct from their male peers that could best be met with treatment designed for women (Covington & Bloom, 2006; Wright et al., 2012). This chapter describes, given the current knowledge base, the patterns of offending and arrests for women versus men, the sociodemographics of incarcerated women, the psychopathology exhibited by incarcerated women, and how best to treat incarcerated women and implement this treatment within jails and prisons.

Background

At year end in 2022, there were 1,230,100 people incarcerated in U.S. state and federal prisons; 1,146,400 (93.2%) were men and 87,800 (6.8%) were women (Carson & Kluckow, 2023). An additional 84,000 women were incarcerated in local jails (Kajstura & Sawyer, 2024).

It is not surprising that most incarcerated persons (IPs) are male; men are arrested more often than women for most offenses except embezzlement, truancy, and prostitution. Men are significantly more likely to be arrested for violent crimes, which explains their longer sentences. Men account for more than 96% of all arrests for rape, 87% of all arrests for murder and nonnegligent manslaughter, 85% of all arrests for robbery, and 75% of all aggravated assault arrests (Federal Bureau of Investigation, 2019). In short, violent offending is a predominately male affair. At the end of 2023, a higher percentage of men (64.2%%) were incarcerated for violent offenses than women (45.5%%) in state prisons (Carson & Kluckow, 2023). Women who commit violent offenses are more likely than men to have male accomplices, to victimize someone they know, and to offend at the victim's home or school. Women are less likely to use weapons and to injure their victims seriously (Greenfeld & Snell, 1999). Most women (55.5%) are incarcerated for nonviolent offenses, including property crimes (18.6%), drug-related charges (24.6%), and public order/other charges (11.3%; Carson & Kluckow, 2023).

Minorities are overrepresented in correctional populations. At year end of 2021, the incarceration rate for Black women stood at 62 per 100,000; Hispanic women, 49 per 100,000; and White women, 38 per 100,000 (Kajstura & Sawyer, 2024). These numbers stand in contrast to those of the U.S. population, where White women outnumber women of color (13.6% Black, 19.1% Hispanic, 58.9% White; U.S. Census Bureau, 2023). The disparity in race among incarcerated women, while notable, decreased by 30.7% for Black women from 2000 to 2009 (Mauer, 2013) and has continued to decrease steadily from 2013 to the present (Monazam & Budd, 2023).

Incarcerated women are likely to be in their early 30s and never to have been married despite having lived with at least one common-law partner for a year or more. They have borne an average of two children and are most often responsible for them. This statistic is striking and important; current data suggest that close to a quarter of a million children have incarcerated mothers (Greenfeld & Snell, 1999; Van Voorhis et al., 2010). Most of these mothers (60%) had custody of their children at the time of arrest. Incarcerated women are more likely to have a high school education than their male counterparts but more often live below the poverty line and lack legal means of support. Most were not seeking work at the time of arrest. They are generally less likely to recidivate than their male peers; 51% of incarcerated women have one or no prior offenses, versus 39% of incarcerated men (Greenfeld & Snell, 1999; Wright et al., 2012).

Incarcerated women report victimization more often than men (Browne et al., 1999). One survey of approximately 40,000 women in prison found that close to half had been assaulted, a third physically abused, and a third sexually abused before incarceration (Snell & Morton, 1991). A similar study of 2,000 incarcerated women found that more than half reported physical abuse, and more than a third reported sexual abuse (American Correctional Association, 1990). Those who were sexually abused were most often victimized for the first time during childhood (at ages 5 to 14). The rates for abuse and victimization exceed those reported by women in community samples and are triple that of incarcerated men (American Correctional Association, 1990). All these factors have a critical impact on the psychopathology observed in this population, how it manifests, and how treatment should be approached.

Psychiatric epidemiology of incarcerated women

Incarcerated women are more likely to have psychiatric disorders than incarcerated men and are more likely to have comorbid diagnoses (DiCataldo et al., 1995; Maden et al., 1994; Trestman et al., 2007). Multiple studies now exist that used different validated and reliable research interviews to determine the prevalence of psychiatric disorders among incarcerated women. Some of these studies focused on women in jail, others on women in prison, and others on mixed populations; one summarized multiple studies (Fazel & Danesh, 2002; Jordan et al., 1996; Lewis, 2006; Lynch et al., 2014; Steadman et al., 2009; Teplin, 1994; Trestman et al., 2007). Table 55.1 summarizes the results of several studies regarding the prevalence of psychiatric disorders in incarcerated women.

Substance use disorders

Substance use disorders (SUDs) are the most common disorders among female correctional populations. This point is critical to remember because treatment for other disorders may be seriously compromised if substance use is not addressed. Women are more likely than men to be intravenous drug users, to have been introduced to substance use by men, to have partners who use substances, and to engage in sex work for drugs (Greenfeld & Snell, 1999; Hammett, 2001). The use of intravenous drugs places women at high risk for contracting infectious diseases. Women are also more likely to use "hard drugs" (e.g., heroin, cocaine) and to use a greater number of drugs than men (Greenfeld & Snell, 1999). With respect to alcohol, women experience a phenomenon called "telescoping" in which their symptom severity proceeds at a much more rapid rate than their male peers. This puts them at higher risk for physical effects earlier during addiction than men (Schuckit et al., 1995).

Figure 55.1 shows the prevalence of SUDs for clinical populations and incarcerated populations of men and women. What is clear is that as the severity of illness worsens, the gender gap erodes—that is, incarcerated women use substances at a level at least as high as incarcerated men (Jordan et al., 1996; Lewis, 2006; Teplin et al., 1996). This is a striking contrast from the data from the general population (Kessler et al., 1994). Incarcerated women use multiple substances as a rule, and the load of symptoms for substance dependence is high

Table 55.1 Psychiatric diagnosis: women in community versus female offenders—lifetime prevalence

Disorder (%)	Kessler et al., 1994*	Lewis 2006[†]	Teplin et al., 1994[‡]	Jordan et al., 1996[§]	Lynch et al., 2014[‖]
Substance use disorder	17.9	65.4	70.2	NR	82
Alcohol use disorder	8.2	43.8	32.3	38.0	NR
Drug use disorder	5.9	56.6	63.6	44.2	NR
Antisocial personality disorder	1.2	32.3	13.8	11.9	NR
Posttraumatic stress disorder	10.4	40.8	33.5	30.0	53
Major depressive disorder	21.3	36.2	16.9	13.0	28.0

* National Comorbidity Survey; a sample of women in the community.
[†] Midsentence female felons (*N* = 136).
[‡] Pretrial female detainees (*N* = 1,272).
[§] Convicted female felons entering prison (*N* = 805).
[‖] Female jail detainees, multisite (*N* = 491).

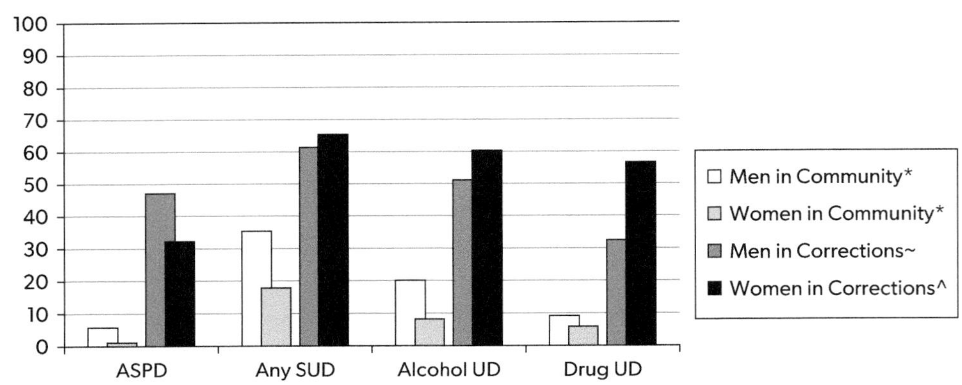

Figure 55.1 Community and correctional mental illness prevalences are different: lifetime prevalence, by gender. *, National Comorbidity Survey (Kessler et al., 1994); ~, 728 jail detainees (Teplin et al., 1996); ^, 136 midsentence female felons (Lewis, 2006). ASPD = antisocial personality disorder; SUD = substance use disorder; UD = use disorder.

(Lewis, 2006, 2010). Two thirds of women who enter the correctional system had used drugs in the months preceding incarceration, 50% were using daily, and 40% were using at the time of their alleged offense (Greenfeld & Snell, 1999).

In summary, SUDs are the most common diagnoses in incarcerated women. When present, the disorder is often severe, as evidenced by high symptom counts, early age of onset, and multiple substances used (Lewis, 2006, 2010). SUDs are associated with higher health service use, worsened prognosis for comorbid disorders, physical problems, comorbidity, and death by completed suicide (Kessler et al., 1999; Roy, 2003; Teplin et al., 1997; Wu et al., 1999).

Posttraumatic stress disorder

Posttraumatic stress disorder (PTSD) is increasingly recognized as a highly prevalent diagnosis among incarcerated women. In many instances, their abuse occurred early in life (i.e., during childhood) and was severe and enduring. Exposure to severe trauma in childhood may result in repeated revictimization in adulthood after high-risk behaviors including sex work and intravenous drug use, with resultant interaction with dangerous people and situations (Zlotnick, 1997). PTSD is also a potent risk factor for suicide and has a synergistic effect in the presence of major depression (Brodsky et al., 2001). Perhaps more importantly, women with comorbid PTSD and SUDs have more inpatient admissions, higher symptom counts, higher service use, and more psychosocial problems (e.g., homelessness, domestic violence, loss of child custody) than women with either problem alone (Najavits, 1998; Zlotnick, 1997).

The importance of sustained, repetitive trauma from which someone cannot escape is particularly important in determining the course of PTSD (Herman, 1992). Many women who are incarcerated have experienced such situations in their childhood homes, as adults in abusive relationships, and as sex workers engaging in high-risk behavior. They can have symptoms of PTSD that are more tenacious than usual and less responsive to treatment (e.g., somatization, dissociation, chronic suicidality). They can also have pathological changes in the ability to form relationships (e.g., intense, unstable relationships; boundary violations; formation of dependent relationships that place them at high risk for exploitation). Women who have been victimized as children are at risk for rape in adulthood, sexual harassment, battering, self-harm (e.g., cutting), and suicidality. While this construct of complex PTSD is an evolving one and conceptualized as a research category, it is important to consider for incarcerated women. Specifically, failure to correctly diagnose PTSD can lead to misapplication of a diagnosis of personality disorder, stigmatization, and incorrect treatment (see Chapter 36).

Antisocial personality disorder

Antisocial personality disorder (ASPD) is prevalent among incarcerated women, particularly convicted felons (Lewis, 2006; Warren et al., 2002; Zlotnick, 1999). ASPD is rare in clinical populations of women. As seen in Table 55.1 and Figure 55.1, the prevalence of ASPD in female correctional populations is much higher than that of women or men in the community. Among felons, the rate approaches that of men (Lewis, 2010; Lynch et al., 2014; Warren et al., 2002; Zlotnick, 1999). Once again, the severity of pathology erodes an expected gender gap. Women with ASPD (with onset of conduct disorder before age 10) have more severe addiction, higher risk of suicide, increased risk of violence, and poorer outcomes with treatment than do men in the community; they approach the profile of incarcerated men with ASPD (Lewis, 2006).

Psychopathy has been found among female felons at prevalences approaching that of male felons (Warren et al., 2002). Psychopathy, which is refractory to treatment and an ominous prognosticator of outcomes, is rarely measured among incarcerated women. Despite this, when assessed for the presence of psychopathy, female felons have shown similar statistics as their male counterparts. These data are important because of implications for treatment.

Gender-responsive treatment

Examination of women within the correctional system as a discrete group is a relatively new phenomenon. In 1978, only 10,918 women were under the jurisdiction of correctional authorities in state and federal facilities; in 2022, there were 87, 800 (Carson & Kluckow, 2023). Given the inflow of women into the correctional system and their complex needs, it is not surprising that it has taken some time to reflect on the correct way to address mental health issues for incarcerated women. A one-size-fits-all approach will not likely be the most feasible or efficacious strategy for a population with such complex needs. Indeed, some of the most severely ill women appear to have psychopathology resembling that of men, and it remains unclear what the full implications of this finding are. While gender should be a consideration in treatment for men and women, it is not yet time to call for "gender-responsive programming" for all women in corrections until there is evidence-based literature suggesting better outcomes (e.g., recidivism, morbidity, mortality) from the treatment. Gender-responsive treatment cannot and should not be the goal in and of itself. With these substantial caveats in mind, several basic tenets that could form a core to inform the treatment of incarcerated women are outlined here.

Steps toward a model treatment program for incarcerated women

Safety first: no treatment can occur in dangerous environments

A prerequisite for successful psychiatric treatment anywhere, but particularly salient in jails and prisons, is physical and emotional safety. Psychiatric staff working in correctional environments must recognize that there are times and situations that place safety and security above treatment (e.g., a patient may need to be strip-searched by custody personnel, treatment may not be able to occur because of a lockdown). Women with PTSD are at heightened risk for revictimization by peers and staff. Management should include specific training for staff who work with incarcerated women, a mechanism for anonymous reporting of violations by staff, structured investigation procedures, provision of supervision to staff to assuage frustration and countertransference, and frequent external oversight of staff interactions with incarcerated persons.

Recognize psychopathy: women can victimize each other

Recent studies have shown that a high percentage of female felons meet the criteria for psychopathy (Lewis, 2006; Warren et al., 2002; Zlotnick, 1999). This subgroup is resistant to treatment and can disrupt groups and treatment units through contagion. While controversial, it is likely that these women would best be housed in a unit that addresses their specific issues. The emphasis in treatment should be on SUDs (often a harm reduction rather than an abstinence model is most realistic), behavior management, addressing comorbid diagnoses such as major depression and PTSD, and offering support through case management. Women without significant levels of traditional mental illness in these units would benefit from vocational programs with close oversight.

Concede limitations: equality is not equivalence

Research on women within the correctional system has grown significantly over the past 30 years. As appreciation of their complex comorbidity has grown, interest has logically risen in applying models successful in the community. The conundrum is that women who are incarcerated differ in many critical ways from their community peers, and most well-studied and validated treatment modules come from community samples. Currently, a variety of approaches are being attempted with incarcerated women, and evidence-based literature has modestly begun to emerge. As programs are evaluated, it is critical to recognize that incarcerated women have specialized profiles that set them apart from women in the community. Similarly, applications that appear to work in the community (e.g., motivational enhancement, contingency management, dialectical behavior therapy) would be and are intriguing to integrate into correctional settings. The caveats to consider have most to do with treatment matching; selecting patients who are appropriate candidates for the therapy in question by appropriately diagnosing them to begin with takes on critical importance in a correctional setting.

Don't discriminate: all qualified staff can treat incarcerated women

Women who have experienced trauma do not necessarily require treatment and contact restricted only to women. Gender-responsive programming should not mean that women can demand only female treatment providers. That would be disruptive, unworkable, and not useful to ultimate recovery. In essence, it would also limit their access to providers, which is a bad idea. There is no robust literature that supports a claim that incarcerated women have better outcomes with female treatment providers. It is therefore important not to exclude male providers who are as likely to be effective, qualified, and helpful as female ones. It is also unworkable to insist upon racial matching because, by doing so, one limits access to treatment for patients. Conflicts based on gender and racial preferences can form the basis of solid therapeutic conversations and working through issues in treatment. Training staff about minority cultures commonly found in correctional settings and encouraging cultural humility among providers can help to navigate these conflicts (see Chapter 22).

Coordinate your effort: have a case manager be "quarterback"

Incarcerated women have often struggled to receive services while in the community. They are not generally skilled self-advocates, and some do not know when to seek mental health or medical care. They have a host of worries outside of corrections, the most important of which can be their children and financial situation upon release. Financial issues including housing can erase mental and medical health gains made within correctional systems upon release if not addressed. Each woman in the system should ideally have a case manager, or "quarterback" (Lewis, 2006), whose job might include help with obtaining services while incarcerated and entitlements upon release (e.g., medical needs, mental health needs, vocational needs, concrete needs such as clothing/phone calls, contact with department of children and families).

Remember the next generation: motherhood is important

Because most incarcerated women are mothers, it is helpful to integrate parenting classes and vocational classes into treatment. Ideally, there would be child-friendly facilities for visits. For mothers incarcerated at a distance from their children, video visitation enabled by computer and appropriately supervised by correctional staff may be an option for maintaining and building these critical relationships. Keeping mothers in contact with children's schools assists both parent and child, particularly with shorter incarcerations. The rise in the ability of schools and correctional systems to teleconference since the COVID-19 pandemic makes parent–teacher conferences a potential reality for incarcerated mothers who are still custodial parents.

Identify what you are treating: obtain detailed criterion-based diagnoses

Other than nonadherence, a major reason for treatment failure concerns inaccurate diagnosis or unrecognized comorbidity. This comorbidity includes other psychiatric diagnoses, medical conditions, and side effects from medications. Incarcerated women have complex pathology, which at times can overwhelm clinicians. During a short, nonstructured interview, it is difficult to correctly diagnose women who have multiple issues. A structured interview offers the opportunity to assess the patient objectively, consider diagnoses that might not arise during an open-ended interview, quantify symptom counts, identify how many substances are used and the severity of use, and have a reasoned assessment of often provocative, complex patients.

Use medication for a reason: adhere to practice guidelines whenever possible and practical

While there are best practice guidelines for many disorders, one of the difficulties confronting the clinician who treats an incarcerated woman is that she may have many disorders. One woman may have PTSD, major depression, panic disorder, multiple SUDs, ASPD, and side effects from medications for the treatment of HIV or hepatitis C, along with uncontrolled diabetes. In these instances, it is not appropriate to withhold therapy because of a substance use history. The myth that "when they stop using, they will not be depressed" is not correct (see Chapter 48). Large prospective studies have shown definitively that women and men who use drugs and/or alcohol tend to have episodes of "clean" and "dirty" (i.e., when they are using) depression. Those with episodes of "dirty depression" are more likely to die by suicide and have higher morbidity (Schuckit et al., 1995). Thus, the history of addiction should not preclude aggressive treatment for depression. Other important issues in treating women are to be aware of body image issues (e.g., avoid medications that cause weight gain; avoid prescribing medications that women may abuse to lose weight) and always know pregnancy status before prescribing.

Address comorbidity head on: use integrated treatment

Treatments for SUDs are best integrated completely with treatment of other mental health disorders. The idea of integrated treatment for PTSD and SUD (the most common diagnoses for incarcerated women) has resulted in several programs, including Seeking Safety (Najavits, 2002), Helping Women Recover (Messina et al., 2010), and the Trauma Recovery and Empowerment Model (Fallot & Harris, 2002). Emerging literature suggests positive outcomes in correctional settings (McHugo et al., 2005; Zlotnick et al., 2003) and within the community (Messina et al., 2010).

Give women with the most severe disorders a "home base": use the therapeutic community

Many incarcerated women would benefit from highly structured housing with an integrated treatment program that addresses addiction, trauma, personality disorders (including ASPD), and depression. The major advantage to a therapeutic community, coupled with personal case management, is a move toward stable, predictable, ongoing care rather than crisis-driven interventions in response to problem behaviors (e.g., cutting, attempting suicide, using drugs). Ideally, medical visits are coordinated for the therapeutic community so that physical problems are addressed. Few studies have formally examined health service use within prisons, but it is likely that a therapeutic community, as outlined here, would increase treatment adherence, decrease crisis-driven work, decrease exigent visits, and afford better outcomes (De Leon, 1995; Farabee et al., 1999; Roth & Presse, 2003).

Don't drop the ball: coordinate discharge care with an eagle eye

Discharge is a critical time for women who have been incarcerated. Many have limited resources (e.g., no home, no car, little money, no job), and some will have had entitlements cut off while incarcerated. The case manager is critical in ensuring that appointments are made that women can attend, that paperwork is filled out if necessary to reinstate entitlements, that medications for the waiting period before seeing a new provider are disbursed, and that appointments with new providers are made. If a woman has children, consideration should be given to a center that offers primary care, including pediatrics and dentistry, as well as mental health to make attendance at appointments more likely.

Summary

Incarcerated women are a group with a high degree of psychiatric comorbidity. The most common diagnoses are SUD, PTSD, major depression, and ASPD. The profile of women in corrections is unique; it differs both from women in the community and from men in corrections. This renders the treatment mission difficult. There is little evidence-based literature on how to treat incarcerated women, in large part because there are so many more incarcerated men. Once the pathology of SUD and ASPD becomes severe, women have behaviors and outcomes like their male peers (e.g., suicidal behavior, violence, more severe substance use, recidivism). Applications of interventions developed in the community may be an imperfect fit for women in carceral settings. Consequently, a therapeutic community for women with the most severe disorders (e.g., SUD, PTSD, self-injurious behavior) that is focused on treatment for trauma and SUD with a strong focus on case management, cognitive-based psychotherapy, appropriate diagnoses, and evidence-based psychopharmacological treatment when necessary is potentially the best and most effective structure for service delivery to this challenging population (De Leon, 1995; Farabee et al., 1999; Roth & Presse, 2003).

REFERENCES

American Correctional Association. (1990). *The female offender*. St. Mary's Press.

Brodsky, B. S., Oquendo, M., Ellis, S. P., et al. (2001). The relationship of childhood abuse of impulsivity and suicidal behavior in adults with major depression. *American Journal of Psychiatry, 158*, 1871–1877.

Browne, A., Miller, B., & Maguin, E. (1999). Prevalence and severity of lifetime physical and sexual victimization among incarcerated women. *International Journal of the Law and Psychiatry, 22*, 2301–2322.

Carson, E. A., & Kluckow, R. (2023). *Prisoners in 2022—Statistical tables*. https://bjs.ojp.gov/document/p22st.pdf

Covington, S., & Bloom, B. (2006). Gender-responsive treatment and services in correctional settings. *Women and Therapy, 29*, 9–33.

De Leon, G. (1995). Therapeutic communities for addictions: A theoretical framework. *International Journal of Addiction, 30*, 1603–1645.

DiCataldo, F., Greer, A., & Profit, W. E. (1995). Screening prison inmates for mental disorder: An examination of the relationship between mental disorders and prison adjustment. *Bulletin of the American Academy of Psychiatry and the Law, 23*, 573–585.

Fallot, R. D., & Harris, M. (2002). The Trauma Recovery and Empowerment Model (TREM): Conceptual and practical issues in a group intervention for women. *Community Mental Health Journal, 38*, 475–485.

Farabee, D., Prendergast, M., Cartier, J., et al. (1999). Barriers to implementing effective correctional drug treatment programs. *Prison Journal, 79*, 150–162.

Fazel, S., & Danesh, J. (2002). Serious mental disorder in 23,000 prisoners: A systemic review of 62 surveys. *The Lancet, 359*, 545–550.

Federal Bureau of Investigation. (2019). Crime in the U.S. https://ucr.fbi.gov/crime-in-the-u.s/2019/crime-in-the-u.s.-2019/topic-pages

Greenfeld, L. A., & Snell, T. L. (1999). *Bureau of Justice Statistics special report: Women offenders*. Bureau of Justice Statistics.

Hammett, T. M. (2001). Making the case for health interventions in correctional facilities. *Journal of Urban Health, 78*, 236–240.

Herman, J. L. (1992). Complex PTSD: A syndrome in survivors of prolonged and repeated trauma. *Journal of Traumatic Stress, 5*(3), 377–391.

Jordan, B. K., Schlenger, W. E., Fairbanks, J. A., et al. (1996). Prevalence of psychiatric disorders among incarcerated women, II: Convicted felons entering prison. *Archives of General Psychiatry, 55*, 513–519.

Kajstura, A., & Sawyer, W. (2024). *Women's mass incarceration: The whole pie*. https://www.prisonpolicy.org/reports/pie2024women.html

Kessler, R. C., Borges, G., & Walters, E. E. (1999). Prevalence of and risk factors for lifetime suicide attempts in the National Comorbidity Survey. *Archives of General Psychiatry, 56*, 617–626.

Kessler, R. C., McGonagle, K. A., Zhao, S., et al. (1994). Lifetime and twelve-month prevalence of DSM-III-R psychiatric disorders in the United States: Results from the National Comorbidity Survey. *Archives of General Psychiatry, 51*, 8–19.

Lewis, C. F. (2006). Treating incarcerated women: gender matters. *Psychiatric Clinics of North America, 29*, 773–789.

Lewis, C. F. (2010). Childhood antecedents of adult violent offending in a group of female felons. *Behavioral Sciences and the Law, 28,* 224–234.

Lynch, S. M., DeHart, D. D., Beknap, J. E., et al. (2014). A multisite study of the prevalence of serious mental illness, PTSD, and substance use disorders of women in jail. *Psychiatric Services in Advance,* February 3, 1–5. Psychiatr Serv. 2014 May 1 *65*(5): 670–4. doi: 10.1176/appips.20300172.PMID:24487481

Maden, T., Swinton, M., & Gunn, J. (1994). Psychiatric disorder in women serving a prison sentence. *British Journal of Psychiatry, 164,* 44–54.

Mauer, M. (2013). *The changing racial dynamics of women's incarceration.* https://www.sentencingproject.org

Mauer, M., Potler, C., & Wolf, R. (1999). *Gender and trust: Women, drugs and the sentencing policy.* The Sentencing Project.

McHugo, G. J., Caspi, Y., Kammerer, N., et al. (2005). The assessment of trauma history in women with co-occurring substance abuse and mental disorders and a history of interpersonal violence. *Journal of Behavioral Health Services Research, 32,* 113–127.

Messina, N., Grella, C., Cartier, J., et al. (2010). A randomized experimental study of gender-responsive substance abuse treatment for women in prison. *Journal of Substance Abuse Treatment, 38,* 97–107.

Monazam, N., & Budd, K. M. (2023). *Incarcerated women and girls.* https://www.sentencingproject.org/app/uploads/2023/05/Incarcerated-Women-and-Girls-1.pdf

Najavits, L. M. (2002). Seeking Safety: Therapy for trauma and substance abuse. *Corrections Today, 64,* 136–141.

Najavits, L. M., Weiss, R. D., Shaw, S. R., et al. (1998). Seeking Safety: Outcome of a new cognitive-behavioral psychotherapy for women with PTSD and substance use disorder. *Journal of Trauma and Stress, 11,* 437–456.

Roth, B., & Presse, L. (2003). Nursing interventions for parasuicidal behaviors in female offenders. *Journal of Psychosocial Nursing Mental Health Services, 41,* 20–29.

Roy, A. (2003). Characteristics of drug addicts who attempt suicide. *Psychiatry Research, 103,* 121–199.

Schuckit, M. A., Andthenelli, R. M., Bucholz, K. K., et al. (1995). The time course and development of alcohol-related problems in men and women. *Journal of Studies on Alcohol, 56,* 218–225.

Snell, T. L., & Morton, D. C. (1991). *Survey of our state prison inmates 1991: Women in prison.* Bureau of Justice, Office of Justice Programs.

Steadman, H. J., Osher, F. C., Robbins, P. C., et al. (2009). Prevalence of serious mental illness among jail inmates. *Psychiatric Services, 60*(6), 761–765.

Teplin, L. A. (1994). Psychiatric and substance abuse disorders among urban jail detainees. *American Journal of Public Health, 84*(2), 290–293.

Teplin, L. A., Abram, K. M., & McClelland, G. M. (1996). Prevalence of psychiatric disorders among incarcerated women, 1: Pre-trial jail detainees. *Archives of General Psychiatry, 53,* 505–512.

Teplin, L. A., Abram, K. M., & McClelland, G. M. (1997). Mentally disordered women in jail: Who receives services? *American Journal of Public Health, 87,* 604–609.

Trestman, R. L., Ford, J., Zhang, W. Z., et al. (2007). Current and lifetime psychiatric illness among inmates not identified as mentally ill at intake in Connecticut's jails. *Journal of the American Academy of Psychiatry and the Law, 35,* 490–500.

U.S. Census Bureau. (2023). *QuickFacts.* https://www.census.gov/quickfacts/fact/table/US/PST045222

Van Voorhis, P., Salisbury, E. J., Wright, E. M., & Bauman, A. (2010). Women's risk factors and their contributions to existing risk/needs assessment: The current status of gender-responsive supplement. *Criminal Justice and Behavior, 37,* 261–288.

Warren, J. I., Hurt, S., Lopez, A. B., et al. (2002). Psychiatric symptoms, history of victimization, and violent behavior among incarcerated female felons: An American perspective. *International Journal of Law and Psychiatry, 25,* 129–149.

Wright, E., Van Voorhis, P., Salisbury, E. J., & Bauman, A. (2012). Gender-responsive lessons learned and policy implications for women in prison: A review. *Criminal Justice and Behavior, 39,* 1612–1632.

Wu, L. T., Kouzis, A. C., & Leaf, P. J. (1999). Influence of co-morbid alcohol and psychiatric disorders on utilization of mental health services in the National Comorbidity Survey. *American Journal of Psychiatry, 56*(8), 1230–1236.

Zlotnick, C. (1997). PTSD comorbidity and childhood abuse among incarcerated women. *Journal of Nervous and Mental Disorders, 185,* 761–763.

Zlotnick, C. (1999). Antisocial personality disorder, affective dysregulation and childhood abuse among incarcerated women. *Journal of Personality Disorders, 13,* 90–95.

Zlotnick, C., Najavits, L. M., Rohsenow, D. J., et al. (2003). A cognitive-behavioral treatment for incarcerated women with substance abuse disorder and posttraumatic stress disorder: Findings from a pilot study. *Journal of Substance Abuse Treatment, 25,* 99–105.

56

Lesbian, gay, bisexual, and transgender individuals

Elie G. Aoun and Lama Bazzi[1]

Introduction

The lesbian, gay, bisexual, and transgender (LGBT) population has been, and remains, disenfranchised in many ways. Despite increasing acceptance of nonheterosexual sexual orientation, evidenced by legalizing gay marriage at the national level (*Obergefell v. Hodges*, 2015; Respect for Marriage Act, 2022), LGBT people continue to have a higher prevalence of mental illness due to minority stress than heterosexuals (Meyer, 2003). Factors such as stigma, prejudice, and discrimination lead to an increased incidence of mental suffering as a result of stressful, hostile, and often unsafe environments. The stressors that LGBT individuals face likely contribute to their disproportionate risk of contact with the criminal justice system, beginning in adolescence and extending into adulthood (National Institute of Corrections, 2014). Transgender individuals, in particular, have a risk for incarceration, for reasons including the need to earn money through the underground economy due to difficulty finding employment (Grant et al., 2011).

The unique needs of incarcerated LGBT individuals with mental illness are often invisible and generally misunderstood and underserved. This chapter seeks to add to the clinical knowledge of practitioners who work with this population, clarify legal precedent, and establish best practices.

Understanding the differences in L, G, B, and T

Mental health issues of LGBT individuals have formerly been studied as if lesbians, gays, bisexuals, and transgender individuals are a homogeneous group. While LGB includes sexual orientation only, LGBT includes gender identity. Although homophobia and transphobia have similar effects, each group also faces unique issues and experiences. Similarly, the lack of familiarity with transgender people and their issues among professionals and the general public alike puts them at much higher risk for societal discrimination and lack of access to appropriate and informed medical and mental health care.

Lesbians

Lesbians, cis or transgender women attracted romantically and sexually to other women, frequently contend with sexism, as well as homophobia. Although they face typical women's health issues, the additional stressor of homophobia puts them at greater risk for mental health problems. They experience higher rates of depression and use more mental health services than the general population (Cochran & Mays, 2009; Cochran et al., 2003; Koh & Ross, 2006). Lesbian women who are more open about their sexual orientation have lower rates of psychological distress compared to those who remain "in the closet" (Koh & Ross, 2006).

Gay men

Gay individuals are cis or transgender men who are attracted romantically and sexually to other men. Gay men live with the specter of HIV due to the historical epidemiological linkage of the AIDS epidemic with gay men in the 1980s and 1990s. The slow progress in HIV research and similarly slow development of effective treatments in the 1980s and 1990s left many gay men feeling purposely left to die, which resulted in an enduring sense of distrust in sources of authority. Older generations dealt with the devastating impact of the AIDS epidemic at a time when little was known, a diagnosis of AIDS was often a death sentence, and friends and partners died due to the absence of effective antiviral therapy. Younger gay men now cope with the reality that sexual exploration could result in a serious medical illness.

Bisexuals

Bisexual individuals experience emotional, romantic, and physical attraction to partners of more than one gender. They frequently contend with incomplete acceptance by the heterosexual, lesbian, or gay communities. They are often incorrectly seen either as heterosexuals who want to appear edgy or trendy or as homosexuals unwilling to admit to being gay. They often do not volunteer their sexual orientation (Pompili et al., 2014), allowing others to make assumptions. Although bisexuals have been part of the LGBT movement, their

1. The authors acknowledge the contributions of Randi Kaufman, Kevin Kapila, and Kenneth L. Appelbaum, who authored this chapter in the textbook's first edition.

needs may go unaddressed, with negative health consequences (San Francisco Human Rights Commission, 2011) including higher rates of depression, anxiety, and suicidal ideation (Brennan et al., 2010; Koh & Ross, 2006; Russell & Fish, 2016). Resources appropriate for gays and lesbians frequently do not meet the needs of bisexuals.

Transgender individuals

"Transgender" is an umbrella term for people who experience or present their gender differently from their natal, or assigned, gender. Gender dysphoria, the *Diagnostic and Statistical Manual of Mental Disorders*, fifth edition, text revision (American Psychiatric Association, 2022) diagnosis that replaced the previous diagnosis of gender identity disorder, describes emotional or cognitive discontent with one's assigned gender. Transgender individuals exist on a spectrum of gender identities and gender expression, with significant variability in one's desire, willingness, or ability to pursue gender-affirming changes. Such changes may occur at a social or interpersonal level (e.g., coming out to others and/or changing clothing, hairstyle, grooming, name, or pronoun) or at a medical level (e.g., puberty blockers and/or hormone therapy, gender-affirming surgeries).

Transgender people commonly encounter discrimination, rejection, and isolation. They face personal intrusiveness when others stare, point, or laugh at them; purposely misgender them; call them names; or ask them inappropriate questions (such as by questioning their transgender identity or their surgical status or asking about genitalia). Not all transgender individuals desire gender-affirming surgical interventions. Reasons for not having surgery include concern about a loss of sensation postoperatively, poor cosmetic results, desire to please a partner, fear of medical procedures, fear of losing custody of children, cost, access to the procedures, or enjoyment of one's original genitalia. Some individuals cannot afford surgery, have medical contraindications, have no one to assist them after surgery, or cannot take time off from work for recovery. Similarly, individuals differ regarding their preferred name and pronouns. Following their preferences helps create a safe and empathic alliance by indicating respect, a nonjudgmental attitude, and acceptance of the person's gender.

General considerations of the lesbian, gay, bisexual, and transgender experience in prison

A 2015 survey of LGBT prisoners found that 58% had their first arrest before the age of 18—a strikingly larger proportion than the overall pool of prisoners (Lydon et al., 2015). The same survey noted that these findings were particularly true among racial minority LGBT individuals. The study postulated that, as a result of the discrimination LGBT individuals experienced, they were more likely to engage in high-risk or illegal behaviors and more likely to have police encounters and be criminalized. Although all incarcerated persons (IPs) experience loss of freedom and separation from loved ones, LGBT IPs may face added burdens of discrimination, marginalization, and physical and sexual abuse. Important considerations that affect their incarceration experience include self-comfort with sexual orientation or gender identity, whether they are out or closeted, whether their appearance reveals sexual orientation or gender nonconformity, and their ability to portray the gender with which they identify (Yap et al., 2020). Correctional psychiatrists should inquire without assumption about these issues and let the patient lead the discussion. No uniform approach can address the mental health needs of all LGBT IPs.

IPs with sexual or gender minority status should have an evaluation of medical and mental health needs, as well as an assessment of victimization risk, at initial reception and whenever transferred to another facility. Approximately 3.5% of heterosexual male IPs report being sexually victimized by another IP, but those rates soar to 34% for bisexual and 39% for homosexual or gay male IPs (Beck et al., 2012). Reported rates of victimization by staff were at least 2 to 3 times higher for gay, lesbian, and bisexual IPs compared to heterosexual counterparts. Fifteen percent of transgender IPs report sexual assault, with Black transgender IPs reporting much higher assault rates by both other IPs and staff than their counterparts (Grant et al., 2011). Nevertheless, isolation for safety or placement in an LGBT segregated unit should occur only when individually necessary and not as a substitute for other protective interventions. According to the National Prison Rape Elimination Commission, any form of isolation should remain a "last resort and interim measure only." The National Prison Rape Elimination Commission (2009, p. 8) also "specifically prohibits housing prisoners based solely on their sexual orientation or gender identity because it can lead to demoralizing and dangerous labeling."

Carceral settings are believed to be highly heteronormative and more homophobic and transphobic than the general outside community. Furthermore, correctional staff's familiarity with the specific needs of LGBT IPs is limited (Donohue et al., 2021). This contributes to the sense of marginalization of LGBT IPs and contributes to their poorer health outcomes. One frequently noted unexpected concern for transgender women IPs relates to the pressure they experience to "pass" as a feminine woman in a male prison to obtain positive affirmation of their feminine identity (Jenness & Fenstermaker, 2014; Yap et al., 2020). Understanding the relationship between the risk of sexual assault and the pursuit of affirmation of femininity for transgender IPs in male prisons requires a nuanced analysis of this complex dynamic. The National Institute of Corrections (2014) issued guidelines and resources to help correctional institutions provide care and develop LGBT treatment policies. Initial steps may involve assessment of staff attitudes and knowledge, open and noncritical dialogue about knowledge gaps, and education for all members of the custody and clinical team.

Minority stress and resilience

Social stress theory posits that, as a result of the general challenges associated with living in society, individuals experience emotional and somatic illness, rendering them more vulnerable to illness. The application of social stress theory to minority populations is known as minority stress theory. Indeed, in this circumstance, the specific stressor relates to identified differences from the majority, with consequent alienation from the norms and values of the majority, prejudice, and stigma (Meyer, 2003). Minority stress theory applies squarely to LGBT individuals whose chronic stressor relates to their status as a sexual or gender minority and manifests as external stressors (how one is perceived and treated by others with elements of prejudice and discrimination including possible parental rejection) or internal stressors (how one processes their minority identity and experiences internalized stigma). Such internal stressors are of particular import due to their devastating effect on one's sense of self. They result in a need to conceal their identity due to a real or imagined expectation of rejection, internalized homophobia/transphobia, and hypervigilance. The deep-rooted impact of these internal stressors is linked to the compounded effect of having to navigate LGBT-specific stressors, in addition to the typical developmental stress associated with puberty and social individualization/intimacy that their heterosexual peers experience (Yarbrough et al., 2024). Minority stress is believed to be a major contributor to the increased risk of victimization, mood or anxiety disorders, substance use, and suicidal behaviors seen in the LGBT community (Friedman et al., 2011; Huebner et al., 2004).

The concept of resiliency stands in clear contrast and as an adaptive response to that of minority stress. Resiliency supplies LGBT individuals the tools to counter the weight of the stressors they face and protects them from functional impairment. Resiliency develops as an alternative mechanism and value system relating to a person's ability to adapt in the face of social and cultural difficulties, and it is believed to be the best predictor of social and mental health outcomes in LGBT communities (Meyer, 2003). Resiliency in the LBGT population is understood to build the sense of shamelessness or pride in one's community needed to counter bullying, marginalization, and institutional homophobia (Herrick et al., 2011). In addition, resiliency relies on social support and social creativity to counter social isolation, altruism and activism to counter communal vulnerability and the risk of victimization, and self-monitoring to instill personal empowerment and a sense of personal control (Aoun & Chao, 2018).

Coming out

Coming out refers to the process where the LGBT person accepts and discloses their sexual orientation or gender identity. How, when, and why to disclose is a highly personal decision. The process is not sequential and can be lifelong (Yarbrough et al., 2024). Incarceration represents a new situation in which to come out or stay closeted. Despite previous choices, some people may choose differently in prison for reasons of safety, mental and emotional well-being, or fear of rejection. Remaining closeted can further isolate LGBT IPs by cutting them off from supports.

Challenges around coming out for transgender IPs include restricted access to clothing, makeup, accoutrements, hairstyle, and ability to "pass" (i.e., being seen as one's identified, not natal, gender) when housed in a prison that does not correspond to the person's gender identity. Inability to express gender identity may cause mental and emotional distress; however, being identified as transgender in prison may put the IP at greater risk for physical or sexual assault.

Behavior versus identity

Complicating the picture, someone in prison might make different behavioral choices that may not be based on their identity. Evidence suggests that the longer one spends in prison and the higher the security level, the greater the inclination to engage in same-sex sexual behavior, even for those who had not done so before incarceration (Garland et al., 2005). This can create confusion for IPs who have never considered themselves as gay, lesbian, or bisexual. They might question their sexual orientation for the first time and confront feelings of internalized homophobia. Behavior and identity, however, do not necessarily correspond.

Substance use in lesbian, gay, bisexual, and transgender communities

Substance use and substance use disorders are more common in the LGBT community than in the general population (Aoun & Chao, 2018). Given the well-documented relationship between substance use and criminal behaviors (Bronson, 2017; Rand, 2008) and the consequent overrepresentation of individuals with substance use disorders in the criminal justice system, it becomes evident why understanding the specificities of LGBT substance use is highly important to any correctional psychiatrist. Given our understanding of the minority stress theory, substance use and the pursuit of intoxication is believed to afford LGBT individuals navigating discrimination and/or internalized homophobia or transphobia a state of temporary emotional dissociation and emotional numbness. Although a maladaptive mechanism, intoxication affords one the ability to suppress emotional distress, feel disinhibited, and exist as one whose identity is seen by others and not infrequently by oneself as unacceptable (Cabaj, 2014; Polak et al., 2015). For some members of the LGBT community, internal stressors leading to a sense of self-hatred related to one's identity is so intense that existing as an LGBT person or socializing with other LGBT persons feels overwhelmingly shameful unless one is intoxicated. Moreover, substance use allows LGBT persons to "fit into" the LGBT community, countering concerns related to ageism, physical appearance expectations, or engaging in LGBT events, including circuit parties where drug and alcohol use may be highly prevalent (Ostrow & Shelby, 2000). One additional factor contributing to substance use in the LGBT community relates to the emotional, physical, and sexual disinhibition resulting from drug or alcohol use, all of which are necessary for one's ability to express oneself sexually or engage with others intimately. Despite the "benefit" of drug use as a sexual lubricant, it is worth noting that drug use and intoxication hinder the user's ability to build substantive emotional connections and enduring relationships, both of which are essential to combat the underlying emotional needs and insecurities leading to the drug use in the first place.

Among gay men, the most commonly used intoxicating substances include alcohol, methamphetamine, methylenedioxymethamphetamine (MDMA, ecstasy or molly) and other stimulants, gamma-hydroxybutyrate (GHB), ketamine, inhaled nitrites such as poppers, and certain hallucinogens (Aoun & Chao, 2018). It is worth noting that a significant positive correlation is found between HIV positivity and methamphetamine use (Semple et al., 2012). It is believed that the introduction of phosphodiesterase inhibitor medications for erectile dysfunction such as sildenafil to the U.S. markets contributed heavily to this correlation. While drugs such as methamphetamines are known to diminish penile erections, erectile dysfunction medications may allow users to overcome the erectile dysfunction related to methamphetamines.

Less data are available regarding lesbian women drug use. Overall, alcohol use and the prevalence of alcohol use disorder appears to be more common among lesbians (Roberts et al., 2004). Interestingly, whereas alcohol use is known to decrease with age among heterosexual women, no such patterns were found among lesbian women (Hughes et al., 2006). Among bisexual individuals, studies have demonstrated a correlation between being out and an increased likelihood for using illicit drugs (Marshal et al., 2008). This is believed to relate to the need to suppress the emotional impact of internal and external stressors, as noted earlier (TolouShams et al., 2013). Even fewer data are available regarding drug and alcohol use in transgender populations. Overall, it appears that substance use disorders are significantly more prevalent among transgender individuals compared to the general population, with transgender women being at an even higher risk than transgender men (Rowe et al., 2015; Santos et al., 2014).

Assessment of lesbian, gay, and bisexual incarcerated persons

The correctional psychiatrist should be aware of personal biases, which might manifest through body language, nervousness in taking a sexual history, or poor eye contact. If necessary, the psychiatrist should seek supervision. It is best to use gender-neutral terminology when inquiring about sexual partners and to avoid assumptions about sexual orientation, even if an IP discloses a same-sex relationship. The provider can express interest regarding how the IP's sexual orientation influences the chief complaint without assuming that this orientation accounts for the presenting problem. Social history should explore the effect sexual orientation has had on the IP's relationship with family and friends or with experiences of discrimination. It is important for correctional psychiatrists to screen for drug use, inquire about the desired effect pursued from drug use, and explore any perceived benefits that drugs have had for the individual. Lesbian, gay, and bisexual IPs who have symptoms of depression or anxiety will respond best to a therapist who understands how homophobia may affect their symptoms.

The diagnosis of bipolar disorder can be made inappropriately in lesbian, gay, and bisexual IPs. A person who has repressed their sexual orientation and finally comes out and starts to accept it may do so with a mix of euphoria and shame, as if they are on an emotional roller coaster. This coming-out process may be mistaken for a manic or mixed state. A person who finally acts on sexual feelings they have long repressed may have multiple partners, which should not be interpreted as mania-driven hypersexuality. When evaluating a lesbian, gay, or bisexual IP's sexual history, it is essential to assess the propriety of their past sexual behaviors, including the number of past sexual partners relative to the same lesbian, gay, or bisexual groups rather than in comparison to their heterosexual peers. Failing to do so could result in an erroneous determination that they are sexually promiscuous, leading to an inaccurate finding of having a history of mania based on their preincarceration sexual history.

Transgender incarcerated persons

Survey data document the higher rates of incarceration of transgender individuals, particularly those who belong to racial minority groups, compared to the general population of the United States. A large 2011 survey found that 16% of transgender respondents had a history of incarceration (including 47% of Black transgender respondents), compared to 2.7% of the general population (Grant et al., 2011). Numerous studies have confirmed that justice-involved transgender individuals fare more poorly than the general population with regard to their physical and mental health (Brown & Jones, 2015).

Assessment of transgender incarcerated persons

When assessing a transgender person, the correctional psychiatrist would ideally have either expertise in gender dysphoria or appropriate supervision. The correctional psychiatrist should demonstrate humility in recognizing aspects of transgender health where they may not have proficiency. If negative stereotypes or bias interfere with their ability to assess or treat the patient, regular supervision or even referral to another clinician may be necessary. Assessment of a gender-nonconforming individual includes a thorough gender history. A helpful approach involves beginning with broad and general inquiries, with focused follow-up questions as indicated. The history includes questions about gender-related distress and how the person has dealt with it. Puberty represents a critical time for many transgender individuals, as they begin to have unwanted physical changes.

Self-harm can result, especially focused on body parts that cause dysphoria. IPs may have confusion about whether they are gay or transgender. The history should explore their understanding of their gender and any desire to transition. Individuals may differ regarding which social, medical, and surgical options they seek. In working with IPs who identify as transgender, the correctional psychiatrist should clarify the purpose. It will be helpful to distinguish between IPs who require evaluation to assess their transgender status and established transgender IPs who require psychiatric treatment provision. In the latter situation, questioning a transgender IP's gender status may result in unnecessary distress to the individual. Although rare, symptoms of gender dysphoria can derive from other mental health disorders. The differential diagnosis includes psychotic disorders, manic states, body dysmorphic disorder, trauma, transvestic fetishism, eating disorders, borderline personality disorder, obsessive–compulsive disorder, and nonconformity to stereotypical gender roles.

Transgender health in prison

Most state and federal prison systems in the United States have policies or other directives regarding health care for transgender IPs. They vary, however, in whether they allow continuation or initiation of hormones, and access to gender-affirming surgical interventions remains extremely limited (Aldrich et al., 2023; Brown & McDuffie, 2009). Blanket restrictions on access to recognized medical care lack parallels with other medical conditions. Professional organizations such as the American Medical Association (2022), the American Psychiatric Association (2018), and the National Commission on Correctional Health Care (2020) have approved policies that support insurance coverage for gender-affirming treatment as recommended by a physician. Policies also need to ensure respect when conducting strip searches (e.g., using officers of the IP's self-identified gender), privacy in bathrooms and showers, and appropriate access to gender-preferred canteen and toiletry items. Meeting a transgender individual's medical and mental health needs in a manner that allows gender expression represents good clinical care, whether in a carceral setting or not.

In recent years, lawsuits by transgender IPs have resulted in expanded access to treatment. Courts in the United States have recognized gender dysphoria as a serious medical condition, and they generally defer to medical staff recommendations in determining Eighth Amendment violations for failure to treat (*Edmo v. Corizon, Inc.*, 2019; Estime, 2021; *Gibson v. Collier*, 2019; National Institute of Corrections, 2014; *Quine v. Beard*, 2017). Courts have increasingly rejected policies that have blanket prohibitions on continuation or initiation of hormones, restrict the professional judgment of clinical staff with expertise in gender dysphoria, or deny treatment based on unsubstantiated security concerns, expense, or public disfavor. *Fields v. Smith* (2011) was the first major court decision expanding access to care for incarcerated transgender individuals. In that decision, the U.S. Court of Appeals for the Seventh Circuit struck down a law preventing access to gender-affirming care for transgender IPs. In 2012, a district court in Massachusetts set precedent and ordered gender-affirming surgery for an IP in the matter of *Kosilek v. Spencer* (2012); the decision was later reversed by the U.S. Court of Appeals for the First Circuit (*Kosilek v. Spencer*, 2014). Ms. Kosilek ultimately received surgical treatment in 2021 after her case was heavily scrutinized (Aldrich et al., 2023). In 2015, in the matter of *Diamond v. Owens* (2015), the Department of Justice issued a directive for all state prisons to continue hormone treatment for all transgender IPs who were already receiving it at the time of incarceration and to evaluate other transgender IPs to assess their clinical need for hormone treatment. At present, requests for surgical treatment of gender dysphoria have been approved only in a handful of cases where the risk of self-harm without surgery was determined to be very high, and only after extensive litigation (*Campbell v. Kallas*, 2018; *Edmo v. Corizon, Inc.*, 2019; *Iglesias v. Federal Bureau of Prisons*, 2022; *Quine v. Beard*, 2017). This area of the law continues to evolve, with ongoing litigation around the country.

Summary

Correctional psychiatrists must understand the challenges faced by LGBT IPs, including the challenges of each unique subgroup. Knowledgeable and sensitive clinical assessment can assist this population with their adjustment, safety, and mental health while incarcerated. Psychiatrists can also aid other correctional staff with their awareness of these issues and help ensure that these IPs have access to appropriate medical and mental health services consistent with prevailing standards. The care of transgender IPs in prisons continues to evolve toward community standards, with courts increasingly rejecting blanket prohibitions on the provision of gender-affirming care in correctional settings.

REFERENCES

Aldrich, J., Kant, J., & Gramszlo, E. (2023). Gender-affirming care, incarceration, and the eighth amendment. *AMA Journal of Ethics*, *25*(6), E407–E413.

American Medical Association. (2022). *Removing financial barriers to care for transgender patients* (H-185.950). https://policysearch.ama-assn.org/policyfinder/detail/H-185.950?uri=%2FAMADoc%2FHOD.xml-0-1128.xml

American Psychiatric Association. (2018). *Position statement on access to care for transgender and gender variant individuals.* https://www.psychiatry.org/getattachment/d3ef4763-8a0e-4da3-ab01-efe932ca9478/Position-2018-Access-to-Care-for-Transgender-and-Gender-Diverse-Individuals.pdf

American Psychiatric Association. (2022). *Diagnostic and statistical manual of mental disorders* (5th ed., text rev.).

Aoun, E. G., & Chao, F. (2018). Substance use disorders in the LGBT community. In J. S. Schneider, V. M. B. Silenzio, & L. Erickson-Schroth (Eds.), *The GLMA handbook on LGBT health* (pp. 57–82). ABC-CLIO.

Beck, A. J., Johnson, C., & U.S. Bureau of Justice Statistics. (2012). *Sexual victimization reported by former state prisoners, 2008.* http://purl.fdlp.gov/GPO/gpo29057

Brennan, D. J., Ross, L. E., Dobinson, C., et al. (2010). Men's sexual orientation and health in Canada. *Canadian Journal of Public Health*, *101*, 255–258.

Bronson, J., & Stroop, J. (2017). *Drug use, dependence, and abuse among state prisoners and jail inmates, 2007–2009.* Bureau of Justice Statistics. https://bjs.ojp.gov/content/pub/pdf/dudaspji0709.pdf

Brown, G. R., & Jones, K. T. (2015). Health correlates of criminal justice involvement in 4,793 transgender veterans. *LGBT Health*, *2*(4), 297–305.

Brown, G. R., & McDuffie, E. (2009). Health care policies addressing transgender inmates in prison systems in the United States. *Journal of Correctional Health Care*, *15*, 280–291.

Cabaj, R. P. (2014). Substance use issues among gay, lesbian, bisexual, and transgender people. In M. Galanter, H. Kleber, & K. Brady (Eds.), *The American Psychiatric Publishing textbook of substance abuse treatment* (pp. 702–722). American Psychiatric Press.

Campbell v. Kallas, 936 F.3d 536 (7th Cir. 2018).

Cochran, S. D., & Mays, V. M. (2009). Burden of psychiatric morbidity among lesbian, gay, and bisexual individuals in the California Quality of Life Survey. *Journal of Abnormal Psychology*, *118*, 647–658.

Cochran, S. D., Mays, V. M., & Sullivan, J. G. (2003). Prevalence of mental disorders, psychological distress, and mental health services use among lesbian, gay, and bisexual adults in the United States. *Journal of Consulting and Clinical Psychology*, *71*, 53–61.

Diamond v. Owens, 131 F. Supp. 3d 1346 (M.D. Ga. 2015).

Donohue, G., McCann, E., & Brown, M. (2021). Views and experiences of LGBTQ+ people in prison regarding their psychosocial needs: A systematic review of the qualitative research evidence. *International Journal of Environmental Research and Public Health*, *18*(17), 9335.

Edmo v. Corizon, Inc., 935 F.3d 757 (9th Cir. 2019).

Estime, E. (2021). Transgender inmates and sex reassignment surgery in Florida: Why failing to provide this standard of care is cruel and unusual punishment under the 8th amendment. *Nova Law Review*, *46*, 59.

Fields v. Smith, 653 F.3d 550 (7th Cir. 2011).

Friedman, M. S., Marshal, M. P., Guadamuz, T. E., et al. (2011). A meta-analysis of disparities in childhood sexual abuse, parental physical abuse, and peer victimization among sexual minority and sexual nonminority individuals. *American Journal of Public Health*, *101*(8), 1481–1494.

Garland, J. T., Morgan, R. D., & Beer, A. M. (2005). Impact of time in prison and security level on inmates' sexual attitude, behavior, and identity. *Psychological Services*, *2*, 151–162.

Gibson v. Collier, 920 F.3d 212 (5th Cir. 2019).

Grant, J. M., Mottet, L. A., Tanis, J., Harrison, J., Herman, J. L., & Keisling, M. (2011). *Injustice at every turn: A report of the national transgender discrimination survey.* National Center for Transgender Equality. https://transequality.org/sites/default/files/docs/resources/NTDS_Report.pdf

Herrick, A. L., Lim, S. H., Wei, C., et al. (2011). Resilience as an untapped resource in behavioral intervention design for gay men. *Journal of AIDS and Behavior*, *15*(Suppl. 1), 25–30.

Huebner, D. M., Rebchook, G. M., & Kegeles, S. M. (2004). Experiences of harassment, discrimination, and physical violence among young gay and bisexual men. *American Journal of Public Health, 94*(7), 1200–1203.

Hughes, T. L., Wilsnack, S. C., Szalacha, L. A., et al. (2006). Age and racial/ethnic differences in drinking and drinkingrelated problems in a community sample of lesbians. *Journal on Studies on Alcohol, 67*(4), 579–590.

Iglesias v. Federal Bureau of Prisons, 598 F. Supp. 3d 689 (S.D. Ill. 2022).

Jenness, V., & Fenstermaker, S. (2014). Agnes goes to prison: Gender authenticity, transgender inmates in prisons for men, and pursuit of "the real deal." *Gender & Society, 28*(1), 5–31.

Koh, A. S., & Ross, L. K. (2006). Mental health issues: A comparison of lesbian, bisexual and heterosexual women. *Journal of Homosexuality, 51*, 33–57.

Kosilek v. Spencer, 889 F. Supp. 2d 190 (D. Mass. 2012).

Kosilek v. Spencer, 774 F.3d 63 (1st Cir. 2014).

Lydon, J., Carrington, K., Low, H., Miller, H., & Yazdy, M. (2015). *Coming out of concrete closets: A report on Black & Pink's national LGBTQ prisoner survey*. https://www.blackandpink.org/wp-content/uploads/2020/03/Coming-Out-of-Concrete-Closets-incorcporated-Executive-summary102115.pdf

Marshal, M. P., Friedman, M. S., Stall, R., et al. (2008). Sexual orientation and adolescent substance use: A meta-analysis and methodological review. *Addiction, 103*(4), 546–556.

Meyer, I. H. (2003). Prejudice, social stress, and mental health in lesbian, gay, and bisexual populations: Conceptual issues and research evidence. *Psychological Bulletin, 129*, 674–697.

National Commission on Correctional Health Care. (2020). *Transgender and gender diverse health care in correctional settings*. https://www.ncchc.org/position-statements/transgender-and-gender-diverse-health-care-in-correctional-settings-2020

National Institute of Corrections. (2014). *Policy review and development guide: Lesbian, gay, bisexual, transgender, and intersex persons in custodial settings* (2nd ed.). https://info.nicic.gov/lgbti/

National Prison Rape Elimination Commission. (2009). *National Prison Rape Elimination Commission Report*. P.8. https://www.ncjrs.gov/pdffiles1/226680.pdf

Obergefell v. Hodges, 576 U.S. 644 (2015).

Ostrow, D., & Shelby, D. (2000). Psychoanalytic and behavioral approaches to drug-related sexual risk taking. *Journal of Gay & Lesbian Psychotherapy, 3*(3–4), 123–139.

Polak, K., Haug, N., Drachenberg, H., & Svikis, D. (2015). Gender considerations in addiction: Implications for treatment. *Current Treatment Options Psychiatry, 2*, 326–338.

Pompili, M., Lester, D., Forte, A., et al. (2014). Bisexuality and suicide: A systematic review of the current literature. *Journal of Sexual Medicine, 11*(8), 1903–1913.

Quine v. Beard, No. 14-cv-02726-JST (N.D. Cal. 2017).

Rand, M. R. (2008). *Criminal victimization in the United States, 2007*. https://bjs.ojp.gov/content/pub/pdf/cv07.pdf

Respect for Marriage Act, Pub. L. No. 117-228 (2022).

Roberts, S. J., Grindel, C. G., Patsdaughter, C. A., et al. (2004). Lesbian use and abuse of alcohol: Results of the Boston Lesbian Health Project II. *Substance Abuse, 25*(4), 1–9.

Rowe, C., Santos, G. M., McFarland, W., et al. (2015). Prevalence and correlates of substance use among trans female youth ages 16–24 years in the San Francisco Bay Area. *Drug and Alcohol Dependence, 147*, 160–166.

Russell, S. T., & Fish, J. N. (2016). Mental health in lesbian, gay, bisexual, and transgender (LGBT) youth. *Annual Review of Clinical Psychology, 12*, 465–487.

San Francisco Human Rights Commission. (2011). *Bisexual invisibility: Impacts and recommendations*. http://www.sf-hrc.org/modules/showdocument.aspx?documentid=989

Santos, G. M., Rapues, J., Wilson, E. C., et al. (2014). Alcohol and substance use among transgender women in San Francisco: Prevalence and association with human immunodeficiency virus infection. *Drug and Alcohol Review, 33*(3), 287–295.

Semple, S. J., Strathdee, S. A., Zians, J., et al. (2012). Factors associated with experiences of stigma in a sample of HIV-positive, methamphetamine-using men who have sex with men. *Drug and Alcohol Dependence, 125*(1–2), 154–159.

TolouShams, M., Tarantino, N., McKirnan, D. J., et al. (2013). Depressive symptoms, illicit drug use and HIV/STI risk among sexual minority young adults. *Journal of Gay and Lesbian Mental Health, 17*(1), 96–102.

Yap, L., Simpson, P., Richters, J., Donovan, B., Grant, L., & Butler, T. (2020). Disclosing sexuality: Gay and bisexual men's experiences of coming out, forced out, going back in and staying out of the "closet" in prison. *Culture, Health & Sexuality, 22*(11), 1222–1234.

Yarbrough, E., Aoun, E. G., & Drescher, J. (2024). LGBTQ individuals. In A. Tasman, M. Riba, T. Schulze, C. Ng, C. Alfonso, R. Alarcon, D. Tosevski, S. Kanba, & D. Ndetei (Eds.), *Tasman's psychiatry* (5th ed.). Springer.

57

Developmental disabilities

Barbara E. McDermott and George W. Hebert

Introduction

The U.S. correctional system is vast and includes individuals incarcerated in jails and prisons, as well as those under the supervision of probation and parole. At the end of 2021, slightly less than 5.5 million individuals were under the supervision of the adult correctional system, representing a decline of over 60,000 individuals from the previous year (Carson & Kluckow, 2023). Regardless of size, the purpose of the correctional system has remained unchanged and includes not just punishment and containment but also rehabilitation. Rehabilitation services seem more relevant in individuals with developmental disabilities than in any other group. Although research is inconsistent, most studies suggest that individuals with developmental disabilities commit less serious offenses yet serve more time in prison than those without such disabilities (MacEachron, 1979; Petersilia, 2000a). In 1975, Talent and Keldgord suggested that efforts at rehabilitating offenders with ID were lacking (Talent & Keldgord, 1975). In 2000, Petersilia (2000a) noted that, 25 years later, this situation remained essentially unchanged. This chapter outlines the progress that has been made in the identification and habilitation of individuals with developmental disabilities, specifically IDs, in the criminal justice system. Definitions, legal issues, and prevalence rates are discussed, as well as the specific vulnerabilities individuals with developmental delays present to the criminal justice system. Finally, screening, management, and habilitation in corrections arising directly from these vulnerabilities are discussed.

Definitions

Federal law defined the term "developmental disability" via the Developmental Disabilities Assistance and Bill of Rights Act of 2000 (42 U.S.C. §§ 15001–15115), which has remained unchanged in the last 2 decades. The legal standard required for an individual to be designated as having a developmental disorder includes the following:

1. The disability is attributed to a mental or physical impairment or combination of the two;
2. The disability manifested before the age of 22;
3. The disability is likely to continue indefinitely;
4. The disability results in functional limitations in *three or more* of the following areas:
   a. Self-care,
   b. Receptive or expressive language,
   c. Mobility,
   d. Self-direction,
   e. Capacity for independent living,
   f. Economic self-sufficiency; and
5. Individualized support is of a lifelong or extended duration and is individually planned.

Many disorders meet these criteria and can include physical disorders, such as cerebral palsy, and mental health disorders, such as autism spectrum disorder. However, according to the Centers for Disease Control and Prevention (1996), intellectual disability (ID) is the most common developmental disability, and individuals with IDs are the most likely (of those with any developmental disability) to be involved with the criminal justice system. For this reason, persons with IDs will be the primary focus of this chapter.

In 2013, the *Diagnostic and Statistical Manual of Mental Disorders*, fifth edition (DSM-5; American Psychiatric Association [APA], 2013) replaced the diagnosis of mental retardation with ID to be consistent with Rosa's Law (Public Law 111–256, 2010), which changed all references to "mental retardation" in federal law to "intellectual disability." The diagnostic criteria were essentially unchanged, although the focus shifted from intelligence to adaptive skills and level of support necessary resulting from any identified skills deficits. More recently, the DSM, fifth edition, text revision (DSM-5-TR; APA, 2022) opted for the diagnosis "intellectual developmental disorder" to provide consistency with the International Statistical Classification of Diseases and Related Health Problems, 11th revision, terminology, although "intellectual disability" was parenthetical to allow for continued use. The criteria were unchanged in the text revision and include the following:

1. Deficits in intellectual functions confirmed by clinical assessment and standardized testing;
2. Deficits in adaptive functioning requiring ongoing support in one or more activities of daily living; and
3. Onset during the developmental period.

The severity of ID is based on functioning in three domains: conceptual (problem solving, reasoning ability), social

(social and communicative behavior), and practical (self-care). The DSM-5-TR defines four categories of ID—mild, moderate, severe, and profound—based on the extent of deficits in the above domains, noting that adaptive skills deficits (rather than IQ scores) dictate the level of support needed.

Prevalence

Although reported prevalence rates of ID in the general population vary depending on the method of assessment and age of the sample, the DSM-5-TR (APA, 2022) estimated the prevalence rate at approximately 1% of the population, noting that the global rates may vary by country based on level of development. Larson (2001), using the National Health Interview Survey—Disability supplement, estimated that approximately 1.5% of noninstitutionalized Americans met criteria for either mental retardation or developmental disability. A more recent study (Patrick et al., 2021) found a similar prevalence rate (1.2%) in a sample of 8-year-olds from nine states in the United States, although they described differing rates based on socioeconomic status, gender, and ethnicity. For example, in this study, boys evidenced double the prevalence of ID as compared to girls (1.58% and 0.77%, respectively). Gonzalez and colleagues (2016) also found disparities in ID in individuals with lower socioeconomic status and disadvantaged backgrounds. Given what we know about offenders in general (higher percentage male, overrepresentation of minorities, more frequently from disadvantaged backgrounds), it is not surprising that the prevalence of ID in the correctional system is typically reported as higher than in the general population (e.g., Garcia-Largo et al., 2020).

Unfortunately, the literature documenting the prevalence rates of incarcerated persons (IPs) with ID contain many methodological problems. Differences in assessment, definition, and methodology, as well as regional differences, affect prevalence reports. Historically, research has indicated that individuals with ID are overrepresented within the criminal justice system (e.g., Cockram, 1998; Petersilia, 1997; Santamour & West, 1982a), although some authors have found no differences from the general population (Conley et al., 1992; Fazel et al., 2008; MacEachron, 1979; New York State Commission on Quality of Care for the Mentally Disabled, 1991).

Santamour and West (1982a) reported that the rate of adults with ID in prison ranged from 8% to almost 30%. Petersilia (2000a) estimated that 4% to 10% of individuals in prison or jail in California are developmentally disabled. However, in a review of 10 studies representing almost 12,000 incarcerated persons, Fazel and colleagues (2008) determined that a prevalence rate of 0.5% to 1.5% was typical. A more recent international study (Garcia-Largo et al., 2020) documented vastly different rates in 13 studies of over 15,000 IPs. The authors found that prevalence rates varied greatly from a low of 1% to a high of almost 70%. They noted that rates varied secondary to methodological issues, primarily method of measurement. Not surprisingly, screening measures yielded higher rates as compared to more comprehensive assessments, such as the Weschler intelligence tests (see Chapter 67). It also is noteworthy that intelligence was used as the estimate of prevalence of ID rather than adaptive skills deficits.

Previous data indicated that in the general population, approximately 89% of all individuals with IDs fall within the mild range based on the IQ criterion (Ellis & Luckasson 1985). With the revision of the DSM to categorize severity based on adaptive skills deficits, the current estimate is that 85% of individuals with IDs fall in the mild range (Boat & Wu, 2015). Consistent with the general population, offenders with mild deficits are most common, as those with moderate to profound IDs are unlikely to remain in the criminal justice system (Conley et al., 1992; Holland et al., 2002; Petrella, 1992). Therefore, the vulnerabilities and habilitation issues present in an individual with mild IDs are most relevant to those working in the correctional system.

Legal issues

One significant problem that has hampered the development of appropriate approaches with individuals with IDs is the lack of distinction in the legal system between mental illness and developmental disabilities. For example, in a study of the attorneys general of the United States and four territories (McAfee & Gural, 1988), the results suggest that the identification of individuals with developmental disabilities in the criminal justice system is unlikely to occur and that most protections for such individuals are contained in statutes pertaining to mental illness. Only in one reporting state did the attorney general (South Carolina) report that judges routinely inquire about a defendant's IQ when a guilty plea is entered. Although many of the attorneys general described that special postconviction protections were in place for defendants with developmental disabilities, several reported that these protections were inconsistently employed. Eighty-six percent reported the use of a postconviction psychological evaluation, although no other named protection (e.g., reduced sentence, incarceration in a specialized unit, special training or education) was utilized in more than 50% of the respondent states.

Various courts in the United States have provided guidance to the correctional system in the management of individuals with developmental disabilities. The U.S. District Court for the Southern District of Texas in *Ruiz v. Estelle* (1980) made specific references to "retarded inmates," noting repeatedly the injustices replete in the correctional system for these individuals, although reparative measures suggested were generic to mental disorders. Federal legislation has been interpreted to include the criminal justice system. For example, in *Pennsylvania Department of Corrections v. Yeskey* (1998), the U.S. Supreme Court held that the Americans With Disabilities Act of 1990 (42 U.S.C. §§ 12101–12213) applies to state prisoners; IPs with disabilities cannot be excluded from prison programs on the basis of their disability. In *Clark v. State of California* (1998), a class action lawsuit was filed alleging that IPs suffered discrimination as a result of their developmental disabilities and sought injunctive relief under the Americans With Disabilities Act. As a result of the *Yeskey* decision, California prison officials agreed to a settlement requiring the development and implementation of a plan to screen IPs for developmental disabilities and to provide these IPs with safe housing and supportive services.

Disproportionate representation in the criminal justice system

The definitions of ID and developmental disability require that the individual evidence impairments in adaptive functioning. These impairments can span numerous areas, often resulting in cognitive limitations that affect their decision-making skills, communication skills, social understanding, moral reasoning, and ability to learn from past mistakes (McGee & Menolascino, 1992; Seay, 2006). Deficits in these areas may lead to increased criminal behavior. Individuals with developmental disabilities may often be manipulated into committing criminal acts by more functional friends and family members (Ebert & Long, 2008; Jones, 2007; Linhorst et al., 2002).

Once arrested, individuals with IDs may not understand their rights. For example, studies have shown that people with IDs often do not understand the Miranda warning against self-incrimination (Cloud et al., 2002; Ellis & Luckasson, 1985; Everington & Fulero, 1999; Fulero & Everington, 1995; Petersilia, 2000a). Given this lack of knowledge, an individual with ID is more likely to waive their rights and provide incriminating information, increasing the likelihood of conviction and incarceration. Individuals with ID are more vulnerable in interrogations because they are more susceptible to suggestion, acquiesce more often, and have a desire to please authority figures (Cloud et al., 2002; Everington & Fulero, 1999; Jones, 2007; Matikka & Vesala, 1997; Pelka, 1997; Petersilia, 1997). These characteristics increase the likelihood of both false and legitimate confessions, increasing the likelihood of conviction. For example, research has indicated that individuals with IDs may not understand the differences between pleading guilty versus not guilty (S. A. Smith, 1993).

The impairments in decision-making, communication, and moral reasoning and the susceptibility to suggestion and willingness to acquiesce, coupled with a system that may be less inclined to release individuals with IDs, impact the number of individuals who are in prison. Taken together, these factors may explain the research that indicates a higher prevalence of individuals with IDs in prisons as compared to the general population. Clearly, the deficits described impair the ability of individuals with IDs to successfully navigate the criminal justice system prior to incarceration. These same vulnerabilities lead to predictable problems in the prison system.

Vulnerability of individuals with intellectual disabilities in corrections

People with developmental disabilities are 4 to 10 times more likely to be victims of crime than those who do not have disabilities, and this trend holds true for persons with developmental disabilities in prison (Petersilia, 2000b). Linhorst and colleagues (2018) noted that IPs with IDs are often the victims of sexual and physical abuse. Prisoners with IDs are more likely to be exploited, victimized, abused, and injured secondary to cognitive deficits (Ellis & Luckasson, 1985; Giamp & West, 2003; Müller-Isberner & Hodgins, 2000; Petersilia, 1997; C. Smith et al., 1990; Stavis, 1991). Petersilia (1997) reported that individuals with IDs who are housed within the general population are victimized in such ways as having their property stolen, being raped, or being manipulated by other IPs to violate the rules. They have difficulty understanding the rules, which also increases the likelihood of disciplinary action. In *Ruiz v. Estelle* (1980, p. 81), the court opined:

> Mentally retarded persons meet with unremitting hardships in prison. They are slow to adjust to prison life and its requirements, principally because they have almost insurmountable difficulties in comprehending what is expected of them. Not understanding or remembering disciplinary rules, they tend to commit a large number of disciplinary infractions.

Table 57.1 Vulnerabilities of individuals with developmental disabilities in the correctional setting

Cognitive limitations
• Difficulty understanding/following rules
Adaptive skills deficits
• Difficulty following guidelines/routines
• More hygiene infractions
Impaired social understanding
• Vulnerable to manipulation/victimization
• May resolve conflicts with aggression
Lower educational/occupational functioning
• Less likelihood of parole

Table 57.1 illustrates common challenges faced by individuals with IDs in correctional settings.

Aside from the obvious consequences of such maltreatment (e.g., physical injury, emotional turmoil), there are more subtle consequences. IPs who are developmentally disabled are likely to resolve conflicts with others by using physical aggression due, in part, to limitations in communication skills (Petersilia, 1997; C. Smith et al., 1990). Individuals with IDs are more likely to have low frustration tolerance (Day, 1990) and poor self-control (Benson, 1994; Cullen, 1993), increasing the likelihood of more disciplinary problems. C. Smith and colleagues (1990) found that youthful IPs with IDs received approximately 3 times as many disciplinary reports for noncompliant behavior and hygiene offenses (e.g., not showering), and they assaulted other IPs or correctional staff over twice as often as other IPs. As a result of such disciplinary problems, IPs with IDs may serve longer prison sentences, be denied parole, or be transferred to a more secure prison (Butwell et al., 2000; Ellis & Luckasson, 1985; Giamp & West, 2003; Petersilia, 1997; Santamour & West, 1982a; Stavis, 1991). In *Ruiz v. Estelle* (1980, p. 81), the court noted, "It is common for mentally retarded inmates in [the Texas Department of Corrections] to serve longer sentences than inmates not fitting this category."

Reception and assessment procedures

In 2010, the International Association for Correctional and Forensic Psychology published standards for psychological services provided in jails, prisons, and other correctional facilities (International Association for Correctional and Forensic Psychology, 2010). Included in these standards are that all IPs receive reception screening that includes assessments of mental illness and cognitive function. The standards further stated that all IPs receiving sentences of longer than 1 year be administered a psychological evaluation early in their admission, which may include group-administered intelligence assessments. IPs requiring further assessment should be evaluated within 2 weeks of the initial assessment. Although these standards were replaced in 2015 with those published by the National Commission on Correctional Health Care, the recommendations remained the same: timeliness of access to appropriate services, including for individuals with ID (National Commission on Correctional Health Care, 2015). While these standards are applicable to both jails and prisons, Scheyett (2009) found that in North Carolina, only 6% of surveyed jails employed screening instruments for intellectual/developmental disabilities, suggesting that reception screening is less comprehensive in these facilities. In contrast, most prison systems employ reception and assessment procedures to identify any circumstance that would require specialized housing for the incoming IP, likely related to lengthier commitments. The National Commission on Correctional Health Care (2008) prison standards suggest that all IPs receive a brief intellectual assessment on admission. Various instruments for this purpose have been suggested as appropriate (Giamp & West, 2003, Megargee, 2013). Unfortunately, many of these instruments are administered in groups. MacEachron (1979) found that the prevalence of offenders with IDs dropped significantly when individual (rather than group) assessments of intelligence were administered. McGee and Menolascino (1992) argue that even screening assessments should be administered individually and only by professionals trained in such administration.

The above assessments are used primarily as a method for identification of IPs with deficits. Critical in formulating an individualized habilitation plan is a more comprehensive assessment that includes both strengths and deficit areas that may be most amenable to habilitation. Many jurisdictions use their own assessments to identify functional deficits (e.g., California, North Carolina), but rarely are these assessments normed or standardized. The American Association on Intellectual and Developmental Disabilities has published a comprehensive assessment called the Supports Intensity Scale (SIS; Tassé et al., 2005). This instrument was developed over a period of 5 years and included an extensive literature review, a Q-sort, and three field tests. It is purported to have "excellent psychometric properties." The SIS is designed to identify deficits in 57 specific life activities, 15 medical conditions, and 13 problem behaviors. Research has indicated that the SIS possesses good interrater reliability, especially if the raters are trained (Thompson et al., 2008). McKenzie and colleagues (2012) determined that the Learning Disability Screening Questionnaire evidences a positive correlation with measures of full-scale intelligence, lending support for its use as a screening tool. More recently, Aparcero and colleagues (2024) described an adaptive functioning scale that held some utility in identifying adult jail IPs with possible intellectual deficiencies.

Habilitation issues

The management of IPs with developmental disabilities has presented correctional systems with significant problems. One controversy has been whether IPs with developmental disabilities should be housed in the general prison population. Those in favor of housing with the general prison population adhere to the principle of normalization, suggesting that individuals with IDs should be treated like others as much as possible (Santamour & West 1982a). However, as previously noted, much has been published on the disadvantages and risks to the prisoner with ID when placed in the general prison population. Critics argue that normalization does not take these disadvantages into account. According to Petersilia (1997, p. 6), "The emerging consensus within the profession seems to be that there are highly unique aspects to the correctional environment and that the normalization goals for the mentally retarded should not fully apply in this setting." Her statement suggests that specialized units may be more appropriate for such individuals.

Although legal decisions such as *Ruiz v. Estelle* (1980) established that individuals with IDs or developmental disabilities have the right to treatment, Hall (1992) estimated that fewer than 10% of IPs with such deficits receive specialized services. Unlike programs for individuals with mental illness, the goals of specialized programs for individuals with developmental disabilities are not remediation of their disability. The goal of most programs is education, training, and skills enhancement tailored to the specific needs of the IP. As with any other disorder, the diagnosis of ID provides no information about the needs of the specific individual. For these reasons, assessment is a critical component in any specialized program. Programs for individuals with IDs generally focus on improving the functioning and adaptation of the IP while incarcerated and upon release (Santamour, 1987). The vulnerabilities outlined in the previous sections lead to logical interventions and include the following:

1. Skills training;
2. Educational/vocational rehabilitation;
3. Treatment specific to the needs of each individual;
4. Strengths-based person-centered treatment planning.

Skills training

Skills training for the offender with ID can encompass a wide variety of areas. The assessment process will guide the areas most necessary for each individual but may include social skills training or training in areas of adaptive functioning. Corrigan (1991) conducted a meta-analysis of social skills training programs and found that individuals with developmental disabilities evidenced the greatest improvement. However, generalization of skills learned was lowest for this group. Social skills training was least effective for the offender group. Interestingly, although the offenders acquired the requisite skills, these skills did not translate into behavior change. This study suggests that social skills training may improve institutional behavior, at least with individuals with developmental disabilities, but may not generalize to other settings.

Educational and vocational rehabilitation

Vocational training is an important aspect of a comprehensive program to treat IPs with developmental disabilities for several reasons. Vocational training teaches IPs the skills and information necessary to perform a job upon release and allows the IP to work in a sheltered environment before reentry into the community (Santamour & West, 1982b). Vocational training also provides IPs with developmental disabilities the opportunity to engage in meaningful, productive work, which decreases behavioral issues and increases feelings of self-worth (Shively, 2004).

Needs-specific treatment: anger management

Lindsay and Taylor (2018) provide a comprehensive review of treatment strategies for specific problems or disorders for offenders with IDs. For example, an entire chapter describes approaches to managing and treating individuals with IDs who have committed sexual offenses (Lindsay et al., 2018). In contrast, this section focuses on examples of treatment approaches associated with improved functioning in the correctional system, rather than improvement in specific disordered behaviors.

Anger management is an important component in a treatment program for prisoners with IDs (Hall, 1992). As previously noted, self-control and aggression can be a problem for some IPs (Shively, 2004). Lack of self-control in a prison environment can lead to negative consequences, such as increased disciplinary reports (C. Smith et al., 1990). The lack of communication and interpersonal skills can lead to frustration and an increased likelihood of acting-out conflicts (C. Smith et al., 1990). Benson (1994) modified an anger management program for use with adults with IDs. Although this program was not developed specifically for offenders, it may be useful in an overall habilitation program that includes individualized treatment. As Benson points out, self-control training may generalize more easily from one situation to another and can reduce incidents of aggression while incarcerated and enable the IP to control their anger in the community.

Strengths-based, person-centered treatment planning

Strengths-based, person-centered treatment planning is a therapeutic strategy that blends the major tenets of positive psychology with a collaborative (as opposed to an expert) model of consultation. It has been implemented successfully in the criminal justice system via risk assessments and the development of interventions to manage risk (e.g., the Short-Term Assessment of Risk and Treatability; Nicholls et al. 2021). However, the utility of this approach with prisoners with IDs is unclear. Despite the lack of research, the benefits of such an approach merit consideration. Bird and colleagues (2012) highlighted that a strengths-based approach for the treatment of mental disorders became prominent with the seminal work of Abraham Maslow and Carl Rogers, both of whom emphasized the attainment of a person's full potential as a therapeutic outcome. More recently, Seligman and colleagues (2006) introduced positive psychotherapy as a further means of capitalizing on existing skills, rather than focusing on deficits, to help patients.

Person-centered planning, in a similar fashion, emerged circa 1985 to assist individuals with intellectual and developmental disabilities in promoting positive integration into the community. These person-centered programs focus on the use of community supports to promote the development of positive behaviors and relationships (Claes et al., 2010). In their review of 15 studies, the authors found support for the effectiveness of these interventions in improving social networks and engagement. Although untested, the use of this model may hold some utility for the incarcerated population with ID via the promotion of positive behaviors. A strengths-based, person-centered approach can readily incorporate adaptive behavior levels as beginning areas of strength, even in a prison setting. The individual with ID can be carefully included in the development of a positive support plan and build on identified strengths, with social and practical competencies as the behavioral targets. To that end, Close and Walker (2010) have advocated for a "forensic special educator" to help individuals with developmental disabilities navigate the criminal justice system.

Summary

Case law and extant literature have made it clear that the habilitation of individuals with developmental disabilities in the correctional system can no longer be ignored. While Hall (1992) noted that correctional facilities should not be viewed as treatment facilities, such institutions can no longer be "deliberately indifferent" to the needs of these individuals. IPs with developmental delays may be more easily led, suggestible, and dependent. Lower levels of comprehension and poor adaptive skills can lead to more rule infractions and disciplinary action, resulting in a decreased likelihood for parole. Research has indicated that these individuals serve more time for the same crime than do individuals without developmental disabilities (Petersilia, 2000a).

Opinions are mixed on whether appropriate services for such individuals should be provided in specialized units. Proponents of this approach cite the vulnerabilities of these individuals. However, all agree that specialized services must include appropriate assessments that consider culture and individualized approaches to habilitation. It cannot be presumed that services designed for the individual with mental illness will be appropriate for IPs with developmental disabilities.

Little research has been conducted on the efficacy of specialized services for offenders with developmental disabilities. As such, correctional facilities must necessarily take guidance from research based on nonoffending samples. An active collaboration between departments of corrections and agencies providing services for individuals with developmental disabilities can enhance service delivery and improve the integration of the individual into the community. As courts continue to protect the rights of individuals with developmental disabilities, correctional facilities must explore creative ways to deliver appropriate services.

REFERENCES

American Psychiatric Association. (2013). *Diagnostic and statistical manual of mental disorders* (5th ed.).

American Psychiatric Association. (2022). *Diagnostic and statistical manual of mental disorders* (5th ed. text rev.).

Americans With Disabilities Act of 1990, 42 U.S.C. §§ 12101–12213 (1990).

Aparcero, M., Lee, H., Wijetunga, C., Conley, E. E., Rosenfeld, B., & Cham, H. (2024, March 22). *Evaluating the utility of the problems in everyday living test (PEDL) to identify adult jail detainees with possible intellectual disability.* Presented at the American Psychology Law Society Annual Meeting, Los Angeles, CA.

Benson, B. A. (1994). Anger management training: A self-control programme for persons with mild mental retardation. In N. Bouras (Ed.), *Mental health in mental retardation: Recent advances and practices* (pp. 224–232). Cambridge University Press.

Bird, V., Boutillier, C. L., Leamy, M., et al. (2012). Assessing the strengths of mental health consumers: A systematic review. *Psychological Assessment, 24*, 1024–1033.

Boat, T. F., & Wu, J. T. (2015). Clinical characteristics of intellectual disabilities. In T. F. Boat & J. T. Wu (Eds.), *Mental disorders and disabilities among low-income children* (pp. 169–178). National Academies Press.

Butwell, M., Jamieson, E., Leese, M., & Taylor, P. (2000). Trends in special (high security) hospitals 2: Residency and discharge episodes, 1986–1995. *British Journal of Psychiatry, 176*, 260–265.

Carson, E. A., & Kluckow, R. (2023). *Correctional populations in the United States, 2021* (NCJ 305542). https://bjs.ojp.gov/library/publications/correctional-populations-united-states-2021-statistical-tables

Centers for Disease Control and Prevention. (1996). State-specific rates of mental retardation—United States, 1993. *Morbidity and Mortality Weekly Report, 45*, 61–65. http://www.cdc.gov/mmwr/preview/mmwrhtml/00040023.htm

Claes, C., Van Hove, G., Vandevelde, S., Van Loon, J., & Schalock, R. L. (2010). Person-centered planning: Analysis of research and effectiveness. *Intellectual and Developmental Disabilities, 48*, 432–453.

Clark v. State of California, United States District Court of Northern California, No. C96-1486 FMS (1998).

Close, D. W., & Walker, H. M. (2010). Navigating the criminal justice system for youth and adults with developmental disabilities: Role of the forensic special educator. *Journal of Behavioral Analysis of Offender and Victim: Treatment and Prevention, 2*, 74–103.

Cloud, M., Shepherd, G. B., Barkoff, A., & Shur, J. V. (2002). Words without meaning: The constitution, confessions, and mentally retarded suspects. *University of Chicago Law Review, 69*, 495–624.

Cockram, J., Jackson, R., & Underwood, R. (1998). People with an intellectual disability and the criminal justice system: The family perspective. *Journal of Intellectual & Developmental Disability, 23*, 41–56.

Conley, R. W., Luckasson, R., & Bouthilet, G. N. (1992). *The criminal justice system and mental retardation*. Paul H. Brookes Publishing.

Corrigan, P. W. (1991). Social skills training in adult psychiatric populations: A meta-analysis. *Journal of Behavior Therapy and Experimental Psychiatry, 22*, 203–210.

Cullen, C. (1993). The treatment of people with learning disabilities who offend. In K. Howells & C. R. Hollin (Eds.), *Clinical approaches to the mentally disordered offender* (pp. 145–162). John Wiley & Sons.

Day, K. (1990). Mental retardation: Clinical aspects and management. In R. Bluglass & P. Bowden (Eds.), *Principles and practice of forensic psychiatry* (pp. 399–418). Churchill Livingstone.

Developmental Disabilities Assistance and Bill of Rights Act of 2000, 42 U.S.C. §§ 15001–15115 (2000).

Ebert, R. S., & Long, J. S. (2008). Mental retardation and the criminal justice system: Forensic issues. In H. V. Hall (Ed.), *Forensic psychology and neuropsychology for criminal and civil cases* (pp. 375–392). CRC Press.

Ellis, J. W., & Luckasson, R. A. (1985). Mentally retarded criminal defendants. *George Washington Law Review, 53*, 414–493.

Everington, C., & Fulero, S. M. (1999). Competence to confess: Measuring understanding and suggestibility of defendants with mental retardation. *Mental Retardation, 37*, 212–220.

Fazel, S., Xenitidis, K., & Powell, J. (2008). The prevalence of intellectual disabilities among 12,000 prisoners—A systematic review. *International Journal of Law and Psychiatry, 31*, 369–373.

Fulero, S. M., & Everington, C. (1995). Assessing competency to waive Miranda rights in defendants with mental retardation. *Law and Human Behavior, 19*, 533–543.

Garcia-Largo, L. M., Marti-Agusti, G., Martin-Fumado, C. M., & Gomez-Guran, E. L. (2020). Intellectual disability rates among male prison inmates. *International Journal of Law and Psychiatry, 70*, 1–9.

Giamp, J. S., & West, M. E. (2003). Delivering psychological services to incarcerated men with developmental disabilities. In B. K. Schwartz (Ed.), *Correctional psychology: Practice, programming, and administration* (pp. 8.1–8.29). Civic Research Institute.

Gonzalez, J. M. R., Cannell, M. B., Jetelina, K. K., & Froehlich-Grobe, K. (2016). Disproportionate prevalence rate of prisoners with disabilities: Evidence from a nationally representative sample. *Journal of Disability Policy Studies, 27*, 106–115.

Hall, J. N. (1992). Correctional services for inmates with mental retardation. In R. W. Conley, R. Luckasson, & G. N. Bouthilet (Eds.), *The criminal justice system and mental retardation: Defendants and victims* (pp. 167–190). Paul H. Brookes Publishing.

Holland, A. J., Clare, I. C. H., & Mukhopadhyay, T. (2002). Prevalence of "criminal offending" by men and women with intellectual disability and the characteristics of the "offenders": Implications for research and service development. *Journal of Intellectual Disability Research, 46*, 6–20.

International Association for Correctional and Forensic Psychology. (2010). Standards for psychology services in jails, prisons, correctional facilities, and agencies. *Criminal Justice and Behaviour, 37*, 749–808.

Jones, J. (2007). Persons with intellectual disabilities in the criminal justice system: Review of issues. *International Journal of Offender Therapy and Comparative Criminology, 51*, 723–733.

Larson, S. A., Lakin, K. C., Anderson, L., Kwak, L., Lee, J. H., & Anderson, D. (2001). Prevalence of mental retardation and developmental disabilities: Evidence from the National Health Interview Survey disability supplement. *American Journal on Mental Retardation, 106*, 231–252.

Lindsay, W. R., & Taylor, J. L. (Eds.). (2018). *The Wiley handbook on offenders with intellectual and developmental disabilities: Research, training, and practice*. Wiley Blackwell.

Lindsay, W., Taylor, J. L., & Murphy, G. H. (2018). The treatment and management of sex offenders. In W. R. Lindsay & J. L. Taylor (Eds.), *The Wiley handbook on offenders with intellectual and developmental disabilities* (pp. 38–55). Wiley Blackwell.

Linhorst, D. M., Bennett, L., & McCutchen, T. (2002). Development and implementation of a program for offenders with developmental disabilities. *Mental Retardation, 40*, 41–50.

Linhorst, D. M., Dirks-Linhorst, P. A., & Sy, J. (2018). Criminal justice responses to offenders with intellectual and developmental disabilities. In W. R. Lindsay & J. L. Taylor (Eds.), *The Wiley handbook on offenders with intellectual and developmental disabilities* (pp. 86–104). Wiley Blackwell.

MacEachron, A. E. (1979). Mentally retarded offenders: Prevalence and characteristics. *American Journal of Mental Deficiency, 84*, 165–176.

Matikka, L. M., & Vesala, H. T. (1997). Acquiescence in quality-of-life interviews with adults who have mental retardation. *Mental Retardation, 35*, 75–82.

McAfee, J. K., & Gural, M. (1988). Individuals with mental retardation and the criminal justice system: The view from states' attorneys general. *Mental Retardation, 26*, 5–12.

McGee, J. J., & Menolascino, F. J. (1992). The evaluation of defendants with mental retardation in the criminal justice system. In R. W. Conley, R. Luckasson, & G. N. Bouthilet (Eds.), *The criminal justice system and mental retardation: defendants and victims* (pp. 55–77). Paul H. Brookes Publishing.

McKenzie, K., Michie, A., Murray, A., & Hales, C. (2012). Screening for offenders with an intellectual disability: The validity of the Learning Disability Screening Questionnaire. *Research in Developmental Disabilities, 33*, 791–795.

Megargee, E. I. (2013). Psychological assessment in correctional settings. In J. R. Graham & J. A. Naglieri (Eds.), *Handbook of psychology, Vol. 10: Assessment psychology* (pp. 394–424). John Wiley and Sons.

Müller-Isberner, R., & Hodgins, S. (2000). Evidence-based treatment for mentally disordered offenders. In S. Hodgins & R. Müller-Isberner (Eds.), *Violence, crime and mentally disordered offenders* (pp. 7–38). John Wiley & Sons.

National Commission on Correctional Health Care. (2008). *Standards for health services in prisons*.

National Commission on Correctional Health Care. (2015). *Standards for mental health services in correctional facilities*.

New York State Commission on Quality of Care for the Mentally Disabled. (1992). *Inmates with developmental disabilities in NYS correctional facilities, March 1991*. http://www.justicecenter.ny.gov/sites/default/files/archivereports/Publications/00067.pdf

Nicholls, T. L., Petersen, K., Almond, M., & Geddes, C. (2021). Short-Term Assessment of Risk and Treatability (START): Rationale, application, and empirical overview. In K. S. Douglas & R. K. Otto (Eds.), *Handbook of violence risk assessment* (2nd ed., pp. 359–388). Routledge/Taylor & Francis Group.

Patrick, M. E., Shaw, K. A., Dietz, P. M., et al. (2021). Prevalence of intellectual disability among eight-year-old children from selected communities in the United States. *Disability and Health Journal, 14*, 1–7.

Pelka, F. (1997). Unequal justice: Preserving the rights of the mentally retarded in the criminal justice system. *Humanist, 57*, 28–32.

Pennsylvania Department of Corrections v. Yeskey, 524 U.S. 206 (1998).

Petersilia, J. (1997). Justice for all? Offenders with mental retardation and the California corrections system. *Prison Journal, 77*, 358–381.

Petersilia, J. (2000a). *Doing justice? Criminal offenders with developmental disabilities.* California Policy Research Center Brief (Vol. 12, No. 4). University of California.

Petersilia, J. (2000b). Invisible victims: Violence against persons with developmental disabilities. *Human Rights, 27*, 9–13.

Petrella, R. C. (1992). Defendants with mental retardation in the forensic services system. In R. W. Conley, R. Luckasson, & G. N. Bouthilet (Eds.), *The criminal justice system and mental retardation: defendants and victims* (pp. 79–96). Paul H. Brookes Publishing.

Rosa's Law, Pub. L. 111–256 (October 5, 2010).

Ruiz v. Estelle, 503 F. Supp. 1265 (S.D. Tex. 1980), cert denied, 103 Ct 1438.

Santamour, M. B. (1987). The offender with mental retardation. *Prison Journal, 66*, 3–18.

Santamour, M. B., & West, B. (1982a). The mentally retarded offender: Presentation of the facts and a discussion of issues. In M. B. Santamour & P. S. Watson (Eds.), *The retarded offender* (pp. 7–36). Praeger Publishers.

Santamour, M. B., & West, B. (1982b). Retarded offenders: Habilitative program development. In M. B. Santamour & P. S. Watson (Eds.), *The retarded offender* (pp. 272–296). Praeger Publishers.

Scheyett, A., Vaughn, J., Taylor, M., & Parish, S. (2009). Are we there yet? Screening processes for intellectual and developmental disabilities in jail settings. *Intellectual and Developmental Disabilities, 47*, 13–23.

Seay, O. J. (2006). Evaluating mental retardation for forensic purposes. *Applied Psychology in Criminal Justice, 2*, 52–81.

Seligman, M. E. P., Rashid, T., & Parks, A. C. (2006). Positive psychotherapy. *American Psychologist, 61*, 774–788.

Shively, R. (2004). Treating offenders with mental retardation and developmental disabilities. *Corrections Today, 66*, 84–87.

Smith, S. A. (1993). Confusing the terms "guilty" and "not guilty": Implications for alleged offenders with mental retardation. *Psychological Reports, 73*(3), 675–678.

Smith, C., Algozzine, B., Schmid, R. E., & Hennly, T. (1990). Prison adjustment of youthful inmates with mental retardation. *Mental Retardation, 28*, 177–181.

Stavis, P. F. (1991, January–February). Doing justice? The criminal justice system and persons with mental retardation. *New York State Commission on Quality of Care for the Mentally Disabled, Quality of Care Newsletter*, (47).

Talent, A., & Keldgord, R. (1975). The mentally retarded probationer. *Federal Probation, 39*, 39–46.

Tassé, M. J., Schalock, R., Thompson, J. R., & Wehmeyer, M. (2005). *Guidelines for interviewing people with disabilities: Support Intensity Scale.* AAMR.

Thompson, J. R., Tassé, M. J., & McLaughlin, C. A. (2008). Interrater reliability of the Supports Intensity Scale (SIS). *American Journal of Mental Retardation, 113*, 231–237.

58

Traumatic brain injury

William R. McBride and Anthony C. Tamburello[1]

Introduction

Traumatic brain injuries (TBIs) are an increasingly recognized phenomenon in the United States and abroad. They are perennially responsible for a high number of emergency department visits, hospitalizations, and deaths in the United States (Faul et al., 2010). Improved public understanding of TBI-related signs and symptoms, the high direct costs associated with TBI, increased media and political attention, improved technology relating to TBI detection, and increased access to such technology are all partially responsible for society's increased awareness of TBI.

Despite this increasing recognition, many people who suffer a TBI either do not pursue treatment or present for medical care only after a significant delay. This phenomenon can be partially explained by the observation that most (75%) TBIs are mild (Centers for Disease Control and Prevention [CDC], National Center for Injury Prevention and Control, 2003). This typically means that the individual will experience milder and relatively shorter lived symptoms compared to those who have experienced a more severe TBI. Despite this, TBIs are still estimated to be responsible for substantial mortality, long-term disability, and direct costs: approximately $400 billion each year worldwide (Maas et al., 2022; Thurman et al., 1999).

TBIs are increasingly observed in a variety of cohorts, including but not limited to those involved in contact sports, persons serving in the armed forces, and civilians who are not involved in either endeavor. There are many reasons for this phenomenon. In the 1960s, increased availability of high-speed vehicles led to an increase in high-speed collisions and more demand for TBI-related health care services in the United States (Cifu et al., 2010; Lewin, 1968). Many contact sports have become increasingly fast-paced, causing participants to be exposed to impact events of greater velocity. Among active-duty military and veteran U.S. military personnel, TBI was described as the "signature wound" of the Gulf War, Operation Iraqi Freedom, and Operation Enduring Freedom due to its high prevalence during these conflicts (Cifu et al., 2010; Guillamondegui et al., 2011; Hoge et al., 2008; Sayer et al., 2009).

Incarcerated individuals are another population with a significantly elevated lifetime exposure to TBI. The presence of TBI complicates the capacity of incarcerated persons (IPs) to function in a carceral setting and to benefit from programming. TBI may be related to the incidence of criminal conduct, as well as to recidivism. This chapter reviews the prevalence of TBI within correctional settings, its influence upon comorbid substance use disorders and psychiatric illnesses, and ways to better identify and medically manage patients who have suffered a TBI.

Prevalence

In the community, TBI mortality rates are nearly 3 times greater for men than for women (CDC, 2022). TBI incidence is also elevated among low-income groups in the United States (Hanks et al., 2003; Turkstra et al., 2003). Among young men, one of the principal causes of TBI is violence (Thurman et al., 1999). Substance use also has a significant impact on both the incidence of TBI and rehabilitation outcomes (Corrigan, 1995; Parry-Jones et al., 2006).

IPs are more likely to have engaged in substance use and to have been involved in activities that increase their risk of both intentional and unintentional injury (Carson & Golinelli, 2013). Frequently reported examples of high-risk situations experienced by IPs include fights, vehicular collisions, intimate partner violence, and gang violence, among others. Substance use during these incidents is often a factor and, if not the root cause, may exacerbate the risk of injury. In addition, many IPs have experienced financially impoverished conditions, with reduced access to health care, so previous TBIs may have been undertreated or not addressed at all. A previous TBI is a risk factor for a future TBI (Lasry et al., 2017). Timonen and colleagues (2002) found that subjects who had suffered a TBI prior to the age of 12 began engaging in criminal behavior considerably earlier than those who suffered a TBI later in their childhood, suggesting a relationship between earlier TBI and criminal behavior (Timonen et al., 2002). Since many of the risk factors for TBI (male gender, substance use, exposure to violence, economic marginalization) overlap risk factors for incarceration, a higher prevalence of TBI is expected within jails and prisons.

In the early 2000s, the CDC began an initiative to determine TBI prevalence among institutionalized populations, including those who are incarcerated. Early prevalence studies were criticized for

1. The authors acknowledge the contributions of Pamela M. Diamond, who authored this chapter in the first edition of this textbook.

their focus on specialized groups (e.g., death row, persons with substance use disorders), studying a single gender, making comparisons between noncomparable facilities, comparing disparate countries, and having small sample sizes. Perhaps more problematic, these studies were done without standardization of TBI definition or measurement (Diamond et al., 2007). Moynan and McMillan (2018) conducted a systematic review of studies of the prevalence of head injuries and associated disability of adult prisoners, with rates reported ranging from 25% to 86%. Even at the lower end of this range, the prevalence of TBI in carceral settings is much higher than the estimated 8.5% in the nonincarcerated population (Wald et al., 2014). However, the methodology of these studies, including many of the concerns above, suggests that these estimates may not be generalizable (Moynan & McMillan, 2018).

Shiroma and colleagues (2010) conducted a meta-analysis of 20 studies that investigated lifetime TBI prevalence among incarcerated adults. Each study had a clear definition of TBI and described their assessment methods. The rate of TBI was approximately 60%, while the rate of TBI with associated loss of consciousness was somewhat lower, at approximately 50% (Shiroma et al., 2010). These estimates are consistent with the findings of a CDC-funded epidemiological study conducted in the South Carolina prison system using a validated instrument to assess TBI among a stratified sample representative of the prison population. Rates of TBI in that study ranged from 50% to 70%, depending on gender and release status (higher for men and those not eligible for release). Most IPs reported a history of multiple TBIs over the course of their lifetime, with an average age at first TBI of approximately 16 years. Ongoing symptoms related to TBI were commonly reported and covaried with the severity of the injury experienced (Ferguson et al., 2012).

Symptoms and sequelae

TBI may result in cognitive, motor, or emotional dysfunction that can impact an individual's ability to interact appropriately with their environment. These sequelae can vary from minor memory lapses to a complete inability to speak or navigate without assistance. Common examples of cognitive deficits include difficulty processing information or remembering what one has read or heard, complex task management, understanding incoming messages, difficulties with judgment, and trouble with social interactions, among others. The extent and nature of these symptoms are often associated with the severity of the injury and the location of the insult to the brain (Silver et al., 2005). Many who experience TBI do not survive; others may need long-term inpatient rehabilitation or even lifelong care (Thurman et al., 1999). IPs often fall into another group: those who have survived a TBI but suffer sequelae of a more diffuse nature. Their symptoms may be temporary, delayed, or long-lasting. Behavior and cognition are often affected. Acquaintances, loved ones, and sometimes even the affected individual may lack an awareness of the relationship between what was thought to be a minor head injury and the problems they develop with motor skills, attention, impulse control, or other symptoms (CDC, 2023; Langlois et al., 2005). The injuries and their sequelae can result in an increased risk of interactions with the legal system, homelessness, tumultuous relationships, or other unfavorable outcomes.

Due to the heterogeneity of TBI, whether aggression or impulsivity will occur as a result is unpredictable. It is possible that a reduction in impulse control or an increase in aggressive tendencies could play a role in the commitment of violent crime (Martin et al., 2019). Multiple studies have indicated that the likelihood of arrest increases post-TBI and that the prevalence of head injury is higher among individuals incarcerated for violent crimes (Brewer-Smyth et al., 2004; Cohen et al., 1999; Miller, 1999). These findings may be linked to the changes in psychological functioning often seen among those who have previously suffered a TBI, such as increased verbal and physical aggression, low tolerance for frustration, and poor impulse control (Miller, 1999).

Among those currently incarcerated, these impairments can have substantial effects on their adjustment to, and interaction with, the demands of functioning and living in an incarcerated setting. The potential behavioral and cognitive sequelae of TBI in carceral settings may be neither understood nor tolerated by correctional, medical, and administrative staff. Cognitive dysfunction carries a greater risk of poor adjustment to incarceration. For example, persons with TBI may misremember rules or may be slow in responding to instructions from custody staff (Harmon, 2012). In a recent study of young incarcerated men, those with TBI had significantly worse behavioral control, higher aggression, and higher levels of hopelessness (Linden et al., 2020). Untreated or undertreated symptoms of TBI and comorbidities are an additional challenge in the effective reintegration of IPs into the community following their release. Because TBI can have such a wide-ranging impact on those who have been incarcerated, enhancing our understanding of and ability to address the needs of this population has become more important for health care professionals in both community and correctional settings (National Commission on Correctional Health Care, 2002).

Comorbidity

Complex, multidirectional relationships exist between TBI, mental illness, substance use disorders, and criminal behavior. Multiple studies support an elevated risk for postinjury mood and behavioral disorders for those who experience a TBI. These disturbances can complicate recovery of TBI and vice versa. Depression is especially common following TBI (Deb et al., 1999; Mooney & Speed, 2001; Rapoport et al., 2003; Seel et al., 2003; Seel & Kreutzer, 2003). Furthermore, those who experience depression following a TBI often have increased difficulty with their day-to-day functioning and worse overall outcomes (Rosenthal et al., 1998). Research has also identified higher rates of comorbid personality disorders (Hibbard et al., 2000), posttraumatic stress disorder (Weil et al., 2016), and other anxiety disorders (Mooney & Speed, 2001) following a head trauma. In a recent study investigating the effects of posttraumatic stress disorder and TBI on subsequent arrests, TBI was found to be predictive of future violent offending but not general reoffending (Lattermore et al., 2022).

Multiple studies have found that those who have suffered a mild TBI are more likely to engage in binge drinking or to suffer from an alcohol use disorder. Researchers have repeatedly identified alcohol intoxication as a proximate cause of TBIs (Corrigan, 1995; Moore et al., 1994; Parry-Jones et al., 2006; Silver et al., 2001; Weil et al., 2016).

Felde and colleagues (2006) found that 40% of 550 voluntary participants in substance use treatment reported a history of TBI. Those who had previously suffered a TBI were more likely to suffer from more severe substance use–related disorders and also exhibited higher rates of comorbid depression and anxiety-related disorders. Those engaged in integrated, dual diagnosis treatment for mental illness and substance use disorders exhibited higher rates of TBI as well (Felde et al., 2006). Corrigan and Deutschle (2008) found that 72% of the patients studied within a dual diagnosis program had a history of at least one TBI. They also found that the individuals who were diagnosed with disorders related to substance use, mental disorders, and TBI had worse current functioning, had initiated their substance use at a younger age, and were more likely to have a comorbid personality disorder (Corrigan & Deutschle, 2008).

A history of alcohol or illicit substance use has also been associated with worse functional, neuropsychological, and medical outcomes (Corrigan, 1995; Parry-Jones et al., 2006). Multiple studies have also suggested that a history of TBI could negatively impact the ability of IPs to recover from substance use–related disorders, avoid recidivism, and effectively reintegrate back into the community upon release (Center for Substance Abuse Treatment, 1998; Corrigan, 1995; Valliant et al., 2003).

Screening

Several screening instruments for TBI have been developed and validated for use in the correctional setting. These include the Traumatic Brain Injury Questionnaire (TBIQ; Diamond et al., 2007), the Ohio State University Traumatic Brain Injury Identification Method (Bogner & Corrigan, 2009), and the Brain Injury Screening Questionnaire (BISQ; Cantor et al., 2004). Each instrument assesses for lifetime history of TBI, provides an indication of severity, allows for the reporting of multiple injuries, and differentiates among those injuries associated with loss of consciousness or posttraumatic amnesia. While they differ somewhat in their scoring and reporting, all have been validated psychometrically. Although shorter screening instruments are easier to administer, research has consistently demonstrated that shorter TBI screening tools embedded within a more broad interview tend to underestimate TBI prevalence significantly. Diamond and colleagues (2007) compared results from the TBIQ, an interview-based instrument, to IPs' responses to an item asking about head injury on a standard screening tool used in the federal prison system. Only 19% of the IPs who reported a TBI on the TBIQ had responded positively to the embedded screening question (Diamond et al., 2007).

Screening for TBI among incarcerated populations is not routinely done in most correctional systems despite the increased availability of validated tools. The Health Resources Services Administration has supported pilot screening programs in multiple states. For example, one program in Minnesota used the TBIQ to screen approximately 1,000 individuals for TBI, while another in Wyoming utilized the BISQ. These studies found prevalence rates consistent with the studies previously described in this chapter (Brain Injury Association of Wyoming, 2008; Wald et al., 2014).

The cost of both screening and treatment is a common concern expressed by prison administrators when asked about implementation of routine screening for TBI. Considering the significantly elevated prevalence of TBI among IPs as compared to the nonincarcerated population, it will be important to develop and adapt treatment programs already used within the correctional setting to provide adequate medical and mental health care. Notably, IPs with a history of at least one TBI are more likely to sustain serious disciplinary charges and to incur behavioral infractions (Chan et al., 2023; Matheson et al., 2020; Piccolino & Solberg, 2014; Shiroma et al., 2010). Since people who suffer from cognitive deficits are more likely to have difficulty following directions or staying on task, staff could interpret these actions as oppositional or confrontational and thus react with frustration. Increasing awareness and understanding of these impairments among staff, as well as the affected individuals, could lead to fewer misunderstandings between all parties, enhanced safety within the prison, and improved overall outcomes for the affected individuals. To the authors' knowledge, a relevant cost analysis in correctional systems has not been done; however, reduced costs related to discipline, staff injuries, and recidivism would be expected to offset the expenses related to TBI-related screening and treatment. Broadly, interventions that aim to optimize functioning and reduce disability within the environment of the affected individual are integral to recovery from TBI and its related sequelae (Chan et al., 2023). Within the incarcerated setting, it may be most cost-effective to focus efforts on adjusting programs that are ordinarily provided within this setting so that these programs satisfy the needs of individuals with cognitive deficits, irrespective of the source of these deficits.

Programming

Much of the research related to TBI rehabilitation is focused on moderate to severe TBI and may not be applicable to those with less conspicuous presentations, as is often observed in persons housed in secure facilities. Cognitive impairment related to TBI may be difficult to distinguish from symptoms referable to other mental health conditions common in correctional settings, like major depressive disorder or attention-deficit/hyperactivity disorder. Given the frequent overlap in symptomatic presentation and comorbid disorders within the incarcerated population, it would likely be beneficial to adapt current programming to target the deficits shared by those with TBI, mental illness, and substance use–related disorders.

Education and training of staff, including correctional officers, who interact with IPs on a day-to-day basis is essential. Misconceptions about TBI, such as believing that patients are unable to recover from their injuries or that TBIs are of low prevalence, are common even among nonspecialist health care providers working in a correctional setting (Yuhasz, 2013). Both staff and IPs will benefit from staff having a better understanding of the potential cognitive and emotional sequelae of TBI and better ways to approach their work with these individuals.

Contemporary approaches to mental health and substance use psychotherapies are regularly grounded in the principles of cognitive-behavioral therapy (CBT; see Chapters 43 and 47). These programs often use protocols developed for use with individuals who do not have limitations in cognitive functioning, frequently relying on the patient's ability to consider their circumstances carefully and participate in developing personalized solutions. Modest modifications to CBT-based programming, like shorter sessions, increased repetition, and the provision of simplified instructions, will significantly enhance treatment efficacy and reduce treatment dropout. A recent pilot study on a modified CBT/mindfulness-based stress reduction intervention for persons incarcerated in a high-security New Zealand prison was encouraging in terms of the development of positive coping strategies (Mitchell et al., 2021). More study is needed of carceral programs that are specifically created or adapted for IPs who struggle with cognitive impairment, including from TBI.

Medication

No medications have been approved by the U.S. Food and Drug Administration specifically to manage psychiatric symptoms secondary to TBI. Some research supports the off-label use of selective serotonin reuptake inhibitors to manage aggression related to TBI (Arciniegas & Wortzel, 2014). Interested readers are referred to the chapters in this text on aggression and behavior management plans (Chapters 53 and 54).

Summary

Recent systematic reviews indicate that up to 86% of IPs have a history of at least one TBI (Chan et al., 2023; Moynan & McMillan, 2018). This prevalence greatly exceeds that reported among the nonincarcerated population (Chan et al., 2023; Farrer & Hedges, 2011). Routine screening for TBI is rarely done in these settings despite the availability of validated instruments and the high number of individuals within this population who have suffered at least one TBI in their lifetime. Residual cognitive deficits secondary to TBI can be difficult to differentiate from those associated with various mental illness or substance use disorders. The etiology of the pertinent cognitive deficits is often challenging to ascertain; nonetheless, these symptoms often make day-to-day life within the incarcerated setting significantly more difficult. Modified programming for IPs with cognitive deficits secondary to TBI or another etiology would likely benefit those suffering from related symptoms. Furthermore, educational interventions intended to improve staff understanding of TBI and its various sequelae, as well as how best to interact with individuals who have a history of TBI, could decrease incidents of misunderstanding and reduce conflict within the carceral setting.

REFERENCES

Arciniegas, D. B., & Wortzel, H. S. (2014). Emotional and behavioral dyscontrol after traumatic brain injury. *Psychiatric Clinics of North America, 37*(1), 31–53.

Bogner, J., & Corrigan, J. D. (2009). Reliability and predictive validity of the Ohio State University TBI identification method with prisoners. *Journal of Head Trauma Rehabilitation, 24*(4), 279–291.

Brain Injury Association of Wyoming. (2008). *Study of undiagnosed brain injuries in Wyoming's prison population.* Wyoming Department of Health Division of Developmental Disabilities, Wyoming. https://docplayer.net/99777465-Study-of-undiagnosed-brain-injuries-in-wyoming-s-prison-population.html

Brewer-Smyth, K., Burgess, A. W., & Shults, J. (2004). Physical and sexual abuse, salivary cortisol, and neurologic correlates of violent criminal behavior in female prison inmates. *Biological Psychiatry, 55*, 21–31.

Cantor, J. B., Gordon, W. A., Schwartz, M. E., Charatz, H. J., Ashman, T. A., & Abramowitz, S. (2004). Child and parent responses to a brain injury screening questionnaire. *Archives of Physical Medicine and Rehabilitation, 85*(4 Suppl. 2), S54–S60.

Carson, E., & Golinelli, D. (2013). *Prisoners in 2012: Trends in admissions and releases, 1991–2012* (NCJ 243920). Bureau of Justice Statistics.

Centers for Disease Control and Prevention. (2022). *Surveillance report on traumatic brain-injury related deaths by age group, sex, and mechanism of injury—United States, 2018 and 2019.* https://www.cdc.gov/traumaticbraininjury/pdf/TBI-surveillance-report-2018-2019-508.pdf

Centers for Disease Control and Prevention. (2023). *Traumatic brain injury (TBI): Topic home.* http://www.cdc.gov/TraumaticBrainInjury/index.html

Centers for Disease Control and Prevention, National Center for Injury Prevention and Control. (2003). *Report to Congress on mild traumatic brain injury in the United States: Steps to prevent a serious public health problem.* U.S. Department of Health and Human Services. https://www.cdc.gov/traumaticbraininjury/pdf/mtbireport-a.pdf

Center for Substance Abuse Treatment. (1998). *Substance use disorder treatment for people with physical and cognitive disabilities.* Treatment Improvement Protocol (TIP) Series, No. 29.: HHS Publication No. (SMA) 12-4078. Substance Abuse and Mental Health Services Administration. https://www.ncbi.nlm.nih.gov/books/NBK64879/

Chan, V., Estrella, M. J., Syed, S., et al. (2023). Rehabilitation among individuals with traumatic brain injury who intersect with the criminal justice system: A scoping review. *Frontiers in Neurology, 13*, 1052294.

Cifu, D. X., Cohen, S. I., Lew, H. L., Jaffee, M., & Sigford, B. (2010). The history and evolution of traumatic brain injury rehabilitation in military service members and veterans. *American Journal of Physical Medicine & Rehabilitation, 89*(8), 688–694.

Cohen, R. A., Rosenbaum, A., Kane, R. L., Warnken, W. J., & Benjamin, S. (1999). Neuropsychological correlates of domestic violence. *Violence and Victims, 14*(4), 397–411.

Corrigan, J. D. (1995). Substance abuse as a mediating factor in outcome from traumatic brain injury. *Archives of Physical Medicine and Rehabilitation, 76*(4), 302–309.

Corrigan, J. D., & Deutschle, J. J., Jr. (2008). The presence and impact of traumatic brain injury among clients in treatment for co-occurring mental illness and substance abuse. *Brain Injury, 22*(3), 223–231.

Deb, S., Lyons, I., Ali, I., & McCarthy, G. (1999). Rate of psychiatric illness 1 year after traumatic brain injury. *American Journal of Psychiatry, 156*, 374–378.

Diamond, P. M., Harzke, A. J., Magaletta, P. R., Cummins, A. G., & Frankowski, R. (2007). Screening for traumatic brain injury in an offender sample: A first look at the reliability and validity of the Traumatic Brain Injury Questionnaire. *Journal of Head Trauma Rehabilitation, 22*(6), 330–338.

Farrer, T. J., & Hedges, D. W. (2011). Prevalence of traumatic brain injury in incarcerated groups compared to the general population: A meta-analysis. *Progress in Neuro-Psychopharmacology & Biological Psychiatry, 35*(2), 390–4.

Faul, M., Xu, L., Wald, M. M., & Coronado, V. G. (2010). *Traumatic brain injury in the United States: Emergency department visits, hospitalizations and deaths 2002–2006.* Centers for Disease Control and Prevention, National Center for Injury Prevention and Control.

Felde, A. B., Westermeyer, J., & Thuras, P. (2006). Co-morbid traumatic brain injury and substance use disorder: Childhood predictors and adult correlates. *Brain Injury, 20*(1), 41–49.

Ferguson, P. L., Pickelsimer, E. E., Corrigan, J. D., Bogner, J. A., & Wald, M. (2012). Prevalence of traumatic brain injury among prisoners in South Carolina. *Journal of Head Trauma Rehabilitation, 27*(3), E11–E20.

Guillamondegui, O. D., Montgomery, S. A., Phibbs, F. T., et al. (2011). *Traumatic brain injury and depression.* Agency for Healthcare Research and Quality.

Hanks, R. A., Wood, D. L., Millis, S., et al. (2003). Violent traumatic brain injury: Occurrence, patient characteristics, and risk factors from the Traumatic Brain Injury Model Systems project. *Archives of Physical Medicine and Rehabilitation, 84*(2), 249–254.

Harmon, K. (2012, February 4). Brain injury rate 7 times greater among U.S. prisoners. *Scientific American.*

Hibbard, M. R., Bogdany, J., Uysal, S., et al. (2000). Axis II psychopathology in individuals with traumatic brain injury. *Brain Injury, 14*(1), 45–61.

Hoge, C. W., McGurk, D., Thomas, J. L., Cox, A. L., Engel, C. C., & Castro, C. A. (2008). Mild traumatic brain injury in U.S. Soldiers returning from Iraq. *New England Journal of Medicine, 358*, 453–463.

Langlois, J. A., Marr, A., Mitchko, J., & Johnson, R. L. (2005). Tracking the silent epidemic and educating the public: CDC's traumatic brain injury-associated activities under the TBI Act of 1996 and the Children's Health Act of 2000. *Journal of Head Trauma Rehabilitation, 20*(3), 196–204.

Lasry, O., Liu, E. Y., Powell, G. A., Ruel-Laliberté, J., Marcoux, J., & Buckeridge, D. L. (2017). Epidemiology of recurrent traumatic brain injury in the general population: A systematic review. *Neurology, 89*(21), 2198–2209.

Lattimore, P. K., Richardson, N. J., Ferguson, P. L., & Pickelsimer, E. E. (2022). The Association of Traumatic Brain Injury, post-traumatic stress disorder, and criminal recidivism. *Health & Justice, 10*(1), 7.

Lewin, W. (1968). Rehabilitation after head injury. *British Medical Journal, 1*(5590), 465–470.

Linden, M. A., O'Rourke, C., & Lohan, M. (2020). Traumatic brain injury and social competence among young male offenders. *Disability and Rehabilitation, 42*(17), 2422–2429.

Maas, A. I. R., Menon, D. K., Manley, G. T., et al. (2022). Traumatic brain injury: Progress and challenges in prevention, clinical care, and research. *Lancet Neurology, 21*, 1004–1060.

Martin, S., Zabala, C., Del-Monte, J., et al. (2019). Examining the relationships between impulsivity, aggression, and recidivism for prisoners with antisocial personality disorder. *Aggression and Violent Behavior, 49*(6), 101314.

Matheson, F. I., McIsaac, K. E., Fung, K., et al. (2020). Association between traumatic brain injury and prison charges: A population-based cohort study. *Brain Injury, 34*, 757–763.

Miller, E. (1999). Head injury and offending. *Journal of Forensic Psychiatry, 10*(1), 157–166.

Mitchell, T., du Preez, E., & Theadom, A. (2021). An intervention to improve coping strategies in adult male prisoners with a history of traumatic brain injury: A pilot randomised clinical trial. *Clinical Rehabilitation, 35*(8), 1185–1195.

Mooney, G., & Speed, J. (2001). The association between mild traumatic brain injury and psychiatric conditions. *Brain Injury, 15*(10), 865–877.

Moore, D., Greer, B. G., & Li, L. (1994). Alcohol and other substance use/abuse among people with disabilities. *Journal of Social Behavior and Personality, 9*(5), 369–382.

Moynan, C. R., & McMillan, T. M. (2018). Prevalence of head injury and associated disability in prison populations: A systematic review. *Journal of head trauma rehabilitation, 33*(4), 275–282.

National Commission on Correctional Health Care. (2002). *The health status of soon-to-be-released inmates: A report to Congress* (Vol. 1). https://www.ojp.gov/pdffiles1/nij/grants/189735.pdf

Parry-Jones, B. L., Vaughan, F. L., & Miles Cox, W. (2006). Traumatic brain injury and substance misuse: A systematic review of prevalence and outcomes research (1994–2004). *Neuropsychological Rehabilitation, 16*(5), 537–560.

Piccolino, A. L., & Solberg, K. B. (2014). The impact of traumatic brain injury on prison health services and offender management. *Journal of Correctional Health Care, 20*, 203–212.

Rapoport, M., McCullagh, S., Streiner, D., & Feinstein, A. (2003). The clinical significance of major depression following mild traumatic brain injury. *Psychosomatics, 44*, 31–37.

Rosenthal, M., Christensen, B. K., & Ross, T. P. (1998). Depression following traumatic brain injury. *Archives of Physical Medicine and Rehabilitation, 79*(1), 90–103.

Sayer, N. A., Cifu, D. X., McNamee, S., et al. (2009). Rehabilitation needs of combat-injured service members admitted to the VA Polytrauma Rehabilitation Centers: The role of PM&R in the care of wounded warriors. *PM & R: The Journal of Injury, Function, and Rehabilitation, 1*(1), 23–28.

Seel, R. T., & Kreutzer, J. S. (2003). Depression assessment after traumatic brain injury: An empirically based classification method. *Archives of Physical Medicine and Rehabilitation, 84*(11), 1621–1628. https://doi.org/10.1053/s0003-9993(03)00270-3

Seel, R. T., Kreutzer, J. S., Rosenthal, M., Hammond, F. M., Corrigan, J. D., & Black, K. (2003). Depression after traumatic brain injury: A National Institute on Disability and Rehabilitation Research Model Systems multicenter investigation. *Archives of Physical Medicine and Rehabilitation, 84*(2), 177–184.

Shiroma, E. J., Ferguson, P. L., & Pickelsimer, E. E. (2010). Prevalence of traumatic brain injury in an offender population: A meta-analysis. *Journal of Correctional Health Care, 16*(2), 147–159.

Silver, J. M., Kramer, R., Greenwald, S., & Weissman, M. (2001). The association between head injuries and psychiatric disorders: Findings from the New Haven NIMH Epidemiologic Catchment Area Study. *Brain Injury, 15*(11), 935–945.

Silver, J. M., McAllister, T. W., & Yudofsky, S. C. (2005). *Textbook of traumatic brain injury* (2nd ed.). American Psychiatric Publishing.

Timonen, M., Miettunen, J., Hakko, H., et al. (2002). The association of preceding traumatic brain injury with mental disorders, alcoholism and criminality: The Northern Finland 1966 Birth Cohort Study. *Psychiatry Research, 113*(3), 217–226.

Thurman, D. J., Alverson, C., Dunn, K. A., Guerrero, J., & Sniezek, J. E. (1999). Traumatic brain injury in the United States: A public health perspective. *Journal of Head Trauma Rehabilitation, 14*(6), 602–615.

Turkstra, L., Jones, D., & Toler, H. L. (2003). Brain injury and violent crime. *Brain Injury, 17*(1), 39–47.

Valliant, P. M., Freeston, A., Pottier, D., & Kosmyna, R. (2003). Personality and executive functioning as risk factors in recidivists. *Psychological Reports, 92*, 299–306.

Wald, M. M., Helgeson, S. R., & Langlois, J. A. (2014). *Traumatic brain injury among prisoners.* Brain Injury Professional. http://www.brainline.org/content/2008/11/traumatic-brain-injury-among-prisoners_pageall.html

Weil, Z. M., Corrigan, J. D., & Karelina, K. (2016). Alcohol abuse after traumatic brain injury: Experimental and clinical evidence. *Neuroscience and Biobehavioral Reviews, 62*, 89–99.

Yuhasz, J. E. (2013). Misconceptions about traumatic brain injury among correctional health care professionals. *Journal of Correctional Health Care, 9*(2), 135–143.

59

Justice-involved youth

Rosa E. Negrón Muñoz[1]

Introduction

The incarceration of minors occurs in both juvenile and adult correctional systems, depending on jurisdiction, age, and criminal charges. This chapter reviews the history and current evidence-based or best practices in the management and treatment of incarcerated youth. The terms "juvenile" and "delinquency" are used to describe justice-involved persons under the age of 18 when historically relevant or otherwise necessary.

History of the juvenile court and juvenile detention centers

The concept of responsibility of underaged persons dates to over 4,000 years ago with the Code of Hammurabi, which referenced runaway and disobedient children. About 2,000 years later, Roman civil and church law introduced the concept of age of responsibility. Jewish law in the Talmud set forth conditions under which immaturity was to be considered in imposing punishment. Muslim law called for standards of leniency where persons younger than 17 years were exempt from the death penalty.

Eighteenth-century scholars contemplated the distinction between children and adults with regard to assessing criminal culpability. In 1765, Sir William Blackstone coined the term "*malitia supplet aetatem*," which translates to "*malice supplies the* [want of] *age*" (Blackstone, 1765). This was a legal doctrine that allowed a minor to be held responsible for their actions as an adult if they acted with malicious intent.

In the United States, the juvenile justice system has its roots in English common law and the concept of *parens patriae*. Under common law, children younger than age 7 were classified as infants and determined incapable of committing a crime because they were too young to fully understand their actions and unable to form criminal *mens rea*. Children older than 14 were classified as adults and were considered fully capable of knowing right from wrong. Children between 7 and 14 were presumed to lack capacity unless proven otherwise by a prosecutor.

In the 16th century, an educational reform movement in England perceived juveniles to be underdeveloped in terms of their moral and cognitive abilities. This fueled a shift toward the reform of juvenile justice in America.

As early as the 17th century, the notion that children were not "little adults" and were cognitively and emotionally different began to take hold (Thompson & Morris, 2016). This new awareness led to the implementation of different methods to manage justice-involved youth. Operating under the concept of *parens patriae*, some of the goals were to separate youth from adults, remove them from adverse home environments "for their own good," minimize court proceedings, provide indeterminate sentences until they were reformed, and use punishment only if other alternatives proved futile. Other goals were to help youth avoid idleness through military drills, physical exercise, and supervision.

The concept of using therapeutic approaches was introduced in the early 19th century. Retrospectively, the early juvenile court and detention center philosophy centered on reforming youth by focusing on education (preferably vocational and religious) and by teaching sobriety, thrift, industry, and prudence. The early court also sought to provide protective factors by increasing the social fabric around justice-involved youth, increasing connectedness and social bonds between them and adults, providing them with opportunities (often in the form of vocational training) to develop self-esteem and social and emotional skills, providing an adult protective shield to monitor situations that could result in risky behaviors, and helping youth transform traumatic life experiences into constructive energy. Some of these early goals continue to be influential today.

The first "House of Refuge" was created by the legislature in New York in 1825, with the purpose of bringing care and education to those juveniles who lacked supervision or who had been referred by the courts (Center on Juvenile and Criminal Justice, 2024). Houses of Refuge became the primary institutions for poor and delinquent youth. Despite the intent of these facilities to help children without incarcerating them, their conditions sometimes included punishments like solitary confinement and lashings (Kopaczewski, 2016).

In 1889, Jane Addams founded Hull House on Chicago's Near West Side as a social settlement house "to aid in the solution of the social and industrial problems which are engendered by the modern

1. The author acknowledges the contributions of Carl C. Bell, who authored this chapter in the first edition of this textbook.

conditions of life in a great city" (Beuttler & Bell, 2010, p. 5). Addams observed:

> Children over ten years of age were arrested, held in the police stations, tried in the police courts. If convicted they were usually fined and if the fine was not paid sent to the city prison. However, often they were let off because justices could neither tolerate sending children to Bridewell nor bear to be themselves guilty of the harsh folly of compelling poverty-stricken parents to pay fines. No exchange of court records existed and the same children could be in and out of various police stations an indefinite number of times, more hardened and more skillful with each experience. (Addams, 2004, p. 133)

In their efforts to change the harsh conditions besetting Chicago's European immigrant youth, in 1899, Addams and her colleagues worked to establish the first juvenile court in Illinois.

The juvenile court system oversaw innovative approaches to justice-involved youth, including smaller cottage institutions, probation, and out-of-home placement. The procedures of the juvenile court were designed to be "primarily protective and educational rather than punitive, and the commission of a child to a correctional institution is deemed to be for his welfare and not for the sole purpose of inflicting penalty" (Beuttler & Bell, 2010, p. 5). By 1925, all but two states had established juvenile courts.

In 1909, the Juvenile Psychopathic Institute (later called the Institute for Juvenile Research [IJR]) was created in Illinois. Neurologist William Healy, MD, the first director, was charged with studying the biological aspects of brain functioning and intelligence, social factors, attitudes, and motivations of justice-involved youth. The IJR is considered the birthplace of child psychiatry (Schowalter, 2000). The IJR's initial goal was to develop an understanding of the causes of behavioral disturbances in children and adolescents by doing research and providing services for justice-involved youth while also developing strategies to prevent delinquency. Early studies found no relationship between genetics and criminality. IJR researchers Shaw and McKay (1942) noted that delinquency was less due to genetic, ethnic, or cultural factors and more due to social disruption, which eroded formal and informal social control in specific transitional neighborhoods (i.e., "delinquency areas") in a city. The research designs at the time were empirical and qualitative rather than quantitative, and much of the IJR's research was biographical. The statistical methodology was very primitive by today's standards, and multivariate influences could not be adequately studied. In this century, research has shown that both sociological and genetic factors are related to lawbreaking in youth (Connolly & Kavish, 2019; Yun et al., 2011).

Unfortunately, the effective century-old habilitative approach to justice-involved youth slowly eroded. The movement from habilitation to retribution was accelerated following the case *In re Gault* (1967). Gerald Gault was a 15-year-old boy adjudicated delinquent by an Arizona juvenile court for making "lewd" phone calls. As a result, he was committed to the Arizona State Industrial School until he turned 21. The maximum penalty Gault would have received if he were an adult was a $50 fine or 2 months in jail. As was typical of juvenile court in those days, he was not afforded counsel or an opportunity to confront or cross-examine his accuser, nor was he offered privilege against self-incrimination. Had he been 18, he would have had substantial constitutional and state statutory rights. After the hearing, although he had no right to appeal to a higher court, Gault's case reached the U.S. Supreme Court, which chided the juvenile court for its pretension of paternalism and blasted the juvenile court model as inadequate to dispense justice.

As a result of the *Gault* decision, justice-involved youth began to be given their Miranda rights and access to counsel. Gradually, the juvenile court moved away from a system of habilitation to one of due process, blurring its distinction from the adult system. The *Gault* decision, combined with public misperceptions of youthful "superpredators" and a perceived upsurge in violent crimes by minors, created pressure to protect society that challenged the habilitation model and favored punishment.

The Juvenile Delinquency Prevention Act of 1968 provided funding to help reduce youthful lawbreaking by emphasizing prevention and rehabilitation. In 1974, the Juvenile Delinquency Prevention Act was replaced by the Juvenile Justice and Delinquency Prevention Act. It is now called the Office of Juvenile Justice and Delinquency Prevention (OJJDP, 2024), which continues to provide guidance for juvenile justice systems and services for justice-involved youth.

The existing juvenile justice system

An American Academy of Pediatrics Committee on Adolescence Policy Statement (Owen et al., 2020) makes it clear that youth in the juvenile system are a high-risk population that has unmet physical, developmental, and mental health needs and that these needs emerge at higher rates than in the general adolescent population. Trauma and adverse childhood experiences also have a significant impact on both the mental and physical well-being of developing youth (Connolly & Kavish, 2019). Justice-involved youth also experience significant barriers such as those related to race and ethnic bias. These concerns have far-reaching effects on families and communities. "Mental, emotional and behavioral disorders among young people burden … juvenile justice systems and, according to one estimate, more than a quarter of total service costs for children who have these disorders are incurred in the school and juvenile justice systems" (National Research Council and Institute of Medicine, 2009, p. 5). Accordingly, mental health practitioners involved with juvenile confinement need to be acutely aware of these realities and take them into consideration to practice health care ethically (McBride & Bell, 2011).

Cases adjudicated delinquent reached a peak in 1997 at 1,855,500 cases, and they have steadily decreased since (Hockenberry, 2023). OJJDP statistics from 2020 show that juvenile courts in the United States handled 508,400 delinquency cases that involved youth charged with criminal law violations: 34.5% were violent offenses, 31.7% were property crimes, and 11.2% were substance related, with the remainder being public order offenses (OJJDP, 2023). Formal probation was the disposition ordered in 66% of cases, and 27% of cases were ordered to residential placement. These dispositional proportions have not significantly changed since 2009. An exception was homicide cases, which increased 47% (OJJDP, 2023). The decline in total cases may be due in part to the use of diversion programs such as mental health courts, drug courts, truancy courts, and others (see Chapter 6).

Justice-involved youth have high rates of mental health disorders (Burke et al., 2015; Cauffman & Grisso, 2005; Illinois Models for Change Behavioral Health Assessment Team, 2010; Owen et al., 2020; Shufelt & Cocozza, 2006; Tamburello et al., 2023; Teplin et al., 2002). The estimated percentage of incarcerated youth with at least one diagnosable mental disorder is between 40% and 80% (Underwood & Washington 2016). According to the National Child Traumatic Stress Network (2024, para. 1), "More than 80% of juvenile justice-involved youth report experiencing trauma, with many having experienced multiple, chronic and pervasive interpersonal traumas." The most prevalent diagnoses among youth in the juvenile justice system are substance use disorders; anxiety disorders; attention-deficit/hyperactivity disorders; mood disorders; trauma-related disorders; and disruptive, impulse control, and conduct disorders. Considering the high rates of trauma, neurodevelopmental disorders, and mental illness in corrections, current science and older wisdom suggest that a strengths-based, prevention approach to the problem should be taken.

The National Commission on Correctional Health Care (2022) Standards for Health Services in Juvenile Detention and Confinement Facilities address the day-to-day physical and mental health care practices for quality care in these facilities. These standards require that all incarcerated youth be screened for physical and mental health problems on admission, including a health assessment within a specific period, with information provided about how to access health care (see Chapter 15). Further, the standards require that regular sick-call services are in place, that correctional staff have first aid and cardiopulmonary resuscitation training, and that the facility can respond to emergency health concerns.

The criminalization of the juvenile justice system has made questions about juvenile competency to stand trial more salient (National Research Council [NRC], 2013). It has become increasingly clear that adolescents are at greater risk for this concern. The MacArthur Foundation's 15-year research endeavor found that about a third of 11- to 13-year-olds and about a fifth of 14- to 15-year-olds were not competent to stand trial when adult criteria are used. Furthermore, age strongly influences one's ability to consider consequences and resist peer pressure, with adolescents being more likely to confess to an authority figure and more willing to accept a plea agreement than adults, regardless of gender or ethnicity (Steinberg, 2003).

A developmental approach to juvenile justice

Since the subjects of the juvenile justice system are children, its overarching goal should be to support the positive social, emotional, and intellectual development of its charges. In turn, this approach would enhance the safety of communities. Other important objectives are to hold youth accountable for wrongdoing and prevent further offending while at the same time treating them fairly and justly. Holding adolescents responsible for behaviors that can lead to crimes ensures accountability and provides justice to victims, though a positive development approach does not conflict with safety (Casey et al., 2020).

The brains of adolescents are still developing. Their flight, fight, or freeze (limbic) systems are fully engaged before their judgment and wisdom (frontal lobe) systems are in place to mediate their behavior (Bell & McBride, 2010). Accordingly, the mechanisms of accountability for justice-involved youth should not mimic adult punishments (NRC, 2013). Condemnation, control, and lengthy confinement are not ordinarily needed to promote positive behavior changes. Juvenile courts should provide an opportunity for youth to accept responsibility for their actions, make amends to victims and the community, and participate in programs that give them a sense of purpose, such as community service (NRC, 2013).

The efficacy of recidivism prevention depends, in part, on how youth are treated while justice involved. Well-organized community-based interventions show greater reductions in rearrests than programs offered in institutional settings, and there is no convincing evidence that confinement of youth beyond 6 months appreciably reduces the likelihood of subsequent offending (NRC, 2013). A few younger individuals are prone to commit serious, chronic, or violent offenses (Department of Health and Human Services, 2001). To identify those at risk for these offenses, courts need to implement risk and needs assessments (Brogan et al., 2015). These tools provide some guidance in determining whether a youth is at a low, medium, or high risk of reoffending based on factors such as prior legal history and school performance. Someone who presents with a high-risk profile can be effectively supported to reduce this risk with evidence-based interventions, community monitoring, or changes in life situation (Lipsey et al., 2010). Further, use of such interventions allows for better targeting of resources, focusing the more intense and costly interventions on those at greater risk of recidivism. Effectively implemented, evidence-based interventions such as the Good Behavior Game (Kellam et al., 2008) or certain psychotherapies such as Aggression Replacement Training and cognitive-behavioral therapy have been shown to reduce reoffending (Desai et al., 2006; Mendel, 2000; Sherman et al., 2006).

Treating youth fairly and with dignity can enhance moral development, legal behavior, and appropriate social control during adolescence. Although the judicial ideal is to have youth represented by properly trained counsel and to have an opportunity to participate in the proceedings, the reality is often different. Attorneys in juvenile courts are often poorly prepared and poorly resourced (OJJDP, 2017). Of course, if racial and ethnic disparities could be addressed, justice-involved youth and their families would feel more inclined to believe in the fairness of the U.S. justice system (Alexander, 2010). Gender-related disparities must also be considered, not only as they relate to boys and girls but also as they relate to gender-nonconforming youth.

Assessment and treatment—best practices

Considering the complexity of the mental, emotional, and behavioral disorders of youth in corrections, there are several best practice approaches to assessment and treatment. First, all juvenile correctional facilities should have procedures for intake health and mental health screening. The Massachusetts Youth Screening Instrument—Second Version (MAYSI-2) is a brief behavioral health screening tool designed especially for juvenile justice programs and facilities. The MAYSI-2 provides scores on seven different areas—alcohol/drug use, angry–irritable, depressed–anxious, somatic complaints, suicide ideation, thought disturbance, and traumatic experiences—and can be used in youth aged 12 to 17 to identify acute or pressing behavioral needs that may need immediate attention. The MAYSI-2 is primarily used in juvenile probation, diversion programs, and intake in juvenile detention or corrections, and it has been validated in juvenile justice settings (Archer et al., 2010; Soulier & McBride, 2016). When assessing justice-involved youth, it is important to include specific screening for neurodevelopmental disorders such as autism spectrum disorder, intellectual disabilities, learning disabilities, fetal alcohol spectrum disorder, and other genetic and medical conditions that may have an impact on behaviors and mental health (Woods et al., 2012).

Screening for suicidal ideation is especially important, though this needs to be an ongoing process (see Chapter 51). Reporting on a national survey on suicides in juvenile facilities, Hayes (2009) found that, unlike in adult corrections, suicide was just as likely to occur later as it was earlier during confinement. Important risk factors for suicide in justice-involved youth include major life events (e.g., a court hearing or a death of a family member), poor social connectedness, impulsivity, and room confinement. Swank and Gagnon (2017) surveyed staff at juvenile correctional facilities and found that only 46% continued to assess for suicidality beyond intake.

Cognitive-behavioral therapy as a means of changing unhealthy ways of thinking, feeling, and behaving is the psychotherapeutic modality best studied in justice-involved youth. Research supports cognitive-behavioral therapy for reducing violence in juvenile detention facilities (Desai et al., 2006). Other psychotherapies have also shown promise. Aggression Replacement Training helps youth improve social skills, moral reasoning, and anger management (Mendel, 2000; Sherman et al., 2006). Life Skills Training is a practice that reduces the risk of substance use and violence by targeting the major social and psychological factors that promote risky behaviors in adolescents (Mackillop et al., 2006).

Medication management in these settings can be complicated. Psychiatrists working with justice-involved youth may find concerns related to incomplete histories, not confirming community medications, limited accessibility of primary caregivers and other collateral informants, lack of informed consent, off-label prescribing, and polypharmacy to be particularly challenging (Tamburello et al., 2023). While research does not support medication to reduce unlawful behavior in youth (Armstrong-Hoskowitz et al., 2020), pharmacotherapy may be indicated for diagnosed disorders (e.g., attention-deficit/hyperactivity disorder; depressive, anxiety, or psychotic disorders; and opioid use disorder), with adequate consideration of risks and benefits, as well as informed consent (American Psychiatric Association, 2022; Shahidullah et al., 2023; Tamburello et al., 2023). Little, if any, research has been done on psychotropic medications specifically involving justice-involved youth as subjects (Desai et al., 2006; Tamburello et al., 2023). Prescribing medication without target symptoms associated with distress or impairment of functioning to justice-involved youth is of unclear benefit (Tamburello et al., 2023). Assessing the patient's motivations for and perceptions about psychotropic medication can be useful for decision-making and to promote adherence (Jensen-Doss et al., 2020).

Proper identification of each individual's needs from a biopsychosocial perspective will allow for better treatment and outcomes. It is also important that staff consider the prevalence and influence of trauma on justice-involved youth. Many facilities are adopting trauma-informed practices to improve engagement, treatment, adherence, and health outcomes (see Chapter 36).

Summary

The population of confined youth is shrinking. Detention and residential facilities have been closing, and administrators are facing decreasing budgets. Nevertheless, the mental health needs of justice-involved youth are prominent and complex. As the knowledge base of these needs continues to increase, so will demand for respectful and effective care of those in custody, as well as appropriate education and training of staff.

As our understanding of youth development becomes more sophisticated and our information technology more interconnected, we will be in a better position to coordinate the services that troubled youth need (e.g., special education, foster care, prosocial programming, and treatment for mental health and substance use disorders). The hope is that community systems can identify early warning signs and intervene before youth become involved in the justice system. Research and centuries of experience have identified risk factors such as trauma, educational difficulties, and family disruptions, among many others. Early identification and sufficient developmental support will make the incarceration of justice-involved youth increasingly rare.

REFERENCES

Addams, J. (2004). *My friend, Julia Lathrop*. University of Illinois Press.

Alexander, M. (2010). *The new Jim Crow*. New Press.

American Psychiatric Association. (2022). *Diagnostic and statistical manual of mental disorders* (5th ed., text rev.).

Archer, R. P., Simonds-Bisbee, E. C., Spiegel, D. R., Handel, R. W., & Elkins, D. E. (2010). Validity of the Massachusetts Youth Screening Instrument-2 (MAYSI-2) scales in juvenile justice settings. *Journal of Personality Assessment*, *92*(4), 337–348.

Armstrong-Hoskowitz, N., Schmidt, A. T., Henderson, C. E., Nelson, D. V., & Allen, B. J. (2020). A field study of the impact of psychotropic medication on delinquency and juvenile justice system involvement among a high-risk sample of children and adolescents. *Journal of Offender Rehabilitation*, *59*(6), 334–353.

Bell, C. C., & McBride, D. F. (2010). Affect regulation and the prevention of risky behaviors. *Journal of the American Medical Association*, *304*(5), 565–566.

Beuttler, F. W., & Bell, C. C. (2010). *For the welfare of every child—A brief history of the Institute for Juvenile Research, 1909–2010*. University of Illinois.

Blackstone, W. (1765). Of the persons capable of committing crimes. In *Commentaries on the Laws of England* (Book 4, Chapter 2). https://lonang.com/library/reference/blackstone-commentaries-law-england/bla-402/

Brogan, L., Haney-Caron, E., NeMoyer, A., & DeMatteo, D. (2015). Applying the risk-needs-responsivity (RNR) model to juvenile justice. *Criminal Justice Review*, *40*(3), 277–302.

Burke, J. D., Mulvey, E. P., & Schubert, C. A. (2015). Prevalence of mental health problems and service use among first-time juvenile offenders. *Journal of Child and Family Studies*, *24*(12), 3774–3781.

Casey, B. J., Taylor-Thompson, K., Rubien-Thomas, E., Robbins, M., & Baskin-Sommers, A. (2020). Healthy development as a human right: Insights from developmental neuroscience for youth justice. *Annual Review of Law and Social Science*, *16*, 203–222.

Cauffman, E., & Grisso, T. (2005). Mental health issues among minority offenders in the juvenile justice system. In D. F. Hawkins & K. Kempf-Leonard (Eds.), *Our children, their children: Confronting racial and ethnic differences in American juvenile justice* (pp. 390–412). University of Chicago Press.

Center on Juvenile and Criminal Justice. (2024). *Juvenile justice history*. https://www.cjcj.org/history-education/juvenile-justice-history.

Connolly, E. J., & Kavish, N. (2019). The causal relationship between childhood adversity and developmental trajectories of delinquency: A consideration of genetic and environmental confounds. *Journal of Youth and Adolescence, 48*(2), 199–211.

Department of Health and Human Services. (2001). *Youth violence: A report of the Surgeon General.* https://www.ojp.gov/ncjrs/virtual-library/abstracts/youth-violence-report-surgeon-general

Desai, R. A., Goulet, J. L., Robbins, J., Chapman, J. F., Migdole, S. J., & Hoge, M. A. (2006). Mental health care in juvenile detention facilities: A review. *Journal of the American Academy of Psychiatry and the Law, 34*(2), 204–214.

Hayes, L. M. (2009). Juvenile suicide in confinement—Findings from the first national survey. *Suicide and Life-Threatening Behavior, 39*(4), 353–462.

Hockenberry, S. (2023). *Delinquency cases in juvenile court, 2020.* https://ojjdp.ojp.gov/publications/delinquency-cases-in-juvenile-court-2020.pdf

Illinois Models for Change Behavioral Health Assessment Team. (2010). *Report on the behavioral health program for youth committed to Illinois' Department of Juvenile Justice.* http://www.modelsforchange.net/publications/271

In re Gault, 387 U.S. 1 (1967).

Jensen-Doss, A., Douglas, S., Phillips, D. A., Gencdur, O., Zalman, A., & Gomez, N. E. (2020). Measurement-based care as a practice improvement tool: Clinical and organizational applications in youth mental health. *Evidence-Based Practice in Child and Adolescent Mental Health, 5*(3), 233–250.

Kellam, S. G., Brown, C. H., Poduska, J. M., et al. (2008). Effects of a universal classroom behavior management program in first and second grades on young adult behavioral, psychiatric, and social outcomes. *Drug and Alcohol Dependence, 95*, S5–S28.

Kopaczewski, J. (2016). *House of Refuge.* https://philadelphiaencyclopedia.org/essays/house-of-refuge/

Lipsey, M. W., Howell, J. C., Kelly, M. R., Chapman, G., & Carver, D. (2010). *Improving the effectiveness of juvenile justice programs: A new perspective on evidence-based practice.* https://www.ojp.gov/ncjrs/virtual-library/abstracts/improving-effectiveness-juvenile-justice-programs-new-perspective

Mackillop, J., Ryabchenko, K. A., & Lisman, S. A. (2006). Life Skills Training outcomes and potential mechanisms in a community implementation: A preliminary investigation. *Substance Use and Misuse, 41*(14), 1921–1935.

McBride, D. F., & Bell, C. C. (2011). Guest editorial: Is denial of evidence-based prevention a violation of human rights? *Journal of the National Medical Association, 103*(7), 618–619.

Mendel, R. A. (2000). *Less hype, more help: Reducing juvenile crime, what works—and what doesn't.* https://files.eric.ed.gov/fulltext/ED445285.pdf

National Child Traumatic Stress Network. (2024). *Essential elements.* https://www.nctsn.org/trauma-informed-care/trauma-informed-systems/justice/essential-elements

National Commission on Correctional Health Care. (2022). *Standards for health services in juvenile detention and confinement facilities.*

National Research Council. (2013). *Reforming juvenile justice: A developmental approach* (R. J. Bonnie, B. M. Chemers, et al., Eds.). https://nap.nationalacademies.org/read/14685

National Research Council and Institute of Medicine. (2009). *Preventing mental, emotional, and behavioral disorders among young people: Progress and possibilities* (M. E. O'Connell, T. Boat, & K. E. Warner, Eds.). https://nap.nationalacademies.org/catalog/12480/preventing-mental-emotional-and-behavioral-disorders-among-young-people-progress

Office of Juvenile Justice and Delinquency Prevention. (2017). *Literature review: A product of the model programs guide—Intersection between mental health and the juvenile justice system.* https://ojjdp.ojp.gov/model-programs-guide/literature- reviews/intsection_between_mental_health_and_the_juvenile_justice_system.pdf

Office of Juvenile Justice and Delinquency Prevention. (2024). *The Juvenile Justice and Delinquency Prevention Act of 1974 chronology.* https://ojjdp.ojp.gov/sites/g/files/xyckuh176/files/media/document/jjdpchronology.pdf

Owen, M. C., Wallace, S. B., Committee on Adolescence, et al. (2020). Advocacy and collaborative health care for justice-involved youth. *Pediatrics, 146*(1), e20201755.

Schowalter, J. E. (2000). Child and adolescent psychiatry comes of age, 1944–1994. In R. W. Menninger & J. C. Nemiah (Eds.), *American psychiatry after World War II, 1944–1994* (pp. 461–480). American Psychiatric Press.

Shahidullah, J. D., Roberts, H., Parkhurst, J., Ballard, R., Mautone, J. A., & Carlson, J. S. (2023). State of the evidence for use of psychotropic medications in school-age youth. *Children (Basel, Switzerland), 10*(9), 1454.

Shaw, C. R., & McKay, H. (1942). *Juvenile delinquency and urban areas.* University of Chicago Press.

Sherman, L. W., Farrington, D. P., MacKenzie, D. L., & Welsh, B. C. (2006). *Evidence-based crime prevention* (rev. ed.). Routledge.

Shufelt, J., & Cocozza, J. (2006). *Youth with mental health disorders in the juvenile justice system: Results from a multi-state prevalence study.* https://www.ojp.gov/ncjrs/virtual-library/abstracts/youth-mental-health-disorders-juvenile-justice-system-results-multi

Soulier, M., & McBride, A. (2016). Mental health screening and assessment of detained youth. *Child and Adolescent Psychiatric Clinics of North America, 25*(1), 27–39.

Steinberg, L. (2003). Juveniles on trial: MacArthur Foundation study calls competency into question. *Criminal Justice, 18*(3), 20–25.

Swank, J. M., & Gagnon, J. C. (2017). A national survey of mental health screening and assessment practices in juvenile correctional facilities. *Child & Youth Care Forum, 46*(3), 379–393.

Tamburello, A., Penn, J., Negron-Muñoz, R., & Kaliebe, K. (2023). Prescribing psychotropic medications for justice-involved juveniles. *Journal of Correctional Health Care: Official Journal of The National Commission on Correctional Health Care, 29*(2), 94–108.

Teplin, L. A., Abram, K. M., McClelland, G. M., et al. (2002). Psychiatric disorders in youth in juvenile detention. *Archives of General Psychiatry, 59*(12), 1133–1143.

Thompson, K. C., & Morris, R. J. (2016). History of the juvenile justice system. In K. C. Thompson & R. J. Morris (Eds.), *Juvenile delinquency and disability* (pp. 55–72). Springer.

Underwood, L. A., & Washington, A. (2016). Mental illness and juvenile offenders. *International Journal of Environmental Research and Public Health, 13*(2), 228.

Woods, G. W., Freedman, D., & Greenspan, S. (2012). Neurobehavioral assessment in forensic practice. *International Journal of Law and Psychiatry, 35*(5–6), 432–439.

Yun, I., Cheong, J., & Walsh, A. (2011). Genetic and environmental influences in delinquent peer affiliation: From the peer network approach. *Youth Violence and Juvenile Justice, 9*(3), 241–258.

60

Aging incarcerated persons

Nicole Mushero and Lisa C. Barry[1]

Introduction

The incarcerated population in the United States is aging rapidly. The prevalence of older incarcerated persons (IPs), defined as aged 55 or older, in U.S. state and federal prisons was approximately 3% in 1993 (Georgoulas-Sherry & Hernandez, 2021). That rose to 20% in 2017, and predictive analyses suggest that by 2030, one third of all IPs in U.S. prisons will be "geriatric" (Bor, 2022; Dayanim et al., 2023; Washington, 2022). Other countries are experiencing similar trends (Australian Bureau of Statistics, n.d.; House of Commons, 2013). Multiple factors contribute to this phenomenon, including harsher minimum sentencing laws, limitations on parole options, a growing number of arrests in later age, and overall population aging (Luallen & Cutler, 2017; Widra, 2023).

IPs experience "accelerated aging" such that their chronological age does not necessarily match their health age. They are more likely to develop medical problems at younger ages than their community counterparts and are considered "geriatric" by age 55, and sometimes earlier (Chiu, 2010; Greene et al., 2018). Accelerated aging is likely caused by life experiences that increase the risk of poor future health (e.g., substance use disorders [SUDs], homelessness, and history of trauma), limited access to health-promoting factors (e.g., poor diet and minimal exercise), limited lifetime access to preventive health care, and chronic stress during incarceration. Consequently, older IPs are, on average, significantly more expensive to care for than younger IPs, and the lack of geriatric expertise in jails and prisons further complicates their care (Garrido & Frakt, 2020; Skarupski et al., 2018). With a higher burden of health needs, limited access to age-specific health care, and shrinking health care budgets, geriatric IPs present a unique challenge to correctional systems (Garrido & Frakt, 2020; Williams et al., 2009).

Aging and life transitions during incarceration

Some older IPs have life sentences ("lifers"), entered prison at an early age, and have aged in place; others have been in and out for repeated convictions over the course of their lives; and still others entered for the first time when already older (Nowotny et al., 2016). Older IPs have fewer visitors and tend to be more isolated than younger IPs (Bond et al., 2005). Lack of social support may be a significant source of anxiety among older IPs returning to the community (Williams et al., 2010) and may be particularly challenging for those incarcerated for the first time, as adapting to the prison environment can be challenging. IPs entering the system for the first time after age 50 are often admitted for serious crimes such as sexual offenses involving minors and are subsequently poised for victimization by peers.

The prospect of dying in prison or having someone in their close network die while in prison may be anxiety producing and can exacerbate older IPs' physical and mental health problems. A 2022 study of men aged 50 or older who had been incarcerated for at least 20 consecutive years found that those who would not be released (i.e., "lifers") had higher rates of functional impairment and suicidal ideation compared with IPs expected to be released (Li et al., 2021).

Medical conditions and disability

Older IPs are more likely to have chronic health conditions and to experience them at earlier ages than their community or younger counterparts, including arthritis, hypertension, chronic obstructive pulmonary disease, hepatitis C, heart disease, and diabetes (Skarupski et al., 2018; Williams et al., 2006). They also experience high rates of geriatric conditions such as hearing impairment (which can result in disciplinary charges when orders from corrections staff are not heard or followed) and incontinence (which can lead to physical confrontations if the resulting unsanitary conditions or odors offend a peer) (Greene et al., 2018). Older IPs also have difficulty completing prison-specific activities of daily living (pADLs) such as getting down to the floor for alarms, climbing on and off a top bunk, and standing in line for medications (Barry et al., 2017; Skarupski et al., 2018; Williams et al., 2006).

1. The authors acknowledge the contributions of Kristin G. Cloyes and Kathryn A. Burns, who were the authors of this chapter in the first edition of this textbook.

Co-occurring mental illness

The prevalence of mental health conditions is considerably higher among IPs compared to the community, regardless of age (Di Lorito et al., 2018; Haesen et al., 2019). Separation from families, limited personal space, risk of violence, loss of social status, loss of physical and social autonomy, and uncertainty about the future predictably result in psychological distress (Bedaso et al., 2020). Compared with younger peers, older IPs have a higher likelihood of previous alcohol use disorders, lower rates of personality disorders, and higher rates of depression (the most common mental health condition in this group). Nearly one third (28.3%) of older IPs have depression, which is almost threefold higher than their community counterparts (Bedaso et al., 2020; Di Lorito et al., 2018). In addition, the prevalence of serious mental illness among older IPs, including psychosis, can be 5 to 10 times higher than in the community (Bedaso et al., 2020; Di Lorito et al., 2018). Mirroring trends seen in older community-dwelling individuals, older IPs have the highest rates of suicide among IPs, with the U.S. Bureau of Justice Statistics indicating a rate of 19 per 100,000 for those over the age of 50 (Carson, 2021).

One study of nearly 11,000 older IPs in the United States found that 70% reported a history of substance misuse. While most used substances for more than 4 decades, over one third never received treatment (Arndt et al., 2002). While younger IPs are more likely to have a history of using cocaine or opioids, their older peers are more likely to have alcohol use disorders (Haesen et al., 2019). SUD rates among IPs are growing most rapidly among those aged 50 and older (Bronson et al., 2017). This trend likely reflects steeper increases in rates of SUDs, SUD-related admissions, and overdose deaths over the past 2 decades experienced by persons in mid- to late life (Mattson et al., 2017). Interactions between SUDs, chronic physical health conditions, mental health disorders, disabilities, cognitive dysfunction, and psychosocial stressors related to aging all complicate assessment and treatment for IPs.

Neurocognitive disorders

Although justice-involved persons are aging rapidly and often experience disease and disability at younger ages, the burden of neurocognitive disorders (i.e., dementia) in this population is largely unknown. A review of international studies found rates of dementia in IPs ranging from 0.8% to 18.8% (Blundell-White et al., 2023). This wide range, at least in part, may be attributed to differences in how dementia was defined and the various screening and diagnostic tools used. The Diagnostic and Statistical Manual of Mental Disorders, fifth edition, text revision (DSM-5-TR; American Psychiatric Association [APA], 2022) defines major neurocognitive disorder as an impairment in one or more cognitive domains that is sufficient to interfere with independence in everyday activities. The diagnosis of mild neurocognitive disorder, corresponding to the DSM-IV-TR diagnosis of mild cognitive impairment (MCI), is made when there is modest impairment in one or more cognitive domains and the individual is still independent in everyday activities (APA, 2022). The Montreal Cognitive Assessment (MoCA), while not a diagnostic measure, is frequently used in clinical settings and research studies to assess cognitive impairment. Several studies have administered the MoCA to older IPs, but the cut-points used as indicators of cognitive impairment, inclusion criteria differences, and differences in functional impairment at similar test scores for White versus Black test takers make it hard to draw conclusions regarding the prevalence of dementia or cognitive impairment (Ahalt et al., 2018; Baillargeon et al., 2023; Washington, 2022). A study of persons aged 55 and older who were incarcerated in one U.S. urban jail system found that 78% scored below the standard cutoff of 26 (out of 30 points), and 49% scored less than 20 (Ahalt et al., 2018).

In prisons, a study of IPs aged 55 and older found that 35% met criteria for MCI with a MoCA threshold score of less than 23, and 9% met criteria for dementia with a MoCA threshold score of less than 18 (Baillargeon et al., 2023). Perez and colleagues (2021) studied male IPs aged 50 and older and applied both education- and race-specific norms to account for social determinants of health and found that 38.5% of participants met criteria for cognitive impairment. Because the percentage of older IPs identifying as non-Hispanic Black is rising twice as fast as older White IPs, and because Black individuals in the community are more likely than White counterparts to develop dementia, it is important to consider how social determinants of health impact cognition (Georgoulas-Sherry & Hernandez, 2021; Washington, 2022; Williams et al., 2021). Depression and suicidal ideation have been found to be correlated with functional disability, as measured by pADLs. Thus, functional assessments related to cognitive impairment should also consider comorbid psychiatric disorders (Barry et al., 2020).

Dementia is associated with an increased likelihood of engaging in law-violating behaviors that could potentially lead to incarceration (Yu et al., 2019). One national study of previously incarcerated U.S. veterans aged 50 and older found that 3.3% had a diagnosis of either dementia or MCI that preceded their most recent incarceration (Kuffel et al., 2022). As dementia becomes more prevalent in the community, more individuals with dementia or MCI may interact with the justice system.

Routine testing for dementia or cognitive impairment is generally not performed in carceral settings; therefore, many living with MCI or dementia in prisons and jails may be undiagnosed. Early stages of cognitive impairment and dementia may be difficult to detect in the structured prison or jail environment because of limited opportunities for IPs to make decisions, make plans, or engage in complex tasks such as using transportation (Brooke & Rybacka, 2020). Unrecognized cognitive impairment can be misinterpreted as behavioral defiance in carceral settings and puts IPs at risk for disciplinary infractions, violence from peers, and being taken advantage of (Washington, 2022).

Mental health assessment

Depression should be routinely assessed using validated tools such as the Patient Health Questionnaire–9 or the Geriatric Depression Scale (GDS). The GDS, for example, is a well-validated screening tool for depression in older persons (Blackburn et al., 2017).

A key area of need is routine assessment of cognitive impairment. While the MoCA is the most widely used and validated screening instrument in the community, it requires certification to use. Other screening tools validated in the community include the Mini Mental State Exam (MMSE), the RUDAS (Rowland Universal Dementia Assessment Scale), and the SLUMS (St. Louis University Mental Status; Ranjit et al., 2020). No cognitive assessment tools have been widely validated in correctional settings, although some early work has been done to close this knowledge gap (Lima Pereira, 2023).

Instruments can be used at periodic intervals to document and monitor for decline over time, and one instrument should be chosen and used consistently. Annual mental health assessments for those over age 50 can be used to document change from baseline, which may provide opportunities for early detection of cognitive difficulties (Washington, 2022; Williams et al., 2012).

Screening for functional disability is recommended, given its importance in navigating day-to-day life while incarcerated. Self-reported functional disability can be assessed using a pADL disability index (Barry et al., 2017; Williams et al., 2006). IPs are asked about six activities: dropping to the floor for alarms, climbing on or off the top bunk, hearing orders from staff, walking while wearing handcuffs, standing in line for medications, and walking to meals. If patients describe these tasks as "very difficult" or "cannot do," they are considered to have a pADL disability (Barry et al., 2017). Further, including laboratory testing to evaluate physical causes of cognitive decline (e.g., thyroid imbalance, infection, hypo- or hyperglycemia, and hypoxia) can be especially important for older adults. Comprehensive assessment may also require neurological consultation and brain imaging.

Medication management

Treatment for mental illness

Depression is common among older IPs, is often treatable, and is important to distinguish from dementia. First-line treatment for depression remains selective serotonin reuptake inhibitor (SSRI) medications because of their overall effectiveness and safety profile. SSRIs with the best safety profile include citalopram, escitalopram, and sertraline. Other medications with favorable safety profiles for older adults include venlafaxine, mirtazapine, and bupropion. Fluoxetine, paroxetine, and fluvoxamine have higher risks of drug–drug interactions and side effects (Avasthi & Grover, 2018; Wiese, 2017).

Starting doses are typically half those of a younger adult, consistent with the adage to "start low and go slow," and maximum doses are often half those of younger adults. Dose adjustments commonly occur over weeks to months. Although it will often take longer to achieve a therapeutic dose, the medication will be better tolerated in the long run. Because of mirtazapine's side effects of somnolence and increased appetite, it can be a good choice for patients reporting insomnia and anorexia. Medications should not be stopped abruptly due the risk of withdrawal (i.e., discontinuation symptoms) but should be titrated off gradually. Hyponatremia is a common side effects of SSRI and serotonin–norepinephrine reuptake inhibitor (SNRI) medications, and sodium levels should be checked about a month after initiation or if a patient develops fatigue, malaise, or delirium (Wiese, 2011).

Antidepressant medications with anticholinergic side effects, like tricyclic antidepressants (TCAs), should be avoided because they cause or increase confusion in older persons, among other serious side effects (Fulone & Lopes, 2017). Treatment response may improve by combining antidepressant medication with cognitive-behavioral therapy, an effective, evidence-based psychotherapy for older persons with depression. Cognitive-behavioral therapy may also be provided as the primary treatment for patients who cannot take medication due to intolerable side effects or when medical contraindications preclude antidepressant use (Thompson et al., 2001). Given that older adults are often prescribed multiple medications to treat comorbidities, psychotropic medication management should be approached in consultation with physical health care providers and a pharmacist to avoid drug–drug interactions.

For patients with a history of serious mental illnesses such as bipolar disorder or schizophrenia, previously effective medications can be continued or restarted. It may, however, be possible to reduce doses because the severity and intensity of symptoms often remit with older age (Horowitz et al., 2021).

Cognitive enhancers

Donepezil, galantamine, and rivastigmine are the most used cholinesterase inhibitors prescribed as first-line medication treatment for people with mild to moderate dementia. Their effect is modest but demonstrated (Birks, 2006). Their most common side effects are gastrointestinal and include nausea, vomiting, and diarrhea. Donepezil and galantamine are often better tolerated than rivastigmine, although rivastigmine comes in a transdermal preparation, which can avoid many of the gastrointestinal side effects (Birks, 2006). Donepezil is also now available in a patch formulation, but its high price makes it cost-prohibitive in many correctional settings.

Memantine, a glutamate antagonist, is approved for use in moderate to severe dementia and is typically prescribed as an adjunct for a cholinesterase inhibitor. Although the demonstrated benefit is modest, memantine is typically well tolerated. Side effects include nausea, dizziness, diarrhea, and agitation (Raina et al., 2008).

Newer therapies are emerging for Alzheimer's disease. Lecanemab is a humanized IgG1 monoclonal antibody that is administered as a 1-hour infusion every 2 weeks, with demonstrated effect in slowing the progression of cognitive decline. It is approved for use in MCI or early-stage dementia (Leqembi, 2023; Van Dyck et al., 2023). However, these medications are likely to be prohibitively expensive and come with serious side-effect profiles, including ARIA, or amyloid-related imaging abnormalities, which may include micro- or macro-hemorrhages, that require frequent monitoring with MRI, another expense and logistical barrier for IPs. Given their limited demonstrated benefit, expense, administration challenges, and safety profile, these medications are unlikely to be adopted in correctional settings anytime soon.

Treatment of behavioral disturbance

Behavioral disturbances are common in dementia and can manifest as psychosis, agitation, mood disorders, disinhibited behavior, or impairment in sleep–wake cycles (Masopust et al., 2018). When these symptoms manifest, a thorough medical review should be undertaken to rule out infection, electrolyte abnormalities, untreated pain, visual or hearing deficits, or other underlying causes. A thorough medication review should be conducted, with tapering or stopping of medications that can cause or exacerbate delirium, such as benzodiazepines or anticholinergics.

There are no medications approved for the treatment of behavioral disturbances and psychotic symptoms in patients with dementia, although these symptoms are common and can often be misinterpreted as willful behavioral issues in IPs. Citalopram, at a maximum of 20 mg, and other well-tolerated SSRIs are often considered first line for agitation because of data supporting their effectiveness, safety profile, and ability to treat comorbid depression (Porsteinsson et al., 2014).

Anticonvulsants, especially valproic acid, are frequently used for behavioral disturbance, although the evidence for effectiveness is limited, while its side-effect burden, particularly at higher doses, can be significant (Baillon et al., 2018). Although not approved for treatment of agitation or psychotic symptoms in patients with dementia, antipsychotics remain commonly used and have some evidence of efficacy. The strongest evidence base is for second-generation antipsychotics such as risperidone and olanzapine. However, side effects of these medications include extrapyramidal symptoms and increased risk of mortality. Thus, they should be prescribed at the lowest possible dose and only if other methods have failed.

Environmental and systems-level interventions

In jails and prisons, lack of infrastructure, staff shortages, and staffing models often do not meet the growing demand for geriatric care (Ahalt et al., 2013). Typical correctional practices related to housing, movement, meals, and daily schedules also introduce barriers for effective care and other risks for older IPs, including the risk of victimization (Washington, 2022). Environment-related dysfunction may occur secondary to lack of adaptive equipment or the inability to accommodate changing physical needs.

Long-term care units

A growing number of reports and position papers have called attention to the problematic nature of housing older, frail, medically or cognitively impaired people in jails and prisons (Bor, 2022; Kodama et al., 2023). Most states and the federal system have a compassionate release process for these types of individuals. Compassionate release is frequently underutilized despite growing calls to increase the number of IPs released due to medical needs (Kanbergs et al., 2023; Mitchell & Williams, 2017). Even if compassionate releases increase, community settings like skilled nursing facilities are often hesitant to accept formerly incarcerated people (Dayanim et al., 2023). The number of IPs meeting preadmission criteria for requiring skilled nursing facility–level care has continued, and likely will continue, to increase. Approaches to accommodate long-term care needs have included establishing separate facilities within prisons, building prison facilities specifically to house older adults with dementia, and releasing them to a department of corrections–partnered skilled nursing facility (Engelhart, 2023; Marchant, 2022). However, this type of care requires increased staffing, policies adapted for more flexibility in daily structure (e.g., time allowed for movement, meals, or daily hygiene), and peer volunteer programs to provide direct care, support, and protection (Mara, 2002; Williams et al., 2012). As the need for these types of specialized units or facilities increases, systems must decide whether to expand or greatly modify current accommodations, create a continuum of care, or further refer these individuals to outside institutions. These decisions must often be made in the context of shrinking budgets and aging carceral facilities.

Palliative and end-of-life care

Many IPs will die in prisons, creating a need for palliative and end-of-life care (Linder & Meyers, 2007). Current programs are a mix of formal and informal, with many prison systems using peers as hospice volunteers. Facilities' physical environments and conflicting priorities between care and custody can present barriers to this care (McParland et al., 2023; McParland & Johnston, 2019). While allowing and fostering close relationships, particularly with family members and peers, facilitates good palliative and end-of-life care, this may conflict with safety priorities. Compassionate release also facilitates access to palliative and end-of-life care, and prison health care staff can help to enable that process (McParland et al., 2023). Currently, standards of excellence in prison-based palliative and end-of-life care are lacking, though access to consistently implemented, specialist palliative care services is widely recognized as important (Schaefer et al., 2023).

Adaptive equipment, practices, and policies

Access to adaptive equipment and environmental changes are needed for older IPs. Examples include modified bed and commode height and installing handrails in hallways and showers. Centralized medication administration and sick calls may help to accommodate those with less mobility. IPs will need adequate access to mobility devices like canes, walkers, and wheelchairs, with policies and staffing levels sufficient to accommodate these.

Training for staff

Little, if any, corrections-specific training for geriatric management exists. Training adapted from community educational resources must include discussion of changes in functional health status and how underlying disease processes may affect behavior, especially as it relates to interactions with custodial staff (Aday & Krabill, 2013). Design and implementation of new programs or units, adaptation of existing norms, development of related policies, and delivery of specialized training all require balancing both sides of the custody-versus-care dynamic within which services are provided.

Summary

Given the increased physical and mental health needs of older IPs, optimizing their health care should be evidence based and consider their unique needs and vulnerabilities (Ahalt et al., 2013; Washington, 2022; Williams et al., 2021). Most current correctional environments require improvements in health care resources, physical plant features, equipment, staffing, and training to meet the needs of aging IPs. As the number of older IPs increases, shortcomings in these regards will become increasingly problematic. More research is needed, along with the dissemination of best practice models specific to geriatric care in the correctional context.

REFERENCES

Aday, R. H., & Krabill, J. J. (2013). Older and geriatric offenders: Critical issues for the 21st century. In L. Gideon (Ed.), *Special needs offenders in correctional institutions* (pp. 203–232). Sage Publications.

Ahalt, C., Stijacic-Cenzer, I., Miller, B. L., Rosen, H. J., Barnes, D. E., & Williams, B. A. (2018). Cognition and incarceration: Cognitive impairment and its associated outcomes in older adults in jail. *Journal of the American Geriatrics Society*, *66*(11), 2065–2071.

Ahalt, C., Trestman, R. L., Rich, J. D., Greifinger, R. B., & Williams, B. A. (2013). Paying the price: The pressing need for quality, cost, and outcomes data to improve correctional health care for older prisoners. *Journal of the American Geriatrics Society*, *61*(11), 2013–2019.

American Psychiatric Association. (2022). *Diagnostic and statistical manual of mental disorders* (5th ed., text rev.).

Arndt, S., Turvey, C. L., & Flaum, M. (2002). Older offenders, substance abuse, and treatment. *American Journal of Geriatric Psychiatry, 10*(6), 733–739.

Australian Bureau of Statistics. (n.d.). *Prisoners in Australia, 2023.* https://www.abs.gov.au/statistics/people/crime-and-justice/prisoners-australia.

Avasthi, A., & Grover, S. (2018). Clinical practice guidelines for management of depression in elderly. *Indian Journal of Psychiatry, 60*(Suppl. 3), S341–S362.

Baillargeon, J., Linthicum, L. C., Murray, O. J., et al. (2023). The prevalence of cognitive impairment and dementia in incarcerated older adults. *Journals of Gerontology: Series B, 78*(12), 2141–2146.

Baillon, S. F., Narayana, U., Luxenberg, J. S., & Clifton, A. V. (2018). Valproate preparations for agitation in dementia. *Cochrane Database of Systematic Reviews, 10*(10), CD003945.

Barry, L. C., Coman, E., Wakefield, D., Trestman, R. L., Conwell, Y., & Steffens, D. C. (2020). Functional disability, depression, and suicidal ideation in older prisoners. *Journal of Affective Disorders, 266*, 366–373.

Barry, L. C., Wakefield, D. B., Trestman, R. L., & Conwell, Y. (2017). Disability in prison activities of daily living and likelihood of depression and suicidal ideation in older prisoners. *International Journal of Geriatric Psychiatry, 32*(10), 1141–1149.

Bedaso, A., Ayalew, M., Mekonnen, N., & Duko, B. (2020). Global estimates of the prevalence of depression among prisoners: A systematic review and meta-analysis. *Depression Research and Treatment, 2020*, 3695209.

Birks, J. S. (2006). Cholinesterase inhibitors for Alzheimer's disease. *Cochrane Database of Systematic Reviews, 2006*(1), CD005593.

Blackburn, P., Wilkins-Ho, M., & Wiese, B. S. (2017). Depression in older adults: Diagnosis and management. *British Columbia Medical Journal, 59*(3), 171–177.

Blundell-White, V., Harrison, J., & Hill, J. E. (2023). Dementia and the prison population: Identifying need. *British Journal of Neuroscience Nursing, 19*(5), 178.

Bond, G. D., Thompson, L. A., & Malloy, D. M. (2005). Lifespan differences in the social networks of prison inmates. *International Journal of Aging and Human Development, 61*(3), 161–178.

Bor, J. S. (2022). The aging of the US prison population: A public health crisis. *Health Affairs, 41*(5), 622–627.

Bronson, J., Stroop, J., Zimmer, S., & Berzofsky, M. (2017). *Drug use, dependence, and abuse among state prisoners and jail inmates, 2007–2009.* https://bjs.ojp.gov/library/publications/drug-use-dependence-and-abuse-among-state-prisoners-and-jail-inmates-2007-2009

Brooke, J., & Rybacka, M. (2020). Development of a dementia education workshop for prison staff, prisoners, and health and social care professionals to enable them to support prisoners with dementia. *Journal of Correctional Health Care, 26*(2), 159–167.

Carson, E. A. (2021). *Suicide in local jails and state and federal prisons, 2000–2019.* https://bjs.ojp.gov/sites/g/files/xyckuh236/files/media/document/sljsfp0019st.pdf

Chiu, T. (2010). *It's about time: Aging prisoners, increasing costs and geriatric release.* https://www.vera.org/publications/its-about-time-aging-prisoners-increasing-costs-and-geriatric-release

Dayanim, G., Mushero, N., & Berk, J. (2023). *Access to long-term nursing care for justice-involved elderly.* Health Affairs Forefront. https://www.healthaffairs.org/content/forefront/access-long-term-nursing-care-justice-involved-elderly

Di Lorito, C., Völlm, B., & Dening, T. (2018). Psychiatric disorders among older prisoners: A systematic review and comparison study against older people in the community. *Aging & Mental Health, 22*(1), 1–10.

Engelhart, K. (2023, August 11). I've reported on dementia for years, and one image of a prisoner keeps haunting me. *The New York Times.* https://www.nytimes.com/2023/08/11/opinion/dementia-prisons.html

Fulone, I., & Lopes, L. C. (2017). Potentially inappropriate prescriptions for elderly people taking antidepressant: Comparative tools. *BMC Geriatrics, 17*(1), 278.

Garrido, M., & Frakt, A. B. (2020). Challenges of aging population are intensified in prison. *JAMA Health Forum, 1*(2), e200170.

Georgoulas-Sherry, V., & Hernandez, H. G. (2021). The aging incarcerated population: Evaluating two decades of upward trends. *Current Research in Psychology and Behavioral Science, 2*, 1031.

Greene, M., Ahalt, C., Stijacic-Cenzer, I., Metzger, L., & Williams, B. (2018). Older adults in jail: High rates and early onset of geriatric conditions. *Health & Justice, 6*(1), 1–9.

Haesen, S., Merkt, H., Imber, A., Elger, B., & Wangmo, T. (2019). Substance use and other mental health disorders among older prisoners. *International Journal of Law and Psychiatry, 62*, 20–31.

Horowitz, M. A., Murray, R. M., & Taylor, D. (2021). Tapering antipsychotic treatment. *JAMA Psychiatry, 78*(2), 125–126.

House of Commons. (2013). *Justice Committee—Fifth report: Older prisoners.* https://publications.parliament.uk/pa/cm201314/cmselect/cmjust/89/8902.htm

Kanbergs, A., Garcia-Grossman, I., Ahalt, C., DiTomas, M., Bedard, R., & Williams, B. (2023). A stepwise guide for healthcare professionals requesting compassionate release for patients who are incarcerated. *International Journal of Prisoner Health, 19*(1), 77–87.

Kodama, L., Williams, B., & Morris, N. P. (2023). Prioritizing diversion and decarceration of people with dementia. *AMA Journal of Ethics, 25*(10), 783–790.

Kuffel, R. L., Byers, A. L., Williams, B., et al. (2022). Prevalence of dementia and mild cognitive impairment before incarceration. *Journal of the American Geriatrics Society, 70*(6), 1792–1799.

Leqembi. (2023). *Prescribing information.* https://www.leqembi.com/-/media/Files/Leqembi/Prescribing-Information.pdf

Li, A., Williams, B., & Barry, L. C. (2021). Mental and physical health of older incarcerated persons who have aged in place in prison. *Journal of Applied Gerontology, 41*(4), 1101–1110.

Lima Pereira, V., Freitas, S., Simões, M. R., & Gerardo, B. (2023). Montreal Cognitive Assessment (MoCA): A validation study among prisoners. *Criminal Behaviour and Mental Health: CBMH, 33*(5), 330–341.

Linder, J. F., & Meyers, F. J. (2007). Palliative care for prison inmates: "Don't let me die in prison." *JAMA, 298*(8), 894–901.

Luallen, J., & Cutler, C. (2017). Growth of older inmate populations: How population aging explains rising age at admission. *Journals of Gerontology Series B: Psychological Sciences and Social Sciences, 72*(5), 888–900.

Mara, C. M. (2002). Expansion of long-term care in the prison system. *Journal of Aging & Social Policy, 14*(2), 43–61.

Marchant, R. (2022, March 21). Longest-serving CT prisoner, now 97, released 72 years after Greenwich yacht club murder. *Greenwich Time.* https://www.greenwichtime.com/news/article/Francis-Smith-longest-serving-prisoner-released-17017465.php

Masopust, J., Protopopová, D., Vališ, M., Pavelek, Z., & Klímová, B. (2018). Treatment of behavioral and psychological symptoms of dementias with psychopharmaceuticals: A review. *Neuropsychiatric Disease and Treatment, 14*, 1211–1220.

Mattson, M., Lipari, R., Hays, C., & Van Horn, S. (2017). *A day in the life of older adults: Substance use facts.* https://www.samhsa.gov/data/sites/default/files/report_2792/ShortReport-2792.html

McParland, C., & Johnston, B. M. (2019). Palliative and end of life care in prisons: A mixed-methods rapid review of the literature from 2014–2018. *BMJ Open*, *9*(12), e033905.

McParland, C., Johnston, B., & Ouwehand, I. E. I. (2023). Caring for people in prison with palliative and end-of-life care needs. *Current Opinion in Supportive and Palliative Care*, *17*(3), 224–230.

Mitchell, A., & Williams, B. (2017). Compassionate release policy reform: Physicians as advocates for human dignity. *AMA Journal of Ethics*, *19*(9), 854–861.

Nowotny, K. M., Cepeda, A., James-Hawkins, L., & Boardman, J. D. (2016). Growing old behind bars: Health profiles of the older male inmate population in the United States. *Journal of Aging and Health*, *28*(6), 935–956.

Perez, A., Manning, K. J., Powell, W., & Barry, L. C. (2021). Cognitive impairment in older incarcerated males: Education and race considerations. *American Journal of Geriatric Psychiatry*, *29*(10), 1062–1073.

Porsteinsson, A. P., Drye, L. T., Pollock, B. G., et al. (2014). Effect of citalopram on agitation in Alzheimer's disease: The CitAD randomized controlled trial. *JAMA*, *311*(7), 682–691.

Raina, P., Santaguida, P., Ismaila, A., et al. (2008). Effectiveness of cholinesterase inhibitors and memantine for treating dementia: Evidence review for a clinical practice guideline. *Annals of Internal Medicine*, *148*(5), 379–397.

Ranjit, E., Sapra, A., Bhandari, P., Albers, C. E., & Ajmeri, M. S. (2020). Cognitive assessment of geriatric patients in primary care settings. *Cureus*, *12*, e10443.

Schaefer, I., Heneka, N., DiGiacomo, M., Panozzo, S., & Phillips, J. L. (2023). The importance of developing palliative care quality indicators for the prison setting: Why now, and next steps. *BMC Palliative Care*, *22*, 69.

Skarupski, K. A., Gross, A., Schrack, J. A., Deal, J. A., & Eber, G. B. (2018). The health of America's aging prison population. *Epidemiologic Reviews*, *40*(1), 157–165.

Thompson, L. W., Coon, D. W., Gallagher-Thompson, D., Sommer, B. R., & Koin, D. (2001). Comparison of desipramine and cognitive/behavioral therapy in the treatment of elderly outpatients with mild-to-moderate depression. *American Journal of Geriatric Psychiatry*, *9*(3), 225–240.

Van Dyck, C. H., Swanson, C. J., Aisen, P., et al. (2023). Lecanemab in early Alzheimer's Disease. *New England Journal of Medicine*, *388*(1), 9–21.

Washington, L. (2022). Dementia and the aging population: Cognitive screening within correctional health. *International Journal of Prisoner Health*, *19*, 63–76.

Widra, E. (2023). *The aging prison population: Causes, costs, and consequences*. Prison Policy Initiative. https://www.prisonpolicy.org/blog/2023/08/02/aging/.

Wiese, B. S. (2011). Geriatric depression: The use of antidepressants in the Elderly. *British Columbia Medical Journal*, *53*(47), 341–347.

Williams, B., DiTomas, M., & Pachynski, A. (2021). The growing geriatric prison population: A dire public health consequence of mass incarceration. *Journal of the American Geriatrics Society*, *69*(12), 3407–3409.

Williams, B. A., Lindquist, K., Hill, T., et al. (2009). Caregiving behind bars: Correctional officer reports of disability in geriatric prisoners. *Journal of the American Geriatrics Society*, *57*(7), 1286–1292.

Williams, B. A., Lindquist, K., Sudore, R. L., Strupp, H. M., Willmott, D. J., & Walter, L. C. (2006). Being old and doing time: Functional impairment and adverse experiences of geriatric female prisoners. *Journal of the American Geriatrics Society*, *54*(4), 702–707.

Williams, B. A., McGuire, J., Lindsay, R. G., et al. (2010). Coming home: Health status and homelessness risk of older pre-release prisoners. *Journal of General Internal Medicine*, *25*(10), 1038–1044.

Williams, B. A., Stern, M. F., Mellow, J., Safer, M., & Greifinger, R. B. (2012). Aging in correctional custody: Setting a policy agenda for older prisoner health care. *American Journal of Public Health*, *102*(8), 1475–1481.

Yu, R., Topiwala, A., Jacoby, R., & Fazel, S. (2019) Aggressive behaviors in Alzheimer disease and mild cognitive impairment: Systematic review and meta-analysis. *American Journal of Geriatric Psychiatry*, *27*(3), 290–300.

61

Incarcerated veterans

James F. DeGroot, Sarah Shelton, John Penezic, and Savannah Shaw

Introduction

The field of correctional psychiatry had continued to grow as rates of incarceration rose for 40 years. This trend was interrupted by the onset of the COVID-19 global pandemic in 2020, which caused incarceration rates to decline and ultimately reach their lowest level in 25 years. However, as the world started to return to its prepandemic state, so did the criminal justice system, with rates of incarceration rising again in 2022. Significant subgroups within incarcerated populations formed, including an increasing number of veterans with issues specific to military service. The correctional landscape was transformed from a somewhat homogeneous group to a more heterogeneous group of many traumatized men, women, and adolescents. Due in part to civil rights litigation, correctional budgets ballooned to pay not only for correction's core mission of security but also for required medical and mental health care services (see Chapters 3 and 11).

Several subspecialties emerged because of this expansion, even in the wake of the COVID-19 pandemic. One of these subspecialties is the provision of mental health services to incarcerated veterans. The success of mental health care with this population depends on understanding where these traumatized veterans "come from and are going to," as well as recognizing that military and correctional cultures have distinct languages, laws, and ethical standards. For example, providers should realize that both military and correctional cultures are dominated by men who value physical strength, independence, and courage while devaluing cowardice, dependence, and help-seeking behavior. Both worlds also value the ability to defend oneself and devalue violence against women and children. Nonveteran incarcerated persons (IPs) tend to be undisciplined and stigmatized, while military IPs tend to be disciplined and admired.

Historically, the correctional and military worlds rarely interacted except during times of war, when some military veterans were convicted of felonies and incarcerated. These veterans "fall from grace" and become disenfranchised IPs who struggle to explain their behavior. Society also struggles with the ambivalence of wanting to punish and rescue them simultaneously, and mental health providers struggle with their own emotional responses as they treat these distressed individuals.

To help mental health care providers meet their personal and professional challenges in working with this complex population, an informational roadmap is presented in this chapter to navigate difficult terrain. The goal in using this map is to help providers avoid potholes (i.e., burnout, cynicism, and malevolence) and head-on collisions with prison leadership and/or incarcerated veterans, resulting in a loss of credibility.

Incarcerated veteran trends and demographics

Population trends

A review of data from the Bureau of Justice Statistics (BJS) revealed that the percentage of IPs who were veterans increased during and after the Vietnam War (1955–1975) until 1978, when it peaked at 24%. During the next 40 years, it steadily declined to 20% in 1985, 10% in 2004, and 7% in 2016. In 1985, 1,971 veterans were incarcerated per 100,000 veteran residents (BJS, 2000). In 1998, the number of incarcerated veterans declined to 937, and in 2004, it fell to 630 (BJS, 2007). Although veterans never seemed to be overrepresented in the criminal justice system, Vietnam veteran trendlines suggested the presence of a gap between time of military discharge and time of incarceration. These trendlines were concerning because, with more than 2 million personnel having served in Iraq (2003–2011) and Afghanistan (2001–2021), the number of incarcerated veterans was expected to rise unless community resources were increased (U.S. Institute for Veteran Policy, 2011). Surprisingly, 12 years after the war in Iraq, and during the 20-year war in Afghanistan, the number of incarcerated veterans continued to decline rather than rise, likely due to increased veterans' services.

Incarcerated veteran data from the Georgia Department of Corrections (GDC) mirrored national trends, revealing a decline in incarcerated veterans from 3,569 in December 2013 (GDC, 2014a) to 2,100 in December 2023 (GDC, 2024a) due to several initiatives (e.g., criminal justice reform, diversion programs, U.S. Department of Veterans Affairs (VA) programs for justice-involved veterans, and specialty courts such as veterans, mental health, and drug courts). During the 10 years between 2013 and 2023, the GDC's total census fell from 54,148 IPs (GDC, 2014b) to 50,674 (GDC, 2024b), a decrease of 6.8%, while its veteran census decreased by a dramatic 39.1%.

That said, the number of veterans in the GDC and several other studies may be an underestimation of the actual number of incarcerated veterans. In the studies, it was difficult to identify veterans because many did not believe they were veterans unless they served in combat. Others denied having been in the military because they did not want to lose their service-connected disability checks. Some did not want their families to lose their benefits while they were in prison, and some were embarrassed by their situation.

Demographics

The demographics of incarcerated veterans differ from those of the general incarcerated population in several ways. For example, the average male veteran was 52 years old in state prison (14 years older than nonveterans) and 51 years old in federal prison (11 years older than nonveterans). In state prison, half of the male veterans were White, 27% were Black, and 11% were Hispanic, while 27% of the male nonveterans were White, 37% were Black, and 26% were Hispanic (BJS, 2015). Male veterans in state prison were twice as likely as male nonveterans in state prison to be serving time for a violent sexual offense (26% and 12%, respectively). Among federally incarcerated populations, 7% of male veterans and 1% of male nonveterans were serving time for a violent sex offense. In state prisons, male veterans were less likely to be serving time for a property or drug offense than male nonveterans (9% and 15%, respectively). Additionally, federally incarcerated male veterans had an average sentence length of approximately 14 years, while nonveterans had an average sentence length of 12 years. In state prison, male veterans were almost twice as likely as male nonveterans to receive a life or death sentence (24% and 13%, respectively). Male veterans in state and federal prisons were also more likely to have no prior incarcerations (35% and 44%, respectively) than male nonveterans in state or federal prisons (19% and 28%, respectively; BJS, 2021).

Intimate partner violence was a common problem among veterans, especially those who had been deployed for an extended period and were having difficulty reintegrating into their family. Data revealed that four in 10 veterans felt as if they were "a guest in their own home." One in four believed their children were afraid of them, while three in five disagreed with their spouse about their family responsibilities and believed their marital relationship was in trouble. The number of veterans convicted of assaulting women was significantly higher than nonveterans: 60% and 41%, respectively (BJS, 2004). Likewise, veterans were convicted at a higher rate than nonveterans for assaulting minors (40% and 24%, respectively) and for sex crimes (23% and 9%, respectively; Substance Abuse and Mental Health Services Administration, 2013).

Veterans in prisons and jails were likely to report having been told they had posttraumatic stress disorder (PTSD). Approximately 48% of veterans and 36% of nonveterans in prison were told they had a mental disorder. Veterans in prison were twice as likely as nonveterans to report that a mental health professional told them they had PTSD (23% and 11%, respectively). Incarcerated combat veterans were more likely than noncombat veterans to have been told they had a mental disorder (60% and 44%, respectively). The most common disorder for veterans and nonveterans was a major depressive disorder (34% and 30%, respectively). The proportion of veterans in jail who were told they had PTSD was twice as high as nonveterans (31% and 15%, respectively; BJS, 2015).

Prevalence and impact of trauma and stress

Prevalence of trauma

Trauma is a common phenomenon, with 87% of veterans reporting exposure to at least one potentially traumatic event (Wisco et al., 2014). Traumas differ in that they may be experienced directly, indirectly, or vicariously. People's vulnerability to trauma and the expression of their distress is variable. Vulnerability to trauma-based disorders varies as a function of risk and protective factors, the intensity of the trauma, and its duration. Risk factors include prior trauma, mental health problems, little support from family and friends, the recent loss of a loved one, recent stressful life changes, a history of alcohol and/or drug misuse, limited education, and older age. Protective factors include the absence of early life-threatening events, an optimistic outlook on life, resourcefulness, and a strong social support network (Clark, 2013). Expressions of distress include internalizing symptoms such as anxiety, dysphoria, and isolating behavior and externalizing symptoms such as disinhibition, anger, and aggressive/impulsive behavior. Most people who experience trauma and become symptomatic do not develop PTSD. The National Comorbidity Survey Replication revealed that 7 to 8% of the population will develop PTSD at some point in their lives. Approximately 10% of the female population, in comparison to 5% of the male population, develops PTSD, often accompanied by depression, substance misuse, emotional dysregulation, and behavioral problems (Kessler et al., 2005).

The prevalence of trauma among IPs in U.S. jails, state prisons, and federal prisons is high. The BJS (1999) reported that 19% of IPs in state prisons, 10% of IPs in federal prisons, and 16% of IPs in local jails report a history of physical and/or sexual abuse. Histories of childhood abuse are more common among incarcerated men and women than in the community. More than half of male IPs (56%) reported a history of childhood physical trauma (Wolff & Shi, 2012). The BJS (2006) reported that 5% to 8% of adult men and 12% to 17% of adult women in the community reported a history of childhood abuse; in prison, 6% to 14% of adult men and 23% to 37% of adult women reported a history of childhood abuse. A review of the GDC's database during a class action lawsuit (*Cason v. Seckinger*, 1984), which included allegations of sexual misconduct, revealed that IPs with mental illness had a much higher incidence of childhood abuse than IPs who were not receiving mental health services. The database also revealed that the incidence of abuse increased with the severity of mental illness for both men and women.

Active-duty military personnel and veterans are at increased risk of developing posttraumatic stress symptoms and PTSD because of wartime stressors and sexual misconduct (Litz & Schlenger, 2009; Wood, 2012a). The VA estimated that 29% of veterans of the Iraq and Afghanistan wars developed PTSD, similar to the 30% of Vietnam veterans who developed PTSD (National Center for PTSD, Veterans Affairs, 2024). Among Iraq and Afghanistan veterans, PTSD is often linked to traumatic brain injury caused by blast waves from explosions (NIH Medline Plus, 2009). The VA also noted that among veterans using VA health care, 23% and 55% of the women reported being sexually assaulted or harassed, respectively, while on active duty. Additionally, 38% of the men experienced sexual harassment while on active duty (New York State Office of Mental Health, 2008).

Impact of trauma

Research on adverse childhood experiences (ACEs) was conducted by the Centers for Disease Control and Prevention (CDC) in collaboration with Kaiser Permanente. Over a 10-year period, 17,421 people were screened to identify the effects of ACEs (trauma) over the lifespan. The adverse experiences consisted of five household categories (substance abuse, divorce, mental illness, domestic violence, and criminal behavior), three abuse categories (emotional, physical, and sexual), and two neglect categories (emotional and physical). The results revealed that as the number of adverse events increases, the probability of medical, emotional, behavioral, interpersonal, educational, and arousal problems also increases (CDC, 2013).

The impact of these ACEs is reflected in subsequent risk of attempting suicide. The ACE study discovered that 1% of people who have no ACEs attempt suicide, 10% of people who have three ACEs attempt suicide, and 20% of people who have seven ACEs attempt suicide (CDC, 2008). The impact of trauma on veterans may be similarly illustrated (Wood, 2012b; Wortzel et al., 2009). During 2020, there were an average of 16.8 military veteran suicides per day, a rate that was 57.3% greater than that for nonveteran U.S. adults (U.S. Department of Veterans Affairs, 2022). The number of attempted and completed suicides is higher in jails and prisons than in the community, which should come as no surprise, given the high incidence of trauma among IPs (BJS, 2005).

Challenges and strategies in the provision of services to incarcerated veterans

Challenges

Reducing the number of IPs remains among the primary challenges facing the criminal justice system. Criminal justice reinvestment and justice reform initiatives focus on diverting and releasing nonviolent individuals who could receive more cost-effective treatment in the community (see Chapter 6). Examples of such initiatives include mental health courts and drug courts. Initiatives for veterans include veterans treatment courts, which divert nonviolent veterans from incarceration to community-based mental health programs, and substance use disorder (SUD) programs in a judicially supervised court setting. As of 2018, there were more than 400 veterans treatment courts nationwide that have diverted more than 7,000 veterans to community-based treatment (Tsai et al., 2018). While there is substantial variability in policy and practice, which makes comparison between the programs difficult (Douds et al., 2017), there is promise in the findings. Some estimates indicate recidivism rates as low as 2.5% (McCall et al., 2018). Other diversion programs include day reporting centers and integrated treatment facilities that were created for probationers who are on the verge of having their probation revoked. Veterans treatment courts, primarily used to divert nonviolent combat veterans from prison, have continued to grow over the past decade. Between fiscal years 2019 and 2023, more than 20 states were able to secure grant funding through the Veterans Treatment Court Coordination Act of 2019 (Bureau of Justice Assistance, 2024).

Over the last 30 years, treatment programs have been developed for IPs with mental illness and SUD whose crimes are related to their illness. Programs for incarcerated veterans with trauma histories are also being developed. Several federal, state, and local correctional facilities created veterans dorms/units where combat and noncombat veterans can experience camaraderie and structured daily programs that help them adapt and prepare to reenter the community. Some of these programs, such as one in Muscogee County Jail—just a few miles away from Fort Moore (previously Fort Benning)—worked closely with the community to connect convicted veterans with services such as the VA, Community Service Board, Alcoholics Anonymous, and supportive housing and employment agencies (Correctional News, 2012). Similarly, the GDC was actively involved in developing and maintaining diversion and reentry programs prior to the COVID-19 pandemic. The previously collected data revealed that a higher percentage of veterans received mental health services than nonveterans (i.e., 19.2% and 15.5% for men and 52.1% and 48.7% for women, respectively). It also revealed that male veterans were more often diagnosed with PTSD than nonveterans; however, incarcerated female veterans were less likely to be diagnosed with PTSD than nonveterans. Additionally, veterans were more likely to have comorbid diagnoses, including SUD, major depressive disorder, and personality disorder.

Many treatment programs met with early termination or were unable to adapt to telehealth during the COVID-19 pandemic. The CDC gave broad guidance against in-person treatment during the COVID-19 pandemic, which continued through 2021 and later in some locations (Galietti et al., 2021). Programs within the GDC were scaled back or terminated. Veterans dorms and clubs within the Kentucky Department of Corrections ceased, as did many nonveteran-related social organizations, to minimize disease transmission. Concurrently, staffing challenges became barriers to restarting programs. For instance, the Kentucky Correctional Psychiatric Treatment Unit had no remaining staff from prior to the COVID-19 pandemic to reincorporate their previous programs, despite data suggesting that they were vital for veterans' reintegration into the community.

Correctional facilities will benefit from these models as they reconstitute services and expand offerings to incarcerated veterans with mental health and SUD recovery needs. The New York Department of Corrections and Community Supervision offers a multitier, comprehensive service model within the correctional setting (New York Department of Corrections and Community Supervision, 2020). The model provides services for veterans across three progressive levels of need. Level I services are provided at all state facilities and include access to records such as copies of the IP's military record and appropriate referrals through the VA for ongoing treatment, education, housing, and employment. A facility veterans liaison is available to assist with readjustment and reentry needs. Level II services, at select facilities, offer veterans inmate organizations or veterans education groups to facilitate education, camaraderie, and support. These facilities may host special events and incorporate local community groups such as Veterans of Foreign Wars or American Legion posts. In addition, these facilities provide curriculum-based programming opportunities that are designed for peer-to-peer facilitation. Level III services, strategically located throughout the state, are designed to provide optimal services to meet veterans' needs. Veteran residential therapeutic programs are 6-month treatment programs to address readjustment issues, including substance use, anger and aggression management, PTSD treatment, and personal enhancement.

Mental health evaluation and diagnosis within correctional settings remain challenging for several reasons. Studies indicate a high prevalence of mental health problems among prison populations (Fazel & Danesh, 2002; see Chapter 31). While many psychological assessment instruments have been developed and tested in community settings, most have not been well studied in correctional settings (Megargee, 2012; see Chapter 67). More research is needed for this population, especially in terms of personality, ability, and educational measures. Some instruments, such as performance validity measures, may recommend more conservative cutoff scores to account for issues unique to psycho-legal cases (Wisdom et al., 2010). The evaluation and diagnosis of veterans are further complicated in that the clinician may need to distinguish emotional symptoms from those of traumatic brain injury, personality disorder, other comorbid disorders, and cultural factors distinct to veterans. For example, many clinicians may overdiagnose PTSD when evaluating combat veterans who have multiple "military" risk factors, while underdiagnosing noncombat veterans due to having few risk factors. It is paramount for clinicians to maintain objectivity in diagnosing veterans with PTSD and not overemphasize "military" risk factors, direct exposure to combat, or externalizing symptoms while minimizing indirect exposure to combat and internalizing symptoms.

Strategies

Many strategies exist to address the treatment needs of veterans with trauma or other mental health disorders. States may elect to implement specialty treatment programs like the New York Department of Corrections and Community Supervision multitier strategy, or they may continue to treat veterans while they are integrated with the general population. Veterans tend to prefer treatment that is more frequent, intense, and delivered by clinicians who are themselves veterans (U.S. Department of Veterans Affairs, 2012; Karlin & Cross, 2014). Additionally, research indicates a significantly stronger preference for cognitive processing therapy (CPT) as compared to other psychotherapies (Schumm et al., 2015).

CPT—veteran/military version (U.S. Department of Veterans Affairs, 2008) has the goal of reducing PTSD symptoms through emotional processing and cognitive restructuring of traumatic emotions and thoughts. The treatment entails 12 weekly individual or group sessions of approximately 60 minutes each. The modality is grounded in social cognitive theory. CPT assists veterans to process trauma-related emotions through the identification and resolution of cognitive "stuck points." Among the many benefits of CPT as a treatment strategy for veterans is its flexible utility and safety. CPT has been shown to be effective with personality disorders and co-occurring conditions, as well as with PTSD. Galovski and colleagues (2024) noted that a written impact statement, which details the impacts of the trauma as compared to an actual trauma retelling, can be optional, with minimal impact to therapy outcome. This may enhance safety for veterans in general population who do not wish to engage in in-depth personal writing while incarcerated.

CPT provides a framework for brief encounters, which may be especially conducive to the needs of the incarceration environment. The format is flexible with regard to modality (individual, group, combined) and number of sessions. Galovski and colleagues (2012) found that 92% of participants who had a variable-length version of CPT, rather than the full course, no longer met diagnostic criteria for PTSD. This may be especially useful when time, access to IPs, or clinical presentation warrants a focus on selected domains. For instance, CPT may be incorporated with other modalities, such as the Collaborative Assessment and Management of Suicidality (CAMS; Jobes, 2023), to address drivers of self-injurious behaviors. Clinicians may incorporate sessions on safety, trust, control, esteem, or intimacy. Once identified in the CAMS, these drivers of self-harm/suicidality originating in "stuck points" (i.e., cognitive distortions rooted in trauma) may be further explored and challenged.

Lessons learned

Several important lessons from veteran-specific treatment programs in correctional settings have been learned:

- Programs need to be resilient to systemic influences and flexible to the needs of individual veterans;
- Procedures should be responsive to challenges faced in the health care community; and
- Safety, which is important for anyone in therapy, should be emphasized, especially for traumatized veterans who left an unsafe environment and entered another threatening environment.

Following these principles enhances the likelihood of successful program implementation.

Summary

The demographics and life experiences of incarcerated veterans, both combat and noncombat, differ substantially from those of nonveterans. Additionally, their criminogenic risk factors and mental health needs differ from other mental health consumers. Nonveterans are being treated with evidence-based correctional mental health and SUD treatment programs, but programs with the unique characteristics of veterans in mind have not been perfected or achieved widespread use. There is a critical need to create and implement evidence-based programs to treat the emotional, behavioral, and neurological needs of veterans with mental illness and histories of trauma. Psychiatry is needed as part of an interdisciplinary team to ensure the best possible treatment for these men and women who were injured while fighting for their country.

REFERENCES

Bureau of Justice Assistance. (2024, February 7). *Veterans treatment court program*. https://www.bja.ojp.gov/program/veterans-treatment-court-program/funding

Bureau of Justice Statistics. (1999). *Prior abuse reported by inmates and probationers*. http://www.wcl.american.edu/faculty/smith/0303conf/article2.pdf

Bureau of Justice Statistics. (2000, January). *Veterans in prison and jail*. https://bjs.ojp.gov/content/pub/pdf/vpj.pdf

Bureau of Justice Statistics. (2004). *Compendium of federal justice statistics, 2004*.

Bureau of Justice Statistics. (2005). *Suicide and homicide in state prisons and local jails*. http://www.bjs.gov/content/pub/pdf/shsply:pdf

Bureau of Justice Statistics. (2006). *Mental health problems of prison and jail inmates*. http://www.bjs.ojp.gov/content/pub/pdf/mhppji.pdf

Bureau of Justice Statistics. (2007, May). *Veterans in state and federal prison, 2004*. https://bjs.ojp.gov/content/pub/pdf/vsfp04.pdf

Bureau of Justice Statistics. (2015, December). *Veterans in prison and jail, 2011–2012*. https://bjs.ojp.gov/content/pub/pdf/vpj1112.pdf

Bureau of Justice Statistics. (2021, March). *Veterans in prison*. https://bjs.ojp.gov/content/pub/pdf/vpspi16st.pdf

Cason v Seckinger, 5:84-cv-00313, U.S. District Court for the Middle District of Georgia (1984).

Centers for Disease Control and Prevention. (2008). *The effects of childhood stress on health across the lifespan*. http://www.cdc.gov/ncipc/pub-res/pdf/childhood_stress.pdf

Centers for Disease Control and Prevention. (2013). *Adverse Childhood Experiences (ACE) Study*. http://www.cdc.gov/ace/

Clark, J. (2013). *How post-traumatic stress disorder works. How Stuff Works*. http://science.howstuffworks.com/ptsd7.htm

Correctional News. (2012, June 14). *Georgia creates nation's first veterans dorm*.

Department of Corrections and Community Services. (2020). *Incarcerated Veterans Program*. https://doccs.ny.gov/incarcerated-veterans-program

Douds, A. S., Ahlin, A. M., Howard, D., & Stigerwalt, S. (2017). Varieties of veterans' courts: A statewide assessment of veterans' treatment court components. *Criminal Justice Policy Review, 28*, 8.

Fazel, S., & Danesh, J. (2002). Serious mental disorder in 23000 prisoners: A systematic review of 62 surveys. *Lancet, 359*(9306), 545–550.

Galietti, C., Wright, V., Higuchi, S. A., & Bufka, L. (2021, May 5). *COVID-19: When is it OK to provide more in-person services?* https://www.apaservices.org/practice/news/in-person-services-covid-19

Galovski, T. E., Blain, L. M., Mott, J. M., Elwood, L., & Houle, T. (2012). Manualized therapy for PTSD: Flexing the structure of Cognitive Processing Therapy. *Journal of Consulting and Clinical Psychology, 80*(6), 968–981.

Galovski, T. E., Norman, S. B., & Hamblen, J. L. (2024). *Cognitive processing therapy for PTSD*. PTSD: National Center for PTSD. http://ptsd.va.gov/professional/treat/txessentials/cpt_for_ptsd_pro.asp

Georgia Department of Corrections. (2014a). *Inmate statistical profile: Inmate validated veterans*. https://gdc.georgia.gov/document/monthly-statistical-reports profile-all-veterans-2013-12/download

Georgia Department of Corrections. (2014b). *Inmate statistical profile: All active inmates*. https://gdc.georgia.gov/document/monthly-statistical-reports/profile-all-inmates-2013-12/download

Georgia Department of Corrections. (2024a). *Inmate statistical profile: Inmate validated veterans*. https://gdc.georgia.gov/document/monthly-statistical-reports/profile-all-veterans-2023-12/download

Georgia Department of Corrections. (2024b). *Inmate statistical profile: All active inmates*. https://gdc.georgia.gov/document/monthly-statistical-reports/profile-all-inmates-2023-12/download

Jobes, D. A. (2023). *Managing suicidal risk: A collaborative approach* (3rd ed.). Guilford Press.

Karlin, B. E., & Cross, G. (2014). From the laboratory to the therapy room: National dissemination and implementation of evidence-based psychotherapies in the US Department of Veterans Affairs Health Care System. *American Psychologist, 69*, 19–33.

Kessler, R. C., Berglund, P., Demler, O., et al. (2005). Lifetime prevalence and age-of-onset distributions of DSM-IV disorders in the National Comorbidity Survey Replication. *Archives of General Psychiatry, 62*, 593–602.

Litz, B., & Schlenger, W. (2009). PTSD in service members and new veterans of the Iraq and Afghanistan wars: A bibliography and critique. *PTSD Research Quarterly, 20*(1), 1050–1835.

McCall, J. D., Tsai, J., & Gordon, A. J. (2018). Veterans treatment court research: Participant characteristics, outcomes, and gaps in the literature. *Journal of Offender Rehabilitation, 57*, 6.

Megargee, E. I. (2012). Psychological assessment in correctional settings. In J. R. Graham, J. A. Naglieri, & I. B. Weiner (Eds.), *Handbook of psychology* (2nd ed.): *Vol. 10: Assessment psychology* (pp. 394–424). John Wiley & Sons.

National Center for PTSD, Veterans Affairs. (2024). *How common is PTSD in veterans?* https://www.ptsd.va.gov/understand/common/common_veterans.asp

New York State Office of Mental Health. (2008). *Post-traumatic stress disorder*. http://www.omh.ny.gov/omhweb/booklets/ptsd.htm

NIH Medline Plus. (2009). *PTSD: A growing epidemic*. http://www.nlm.nih.gov/medlineplus/magazine/issues/winter09/articles/winter09pg10- 14.html

Schumm, J. A., Walter, K. H., Barone, A. S., & Chard, K. M. (2015). Veteran satisfaction and treatment preferences in response to a posttraumatic stress disorder specialty clinic orientation group. *Behavior Research and Therapy, 69*, 75–82.

Substance Abuse and Mental Health Services Administration. (2013). *Co-occurring disorders in veterans and military service members*. http://www.samhsa.gov/co-occurring/topics/military/impact-of-deployment.aspx

Tsai, J., Finlay, A., Flatley, B., Kasprow, W. J., & Clark, S. (2018). A national study of veterans treatment court participants: Who benefits and who recidivates. *Administration and Policy in Mental Health, 45*(2), 236–244.

U.S. Department of Veterans Affairs. (2008). *Cognitive processing therapy veteran/military version: Therapist's manual*.

U.S. Department of Veterans Affairs. (2012). *VHA handbook 1160.05: Local implementation of evidence-based psychotherapies for mental and behavioural health conditions*.

U.S. Department of Veteran Affairs. (2022, September). *National veteran suicide prevention annual report*. https://www.mentalhealth.va.gov/docs/data-sheets/2022/2022-National-Veteran-Suicide-Prevention-Annual-Report-FINAL-508.pdf

U.S. Institute for Veteran Policy. (2011). *Veterans and criminal justice: A review of the literature*. http://www.swords-to-plowshares.org/wp-content/uploads/Veterans-and-Criminal-Justice-Literature-Review.pdf

Wisco, B. E., Marx, B. P., Wolf, E. J., Miller, M. W., Southwick, S. M., & Pietrzak, R. H. (2014). Posttraumatic stress disorder in the US veteran population: Results from the National Health and Resilience in Veterans Study. *Journal of Clinical Psychiatry, 75*(12), 1338–1346.

Wisdom, N. M., Callahan, J. L., & Shaw, T. G. (2010). Diagnostic utility of the structured inventory of malingered symptomatology to detect malingering in a forensic sample. *Archives of Clinical Neuropsychology, 25*(2), 118–125.

Wolff, N., & Shi, J. (2012). Childhood and adult trauma experiences of incarcerated persons and their relationship to adult behavioral health problems and treatment. *International Journal of Environmental Research and Public Health, 9*(5), 1908–1926.

Wood, D. (2012a, July 4). *Iraq, Afghanistan war veterans struggle with combat trauma*. Huffington Post. http://www.huffingtonpost.com/2012/07/04/iraq-afghanistan-war-veterans-combat-trauma_n_1645701.html

Wood, D. (2012b, October 2). *Veterans: Coming home*. Huffington Post. http://www.huffingtonpost.com/2012/10/02/veterans-coming-home_n_1932366.html

Wortzel, H., Binswanger, I. A., Anderson, C. A., et al. (2009). Suicide among incarcerated veterans. *Journal of the American Academy of Psychiatry and the Law, 37*, 82–91.

62

Immigrants in detention

Maria Masotta and Rose Kleman

Introduction

The goal of this chapter is to provide an overview of immigration to the United States, with a focus on incarcerated persons (IPs) who are held in detention facilities. While these noncitizen IPs have entered the United States illegally, unlike U.S. citizen IPs who are incarcerated pending a criminal proceeding or to serve a criminal sentence, the majority of these IPs have not committed a crime other than being in the United States illegally. The reader will gain an understanding of immigration in the United States, the facilities used to detain unauthorized immigrants, and standards of care that govern these facilities. Challenges encountered in detention, treatment needs, and available mental health services are also discussed.

An overview of immigration

Immigrants come to the United States for multiple reasons. Immigrants include people seeking a permanent life in the United States, whether through authorized or unauthorized means, and those who come to the United States for temporary purposes. In 2022, there were 46.2 million immigrants living in the United States (Batalova, 2024).

U.S. immigration law is based on the following principles: family reunification, value to the U.S. economy, refugee protection, and promotion of diversity (American Immigration Council, 2021). U.S. immigration is a complex process accomplished by an array of government agencies that play a role in enacting and enforcing immigration policy. Processes associated with becoming a U.S. citizen are managed by the U.S. Department of Homeland Security's Citizenship and Immigration Services, which oversees the process of lawful entry into the United States.

Visas, issued by the U.S. Department of State, allow legal entry to the United States. Visas are required when a foreign citizen wants to visit the United States temporarily for work, education, or tourism or to begin the process of permanent residency. In fiscal year (FY) 2023, the U.S. Department of State issued 10.4 million temporary visas for tourists, international students, and others (Batalova, 2024).

Once a visa is granted, an immigrant can apply for a "green card," the first step in becoming a U.S. citizen. There are four pathways to obtain a green card and become a lawful permanent resident: family relationships, sponsorship by an employer, protection for refugees and asylees, and the Diversity Visa lottery. Of the 1 million immigrants receiving a green card in FY22, 58% had familial relationships with U.S. citizens, 27% were sponsored by an employer, 8% were accepted as refugees or asylees, and 4% were selected through the lottery (Batalova, 2024). To become a U.S. citizen, an immigrant must hold a green card continuously for at least 5 years while residing in the United States, be at least 18 years of age, and pass English and civics exams. According to Batalova (2024), the average length of time between receiving a green card and becoming a citizen is 7 years.

Unauthorized immigrants at a glance

The U.S. Department of Homeland Security's Office of Homeland Security Statistics estimates that there were 11 million unauthorized immigrants living in the United States in January 2022 (Baker & Warren, 2024). Between FY17 and FY23, less than 1% (79,000) of unauthorized immigrants had criminal convictions. Further, just under half of criminal convictions were attributed to illegal entry to the United States (U.S. Customs and Border Protection, n.d.). As many as 45% of unauthorized immigrants arrived at legal points of entry, received visas allowing them to visit or reside in the United States for a specific amount of time, and then overstayed their visa expiration date (Passel & Krogstad, 2023). Most of the remaining unauthorized immigrants entered the country illegally. Some evaded customs inspection by hiding in vehicles, while others waded across the Rio Grande River or crossed the desert to avoid inspectors and Border Patrol.

Mexico is the country of origin for the largest number of unauthorized immigrants, with more than 4.8 million in 2022. Guatemala (750,000), El Salvador (710,000), and Honduras (560,000) were the next largest countries. Other countries with significant numbers of unauthorized immigrants include the Philippines (350,000), Venezuela (210,000), Columbia (240,000), Brazil (230,000), India (220,000), and China (210,000). All other countries combined account for 2.6 million unauthorized immigrants (Baker & Warren, 2024). Almost every region of the world has shown an increase in the number of unauthorized immigrants in the United States.

Immigrants attempt unauthorized entry into the United States for many reasons. The Congressional Research Service (2023) notes that immigrants from Guatemala, Honduras, and El Salvador migrate due to financial inequity in their home countries, fleeing widespread poverty. Natural disasters including extreme temperatures, crop loss, and decreasing employment opportunities lead to food insecurity. Violence, including that targeting sexual orientation and gender identity; trafficking of narcotics to the United States; and increases in gang activity are critical reasons for leaving home countries. Unauthorized immigrants enter the United States in search of financial and employment opportunities, family stability, and the relative safety of U.S. communities.

Traveling to the U.S. border is long and treacherous. The Council on Foreign Relations (2024) reports that in 2023, more than 500,000 immigrants from South and Central America traveled through a dangerous stretch of jungle called the Darien Gap on the border of Columbia and Panama, walking 10 or more days with the help of paid guides. En route, they faced smugglers and criminal groups who often extorted and sexually assaulted them. The migrants' willingness to potentially encounter these risks speaks to the desperation they experience when embarking on this journey and the level of trauma to which they are exposed throughout. Young children get separated from their families during the trek. Once they complete the hike through the Darien Gap, the United States is still 2,500 miles away. During this additional 2,500-mile journey, they continue to face uncertainty and safety concerns.

U.S. immigration detention

There are two government agencies responsible for identifying, apprehending, and detaining unauthorized immigrants: U.S. Customs and Border Protection (CBP) and U.S. Immigration and Customs Enforcement (ICE). Both agencies work under the umbrella of U.S. Department of Homeland Security and were formed in 2003.

CBP, a comprehensive border security agency, apprehends individuals at ports of entry, such as borders, airports, and seaports. CBP reported more than 3.2 million encounters at U.S. borders, airports, and seaports in FY23, a record high and up from the nearly 2.8 million in FY22 and 2 million in FY21 (Batalova, 2024).

Unauthorized immigrants are taken to CBP stations and processing centers, which are intended for short stays. Some facilities use cement holding cells to house multiple people. Others house people outside within chain link fencing. Medical and mental health care is sparse. Hot meals, religious and dietary accommodations, and showers are inconsistent. The U.S. CBP National Standards on Transport, Escort, Detention, and Search, which direct CBP detention, states that "every effort must be made to hold detainees for the least amount of time required for their processing, transfer, release, or repatriation as appropriate and as operationally feasible … should generally not be held for longer than 72 hours" (U.S. CBP, 2015, p. 14). After an unauthorized immigrant is processed by CBP at or near the border, the immigrant is transferred to ICE custody and moved to an ICE detention facility.

ICE uses a variety of facilities to detain noncitizens, including county jails, state and federal prisons, private detention centers, and hotels. There are five types of ICE facilities (American Immigration Council, 2024):

1. Service processing centers are owned by ICE;
2. Contract detention facilities are owned and operated by private prison companies;
3. Nondedicated intergovernmental service agreements are city or county jails with some bed space reserved for individuals in ICE custody;
4. Dedicated intergovernmental service agreements are owned by local governments and only house individuals in ICE custody; and
5. U.S. Marshals Service intergovernmental agreements are owned by local governments and house ICE detainees and others in U.S. Marshals Service custody.

The average length of stay at ICE facilities is often dependent on the individual's case. IPs may request expedited deportation, which may shorten their stay in detention. IPs seeking asylum may remain in a detention facility for 2 years or more while waiting for a hearing (American Immigration Council, 2024).

Standards of care

There are various applicable standards of care for mental health services with noncitizen IPs in detention facilities. As discussed in depth in Chapter 73, applicable detention facility standards include those by the American Correctional Association (ACA) and National Commission on Correctional Health Care (NCCHC). The ACA focuses on the safety, security, and operations of correctional facilities (although health services are addressed), while the NCCHC focuses on health care and suicide prevention. The NCCHC "recommend[s] requirements for the proper management of a correctional mental health services delivery system" and for a "correctional health services delivery system" (NCCHC, 2015, p. vii; NCCHC, 2018, p. vi). In a task force report, the American Psychiatric Association (2016, p. 5) stated, "The fundamental policy goal for correctional mental health care is to provide the same level of mental health services to each patient in the criminal justice process that should be available in the community."

Detention facilities that maintain a contract with ICE are required to follow one of three ICE National Detention Standards (NDS). The NDS were developed in 2000 and updated in 2019 (ICE, 2022). The Performance-Based National Detention Standards (PBNDS) were developed in 2008 and updated in 2011 (ICE, 2011). The Family Residential Standards were developed in 2007 and revised in 2020 (U.S. Immigration and Customs Enforcement, 2020). After March 2021, ICE converted family residential centers, which allowed families to live for more than 72 hours, to family staging centers that could not be used for more than 72 hours. ICE discontinued the practice of housing families in December 2021 (ICE, 2024).

The NDS (ICE, 2022) and PBNDS (ICE, 2011) direct all facets of a detention facility's operations, including safety and security; discipline; access to legal services, libraries, and religious services; daily food and sanitation operations; visitation and phone call processes; suicide prevention; and medical and mental health care. The ACA and NCCHC standards are generally broader and more comprehensive than the NDS and PBNDS.

Mental health professionals who work at detention facilities may be guided by their professional ethical guidelines. When standards conflict with each other or one's ethical guidelines, it is recommended that the higher standard be followed.

Challenges

Living in a detention facility as an IP poses a host of challenges, which include engaging in basic communication with staff and others who do not share a common language, accessing legal and support services to address the logistics of the immigration system, and maintaining communication with family.

Living in a detention center

While detention centers vary in physical plant layout and procedures, their operations share many features with jails and prisons. The facilities are locked and have a secure perimeter. IPs live in housing units where a custody officer maintains supervision of them 24 hours a day, 7 days a week. Detention facilities have designated times when each individual is accounted for, known as "count time." During that time, IPs must be in their assigned sleep area.

IPs can socialize in a dayroom or watch television. Personal space is limited, as IPs may share a small cell with a toilet and sink with one or more peers. Alternatively, at some facilities, IPs are assigned to a large room, or "dorm," that includes a sleeping area, typically multiple bunk beds; the officer's workstation; and a dayroom. Regardless of housing layout, showers in the housing unit are located in a private area. Institutional rules dictate every aspect of daily life, including such basic activities as leaving the cell, showering, using the phone, and eating meals.

Ability to communicate

The primary challenge IPs experience is the language barrier. Few IPs are proficient in English, and most have little understanding of English. This language barrier impacts IPs' ability to function in the correctional environment and follow institutional rules and norms. Rules are communicated in an institutional handbook or by video, but not every spoken language is represented. Written materials are generally provided in Spanish, as per the NDS (ICE, 2022) and PBNDS (ICE, 2011).

Language barriers also impact IPs' ability to access health care. Once IPs learn the process of how to access care (often via a written form or via an application on a tablet), the next step is to communicate their needs to staff, which may or may not be feasible in their native language. Staff use professional interpretation services when needed, often via a designated phone line that provides a more objective perspective than a bilingual staff person. If a staff member must be used, health care personnel are preferred over custody staff, who should only be used as a last resort. The NDS (ICE, 2022) permit the use of a peer during an emergency, which raises confidentiality and safety concerns. In contrast, the PBNDS (ICE, 2011) explicitly state that peers should not be used for health care and mental health care.

The language barrier also impacts IPs' ability to communicate effectively with peers. IPs tend to socialize with peers who speak the same language. IPs who do not speak the same language as their peers can experience social isolation and boredom, as television programs and books are often not available in all IPs' native languages. This inability to distract oneself can exacerbate situational stressors and underlying mental health conditions.

Legal access

A primary concern for IPs is the status of their immigration case, which is exacerbated by challenges with legal access. In contrast to their criminally committed counterparts, noncitizen IPs do not have the right to free legal representation, but they are allowed to have representation at their own expense. According to the *Harvard Law Review* ("The Right to Be Heard From Immigration Prisons," 2018), legal representation is rare, primarily due to cost and lack of attorneys. Thirty-six percent of IPs who sought an attorney located one. Fourteen percent of IPs had legal representation for removal proceedings. Even after an attorney is secured, access to them can be difficult due to the remote location of detention facilities and transfer of detainees to a different facility in another state without attorney notification. Attorneys may face delays in seeing the IP despite a prescheduled visit. Phone calls can only be initiated by the IP and are complicated by time-limited and costly phone access. Some facilities allow communication via tablets, which improves access. IPs have access to the detention facility law library; however, available documentation is not routinely available in all IPs' native language.

Family separation

IPs often leave family members behind when leaving their country of origin. In addition to the impact this has on their support system, IPs may be concerned about the safety of those they left behind, increasing their anxiety. They may also lose contact when transferred to new detention facilities, taking away their support systems and increasing stress.

In 2018, an estimated 5,000 families that traveled to the United States with children were separated. Adults were held in detention centers, and children were brought to shelters. This impacted the mental health of the parents as well as the children. A class action lawsuit, Ms. L., et al., v. ICE, et al. (2018), was filed and resulted in a nationwide injunction. In December 2023, a federal judge approved the settlement and prohibited the practice of separating families at the border for the next 8 years and aided in reuniting separated families (American Civil Liberties Union, 2023).

Trauma

Whether hiking the Darien Gap, riding in the back of closed trucks, walking through deserts, riding atop or in freight train railcars through Mexico, or taking boats from Haiti, the challenge of escaping violence, poverty, hunger, and instability to reach the United States can be traumatizing and contribute to health and mental health concerns. Women face additional risk for trauma, given the risk of sexual violence that can occur during the journey. In addition to the treacherous journey, the American Psychiatric Association (n.d.) notes that unauthorized immigrants are often profiled as gang members or criminals, leading to fear, anxiety, and isolation.

The American Psychiatric Association (n.d.) concluded that many unauthorized immigrants are at higher overall risk for mental health concerns due to exposure to trauma that occurs in their countries of origin and during travel to the United States. Often, trauma symptoms can be triggered by the conditions of confinement, whether through exposure to the daily detention routine that includes being locked in a cell, large peer groups, and loud noises during daily institutional operations such as operation of heavy cell and facility doors, keys, and overhead announcements or through potential exposure to peers and staff using raised voices, placement in restrictive housing, or witnessing violence between peers.

Facility admission

IPs are often transferred to the detention facility on a bus with up to 50 other individuals they do not know. The group is escorted into the admission area to undergo the booking process. The admission area is often chaotic, and space is limited. The area is generally loud due to many staff and other newly admitted IPs talking, yelling, and moving throughout the area. In addition to the language barrier, the confidentiality of initial assessments is often a concern, particularly with assessments completed by custody staff. IPs may not self-disclose mental health needs due to the perceived stigma and lack of confidentiality. IPs may also be reluctant to disclose mental health needs given concerns that mental health treatment could impact their legal case and result in deportation. Transgender status and sexual orientation are asked as part of the assessment; vulnerability to sexual assault is also explored. IPs may be reluctant to share such sensitive information. Thus, treatment needs may be missed, and in turn, symptoms can worsen. In these cases, IPs may come to the attention of mental health staff through a self- or staff-initiated referral. Staff should consider the potential that the initial denial of mental health needs was based on other factors. It should not be considered exaggerating or lying; the report of symptoms must be fully assessed and information from prior facilities sought when appropriate.

In facilities where there is a pattern of denial of mental health symptoms during the booking process followed by a mental health referral (self or staff), a quality improvement project is worth considering to address barriers and increase the potential that a future IP will share information.

Transfer and release

IPs may be transferred to another ICE facility in a different state with minimal advance notice. In addition to the emotional impact of a sudden unexpected move, the need to learn how to function in another institutional environment is added stress for the IP. Further, abrupt transfers do not allow for appropriate termination of the therapeutic relationship and are disruptive to continuity of care.

Once at the new facility, the IP undergoes an identical booking process to the one during the previous facility admission. However, minimal mental health information from the sending institution typically accompanies the IP. This limited information, coupled with the language barrier, complicates the ability for mental health staff to obtain a complete assessment of the IP's mental health history and current treatment needs. At a minimum, diagnoses and medication names and dosages are provided. Psychotropic medications are continued at the new facility; however, depending on pharmacy availability, there may be a delay in medication receipt. During this time of transition, the language barrier can also impact access to care, as IPs need to learn when and where medication distribution occurs.

Facility release can occur just as suddenly as facility transfers, with limited time to prepare. IPs may be deported to their country of origin, or they could be released to a community that is a great distance from where they were apprehended and where their social supports reside. This may result in emotional reactions that warrant mental health intervention. To aid the IP in preparing for the change, mental health professionals can assist with symptom management and develop a plan to continue treatment as needed, regardless of the release plan.

IPs are often released with a supply of psychotropic medication. Medications offered in the detention facility may not always be available in the home country, or they may be too expensive for the IP to purchase. Efforts should be made to use medications that will be available to the IP upon discharge. When possible, mental health staff should assist with scheduling an appointment with a community provider for medication management and counseling.

IPs who are identified as at risk of harm to self or others, acutely psychotic, or unable to function in the community due to a mental illness should be assessed by a mental health clinician prior to discharge. Mental health staff should alert the correctional authority to address concerns with stakeholders and develop a safe discharge plan.

Restrictive housing

Noncitizen IPs are held to the same rules as their citizen counterparts who are detained on criminal charges. Staff do not distinguish between populations; interactions with and treatment of IPs do not vary. A rule violation due to a language barrier can result in a disciplinary infraction and ultimately to restrictive housing placement, referred to as special management units in the NDS (ICE, 2022) and PBNDS (ICE, 2011). Restrictive housing, discussed more in Chapter 10, can have detrimental effects on one's mental health, particularly those with mental illness. In recognition of the impact restrictive housing can have, special monitoring of IPs with mental health concerns is mandated by the NDS (ICE, 2022), PBNDS (ICE, 2011), and a directive issued by ICE (ICE, n.d.).

IPs can request separation from the general population based on protective housing needs. Transgender IPs who report feeling unsafe in their assigned housing units may be kept in protective custody at their request. In these cases, the protective setting should afford the same access to out-of-cell activities, legal services, visitation, and other privileges as is available in general population settings.

Mental health care

With the dangerous and traumatic journey to the U.S. border, it is not surprising that IPs may have mental health needs upon arrival to the detention center or develop mental health needs at any time during detainment. The noncitizen IP has mental health needs that vary from adjustment to detainment to the need for treatment for trauma and serious mental illness. Common clinical presentations include stress associated with detention, inability to sleep due to a new and crowded environment, anxiety related to potential deportation, depression and grief after leaving family, and trauma from turmoil in the home country or occurring on the trek to the U.S. border. Psychiatric medication and counseling may be necessary to assist the IP in symptom management and psychiatric decompensation.

Staffing

Mental health care is often dependent on space and staffing. Staff in detention facilities routinely share offices. Despite confidentiality requirements (NCCHC, 2015, 2018), mental health consultations may occur at cell doors or in areas of the facility that limit confidentiality. Mental health staff can be employed by the facility, provided by ICE via the ICE Health Services Corps, or accessed through a local community provider agreement between the facility and a local community provider or hospital. The PBNDS (ICE, 2011) and NDS (ICE, 2022) require that facilities have psychiatric providers. These providers can be physicians, nurse prescribers, or, in rare cases as permitted by state law, psychologists who have additional psychiatric expertise. Often psychiatric care is accomplished via telemedicine. Some facilities also utilize psychologists as individual and group mental health providers, while others use master's-level counselors.

Treatment planning

Treatment plans are an essential component of mental health care. Treatment plans should be developed collaboratively with input from the assigned psychiatric provider, mental health clinician, and IP. Measurable and objective treatment goals should be individualized to the IP's treatment needs. Interventions provided via routine psychotherapy and medication management should be evidence based and individualized to the IP's treatment needs. This may require more frequent contacts than is typical, which is generally every 30 to 90 days.

Individual psychotherapy

As noted by the NCCHC (2018, p. 6), "mental health treatment is more than prescribing medication." Individual psychotherapy is an integral part of mental health care (see Chapter 42). Well-rounded clinicians with various skill sets will be able to adjust to IPs' various treatment needs. In addition to being a source of support, individual psychotherapy can be a forum to learn skills to manage symptoms such as anxiety or depression that may be related to a mental illness or due to situational stressors. Skills to manage trauma symptoms, likely exacerbated by life in the correctional environment, are necessary. Clinicians are also responsible for monitoring IPs' mental status for any signs of decompensation and encouraging healthy coping and medication adherence.

Individual therapy is typically short term and focused on symptom management rather than the long-term therapy that may be available in the broader community. Currently, available treatment in detention facilities is not typically aimed at addressing the underlying causes of mental health disorders such as trauma, despite its significant impact on the broader population of IPs.

Group treatments and psychoeducation

Psychoeducation using worksheets, reading materials, and small group discussion is available at some detention facilities. These interventions are cost-effective and useful for mild mental health conditions, such as sleep disturbance, difficulty adjusting to detention, and interpersonal challenges. Group programs and psychoeducation can provide short- and long-term benefits. In addition, an assessment by mental health staff is warranted to determine whether symptoms are secondary to a mental illness or due to situational stressors and whether psychiatric medications can be considered.

Access to higher levels of care

As in jails and prisons, IPs determined to be at risk of harm to themselves or others or who are gravely disabled are placed in suicide-resistant rooms for additional safety and monitoring. A lack of improvement within 72 hours warrants consideration for a higher level of care, which can include transfer to an ICE dedicated inpatient psychiatric facility. Alternatively, facilities can utilize a local emergency room or inpatient psychiatric hospital (see Chapter 26), which may warrant the need for an official agreement or memorandum of understanding. If IPs engage in self-harm while in a detention facility, the least restrictive clinical interventions should be utilized, which may include verbal de-escalation, increased observation, emergency psychiatric medication, or utilization of therapeutic restraints (see Chapters 24 and 25).

Summary

Noncitizen IPs face unique challenges compared to their citizen counterparts, including language barriers, trauma experienced in the home country and during travel to the United States, and separation from family. Assessment of an IP's trauma history is imperative, and awareness of how trauma and other mental health needs can be exacerbated in a detention facility is crucial. Access to individualized, goal-directed treatment, including individual therapy, psychotropic medication, crisis stabilization, and discharge planning, is ethically necessary. Currently, many detention facilities lack these services despite mental health professionals' essential role in facilitating immigrants' safe adjustment to detention and, eventually, transition to the community.

REFERENCES

American Civil Liberties Union. (2023, December 8). *Court approves historic settlement in ACLU's family separation lawsuit.* https://www.aclu.org/press-releases/court-approves-historic-settlement-in-aclus-family-separation-lawsuit

American Immigration Council. (2021). *How the United States immigration system works.*http://live-americanimmigrationcouncil.pantheonsite.io/research/how-united-states-immigration-system-works

American Immigration Council. (2024). *Immigration detention in the United States by agency.* https://www.americanimmigrationcouncil.org/research/immigration-detention-united-states-agency

American Psychiatric Association. (n.d.). *Stress and trauma toolkit for treating undocumented immigrants in a changing political and social environment.* https://www.psychiatry.org/psychiatrists/diversity/education/stress-and-trauma/undocumented-immigrants

American Psychiatric Association. (2016). *Psychiatric services in correctional facilities* (3rd ed.).

Baker, B., & Warren, R. (2024, April). *Estimates of the unauthorized immigrant population residing in the United States: January 2018–January 2022.* Office of Homeland Security Statistics, U.S. Department of Homeland Security.

Batalova, J. (2024, March 13). *Frequently requested statistics on immigrants and immigration in the United States.* Migration Policy Institute. https://www.migrationpolicy.org/article/frequently-requested-statistics-immigrants-and-immigration-united-states-2024

Congressional Research Service. (2023). *Central American migration: Root causes and US policy.* https://crsreports.congress.gov/product/pdf/IF/IF11151

Council on Foreign Relations. (2024). *Crossing the Darien Gap: Migrants risk death on the journey to the US.* https://www.cfr.org/article/crossing-darien-gap-migrants-risk-death-journey-us

The right to be heard from immigration prisons: Locating a right of access to counsel for immigration detainees in the right of access to courts. (2018, December 10). *Harvard Law Review*. https://harvardlawreview.org/print/vol-132/the-right-to-be-heard-from-immigration-prisons-locating-a-right-of-access-to-counsel-for-immigration-detainees-in-the-right-of-access-to-courts/

Ms. L.; et al., v. U.S. Immigration and Customs Enforcement ("ICE"); et al. (2018). United States District Court Southern District of California. Case No: 18cv0428 DMS (MDD). https://assets.aclu.org/live/uploads/legal-documents/83_Order_Granting_PI.pdf

National Commission on Correctional Health Care. (2015). *Standards for mental health services in correctional facilities.*

National Commission on Correctional Health Care. (2018). *Standards for health services in jails.*

Passel, J., & Krogstad, J. M. (2023, November 16). *What we know about unauthorized immigrants living in the US.* Pew Research Center. https://www.pewresearch.org/short-reads/2023/11/16/what-we-know-about-unauthorized-immigrants-living-in-the-us/

U.S. Customs and Border Protection. (n.d.). *Criminal noncitizen statistics.* https://www.cbp.gov/newsroom/stats/cbp-enforcement-statistics/criminal-noncitizen-statistics

U.S. Customs and Border Protection. (2015, October). *National standards on transport, escort, detention, and search.* https://www.cbp.gov/sites/default/files/assets/documents/2020-Feb/cbp-teds-policy-october2015.pdf

U.S. Immigration and Customs Enforcement. (n.d.). *Review of the use of segregation for ICE detainees.* https://www.ice.gov/doclib/detention-reform/pdf/segregation_directive.pdf

U.S. Immigration and Customs Enforcement. (2011). *Performance-based national detention standards 2011.* https://www.ice.gov/doclib/detention-standards/2011/pbnds2011r2016.pdf

U.S. Immigration and Customs Enforcement. (2020). *Family residential standards: Program philosophy, goals and expected outcomes.* https://www.ice.gov/doclib/frs/2020/2020family-residential-standards.pdf

U.S. Immigration and Customs Enforcement. (2022, February 18). *2019 national detention standards for non-dedicated facilities.* https://www.ice.gov/doclib/detention-standards/2019/nds2019.pdf

U.S. Immigration and Customs Enforcement. (2024, June 6). *Detention management.* https://www.ice.gov/detain/detention-management#

63

Sex offenders

Fabian M. Saleh and Reena Kapoor[1]

Introduction

The treatment of sex offenders in correctional contexts is arguably one of the most challenging undertakings for psychiatrists. Sex offenders are highly stigmatized and typically engender intense negative feelings in both the professional and lay communities. This chapter reviews some of the clinical and legal issues relevant to the care of convicted sex offenders in correctional settings.

Incidence of sex offending

The growing number of publicized sex offenses, "overdramatized by print and video media that overvalue sensationalism" (LaFond & Winick, 1998, p. 3), has had a profound impact on public perception. While the number of sex offenses committed in the United States on an annual basis is significant, the figure is not astronomical. According to Federal Bureau of Investigation (FBI) statistics, in 2019, there were 121,333 sex offenses against persons in the United States reported to the National Incident-Based Reporting System (NIBRS; FBI, 2019). In 2019, all sex crimes against persons or society accounted for about 1.7% of the approximately 7.6 million incidents of crime reported to the NIBRS, and sex crimes against persons accounted for about 6.4% of the 1.9 million reported crimes against persons (FBI, 2019). Comparisons over time are difficult because of changing crime definitions and data collection methodologies, but FBI data indicate that rape charges have increased in the past decade, from 9,129 cases in 2014 to 16,413 in 2023 (FBI, 2024), possibly reflecting an increase in law enforcement agencies reporting to the NIBRS. According to the U.S. Sentencing Commission (2021), which tracks federal sex crimes, in fiscal year 2021, 57,287 cases were reported to the U.S. Sentencing Commission, with a reduction of sexual abuse offenses by 3.2% since fiscal year 2017. These offenses included rape (§ 2A3.1), statutory rape (§ 2A3.2), criminal sexual abuse of a ward (§ 2a3.3), abusive sexual contact (§ 2a3.4), promoting a commercial sex act (§ 2g1.1), travel to engage in prohibited sexual conduct with a minor (§ 2g1.3), production of child pornography (§ 2g2.1), and child exploitation enterprises (§ 2g2.6).

The rate of recidivism over 25 years among sex offenders has been estimated to be as high as 52% (Prentky et al., 1997, p. 11). However, another analysis of the data has shown that while persons incarcerated for sex offenses are rearrested at high rates, it is (with a few notable exceptions) seldom for a new sexual offense. In a large study of 272,111 prisoners, 68% of whom were rearrested during a 3-year follow-up, 43% of the 9,691 male sex offenders released (two thirds of all male sex offenders released in 1994) were rearrested for another crime within 3 years of release. More specifically, the released sex offenders were rearrested for a new sex crime at a rate of 5.3%, only 10% of the overall recidivism rate (Langan et al., 2003).

The law, however, is "a reflection of the society that generates it. The current attitudes, fears, and beliefs of the community about the world around it, accurate or not, are reflected in the law that governs at any given time" (Hafemeister & Petrila, 1994, p. 731). For example, in 1997, child pornography offenders who possessed, received, or distributed child pornography but did not produce or attempt production received a mean sentence of 20.59 months of confinement (Stabenow, 2009). In 2023, defendants sentenced for possession of child pornography received an average sentence of 70 months, while those convicted of receiving child pornography were sentenced to an average of 101 months (U.S. Sentencing Commission, 2023). The behaviors did not change; society's perception of and response to them did.

Medical-legal considerations

Sex offenders are a heterogeneous clinical population. Mental health professionals must not conflate whatever psychiatric diagnoses might be assigned to a given patient with the legal designation of that same patient as a "sex offender." The legal designation is based on the fact that the patient has transgressed against society and/or one or more of its members by violating culturally defined rules governing permissible sexual behavior. The psychiatric diagnosis addresses the issue of what underlying vulnerabilities might be causative or contributory to such transgression.

1. The authors acknowledge Albert J. Grudzinskas and H. Martin Malin, who contributed to the manuscript of this chapter in the textbook's first edition.

Sex offending is a legal construct without clinical significance, and debate surrounding the management of the "sex offender" is seldom well informed by medical knowledge. The lay perception and, to some degree, the legal construct of the sex offender is one of an evil person, or at least a person who has done evil things, causing undeserved pain to others by behaving badly.

Society's understanding of sex offending is further clouded by the use of such pseudo-psychiatric terminology as "mentally disordered sex offender," "sexually violent person," and the more commonly used pejorative, "sexual predator." Such terms are in widespread parlance and frequently encountered in judicial proceedings. These terms may be seen to justify the civil commitment of sex offenders who have served their penal sentences. "Sexually violent person" laws take it as a given that many sex offenders have a mental condition that predisposes them to commit sex offenses. Indefinite civil commitment might then be justifiable since they are perceived as being at high risk of reoffending due to a serious impairment in the ability to control their dangerous behavior (Elwood, 2009).

The legality of any given sexual behavior is culture bound—what is legal at one time may not be legal at another. What constitutes a sex offense also differs from jurisdiction to jurisdiction. The term provides no context regarding the individual's motivation and does not, by itself, indicate any underlying psychopathology. Illegal sexual behavior, however, is different from most other illegal behavior in that it may occur in the context of a strong, biologically mediated drive (Saleh et al., 2010).

There is no single motivation for engaging in sexual behavior or committing sex offenses. The psychiatrist, as part of assessment for treatment, wants to know what has motivated a patient who may otherwise be a law-abiding citizen to engage in illegal behavior. Conversely, the psychiatrist who encounters a patient who has made a life career of antisocial behavior will not be greatly surprised to learn that the patient has simply added illegal sexual behavior to their repertoire (Saleh et al., 2010).

Sex offenders and mental illness

People may commit sex offenses in the context of a psychiatric condition. These conditions include developmental disorders, depression, mania, intoxication with psychoactive substances, and altered mental states associated with delusions, hallucinations, and compulsions. While there are clearly sex offenders whose illegal behavior is rooted in refractory personality disorders, others just as clearly commit their offenses in the context of serious mood or psychotic disorders (Saleh et al., 2010). An altered state of consciousness with impaired reality testing appears to be an important contributor to illegal behavior in some sex offenders. For example, Berlin (1986) documented the case of a patient with bipolar disorder who raped several women during a prolonged manic episode; he believed they were seeking him out, having been sent as sacrificial lambs in a cosmic battle between good and evil. While he had previously run naked through a canteen during a similar manic state while stationed overseas in the military, he had no prior history of criminal behavior outside of such altered mental states. While the cognitive-behavioral and moral habilitation strategies that form the core of typical offender treatment programs may be adjunctively useful in such cases, pharmacotherapy clearly plays a central role for individuals who suffer from perceptual disorders.

The same can likely be said for sex offenses committed in the context of paraphilic disorders. The imagery pathognomonic of the paraphilic disorders is enmeshed with the biology of sexual desire and may impair the ability to conform sexual behavior to accepted norms. Paraphilias therefore form a class of disorders qualitatively different from other mental disorders (Fagan et al., 2005). As is the case with perceptual disorders, treatment strategies that involve pharmacological blunting of the sex drive may enhance the effectiveness of more conventional cognitive-behavioral treatment strategies. In addition, paraphilic-like behavior that results from general medical disorders, including traumatic brain injury, is sometimes ameliorated by medical therapy (Lehne, 1986).

Of course, not all sex offenders present with paraphilic disorders, and not all patients with paraphilic disorders commit sex offenses. In addition, the consensual expression of some paraphilias (e.g., the cross-dressing associated with transvestic disorder) is not currently illegal in the United States but may be in some other countries. Similarly, until the mid-1970s, child pornography was openly and legally displayed for sale on the shelves of adult booksellers in most major U.S. cities. Such a practice today would certainly lead to prosecution.

Ethical concerns with sex offender treatment

As noted earlier, sex offenders are an exceptionally heterogeneous group. Some, but not all, will eventually come to be seen as legitimate psychiatric patients. Some of those will be treated while incarcerated. Incarcerated persons are owed a basic duty of care, including mental health care (see Chapter 3). The U.S. Supreme Court has grounded this right in the Eighth Amendment proscription on cruel and unusual punishment (*Estelle v. Gamble*, 1976) and the 14th Amendment due process clause (*Bell v. Wolfish*, 1979). The duty to "avoid deliberate indifference" (*Farmer v. Brennan*, 1994) to the incarcerated person's (IP's) medical or psychological needs is seen as an obligation to "avoid the needless infliction or prolongation of pain and suffering" (Cohen, 2003, p. 120). Although the civil rights of persons being treated while incarcerated are similar to the rights of other persons in treatment and are protected by the U.S. Constitution (and, in many instances, by additional state laws and judicial decisions), there are differences.

The nature of the prison environment and the need to secure the safety of staff, visitors, and IPs affect mental health care in important ways. The American Psychiatric Association's (APA's) task force on jails and prisons recognizes, for example, that there are numerous instances where confidentiality might be limited because of institutional needs for safety and security (APA, 2016). The concepts of confidentiality and privilege are grounded in a person's expectation of privacy. Full disclosure of the limits of privacy and the nature of the clinician's agency, particularly in instances of diagnosis, evaluation, and classification in incarcerated settings, helps clinicians avoid conflicts as treatment proceeds.

Additional privacy issues arise in the treatment of sex offenders since treatment is often mandated (Clayton, 2002). This can lead to significant risks for the patient when coupled with the belief among many clinicians that sex offenders must "acknowledge their responsibility for the offense and their problematic sexual behavior before they can fully participate in treatment and work toward change" (Farkas & Miller, 2008, pp. 78–79). Such risks for the IP may go beyond concerns of threats from other IPs if their sex offender status becomes known. The U.S. Supreme Court in *McKune v. Lile* (2002) found that the admission of guilt required for participation in treatment programs, even when coupled with loss of privileges and transfer to a higher security level, was not "compelling enough" to be unconstitutional.

Assessment

The clinical response to sex offending properly begins with a thorough and accurate differential diagnosis. In the differential diagnostic process, the clinician will collect the usual medical and psychosocial historical data and attempt to synthesize an explanation for the behavior as a function of the patient's life story (Fagan et al., 2005). While terms having legal significance may well be left to the legislature (see *Kansas v. Hendricks*, 1997), without a medical diagnosis to inform the specific treatment needs of a specific patient, there can be no treatment. The days of relying on the "great professor principle" paradigm of psychiatric nosology described by Kendler (1990) have given way to the "consensus of the experts" paradigm of diagnosis for the *Diagnostic and Statistical Manual of Mental Disorders*, fifth edition, text revision (APA, 2022). Today, a differential diagnosis should take into account global patterns of behavioral problems; pervasive impairments in interpersonal relationships; isolated, opportunistic, or impulsive sexual problem behaviors; time-limited, reactive patterns of oversexualized behaviors; and psychiatric, neuropsychiatric, and/or neurological disorders, including paraphilic disorders such as pedophilic disorder. Only then can treatment goals be established. Such goals typically include risk reduction/mitigation of future sexual misconduct/sexual offending behavior, improvement in quality of life, decreased personal distress, increased autonomy and independence, and reintegration into the community, if appropriate and possible.

Psychotherapeutic interventions

Psychotherapy with sex offenders traditionally involves some form of highly structured cognitive-behavioral therapy program. Some states (e.g., California, Texas) prohibit general psychotherapists without specialized training, certification, or subspecialty licensure in sex offender management from treating convicted sex offenders. It has become common to refer to mental health interventions with sex offenders as "treatment" or "management" rather than "psychotherapy." The underlying assumption of this philosophy is that the primary beneficiary of sex offender treatment should be society, not the individual offender, and that community safety takes precedence over the mental health needs of any individual offender. To that end, treatment is highly directive and focuses on taking full responsibility for the offending behavior and the cognitive restructuring of thinking errors and deficiencies in moral judgment that may have led to the behavior. Such treatment seeks to identify high-risk situations in which behavioral control might fail and attempts to teach cognitive and behavioral strategies that would help the offender avoid high-risk situations that could lead to reoffending.

More recently, treatment of problematic sexual behavior has incorporated the needs of the individual patient in addition to considering the needs of society (i.e., to reduce recidivism). For example, the Good Lives Model (Ward, 2002), a commonly used treatment program in prison and forensic hospital settings, adopts a strengths-based approach, acknowledging that all human beings desire a sense of happiness and fulfillment in their lives. Therapeutic interventions are aimed at building skills and encouraging individuals to find prosocial pathways to a "good life." The Good Lives Model has been integrated with the risk–needs–responsivity framework in some correctional settings (Ward & Fortune, 2013), with the goal of overcoming barriers that prevent individuals from engaging in treatment.

Sex offender treatment is not typically aimed at reducing sexual arousal, although it may address deviant arousal patterns through such cognitive-behavioral strategies as covert sensitization and olfactory conditioning (Corabian et al., 2011). It is more common to teach techniques for behavioral management of sexual arousal patterns or to prescribe medications, as described in the next section.

Treatment with testosterone-lowering medications

Androgen-lowering medications should be considered the treatment of choice for symptomatic paraphilic sex offenders (Bradford & Saleh, 2021; Saleh et al., 2010; Thibaut et al., 2020). Consistent with community treatment standards, incarcerated and symptomatic sex offenders should be afforded treatment with a testosterone-lowering agent to decrease the likelihood of sexual recidivism while decreasing paraphilic symptomatology. The World Federation of Societies of Biological Psychiatry creates guidelines and algorithms that could help clinicians to match an individual's clinical needs and risk with appropriate pharmacologic agents (Thibaut et al., 2020).

Prescribing androgen-lowering medications to incarcerated individuals raises complex legal and ethical concerns (Mellela et al., 1989; Miller, 1998; Ward et al., 2007). In the United States, as of 2015, nine states authorized some form of mandated surgical or pharmacological sex drive reduction treatment (commonly but erroneously referred to as "castration") as an adjunct to parole or probation supervision for certain sex offenders for whom release to the community from incarceration is being contemplated. The term "chemical castration" is a misnomer since "castration" necessarily refers to the surgical removal of gonads. Thus, in sex offenders, castration involves mutilation, including the irreversible destruction of healthy reproductive tissue, and renders the patient sterile as well as hormonally altered. Pharmacotherapy, by contrast, is nonmutilating and preserves healthy gonadal tissue while altering hormonal balance with the aim to decrease sexual drive. Pharmacological drive reduction does not typically interfere with spermatogenesis or the ability to reproduce. That being said, testosterone-lowering agents are not devoid of side effects, and proper informed consent should be obtained prior to commencement of treatment.

Jurisdictions vary in the permissibility of surgical or pharmacological drive reduction (Scott & Holmberg, 2003). Texas (Texas Government Code Annotated § 501.061 and § 508.226) provides for voluntary surgical castration as the only treatment option. California (California Penal Code § 645), Florida (Florida Statutes Annotated § 794.011-0235), Iowa (Iowa Code § 903B.1), and Louisiana (Louisiana Revised Statutes Annotated § 15:538) allow for some provision of either pharmacotherapy or voluntary surgical castration. Georgia (Georgia Code Annotated § 16-6-4 and §42-9-44.2), Montana (Montana Code Annotated § 45-5-512), Oregon (Oregon Revised Statutes §144.625–631), and Wisconsin (Wisconsin Statutes Annotated § 304.06 and § 980.08-12) permit the use of pharmacotherapy only. Numerous other states either have considered such laws or have judicial decisions that address the process without legislative authority (see *People v. Gauntlett*, 1984; *State v. Brown*, 1985). The practice has also been sanctioned in Canada and, at various times, in Denmark, Germany, Norway, Sweden, and Switzerland (Druhm, 1997).

In the various state actions and in numerous commentaries (see Druhm, 1997; Miller, 1998; Rice & Harris, 2011; Winslade et al., 1998), challenges are usually organized on Eighth Amendment (i.e., that the forced treatment is cruel and unusual punishment) or 14th Amendment grounds (i.e., the process is not sufficiently spelled out to satisfy due process concerns). These are usually counter to the argument that pharmacotherapy is a treatment with therapeutic value. Further complicating the issue is the fact that the medications have demonstrated efficacy only for individuals whose problematic behavior is based on sex drive; they have not shown efficacy for individuals whose behavior derives from anger or a hostile disposition.

Finally, the courts will have to resolve the issue that the statutes mentioned do not all provide for discrimination among offenders to ensure that only those who would benefit from treatment are actually receiving the treatment. To that end, the APA issued a position statement in 2021 against mandated "castration" laws without proper clinical assessment:

> The APA opposes laws that require orchiectomy (i.e., surgical removal of the testicles) or treatment with anti-androgen medications as a condition of release from incarceration. Orchiectomy or treatment with anti-androgen medications is appropriate only in cases where a psychiatrist has diagnosed a paraphilic disorder for which such treatment is indicated and where the patient has provided informed consent. (APA, 2021)

Clinicians also have to consider the consequences of withholding a medication that may help decrease a person's tormented, out-of-control feelings or impulses; lessen the intensity of paraphilic fantasies and urges, in turn facilitating fuller participation in a cognitive-behavioral program; and reduce the risk of reoffending.

Summary

The potential contributions of psychiatry to sex offender management span a considerable segment of the patient's life, from postarrest evaluation and emergent care through adjudication in the courts, incarceration, possible civil commitment, and supervised release. Nevertheless, as physicians and treaters, psychiatrists bring much-needed medical expertise to the discussion. Foremost is the ability of psychiatry to demonstrate that sex offenders are not a homogeneous population. Further, a rational, effective, and humane approach to the social problem of sex offending depends on accurate assessment, diagnosis, and treatment approaches for the individual. Psychiatrists can also inform the ongoing debate about competency, dangerousness, the appropriateness of civil commitment, lifelong sex offender registration, compulsory medication, and other medically relevant issues in sex offender management.

REFERENCES

American Psychiatric Association. (2016). *Psychiatric services in correctional facilities* (3rd ed.).

American Psychiatric Association. (2021). *Position statement orchiectomy or treatment with anti-androgen medications as a condition of release from incarceration.* https://www.psychiatry.org/getattachment/35b0c2aa-313a-4d53-893d-5c569c7dc286/Position-Orchiectomy-Anti-Androgen-Medication-Incarceration-Release-Condition.pdf

American Psychiatric Association. (2022). *Diagnostic and statistical manual of mental disorders* (5th ed., text rev.).

Bell v. Wolfish, 441 U.S. 520 (1979).

Berlin, F. (1986). Interviews with five rapists. *American Journal of Forensic Psychiatry, 41*, 11–41.

Bradford, J. M., & Saleh, F. M. (2021). Pharmacological treatment of paraphilic sex offenders. In F. M. Saleh Jr., J. M. Bradford, & D. J. Brodsky (Eds.), *Sex offenders: Identification, risk assessment, treatment, and legal issues* (2nd ed., Chapter 14). Oxford University Press.

California Penal Code § 645.

Clayton, S. L. (2002). Sex offenders. *Corrections Compendium, 27*, 8.

Cohen, F. (2003). Correctional mental health law & policy: A primer. *District of Columbia Law Review, 7*(1), 117–142.

Corabian, P., Dennett, L., & Harstall, C. (2011). Treatment for convicted adult male sex offenders: An overview of systematic reviews. *Sexual Offender Treatment, 6*, 1.

Druhm, K. W. (1997). Comment: A welcome return to Draconia: California Penal Law 645, the castration of sex offenders and the Constitution. *Albany Law Review, 61*, 285.

Elwood, R. W. (2009). Mental disorder, predisposition, prediction, and ability to control: Evaluating sex offenders for civil commitment. *Sexual Abuse: A Journal of Research and Treatment, 21*(4), 395–411.

Estelle v. Gamble, 429 U.S. 97 (1976).

Fagan, P. J., Lehne, G., Strand, J., & Berlin, F. (2005). Paraphilias. In G. O. Gabbard, J. S. Beck, & J. Holmes (Eds.), *Oxford textbook of psychotherapy* (pp. 215–227). Oxford University Press.

Farkas, M. A., & Miller, G. (2008). Sex offender treatment: Reconciling criminal justice priorities and therapeutic goals. *Federal Sentencing Reporter, 21*, 78.

Farmer v. Brennan, 511 U.S. 825 (1994).

Federal Bureau of Investigation. (2019). *Data tables: Crimes against persons offenses.* https://ucr.fbi.gov/nibrs/2019/tables/pdfs/crimes_against_persons_offenses_offense_category_by_state_2019.pdf

Federal Bureau of Investigation. (2024). *FBI crime data explorer.* https://cde.ucr.cjis.gov/LATEST/webapp/#/pages/explorer/crime/crime-trend

Florida Statutes Annotated § 794.011-0235.

Georgia Code Annotated § 16-6-4 and §42-9-44.2.

Hafemeister, T. L., & Petrila, J. (1994). Treating the mentally disordered offender: Society's uncertain, conflicted, and changing views. *Florida State University Law Review, 21*, 731-869.

Iowa Code § 903B.1.

Kansas v. Hendricks, 521 U.S. 346, 359 (1997).

Kendler, K. S. (1990). Toward a scientific psychiatric nosology. *Archives of General Psychiatry, 47*, 969–973.

LaFond, J. Q., & Winick, B.J. (1998). Special theme: Sex offenders: Scientific, legal, and policy perspective. Foreword: Sex offenders and the law. *Psychology, Public Policy, and Law, 3*, 3.

Langan, P. A., Schmitt, E. L., & Durose M. R. (2003). *Recidivism of sex offenders released from prison in 1994.* U.S. Department of Justice.

Lehne, G. K. (1986). Brain damage and paraphilia: Treated with medroxyprogesterone acetate. *Sexuality and Disability, 7,* 145–158.

Louisiana Revised Statutes Annotated § 15:538.

McKune v. Lile, 536 U.S. 24 (2002).

Mellela, J. T., Travin, S., & Cullen, K. (1989). Legal and ethical issues in the use of antiandrogens in treating sex offenders. *Bulletin of American Academy of Psychiatry and Law, 17*(3), 222–233.

Miller, R. D. (1998). Forced administration of sex-drive-reducing medication to sex offenders: Treatment or punishment? *Psychology, Public Policy, and Law, 4*(1–2), 175–199.

Montana Code Annotated § 45-5-512.

Oregon Revised Statutes §144.625–631.

People v. Gauntlett, 352 N.W.2d 310 (Mich. Ct. App. 1984).

Prentky, R., Knight, R., & Lee, A. (1997). *Child sexual molestation: Research issues.* U.S. Department of Justice.

Rice, M. E., & Harris, G. T. (2011). Is androgen deprivation therapy effective in the treatment of sex offenders? *Psychology, Public Policy, and Law, 17,* 315.

Saleh, F. M., Grudzinskas, A. J., Malin, H. M., & Dwyer, G. (2010). The management of sex offenders: Perspectives for psychiatry. *Harvard Review of Psychiatry, 18*(6), 359–368.

Scott, C. L., & Holmberg, T. (2003). Castration of sex offenders: Prisoners' right versus public safety. *Journal of the American Academy of Psychiatry and the Law, 31,* 502–509.

Stabenow, T. (2009). *Deconstructing the myth of careful study: A primer on the flawed progression of the child pornography guidelines 2-3.* Retrieved January 16, 2014, from http://www.fd.org/pdf_lib/child%20porn%20 july%20revision.pdf

State v. Brown, 326 S.E.2d 410 (S.C. 1985).

Texas Government Code Annotated § 501.061 and § 508.226.

Thibaut, F., Cosyns, P., Fedoroff, J. P., Briken, P., Goethals, K., & Bradford, J. M. W. (2020). The World Federation of Societies of Biological Psychiatry (WFSBP) 2020 guidelines for the pharmacological treatment of paraphilic disorders. *World Journal of Biological Psychiatry, 21*(6), 412–490.

U.S. Sentencing Commission. (2021). *FY 2017 through FY 2021 datafiles, USSCFY17–USSCFY21.* https://www.ussc.gov/research/datafiles/commission-datafiles

U.S. Sentencing Commission. (2023). *QuickFacts: Child pornography offenses.* https://www.ussc.gov/research/quick-facts/child-pornography#:~:text=Punishment,average%20sentence%20was%20114%20months.&text=87.3%25%20of%20these%20individuals%20were,average%20sentence%20was%20135%20months

Ward, T. (2002). The management of risk and the design of good lives. *Australian Psychologist, 37*(3), 172–179.

Ward, T., & Fortune, C.-A. (2013). The Good Lives Model: Aligning risk reduction with promoting offenders' personal goals. *European Journal of Probation, 5*(2), 29–46.

Ward, T., Gannon, T. A., & Birgden, A. (2007). Human rights and the treatment of sex offenders. *Sexual Abuse, 19*(3), 195–216.

Winslade, W., Stone, T. H., Smith-Bell, M., & Webb, D. M. (1998). Castrating pedophiles convicted of sex offenses against children: New treatment or old punishment? *SMU Law Review, 51,* 349.

Wisconsin Statutes § 304.06 and § 980.08-12.

64

Clinical and legal implications of gangs

Annette L. Hanson

Introduction

Gangs are a fact of life in jails and prisons. Psychiatrists need to be aware of the dynamics of gang leadership, membership, and involvement when working with any gang member, as that may affect their ability to participate in and interest in collaborative treatment. This chapter presents a review of gang prevalence and the roles gangs play in the community and in correctional settings and then discusses historical context, institutional management techniques, and approaches to therapeutic intervention.

History and prevalence of gangs

A gang has commonly been defined as a group of three or more individuals who engage in criminal activity and that identifies itself with a common name or sign (Martin et al., 2011). Under federal law, a gang has been defined as an ongoing association of five or more persons whose primary purpose is to commit one or more interstate criminal offenses in the previous 5 years (18 U.S.C. § 521). Within correctional facilities, the more generic term "security threat group" (STG) has been used to denote a group of two or more individuals who represent a threat to the security or orderly management of the facility and who act in concert to disrupt programs and activities. The STG designation recognizes that certain organized activities such as possession and distribution of tobacco would not be considered a crime in free society but would be considered a violation of correctional rules in some facilities. Regardless of designation, both prison gangs and STGs are often bound by common ideological, ethnic, or racial ties. They have an organizational structure that includes a leader, a council, a code of conduct, and oaths of loyalty and secrecy. Violence is a common price of admission to membership, as well as a consequence of disloyalty or withdrawal (Pyrooz, 2020).

The first prison gangs arose in California in the 1950s and 1960s, and many of these early gangs are nationally known today, including the Crips, Bloods, Aryan Brotherhood, Black Guerrilla Family, MS-13, and Black Gangster Disciples. The boundaries of any given gang are fluid, and they may blend with regional chapters or groups that assume the name of a national organization but have no formal or official ties to it. New gangs have formed due to the resettlement of refugees, such as Somalian and Vietnamese street gangs in the Upper Midwest (Ellis et al., 2022). Finally, gangs may form within a prison system for protection from a larger gang. For example, in 2000, a group of White prisoners banded together in the Maryland prison system to form Dead Man Inc., which now has a national presence (Howell & Moore, 2010).

According to the National Gang Intelligence Center, in 2010 there were approximately 1.4 million members of 33,000 street and prison gangs in the United States. This represents a 40% increase over gang membership reported by federal, state, and local law enforcement and correctional systems in 2009 (National Gang Intelligence Center, 2011). While the exact prevalence of gang affiliation in correctional facilities is not known, studies have shown that between 9% and 24% of prisoners have affiliations to street or prison gangs (Gaes et al., 2002; Griffin & Hepburn, 2006; Jackson & Sharpe, 1997; New Jersey Commission of Investigation, 2013). As many as 480 active prison gangs in the United States have been identified, including at least five that operate nationally (Boyd, 2010).

Prison gangs and the challenges they present are not unique to the United States (Coid et al., 2013). In 2011, the Inter-American Commission on Human Rights called for reform after a clash between gangs in one Venezuelan prison left 19 prisoners dead and 25 seriously injured (Inter-American Commission on Human Rights, 2011). Similarly, a gang war in Brazil's fourth largest prison caused the deaths of 59 prisoners in a single year, some killed through beheading or torture (BBC, 2013). American prison and street gangs with Mexican, Caribbean, and South American connections such as MS-13, La Eme, Latin, Surenos, and Nortenos also have ties to international drug trafficking organizations (Hull, 2020).

Although there has been an increase in gang-affiliated female prisoners, relatively less is known about this group than about male gang members. In one of the few studies of female prisoners, Scott and Ruddell (2011) found that female gang members had more past convictions, were more likely to be assigned to a higher security level, and were more likely to have been incarcerated in the juvenile justice system than nongang members. There are several social theories to explain the motivation for joining a gang. One large random sample of 7,212 adolescents drawn from a national longitudinal health study found little evidence that risk factors for gang involvement differed between male and female teenagers. Neighborhood disadvantage, parent–child relationship factors, school safety, and exposure to violent peers were risk factors for both genders (Bell, 2009). Of more concern is the observation that female gang members are more likely to serve an intelligence-gathering function and may seek employment in law enforcement or government agencies for this purpose (Scott & Ruddell, 2011).

Sexual orientation plays a role in both gang affiliation and desistance. Panfil (2020) found in an interview with 48 gay street gang members that some left the gang to establish life more authentically as a gay individual. Gangs composed solely of homosexual members maintained their gang affiliation because the gang provided psychological support as a "chosen family."

Community-based gangs are bound by a common antisocial interest or criminal activity, including drug distribution, weapons trafficking, prostitution, human smuggling, and violent crimes such as robbery. In jail and prison, by virtue of the more controlled environment, there is a shift toward acquisition of property or other privileges, such as cell phones, tobacco, sex, drugs, and extra food or clothing. Gangs have also been known to direct loan shark and gambling operations within a jail or prison. Gang-related violence is generally intended to protect territory and distribution channels rather than for direct financial gain. Gangs have been known to plan and carry out assaults on other prisoners and to contract with another gang to carry out "hits" on officers, prisoners, or witnesses outside the facility. Witness intimidation is a necessary aspect of gang life, and a newly recruited member may be asked to take part in this as an initiation ritual. The financial side of gang business takes place mainly outside the facility between associates of the prison gang (typically the buyer) and the community-based gang (the seller or provider).

The extent and impact of gang activity on a facility will depend on the size and geographic location of the facility. Smaller jails and prisons and facilities in rural areas are more likely to be involved with local or regional groups, also known as street gangs, while large facilities in urban areas will be affected more by nationally known or connected gangs.

The impact of gangs within a facility is considerable. One survey of Florida prisoners found that prisoners who were suspected or confirmed gang members were 35% more likely to commit violent acts than nonmembers (Cunningham & Sorensen, 2007). Similarly, a study of 82,504 individuals in the Federal Bureau of Prisons found that gang membership was associated with increased violent behavior as well as less serious rule infractions. Further, the likelihood of violent misconduct was higher for members who were core to the organization rather than peripheral. However, even peripheral members were more likely to commit violence than nonmembers (Gaes et al., 2002). In a study of 2,158 male prisoners in the Arizona Department of Corrections, gang-affiliated individuals were more than twice as likely as nonaffiliated prisoners to commit an assault during the first 3 years of confinement, even when controlled for age, ethnicity, commitment offense, prior incarceration, sentence length, and security level (Griffin & Hepburn, 2006).

Since the terrorist attacks on September 11, 2001, prison gangs have also become a potential national security risk. Gangs espousing strong antigovernment, prorevolutionary views have drawn the attention of counterterrorism experts, particularly since some domestic terrorists are now housed in federal prison. The "radicalization" of prison gangs is an ongoing concern. To address this issue, the National Gang Intelligence Center was created in 2005 to establish information-sharing networks between the Federal Bureau of Investigation; the Drug Enforcement Administration; the Bureau of Alcohol, Tobacco, Firearms and Explosives; the Federal Bureau of Prisons; Immigrations and Customs Enforcement; and the Department of Defense. Law enforcement databases share information between these agencies and typically include identifying information, gang affiliation, known associates, and tattoos or other identifying characteristics of any confirmed gang member. The National Gang Intelligence Center issues regular threat assessment reports to track gang trends and networks nationally. The Federal Bureau of Investigation's Cryptanalysis and Racketeering Records Unit has a Tattoo and Graffiti team that aids investigation of prison gangs by breaking coded messages between prisoners and outside gang members (Foundos & Hirschfield, 2019).

Institutional management

The National Gang Intelligence Center maintains a list of confirmed prison gangs and provides support for gang-related investigations within facilities. For more regionalized gangs, many institutions have a policy for establishing which group of individuals should be deemed an STG. An STG designation can be given based on involvement with or connection to a known, established organization, or it may be an internal group identified by institutional intelligence-gathering methods. Policies regarding the identification and management of gang members vary significantly between states (Li, 2023).

Once a group is designated as an established gang or STG, newly received detainees are assessed for affiliation. The facility may have an STG specialist who interviews the detainee to determine if they actually are a gang member and to gather intelligence about gang structure, involved members, distribution, and activities. The STG officer may ask if the prisoner knows certain basic principles of a given gang, such as a gang credo, hand symbol, or other signs. They may be asked about participation in gang-related violence or institutional misconduct. Once this determination is made, the person is said to be a "validated" gang member. Validation allows the institution to manage the detainee with special security measures such as placing them in a higher security facility or in restricted housing or to restrict liberty within the facility. Thirteen states segregate prisoners who are validated gang members (Columbia Human Rights Law Review, 2021). Most prison systems use a variety of gang control and suppression strategies such as sharing intelligence with law enforcement, monitoring institutional mail and phone calls, and using modern data-mining approaches (Winterdyk & Ruddell, 2010). Jail and prison policies typically consider any attempt to recruit for a gang as a violation of institutional rules.

For detainees or sentenced prisoners not identified at intake, gang validation may be made later during incarceration if the person participates in a gang-related crime or rule violation or is identified as an associate of a validated gang member. They could also be identified later through inclusion in a law enforcement gang database. Other identifiers could be authorship or possession of gang-related documents, pictures with validated members, or possession of gang-related books.

Over time, correctional strategies to control gangs have alternated between gang suppression and gang dispersal efforts. Dispersion, or transfer of gang leaders to out-of-state systems, eventually was shown to be ineffective in that it inadvertently provided an opportunity for a gang to establish itself in new territory (Pyrooz, 2022). Suppression involved placing leaders in isolation through long-term segregation (i.e., restrictive housing). Advocacy groups challenged this practice as being arbitrary and inhumane (Columbia Human Rights Law Review, 2021). More recently, prison systems have created policies that allow gang members to work their way out of long-term segregation or avoid it completely through a gang renunciation program.

The renunciation program used in the Texas prison system requires the prisoner to be housed in a specialized unit for several weeks while completing several modules designed to help them manage life without a gang (Mandeville, 2004). Other renunciation programs provide anger management training, treatment for substance use disorders, and job skills training. During renunciation, the prisoner is required to live on a tier with members of competing gangs for a period of time without sustaining any infractions. Once this process is complete, they are allowed to transfer to the general prison population in a regular facility without a gang-labeled status. Unfortunately, some who renounce gang membership may rejoin later, and there are few outcome studies to prove the effectiveness of any particular gang management policy (Pyrooz, 2022).

Legal challenges to gang management

Initially, street and prison gangs were prosecuted under the federal Racketeer Influenced and Corrupt Organizations Act (RICO), which designated certain crimes as racketeering offenses when committed for the purpose of furthering or supporting an existing criminal enterprise (RICO, 1970). Any money gained through this organized illegal activity was considered "unlawful debt" subject to seizure, and the participant could be sentenced to 20 years to a life sentence depending on the underlying offense. RICO was used to prosecute mafia families in the 1970s, as well as certain outlaw motorcycle gangs involved in interstate trafficking of weapons.

The limitation of RICO for prison gang prosecution was that the law could only be used if there was proof of money-laundering activities or interstate crime. For a prison-based gang, financial transactions are often conducted through the use of disposable prepaid cell phones or through cash transfers made by phone applications.

To address this problem, many states adapted variations of RICO in local antigang legislation. The goal of state legislation was to punish recruitment of youth into gangs, as well as the gang's criminal activity. Antigang legislation allowed prosecution for a criminal act with additional criminal liability under state racketeering laws if the act was committed to further the goals of the organization. The laws allowed for enhanced sentencing and for expert testimony at trial regarding the nature, culture, and symbols or signs of known gangs. Presently, all 50 states and the District of Columbia, as well as the federal government, have laws to target and enhance sentencing for those convicted of gang-related criminal activity (Hildebrand, 2022).

Legal efforts to break up and control gangs have not gone unchallenged. Sentence enhancements based on a single gang-related offense may be considered a violation of double jeopardy, and there have been challenges to the admissibility of law enforcement expert testimony about gang culture (Hayat, 2021; Hildebrand, 2022).

Since institutional management often involves restriction of privileges, placement in long-term restrictive housing, or transfer to a control unit prison, advocacy groups and individual prisoners have filed suit against these policies based on First and Eighth Amendment, religious freedom, and antidiscrimination claims (Columbia Human Rights Law Review, 2021). Gang validation procedures have been challenged as arbitrary and inaccurate, leading to inappropriate segregation or restrictions on prisoners who have exhibited no institutional violence.

Unfortunately, religious services have been used to facilitate gang meetings, promote extremism, and plan criminal activity. The Civil Rights of Institutionalized Persons Act protects the religious freedom of prisoners under the section known as the Protection of Religious Exercise in Land Use and by Institutionalized Persons Act (RLUIPA, 2000). Any effort to investigate gang activity by monitoring religious services or to control gang communication by restricting religious services or practices would likely fall within the reach of an RLUIPA claim. Religious affiliation alone has also been barred as a basis for gang validation.

Housing assignments used to prevent intragang violence or to suppress gang leadership have been challenged under both Eighth Amendment and antidiscrimination laws. In *Johnson v. California* (2005), a prisoner sued the California Department of Corrections over a policy that segregated prisoners by race temporarily, pending a regular housing assignment. This policy was defended as nondiscriminatory since all prisoners were subject to it and because it was reasonably related to institutional security. The U.S. Supreme Court reversed the lower court's judgment that upheld the policy and ruled that any prison policy based solely on race should be held to a strict scrutiny standard rather than following traditional deference to the judgment of prison officials. Similarly, Eighth Amendment claims against the use of long-term solitary confinement have been brought when the sole reason for the restrictive housing placement was to separate a gang leader from the general population, absent proof of institutional rule breaking or violence (Columbia Human Rights Law Review, 2021).

Aside from body cavity searches, courts have generally held that prisoners do not have a right to privacy. Gang control policies often include the examination of mail for coded communication and the monitoring of phone calls between identified gang members. Property such as gang-related reading material may be seized if the seizure is reasonably related to a legitimate penological purpose. Since some gangs are based on religious affiliation, reading material can only be banned if it encourages violence, undermines rehabilitation, or represents a threat to institutional security.

Implications for the clinician

CASE VIGNETTE

The patient is a 23-year-old man incarcerated for a misdemeanor theft. As a prison maintenance worker, he had access to tools and locations in the facility that would allow for an escape. Gang members on the tier attempted to coerce him into the escape plan, but he resisted and reported the plan to the security chief. While the investigation was pending, he was moved to a restrictive housing unit for protective custody. Gang-affiliated officers there made implied threats and warned him not to cooperate with the investigation. On segregation rounds, he asked to be seen in the mental health department, where he expressed fear for his safety but exhibited no signs of clinical depression or other evidence of mental illness. He asked the institutional clinician to contact the security chief so that he could reveal the names of the gang-involved officers. He had no external family or relationships to rely on for support.

Discussion

In this vignette, the patient revealed the presence of gangs to the correctional psychiatrist. While at present it is not a standard of clinical care to question correctional patients about gang involvement or gang activity on a tier, this knowledge can inform the clinician's assessment of a patient's mental state and safety risk. Unfortunately, there is little information available in the literature regarding how to do this, and gang assessment is not part of traditional psychiatric training or orientation to correctional facilities.

In most situations, information can be obtained by directly questioning patients periodically about safety concerns on the tier and about their own observations. A prison or jail patient may observe that access to the telephone is controlled by a group of prisoners or that there are rivalries on the unit between factions of those on the tier. A prisoner or detainee may report that they have been asked to hold contraband or keep quiet about smuggling or other illicit activity. They may express frustration that volunteer jobs on the unit are given preferentially to gang members, a sign that the gang may be colluding with correctional staff. They may report pressure from others to join a gang. An individual who frequently seeks psychiatric admission or repeatedly requests protective custody should raise a concern about gang influence.

The correctional psychiatrist who learns of gang activity in the facility has a duty to help the patient negotiate the risks this situation poses to them but also has a duty to ensure institutional safety. Reporting gang members to custody could place the patient in danger since an investigation can only take place based on information from an identified reliable informant. The principles of nonmaleficence and respect for patient confidentiality dictate that the clinician explore the potential ramifications of disclosure with the patient and act in accordance with the prisoner or detainee's wishes. An individual who wants to cooperate with an investigation should be offered the option of protective housing, if such an offer is within the clinician's authority. Involuntary protective custody should be avoided since this could bar the patient from jobs, programs, and activities they would normally have access to. If the gang activity presents a serious enough risk of imminent danger to the unit or institution, such as an impending riot or planned violence, the traditional duty to warn or protect third parties would apply. The advantage of cooperation would be to clear the patient of any potential connection or involvement with the gang and to avoid the risk of guilt by association.

There is evidence to suggest that gang members are more likely to suffer from mental disorders and to use psychiatric services than other prisoners. A 2013 study of 4,664 men in Great Britain compared prevalence of mental disorders, mental health service use, and suicide attempts among violent men according to gang membership. The gang members were more likely to have seen a psychiatrist or psychologist, to have been admitted to a psychiatric hospital, and to have attempted suicide (Coid et al., 2013). Gang members are also more likely than non–gang members to exhibit symptoms of anxiety, paranoia, and posttraumatic stress disorder (Wood & Dennard, 2017).

When assessing a correctional patient who is also a gang member, several additional questions should be asked to inform treatment. Table 64.1 includes a list of suggested questions.

Table 64.1 Suggested assessment questions for gang members

1. Which gang are you part of?
2. How long have you been a member?
3. Did you join in the community or in the facility?
4. What led you to join?
5. What role do you play in the gang?
6. Have you ever thought about leaving the gang or have you tried to leave?
7. What happened when you tried to leave?
8. Is anyone harassing you or threatening you here?
9. Do you owe anybody money?
10. Have you been asked to hold contraband?
11. Are you being pressured to do something you don't want to do?
12. What have they said would happen if you don't go along with them?
13. Is your family safe? Do you have concerns about friends, family, or children on the outside?
14. If you move to another facility, will this problem follow you?
15. How long has this been going on?
16. Do you want to report this activity to the security chief?

The answers to these questions will reveal potential vulnerability to victimization or coercion, potential for violence, and the strength of gang affiliation. While a prisoner may join a gang for protection, gang membership actually increases the risk of being a victim of violence. While there are few published studies, fear of retaliatory violence can also be a risk factor for self-injury, particularly when the intended target is an outside family member or loved one. Retaliatory violence can also take place when a member decides to leave a gang, and the risk can carry over into the community following release (Pyrooz, 2020). The strength of gang affiliation and the degree of involvement are relevant in that more peripherally involved gang members are more likely to renounce and leave the group than key members.

Documenting the answers to these questions poses another dilemma for the correctional clinician. In a system that uses a combined medical and psychiatric record system, the correctional psychiatrist should be circumspect about documenting specific information regarding a patient who reports corruption, who cooperates with internal gang prevention efforts, or who frankly acknowledges involvement in illegal gang activities.

Correctional psychiatrists should also be aware that prisoners can use an institutional mental health system to facilitate gang business. In a facility that uses a "pill line" to pass medication, the pharmacy window can become an unofficial gang meeting place. Medication passes have been stolen or forged because they give relative freedom of movement through a facility at specified times of the day. For this reason, a medication pass is sometimes called a "skate" in prison slang. A prisoner may press a psychiatrist to prescribe medication to get a medication pass.

Gangs have also used the psychiatric infirmary. A gang member may seek admission to follow or get close to an intended target. A psychiatric unit may be used as a meeting place for gang members from separate tiers. When a prisoner seeks frequent admission, the clinician should ask the tier officer about any gang-related connections between admitted patients or about gang conflicts that might be a factor in the admission.

Psychiatric medications may be traded and sold as a commodity to support gang business. Any medication with sedative effects has economic value within a jail or prison and will support a gang's underground or black market trade. Also, vulnerable psychiatric patients may be coerced or intimidated into giving up their prescribed medication. Judicious use of medication with abuse potential will decrease the likelihood of this activity (Tamburello et al., 2022).

Gang-led, organized hunger strikes will require the involvement of an institutional psychiatrist. Hunger strike policies typically require that the striker's competency be assessed on a regular basis to determine their understanding of the effects of starvation and determine if the decision to strike is free of coercion. If the tier and the hunger strike were under the control of a gang, an unaffiliated prisoner would likely feel a high degree of coercion to cooperate with the strike.

All gang influence is not negative, however. Some prisoners or detainees organize themselves into protective groups centered on religious studies—a self-labeled "God gang." And in the author's experience, even a hardened gang once banded together to make sure a formerly manic prisoner took his medication when he was known to become violent when ill. Gangs may also coordinate with external civil rights organizations to promote improved prison conditions or progressive criminal justice policies (Li, 2023).

Summary

Gang management is a challenge for correctional institutions; treating gang members with psychiatric illness is a challenge for psychiatry. Understanding the background, motivation, and dynamics of gangs is an important aspect of psychiatric practice in jails and prisons. Psychiatric care is best when it is informed by sensitivity to the culture, environmental effects, and individual impact of gangs on the correctional patient.

REFERENCES

18 U.S.C. § 521(a).

BBC. (2013). *Gang war in Brazil's Pedrinhas jail kills 59 in 2013.* Retrieved January 5, 2014, from http://www.bbc.co.uk/news/world-latin-america-25536187.

Bell, K. (2009). Gender and gangs: A quantitative comparison. *Crime and Delinquency, 55*, 363–387.

Boyd, S. (2010). Implementing the missing peace: Reconsidering prison gang management. *Quinnipiac Law Review, 28*, 969–1018.

Coid, J., Ullrich, S., Keers, R., Bebbington, P., DeStavola, B., Kallis, C., et al. (2013). Gang membership, violence, and psychiatric morbidity. *American Journal of Psychiatry, 170*, 985–993.

Columbia Human Rights Law Review. (2021). *Security classification and gang validation.* https://jlm.law.columbia.edu/files/2021/02/38.-Chapter-31.pdf

Cunningham, M., & Sorensen, J. (2007). Predictive factors for violent misconduct in close custody. *The Prison Journal, 87*, 241–253.

Ellis, B., Decker, H., Abdi, M., Miller, B., Barrett, C., & Lincoln, K. (2022). A qualitative examination of how Somali young adults think about and understand violence in their communities. *Journal of Interpersonal Violence, 37*(1–2), NP803–NP829.

Foundos, N., & Hirschfield, J. (2019, December 9). *Focus on forensics: Tattoo and symbol analysis in the FBI.* https://leb.fbi.gov/articles/focus/focus-on-forensics-tattoo-and-symbol-analysis-in-the-fbi

Gaes, G., Wallace, S., Gilman, E., Klein-Saffran, J., & Suppa, S. (2002). The influence of prison gang affiliation on violence and other prison misconduct. *The Prison Journal, 82*, 359–385.

Griffin, M., & Hepburn, J. (2006). The effect of gang affiliation on violent misconduct among inmates during the early years of confinement. *Criminal Justice and Behavior, 33*, 419–448.

Hayat, F. N. (2021). Preserving due process: Require the Frye and Daubert expert standards in state gang cases. *New Mexico Law Review, 51*(1), 196–233.

Hildebrand, S. (2022). Racialized implications of officer gang expert testimony. *Mississippi Law Journal, 92*(1), 155–194.

Howell, J., & Moore, J. (2010). *History of street gangs in the United States.* https://www.ojp.gov/ncjrs/virtual-library/abstracts/history-street-gangs-united-states

Hull, S. (2020). Jail and prison communications in gang investigations. *Department of Justice Journal of Federal Law and Practice, 68*(5), 9–14.

Inter-American Commission on Human Rights. (2011). *IACHR deplores violent deaths in Venezuelan prison.* http://www.oas.org/en/iachr/media_center/PReleases/2011/057.asp

Jackson, M., & Sharpe, E. (1997). Prison gang research: Preliminary findings in eastern North Carolina. *Journal of Gang Research, 5*, 1–7.

Johnson v. California, 543 U.S. 499 (2005).

Li, G. (2023). Associations in prison. *UC Irvine Law Review, 13*(4), 1119–1186.

Mandeville, M. (2004). *Leaving gang life behind in Texas.* http://www.corrections.com/news/article/3071

Martin, R., Gwynne, J., Parillo, R., Younker, B., & Carter, R. (2011). Alabama prison gang survey. *Journal of Gang Research, 18*, 1–19.

National Gang Intelligence Center. (2011). *National gang threat assessment: Emerging trends 2011.* http://www.fbi.gov/stats-services/publications/2011-national-gang-threat-assessment

New Jersey Commission of Investigation. (2013). *Gangland behind bars: How and why organized criminal street gangs thrive in New Jersey's prisons.* http://nicic.gov/Library/025742

Panfil, V. R. (2020). "I was homo thug, now I'm just homo": Gay gang members' desistance and persistence. *Criminology, 58*(2), 255–279.

Protection of Religious Exercise in Land Use and by Institutionalized Persons Act, Title 42, U.S.C. Section 2000 (2000).

Pyrooz, D. C. (2020, April 3). *We spoke to hundreds of prison gang members—Here's what they said about life behind bars.* https://theconversation.com/we-spoke-to-hundreds-of-prison-gang-members-heres-what-they-said-about-life-behind-bars-132573

Pyrooz, D. C. (2022). The prison and the gang. *Crime and Justice, 51*, 237–306.

Racketeer Influenced and Corrupt Organizations Act (RICO), Title 18, U.S.C. Chapter 96 (1970).

Scott, T., & Ruddell, R. (2011). Canadian female gang inmates: Risks, needs, and the potential for prison rehabilitation. *Journal of Offender Rehabilitation, 50*, 305–326.

Tamburello, A., Penn, J., Ford, E., et al. (2022). Practice resource for prescribing in corrections. *Journal of the American Academy of Psychiatry and the Law, 50*(4 Suppl.), S1–S62.

Winterdyk, J., & Ruddell, R. (2010). Managing prison gangs: Results from a survey of U.S. prison systems. *Journal of Criminal Justice, 38*, 730–736.

Wood, J., & Dennard, S. (2017). Gang membership: Links to violence exposure, paranoia, PTSD, anxiety, and forced control of behavior in prison. *Psychiatry, 80*(1), 30–41.

SECTION XI
Special topics

65
Staff wellness

Elizabeth B. Ford

Introduction

The safety and care of incarcerated people, a marginalized and underprivileged population in the United States with higher rates of mental health disorders (Bureau of Justice Statistics, 2017, 2021) and trauma exposure (Liu et al., 2021) than the general population, is the responsibility of varied staff, including custodial staff such as correctional officers or sheriff's deputies; health care staff such as physicians, nurses, psychologists, social workers, counselors, and dentists; and a range of additional staff that may include religious leaders, employment specialists, teachers, and peer specialists. These staff are exposed to work conditions in facilities that are frequently overcrowded, underresourced, geographically and technologically isolated, and challenging to their mission. To varying degrees based on their roles and supervisory levels, staff face a lack of control over their work environment such as restricted movement, limited privacy, regulations about personal items, and unexpected security concerns that may affect their work hours (Subedi et al., 2023). The physical and emotional health of staff is critical to providing safe care for those in custody.

The National Institute for Occupational Safety and Health (NIOSH) has identified 10 "issues relevant to advancing worker well-being" that track across workplace settings: prevention and control of hazards and exposures, built environment supports, community supports, compensation and benefits, healthy leadership, organization of work, policies, technology, work arrangements, and workforce demographics (NIOSH, 2016). Carceral settings face specific challenges in each of these areas that make the maintenance of staff well-being difficult. As examples, managing risk includes understanding and humanely addressing interpersonal violence. Policy development often involves decisions that are made outside of the facilities because of litigation or legislation. With continued mass incarceration, there is limited ability to match workforce quantity and quality with the volume and needs of people who are incarcerated. Without adequate quantity, quality, and allocation of staff, mental health care in a jail or prison can grind to a halt.

Because of the symbiotic relationship that exists between carceral health care staff and correctional officers, and the impact of one group's well-being on the other, as well as on the health of people who are incarcerated, this chapter will discuss wellness for both groups, identifying several areas where strategies may differ based on role, training, environmental stressors, and agency mission.

Health risks

Individuals who care for traumatized populations are themselves likely to experience trauma symptoms such as intrusion, avoidance, or arousal (Robinson-Keilig et al., 2014). Available data indicate that correctional officers are at high risk for suicide (Bureau of Labor Statistics, 2022); mental health disorders such as mood, anxiety, and trauma-related disorders (Carleton et al., 2020; Ellison & Jaegers, 2022; James & Todak, 2018); substance use (Jayawardene et al., 2024); obesity; hypertension; injury; and early death due to chronic illness (El Ghaziri et al., 2020).

The prevalence of these illnesses in carceral mental health care staff is less well known or studied. However, a survey distributed to correctional officers and health care staff representing a range of disciplines in 78 jails and prisons across four Mid-Atlantic states revealed that 48% of health care staff had depressive symptoms, and 50% had symptoms of posttraumatic stress disorder (Burhanullah et al., 2022). These numbers were higher than for the correctional officers, 32% of whom had depressive symptoms and 45% of whom had symptoms of posttraumatic stress disorder.

Witnessing physical or verbal assaults is a near-universal experience across disciplines that work in carceral settings, and staff are assured of being directly or indirectly exposed to the trauma histories and related behaviors of incarcerated persons (IPs). Correctional officers are among the most at-risk professions for workplace assault, with one study finding that 16% of officers in 18 jails had been physically assaulted in the last year (Ellison & Gainey, 2020). While health care staff are less likely to be direct victims of physical violence than correctional officers, the risk of victimization is a significant source of anxiety and fear for carceral health care staff. For mental health professionals who practice in dangerous or life-threatening situations, such as in prisons, as provider distress increases, professional competence decreases (Johnson et al., 2011).

Burnout

Occupational burnout was defined by Maslach and Jackson (1981) as emotional exhaustion, depersonalization, and a reduced sense of accomplishment. Burnout is especially prevalent in occupations that are "people intensive" and emotionally challenging, particularly public safety, medicine, social work, and education

(Forman-Dolan et al., 2022). Many carceral settings include professionals from all four of these professions. Burnout significantly contributes to reduced staff wellness, staff and patient safety, health care competence, and productivity; it can lead to medical and psychiatric morbidity and mortality (Hanae & Giddings, 2017). A complete discussion of the associated conditions that accompany working with traumatized populations in high-risk settings (e.g., secondary traumatic stress and compassion fatigue; Figley, 1995) is outside the scope of this chapter; burnout will be used to describe these conditions generally.

Armstrong and Griffin's (2004) study of 3,794 employees in adult state prisons in the United States indicated little difference between correctional officers and treatment personnel with respect to contributors to job stress and health. For both groups, longer tenure in the job, safety concerns, role problems (e.g., lack of clarity about responsibility, dual loyalty), and a lack of organizational support contributed to higher levels of stress. Intrinsic rewards and positive coworker support alleviated job stress in both groups.

A more recent systematic review identified five organizational factors that influenced burnout levels among front-line carceral staff: *factors intrinsic to the job role* (e.g., poor physical working conditions, work overload, time pressures, isolation, and meaningfulness of work), *role in the organization* (e.g., role ambiguity and high levels of responsibility with unclear boundaries), *career development* (e.g., over- or underpromotion and job security), *relationships at work* (e.g., threats of violence, unsupportive management, and harassment), and *organizational structure/climate* (e.g., rigid management style and lack of shared decision-making; Forman-Dolan et al., 2022).

Research indicates that correctional officers face higher rates of stress and burnout than the general population and personnel from other law enforcement agencies (El Ghaziri et al., 2020), although barriers remain to understanding the scope of the problem. Continued stigma associated with mental health and help seeking among correctional staff and concern about "tarnishing" an agency's reputation (National Institute of Corrections, 2016) may contribute to underreporting. Officers express distrust of institutional Employee Assistance Programs, confidentiality concerns, a lack of psychological safety, and fear of the impact of help seeking on work privileges such as security clearances and authorization to carry a firearm (Lambert et al., 2015).

Burnout in community mental health professionals is well studied. For example, 73% of American psychiatrists surveyed who completed the Oldenburg Burnout Scale were found to be at risk for burnout (American Psychiatric Association [APA], 2018), with higher risk for female gender, recent medical school graduation, and perceived lack of control over one's schedule. Among psychiatrists without depression, burnout scores are lower in academic settings or those with an academic affiliation. However, limited research has focused on professionals who work in jails and prisons. A systematic review focusing specifically on correctional health care providers (Keller et al., 2022) revealed only 11 studies across five countries that met criteria for inclusion, and six were specific to nursing staff. Three primary themes emerged with respect to environmental stressors contributing to burnout: conflict (e.g., related to correctional policies conflicting with health care roles), fear (e.g., for personal and patient safety), and demands (e.g., high workloads and poor managerial support). There is some evidence that mental health professionals who work in jails and prisons have higher rates of burnout than those who work with forensic patients in community settings (Mivshek & Shriver, 2024).

Strategies to promote wellness

Identifying a one-size-fits-all approach to improving staff wellness in carceral settings is currently unrealistic. National and local systems of incarceration, which are driven by jurisdiction-specific public policy and legislation, contribute to stressors in jails or prisons, all of which may affect the health and well-being of every staff member. Although carceral settings remain relative "black boxes" with respect to data reporting and transparency about policies and operational specifics that could inform quality improvement related to staff wellness, there has been increasing attention to this in recent years.

Examples of NIOSH-developed principles to reduce work-related stress include implementing policies that give workers more control over their schedules, providing training for supervisors about managing stressful work conditions, and providing access to stress reduction skills development for employees (NIOSH, 2016). These principles emphasize that organizational-level change is more feasible, effective, and lasting for the overall health of a workforce than individual-level efforts such as encouraging personal change.

The following sections will discuss systemic, institutional, and individual-level interventions that focus on improving staff wellness in jails and prisons.

Systemic interventions

A society's values with respect to incarceration play a substantial role in the quality of life and risk for poor health outcomes in the staff who work there (Crewe et al., 2014). Systems in which IPs face more deprivation and a higher degree of staff authority and control may lead to more difficult work conditions because of the increased stress-related needs of IPs and increased pressure on correctional staff to maintain strict order. However, a lack of supervision and structure in these settings can also create a dangerous working environment, especially where subgroups or gangs exert the most control. Models of incarceration that are accepted by a society, the staff who work in the carceral settings, and those who are incarcerated as legitimate by virtue of being fair (Smoyer et al., 2015) have demonstrated improved staff satisfaction and lower rates of harm (Cloud et al., 2021; Zhao et al., 2023).

In the United States, efforts are underway to return to the rehabilitative carceral model that existed prior to the 1960s (Ahalt et al., 2020), and multiple state prison and local jail systems have started to closely examine the model of Norway's correctional services, whose vision and approach reflect that "during the serving of a sentence, life inside will resemble life outside as much as possible" (Norwegian Correctional Service, n.d., Principle of Normality section).

Improving access to treatments that are the standard of care for mental health and substance use disorders can play a significant role in both improving the health and safety of people who are incarcerated—which improves the health and safety of the staff caring for them—and directly reducing the feelings of helplessness and reduced agency that are so frequently precursors to health care staff burnout. Examples of standard-of-care treatments that are typically restricted or very difficult to obtain in carceral settings include medications for opioid use disorders, electroconvulsive therapy, clozapine, and nonpharmacological interventions such as manualized psychotherapies, regular exercise programs, and healthy diets (Tamburello et al., 2018).

Reducing employee stigma associated with experiencing mental health difficulties and seeking care for such is a challenge that spans across almost all occupations. These efforts may be particularly difficult in carceral systems that value toughness and bravery in their employees. Individual mental health concerns may be seen as a personal weakness that jeopardizes the safety of the system and the institution. In a sample of over 900 Canadian correctional officers, for example, institutional correctional officers indicated a higher degree of stigma, higher distrust for colleagues with mental illness, and a lower likelihood of seeking professional help for a mental health disorder of their own than officers who worked in a probation (community) setting (Shields et al., 2024).

Institutional interventions

Strategies to increase the quantity and quality of staffing in jails and prisons differ from general staff recruitment and retention principles because of the specific complexity and ethical challenges of the work environment. Increased compensation, for example, has not been shown to consistently overcome the lack of interest psychiatrists have to working in these settings. Morris and Edwards (2022) describe failed efforts by the Federal Bureau of Prisons and the California prison system to recruit psychiatrists despite substantial salary increases. Regardless, appropriate compensation is necessary, while perhaps not always sufficient, to maintain safe staffing levels.

Strategies to increase mental health staffing include offering options that reduce the amount of physical exposure a mental health provider has to the carceral environment. Telepsychiatry in the United States began in the prison system because of limited provider availability and expanded substantially during and following the COVID-19 pandemic (see Chapter 21). While further research is needed to understand the impact of telepsychiatry on the quality of care delivered in carceral settings (APA, 2023), including its potential to further isolate a patient in an already isolated environment, telepsychiatry can expand access to care for IPs while reducing physical stress on providers.

Flexible work schedules, such as part-time and alternate full-time assignments (e.g., four 10-hour days, three 12-hour days), also reduce physical exposure to the environment. However, these arrangements are complicated because individual needs do not always align with staff schedules, and interdisciplinary teamwork and communication are strong components of staff well-being. Alternate schedules have the potential to improve an individual staff member's well-being while worsening the well-being of the remaining staff who must cover in their absence.

Establishing practices for mental health providers in jails and prisons that mirror community health care settings (e.g., regularly scheduled and protected individual or group supervision, interdisciplinary team communication, structured sign-outs at change of shift, consultation, mentorship) can be helpful in mitigating some of the environmental and operational structures that contribute to burnout. Regular supervisory meetings can provide staff with emotional outlets for processing traumatic work experiences and general work-related concerns. Limited studies show a correlation between more clinical supervision and less traumatic stress (Hanae & Giddings, 2017).

There are also opportunities through supervision to emphasize provider resilience and the intrinsic rewards that can come from trying to help a vulnerable patient population in a difficult environment (Nuttman-Schwartz, 2015). Supervision can emphasize some of the ways in which clinical care may not be as constrained as in the community, such as a lack of insurance mandates, the potential for a wider array of creative and innovative treatments, and opportunities to work with and influence policy and practice in meaningful ways (APA, 2016b).

An additional intervention may include supporting more liberal access to paid time off, instead of limiting this to vacation planned well in advance, personal days only in the midst of a crisis, or when an employee is sick. Of course, this relies on a sufficient workforce quantity and quality to support such an initiative. A confidential and skilled Employee Assistance Program is also critical so that staff can safely identify health- and wellness-related concerns in themselves and their colleagues without fearing repercussions in the workplace.

There are limited data about specific training and education proven to be successful in supporting staff wellness in carceral settings. A systematic review of peer-reviewed research examining intervention strategies for front-line staff in adult correctional facilities identified only two studies assessing the efficacy of burnout interventions. One, from Croatia (Bagaric & Markanovic, 2021), demonstrated improved well-being after two 8-hour group training workshops. Another, from Sweden (Norman et al., 2020), demonstrated reduced cynicism among prison employees after training on "everyday conversations" (Forman-Dolan et al., 2022).

Regardless of evidence, it may be reasonable to assume that education related to mindfulness, stress management and prevention, illness and symptom recognition, and healthy lifestyle choices (e.g., substance use, exercise, diet, sleep, and personal relationships) may have some impact on, or at least will not worsen, staff well-being. Any trainings should be provided free of charge and during time when the staff is protected from other responsibilities. There should also be support from the institution for any skills learned. For example, if a jail system is interested in reducing stress levels through mindfulness training, introducing a 3-minute mindfulness exercise into daily roll call can promote real-life application and practice of the skill.

The methods with which staff are allocated to tasks can impact the quality of their work life. For example, establishing expectations that individuals will develop experience with various settings within an institution (e.g., general population, mental health units, infirmary, and restrictive housing units) allows for a variety of work assignments that can relieve staff of setting-specific stressors while also increasing their level of understanding and competency across what are typically complex institutional structures and workflows. A psychiatrist who is working on a mental health unit and then moves to a general population clinic may feel relief at the decreased level of intensity of need, feel more competent about making assessments about patients in general population who may need a mental health unit, and become more efficient in the transfer process because of professional relationships established on that unit. However, rotational work may also reduce staff well-being if they are not able to work long enough to develop agency and competency in a particular setting.

The expectation of participation in quality improvement initiatives as part of work responsibilities can serve to increase staff feelings of agency and control through direct engagement in activities typically reserved only for leadership. This can help the institution establish and implement practices that are more tailored to the needs of the staff and the individuals for whom they provide care. This cannot be done without adequate staffing and strong institutional support. Affiliations with community organizations and academic institutions can often be helpful with these initiatives, and accrediting bodies such as the National Commission on Correctional Health Care offer guidance about implementing continuous quality improvement (see Chapter 73).

Many carceral settings are "academic deserts," with little to no resources devoted to professional education and development (Subedi et al., 2023). This contributes to recruitment challenges in jails and prisons, while also perpetuating the lack of focus in academic communities on carceral work. Psychiatrists and mental health providers typically value work environments that foster their professional growth and education. Academic–carceral facility partnerships have the potential to be widely beneficial, including fulfilling a core mission of most academic centers to care for underserved populations (Trestman, 2015). The presence of trainees, clinical supervision, education, and research activities that accompany affiliations with an academic institution typically bring a level of intellectual curiosity to carceral settings that can strengthen health care providers' resilience and sense of intrinsic reward in the work (Morris & West, 2020).

Although many organizational, facility, and individual interventions may reasonably be expected to improve staff well-being, there are pressures and challenges that affect some groups more than others. For example, psychiatrists may feel particularly ineffective or helpless about available treatment options within a jail or prison as they strive to follow the recommendations of the APA that adult correctional facilities should include "an appropriate range of therapeutic interventions" (APA, 2021), including medications for substance use disorders (APA, 2016a). Depending on the policies and practices of the jail or prison, mental health professionals may also be frustrated by a paramilitary hierarchy that prioritizes security over a patient's health care–related best interests.

Professional organizations that represent correctional officers, social workers, psychiatrists, psychologists, nurses, nurse practitioners, peer specialists, chaplains, and other staff can assist their members by prioritizing awareness of the wellness concerns specific to their members. Multiple organizations have made strides in this regard, including the American Correctional Association (2021), American Correctional Nurses Association (n.d.), and National Sheriffs' Association (n.d.). While there is not enough evidence yet to support particular professional organization interventions, it is reasonable to assume that acknowledgment of the importance of the work individuals do in carceral settings may positively increase a worker's sense of accomplishment and pride.

Professional organizations may also consider establishing peer support or process groups for their members who work in settings where the environment is substantially different from community settings or for which there is little emphasis during one's professional training. It is important to consider the many factors that contribute to successful peer groups, including confidentiality (and rules about when it might be broken for safety), leadership (e.g., ensuring the leader or moderator is not any member's supervisor), protection from retaliation, and consistent attendance. A pilot peer support group for psychiatric providers in jails and prisons across the United States, started by one former (this author) and one current carceral psychiatrist, revealed some of the benefits and challenges of this process. The group was scheduled during the workday to avoid encroachment on members' personal time and to model the importance of wellness as "part of the job." While initial interest was robust, attendance declined over time. The group was conducted over the phone because of various institutions' restrictions on the use of video conferencing. Feedback after the group ended was that it provided a range of perspectives and support for the members but was difficult to attend for staff who had little flexibility with their schedule. Future organizers of such support groups may consider varying the timing of the groups and optimizing the use of technology while respecting local policies.

Individual interventions

Staff who work in carceral settings will be best able to avoid the potentially harmful side effects of their jobs by caring for their personal health as much as possible. This includes prioritizing sleep, healthy eating, regular exercise, supportive relationships, medical care, and minimizing substance use. Often characterized as "self-care," these practices have been shown to improve job satisfaction, which also has benefits for coworkers and patients (Monroe et al., 2021). Many of these activities can be difficult when the expectations of the job—as is the case in many jails and prisons—include mandatory overtime, limited breaks, workload burdens that exceed the time allowed to complete them, and limited food options. Institutions can establish practices and policies to encourage healthy employee habits, but these may have limited impact on an individual's life outside of work. Staff, with institutional support, may consider creating or participating in a wellness committee to promote the well-being of their coworkers through education and other organized activities.

Engaging in personal mental health care that is appropriate for one's level of distress, from "check-ins" with a therapist to treatment for a mental health or substance use disorder, can be helpful in preventing and alleviating some of the health impact of working in a carceral setting. As mentioned earlier, mental health professionals, based on their training and experience, may perceive less stigma and be less hesitant to engage in psychotherapy than other professionals, such as correctional officers.

Summary

Providing care in jails and prisons, while deeply rooted in a mission to care for vulnerable populations, can come with risks to an individual's emotional and physical health. These risks vary in exposure and intensity based on one's specific profession. Increasing attention is being paid to improving staff wellness. However, much more needs to be understood about how to protect this workforce effectively.

REFERENCES

Ahalt, C., Haney, C., Ekhaugen, K., & Williams, B. (2020). Role of a US-Norway exchange in placing health and well-being at the center

of US prison reform. *American Journal of Public Health, 110*(S1), S27–S29.
American Correctional Association. (2021). *Correctional employee wellness: Improving the health of our greatest asset* [White paper]. https://www.aca.org/ACA_Member/ACA/ACA_Member/Staff_Wellness_Prep.aspx
American Correctional Nurses Association. (n.d.). *Duty to self during a crisis* [Brief]. https://s3.amazonaws.com/nursing-network/production/files/107008/original/Brief_234_SelfCare.pdf?1638484374
American Psychiatric Association. (2016a). *Position statement on substance use disorders in the criminal justice system.* https://www.psychiatry.org/getattachment/45b40a54-cf57-4b94-be6c-f03fd5440d0e/Position-2016-Substance-Use-Disorders-in-the-Criminal-Justice-System.pdf
American Psychiatric Association. (2016b). *Psychiatric services in correctional facilities* (3rd ed.). American Psychiatric Publishing.
American Psychiatric Association. (2018). *Psychiatrist well-being and burnout.* https://www.psychiatry.org/getmedia/5f5cf9ac-3de4-42c1-9e89-0d253361f1c6/APA-BOT-Workgroup-Psychiatrist-Wellbeing-and-Burnout.pdf.
American Psychiatric Association. (2021). *Position statement on psychiatric services in adult correctional facilities.* https://www.psychiatry.org/getattachment/af0301db-f33c-495a-861c-35036c8c91ae/Position-Psychiatric-Services-in-Adult-Correctional-Facilities.pdf.
American Psychiatric Association. (2023). *Resource document on telepsychiatry in jails and prisons.* https://www.psychiatry.org/getattachment/00e3f401-0792-4b78-90ba-5985dd791a4e/Resource-Document-on-Telepsychiatry-in-Jails-and-Prisons.pdf
Armstrong, G. S., & Griffin, M. L. (2004). Does the job matter? Comparing correlates of stress among treatment and correctional staff in prisons. *Journal of Criminal Justice, 32,* 577–592.
Bagaric, B., & Markanovic, D. (2021). Application of stress-focused mindfulness-based cognitive therapy with prison system staff. *Kriminologija & Socijalna Integracija, 29*(1), 66–104.
Bureau of Justice Statistics. (2017). *Indicators of mental health problems reported by prisoners and jail inmates, 2011–2012* (NCJ 250612). U.S. Department of Justice, Office of Justice Programs. https://bjs.ojp.gov/content/pub/pdf/imhprpji1112.pdf
Bureau of Justice Statistics. (2021). *Alcohol and drug use and treatment reported by prisoners* (NCJ 252641). U.S. Department of Justice, Office of Justice Programs. https://bjs.ojp.gov/sites/g/files/xyckuh236/files/media/document/adutrpspi16st.pdf
Bureau of Labor Statistics. (2022). *National census of fatal occupational injuries in 2021* (USDL-22-2309). U.S. Department of Labor. https://www.bls.gov/news.release/archives/cfoi_12162022.htm.
Burhanullah, M. H., Rollings-Mazza, P., Galecki, J., Van Wert, M., Weber, T., & Malik, M. (2022). Mental health of staff at correctional facilities in the United States during the COVID-19 pandemic. *Frontiers in Psychiatry, 12,* 767385.
Carleton, R. N., Ricciardelli, R., Taillieu, T., Mitchell, M. M., Andres, E., & Afifi, T. O. (2020). Provincial correctional service workers: The prevalence of mental disorders. *International Journal of Environmental Research and Public Health, 17*(7), Article 2203.
Cloud, D. H., Augustine, D., Ahalt, C., et al. (2021). "We just needed to open the door": A case study of the quest to end solitary confinement in North Dakota. *Health Justice, 9,* 28.
Crewe, B., Liebling, A., & Hulley, S. (2014). Heavy-light, absent-present: Rethinking the "weight" of imprisonment. *British Journal of Sociology, 65*(3), 387–410.
El Ghaziri, M., Jaegers, L. A., Monteiro, C. E., Grubb, P. L., & Cherniack, M. G. (2020). Progress in corrections worker health: The national corrections collaborative utilizing a total worker health® strategy. *Journal of Occupational and Environmental Medicine, 62*(11), 965–972.
Ellison, J. M., & Gainey, R. (2020). An opportunity model of safety risks among jail officers. *Journal of Criminal Justice, 66,* 1–12.
Ellison, J. M., & Jaegers, L. A. (2022). Suffering in silence: Violence exposure and post-traumatic stress disorder among jail correctional officers. *Journal of Occupational and Environmental Medicine, 64*(1), e28–e35.
Figley, C. R. (Ed.). (1995). *Compassion fatigue: Coping with secondary traumatic stress disorder in those who treat the traumatized.* Routledge.
Forman-Dolan, M., Caggiano, C., Anillo, I., & Kennedy, T. D. (2022). Burnout among professionals working in corrections: A two-stage review. *International Journal of Environmental Research and Public Health, 19,* 9954.
Hanae, K., & Giddings, M. M. (2017). Hidden trauma victims: Understanding and preventing traumatic stress in mental health professionals. *Social Work in Mental Health, 15*(3), 331–353.
James, L., & Todak, N. (2018). Prison employment and post-traumatic stress disorder: Risk and protective factors. *American Journal of Industrial Medicine, 61*(9), 725–732.
Jayawardene, W., Kumbalatara, C., Jones, A., & McDaniel, J. (2024). Work stress and psychoactive substance use among correctional officers in the USA. *Psychoactives, 3*(1), 65–77.
Johnson, W. B., Johnson, S. J., Sullivan, G. R., Bongar, B., Miller, L., and Sammons, M. T. (2011). Psychology in extremis: Preventing problems of professional competence in dangerous practice settings. *Professional Psychology: Research and Practice, 42*(1), 94–104.
Keller, E., Boch, S., & Hittle, B. M. (2022). Unsafe and unsettling: An integrative review on correctional nursing work environments and stressors. *Journal of Forensic Nursing, 18*(4), 229–236.
Lambert, E. G., Hogan, N. L, Griffin, M. L., & Kelley, T. (2015). The correctional staff burnout literature. *Criminal Justice Studies, 28*(4), 397–443.
Liu, H., Li, T. W., Liang, L., & Hou, W. K. (2021). Trauma exposure and mental health of prisoners and ex-prisoners: A systematic review and meta-analysis. *Clinical Psychology Review, 89,* 102069.
Maslach, C., & Jackson, S. (1981). The measurement of experienced burnout. *Journal of Organizational Behavior, 2,* 99–113.
Mivshek, M. E., & Schriver, J. L. (2024). Burnout and empathy in mental health professionals working in correctional settings, community settings, and with sex offenders. *Psychology, Crime & Law, 30*(1), 86–100.
Monroe, C., Loresto, F., Horton-Deutsch, S., et al. (2021). The value of intentional self-care practices: The effects of mindfulness on improving job satisfaction, teamwork, and workplace environments. *Archives of Psychiatric Nursing, 35*(2), 189–194.
Morris, N. P., & Edwards, M. L. (2022). Addressing shortages of mental health professionals in U.S. jails and prisons. *Journal of Correctional Health Care, 28*(4), 209–214.
Morris, N. P., & West, S. G. (2020). Misconceptions about working in correctional psychiatry. *Journal of the American Academy of Psychiatry and the Law, 48*(2), 251–258.
National Institute for Occupational Safety and Health. (2016). *Fundamentals of total worker health approaches: Essential elements for advancing worker safety, health, and well-being* (Publication No. 2017-112). https://www.cdc.gov/niosh/docs/2017-112/pdfs/2017_112.pdf?id=10.26616/NIOSHPUB2017112

National Institute of Corrections. (2016). *Correctional officer suicide* (Accession No. 033237). U.S. Department of Justice. https://nicic.gov/resources/nic-library/all-library-items/correctional-officer-suicide-annotated-bibliography

National Sheriffs' Association. (n.d.). *Officer wellness.* https://www.sheriffs.org/ruralresources/officerwellness

Norman, Å., Lundberg, U., Farbring, C. Å., Källmén, H., & Forsberg, L. (2020). The feasibility and potential of training correctional officers in flexible styles of communication to reduce burnout: A multiple baseline trial in real-life settings. *Scandinavian Journal of Work and Organizational Psychology, 5*, 12.

Norwegian Correctional Service. (n.d.). *About the Norwegian Correctional Service.* https://www.kriminalomsorgen.no/informasjon-paa-engelsk.536003.no.html

Nuttman-Shwartz, O. (2015). Shared resilience in a traumatic reality: A new concept for trauma workers exposed personally and professionally to collective disaster. *Trauma, Violence, & Abuse, 16*(4), 466–475.

Robinson-Keilig, R. A. (2014). Secondary traumatic stress and disruptions to interpersonal functioning among mental health therapists. *Journal of Interpersonal Violence, 29*, 1477–1496.

Shields, R. E., Ricciardelli, R., Jamshidi, L., & Carleton, R. N. (2024). Mental health knowledge, stigma, and service use intentions among correctional workers. *Canadian Journal of Behavioural Science, 56*(4), 409–421.

Smoyer, A. B., Kershaw, T. S., & Blankenship, K. M. (2014). Confining legitimacy: The impact of prison experiences on perceptions of criminal justice legitimacy. *Journal of Forensic Social Work, 5*(1–3), 258–270.

Subedi, B., Barber-Rioja, V., & Ford, E. (2023). Recruitment, retention, support and supervision of jail mental health providers in the context of occupational syndromes and work-related trauma. In V. Barber-Rioja, A. Garcia-Mansilla, B. Subedi, & A. B. Batastini (Eds.), *Handbook of mental health assessment and treatment in jail* (pp. 307–322). Oxford University Press.

Tamburello, A., Metzner, J., Fergusen, E., et al. (2018). The American Academy of Psychiatry and the Law practice resource for prescribing in corrections. *Journal of the American Academy of Psychiatry and the Law, 46*(2), 242–243.

Trestman, R. L., Ferguson, W., & Dickert, J. (2015). Behind bars: The compelling case for academic health centers partnering with correctional facilities. *Academic Medicine, 90*(1), 6–9.

Tyler, T. (2006). *Why people obey the law.* Princeton University Press.

Zhao, X., Nylander, P., & Bruhn, A. (2023). Swedish prison officers' perceptions of management and support: Key predictors and subgroups. *Psychology, Crime & Law*, 1–15.

66

Forensic and legal issues

Erik Roskes and Charles D. Cash

Introduction

This chapter focuses on common forensic issues that a psychiatrist working in a correctional setting may have to address, including the management of detainees found incompetent to stand trial (IST) and liability exposures. State and local laws vary widely, and different problems may arise depending on the location where the psychiatrist works. Examples used may not generalize to all settings, so the reader should become familiar with relevant federal, state, and local laws relevant to their specific place of work.

Competency restoration

Because data is not gathered at a national level, it is difficult to estimate the number of competency evaluations that are court ordered. However, recent literature suggests that between approximately 94,000 and 141,000 competency evaluations are ordered in the United States every year (Morris et al., 2021; Murrie et al., 2023; Kois et al., 2024), representing a three- to fivefold increase over the past 50 years. Approximately one fifth of defendants who are evaluated are found IST (Dressel & Burns, 2012). Upon adjudication as IST, a criminal case is stayed while the defendant is treated, with the goal of rendering that person competent to stand trial (CST) so that the case may proceed. In general, this does not involve correctional psychiatrists; in most states, the IST finding permits the court to place the defendant in a clinical setting for treatment to restore competency. Such orders alone, however, do not by themselves permit treatment over the objection of a defendant. In *Sell v. United States* (2003), the U.S. Supreme Court found:

> The Constitution permits the Government involuntarily to administer antipsychotic drugs to render a mentally ill defendant competent to stand trial on serious criminal charges if the treatment is medically appropriate, is substantially unlikely to have side effects that may undermine the trial's fairness, and, taking account of less intrusive alternatives, is necessary significantly to further *important governmental trial-related interests*. This standard will permit forced medication *solely for trial competency purposes* in certain instances. But those instances may be rare. (p. 167, emphasis added)

These instances will be rare because most criminal cases involve minor charges that do not rise to the level of "important governmental trial-related interests." Unfortunately, many detainees found to be IST spend long periods of time incarcerated in local jails awaiting transfer to a state hospital facility due to significant shortages of forensic hospital beds for competency restoration purposes. It is frequently not legally permissible to involuntarily medicate these persons on a nonemergency basis in a jail setting due to state law or regulations (see Chapter 25).

The dicta in *Sell* suggest that the use of *Harper* proceedings, when applicable, is preferred. In *Washington v. Harper* (1990), the U.S. Supreme Court held that the due process clause permits a state to treat an incarcerated person (IP) based solely on determinations by an administrative committee (inclusive of medical professionals) that the IP is dangerous and that treatment is in their medical interest. Some states, however, use stricter criteria, such as full judicial review, findings of incompetence, and the appointment of a guardian or substituted decision-maker. In most jurisdictions, *Harper* is interpreted as applying to prison settings and not jails, which limits the ability to use nonemergency involuntary psychotropic medications in many pretrial scenarios. Correctional psychiatrists need to know the statutory and case law relevant in their own jurisdictions.

Where competency restoration treatment is provided depends entirely on local resources. Ideally, such defendants would be transferred to the most clinically appropriate setting for treatment, and this does occur in many states. Historically, states required such defendants to be admitted to a hospital for treatment; in some states, this is still the case (NRI, 2021). For example, in Maryland, a defendant found IST and dangerous to self, others, or the property of others due to a mental disorder is committed to a state psychiatric hospital until that defendant is no longer IST or dangerous due to a mental disorder or until "there is not a substantial likelihood that the defendant will become competent to stand trial in the foreseeable future" (Annotated Code of Maryland 2022, Crim. Proc., § 3-106(c)(1)(i)(3); *Jackson v. Indiana*, 1972). Alternatively, a defendant found IST and dangerous due to intellectual disability (still known in some state statutes, including Maryland's, as "mental retardation") is committed to a facility for people with intellectual disabilities until reaching similar endpoints (Annotated Code of Maryland 2022, Crim. Proc., § 3-106). Thus, Maryland provides all treatment pursuant to a finding of IST and dangerousness due to mental disorder or intellectual disability in institutional clinical settings.

In many states, though, there are inadequate resources to meet the rising demand, spawning litigation to force states to expand available institutionally based competency restoration programs.

Decisions from the Ninth Circuit Court of Appeals have resulted in numerous lawsuits related to competency restoration, both in the Ninth Circuit and elsewhere, most of which have resulted in consent decrees (Bloom & Kirkorsky, 2021).

In many states, a finding of IST alone is insufficient to commit the defendant to a treatment facility. In Maryland, for example, the dangerousness requirement, and the requirement that the dangerousness be causally connected to mental illness or intellectual disability, leaves a potential gap. Those found IST but not found dangerous, or not found dangerous due to mental illness or intellectual disability, may not be committed to a psychiatric hospital for competency restoration. Such defendants, if remanded or unable to make bail, would remain incarcerated.

For example, consider someone arrested for simple drug possession. The defendant is a young man with an IQ in the mid-70s and with no apparent mental illness. He cooperates with the police, presenting no resistance upon arrest. The court finds that he does not understand the charges and cannot work with his attorney. Yet, he remains cooperative and compliant with all proceedings. This defendant's crime is nonviolent, and even if the crime may be legally presumed to be dangerous (*Jones v. U.S.*, 1983), that dangerousness has no obvious connection to mental illness or intellectual disability. Thus, in Maryland, this defendant could not be admitted to a psychiatric hospital and, unless released on bail or recognizance, would remain incarcerated without an obvious remedy to his finding of incompetency. In some states, such as New York, defendants found IST for misdemeanor crimes cannot be criminally committed and instead must have their charges dismissed; if such defendants do not meet civil commitment criteria, they must be released (New York CPL—Crim. Proc. § 730.70, 2014).

As above, in some states, the available hospital resources do not meet the demand, and defendants found IST are instead managed in detention or sometimes in the community (Policy Research Associates, 2020; see Chapter 71). During the early years of the 21st century, jurisdictions began using nonhospital approaches toward competency restoration. Jennings and Bell (2012) describe the jail-based competency restoration program utilized in one Virginia county. Kapoor (2011) reported that defendants in Texas found IST and committed for treatment waited between 72 and 180 days to be admitted to the hospital. In response, Texas examined alternative strategies toward resolving cases halted due to the defendant's incompetence to proceed. In an issue brief, the Hogg Foundation (2013) compared the costs, length of stay, and restoration rates of four competency restoration models: state psychiatric hospital, community hospital, outpatient, and jail based. The review found that jail-based and community-based restoration programs are generally far less costly for defendants who do not require hospitalization based on either clinical need or the severity of the offense.

More recently, Danzer and colleagues (2019) conducted a review of competency restoration practices and provided a set of best practice recommendations. They concluded that hospital beds (which then cost between $300 and $1,000 per day) should be "best reserved for defendants facing serious and violent charges, with psychotic disorders, cognitive impairment, medication non-adherence, and lesser concern about malingering" (Danzer et al., 2019, p. 80). They viewed jail-based approaches ($42 to $222 per day) as better suited to defendants with a high index of suspicion for feigning, while community-based restoration ($100 to $500 per day)

> may be ideal for defendants charged with nonviolent or … lesser violent crimes … who do not meet criteria for civil commitment, who do not have as significant a history of substance use, who are … more likely to be medication adherent … and who do not have as great a need for hospital-based services. (Danzer et al., 2019, p. 80)

In keeping with long-standing principles of mental health law, defendants who are IST should be managed in the least restrictive setting appropriate for their clinical and forensic needs. Jurisdictions that permit competency restoration in various settings may wish to institute a "triage" process whereby individual defendants are matched to the setting most appropriate to their needs. This would allow jurisdictions to reserve precious hospital beds for those defendants (and other forensic and nonforensic patients) most in need of inpatient treatment, while permitting the restoration of less ill defendants in less intensive settings, including jails (Murrie et al., 2023).

While each venue for competency restoration has its strengths and weaknesses, the utility of jail- or community-based restoration programs is predicated on the availability of adequate and specialized staffing and on the separation of evaluators and treatment staff to avoid conflicts of interest. Thus, in jails already stretched thin due to overcrowding and inadequate staffing, competency restoration is not recommended as a solution to the lack of availability of hospital beds or community-based resources unless new staff and adequate programming space are specifically allocated. If there is adequate staffing, both in numbers and in training and experience, a jail-based competency restoration program can be considered where there are inadequate hospital-based resources and where relevant statutes and regulations permit this approach.

Psychiatrists working in correctional institutions that treat defendants found IST are strongly encouraged to become familiar with competency restoration, education, and therapeutic and habilitation procedures beyond psychopharmacology. In addition, psychiatrists in these situations should advocate for a clear separation between two potentially conflicted roles: the treatment role (which may include restoration techniques) and the forensic evaluation and reporting role that keeps the court apprised of the defendant's competency status. Psychiatrists are encouraged to advocate for adequate resources for defendants found IST and in clinical need of hospitalization. Having adequate jail-based restoration programs does not negate the need for other mental health resources, including hospital-based inpatient programs for those requiring it and community-based competency restoration programs for defendants who do not require institutionalization while undergoing treatment services.

Liability risk in correctional care

Psychiatrists working in correctional settings face specific litigation risks regarding professional negligence and other forms of liability. Psychiatrists need to review the categories of claims covered by their insurance policies. Especially important is understanding whether the insurance carrier covers forensic and correctional work.

Correctional psychiatrists also need to consider the quality of care that they deliver to their patients, as emphasized by the American Psychiatric Association (2016):

> The fundamental policy goal for correctional mental health care is to provide the same level of mental health services to each patient in the criminal justice process that *should be available* in the community. This policy goal is deliberately higher than the "community standard" that is called for in various legal contexts, because resource restrictions on community care can sometimes limit the adequacy of available services. (p. 5, emphasis original)

At times, there may be restrictions on corrections-based care, such as medication formularies or volume-based expectations regarding the number of patients seen per unit time. These are cost and care management strategies common to other settings too and as a matter of principle should be considered in the conceptual standard of care, but they may not be acceptable reasons for failing to provide adequate care. For example, when viewed through the lens of malpractice or other litigation, questions may be raised regarding the psychiatrist's failure to seek a formulary exception or to spend adequate time assessing or treating a patient in crisis. It is imperative to document effectively and completely, to manage known risks of medications, and to engage in and document informed consent discussions with patients when making treatment recommendations. As in all settings, communication with other providers helps ensure appropriate care (see Chapter 14); working with the correctional staff who know the patients well is also advisable. Finally, becoming familiar with relevant guidelines and accreditation standards promulgated by organizations such as the American Psychiatric Association (2016), the American Correctional Association (2010), and the National Commission on Correctional Health Care (2015) can be useful.

Correctional psychiatry is accompanied by increased professional liability exposure when compared with general psychiatric practice in the community, due to unique risks, including:

- **IPs in the United States have a constitutional right to receive medical care (see Chapter 3), allowing them to claim civil rights violations in addition to claims for medical malpractice.** Courts have held that deliberate indifference to serious medical and mental health needs violates the Eighth Amendment. Federal law (42 U.S.C. § 1983, n.d.) imposes liability on government employees—or those linked to the government, such as private contractors—for violation of a citizen's constitutional rights, including those covered by the Eighth Amendment. As discussed in *Estelle v. Gamble* (1976), deliberate indifference to serious medical needs of prisoners constitutes the unnecessary and wanton infliction of pain, proscribed by the Eighth Amendment, which is actionable against correctional psychiatrists under § 1983. Progeny of *Estelle v. Gamble* extended this right to mental health care (*Bowring v. Godwin*, 1977) and jail settings (*Bell v. Wolfish*, 1979).
- **The rate of suicide is high in correctional settings.** In 2019, there were 25 suicides per 100,000 state prisoners, 20 per 100,000 federal prisoners, and 49 per 100,000 people in local jails (Carson 2021a, 2021b). By contrast, the suicide rate in the general population in 2022 was 14.3 per 100,000 (Curtin et al., 2023). Suicide is the most common cause of action against the correctional psychiatrist for medical malpractice and may also result in a claim of deliberate indifference under § 1983 (Tamburello & Azuh-Showole, 2022).
- **There is the potential for class action exposure.** Advocacy groups may file class action litigation against the correctional facility for alleged problems, such as overcrowding, violence, and substandard health care. Correctional psychiatrists may be named in these cases.
- **The correctional psychiatrist lacks full control of the treatment environment.** IPs are in the custody of the corrections staff, who may impede access to necessary treatment. Additionally, there may be disagreements with administration over clinical matters, such as restricted formulary options and the timing and number of medication administrations per day. The correctional environment itself may render it difficult or impossible to maintain confidentiality, making appropriate treatment difficult to provide because of resulting limitations to the quantity and quality of information disclosed by patients. This is especially true in higher security and restrictive housing settings.
- **Many cases by IPs are brought *pro se* (i.e., by someone not represented by counsel).** Typically, courts allow *pro se* litigants more latitude in prosecuting their complaints than they would permit an attorney filing on a litigant's behalf. Processing cases with little merit may take much longer, as trial judges tend to be very accommodating to *pro se* litigants in allowing amended complaints to which defendant psychiatrists and their attorneys must respond, often multiple times.

In general, IPs are more litigious than people in the community, for reasons that may include legitimate grievances regarding the context in which care is delivered. Claims of professional negligence may include common legal theories such as wrongful death or suicide, adverse drug reactions, and failures to obtain informed consent, diagnose, or treat appropriately. Some IPs use their unstructured time to devise unusual legal claims. While many of these claims ultimately will be dismissed as frivolous, they still must be addressed and defended. Health care providers may be named in these claims. IPs may file actions in both state and federal court based on more than one legal theory, including professional negligence claims, ordinary negligence claims, and civil rights claims. An additional avenue exists in the form of an administrative action, such as a state licensing board complaint, which can be filed concurrently with a lawsuit. Thus, litigation in these settings is potentially far more complex than patient complaints in the community.

When an incarcerated plaintiff is represented in a § 1983 lawsuit, the attorney may be motivated to include as many defendants as possible and to keep them in the case as long as possible, because § 1983 actions allow for the recovery of attorneys' fees. This increases the cost of defending even cases that ultimately are dismissed.

In some circumstances, public officials, but not private practitioners or other correctional contractors, are found eligible for qualified immunity, which shields potential defendants from lawsuits. In *Filarsky v. Delia* (2012), however, the U.S. Supreme Court held that, in certain scenarios, even private providers may be entitled to qualified immunity. Given how common it is for departments of corrections to contract with private health and mental health care providers, questions regarding the role of the clinician and the potential for qualified immunity are highly complex and could result in lengthy and costly litigation. That said, qualified immunity will not protect a public official from allegations of reckless or malicious acts.

Litigation outcomes

While the risk of having a claim filed in correctional practice may be higher than in community practice, payouts are generally much fewer and smaller. A review of closed claims data from Professional

Risk Management Services (PRMS, 2023) for the period 2014–2023 revealed that only 4% of claims against PRMS-covered psychiatrists in correctional practice resulted in an indemnity payment, whereas for noncorrectional PRMS-covered psychiatrists, this figure was approximately 25% of claims. Of the correctional claims that resulted in indemnity payment, the average payment was $205,000. For noncorrectional, PRMS-covered psychiatrists, this figure was approximately $300,000.

Although the vast majority of correctional claims close with no indemnity payment, the cost of defending these claims—especially when they include § 1983 complaints—may be quite high. As one example from the reviewed cohort of closed claims, a § 1983 complaint against the psychiatrist eventually was dismissed, but defense costs to obtain that outcome exceeded $50,000 (PRMS, 2023).

Of the entire cohort of correctional psychiatry–related matters reviewed for the period, 79% were claims or lawsuits. Five percent were administrative actions (all licensing board complaints). Administrative actions resulting in a sanction against the psychiatrist were exceedingly rare (PRMS, 2023). In the remainder of the cases, either the outcome of the case was unknown because the defense was taken over by the relevant government entity or the covered psychiatrist reported an untoward event to PRMS that did not result in a claim.

Habeas corpus

The doctrine of *habeas corpus* stems from the common law and is enshrined in the U.S. Constitution: "The Privilege of the Writ of Habeas Corpus shall not be suspended" (U.S. Const. art. I, § 9, n.d.). *Habeas* petitions are primarily used to challenge the legality of continued detentions, and they are occasionally brought by IPs who seek a hearing. For example, a *habeas* petition could be brought to seek medical interventions that are being denied by the detaining institution, and as such, the medical staff could be named defendants. A correctional psychiatrist who is advised that a patient has filed for a *habeas* hearing should notify institutional management and the psychiatrist's attorney and professional liability insurance carrier.

Class action litigation

Many class actions have involved correctional mental health care. Clinicians working in correctional settings may welcome these suits, as they focus the attention of the courts, and at times the media and the public, on deficiencies in care related to inadequate resources. While such lawsuits can be sensitive, especially in the earlier phases when the outcome is in doubt, correctional psychiatrists and other clinicians may also serve as sources of information for each party to the case and to the court.

Class actions may result in remedial court orders (e.g., consent decrees) or private settlement agreements in which the jurisdiction agrees to modify services. During these remediation phases, policies may change, and resources may be added to ensure provision of the enhanced services agreed to by settlement or ordered by the court. Additionally, there may be court monitoring or other oversight of the case during the remediation phase. It is important to be aware of such cases when working in a correctional setting to ensure that the care provided is consonant with the expectations of the court and the parties to the litigation.

External review and investigation

Public and certain private institutions where individuals may be detained are subject to the independent oversight of the U.S. Department of Justice Civil Rights Division pursuant to the Civil Rights of Institutionalized Persons Act (CRIPA). Passed in 1980, this legislation covers institutions designed for people with mental illnesses or disabilities, as well as jails, prisons, and juvenile detention centers. A CRIPA action can be initiated by the attorney general based on "reasonable cause" that a state or county, or the employees of a state or county, are

> subjecting persons residing in or confined to an institution ... to egregious or flagrant conditions which deprive such persons of any rights, privileges, or immunities secured or protected by the Constitution or laws of the United States causing such persons to suffer grievous harm, and that such deprivation is pursuant to a pattern or practice of resistance to the full enjoyment of such rights, privileges, or immunities. (CRIPA, 1980, § 1997a)

These investigations are carried out by the U.S. Department of Justice's Civil Rights Division, Special Litigation Section. At times, the state's Protection and Advocacy for Individuals With Mental Illness or other advocacy-oriented legal groups may join in these investigations. The role of the correctional psychiatrist in such actions is parallel to their role in class action complaints.

Confidentiality

Some typical rules of confidentiality in health care settings may not apply in a correctional setting. For example, the fact that an IP is receiving mental health treatment may not be kept confidential from custody staff for many reasons (e.g., scheduling, managing heat-related risks associated with certain medications, providing mental health input into the disciplinary process) and is apparent to other IPs based on medication passes (i.e., pill call lines) and clinic visits. A balance needs to be maintained between the privacy rights of the IP receiving mental health care and the needs of their peers (e.g., for personal safety or public health concerns), in addition to the security needs of the facility (American Psychiatric Association, 2016). Correctional staff in special mental health units are often considered part of the treatment team and attend treatment team meetings where confidential information is shared with all team members. Other practice variations or exceptions to the usual rules of confidentiality include:

- Parole board evaluators accessing the health care record without requiring consent from the IP (varies by jurisdiction);
- Duty to warn or protect exceptions in many jurisdictions;
- Duty to reveal knowledge of escape plans; and
- In some facilities, a vague "need to know" exception for security purposes.

The mental health clinician should inform their clients of the limitations of and exceptions to confidentiality.

Mental health input into the disciplinary process

Little has been written regarding the provision of mental health input into the disciplinary process. Krelstein (2002) demonstrated that there is considerable diversity among the states in terms of the involvement of mental health personnel in the disciplinary process for IPs. Metzner (2002) recommended that mental health input into the disciplinary process not address issues of responsibility (i.e., "not guilty by reason of insanity") but be limited to identifying mitigating factors related to mental illness when present, dispositional recommendations when clinically appropriate, and competency-to-proceed issues in the context of the disciplinary hearing. This quasi-forensic assessment should be done by an appropriately trained clinician who is not the IP's clinician to minimize dual agency and conflict of interest. More recently, others have argued (Obegi, 2021; Tamburello & Haston, 2021) that there is a role for more complete and definitive forensic assessments of an IP's culpability for infractions, as well as opportunities in these assessments to identify those previously unrecognized as in need of treatment. A psychiatrist working in a correctional setting must have a comprehensive understanding of their role in assessing culpability in disciplinary proceedings, including knowledge of the standard to apply in rendering an opinion (Obegi, 2021).

Prison Rape Elimination Act

The Prison Rape Elimination Act (PREA, 2003) has reshaped correctional attitudes and responses to sexual assault in U.S. jails and prisons (see Chapter 69). While the forensic ramifications continue to unfold, psychiatrists working in U.S. correctional settings need to understand their screening, training, management, and evidentiary responsibilities (National PREA Resource Center, 2013).

Summary

This chapter presented common forensic challenges in correctional psychiatric practice. Numerous defendants are found IST each year, and some jurisdictions have inadequate public mental health resources to handle this burden. Thus, correctional psychiatrists may be expected to both treat illness and restore competency. Correctional psychiatrists may face allegations and investigations in addition to the more usual cases alleging professional negligence or malpractice found in other settings. They should be cautious about limitations of confidentiality, formulary restrictions, avoiding dual agency, and providing adequate care. The forensic and legal context of jails and prisons, including class action litigation, external review and investigations, and other formative law (such as CRIPA and PREA), shapes the work correctional psychiatrists do and is important to understand.

REFERENCES

42 U.S.C. § 1983: Civil action for deprivation of rights. (n.d.). http://www.gpo.gov/fdsys/pkg/USCODE-2009-title42/pdf/USCODE-2009-title42-chap21-subchapI-sec1983.pdf

American Correctional Association. (2010). *Public correctional policy on correctional mental health care.* https://www.criminallegalnews.org/media/publications/aca_public_correctional_policies_aug_2010.pdf

American Psychiatric Association. (2016). *Psychiatric services in correctional facilities* (3rd ed.).

Annotated Code of Maryland, Criminal Procedure Article, § 3-106. (2022). https://casetext.com/statute/code-of-maryland/article-public-safety/title-3-law-enforcement/subtitle-1-police-accountability-and-discipline/section-3-106-adjudication-of-disciplinary-matters

Bell v. Wolfish, 441 U.S. 520 (1979).

Bloom, J. D., & Kirkorsky, S. E. (2021). The Ninth Circuit Court of Appeals and jail-based competency evaluation and restoration. *Journal of the American Academy of Psychiatry and the Law, 49*(3), 415–421.

Bowring v. Godwin, 551 F.2d 44 (1977).

Carson, E. A. (2021a). *Mortality in state and federal prisons, 2001–2019—Statistical tables.* Bureau of Justice Statistics. https://bjs.ojp.gov/content/pub/pdf/msfp0119st.pdf

Carson, E. A. (2021b). *Suicide in local jails and state and federal prisons, 2001–2019—Statistical tables.* Bureau of Justice Statistics. https://bjs.ojp.gov/library/publications/mortality-state-and-federal-prisons-2001-2019-statistical-tables

Civil Rights of Institutionalized Persons Act, 42 U.S.C. § 1997 (1980). http://www.justice.gov/crt/about/spl/cripastat.php

Curtin, S. C., Garnett, M. F., & Ahmad, F. B. (2023). *Provisional estimates of suicide by demographic characteristics: United States, 2022.* https://www.cdc.gov/nchs/data/vsrr/vsrr034.pdf

Danzer, G. S., Wheeler, E. M. A., Alexander, A. A., & Wasser, T. D. (2019). Competency restoration for adult defendants in different treatment environments. *Journal of the American Academy of Psychiatry and the Law, 47*(1), 68–81.

Dressel, W. F., & Burns, D. (2012). The national judicial college and the mental competency best practices model. *Judges' Journal, 51*, 16–19. https://heinonline.org/HOL/LandingPage?handle=hein.journals/judgej51&div=21&id=&page=ttp://mentalcompetency.org/

Estelle v. Gamble, 429 U.S. 97 (1976).

Filarsky v. Delia, 566 U.S. 377 (2012).

Hogg Foundation. (2013). *Issue brief: Restoration of competency to stand trial.* https://utw10282.utweb.utexas.edu/wp-content/uploads/2015/09/Competency-Restoration-Brief.pdf

Jackson v. Indiana, 406 U.S. 715 (1972).

Jennings, J. L., & Bell, J. D. (2012). The "ROC" model: Psychiatric evaluation, stabilization and restoration of competency in a jail setting. In L. Labate (Ed.), *Mental illnesses—Evaluation, treatments and implications.* https://cdn.intechopen.com/pdfs/25947/InTech-The_roc_model_psychiatric_evaluation_stabilization_and_restoration_of_competency_in_a_jail_setting.pdf. *InTech*, 75–88.

Jones v. United States, 463 U.S. 354 (1983).

Kapoor, R. (2011). Commentary: Jail-based competency restoration. *Journal of the American Academy of Psychiatry and the Law, 39*, 311–315.

Kois, L. E., Potts, H., Cox, J., & Zapf, P. (2024). Court-reported competency to proceed data across the United States. *Law and Human Behavior, 48*(3), 182–202.

Krelstein, M. S. (2002). The role of mental health in the inmate disciplinary process: A national survey. *Journal of the American Academy of Psychiatry and the Law, 30*, 488–496.

Metzner, J. L. (2002). Commentary: The role of mental health in the inmate disciplinary process. *Journal of the American Academy of Psychiatry and the Law, 30*(4), 497–499.

Morris, N. P, McNeil, D. E., & Binder, R. L. (2021). Estimating annual numbers of competency to stand trial evaluations across the US. *Journal of the American Academy of Psychiatry and the Law*, *49*(4), 530–539.

Murrie, D. C., Gowensmith, W. N., Kois, L. E., & Packer, I. K. (2023). Evaluations of competence to stand trial are evolving amid a national "competency crisis." *Behavioral Sciences and the Law*, *41*(5), 310–315.

National Commission on Correctional Health Care. (2015). *Standards for mental health services in correctional facilities.*

National PREA Resource Center. (2013). *Prison and jail standards.* http://www.prearesourcecenter.org/training-technical-assistance/prea-101/prisons-and-jail-standards

New York CPL—Criminal Procedure, § 730.70. (2014). *Fitness to proceed: Procedure following termination of custody by commissioner.* https://newyork.public.law/laws/n.y._criminal_procedure_law_section_730.70

NRI. (2021). Competency restoration: Use of state hospitals, community-based, and jail-based approaches 2020–2021. https://www.nri-inc.org/our-work/nri-reports/competency-restoration-use-of-state-hospitals-community-based-and-jail-based-approaches-november-2021/

Obegi, J. H. (2021). Disciplinary responsibility in prison. *Journal of the American Academy of Psychiatry and the Law*, *49*(3), 316–322.

Policy Research Associates. (2020). *Quick fixes for effectively dealing with persons found incompetent to stand trial* (2nd ed). https://documents.ncsl.org/wwwncsl/Summit/2023/Session-Resources/Quick-Fixes-for-Effectively-Dealing-With-Persons-Found-Incompetent-to-Stand-Trial.pdf

Prison Rape Elimination Act of 2003, Pub. L. 108-79 (2003). https://www.congress.gov/108/plaws/publ79/PLAW-108publ79.pdf

Professional Risk Management Services. (2023). *Closed claims database.*

Sell v. United States, 539 U.S. 166 (2003).

Tamburello, A., & Azuh-Showole, C. (2022). Correctional psychiatry. In P. Ash, R. L. Frierson, & S. H. Friedman (Eds.), *Malpractice and liability in psychiatry* (pp. 217–224). Springer.

Tamburello, A. C., & Haston, L. (2021). Mischief, mayhem, and remediation. *Journal of the American Academy of Psychiatry and the Law*, *49*(3), 323–325.

U.S. Const. art. I, § 9, Clause 2. (n.d.). https://www.archives.gov/founding-docs/constitution-transcript.

Washington v. Harper, 494 U.S. 210 (1990).

67

Psychological testing

Virginia Barber Rioja, Tasha R. Phillips, and Ira K. Packer

Introduction

Correctional settings have an overrepresentation of people with different clinical presentations including severe psychopathology, trauma-related symptoms, and substance use and personality disorders (Baranyi et al., 2018; Karberg & James, 2005; Steadman et al., 2009). Early and ongoing identification of behavioral health issues in incarcerated persons (IPs) is important to inform treatment, levels of care/housing, and reentry services. However, identifying the exact diagnoses can be challenging for several reasons, including rapid turnover (particularly in jails), reliance on self-report, motivations to exaggerate or minimize symptoms, and confounding factors such as substance use, trauma, and the stressful environment of incarceration (Barber-Rioja et al., 2023). To better understand IPs' clinical presentations, psychological testing can be a helpful adjunct to standard screening and clinical assessments. In this chapter, we discuss the reasons for using psychological testing, as well as challenges of its use in correctional institutions. We discuss three domains of assessment and briefly describe the most commonly used tests in jails/prisons. We also discuss cultural issues, the forensic use of psychological testing, and the factors to consider when using new instruments. A brief case vignette is presented to illustrate how some tests help with assessment.

Rationales for using psychological testing in correctional settings

The institutional elements of correctional environments make arriving at the right diagnosis difficult. Many IPs have histories of inconsistent mental health care and can have histories of inconsistent or inaccurate diagnoses (Barber-Rioja et al., 2023). For these and other reasons, the rate of incorrect diagnoses in correctional settings is assumed to be higher than in the community (Martin et al., 2016). When diagnoses are not accurate, correctional settings run the risk of underdiagnosing, which can lead to overlooking IPs in need for treatment, or overdiagnosing, which can have other negative consequences such as causing stigma or unnecessary prescription of medications (Martin et al., 2016). Overdiagnosing can occur when the correctional system relies solely on the diagnoses made upon intake, a time when individuals might be experiencing anxiety due to stress or experiencing the effects of intoxication. Psychological testing can be helpful in reducing the likelihood of misdiagnoses. In turn, this allows correctional systems to allocate treatment resources appropriately.

Furthermore, the advantages of using psychological tests in an assessment include (a) standardization, (b) increased objectivity, and (c) comparison to established norms. When choosing to administer a test, it is important to consider whether the test has good psychometric properties and has been found appropriate for a correctional population. Psychometric qualities include reliability in scoring items and interpreting results (i.e., not varying significantly from one rater to another or from one administration to another given close in time), validity (accurately measuring what it purports to), and having well-established normative data (e.g., Weiner, 2012).

Psychological tests employ a standard set of questions or stimuli. This reduces the variability that can typify a clinical assessment. Tests also provide an objective source of information, as they include scoring rules that are applied consistently across administrations. Furthermore, psychometrically validated tests produce norms, which allow comparisons across individuals and time. For example, a test measuring psychopathology allows the psychologist to compare the IP's profile to that of other individuals. If the test is readministered, it allows comparison within the individual to determine whether significant change has occurred (such as improvement with treatment or decompensation).

Challenges of using psychological testing in correctional settings

Although psychological testing can be a valuable adjunct to other assessment procedures, there are limitations to its administration that must be considered. The primary challenge is staffing. Many jails and prisons do not hire licensed psychologists who are trained to administer and interpret psychological tests. Others may hire a small number of psychologists who might not have sufficient time or resources (e.g., testing materials). Given the range of tests, with varying suitability to a correctional population, a qualified doctoral-level psychologist should make the decision about which tests to administer (International Association of Correctional and Forensic Psychology, 2010). The referral should identify the issues and questions to address, instead of requesting specific tests, to allow the psychologist to choose the best instruments. Although technicians may administer many tests, only a qualified psychologist can interpret the results. The psychologist should produce a report that explains the results, their applicability to the referral issues, and any caveats about their validity. The results can then be integrated into the diagnostic assessment and treatment plan for the IP.

Furthermore, psychological testing should be administered in a standardized way and in a private and quiet environment. This is often difficult in correctional settings where security staff might need to be in close proximity to IPs, raising issues about test security and the impact on performance (Eastvold et al., 2012). Lastly, IPs are underrepresented in the normative samples of many psychological tests, which might limit data interpretation. Tests that include IPs in their normative or validation samples should be prioritized.

Three main categories of psychological testing can be useful in correctional settings: (a) cognitive, (b) personality and psychopathology, and (c) symptom or performance validity. Screening and comprehensive measures in each of these areas are discussed in the next sections.

Cognitive testing

Cognitive testing includes measurement of intelligence and assessment of functioning that may indicate neuropsychological impairment. Although the actual rate of intellectual disability (ID) in correctional settings is not known, it is believed to be higher than in the community (Mottram, 2007; see Chapter 57). Furthermore, given the significant increase in the aging population in jails and prisons (Carson & Sabol, 2016), neurocognitive disorders (NDs) are also a concern (see Chapter 60). Individuals with both IDs and NDs can be at risk of experiencing challenges when incarcerated, such as difficulties following institutional rules or an increased vulnerability to being victimized (Garcia-Mansilla & Wijetunga, 2023). For these reasons, correctional settings should briefly screen for IDs and NDs. Of note, thorough measures of neuropsychological functioning require specialized training and expertise to interpret the results. Clinical neuropsychology is a specialty area within psychology, and only those with this specialized training are qualified to interpret neuropsychological batteries and make appropriate recommendations.

Because there are many cognitive measures, with varying purpose, comprehensiveness, and utility, a full review is beyond the scope of this chapter. Rather, we highlight several measures frequently employed in correctional settings.

Screening measures

- *Wechsler Abbreviated Scale of Intelligence, Second Edition (WASI-II; Wechsler, 2011)*: A brief screening measure of general intellectual functioning through measures of verbal comprehension and perceptual reasoning. The WASI-II can be flexibly administered using all four subtests or only two subtests. It is strongly linked to the WAIS-IV (discussed below).
- *Beta-4 (Kellogg & Morton, 2016)*: Brief screening measure of nonverbal intelligence. The Beta-4 can be used with individuals who are non–English speaking, are illiterate, or have limited reading comprehension, and it can be administered in a group format. Although developed and normed on prison populations, very little subsequent research has been done to validate its use.
- *Repeatable Battery for the Assessment of Neuropsychological Status Update (RBANS; Randolph, 2012)*: Screening measure of cognitive status across four domains of neuropsychological functioning: language, attention, visuospatial/constructional, and immediate/delayed memory. The RBANS has been well validated as a screening tool for cognitive status of examinees with dementia, schizophrenia, and acute and postacute traumatic brain injury. Of note, a few authors have cautioned that this measure is not effective in detecting milder cognitive impairments (Duff et al., 2010; McKay et al., 2007).

Other screening cognitive measures that have been studied in correctional settings include the Hayes Ability Screening Index (Hayes, 2000), the Learning Disability Screening Questionnaire (McKenzie & Paxton, 2006), and the Rapid Assessment of Potential Intellectual Disability (Ali & Galloway, 2016).

Comprehensive measures

- *Wechsler Adult Intelligence Scale, Fourth Edition (WAIS-IV; Wechsler, 2008)*: Comprehensive measure of general intellectual functioning in four domains: verbal comprehension, perceptual reasoning, working memory, and processing speed. This instrument is the most widely used measure of general intellectual functioning in correctional, forensic, and community samples. However, because of its comprehensiveness, it can take 60 to 90 minutes to administer (Benson at al., 2010). The fifth version of the WAIS was published in 2024.
- *Wechsler Memory Scale, Fourth Edition (WMS-IV; Wechsler, 2009)*: Comprehensive measure of auditory, visual, and working memory. The WMS-IV is the most recent iteration of the most extensively validated measure of memory impairment. Because of its comprehensiveness, it can take 45 to 60 minutes to administer (Hoelzle et al., 2011). A fifth edition of the WMS is forthcoming according to the publishing company.

Personality and psychopathology testing

There are multiple self-report scales that have been developed to screen for symptoms of mental health or substance use disorders that can be used during the intake process in jails/prisons to flag IPs who require further assessment. A full review of these self-report scales is not within the purview of this chapter. However, it is important to note that few of these scales have been studied in correctional settings.

More comprehensive psychometric tests of psychopathology and personality can be employed in correctional settings (e.g., Boothby & Clements, 2000). These self-report inventories can take over an hour to complete and are not typically administered upon the IP's admission to the facility but rather after an initial mental health screening finds a need for additional data to help clarify the clinical formulation and diagnosis. The most commonly used tests for this purpose are the Minnesota Multiphasic Personality Inventory-2 (MMPI-2; Butcher et al., 2001) and subsequent revisions, the Millon Clinical Multiaxial Inventory-IV (MCMI-IV; Millon et al., 2015) and the Personality Assessment Inventory (PAI; Morey, 1991, 2007). These tests do not provide definitive diagnoses. Instead, they help generate hypotheses about diagnosis and symptom presentation that can be corroborated or disconfirmed by further clinical inquiry, observation, and other collateral courses. They also can serve as a source of convergent validity with clinical diagnoses. In other words, confidence in the diagnostic assessment will increase when the clinically derived diagnosis and the profile on the objectively scored test agree. These tests also include validity scales to assess overreporting and underreporting of problems and consistency of responses. One advantage of self-report measures in correctional facilities is that they can be administered in a group setting, with careful monitoring by qualified staff.

These tests are typically scored by a computer program, which produces a profile. In addition, testing companies offer interpretive reports, including ones specific to correctional settings. We urge caution in using such interpretive reports without review by a qualified psychologist.

In addition to these self-report inventories, projective techniques assess psychopathology and personality styles more indirectly. The best known of these is the Rorschach inkblot test. Considerable controversy exists in the psychology community about this test; some have criticized it, claiming that many of its measures have not been sufficiently validated (Wood et al., 2000), while others dispute these contentions (Meyer & Archer, 2001). Given this controversy, there is no consensus about the utility of this instrument. However, even its detractors acknowledge that the measure of thought disorder has good empirical support (Wood et al., 2000). Thus, the Rorschach may be useful to assess individuals who are guarded in a self-report format or who are in the early stages of a psychotic disorder (e.g., first-break schizophrenia). Other projective techniques, such as the Draw a Person Test or House Tree Person Test, are not widely accepted, as questions have been raised about the reliability and validity of interpretation (e.g., Garb et al. 2002).

- *Minnesota Multiphasic Personality Inventory-2 (MMPI-2; Butcher et al., 2001)*: A 567-item, true–false, self-report inventory that assesses personality traits, psychopathology, and response style. In 2000, Boothby and Clements reported that the MMPI-2 was the most widely used inventory of personality and psychopathology in correctional settings. The MMPI-2 has been extensively validated across correctional populations. However, one limitation is considerable item overlap, which resulted in limited discriminant validity (e.g., Graham, 2011).
- *Minnesota Multiphasic Personality Inventory-2—Restructured Form (MMPI-2-RF; Ben-Porath & Tellegen, 2008/2011)*: A revised 338-item version of the MMPI-2 designed to assess personality traits, psychopathology, and response style, which was developed to improve the convergent and discriminant validity of the instrument. Although this measure has not been as researched in correctional settings as its predecessor (Ben-Porath, 2012), studies have emerged in recent years exploring the construct validity of the MMPI-2-RF in correctional settings (see Tylicki et al., 2020).
- *Minnesota Multiphasic Personality Inventory-3 (MMPI-3; Ben-Porath & Tellegen, 2020)*: A 335-item version of the MMPI that was built on the MMPI-2-RF foundations with the goals of collecting new norms and enhancing content coverage. The MMPI-3 includes new scales. A significant advantage of the MMPI-3 is that, for the first time, the Spanish translation includes norms derived from a sample of U.S. Spanish speakers.
- *Personality Assessment Inventory (PAI; Morey, 2007*: A 344-item self-report inventory to assess personality traits, psychopathology, and response style. Several studies have demonstrated the widespread utility of this measure across correctional settings (Paulino et al., 2024). In addition to tapping constructs of psychopathology, the PAI assesses normative personality traits. However, the 4-point Likert response format can be particularly challenging for examinees with limited comprehension abilities (e.g., Magyar et al., 2012).
- *Millon Clinical Multiaxial Inventory, Fourth Edition (MCMI-IV; Millon* et al., *2015)*: A 195-item self-report inventory to assess *Diagnostic and Statistical Manual of Mental Disorders* categories of personality disorders and general psychopathology. The MCMI-IV focuses on personality disorders, which are prevalent in correctional settings. However, it has been noted that it might be susceptible to overpathologizing (McCann et al., 2001).

Validity testing

The third category of psychological testing relates to measures of symptom and performance validity. Symptom validity refers to the accuracy of self-reported symptoms, whereas performance validity refers to test performance (Larrabee, 2011). Symptom validity tests or embedded indicators (e.g., validity scales of MMPI-2 or PAI) often rely on self-report and structured interviews to gather data about the accuracy of an examinee's reported symptoms. The obtained score is compared to profiles of individuals known to have a genuine disorder or known to be exaggerating (including groups instructed to "fake bad" when taking the test).

Performance validity tests often rely on a forced-choice testing methodology, which was introduced by Pankratz et al. (1975). Forced-choice testing involves a series of trials in which examinees select between two alternatives: the correct response (or target) and the incorrect response (or foil). Significantly below-chance scores provide definitive evidence of intentionally incorrect answers (i.e., even a completely impaired examinee should obtain a 50% score by random guessing). However, because few people who malinger score below chance, performance validity instruments also provide cutoff scores that are above chance but below scores obtained by individuals with genuine impairments.

For a full review on the assessment of malingering in correctional settings, see Chapter 20. We highlight below a few frequently used symptom and performance validity instruments appropriate for correctional settings.

Symptom validity tests

- *Miller Forensic Assessment of Symptoms of Test (M-FAST; Miller, 2001)*: A brief (25-item) structured interview designed to screen for overreported psychopathology. Research has demonstrated that the M-FAST has good clinical utility across racial/ethnic groups and literacy levels. Of note, the M-FAST is not meant to screen for exaggeration of cognitive impairment.
- *Structured Inventory of Malingered Symptomatology (SIMS; Smith, 1998)*: A 75-item instrument to screen for overreporting of psychopathology and neuropsychological impairment. The SIMS has high sensitivity, which is a desirable characteristic for screening measures. However, some research suggests that it has a high false-positive rate—that is, it misclassifies examinees with genuine psychiatric illness as feigners (Edens et al., 2007).
- *Structured Inventory of Reported Symptoms, Second Edition (SIRS-2; Rogers et al., 2010)*: A 172-item structured interview

that uses several methods to assess overreporting. The SIRS-2 is considered the most comprehensive instrument for assessment of overreporting of psychotic symptoms. Because it typically takes 30 to 40 minutes per administration, we recommend use only after an IP has scored above the threshold for overreporting on one of the briefer screening tests described above. The SIRS-2 is a modified version of the original SIRS. The major modifications involve criteria for determining malingering. As a result, it can often result in indeterminate findings, thus limiting its sensitivity (Green et al., 2013). There is some controversy in the literature about the utility of using the SIRS-2 versus the SIRS due to this factor, and some have questioned whether the SIRS, rather than the SIRS-2, is the more useful instrument (e.g., DeClue, 2011; Rogers et al., 2020; Rubenzer, 2010; Tylicki et al., 2021).

Performance validity tests

- *Test of Memory Malingering (TOMM; Tombaugh, 1996)*: A forced-choice visual recognition test for distinguishing between exaggerated and bona fide memory impairments. The TOMM is easy to administer, and it has been adequately validated in criminal forensic samples. However, its established cutoff scores may result in false positives for individuals with dementia and intellectual disability (e.g., Gervais et al., 2004; Ray, 2012).
- *Validity Indicator Profile (VIP; Frederick, 1997; Frederick & Crosby, 2000)*: Assesses motivation and effort during cognitive testing and comprises a verbal and a nonverbal subtest, which can be used independently or as companion measures. The nonverbal subtest can be easily administered to non-English-speaking populations. The VIP is not considered appropriate for examinees with known diagnoses of intellectual disability (Frederick, 2002). Concerns have also been raised about its ability to distinguish cognitive feigning from active psychosis (Hunt et al., 2014).

Forensic use of psychological testing

It is important to remember that anything documented in the correctional medical record can be subpoenaed or requested by the courts. This is particularly relevant for individuals in jails whose cases have not yet been adjudicated. For example, it is common for medical records to be requested by attorneys and used with the purpose of making decisions about appropriateness for diversion programs. Records can also be requested by experts who are conducting evaluations to answer psycho-legal questions (e.g., criminal responsibility, competency to stand trial; see Chapter 66). In prisons, there is also a possibility that psychological testing results, which were meant to inform treatment, might instead be used by parole boards to make release decisions. As a result of the potential forensic use of psychological testing, some cautionary procedures should be followed. First, confidential health care documentation, including psychological testing reports, should be secured separately from corrections records. Second, the raw testing data should be stored separately and should not be part of the medical record. Third, IPs should be informed of all limits of confidentiality prior to beginning psychological testing. Lastly, it is recommended that testing reports include a statement clarifying that the report is not meant to answer psycho-legal questions (Barber-Rioja et al., 2023).

Cultural considerations

It is well known that Black people, Indigenous people, and people of color (BIPOC), including Hispanic people (Carson, 2021), are overrepresented in correctional settings and that racial biases can be a source of misdiagnosing in forensic settings (Pinals et al., 2004). Furthermore, most psychological tests have been developed and validated in Western, educated, industrialized, rich, and democratic (WEIRD) samples, raising concerns about the cultural validity of psychological testing for some IPs (Henrich et al., 2010). Cultural validity in assessment has been defined as the extent to which a measure addresses essential cultural factors to arrive at an accurate clinical diagnosis (Solano-Flores & Nelson-Barber, 2001). The lack of cultural validity can lead not only to misdiagnosis but also to stigmatizing or stereotyping of certain groups (Leong et al., 2020). Therefore, before deciding on the use of any one test, evaluators need to consider the cultural validity of the tests with respect to the IP's group membership. It is also important to note that although some tests are available in more than one language, this does not mean that there is research demonstrating the test's measurement equivalence and psychometrics (Leong et al., 2020). If evaluators decide to use tests with normative samples that differ from the background of the evaluee, they should weight the risks and benefits of using testing, and if the decision is that testing data can still add valuable information, the cultural limitations of the instrument need to be acknowledged in the report and considered when interpreting the data (American Psychological Association, 2013).

Assessing utility of new tests for correctional settings

Although this chapter focuses on a description and assessment of the most commonly used psychological tests in correctional settings, the field is constantly evolving, and new tests are likely to become available. The following guidelines can help determine the usefulness of newly developed tests:

1. Does the test have high reliability?
2. Has the test been validated on the relevant demographic population (factors include gender, race, ethnicity, education, language, acculturation, and age)?
3. Is the test valid for a correctional population? Megargee (2012) noted that the research on psychological tests in correctional settings lags behind the more extensive work in community settings. As new tests are developed and considered for correctional settings, it will be important to verify that they have demonstrated validity for that population.

Case example

Mr. Smith, a 51-year-old man, was convicted of murder and sentenced to 30 years in a maximum-security correctional facility. During intake, he reported a long-standing history of major mental illness and alcohol use. He described his most prominent historical symptoms as paranoid ideation, auditory hallucinations, and affective lability. He had been prescribed psychotropic medications in the community, with variable response. Prior to his incarceration in a state prison, he was detained in the county jail for approximately 8 months, during which he was prescribed a mood-stabilizing medication, a first-generation antipsychotic medication, and an atypical antipsychotic medication. When he arrived at the state facility, he appeared behaviorally stable but exhibited enduring paranoid delusions. Within a few weeks, he began to display confusion, agitation, confabulation, and repetitive verbalizations. His attending psychiatrist referred him for psychological testing to determine the nature and extent of his symptoms and to rule out feigning or exaggeration of symptoms.

Based on the referral information, the psychologist selected two tests to administer: the MMPI-2-RF and the RBANS. The MMPI-2-RF was selected to assess a wide range of clinical symptoms, personality characteristics, behavioral tendencies, and interpersonal functioning that can inform diagnosis and treatment recommendations. In addition, the MMPI-2-RF can provide information about Mr. Smith's response style. The RBANS was selected to screen broadly for potential neurocognitive impairment and to determine the need for further neuropsychological testing. The following is an example of potential findings from the psychologist's report:

> Based on his responses to the validity scales (assessing overreporting and underreporting of symptoms and consistency of responses), Mr. Smith answered MMPI-2-RF items in a seemingly honest and forthright manner. Thus, his scores on the substantive scales likely present an accurate portrayal of his psychological functioning. Mr. Smith's responses indicate serious thought dysfunction. He reports prominent persecutory ideation and is likely to feel alienated and suspicious of others and to have delusional thinking. He also reports unusual perceptions such as auditory hallucinations.
>
> In addition, Mr. Smith has cognitive difficulties including memory problems, poor concentration, and confusion. His cognitive complaints may be associated with his thought disturbance. He is likely to have low frustration tolerance and difficulty coping with stress. Finally, Mr. Smith reports a pattern of externalizing behavior, including antisocial conduct and substance use.
>
> Mr. Smith scored 64 on the RBANS. Compared to other individuals his age, his score is in the severely impaired range of neuropsychological functioning. His most prominent deficits are in immediate and delayed memory. Mr. Smith also has impairment in oral language and auditory and visual attention. He showed no deficits in visuospatial/constructional functioning.
>
> Mr. Smith's test results indicate several concerns and possible diagnoses for follow-up evaluation. Specifically, he has symptoms consistent with a thought disorder, most likely schizophrenia. In addition, Mr. Smith has neurocognitive difficulties. Although his symptoms of psychosis could partially account for these deficits, further specialized neuropsychological testing is recommended to explore other etiologies, such as side effects of his psychotropic medication or early-onset dementia.

After receiving the psychologist's report, the psychiatrist discussed the findings with the clinical team, who revised Mr. Smith's treatment plan accordingly and began investigating options for neuropsychological evaluation.

Summary

Well-validated psychological tests can be an important adjunct to mental health assessment in correctional settings. They can determine the validity of self-reported symptoms and identify psychiatric symptoms and cognitive deficits that may impair functioning. They can also help decrease the rate of misdiagnoses. However, there are significant challenges to the use of psychological testing that must be considered, including the fact that jails and prisons often do not have enough staff who are qualified to administer or interpret testing results, as well as the reduced number of instruments that have been appropriately studied in IPs and therefore are culturally valid. Lastly, it is important to set up policies or procedures to avoid unintended uses of psychological testing data.

REFERENCES

Ali, S., & Galloway, S. (2016). Developing a screening tool for offenders with intellectual disabilities—The RAPID. *Journal of Intellectual Disabilities and Offending Behaviour*, *7*(3), 161–170.

American Psychological Association. (2013). Specialty guidelines for forensic psychology. *American Psychologist*, *68*(1), 7–19.

Baranyi, G., Cassidy, M., Fazel, S., Priebe, S., & Mundt, A. P. (2018). Prevalence of posttraumatic stress disorder in prisoners. *Epidemiologic Reviews*, *40*(1), 134–145.

Barber-Rioja, V., Garcia-Mansilla, A., & Rodriguez, E. (2023). Identification of mental illness in jails: Screening and assessment. In V. Barber-Rioja, A. Garcia-Mansilla, B. Subedi, & A. Batastini (Eds.), *The handbook of mental health assessment and treatment in jails*. Oxford University Press.

Ben-Porath, Y. S. (2012). *Interpreting the MMPI-2-RF*. University of Minnesota Press.

Ben-Porath, Y. S., & Tellegen, A. (2011). *Minnesota Multiphasic Personality Inventory-2-Restructured Form: Manual for administration, scoring, and interpretation*. University of Minnesota Press. (Original work published 2008)

Ben-Porath, Y. S., & Tellegen, A. (2020). *Minnesota Multiphasic Personality Inventory-3. Manual for administration, scoring, and interpretation*. University of Minnesota Press.

Benson, N., Hulac, D., & Kranzler, J. (2010). Independent examination of the Wechsler Adult Intelligence Scale—Fourth Edition (WAIS-IV): What does the WAIS-IV measure? *Psychological Assessment*, *22*(1), 121–130.

Boothby, J. L., & Clements, C. B. (2000). A national survey of correctional psychologists. In C. R. Bartol & A. M. Bartol (Eds.), *Current perspectives in forensic psychology and criminal justice* (pp. 215–222). Sage Publications.

Butcher, J. N., Graham, J. R., Ben-Porath, Y. S., Tellegen, A. T., Dahlstrom, W. G., & Kaemmer, B. (2001). *Minnesota Multiphasic Personality Inventory-2: Manual for administration, scoring, and interpretation, revised edition*. University of Minnesota Press.

Carson, E. A. (2021). *Prisoners in 2020—Statistical tables* (NCJ 302776). Bureau of Justice Statistics, U.S. Department of Justice.

Carson, E. A., & Sabol, W. J. (2016). *Aging of the state prison population* (May report, NCJ 248766). Bureau of Justice Statistics, U.S. Department of Justice.

DeClue, G. (2011). Harry Potter and the Structured Interview of Reported Symptoms? *Open Access Journal of Forensic Psychology*, *3*, 1–18.

Duff, K., Hobson, V., Beglinger, L., & O'Bryant, S. (2010). Diagnostic accuracy of the RBANS in mild cognitive impairment: Limitations on assessing milder impairments. *Archives of Clinical Neuropsychology*, *25*(5), 429–441.

Eastvold, A., Belanger, H., & Vanderploeg, R. (2012). Does a third party observer affect neuropsychological test performance? It depends. *Clinical Neuropsychologist*, *26*(3), 520–541.

Edens, J., Poythress, N., & Watkins-Clay, M. (2007). Detection of malingering in psychiatric unit and general population prison inmates: A comparison of the PAI, SIMS, and SIRS. *Journal of Personality Assessment, 88*(1), 33–42.

Frederick, R. (1997). Review of the Validity Indicator Profile. *Journal of Forensic Neuropsychology, 2*, 125–145.

Frederick, R., & Crosby, R. (2000). Development and validation of the Validity Indicator Profile. *Law and Human Behavior, 24*, 59–82.

Garb, H., Wood, J., Lilienfeld, S., & Nezworski, M. (2002). Effective use of projective techniques in clinical practice: Let the data help with selection and interpretation. *Professional Psychology: Research and Practice, 33*(5), 454–463.

Garcia-Mansilla, A., & Wijetunga, C. (2023). Screening and assessment of intellectual disability and neurocognitive disorder in jails. In V. Barber-Rioja, A. Garcia-Mansilla, B. Subedi, & A. Batastini (Eds.), *The handbook of mental health assessment and treatment in jails*. Oxford University Press.

Gervais, R., Rohling, M. L., Green, P., & Ford, W. (2004). A comparison of WMT, CARB, and TOMM failure rates in non-head-injury disability claimants. *Archives of Clinical Neuropsychology, 19*, 475–487.

Graham, J. R. (2011). *MMPI-2: Assessing personality and psychopathology* (5th ed.). Oxford University Press.

Green, D., Rosenfeld, B., & Belfi, B. (2013). New and improved? A comparison of the original and revised versions of the Structured Interview of Reported Symptoms. *Assessment, 20*, 210–218.

Hayes, S. C. (2000). *The Hayes Ability Screening Index (HASI) manual*. Department of Behavioural Sciences in Medicine, University of Sydney.

Henrich, J., Heine, S. J., & Norenzayan, A. (2010). The weirdest people in the world? *Behavioral and Brain Sciences, 33*(2–3), 61–83.

Hoelzle, J., Nelson, N., & Smith, C. (2011). Comparison of Wechsler Memory Scale-Fourth Edition (WMS-IV) and Third Edition (WMS-III) dimensional structures: Improved ability to evaluate auditory and visual constructs. *Journal of Clinical and Experimental Neuropsychology, 33*(3), 283–291.

Hunt, S., Root, J. C., & Bascetta, B. L. (2014). Effort testing in schizophrenia and schizoaffective disorder: Validity indicator profile and test of memory malingering performance characteristics. *Archives of Clinical Neuropsychology, 29*(2), 164–172.

International Association of Correctional and Forensic Psychology. (2010). Standards for psychology services in jails, prisons, correctional facilities, and agencies, third edition. *Criminal Justice and Behavior, 37*, 749–808.

Joe, S., Woolley, M., Brown, G., Ghahramanlou-Holloway, M., & Beck, A. (2008). Psychometric properties of the Beck Depression Inventory-II in low-income, African American suicide attempters. *Journal or Personality Assessment, 90*(5), 521–523.

Karberg, J. C., & James, D. J. (2005). *Substance dependence, abuse, and treatment of jail inmates, 2002*. U.S. Department of Justice, Office of Justice Programs, Bureau of Justice Statistics.

Kellogg, C. E., & Morton, N. W. (2016). *Beta-4*. Pearson.

Larrabee, G. J. (2011). *Forensic neuropsychology: A scientific approach*. Oxford University Press.

Leong, F. T., Priscilla Lui, P., & Kalibatseva, Z. (2020). Multicultural issues in clinical psychological assessment. In M. Sellbom & J. A. Suhr (Eds.), *The Cambridge handbook of clinical assessment and diagnosis* (pp. 25–37).

Magyar, M., Edens, J., Lilienfeld, S., Douglas, K., Poythress, N., & Skeem, J. (2012). Using the Personality Assessment Inventory to predict male offenders' conduct during and progression through substance abuse treatment. *Psychological Assessment, 24*(1), 216–225.

Martin, M. S., Hynes, K., Hatcher, S., & Colman, I. (2016). Diagnostic error in correctional mental health: Prevalence, causes, and consequences. *Journal of Correctional Health Care, 22*(2), 109–117.

McCann, J. T., Flens, J. R., Campagna, V., Collman, P., Lazzaro, T., & Connor, E. (2001). The MCMI-III in child custody evaluations: A normative study. *Journal of Forensic Psychology Practice, 1*(2), 27–44.

McKay, C., Casey, J., Wertheimer, J., & Fichtenberg, N. (2007). Reliability and validity of the RBANS in a traumatic brain injured sample. *Archives of Clinical Neuropsychology, 22*(1), 91–98.

McKenzie, K., & Paxton, D. (2006). *Learning Disability Screening Questionnaire (LDSQ) manual*. GCM Records.

Megargee, E. I. (2012). Psychological assessment in correctional settings. In I. B. Weiner (Ed.), *Handbook of psychology: Vol. 10, Assessment* (pp. 365–388). Wiley and Sons.

Meyer, G. J., & Archer, R. P. (2001). The hard science of Rorschach research: What do we know and where do we go? *Psychological Assessment, 13*(4), 486–502.

Millon, T., Grossman, S., & Millon, C. (2015). *Millon Clinical Multiaxial Inventory-IV (MCMI-IV) manual*. NCS Pearson.

Morey, L. C. (1991). *Personality Assessment Inventory professional manual*.

Morey, L. C. (2007). *Personality Assessment Inventory professional manual* (2nd ed.).

Mottram, P. G. (2007). *HMP's Liverpool, Styal and Hindley YOI: Preliminary results*. NHS Specialised Services Commissioning Team, University of Liverpool.

Pankratz, L., Fautsi, A., & Peed, S. (1975). A forced-choice technique to evaluate deafness in the hysterical or malingering patient. *Journal of Consulting and Clinical Psychology, 43*, 421–422.

Paulino, M., Edens, J. F., Moniz, M., Moura, O., Rijo, D., & Simões, M. R. (2024). Personality assessment inventory (PAI) in forensic and correctional settings: A comprehensive review. *Journal of Forensic and Legal Medicine, 103*, 102661.

Pinals, D. A., Packer, I. K., Fisher, W., & Roy-Bujnowski, K. (2004). Relationship between race and ethnicity and forensic clinical triage dispositions. *Psychiatric Services, 55*(8), 873–878.

Randolph, C. (2012). *Repeatable battery for the Assessment of Neuropsychological Status Update (RBANS™ update)*. Pearson.

Ray, C. (2012). Assessment of feigned cognitive impairment: A cautious approach to the use of the Test of Memory Malingering for individuals with intellectual disability. *Open Access Journal of Forensic Psychology, 4*, 24–50.

Rogers, R., Sewell, K. W., & Gillard, N. D. (2010). *Structured Interview of Reported Symptoms (SIRS), 2nd Edition, professional manual*. Psychological Assessment Resources.

Rogers, R., Velsor, S. F., & Williams, M. M. (2020). A detailed analysis of SIRS versus SIRS2 critiques. *Psychological Injury and Law, 13*, 275–283.

Rubenzer, S. (2010). Review of the Structured Interview of Reported Symptoms-2 (SIRS-2). *Open Access Journal of Forensic Psychology, 2*, 273–286.

Solano-Flores, G., & Nelson-Barber, S. (2001). On the cultural validity of science assessments. *Journal of Research in Science Teaching: Official Journal of the National Association for Research in Science Teaching, 38*(5), 553–573.

Smith, G. P. (1998). *Structured Interview of Malingered Symptomatology (SIMS)*. PAR.

Steadman, H. J., Osher, F. C., Robbins, P. C., Case, B., & Samuels, S. (2009). Prevalence of serious mental illness among jail inmates. *Psychiatric Services, 60*(7), 61–765.

Tombaugh, T. N. (1996). *Test of Memory Malingering (TOMM)*. Multi-Health Systems.

Tylicki, J. L., Glassmire, D. M., Tarescavage, A. M., Wygant, D. B., & Sellbom, M. (2021). A response to Rogers and colleagues' analysis of a "trio" of SIRS/SIRS-2 comparison studies. *Psychological Injury and the Law, 14*, 281–290.

Tylicki, J. L., Phillips, T. R., Ben-Porath, Y. S., & Sellbom, M. (2020). Construct validity of Minnesota Multiphasic Personality Inventory-2-Restructured Form scale scores in correctional settings. *Personality and Mental Health, 14*(4), 319–335.

Weiner, I. B. (2012). The assessment process. In I. B. Weiner (Ed.), *Handbook of psychology: Vol. 10, Assessment* (pp. 3–25). Wiley and Sons.

Wechsler, D. (2008). *Wechsler Adult Intelligence Scale—Fourth Edition administration and scoring manual*. Pearson.

Wechsler, D. (2009). *Wechsler Memory Scale—Fourth Edition (WMS-IV)*. Pearson.

Wechsler, D. (2011). *Wechsler Abbreviated Scale of Intelligence—Second Edition (WASI-II)*. Pearson.

Wechsler, D., Raiford, S. E., & Presnell, K. (2024). *Wechsler Adult Intelligence Scale–Fifth Edition (WAIS-5)* [Psychological assessment]. Pearson.

Wood, J. M., Lilienfeld, S. O., Garb, H. N., & Nezworski, M. T. (2000). The Rorschach test in clinical diagnosis: A critical review, with a backward look at Garfield (1947). *Journal of Clinical Psychology, 56*, 395–430.

68

Pandemic management

Nathaniel P. Morris

Introduction

Infectious diseases have long posed risks to the health of people in jails and prisons (Beaudry et al., 2020; Fazel & Baillargeon, 2011). High rates of homelessness, poverty, substance use disorders, and other risk factors predispose incarcerated populations to communicable diseases (Fazel & Baillargeon, 2011). Additional structural factors, including overcrowding, confined spaces, inadequate access to health services, and limited ventilation, may further foster the spread of infectious disease behind bars (National Academies of Sciences, Engineering, and Medicine, 2020). Studies in the United States and elsewhere have found that incarcerated populations tend to have a higher prevalence of infectious diseases, such as HIV, tuberculosis, and viral hepatitis, than the general population (Fazel & Baillargeon, 2011; Hammett et al., 2002).

The emergence of a pandemic intensifies these challenges for jails and prisons. Although definitions vary (Morens et al., 2009), one definition of a pandemic is "an outbreak of a disease that occurs over a wide geographic area (such as multiple countries or continents) and typically affects a significant proportion of the population" (Merriam Webster, n.d.). When these types of large-scale outbreaks occur, such as influenza (Stanley, 1919), HIV (Harding, 1987), or COVID-19 (Rayman & Blau, 2023), people inside jails and prisons may face considerable risks of not only contagion but also adverse mental health effects. With a focus on the recent COVID-19 pandemic, this chapter explores the mental health implications of a pandemic for people inside jails and prisons, including deterioration of mental health, barriers to providing mental health services, and opportunities for providing care in these contexts. This chapter also examines strategies moving forward for addressing the mental health needs of people in jails and prisons within the context of the ever-present threat of infectious disease outbreaks.

Mental health effects on people in jails and prisons

While a pandemic can lead to a wide range of mental health effects on the general population (Salanti et al., 2022), people who are incarcerated or working in jails and prisons may be particularly susceptible to adverse mental health outcomes. Jails and prisons are "uniquely suited for the rapid multiplication and broader dissemination of infectious diseases" (Reinhart, 2023, p. 1418), which may heighten the psychological stress of a pandemic for incarcerated persons (IPs) and staff. In addition, incarcerated populations tend to have high rates of mental disorders, including substance use disorders (Fazel & Baillargeon, 2011); as a result, IPs may be especially vulnerable to the psychological stressors and disruptions in mental health services that may occur under these circumstances.

Common reactions, particularly during the early stages of a pandemic, include fear and anxiety about spreading infection, which many people may experience whether behind bars or not (Johnson et al., 2021). Strategies for reducing risks of infection, such as social distancing, hand hygiene, or face masking, may not always be feasible in the overcrowded and confined spaces of jails and prisons (Hawks et al., 2020), which can be stressful or even terrifying. For example, a recent oral history of the Rikers Island jail complex in New York City documented the widespread fear associated with the emergence of COVID-19. One formerly incarcerated person recalled:

> People were freaking out. Anytime there was a new person coming in, basically they would yell at the [correctional officers] not to open the gate for a new person ... that's the main thing that was going on during that time, a paranoia of just letting a new person into the house. That this could be somebody who's going to expose you to the virus. (Rayman & Blau, 2023, p. 340)

According to an attorney, "It was just chaos, and people were calling our phones, crying, freaking out ... the dorms were going under quarantine. Nobody knew what that meant. It was just sheer fear and confusion" (Rayman & Blau, 2023, p. 338).

Deteriorating conditions of confinement may place further psychological stress on IPs and staff in these facilities (Johnson et al., 2021). Infection control measures put in place during a pandemic may lead to near- or total-facility lockdowns for extended periods. IPs infected with or exposed to spreading disease may find themselves separated from others for lengthy periods in conditions resembling solitary confinement (Cloud et al., 2020). More broadly, restrictions on in-person visits, programming, and other out-of-cell activities may adversely affect the mental health of incarcerated populations and staff (Craig et al., 2023). In a survey of IPs in Illinois during the COVID-19 pandemic (John Howard Association, 2020, pp. 3–7), one respondent noted, "We haven't been outside ... everybody's going crazy, fighting and more," whereas another added, "Continued denial of yards, dayrooms, and gym no longer keeps us safe. In fact it endangers our mental health because it is not healthy for human beings to only be allowed to go outside for only 90 minutes every two weeks." Inability to see or communicate with loved ones, delays in court proceedings, and lack of access to up-to-date information can add even more psychological strain for people experiencing incarceration and their families during a pandemic (Charles et al., 2022).

Staffing shortages can compound these adverse mental health effects. Whether because of falling ill, fearing coming to work, or being denied access to entry, staff and volunteers may be less present in jails and prisons during a pandemic (Craig et al., 2023; Rayman & Blau, 2023). An attorney describing Rikers Island during the COVID-19 pandemic stated, "The correction officers were dropping like flies. And I think at one point in time, they had like three thousand or four thousand correction officers sick. So correctional officers were working three shifts at a time and falling asleep on the job" (Rayman & Blau, 2023, pp. 337–338). Due to decreased staff presence, IPs may face more difficulties in not only being let out of their cells but also getting basic needs met (e.g., food, hygiene supplies, phone calls, transportation to appointments; Craig et al., 2023). Pandemic-related staffing crises may also foster dangerous conditions in carceral environments, with media reports of IPs taking over housing areas, violence, and other adverse events during the COVID-19 pandemic (Blakinger et al., 2021; Ransom et al., 2021).

Falling ill with the disease spreading during a pandemic may itself lead to neuropsychiatric symptoms warranting clinical attention. High rates of chronic illness, older age, and other risk factors may place incarcerated populations at increased risk for infection-related morbidity and mortality, including neuropsychiatric sequelae (Hawks et al., 2020; Tronick et al., 2022). Published reports have documented a range of short-term and long-term neuropsychiatric symptoms associated with infectious diseases, such as COVID-19 (Schou et al., 2021), HIV (Knights et al., 2017), and influenza (Mizuguchi, 2013). The types of infection-related neuropsychiatric symptoms that people in jails and prisons might experience depend on the illness spreading during a pandemic; however, common examples of neuropsychiatric symptoms that have been tied to such infectious diseases include mood disturbances, behavioral changes, cognitive dysfunction, and fatigue, among others (Knights et al., 2017; Mizuguchi, 2013; Munjal et al., 2017; Schou et al., 2021). Even if available in jails and prisons, specific treatments for infectious diseases, such as antiviral therapies (Zareifopoulos et al., 2020) or corticosteroids (Warrington & Bostwick, 2006), may be associated with neuropsychiatric side effects that must also be considered.

In a 2021 scoping review of the recent COVID-19 pandemic, Johnson and colleagues (2021, p. 5) summarized that "the reported impacts on the mental health of imprisoned people are overwhelmingly negative, caused not just by fear of COVID-19, but mediated through the regime changes implemented to minimise infection risks." Still, there may be limited examples of positive mental health outcomes for people with criminal legal involvement during a pandemic (Abrams et al., 2023). For instance, the COVID-19 pandemic drew international attention to the risks of contagion in jails and prisons, inspiring decarceration efforts (DLA Piper, 2020; Tronick et al., 2022). One law firm report estimated that more than 1 million people around the world may have been released from incarceration by December 2020 in response to the COVID-19 pandemic (DLA Piper, 2020). For people who otherwise would have been incarcerated, living in the community due to pandemic-related policy shifts may bring some degree of mental health benefits, such as avoiding the trauma of incarceration or reuniting with family and friends (Abrams et al., 2023; McConnell, 2023). People leaving jail and prison settings during a pandemic still face reentry challenges, including risks of homelessness, unemployment, limited access to mental health services, and return to substance use, that must also be considered (Piel, 2020; Tronick et al., 2022). Such decarceration efforts may also be short-lived, as seen in the United States, where many jail and prison populations soon rebounded after the start of the COVID-19 pandemic (Kang-Brown et al., 2023).

Barriers to providing mental health services

This section reviews just a few of the challenges that a pandemic brings for mental health services in jails and prisons. First, institutional responses to a pandemic may affect incarcerated patients' willingness to participate in mental health care. Some patients may not be willing to take the risks of participating in care if infection control measures are unavailable or underutilized (James, Riddle, et al., 2023; Liu, LeBoa, et al., 2022; Suhomlinova et al., 2022). Even when infection control measures are implemented and available, patients may find that these measures (e.g., face masks, social distancing, telepsychiatry services) impede relationships with clinicians and peers (Daou et al., 2023; Erschens et al., 2022; Mitzkovitz et al., 2022). Rapid changes in pandemic-related policies (e.g., masking, testing) may foster confusion among both IPs and staff (Abrams et al., 2023; Rayman & Blau, 2023; Schultz & Ricciardelli, 2023). Mistrust of custody and health staff is common among IPs, and failures of pandemic management may further exacerbate such mistrust, potentially reducing participation in mental health care (Craig et al., 2023; Liu, LeBoa, et al., 2022; Liu, Oto, et al., 2022). Custody and health staff might also mistrust pandemic-related information and interventions (e.g., face masks, vaccines), which can complicate the delivery of mental health services (Craig et al., 2023; James, Riddle, et al., 2023; Saloner et al., 2023). Providing clear and ongoing communication about pandemic-related updates to both staff and IPs is an essential part of addressing such issues.

Second, pandemic-related staffing challenges may reduce the availability of mental health services behind bars (Rayman & Blau, 2023; Wainwright et al., 2023). Jails and prisons face chronic shortages of mental health staff (Morris & Edwards, 2022); however, even fewer mental health staff may be available to work in jails and prisons during a pandemic due to illness, fear of coming to work, restrictions on in-person care, and other logistical challenges (Hewson et al., 2020; Kothari et al., 2020). Decreased availability of custody staff during a pandemic can also complicate the provision of mental health services, preventing the completion of essential tasks such as transporting patients to and from appointments (Kothari et al., 2020; Sherman, 2021). Amid these staffing challenges, custody and health staff who continue working during a pandemic can face increased workloads, stress, and burnout, which may also affect their abilities to function adequately (Burhanullah et al., 2021).

Third, restrictive conditions of confinement can limit the availability of nonpharmacologic options for managing mental health concerns. Virtually every source of support that patients might rely on for mental well-being, from communication with family to in-person visits to educational classes, might be cut off during a pandemic (Charles et al., 2022; Craig et al., 2023; Rayman & Blau, 2023).

Social distancing efforts may lead to decreased availability or the complete suspension of individual and group therapy for incarcerated patients (Burton et al., 2021; Hearty et al., 2023). Patients who rely on physical exercise to maintain mental well-being may not be able to do so amid extended lockdowns because of restrictions on yard or gym access (John Howard Association, 2020). Under these circumstances, mental health professionals may find that medication prescribing is one of the few options available to them for managing the distress of patients behind bars (Izenberg & Morris, 2023).

Opportunities for providing mental health services

A pandemic complicates the delivery of mental health services behind bars; at the same time, such disruptions can allow for some unexpected opportunities for providing care to people with criminal legal involvement. For example, a number of jails and prisons turned to telepsychiatry to facilitate mental health services for IPs during the COVID-19 pandemic (Burton et al., 2021; Kamat et al., 2023). Some carceral systems used telepsychiatry for years preceding the COVID-19 pandemic (Daou et al., 2023; Deslich et al., 2013); still, the recent pandemic brought renewed attention to the potential utility of telepsychiatry behind bars, including the decreased risks of contagion and the ability of clinicians to reach patients from afar (Burton et al., 2021; Daou et al., 2023). Telepsychiatry in carceral settings is not without its challenges, including the costs of equipment upgrades, training requirements for health and custody staff, need for collaboration between on-site and off-site staff, and security considerations (Daou et al., 2023). Telepsychiatry may be a useful option for outpatient mental health services behind bars, although questions remain about the effectiveness of telepsychiatry for providing higher levels of care (e.g., emergency or inpatient) in carceral environments (Daou et al., 2023; see Chapter 21).

Widespread focus on the need for decarceration during a pandemic may also provide opportunities to care for patients in less restrictive settings. As previously discussed, the COVID-19 pandemic led to rapid reductions in incarceration, for example, through decreased arrests or increased releases, in many places around the world (DLA Piper, 2020; James, Dauria, et al., 2023; Tronick et al., 2022). Whether during a pandemic or not, providing mental health services behind bars can entail numerous challenges. In contrast, decarceration efforts during a pandemic might allow some patients to receive mental health services in less restrictive community settings that are better suited to their individual needs (Tronick et al., 2022). When a pandemic is so severe, however, as to inspire such decarceration efforts, court systems and other community resources, such as mental health care, housing services, employment opportunities, and transportation, will also likely face significant disruptions, which can complicate reentry planning (Howell et al., 2020; James, Dauria, et al., 2023; Piel, 2020; Tronick et al., 2022).

Looking forward

Research from this latest pandemic indicates that people behind bars experienced high rates of morbidity and mortality related to COVID-19, with many jails and prisons experiencing significant outbreaks (Burton et al., 2021; Sugie et al., 2023). The degree of infectious disease transmission in carceral environments can also pose risks to surrounding communities by intensifying the spread of disease, including upon release and reentry (Reinhart & Chen, 2020). Not all pandemics are the same, as the type of spreading illness, modes of disease transmission, availability of vaccines and treatments, and other factors can shape the ways in which a pandemic might affect jails and prisons (Morens et al., 2009). Still, scholars have warned that greater global interconnectedness may increase risks of future pandemics (Baker et al., 2022). Jails and prisons face constant challenges related to infectious diseases (Beaudry et al., 2020; Fazel & Baillargeon, 2011) and should have policies in place regarding the management of large-scale infectious disease outbreaks, including the continuation of mental health services (Saloner et al., 2023).

In preparation for such outbreaks, jails and prisons should have clear procedures for implementing new public health measures, communicating with relevant government agencies, and disseminating information updates to IPs, staff, and the broader public (Saloner et al., 2023). As noted by Saloner et al. (2023, p. 847), these guidelines should "allow tailoring for the resources, staffing, and space of individual facilities." To guide decision-making among health and custody staff, jails and prisons must have a defined organizational hierarchy for these situations; in particular, regular collaborative meetings across disciplines (e.g., leadership from health and custody staff) can be essential for coordinating responses to these types of infectious disease outbreaks (Puglisi et al., 2022). Coordination with local and state department of health officials is essential, as well as current knowledge of relevant guidelines from national agencies, such as the Centers for Disease Control and Prevention (Puglisi et al., 2022; Saloner et al., 2023).

Shortages of health and custody staff are chronic problems in many carceral systems, and given that a pandemic may acutely exacerbate these shortages, jails and prisons should develop contingency plans for the continuation of mental health services and other essential functions in the event of such absences (Saloner et al., 2023). Jail and prison leaders also need to recognize and address the adverse mental health effects of a pandemic, including anxiety, depression, and burnout, on health and custody staff (Burhanullah et al., 2022). For example, establishing protocols early on for symptom screening, disease testing, telework, use of sick leave, and other supportive services may be key for balancing the risks of infectious disease spread with the need to support the well-being and presence of staff (Beaudry et al., 2020; Kothari et al., 2020).

The adverse mental health effects of infection control measures need to be carefully weighed against the risks of contagion (Johnson et al., 2021; Saloner et al., 2023). To mitigate these mental health risks, jail and prison leadership should rely on the least restrictive means necessary to prevent and control infection, as well as review the necessity of restrictions placed on conditions of confinement on a regular basis (James, Riddle, et al., 2023; Johnson et al., 2021). For example, jail and prison leadership should not reflexively place people who have been exposed to illness or infected into punitive isolation, which has been referred to as "solitary confinement by another name," but instead "follow community standards of care" for medical isolation and quarantine (Cloud et al., 2020, p. 2741). Facilitating access to digital tools (e.g., email or video calls for communicating with family, electronic tablets for programming and entertainment) may be another approach that can ameliorate some, but not all, of the adverse mental health effects of infection control measures in jails and prisons during a pandemic (Reisdorf, 2023).

The devastating effects that a pandemic can have on people in jails and prisons reinforce the need to reduce unnecessary use of incarceration in the United States and beyond (National Academies of Sciences, Engineering, and Medicine, 2020). Decarceration is possible through a range of policy approaches, such as decreasing inflow into incarceration (e.g., sentencing reforms, developing alternatives to incarceration; see Chapter 6) or increasing outflow from incarceration (e.g., changing release policies; National Academies of Sciences, Engineering, and Medicine, 2020; Tronick et al., 2022). Such approaches are essential for addressing the overcrowding, staffing shortages, and other resource constraints that otherwise turn jails and prisons into such high-risk places during a pandemic (National Academies of Sciences, Engineering, and Medicine, 2020; Tronick et al., 2022). Decarceration policies must be paired with robust reentry planning and investment in community services to meet the mental health and other reentry needs of people who otherwise would have been incarcerated (Howell et al., 2020; Piel, 2020; Tronick et al., 2022; see Chapter 23).

Finally, continued research into the mental health implications of the COVID-19 pandemic and other disease outbreaks is vital for better understanding and meeting the needs of people in jails and prisons. In an article examining infectious disease in prisons from a human rights perspective, Paul Farmer (1999, p. 1492), a physician and anthropologist, once wrote, "We need to listen to the sick and abused and to those most likely to have their rights violated." In addition to the perspectives of staff, the voices of incarcerated and formerly incarcerated people can offer firsthand insights into the failures and successes of pandemic management behind bars (Rayman & Blau, 2023). Including these voices in the studies and practices that arise out of the COVID-19 years is crucial to better prepare jails and prisons for the next pandemic to emerge.

Summary

Pandemics pose considerable risks to people who are incarcerated or working inside jails and prisons. Outbreaks of illness, fear of infection, shortages of custody and health staff, disruptions in correctional mental health services, and challenges to reentry planning, among other factors, may lead to adverse mental health outcomes among IPs and staff. Jails and prisons should have policies in place to mitigate the risks of infectious disease outbreaks and to meet the mental health needs of IPs and staff when these circumstances arise. Reducing unnecessary use of incarceration is essential for addressing the risks that infectious disease poses to people behind bars, particularly during a pandemic.

REFERENCES

Abrams, L. S., Reed, T. A., Bondoc, C., Acosta, D. R., Murillo, M., & Barnert, E. S. (2023). "It was there when I came home": Young adults and jail reentry in the context of COVID-19. *American Journal of Criminal Justice*, *48*(3), 767–785.

Baker, R. E., Mahmud, A. S., Miller, I. F., et al. (2022). Infectious disease in an era of global change. *Nature Reviews Microbiology*, *20*(4), 193–205.

Beaudry, G., Zhong, S., Whiting, D., Javid, B., Frater, J., & Fazel, S. (2020). Managing outbreaks of highly contagious diseases in prisons: A systematic review. *BMJ Global Health*, *5*(11), e003201.

Blakinger, K., Lartey, J., Schwartzapfel, B., Thompson, C., & Sisak, M. R. (2021, November 1). *US prisons face staff shortages as officers quit amid COVID*. AP News and The Marshall Project. https://apnews.com/article/coronavirus-united-states-prisons-staff-shortages-health-dba13f1c6368392be2bc5e7375170a78

Burhanullah, M. H., Rollings-Mazza, P., Galecki, J., Van Wert, M., Weber, T., & Malik, M. (2021). Mental health of staff at correctional facilities in the United States during the COVID-19 pandemic. *Frontiers in Psychiatry*, *12*, 767385.

Burton, P. R. S., Morris, N. P., & Hirschtritt, M. E. (2021). Mental health services in a U.S. prison during the COVID-19 pandemic. *Psychiatric Services*, *72*(4), 458–460.

Charles, P., Muentner, L., Jensen, S., et al. (2022). Incarcerated during a pandemic: Implications of COVID-19 for jailed individuals and their families. *Corrections*, *7*(5), 357–368.

Cloud, D. H., Ahalt, C., Augustine, D., Sears, D., & Williams, B. (2020). Medical isolation and solitary confinement: Balancing health and humanity in US jails and prisons during COVID-19. *Journal of General Internal Medicine*, *35*(9), 2738–2742.

Craig, M. O., Kim, M., & Beichner-Thomas, D. (2023). Incarcerated in a pandemic: How COVID-19 exacerbated the "pains of imprisonment." *Criminal Justice Review*, *49*(2), 244–266.

Daou, M. A. Z., Ford, E., Gandhi, T., et al. (2023). *Resource document on telepsychiatry in jails and prisons*. American Psychiatric Association. https://www.psychiatry.org/getattachment/00e3f401-0792-4b78-90ba5985dd791a4e/Resource-Document-on-Telepsychiatry-in-Jails-and-Prisons.pdf

Deslich, S. A., Thistlethwaite, T., & Coustasse, A. (2013). Telepsychiatry in correctional facilities: Using technology to improve access and decrease costs of mental health care in underserved populations. *Permanente Journal*, *17*(3), 80–86.

DLA Piper. (2020). *A global analysis of prisoner releases in response to COVID-19*. https://www.dlapiper.com/-/media/files/insights/publications/2021/03/dla-piper-prison-population-during-covid-19.pdf

Erschens, R., Adam, S. H., Weisshap, C., et al. (2022). The role of face masks within in-patient psychotherapy: Results of a survey among inpatients and healthcare professionals. *Frontiers in Neuroscience*, *16*, 1030397.

Farmer, P. (1999). Pathologies of power: Rethinking health and human rights. *American Journal of Public Health*, *89*(10), 1486–1496.

Fazel, S., & Baillargeon, J. (2011). The health of prisoners. *The Lancet*, *377*(9769), 956–965.

Hammett, T. M., Harmon, M. P., & Rhodes, W. (2002). The burden of infectious disease among inmates of and releasees from US correctional facilities, 1997. *American Journal of Public Health*, *92*(11), 1789–1794.

Harding, T. W. (1987). AIDS in prison. *The Lancet*, *2*(8570), 1260–1263.

Hawks, L., Woolhandler, S., & McCormick, D. (2020). COVID-19 in prisons and jails in the United States. *JAMA Internal Medicine*, *180*(8), 1041–1042.

Hearty, P., Canvin, K., Bellass, S., Hampton, S., Wright, N., & Sheard, L. (2023). Understanding the impact of Covid-19 on the delivery and receipt of prison healthcare: An international scoping review. *Health & Justice*, *11*, 42.

Hewson, T., Shepherd, A., Hard, J., & Shaw, J. (2020). Effects of the COVID-19 pandemic on the mental health of prisoners. *Lancet Psychiatry*, *7*(7), 568–570.

Howell, B. A., Batlle, H. R., Ahalt, C., et al. (2020). Protecting decarcerated populations in the era of COVID-19: Priorities for emergency discharge planning. Health Affairs. https://www.healthaffairs.org/content/forefront/protecting-decarcerated-populations-era-covid-19-priorities-emergency-discharge

Izenberg, J. M., & Morris, N. P. (2023). The freedom cure—Structural intervention as medicine. *New England Journal of Medicine, 389*, 389–391.

James, J. E., Dauria, E. F., Desai, R., Bell, A., & Izenberg, J. M. (2023). "Good luck, social distance": Rapid decarceration and community care for serious mental illness and substance use disorder during the COVID-19 pandemic. *Health & Justice, 11*(1), 39.

James, J. E., Riddle, L., & Perez-Aguilar, G. (2023). "Prison life is very hard and it's made harder if you're isolated": COVID-19 risk mitigation strategies and the mental health of incarcerated women in California. *International Journal of Prisoner Health, 19*(1), 95–108.

John Howard Association. (2020). *Perceptions and experiences from people inside prison during the pandemic: Yard & out-of-cell time.* https://static1.squarespace.com/static/5beab48285ede1f7e8102102/t/5f9b3e44d3553d44af1ea255/1604009540162/JHA+COVID-19+Prison+Survey+Comment+Report+Yard+and+Out-of-cell+Time+Section.pdf

Johnson, L., Gutridge, K., Parkes, J., Roy, A., & Plugge, E. (2021). Scoping review of mental health in prisons through the COVID-19 pandemic. *BMJ Open, 11*(5), e046547.

Kamat, S. M., Gansa, W., D'Ovidio, T., et al. (2023). Clinician perspectives for mental health delivery following COVID-19 in carceral settings: A pilot study. *Psychiatric Quarterly, 94*(2), 233–242.

Kang-Brown, J., Jones, S., Tagal, J., & Zhang, J. (2023). *People in jail and prison in 2022.* Vera Institute of Justice. https://www.vera.org/downloads/publications/People-in-Jail-and-Prison-in-2022.pdf

Knights, M. J., Chatziagorakis, A., & Kumar Buggineni, S. (2017). HIV infection and its psychiatric manifestations: A clinical overview. *BJPsych Advances, 23*(4), 265–277.

Kothari, R., Forrester, A., Greenberg, N., Sarkissian, N., & Tracy, D. K. (2020). COVID-19 and prisons: Providing mental health care for people in prison, minimising moral injury and psychological distress in mental health staff. *Medicine, Science and the Law, 60*(3), 165–168.

Liu, Y. E., LeBoa, C., Rodriguez, M., et al. (2022). COVID-19 preventive measures in Northern California jails: Perceived deficiencies, barriers, and unintended harms. *Frontiers in Public Health, 10*, 854343.

Liu, Y. E., Oto, J., Will, J., et al. (2022). Factors associated with COVID-19 vaccine acceptance and hesitancy among residents of Northern California jails. *Preventive Medicine Reports, 27*, 101771.

McConnell, S. (2023). Sentenced to prison, not to death: Home confinement during the pandemic and moving beyond COVID-19. *Arkansas Law Review, 75*(4), 929–957.

Merriam-Webster. (n.d.). *Pandemic.* https://www.merriam-webster.com/dictionary/pandemic

Mitzkovitz, C., Dowd, S. M., Cothran, T., & Musil, S. (2022). The eyes have it: Psychotherapy in the era of masks. *Journal of Clinical Psychology in Medical Settings, 29*(4), 886–897.

Mizuguchi, M. (2013). Influenza encephalopathy and related neuropsychiatric syndromes. *Influenza and Other Respiratory Viruses, 7*(s3), 67–71.

Morens, D. M., Folkers, G. K., & Fauci, A. S. (2009). What Is a pandemic? *Journal of Infectious Diseases, 200*(7), 1018–1021.

Morris, N. P., & Edwards, M. L. (2022). Addressing shortages of mental health professionals in U.S. jails and prisons. *Journal of Correctional Health Care, 28*(4), 209–214.

Munjal, S., Ferrando, S. J., & Freyberg, Z. (2017). Neuropsychiatric aspects of infectious diseases. *Critical Care Clinics, 33*(3), 681–712.

National Academies of Sciences, Engineering, and Medicine. (2020). *Decarcerating correctional facilities during COVID-19: Advancing health, equity, and safety.* National Academies Press.

Piel, J. (2020). Letter to the editor—Behavioral health implications of inmate release during COVID-19. *Journal of Forensic Sciences, 65*(4), 1379–1381.

Puglisi, L. B., Rosenberg, A., Credle, M., et al. (2022). Paths to improving pandemic preparedness in jails and prisons: Perspectives of incarcerated people and correctional staff. *American Journal of Public Health, 112*(S9), S869–S873.

Ransom, J., Bromwich, J. E., & O'Brien, R. D. (2021, October 11). Inside Rikers: Dysfunction, lawlessness and detainees in control. *The New York Times.* https://www.nytimes.com/2021/10/11/nyregion/rikers-detainees-correction-officers.html

Rayman, G., & Blau, R. (2023). *Rikers: An oral history.* Random House.

Reinhart, E. (2023). Abolitional public health. *The Lancet, 401*(10386), 1418–1419.

Reinhart, E., & Chen, D. L. (2020). Incarceration and its disseminations: COVID-19 pandemic lessons from Chicago's Cook County Jail. *Health Affairs, 39*(8), 1412–1418.

Reisdorf, B. C. (2023). Locked in and locked out: How COVID-19 is making the case for digital inclusion of incarcerated populations. *American Behavioral Scientist, 68*(9), 1180–1199.

Salanti, G., Peter, N., Tonia, T., et al. (2022). The impact of the COVID-19 pandemic and associated control measures on the mental health of the general population. *Annals of Internal Medicine, 175*(11), 1560–1571.

Saloner, B., Kramer, C., Song, M., et al. (2023). COVID-19 restrictions in jails and prisons: Perspectives from carceral leaders. *Health Affairs, 42*(6), 841–848.

Schou, T. M., Joca, S., Wegener, G., & Bay-Richter, C. (2021). Psychiatric and neuropsychiatric sequelae of COVID-19—A systematic review. *Brain, Behavior, and Immunity, 97*, 328–348.

Schultz, W. J., & Ricciardelli, R. (2023). The floating signifier of "safety": Correctional officer perspectives on COVID-19 restrictions, legitimacy and prison order. *British Journal of Criminology, 63*(5), 1237–1254.

Sherman, R. (2021, August 26). *Rikers staffing crisis limits access to medical care.* THE CITY with New York Focus. http://www.thecity.nyc/2021/08/26/rikers-staffing-crisis-medical-care/

Stanley, L. L. (1919). Influenza at San Quentin prison, California. *Public Health Reports (1896–1970), 34*(19), 996–1008.

Sugie, N. F., Turney, K., Reiter, K., et al. (2023). Excess mortality in U.S. prisons during the COVID-19 pandemic. *Science Advances, 9*(48), eadj8104.

Suhomlinova, O., Ayres, T. C., Tonkin, M. J., O'Reilly, M., Wertans, E., & O'Shea, S. C. (2022). Locked up while locked down: Prisoners' experiences of the COVID-19 pandemic. *British Journal of Criminology, 62*(2), 279–298.

Tronick, L. N., Amendolara, B., Morris, N. P., et al. (2022). Decarceration of older adults with mental illness in the USA—Beyond the COVID-19 pandemic. *International Journal of Prisoner Health, 18*(2), 213–226.

Wainwright, L., Senker, S., Canvin, K., & Sheard, L. (2023). "It was really poor prior to the pandemic. It got really bad after": A qualitative study of the impact of COVID-19 on prison healthcare in England. *Health & Justice, 11*(1), 6.

Warrington, T. P., & Bostwick, J. M. (2006). Psychiatric adverse effects of corticosteroids. *Mayo Clinic Proceedings, 81*(10), 1361–1367.

Zareifopoulos, N., Lagadinou, M., Karela, A., Kyriakopoulou, O., & Velissaris, D. (2020). Neuropsychiatric effects of antiviral drugs. *Cureus, 12*(8), e9536.

69

Hunger strikes

Haseeb Haroon and Emily A. Keram

He has chosen death:
Refusing to eat or drink, that he may bring
Disgrace upon me; for there is a custom,
An old and foolish custom, that if a man
Be wronged, or think that he is wronged, and starve
Upon another's threshold till he die,
The Common People, for all time to come,
Will raise a heavy cry against that threshold,
Even though it be the King's.

—W. B. Yeats, *The King's Threshold* (Yeats & Kiely, 2005)

Introduction

The management of incarcerated persons (IPs) on hunger strikes presents unique clinical and ethical challenges for physicians. A physician's primary considerations are the health of their patient and respect for human life (World Medical Association [WMA], 2022), advanced within an ethical framework of respect for patient autonomy, beneficence, nonmaleficence, and justice (Beauchamp & Childress, 2019). Physicians caring for hunger strikers may be involved in medical decisions that lead to opposite extremes, from death by starvation to force-feeding. The potential for such complex tensions between medical decision-making and ethics rarely exists in other settings.

This chapter provides psychiatrists with a historical, legal, and ethics background for working with incarcerated hunger strikers. The lack of international consensus on the topic is discussed. The psychiatric evaluation and treatment of hunger strikers within the management protocols of correctional institutions are reviewed. The role of psychiatrists as consultants for treatment teams and correctional staff is explored.

Definition

The WMA defines hunger strikes as voluntary refusal of nutrition by a mentally competent person, usually as a form of protest. The extent may vary, with some individuals refusing food but accepting supplements such as vitamins and minerals, whereas others refuse all nutrition except fluids. Food refusal for less than 72 hours is usually excluded from the WMA definition of hunger strikes because it rarely causes medical problems for healthy individuals. Religious fasts are not considered hunger strikes. Dry fasting refers to the refusal of nutrition and hydration (WMA, 2006), which can cause serious harm, as humans cannot survive more than a few days without fluids.

History

Self-starvation as an instrument of nonviolent protest has an ancient history. Hindu scriptures from approximately the 4th century BCE reference hunger strikes. In the Ramayana, Prince Bharata refuses to eat to compel his brother Rama to assume the throne (Menon, 2004; Narayan, 2006). Brehon law, a system of oral law in pre-Christian Ireland, enforced judgments with *troscud*: If a defendant failed to provide the adjudicated compensation, the wronged party would fast at their doorstep to coerce payment (Higgins, 2011). A similar system of justice, sitting *dhurna*, existed in ancient India (Vernon, 2007).

In prisons, hunger strikes have occurred regularly since the early 1900s. The first recorded hunger striker was Marion Wallace-Dunlop, a detained English suffragette. Other suffragettes in Britain and the United States later adopted the practice. The authorities subjected them to force-feeding, which they protested as a form of torture (Sullivan & Romilly, 2000). Public outcry against their maltreatment led to the passage of the Prisoner's Temporary Discharge of Ill Health Act of 1913 in Britain, allowing the temporary release of incarcerated hunger strikers if they became ill.

The vacillating approach of British authorities to political prisoners in the 20th century demonstrates the challenges correctional facilities face in determining how to respond to hunger strikes. When imprisoned proponents of Irish independence adopted hunger strikes in 1917 (Beresford, 1997; O'Malley, 1991), the authorities force-fed them. After Thomas Ashe died of injuries from force-feeding, the practice was suspended. In the 1920s and 1940s, though, dozens of hunger strikers were allowed to die without intervention. Force-feeding intermittently resumed from the 1970s onward. Several hunger strikers, including Michael Gaughan, died, some after force-feeding. Later, 10 prisoners died in a 1981 hunger strike where the authorities did not intervene. The strike only ended after some of the prisoners' demands were met following the deaths.

Contemporary hunger strikes

Hunger strikes continue to occur in prisons around the world. Some capture global attention, such as the mass hunger strikes in South African prisons in the 1980s (Reyes, 1998), while others receive little coverage. In the 2000s and 2010s, the maltreatment of hunger strikers detained in the U.S. Naval Station at Guantanamo Bay drew unanimous criticism from professional medical associations and renewed scrutiny on the management of custodial hunger strikes (Rosenberg, 2014; Rubenstein & Thomson, 2013).

When the COVID-19 pandemic began in 2020, IPs across North America staged collective hunger strikes over conditions in detention facilities (Stern, 2022). Asylum seekers and undocumented immigrants detained in Europe and the United States held mass hunger strikes to protest the conditions of their detention (Strauss, 2021) and were reportedly subjected to retaliatory abusive treatment including force-feeding, involuntary catheterization, and restrictive housing (American Civil Liberties Union, 2021). Amnesty International (2023) provides frequent updates about ongoing hunger strikes around the world.

Ethical and legal frameworks

Regulatory and legal bodies often lack consensus on how to balance competing interests such as the health of IPs, their civil rights, and the safety needs of correctional institutions during hunger strikes. Varying international conceptions of inviolable human rights contribute to disparate approaches that are further complicated by the differing roles and priorities of IPs, custodial personnel, and physicians during hunger strikes.

International medical organizations

The WMA Declaration of Malta (WMA, 2017), supported by most national medical associations, states that when "a prisoner refuses nourishment and is considered by the physician as capable of forming an unimpaired and rational judgment concerning the consequences of such a decision, he or she shall not be fed artificially" (Principle 21). The Declaration further states, "Forced feeding is never ethically acceptable" (Principle 23).

The WMA established additional standards for physicians caring for detained hunger strikers, including the need to ascertain that the fasting is voluntary, to respect the autonomy of competent hunger strikers (even if it may lead to harm), and to transfer care to another physician if they cannot honor the patient's choices. Balancing dual loyalties and acting independently from detaining authorities are emphasized. A physician's primary obligation is always to their patient. Physicians are encouraged to exercise their moral judgment in complex situations, and the WMA pledged to support physicians who refuse to follow the orders of detaining authorities on ethical grounds.

The International Committee of the Red Cross (2013) also considers force-feeding hunger strikers a "gross violation of medical ethics." When invited, the International Committee of the Red Cross monitors facilities with ongoing hunger strikes to ensure that IPs are receiving appropriate medical care that meets ethical standards and that health professionals are not involved in coercive acts like force-feeding.

International views

The United Nations' Standard Minimum Rules for the Treatment of Prisoners were unanimously adopted by the 193 United Nations member states (United Nations, 2015). The rules outline the minimum human rights standards to be guaranteed in detention facilities and prohibit coercive and degrading treatment of IPs. However, they do not specifically address hunger strikes.

The European Court of Human Rights (2022) established binding case law on correctional hunger strikes for member nations. The European Court of Human Rights allows for force-feeding on a case-by-case basis. States must balance their "positive obligation" to protect human life against the prohibition of torture. Detaining authorities may use forced interventions if there is medical evidence of a serious risk of harm to the hunger striker's life or health. Even then, force-feeding is unlawful if it cannot be administered without excessive force or degrading elements. Permitting a mentally competent hunger striker to die from voluntary refusal of nutrition or other care does not violate the European Convention on Human Rights so long as the detaining authority "duly examined and managed the situation" (European Court of Human Rights, 2022, p. 41).

Other continental courts, such as the Inter-American Court of Human Rights and African Court on Human and Peoples' Rights, have the jurisdiction to address human rights issues in their regions. They have not yet established case law on the treatment of detained hunger strikers.

National laws

In the absence of binding international law, nations' approaches to hunger strikers in custody vary. Although a complete discussion of differences between nations' laws is beyond the scope of this chapter, comparing Canada and the United States demonstrates these inconsistencies, even in geographically contiguous, socioeconomically comparable nations.

The Corrections and Conditional Release Act of 1992 governs the treatment of incarcerated persons in Canada (Statutes of Canada, 1992). It states in § 89 that custodial authorities "shall not direct the force-feeding, by any method, of an inmate who had the capacity to understand the consequences of fasting at the time the inmate made the decision to fast."

In contrast, there are no national statutes directly addressing this matter in the United States, though case law supports force-feeding for custodial hunger strikers if medically necessary. The foundational precedent is a Supreme Court verdict (*Turner v. Safley*, 1987) that intrusions on the constitutional rights of prisoners are lawful if they are "reasonably related to legitimate penological interests." This principle also allows prison authorities to medicate IPs forcibly, even in the absence of a determination that they are incompetent (*Washington v. Harper*, 1990). The U.S. Supreme Court has not established a nationwide precedent specifically addressing force-feeding during hunger strikes. The Connecticut Supreme Court held that custodial staff could force-feed a prisoner if medically necessary because the state's interests in the prisoner's health and facility safety outweighed the prisoner's rights to bodily integrity, free speech, and privacy (*Commissioner of Correction v. Coleman*, 2012).

Ethics dilemmas for physicians

Correctional psychiatrists may be asked to serve several roles while managing hunger strikes. They may assess medical decision-making capacity and the voluntariness of food refusal, assist the patient in formulating advance directives, treat co-occurring mental illness, and liaise between different stakeholders. Physicians are also obligated to report any known or suspected torture or abuse and should know the procedures for such reporting, along with policies and laws protecting whistleblowers (Daines, 2007).

Hunger strikers may be distrustful of clinicians, viewing them as agents of the detaining authority who lack impartiality. If clinicians perform forced medical interventions, they may feel that they are violating their patients' trust to meet their employers' demands. Dual loyalty, where physicians experience conflict between duty to their patients and the expectations of their employer, is a major concern. Clinicians of hunger strikers describe feeling "caught between" and "instrumentalized" by the agendas of stakeholders (Haselwarter et al., 2022). Medical personnel may perceive that the authorities pressure them to prematurely declare hunger strikers at risk of death or serious injury to justify the authorities' interventions to end the strike. At the same time, clinicians may feel that hunger strikers are attempting to use them for their political goals.

Medical ethics are unequivocal that a physician's primary obligation is to their patients. However, determining what is best for a patient's well-being may be complicated in the context of a hunger strike. Physicians may have to reckon with conflicting concepts of "benefit" and "harm." The principle of beneficence urges clinicians to resuscitate deteriorating hunger strikers; however, intervening over the person's informed objection constitutes maleficence. Dilemmas around the refusal of life-saving care are emotionally challenging. Further complexity arises when clinicians are asked to provide supportive care (like analgesics) that could prolong the hunger strike and increase health risks for the patient. Clinicians must ensure that their value judgments about the patient's protest and refusal of certain interventions do not prejudice the provision of other appropriate care.

Role of the psychiatrist

Correctional psychiatrists may be vital to the positive resolution of hunger strikes in custody. Around 1% to 3% of prisoners may participate in hunger strikes annually (Daines, 2007; Eichelberger et al., 2014), and as many as 45% of hunger strikers have been reported to have a mental health diagnosis (Reeves et al., 2017).

Decision-making capacity and voluntariness

The assessment of decision-making capacity during hunger strikes is like the process in other settings (Appelbaum & Grisso, 1988). To determine whether to allow an IP's strike to continue, their understanding of the potential effects of the hunger strike on their health must be assessed. They must understand the physical and mental health consequences of refusing food and recommended medical care, and they must have intact reality testing for these concerns. Prisoners lacking this capacity may require interventions including force-feeding. As religious fasts are not considered hunger strikes, they should be respected.

The presence of mental illness is insufficient to establish that the patient lacks capacity; the symptoms must be related to the food refusal. If fasting is a psychiatric symptom (e.g., it is based on delusions or suicidal intent), the underlying cause must be treated. Incapacitated patients should not be allowed to fast to the point that their health is damaged. If the safety of an IP with a mental illness is at risk or their judgment regarding their need for treatment is impaired, psychiatrists should follow institutional guidelines for involuntary treatment (see Chapter 25). Conversely, the initial absence of mental illness does not establish capacity to refuse food indefinitely. The physiologic consequences of starvation may lead to changes in hunger strikers' mental states. Decision-making capacity is not fixed and must be reevaluated periodically. Institutions may codify minimum intervals for reevaluation. Physicians should exercise their discretion and reassess capacity as dictated by the patient's clinical condition.

If the hunger striker is competent, the psychiatrist's next duty is to evaluate the voluntariness of food refusal. To be voluntary, the decision to fast must reflect the individual's own will, preferences, and motives rather than external pressures. Psychiatrists may consider whether the decision is subject to undue influence—a concept often associated with probate law. Factors that suggest the decision-maker may be under undue influence include the vulnerability of the decision-maker (e.g., if they are cognitively or intellectually impaired); if there is an influencer with power over the decision-maker; the overt or covert use of affection, intimidation, or control to influence the decision-maker; and inequities in outcomes (i.e., the consequences are incongruent with the values of the decision-maker or harm them disproportionately, Plotkin et al., 2016).

Psychiatrists should discuss flaws or lack of logic in the IP's decision-making without causing undue pressure. They should be aware of possible sources of coercion such as hunger-striking peers or family members. IPs may fear retribution from the influencer if they accept medical care or end their strike. Inappropriate treatment (e.g., taunting) by staff members or peers may also inhibit hunger strikers from stopping their fast. Clinicians should discuss these possibilities with hunger strikers and attempt to ensure their safety. If the decision to strike appears voluntary, it should be respected. If hunger strikers appear under duress, transferring them to a hospital can be recommended on medical grounds. If duress is confirmed, feeding can be offered and accomplished in the hospital, away from coercive influences. If a psychiatrist cannot gain a hunger striker's trust to conduct a sufficiently detailed evaluation, an external psychiatrist with no relationship to custodial authorities may be invited to perform the evaluation.

Psychiatrists must be able to talk privately with hunger strikers for effective assessment. However, complete privacy may be unattainable in the high-surveillance environments of detention facilities. Even in the absence of actual monitoring, IPs may perceive that they are being observed. These limits to confidentiality should be discussed prior to evaluation and patients' concerns addressed where possible. Reports or recommendations submitted to a decision-making authority should acknowledge the impact a lack of privacy had on the reliability of an evaluation.

If interpreters are used, efforts should be made to ensure they are impartial and unrelated to the authorities or other stakeholders. Significant cultural differences often exist between interpreters and patients. In the context of heightened emotions surrounding a hunger strike, these may contribute to antagonistic interactions that interfere with the patient–physician relationship. Psychiatrists should be aware of these potential interpersonal dynamics and, as necessary, address the working relationship between patient and interpreter or request a different interpreter.

Consideration of hunger strikers' advance directives regarding artificial feeding and resuscitation varies by region. In some jurisdictions, a patient's advance instructions dictate physicians' interventions once they lose consciousness. In others, physicians face prosecution if they do not intervene to save a hunger striker's life. Prior to or early in a hunger strike, physicians should have a frank discussion with patients about whether and when they wish to receive artificial feeding and resuscitation if they become incapacitated. If physicians are legally bound to perform life-saving interventions against the patient's wishes, they should discuss this as well. If physicians cannot accept a patient's competent, legally permissible decision because of their personal values or beliefs, a physician willing to act in accord with the patient's choices should take their place.

It may be beneficial to have a psychiatrist present for discussions about advanced directives between the IP and treating clinicians. This allows the psychiatrist to assess capacity in a context where the IP's questions and concerns can be addressed and provides the responsible medical providers with a contemporaneous opinion of the hunger striker's capacity to understand the risks of food refusal. Psychiatrists can assist both parties with identifying and working through uncomfortable affect generated by such discussions.

Physiological and psychological sequelae

The fasting body initially uses liver and muscle glycogen stores for energy. Later, ketosis occurs, which is evident on the breath and lab studies, and subdues the sensation of hunger (WMA, 2006). Glycogen stores are depleted in 10 to 14 days; at this point, muscle—including cardiac muscle—is catabolized for amino acids used in gluconeogenesis. The WMA recommends close medical monitoring after 10% of body weight is lost, and major health problems may arise around a weight loss of 18%. Dehydration becomes a serious risk as homeostatic hunger and thirst mechanisms are lost.

Hunger strikes involving cessation of fluids pose the most danger, as death is almost certain to occur within a week (WMA, 2006). Patients experience hypovolemia, hypotension, and tachycardia. Peripheral vasoconstriction initially preserves brain, cardiac, and renal perfusion. As dehydration progresses, renal function declines, elevating serum blood urea nitrogen, creatinine, and potassium (Daines, 2007). Severe hyperkalemia can cause fatal arrhythmias.

Most hunger strikers continue to ingest fluids while refusing food (WMA, 2006). Orthostatic hypotension, bradycardia, and hypothermia occur frequently (Gordon et al., 2018). There may be electrocardiogram changes including early repolarization and QTc interval prolongation (Daines, 2007; Hobikoğlu et al., 2019). Early repolarization is typically a benign finding but may elevate the risk of sudden cardiac death for patients with a history of ventricular arrhythmia or a family history of sudden cardiac death. Orthostatic hypotension and QTc prolongation can be exacerbated by psychotropic medications, especially antipsychotics and tricyclic antidepressants, and cause serious adverse events. Dehydration may increase the risk of neuroleptic malignant syndrome. Physicians must account for these changes in treatment decisions.

Hunger strikers often report chest pain, abdominal pain, and dizziness (Gordon et al., 2018). Dyspnea is less common. Leukopenia is frequent, while hemoglobin is typically within normal limits (Gordon et al., 2018). The international normalized ratio is often prolonged and should prompt evaluation for other risk factors for abnormal bleeding (e.g., selective serotonin reuptake inhibitors). Vitamin K supplementation should be considered.

Electrolyte disturbances such as hyponatremia and hypokalemia may be observed and are usually manageable with fluids (Eichelberger et al., 2014; Gordon et al., 2018). Thiamine deficiency may occur after approximately 4 weeks of inadequate intake and cause Wernicke encephalopathy or cardiomyopathy, which can be debilitating and lethal. There should be a low threshold to supplement thiamine.

Hypoalbuminemia and hypoproteinemia may occur with prolonged fasting (Gordon et al., 2018), affecting the serum concentrations of highly protein-bound drugs, such as valproic acid. Patients may need close observation for signs of toxicity. Unbound drug concentrations should be considered for monitoring the therapeutic level of the drug.

Psychiatrists should also be aware of the effects of food refusal on mental state. Early in a hunger strike, anger and irritability may intensify, increasing motivation to continue the strike even as health risks increase (Fessler, 2003). These negative emotions may strengthen the need for instant gratification—in this instance, redress of grievances—and skew the IP's assessment of the risks and benefits of food refusal. Long-term hunger strikers experience significant gaps in memory and an inability to concentrate (WMA, 2006). As the body begins to experience medical and psychiatric consequences, physicians must resume serious discussions with hunger strikers about their wishes (Fessler, 2003).

If IPs end their hunger strike, food must be reintroduced cautiously to avoid refeeding syndrome. Symptoms may include malabsorptive diarrhea, fluid shifts resulting in edema and congestive heart failure, arrhythmias, and cardiac death (Eichelberger et al., 2014). Institutions should implement refeeding protocols for hunger strikers to avoid preventable complications. Empirical supplementation of micronutrients followed by gradual refeeding with fluid restriction reduces adverse outcomes (Eichelberger et al., 2014).

Co-occurring psychiatric illness

Due to the stress of hunger strikes and their precipitants, IPs may develop acute psychiatric problems, and those with chronic conditions may decompensate. Psychiatrists should be vigilant for the emergence of symptoms in patients on strike—which may affect capacity—and offer treatment as indicated.

Nonpharmacologic options such as cognitive and supportive psychotherapy may reduce distress. Pharmacologic options to treat psychiatric symptoms for hunger strikers are generally similar to those for noncustodial patients; however, some important distinctions should be considered for drug selection. The physiological effects of prolonged food refusal may alter the pharmacokinetics or exacerbate side effects of psychotropic medications. For instance, bupropion is associated with seizures in patients with eating disorders, tricyclic antidepressants and antipsychotics cause and exacerbate orthostatic hypotension, and the risk of lithium toxicity is higher with dehydration (Daines, 2007).

Hunger strikers may be willing to accept psychotropic medications while fasting. If suicidality or psychosis become the motivation for continued food refusal, physicians may be ethically obligated to provide involuntary treatment through artificial feeding, fluid resuscitation, and forced medications. Institutional policy and local laws should be followed in determining the need for involuntary treatment. Psychiatrists should be familiar with parenteral agents available at the facility for involuntary medication. Insertion of a nasogastric tube may be necessary to administer nutrition and medications (Daines, 2007).

Mental illness symptoms may be difficult to distinguish from signs of starvation. For instance, depression symptoms include appetite loss, weight loss, impaired concentration, psychomotor retardation, and fatigue. Depressive symptoms not expected solely due to starvation include suicidal ideation, anhedonia, depressed mood, diminished self-worth, and guilt. Conversely, IPs previously overwhelmed by the very real loss of control over their lives in detention may experience a restored sense of self-worth, purpose, and autonomy with participation in a hunger strike. Psychiatrists should be attuned to the possible presence of these dynamics to improve their understanding of the patient's needs.

IPs may have the capacity to refuse nourishment despite having a serious mental illness. Absent flagrant symptoms (e.g., command hallucinations or delusional beliefs regarding the hunger strike), psychiatrists should conduct a detailed evaluation of the patient's decision-making capacity as they would for hunger strikers without psychosis.

Eating disorders can be particularly challenging to diagnose and manage with hunger strikes. They may be overlooked if IPs declare motivations other than caloric restriction for fasting (Daines, 2007). Psychiatrists should routinely assess patients' prestrike nutritional history and inquire about body image to avoid missing an eating disorder. Suspicious physical exam findings (e.g., amenorrhea, hair loss, lanugo, dental enamel erosion, parotid hypertrophy) should prompt further evaluation (Klein et al., 2021).

Consultation and liaison

Psychiatric consultation may be useful in correctional hunger strikes by providing education and improving communication. Psychiatrists can help the treatment team and custodial staff clarify and modulate negative feelings toward hunger strikers. Helping staff understand the psychological effects of starvation, such as anger and irritability, may decrease their perception of being personally attacked by hunger strikers. Explaining IPs' psychiatric symptoms to staff members may assist them in interacting with challenging patients and de-escalating conflict around events such as physical examinations and cell moves.

Custodial personnel might view hunger strikes antagonistically as blackmail. In military custodial settings, hunger strikes may—incorrectly—be perceived as engaging in "asymmetric warfare." Psychiatrists may be able to mediate between hunger strikers and custodial authorities, especially when they have the trust of both parties. They can provide a historical context on hunger strikes in detention and help reframe the hunger strike by emphasizing the goals of the stakeholders. If clinicians treating hunger strikers experience conflicts between their perceived ethical responsibilities and honoring the patient's choices, psychiatrists can provide support to help them navigate these dilemmas.

The WMA suggests that most hunger strikers want to find a way to end their fast and may do so if the authorities make minor concessions. Psychiatrists may be able to negotiate such compromises. If hunger strikers' demands are obviously out of reach, psychiatrists must not pretend otherwise. They should make clear to both parties that their role is to assist in negotiations and that they are not a party to them. During this process, they should continue providing accurate information to patients about their medical condition without interference from the authorities.

Summary

Participating in the management of a hunger-striking IP poses demanding clinical and ethics questions for physicians. Psychiatrists should have a clear understanding of international guidelines for physicians on the ethical management of hunger strikes, as well as their institution's policies and procedures on hunger strikes and force-feeding. They should resolve whether they are willing or able to provide care in a setting where their patients' wishes or the demands of their employer conflict with their beliefs regarding their professional obligations. Consultation with peers and experts in the field may assist in balancing conflicting roles and responsibilities.

REFERENCES

American Civil Liberties Union. (2021). *Behind closed doors: Abuse and retaliation against hunger strikers in U.S. immigration detention.* https://www.aclu.org/publications/report-behind-closed-doors-abuse-retaliation-against-hunger-strikers-us-immigration-detention

Amnesty International. (2023). *Amnesty International report: The state of the world's human rights.* https://www.amnesty.org/en/documents/pol10/5670/2023/en/

Appelbaum, P. S., & Grisso, T. (1988). Assessing patients' capacities to consent to treatment. *New England Journal of Medicine, 319*(25), 1635–1638.

Beauchamp, T. L., & Childress, J. F. (2019). *Principles of biomedical ethics.* Oxford University Press.

Beresford, D. (1997). *Ten men dead: The story of the 1981 Irish hunger strike.* Atlantic Monthly Press.

Commissioner of Correction v. Coleman, 303 Conn. 800 (2012).

Daines, M. K. (2007). Hunger strikes in correctional facilities. In O. J. Thienhaus & M. Piasecki (Eds.*), Correctional psychiatry: Practice guidelines and strategies* (pp. 8–1–8–13). Civic Research Institute.

Eichelberger, M., Joray, M., Perrig, M., Bodmer, M., & Stanga, Z. (2014). Management of patients during hunger strike and refeeding phase. *Nutrition, 30*(11–12), 1372–1378.

European Court of Human Rights. (2022). *Guide on the case-law of the European Convention on Human Rights.* https://www.echr.coe.int/documents/d/echr/Guide_EU_law_in_ECHR_case-law_ENG

Fessler, D. M. T. (2003). The implications of starvation induced changes for the ethical treatment of hunger strikers. *Journal of Medical Ethics, 29*, 243–247.

Gordon, D., Drescher, M., & Shiber, S. (2018). Security hunger-strike prisoners in the emergency department: Physiological and laboratory findings. *Journal of Emergency Medicine, 55*(2), 185–191.

Haselwarter, D., Wild, V., & Kuehlmeyer, K. (2022). Providing health care in politically charged contexts: A qualitative study about experiences during a public collective hunger strike of asylum seekers in Germany. *International Journal of Qualitative Studies on Health and Well-Being, 17*, 2018770.

Higgins, N. (2011). The lost legal system: Pre-common law Ireland and Brehon law. In D Frenkel (Ed.), *Legal theory, practice and education* (pp. 193–205). Atiner.

Hobikoğlu, G., Urumdaş, M., Özkurt, Y., Zehir, R., & Güner, A. (2019). Effect of hunger strike on electrocardiographic parameters. *Archives of the Turkish Society of Cardiology, 47*(5), 379–383.

International Committee of the Red Cross. (2013). *Hunger strikes in prison: The ICRC's position*. https://www.icrc.org/en/document/hunger-strikes-prisons-icrc-position

Klein, D. A., Sylvester, J. E., & Schvey, N. A. (2021). Eating disorders in primary care: Diagnosis and management. *American Family Physician, 103*(1), 22–32.

Menon, R. (2004) *The Ramayana: A modern retelling of the great Indian epic*. North Point Press.

Narayan, R. K. (2006). *The Ramayana*. Penguin Group.

O'Malley, P. (1991). *Biting at the grave: The Irish hunger strikes and the politics of despair*. Beacon Press.

Plotkin, D. A., Spar, J. E., & Horwitz, H. L. (2016). Assessing undue influence. *Journal of the American Academy of Psychiatry and the Law, 44*(3), 344–351.

Reeves, R., Tamburello, A., Platt, J., Tepper, D., & Edelman, K. (2017). Characteristics of inmates who initiate hunger strikes. *Journal of the American Academy of Psychiatry and the Law, 45*(3), 302–310.

Reyes, H. (1998). *Medical and ethical aspects of hunger strikes in custody and the issue of torture*. https://www.icrc.org/en/doc/resources/documents/article/other/health-article-010198.htmRosenberg, C. (2013). *AMA opposes forced feedings at Guantanamo*. https://www.miamiherald.com/news/nation-world/world/americas/guantanamo/article1950859.html

Rubenstein, L., & Thomson, G. (2013). *Ethics abandoned: Medical professionalism and detainee abuse in the "War on Terror."* Institute on Medicine as a Profession.

Statutes of Canada. (1992). *Corrections and Conditional Release Act, § 89*. Amended June 23, 2022. https://canlii.ca/t/55h6k

Stern, G. (2022). *Dozens on hunger strike at Nevada prison over food, health*. https://apnews.com/article/health-hunger-strikes-nevada-covid-reno-1b6dbb97d32ed3890b0cfe0c4ba5ae14

Strauss, M. (2021). *Migrants' hunger strike puts Belgian government in danger*. https://www.reuters.com/world/europe/migrants-hunger-strike-puts-belgian-government-danger-2021-07-21/

Sullivan, D., & Romilly, C. (2009). Hunger strike and food refusal. In S. Wilson & I. Cumming (Eds.), *Psychiatry in prisons: A comprehensive handbook* (pp. 155–171). Jessica Kingsley Publishers.

Turner v. Safley, 482 U.S. 78 (1987).

United Nations. (2015). *Standard minimum rules for the treatment of prisoners*. Amended December 2015. https://www.unodc.org/documents/justice-and-prison-reform/Nelson_Mandela_Rules-E-ebook.pdf

Vernon, J. (2007). *Hunger: A modern history*. Belknap Press.

Washington v. Harper, 494 U.S. 210 (1990).

World Medical Association. (2006). WMA Declaration of Malta—A background paper on the ethical management of hunger strikes. *World Medical Journal, 52*(2), 36–43.

World Medical Association. (2017). *Declaration on hunger strikers (Declaration of Malta)*.Amended October 2017. https://www.wma.net/policies-post/wma-declaration-of-malta-on-hunger-strikers/

World Medical Association. (2022). *International code of medical ethics*. Amended October 2022. https://www.wma.net/policies-post/wma-international-code-of-medical-ethics/

Yeats, W. B., & Kiely, D. (2005). *The king's threshold: Manuscript materials*. Cornell University Press.

70

Responding to sexual abuse of incarcerated persons

Robert W. Dumond and Doris A. Dumond

Introduction

This chapter explores the status of sexual victimization in U.S. correctional settings in the 21st century; examines what is known about sexual victimization in America's jails, prisons, and juvenile facilities; discusses the successes and promising practices facilitated by the Prison Rape Elimination Act (PREA) of 2003; considers the challenges that continue to exist; and makes recommendations for addressing the issues.

Sexual abuse in U.S. jails and prisons has long been known but ignored

At the dawn of the U.S. penitentiary movement, the Reverend Louis Dwight, president of the Boston Discipline Society (1824–1854), decried that "nature and humanity cry aloud for redemption from this dreadful degradation" of sexual abuse (Katz, 1976, p. 27). One hundred years later, Joseph F. Fishman, a federal inspector of prisons who visited 1,500 jails and prisons in the United States before 1920 (Freidman, 1993), found the problem unabated as many boys and young men were "made homosexual, either temporarily or permanently" (Fishman, 1934, p. 5). Unfortunately, it would take nearly 2 centuries for there to be a substantive response to "America's most open secret" (Bell et al., 1999, p. 195), the "plague that persists" (Dumond, 2000, p. 407), and "America's most ignored crime problem" (Lehrer, 2001, p. 24).

March to the Prison Rape Elimination Act of 2003

A series of court cases involving staff sexual misconduct in the 1990s brought attention to the problem of sexual abuse in prisons and jails (*Cason v. Seckinger*, 2000; *Farmer v. Brennan*, 1994; *Women Prisoners v. District of Columbia Department of Corrections*, 1994). In addition, groundbreaking surveys of sexual abuse in several correctional agencies (Struckman-Johnson & Struckman-Johnson, 2000; Struckman-Johnson et al., 1996) and a series of scathing national reports about staff sexual misconduct (Amnesty International, 1999; Coomaraswamy, 1999; Human Rights Watch, 1996, 1998; B. Smith, 1998) led leaders to grapple with this human rights violation at the national level. An innovative, bipartisan coalition of political, religious, human rights, social service, and professional organizations joined together to pursue national legislation to address all sexual violence in prisons and jails in the United States. In the summer of 2003, both houses of Congress unanimously passed PREA (117 Stat. 972-989). PREA was enacted as Public Law 108-79 in September 2003 (Dumond, 2003).

As noted by Dr. Cindy Struckman-Johnson, who served as one of the National Prison Rape Elimination Commission (NPREC) commissioners, "The passage of PREA was an unexpected victory for those who were familiar with the long-standing social and political indifference toward prison rape" (Struckman-Johnson & Struckman-Johnson, 2013, p. 340). PREA demanded a "zero tolerance" standard, focused on prevention as a top priority, and established important priorities for correctional agencies nationwide. These priorities included preventing, deterring, and detecting incidents of prisoner sexual victimization upon incarcerated persons (IPs); identifying and treating survivors; identifying, investigating, and prosecuting perpetrators, whether IP or staff; collecting and reporting data about sexual violence of an IP to the Bureau of Justice Statistics (BJS); establishing comprehensive training for correctional staff; developing national standards and ensuring compliance once the standards are promulgated; and creating safety for staff, IPs, and society (Figure 70.1). Most importantly, PREA assembled the resources of federal agencies within the U.S. Department of Justice to study, address, and manage this problem, including the NPREC, the National Institute of Corrections (NIC), the Bureau of Justice Assistance, the BJS, the National Institute of Justice, the U.S. Attorney General's Review Panel on Prison Rape, and, most recently, the PREA Resource Center (PRC). While each of these agencies has been instrumental in crafting a blueprint for substantive systemic, policy, and programmatic changes in American correctional agencies, the current state of affairs in U.S. corrections suggests that correctional agencies have lagged behind in PREA's proper implementation, leading to continued victimization and suffering for IPs nationwide and the recognition that "many challenges persist" (Marcellin & McCoy, 2021).

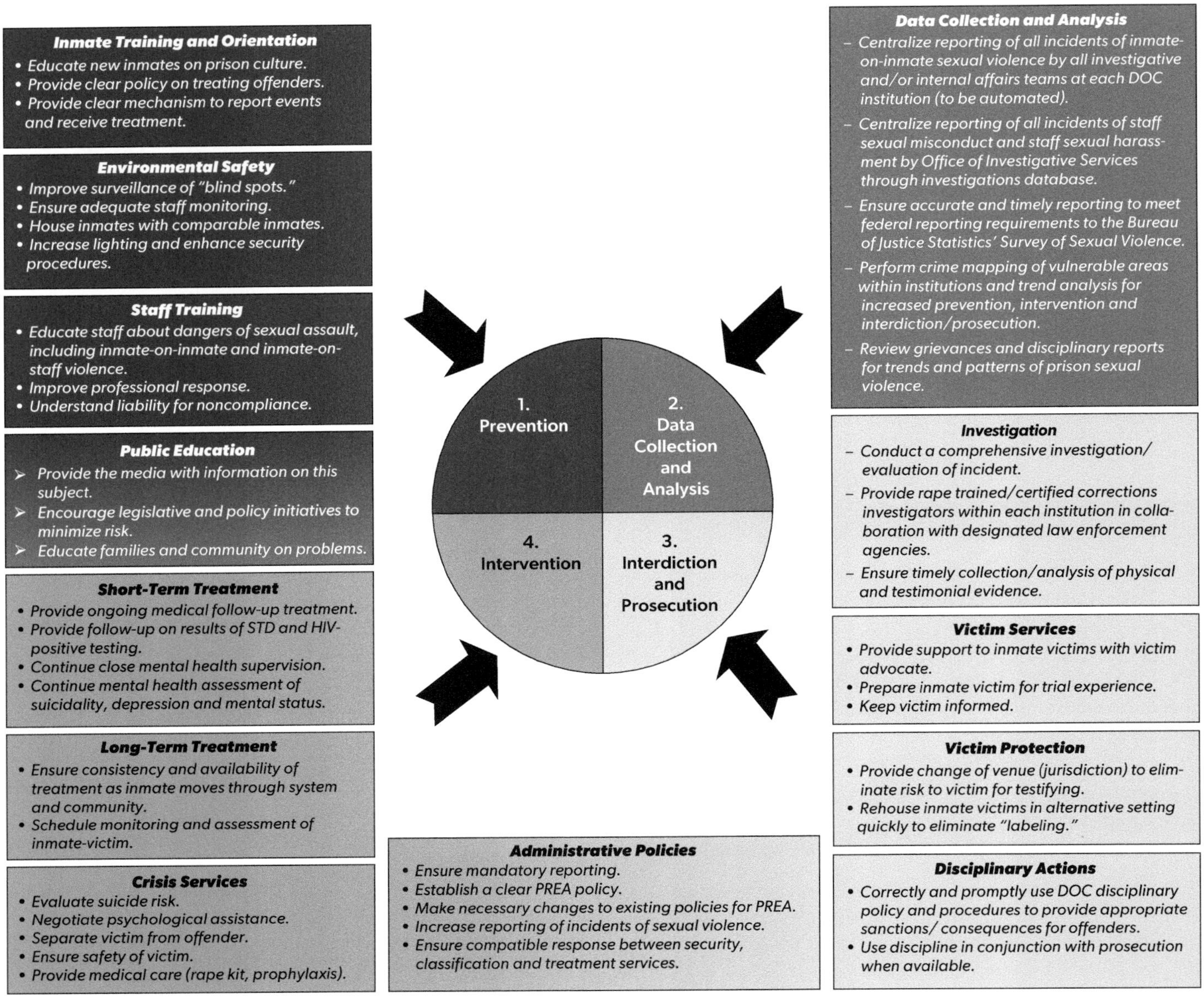

Figure 70.1 Prison Rape Elimination Act Program Model. BJS = Bureau of Justice Statistics; DOC = Department of Corrections; OIS = Office of Investigative Services; PREA = Prison Rape Elimination Act; STD = sexually transmitted disease.
Source: Expanded upon Figure II from Dumond, 1992. Used with Permission of the American Correctional Association, 2024

Successes and promising practices to date

This impressive assembly of federal partners and national initiatives has spawned important successes and promising practices in responding to sexual abuse of IPs.

National Prison Rape Elimination Commission

The NPREC was charged with conducting a thorough analysis of the sexual victimization of IPs in the United States, studying the causes and consequences of sexual abuse in confinement, and developing national standards to eliminate prison rape. Conducting hearings throughout the United States and hearing testimony from hundreds of correctional authorities, researchers, medical and mental health experts, community advocates, and prison rape survivors, the NPREC produced a comprehensive report on prisoner sexual violence (NPREC, 2009a) and accompanying standards for use in adult prisons and jails (NPREC, 2009b), community corrections (NPREC, 2009c), juvenile facilities (NPREC, 2009d), and lockups (NPREC, 2009e).

The NPREC focused on three major themes that oversaw all of its deliberations, as well as the work of community partners: (a) to understand and prevent sexual abuse, one must acknowledge there is problem that must be solved and recognize that leadership matters, that certain IPs have unequal risk for vulnerability and victimization, and that internal and external oversight is necessary; (b) to effectively respond to victims and perpetrators, there must be adequate reporting by victims, investigation of incidents and punishment for perpetrators, and adequate treatment of trauma; and (c) special populations exist with specific needs that must be recognized and addressed, including children, community corrections, and immigrants in detention. Thankfully, all of the hearing transcripts and additional material have been archived (see http://nprec.us/publication/; NPREC, 2009). These documents represent the collective work of the NPREC during the years of its existence

(2003–2009) and provide a comprehensive roadmap and template for substantial change in U.S. correctional practice.

National Institute of Corrections

The NIC became the initial clearinghouse of information for correctional agencies and established two cooperative agreements to advance training and knowledge about PREA. The first agreement involved the Moss Group Inc., founded by Andie Moss, who was the assistant deputy commissioner in the Georgia Department of Corrections, oversaw the department's response to the *Cason v. Seckinger* (2000) class action lawsuit, and was a program specialist with the NIC (1996–2002). The other agreement was with the American University–Washington College of Law. This resulted in End Silence: The Project on Addressing Prison Rape, established by law professor and former NPREC commissioner Brenda Smith (American University/Washington College of Law, 2000) to provide consultation, training, and assistance. The agencies involved with each of these agreements are outstanding resources for correctional practitioners to consult; they have a plethora of print, video, and online research and training resources. Though no longer the major clearinghouse for PREA, the NIC still maintains an impressive list of resources, reports, videos, and trainings on the topic (NIC, 2004).

Bureau of Justice Assistance

The Bureau of Justice Assistance implemented multiple initiatives to assist correctional agencies nationwide in responding to prisoner sexual violence, including rounds of funding to correctional agencies for the Protecting Inmates and Safeguarding Communities initiative, which is now called the Implementing the PREA Standards, Protecting Inmates, and Safeguarding Communities initiative (PREA Resource Center, n.d.). The grants provided funding to dozens of state and local correctional agencies to create and expand "zero-tolerance" cultures around sexual abuse between 2006 and 2020 (PREA Resource Center, n.d.).

Bureau of Justice Statistics

PREA mandated the establishment of the National Prison Rape Statistics Program under the auspices of the BJS to provide a comprehensive national data collection strategy. BJS data confirmed that sexual violence continues to be a major problem that affects thousands of prisoners and juvenile residents nationwide (Beck et al., 2014). The BJS data collection methodologies use a large sample pool and include a large, representative sample of correctional facilities. The BJS also uses four standardized, behaviorally specific definitions: two IP-on-IP definitions ("nonconsensual sexual acts," essentially acts of penetration, considered rape in most jurisdictions, and "abusive sexual contacts," other sexually assaultive behaviors without penetration) and two staff-on-IP definitions ("staff sexual misconduct," sexual contact between a staff and IP, and "staff sexual harassment"). Since 2010, the BJS added several additional clarifying terms, including "sexual victimization," "unwilling activity," and "willing activity" for use with staff (Beck et al., 2010). In addition, the following four possible investigation outcomes of alleged incidents must be reported:

- Substantiated: if the incident was determined to have occurred;
- Unsubstantiated: if the evidence was insufficient to make a final determination;
- Unfounded: if the incident was determined not to have occurred; and
- Investigation ongoing: if a final determination had not been made at the time of data collection.

There had been little previous consensus on what constitutes sexual violence. By creating consistency in identifying prisoner sexual violence and mandating that all correctional agencies use the same definition, the BJS has assembled an accurate national portrait of sexual abuse in prisons, jails, and juvenile facilities. Important prevalence information, developed by using broad, well-constructed national samples and statistically sound methodologies, is now available.

To understand the implications of these studies fully, it is necessary to recognize that, of all crime categories, rape and sexual violence are the most underreported, making an accurate assessment of community-based occurrence rates difficult. There are three major methods to report crime: administrative records of crimes reported to law enforcement agencies (e.g., Uniform Crime Reports), victimization surveys (e.g., National Crime Victimization Survey), and self-report studies (Bartol & Bartol, 2008). The BJS has developed methodologies that incorporate all three strategies. Four national correctional data collection endeavors have provided relevant data: the Survey of Sexual Victimization (BJS, 2024), the National Inmate Survey (BJS, 2023), the National Survey of Youth in Custody (National Archive of Criminal Justice Data, 2022), and the National Former Prisoner Survey (BJS, 2009).

The Survey of Sexual Victimization belongs to the first category of data collection strategies—administrative records. The outcome most often reported upon investigation was unsubstantiated; however, in the years following initial implementation of this methodology, there has been a statistically significant increase in reports of sexual abuse (Beck et al., 2014). This increase suggests that correctional agencies are taking seriously such reports, resulting in greater willingness to report by IP victims.

The other three BJS PREA data collection initiatives (National Inmate Survey, National Survey of Youth in Custody, and National Former Prisoner Survey) have elements of both victimization and self-report surveys. Relevant studies (Beck & Harrison, 2006, 2007, 2008; Beck & Hughes, 2005; Beck & Johnson, 2012; Beck et al., 2007, 2010, 2013, 2014; Buehler, 2021, 2023a, 2023b; Guerino & Beck, 2011; Rantala, 2018; E. L. Smith & Stroop, 2019) have found the following:

- Prisoner sexual violence victimization in all forms is common in correctional settings;
- The formal allegations reported to authorities represent a small fraction of actual incidents of sexual assault victimization in jails, prisons, and juvenile settings;
- The predominant forms of prisoner sexual abuse are staff sexual misconduct, followed by nonconsensual sexual acts;
- Since 2004, an estimated 80,600 adult and juvenile incarcerated and formerly incarcerated persons reported one or more incidents of sexual victimization by another IP or facility staff in the past 12 months of the study periods;
- Since the adoption of the national PREA standards, there have been statistically significant increases in reporting allegations of all forms of prisoner sexual victimization for all U.S. correctional institutions, both adult and juvenile, which suggests that awareness and recognition exist;

- This recognition has not resulted in an increase in substantiated cases following investigations, nor has it ensured that survivors are able to access and actually receive medical examination, prophylactic care, and mental health care;
- Based on the large number of the staff sexual victimization incidents involving IPs who state that contact was "willing," much work needs to be done by correctional agencies to address this issue (Colette & McCoy, 2021);
- Identified perpetrators in most cases of substantiated staff sexual misconduct cases faced prosecution/dismissal in less than 50% of the incidents;
- The collective data does little to describe what efforts, if any, have been made to treat IPs responsible for IP-on-IP victimization; and
- Several studies (Beck & Harrison, 2006; Beck & Johnson, 2012; Buehler, 2021) note with concern that once identified, many survivors fail to be offered or fail to receive medical and/or mental health interventions, which has major implications for carceral management and public health.

National standards to prevent, detect, and respond to prison rape

The national PREA standards are the vehicle to ensure compliance with PREA. These mandatory standards are the benchmark for all U.S. correctional agencies in the elimination of prisoner sexual violence. The final standards were released by the U.S. Department of Justice on May 17, 2012 (28 CFR § 115, 2013). They provide comprehensive guidelines on all aspects of custodial sexual abuse in 11 categories: prevention planning, responsive planning, training and education, screening, reporting, response to report, investigations, discipline, health care, data collection, and audits. These standards include requirements that correctional agencies must:

- Provide a coordinated response upon learning of an incident of sexual abuse;
- Stipulate specific first-responder duties once an incident has been revealed;
- Offer forensic medical exams, access to emergency medical and mental health care, and ongoing medical and mental health care to sexual abuse victims and abusers;
- Attempt to make available a victim advocate from a rape crisis center and confidential outside support systems for IPs and residents including legal representation for juveniles;
- Provide screening for risk of victimization and abusiveness, which includes obtaining information from residents (i.e., youth in juvenile facilities);
- Use the screening information to inform housing, bed, work, education, and program assignments and improve safety for IPs and residents;
- Provide training for custody staff, employees, volunteers, and contractors, including specialized training for investigative, medical, and mental health staff;
- Provide IP education and resident education; and
- Provide multiple reporting avenues for IPs and residents.

The national PREA standards help ensure that prisoners and detainees receive evidence-based, trauma-informed, and gender-responsive care and treatment consistent with community standards to ameliorate the devastating impact of sexual assault (see Chapter 36).

Additional partners in improving the response to prisoner sexual violence

In addition to federal partners, the Moss Group Inc., and the American University–Washington College of Law's Project on Addressing Prison Rape, there are additional partners in the fight to manage sexual assault in prisons and jails more effectively, including Just Detention International (JDI; formerly Stop Prisoner Rape) and the national PRC.

JDI began its work in the 1970s with former prisoners who had been victims of prisoner sexual abuse. JDI has since become an international nonprofit health and human rights organization working to end sexual violence against men, women, and youth in all forms of detention. JDI played a key role in the passage of PREA and in the deliberations of the NPREC. It continues to be involved in the data collection efforts of the BJS and in promulgating national standards to eliminate sexual abuse. JDI continues to advance concerns about safety in correctional settings, including groundbreaking work on violence in U.S. detention facilities (Stop Prisoner Rape, 2006); an innovative guide to help survivors cope (JDI, 2009a); a call to protect the rights of lesbian, gay, bisexual, and transgender individuals (JDI, 2009b); a guide to building a victim services program for IPs (JDI, 2017); and timely, well-researched action updates. Continuing to give voice to survivors, JDI has assembled an impressive array of stories that provide unique insight into the experience of survivors of carceral sexual victimization. Their website has useful resources for survivors, correctional practitioners, victim advocates, sexual assault providers, and all those interested in eliminating sexual violence.

The national PRC has become the central repository for research on trends, prevention, response strategies, and best practices in corrections. The PRC provides technical assistance and resources, collaborates with federal partners, and is taking the lead in implementing the national PREA standards. The PRC has implemented an automated audit process, a revised auditor handbook, and a new policy manual (National PREA Resource Center, 2022), and they continue to offer a variety of trainings and certifications for PREA auditors.

Future challenges and issues of concern

U.S. correctional facilities should make substantive changes to abate sexual abuse and improve management of IPs. The following recommendations should be considered:

There must be a sufficient number of properly trained and carefully vetted corrections security staff in all facilities. Increased numbers of staff alone will not end sexual abuse in detention. As BJS reports demonstrate, staff are reported as the perpetrators in more than half of alleged instances of sexual abuse. Facilities must educate their staff about the dynamics of sexual abuse and the methods for eliminating it. Struckman-Johnson and Struckman-Johnson (2000), in their study of seven midwestern prisons, opined that "the presence of a sufficient number of motivated security staff and tight security measures appeared to limit sexual coercion among IPs" (p. 389). Correctional officers are key to intervening and responding appropriately with IPs who are mentally ill or in distress (Appelbaum, 2010).

All corrections staff must have adequate and appropriate medical and mental health training. Such training will enable staff to recognize IPs with mental illness, adequately manage them, and respond appropriately to threats or incidents of sexual abuse. Ideally, facilities should put in place cross-training (Fagan & Augustin, 2011) with custody staff and mental health professionals (see Chapter 14).

Corrections mental health treatment and services for female prisoners should be trauma informed and gender responsive. Because of the unique pathways to incarceration and the special needs of female IPs, their treatment should be trauma informed and gender responsive (see Chapters 36 and 55; Bloom et al., 2005; Elliott et al., 2005; Harris & Fallot, 2001). Such approaches recognize and address the ubiquitous nature of previous trauma, high rates of mental illness and addiction, and impact of gender bias within the female incarcerated population (Dumond & Dumond, 2010).

Corrections agencies must provide suicide training for all staff and develop strong policies and practices for managing suicide. Medical and mental health staff must recognize that the traditional responses of isolation and observation, while effective for ensuring immediate safety, are often experienced as revictimizing by survivors of sexual abuse (see Chapter 51).

Corrections agencies must ensure that IPs have access to adequate community reentry and reintegration services. As the vast majority of IPs ultimately return to the community, it is especially important that prisoners, especially those with serious, persistent mental illness and those who have experienced sexual abuse, are provided with referrals to community mental health programs (see Chapter 23). Survivors of trauma, in particular, may be more amenable to reaching out for help in the community immediately after being released, reducing the likelihood that they will be arrested again.

Corrections departments should consider developing specialized response teams similar to the crisis intervention teams currently in operation in many jurisdictions. The NIC has developed a noteworthy model for crisis intervention teams (NIC, 2010a, 2010b) that can be adapted to respond to IP sexual assaults.

Agencies must create corrections environments that focus on dignity and respect for all prisoners and ensure that those who are incarcerated are afforded legal, safe, and constitutional care and custody. Staff noncompliance with standards of professional behavior can never be tolerated and must be immediately identified and corrected by agency or facility management and supervisory staff. Corrections environments must have zero tolerance for sexual abuse and for language or behavior that demeans IPs or staff because of their race, ethnicity, religion, sexual orientation, gender, gender identity, or disability. Staff members must also be given tools for effective communication with IPs who are culturally different from them through training, mentoring, and supervision (see Chapter 22).

Continued efforts must be made to help agencies understand how the PREA standards work together. The PREA regulations are a set of groundbreaking standards that, once fully implemented, have the potential to dramatically improve safety in U.S. corrections facilities. However, the standards for adult jails and prisons and juvenile facilities each have more than 50 provisions and run dozens of pages. All agencies must ensure that their staff understand how the standards work together.

Summary

Given the proper tools, training, and resources, correctional systems can and will eliminate prisoner sexual violence. However, corrections is a subset of the body politic itself and hence is subject to budget shortfalls, political pressure, and the broader attitudes of the public. Adequate financial and programmatic resources must be mobilized to ensure appropriate staff skill levels to keep jails and prisons safe. Safe, well-run jails and prisons can, if properly used, help keep communities safe. Together with community partners, correctional systems can, and must, respond with vision and leadership to make prisons and jails safe places where human rights and dignity are protected and the most vulnerable among us can emerge stronger and healthier than they went in.

REFERENCES

28 CFR § 115. (2013). *Part 115—Prison Rape Elimination Act National Standards.* U.S. Department of Justice. https://www.ecfr.gov/current/title-28/part-115

American University/Washington College of Law. (2000). *End Silence: The Project on Addressing Prison Rape.* https://www.american.edu/wcl/impact/initiatives-programs/endsilence/

Amnesty International. (1999). *Not part of my sentence: Violations of the human rights of women in custody.* https://static.prisonpolicy.org/scans/NotPartofMySentence.pdf

Appelbaum, K. L. (2010). The mental health professional in a correctional culture. In C. Scott (Ed.), *Handbook of correctional mental health* (2nd ed., pp. 91–117). American Psychiatric Press.

Bartol, C. R., & Bartol, A. M. (2008). *Introduction to forensic psychology: Research and application* (2nd ed.). Sage Publications.

Beck, A. J., Berzofsky, M., Casper, R., & Krebs, C. (2013, May). *Sexual victimization in prisons and jails reported by inmates. National Inmate Survey, 2011–12* (NCJ 241399). U.S. Department of Justice, Bureau of Justice Statistics. https://www.bjs.gov/content/pub/pdf/svpjri1112.pdf

Beck, A. J., & Harrison, P. M. (2006, July). *BJS Special Report—PREA—Sexual violence reported by correctional authorities, 2005* (NCJ 214646). U.S. Department of Justice, Office of Justice Programs. https://bjs.ojp.gov/library/publications/sexual-violence-reported-correctional-authorities-2005

Beck, A. J., & Harrison, P. M. (2007, December). *BJS Special Report—PREA—Sexual victimization in state and federal prisons reported by inmates, 2007* (NCJ 219414). U.S. Department of Justice, Office of Justice Programs. https://bjs.ojp.gov/library/publications/sexual-victimization-state-and-federal-prisons-reported-inmates-2007

Beck, A. J., & Harrison, P. M. (2008, June). *BJS Special Report—PREA—Sexual victimization in local jails reported by inmates, 2007* (NCJ 221946). U.S. Department of Justice, Office of Justice Programs. https://bjs.ojp.gov/library/publications/sexual-victimization-local-jails-reported-inmates-2007

Beck, A. J., Harrison, P. M., & Adams, D. B. (2007, August). *BJS Special Report—PREA—Sexual violence reported by correctional authorities, 2006* (NCJ 218914). U.S. Department of Justice, Office of

Justice Programs. https://bjs.ojp.gov/library/publications/sexual-violence-reported-correctional-authorities-2006

Beck, A. J., Harrison, P. M., & Guerino, P. (2010, January). *BJS Special Report—PREA—Sexual victimization in juvenile facilities reported by youth, 2008–09* (NCJ 228416). U.S. Department of Justice, Office of Justice Programs. https://bjs.ojp.gov/library/publications/sexual-victimization-juvenile-facilities-reported-youth-2008-09

Beck, A. J., & Hughes, T. A. (2005, July). *BJS Special Report—PREA—Sexual violence reported by correctional authorities, 2004* (NCJ 210333). U.S. Department of Justice, Office of Justice Programs. https://bjs.ojp.gov/library/publications/sexual-violence-reported-correctional-authorities-2004

Beck, A. J., & Johnson, C. (2012). *Sexual victimization reported by former state prisoners, 2008. National Former Prisoner Survey* (NCJ 237363). U.S. Department of Justice, Office of Justice Programs. https://bjs.ojp.gov/content/pub/pdf/svrfsp08.pdf

Beck, A. J., Rantala, R. R., & Rexroat, J. (2014). *Sexual victimization reported by adult correctional authorities, 2009–11* (NCJ 243904). U.S. Department of Justice, Office of Justice Programs. https://bjs.ojp.gov/content/pub/pdf/svraca0911.pdf

Bell, C., Cover, M., Cronan, J. P., Garza, C. A., Guggemos, J., & Storto, L. (1999). Rape and sexual misconduct in the prison system: Analyzing America's most "open" secret. *Yale Law and Policy Review, 18*(1), 195–223.

Bloom, B., Owen, B., & Covington, S. (2005). *Gender-responsive strategies for women offenders: A summary of research, practice, and guiding principles for women offenders* (NIC Accession No. 020418). National Institute of Corrections. https://www.ojp.gov/ncjrs/virtual-library/abstracts/gender-responsive-strategies-research-practice-and-guiding

Buehler, E. D. (2021, June). *BJS Special Report—PREA—Sexual violence reported by adult correctional authorities, 2004* (NCJ 255356). U.S. Department of Justice, Office of Justice Programs. https://bjs.ojp.gov/library/publications/sexual-victimization-reported-adult-correctional-authorities-2016-2018

Buehler, E. D. (2023a, January). *BJS Special Report: Substantiated incidents of sexual victimization reported by correctional authorities, 2016–2018* (NCJ 304834). U.S. Department of Justice, Office of Justice Programs. https://bjs.ojp.gov/document/sisvraca1618.pdf

Buehler, E. D. (2023b, March). *BJS Special Report: Substantiated incidents of sexual victimization reported by juvenile correctional authorities, 2013–2018* (NCJ 305192). U.S. Department of Justice, Office of Justice Programs. https://bjs.ojp.gov/document/sisvrjja1318.pdf

Bureau of Justice Statistics. (2009). *National Former Prisoner Survey.* http://hdl.handle.net/20.500.11990/1452

Bureau of Justice Statistics. (2023). *National Inmate Survey.* https://bjs.ojp.gov/data-collection/national-inmate-survey-nis

Bureau of Justice Statistics. (2024). *Survey of Sexual Victimization (SSV).* https://bjs.ojp.gov/data-collection/survey-sexual-victimization-ssv

Cason v. Seckinger, 231 F.3d 777 (11th Cir. 2000).

Colette, M., & McCoy, E. F. (2021). *Preventing and addressing sexual violence in correctional facilities. Research on the Prison Rape Elimination Act.* Urban Institute. https://www.urban.org/research/publication/preventing-and-addressing-sexual-violence-correctional-facilities

Coomaraswamy, R. (1999). *Report on the mission of the United States of America on the issue of violence against women in state and federal prisons* (E/CN.4/1999/68/Add.2). United Nations High Commissioner. https://digitallibrary.un.org/record/1492561?ln=en&v=pdf

Dumond, R.W. (1992). The sexual assault of male victims in incarcerated settings. *International Journal of the Sociology of Law*, 20 Issue: 2 Dated: (June 1992) Pages: 135–157. NCJ139657. https://www.academia.edu/116271470/The_sexual_assault_of_male_victims_in_incarcerated_settings?uc-g-sw=9124870

Dumond, R. W. (2000). Inmate sexual assault: The plague that persists. *Prison Journal, 80*(4), 407–414. https://citeseerx.ist.psu.edu/document?repid=rep1&type=pdf&doi=9e5cc497ee1365a782a9629d63135683e913d650

Dumond, R. W. (2003). Confronting America's most ignored crime problem: The Prison Rape Elimination Act of 2003. *Journal of the American Academy of Psychiatry and the Law, 31*(3), 354–360. https://jaapl.org/content/jaapl/31/3/354.full.pdf

Dumond, R. W., & Dumond, D. A. (2007). Correctional health care since the passage of the Prison Rape Elimination Act of 2003: Where are we now? *Corrections Today, 69*(5), 76–79. https://www.researchgate.net/publication/313598616_Corrections_Today

Dumond, R. W., & Dumond, D. A. (2010). Working with female offenders: Gender-specific and trauma-informed programming. In S. Stojkovic (Ed.), *Managing special populations in jails and prisons* (Vol. II, part IV, Chapter 13). Civic Research Institute.

Elliott, D., Bjelajac, P., Fallot, R. D., Markoff, L. S., & Reed, B. G. (2005). Trauma-informed or trauma-denied: Principles and implementation of trauma-informed services for women. *Journal of Community Psychology, 33*(4), 461–477. https://www.researchgate.net/publication/227841013_Trauma-informed_or_trauma-denied_Principles_and_implementation_of_trauma-informed_services_for_women

Fagan, T. J., & Augustin, D. (2011). Criminal justice and mental health systems. In T. J. Fagan & R. K. Ax (Eds.), *Correctional mental health: from theory to best practice* (pp. 7–35). Sage.

Farmer v. Brennan, 511 U.S. 825 (1994).

Fishman, J. F. (1934). *Sex in prison: Revealing sex conditions in America's prisons.* National Library Press.

Freidman, L. M. (1993). *Crime and punishment in American history.* Basic Books.

Guerino, P., & Beck, A. J. (2011, January). *BJS Special Report—PREA—Sexual violence reported by adult correctional authorities, 2007–2008* (NCJ 231172). U.S. Department of Justice, Office of Justice Programs. https://bjs.ojp.gov/library/publications/sexual-victimization-reported-adult-correctional-authorities-2007–2008

Harris, M., & Fallot, R. D. (2001). Designing trauma-informed addictions services. In M. Harris & R. D. Fallot (Eds.), *Using trauma theory to design service systems* (pp. 57–74). Jossey-Bass.

Human Rights Watch. (1996). *All too familiar: Sexual abuse of women in U.S. state prisons.* https://www.hrw.org/reports/1996/Us1.htm

Human Rights Watch. (1998). *Nowhere to hide: Retaliation against women in Michigan state prisons.* https://www.hrw.org/legacy/reports98/women/Mich.htm

Just Detention International. (2009a). *Hope for healing: Information for survivors of sexual assault in detention.* https://justdetention.org/wp-content/uploads/2015/10/Hope-for-Healing-Information-for-Survivors-of-Sexual-Assault-in-Detention.pdf

Just Detention International. (2009b). *Call for change: Protecting the rights of LGBTQ detainees.* https://justdetention.org/wp-content/uploads/2015/10/Call-for-Change-Protecting-the-Rights-of-LGBTQ-Detainees.pdf

Just Detention International. (2017). *No one left behind: Building a victim services program for incarcerated survivors of sexual abuse.*

https://justdetention.org/wp-content/uploads/2017/10/jdi-noon eleftbehind-.pdf

Katz, J. (1976). *Gay American history*. Thomas Cromwell.

Lehrer, E. (2001). Hell behind bars: The crime that dares not speak its name. *National Review*, *53*, 24–26.

Marcellin, C., & McCoy, E. F. (2021, May). *Preventing and addressing sexual violence in correctional facilities: Research on the Prison Rape Elimination Act*. Urban Institute, Justice Policy Center. https://www.urban.org/sites/default/files/publication/104230/preventing-and-addressing-sexual-violence-in-correctional-fac ilities.pdf

National Archive of Criminal Justice Data. (2022). *National Survey of Youth in Custody*. https://www.icpsr.umich.edu/web/NACJD/studies/38500/versions/V1

National Institute of Corrections. (2004). *PREA/sexual safety for the incarcerated*. https://nicic.gov/resources/resources-topics-and-roles/topics/preasexual-safety-incarcerated

National Institute of Corrections. (2010a). *Crisis intervention teams: an effective response to mental illness in corrections* [Satellite/Internet broadcast]. http://nicic.gov/Library/024517 https://cybercemet ery.unt.edu/archive/oilspill/20121007102121/http://nicic.gov/Library/024517

National Institute of Corrections. (2010b). *Crisis intervention teams: A frontline response to mental illness in corrections* [Lesson plans and participant's manual]. https://nicic.gov/resources/nic-libr ary/all-library-items/crisis-intervention-teams-frontline-respo nse-mental-illness

National PREA Resource Center. (n.d.). *Grant awards*. https://www.prearesourcecenter.org/implementation/prea-in-action/grant-awards.

National PREA Resource Center. (2022, December). *PREA auditor handbook*. Version 2.1. http://www.prearesourcecenter.org/audit/prea-auditors/auditor-handbook

National Prison Rape Elimination Commission. (2009). *Public hearings*. https://cybercemetery.unt.edu/archive/nprec/20090820154 827/http://nprec.us/home/public_proceedings/

National Prison Rape Elimination Commission. (2009a). *National Prison Rape Elimination Commission report* (NCJ 226680). https://www.ojp.gov/pdffiles1/226680.pdf

National Prison Rape Elimination Commission. (2009b). *Standards for the prevention, detection, response, and monitoring of sexual abuse in adult prisons and jails* (NCJ 22682). https://nij.ojp.gov/library/publications/standards-prevention-detection-response-and-monitoring-sexual-abuse-adult

National Prison Rape Elimination Commission. (2009c). *Standards for the prevention, detection, response, and monitoring of sexual abuse in community corrections* (NCJ 22683). https://www.ojp.gov/library/publications/standards-prevention-detection-respo nse-and-monitoring-sexual-abuse-community

National Prison Rape Elimination Commission. (2009d). *Standards for the prevention, detection, response, and monitoring of sexual abuse in juvenile facilities* (NCJ 22684). https://nij.ojp.gov/library/publi cations/standards-prevention-detection-response-and-monitor ing-sexual-abuse-juvenile

National Prison Rape Elimination Commission. (2009e). *Standards for the prevention, detection, response, and monitoring of sexual abuse in lockups* (NCJ 22685). https://nij.ojp.gov/library/publications/standards-prevention-detection-response-and-monitoring-sex ual-abuse-lockups

Rantala, R. R. (2018, July). *BJS Special Report—PREA—Sexual violence reported by adult correctional authorities, 2012–15* (NCJ 251146). U.S. Department of Justice, Office of Justice Programs. https://bjs.ojp.gov/library/publications/sexual-victimization-reported-adult-correctional-authorities-2012–15

Smith, B. (1998). *An end to silence: Women prisoner's handbook on identifying and addressing sexual misconduct*. National Women's Law Center. https://digitalcommons.wcl.american.edu/cgi/view content.cgi?article=1030&context=fasch_rpt

Smith, E. L., & Stroop, J. (2019, December). *Special Report: National Survey of Youth in Custody, 2018—Sexual victimization in juvenile facilities reported by youth in juvenile facilities, 2018* (NCJ 253042). U.S. Department of Justice, Office of Justice Programs. https://bjs.ojp.gov/library/publications/sexual-victimization-reported-youth-juvenile-facilities-2018

Stop Prisoner Rape. (2006). *In the shadows: Sexual violence in U.S. detention facilities*. https://justdetention.org/wp-content/uploads/2015/10/In-The-Shadows-Sexual-Violence-in-U.S.-Detention-Facilities.pdf

Struckman-Johnson, C., & Struckman-Johnson, D. (2000). Sexual coercion rates in seven Midwestern prison facilities for men. *Prison Journal*, *80*, 379–390. https://citeseerx.ist.psu.edu/docum ent?repid=rep1&type=pdf&doi=fcbb69c37aa411fad986341bc 344769b03713ce6

Struckman-Johnson, C., & Struckman-Johnson, D. (2013). Stopping prison rape: The evolution of standards recommended by PREA's National Prison Rape Elimination Commission. *Prison Journal*, *93*(3), 335–354. https://www.ojp.gov/ncjrs/virtual-library/abstra cts/stopping-prison-rape-evolution-standards-recommended-preas-national

Struckman-Johnson, C. J., Struckman-Johnson, D. L., Rucker, L., Bumby, K., & Donaldson, S. (1996). Sexual coercion reported by men and women in prison. *Journal of Sex Research*, *33*, 67–76.

Women Prisoners vs. District of Columbia Department of Corrections, Women Prisoners I, 877 F. Supp. 634 (D.D.C. 1994). https://law.justia.com/cases/federal/district-courts/FSupp/877/634/1396771/

71

Jail-based competency restoration

Peter Ash and Reema Dedania

Introduction

To proceed to trial or actively resolve a case, a criminal defendant in the United States must be competent to stand trial. The U.S. Supreme Court decision in *Dusky v. United States* (1960) sets out the constitutional floor for competency to stand trial: that the defendant has "sufficient present ability to consult with his lawyer with a reasonable degree of rational understanding and whether he has a rational as well as factual understanding of the proceedings against him" (p. 402). Some states add other factors into the assessment, and subsequent legal cases have provided further clarification on competency in particular circumstances, such as when a defendant wishes to represent themselves rather than use an attorney. When a defendant's competency is in question, legal proceedings are suspended, and typically a court order is issued to evaluate the defendant's competency.

Traditionally, jailed defendants who were adjudicated incompetent to stand trial (IST) were admitted to forensic inpatient units in hospitals for restoration of their competency. Jail-based competency restoration (JBCR), in which restoration services are provided in a jail rather than a hospital, was developed as an alternative to hospitalization. Jail restoration is a relatively recent development and is somewhat controversial. While the first jail restoration unit was developed in 1997, until 2014 there were only a handful of programs in the country. Multiple factors have led to a marked increase in the number of programs in the last 10 years (Jennings & Rice, 2022), and programs vary widely in their structure and approaches. JBCR can be seen as being on a continuum of competency restoration services that includes outpatient restoration programs, JBCR conducted with defendants in the general jail population, specialized JBCR units in which defendants are transferred to a dedicated restoration housing unit in the jail, and inpatient forensic psychiatric units in a hospital. This chapter reviews the development, operation, and outcomes of various types of JBCR programs and explores the individualized approach of jail-based restoration.

Development of jail competency restoration programs

The 1960s ushered in a wave of changes that markedly altered the landscape of psychiatric treatment in the American correctional setting. Stricter civil commitment criteria, coupled with a social movement favoring deinstitutionalization, resulted in fewer state hospital inpatient psychiatric beds and reductions in funding for many state hospitals (Beltrani & Zapf, 2020). The funding reductions for inpatient beds did not result in a parallel increase in funding for outpatient services, and as a result, community programs became increasingly ill-equipped to treat the large numbers of individuals with severe mental illness released from hospitals (Beltrani & Zapf, 2020). This led to a marked increase in people with mental illness being jailed, to the point that in 2014 it was estimated that there were 10 times as many people with mental illness in jail and prisons as there were in state mental hospitals (McCarthy, 2014). Along with the increase in the number of defendants with mental illness, there has been a marked increase in the number of defendants adjudicated IST (Gowensmith et al., 2016; Warburton et al., 2020).

Competent defendants may move forward with legal proceedings, whereas those adjudicated IST are ordered to a period of restoration. State psychiatric hospitals have historically served as the primary site for competency restoration treatment. In 1972, the U.S. Supreme Court ruled in *Jackson v. Indiana* that incompetent defendants cannot be held in a hospital indefinitely and that if restoration is not likely to occur in the foreseeable future, the defendant must be either released or civilly committed. The combination of decreased state hospital beds and an increased number of IST defendants led in many states to increasingly long wait times before a defendant is transferred from a jail to an inpatient hospital forensic unit for restoration. In the case of *Trueblood v. Washington State Department of Social and Health* (2016), the Ninth Circuit Court of Appeals upheld a lower court ruling that a defendant adjudicated IST needed to be transferred to a competency restoration program within 1 week. Subsequent similar cases in other states (Bloom & Kirkorsky, 2021) have put increased pressure on states to transfer IST defendants to restoration programs despite the shortage of inpatient hospital beds and long waitlists for admission.

The origin of the JBCR unit model is traced to a novel program that created a temporary 35-bed acute inpatient forensic unit in a regional jail in Virginia in 1997 (Jennings & Bell, 2012). This jail-based competency unit housed overflow patients from the state forensic hospital undergoing renovation. Implemented and operated by a private behavioral health provider in Virginia from 1997 to 2003, the "Liberty Forensic Unit" succeeded in showing that the competency restoration treatment model could be effective in a jail setting (Jennings et al., 2021). Specifically, the unit achieved an 83%

restoration rate in an average of 77 days for about 484 incompetent defendants.

The Virginia program's success led to the development of other JBCR units around the country, generating controversy about the movement of psychiatric treatment from hospital systems into jail systems. Nonetheless, JBCR programs continued to grow. Motivating factors for the expansion of JBCR units include circumventing hospital waitlists and restoring defendants with mental illness quickly, providing relief to an overburdened mental health system, contributing to a reduction in overall incarceration time due to faster resolution of cases, and creating a less expensive means of restoring competency compared with hospitalization (Ash et al., 2020; Danzer et al., 2019; Jennings & Bell, 2012; Kirkorsky et al., 2020; Rice & Jennings, 2014; Wik, 2018).

Approaches to jail restoration

Although a wide range of mental conditions can cause a defendant to be IST, the most typical impairments are (a) that the defendant is psychotic to a degree that interferes with competency (e.g., the defendant is delusional about their attorney, their charges, or other important aspects of their case or is so disorganized that they cannot attend to the proceedings) and/or (b) the defendant lacks an understanding of the legal process to a degree that interferes with their ability to meet the threshold for competency. Lack of understanding may stem from intellectual limitations but may also result from cognitive impairments due to mental illness that decrease when the mental illness is successfully treated. Thus, the two main classes of intervention are medication to treat the psychosis or underlying mental illness and educational approaches to improve understanding of legal processes.

Jail restoration programs vary widely in their structure and approach. The major variations are listed in Table 71.1. Probably the most significant difference in jail restoration programs is whether defendants are seen individually while housed in the jail general population or are seen in a special housing unit in the jail. When seen in general population, typically medication is handled much as it would be when treating prisoners with mental illness in the jail general population. Additionally, the defendant is seen individually every week or two for monitoring and individualized instruction to enhance their understanding of court proceedings.

On a JBCR unit, the defendant is observed more closely, somewhat similarly to a jail mental health unit. In addition, most JBCR units have individual interventions and active programming designed to improve understanding, consisting of groups that address such subjects as education about legal processes, mock trials, cognitive remediation, psychoeducation, and improvement of general coping skills. These interventions are similar to group interventions offered in forensic hospital inpatient units.

Some programs offer a continuum of services based on the needs of the individual defendant, varying in intensity from outpatient restoration to restoration in general population to a JBCR unit to hospitalization in an inpatient hospital. JBCR units vary widely in their selection criteria. Perhaps the main distinction is between programs that admit only from the jail in which they are located and programs where selection decisions are made by a state agency and defendants may be transferred from other jails. The latter system typically allows for more selectivity along such dimensions as severity and type of impairment, history of medication adherence, and estimated ease of restoration.

Whether and under what conditions a jail-based program can administer involuntary medications to defendants who refuse medication varies widely based on jail policies and state laws (see Psychopharmacology, below). Jail-based restoration programs also vary widely in how they are staffed. Restoration of defendants in general population typically involves a jail psychiatrist or nurse practitioner who prescribes medication and a mental health practitioner who is trained to provide specialized education about the legal processes relevant to the defendant's case. JBCR units usually have their own staff who are separate from regular jail staff who prescribe medication, provide individual treatment, and run groups that have a specialized focus, such as legal education, mock trials, cognitive remediation, and trauma-focused treatment, similar to group interventions that are often provided in inpatient forensic hospital restoration units. Jail restoration units typically also have jail security officers present. With an agitated or threatening defendant, jail deputies have fewer constraints than inpatient hospital staff who are regulated by Joint Commission standards for seclusion and restraint.

The particular mix of services varies from program to program, much as the interventions used in hospital inpatient forensic units vary from hospital to hospital. Because of shortages of psychiatrists

Table 71.1 Variations in jail restoration programs

Variable	Common variations
Housing	Services in general population, specialized jail unit
Selection criteria	Appropriateness for jail-based restoration environment, moved within local jail, transferred from other jails
Involuntary medication	Allowed under various conditions, not allowed
Service providers	General jail mental health staff, specialized independent program staff, or a combination
Service mix	Individual sessions, group interventions, telehealth sessions, in-person sessions
Diversion	Competency restoration only, diversion actively explored
Time limits	Time frame allowed for restoration attempts, jail restoration only while waiting for hospital placement
Jurisdictional variations	Whether misdemeanor defendants included, jail-specific policies, availability of alternatives such as outpatient restoration and waitlist time until inpatient hospitalization
Timing of transfers	Movement to jail-based competency restoration unit prior to incompetent to stand trial (IST) court order (or while IST court order is pending)

in rural areas, many rural jails utilized telehealth services in the prepandemic period. The COVID-19 pandemic increased the use of telehealth services, but there are limited data regarding their use in JBCR units. One study (Lewis et al., 2023) reported higher rates of restoration during the pandemic while utilizing primarily telehealth services, suggesting that such services are effective.

While many inpatient hospitals and jail-based restoration programs focus on competency restoration, some programs also emphasize exploring the possibility of diversion out of the criminal justice system as a way of resolving a case. Ash and colleagues (2020) reported that about a third of defendants in one JBCR unit were diverted out of the criminal justice system rather than being restored. Typically, those diverted were misdemeanor defendants with relatively minor charges (e.g., criminal trespass) who were cooperating with treatment and for whom the prosecutor was willing to dismiss charges when a reasonable mental health aftercare treatment plan was developed.

Competency restoration practices vary widely by jurisdiction, as state laws vary and may differ from federal laws. For example, some jurisdictions do not restore incompetent defendants charged with misdemeanors. Some have specific time periods within which restoration must be begun. Alternatives such as outpatient restoration and the availability of rapid admission to a hospital-based forensic inpatient unit vary. State laws and court holdings regarding involuntary administration or psychoactive medications vary as well.

Interventions

Restoration of competency to stand trial in a hospital typically involves a variety of different approaches, including medication, psychoeducation, cognitive remediation, individual treatment, and specialized interventions for developmental disabilities (Danzer et al., 2019; Wall et al., 2018; Zapf, 2013). Jail restoration programs typically utilize many of these same interventions, but the jail setting leads to some variations.

Psychopharmacology

IST defendants with severe mental illness, particularly those with psychotic disorders, are far more likely to be restored to competency with psychopharmacological intervention (Jennings et al., 2021). Best practices for restoration in the jail setting have not yet been established or standardized due to its novel nature, leaving many potential pathways for treatment delivery but no consensus (Kirkorsky et al., 2020). Others, such as Danzer and colleagues (2019), found that IST defendants in JBCR units had characteristics similar to those in hospital settings and comparable restoration outcomes. The nature of the jail environment (i.e., a security-focused rather than therapeutic approach) and the lack of separation between evaluators and treatment providers (Kirkorsky et al., 2020) were other concerns that were raised in regard to jail-based treatment settings.

Perhaps the most relevant treatment concern regarding competency restoration in the jail setting is restrictions on prescribing involuntary medication (see Chapter 25). The U.S. Supreme Court case *Washington v. Harper* (1990) found it constitutionally permissible to involuntarily medicate a convicted prisoner who is dangerous and when treatment is in his medical interest. Some jails have protocols in place to involuntarily medicate adult incarcerated persons with mental illness when acute safety is of concern and when it is medically appropriate. However, the appropriateness of applying the *Harper* decision to jails often comes into question, as the decision by the U.S. Supreme Court involved a convicted prisoner instead of a pretrial detainee. *Harper* does not permit using forced medications in a defendant who is not dangerous solely to restore competency. In general, psychiatrists working in correctional settings should be familiar with jurisdictional criteria allowing for the use of involuntary medications. While some states allow the determination to be made by a medical professional, others have more complex procedural protections, such as requiring a judicial review or appointing a guardian or substituted decision-maker.

The U.S. Supreme Court decision *Sell v. United States* (2003) gave courts legal authority to mandate the involuntary administration of medications to restore competency if four conditions are met: (a) an important governmental interest is at stake, (b) the forced medication is substantially likely to render the defendant competent and is substantially unlikely to have side effects that will interfere significantly with the defendant's ability to assist counsel in conducting a defense, (c) less intrusive means of restoring competency have been tried and failed, and (d) the medication is medically appropriate. Through a court order, a judge may order that a defendant be involuntarily medicated to restore competency only if the *Sell* criteria are met. These criteria need only be applied when an incarcerated person is not dangerous or gravely disabled.

Even with a *Sell* order in place, jails must still have the capability to carry out the court order and administer medications involuntarily. There is jurisdictional variation with regard to how involuntary medications can be given in jail-based restoration settings; how the medication is actually administered is contingent upon each facility's policies. Recent legislation in California (California Penal Code § 2603, 2022), for instance, grants providers in jail settings the ability to prescribe medication without consent when medically indicated. Many county jails have determined that it is problematic from an ethical and monitoring standpoint to allow for involuntary medications and avoid it entirely except for emergency medications allowed on a very short-term basis (Ash et al., 2020). Further, medication administration in a JBCR program may be largely managed by correctional mental health providers who, as a matter of facility policy, may not be allowed to involuntarily medicate incarcerated persons. Some programs, however, do have dedicated nurses who will administer involuntary medications to defendants undergoing competency restoration (Kirkorsky et al., 2020). As Felthous and Bloom (2018) discuss, the ability of an institution—whether a hospital or a jail—to effectively implement a *Sell* order is contingent upon adequate staffing, programming, and facilities to ensure that the medical component of *Sell* is applied in accordance with professional standards. They contend that most jails are ill-equipped to meet the standard of medical care that would make the *Sell* criteria meaningful.

Psychosocial interventions

Competency restoration conducted with defendants in the jail general population is often done in one-to-one sessions by mental health professionals who typically are not regular jail staff but are specially trained in competency restoration. Their techniques tend to be those used in outpatient competency restoration programs, in which remediation is tailored to the cognitive deficits of the defendant. Interventions typically include education about the defendant's particular case, such as the defendant's charges, and education about the relevant legal processes, including such issues as plea bargaining, trial procedure, and roles of trial participants. Patients are informally assessed for improvement in legal knowledge at regular intervals, usually on a weekly or biweekly basis, so that treatment plans can be adjusted accordingly.

In JBCR units, psychosocial treatments include similar individual interventions but also include many interventions utilized in hospital competency restoration units. There is no detailed consensus as to which specific interventions are most effective (Wall et al., 2018, pp. S63–S72; Zapf, 2013), but in addition to medication and individual treatment, they often include group interventions that focus on such topics as medication compliance, cognitive remediation, mock trials, and education about legal processes. These units strive to provide a milieu and services similar to a hospital-based restoration unit, although jail security issues often affect the milieu because of such factors as limiting time out of cell, limiting time outside, decreased recreational activities, and reduced staffing. Finally, JBCR units often operate only as day programs, reverting to jail security units during evening and night shifts.

Restoration outcomes

JBCR programs that have reported restoration outcomes have, with few exceptions, reported restoring or diverting a majority of defendants within 3 months (Ash et al., 2020; Jennings et al., 2021; Wik, 2018). Some programs have reported high rates of restoration, greater than 70%, which are comparable with inpatient restoration rates (Bloom & Kirkorsky, 2019). Because of the wide variations in the structure, selectivity, and laws pertaining to JBCR, programs operate quite differently, so it is difficult to link specific procedures to the variations in outcomes. While one would expect that a jail-based unit would be more effective than restoration in the jail general population, given the higher intensity of services on a dedicated unit, at the time of this writing, there are no published studies that randomly assign IST defendants to the two alternatives in the same jurisdiction.

Controversies

The two main drivers of JBCR have been the reduced cost of restoring defendants in jail and, given the long waitlists for admission to state forensic hospital units, that JBCR can begin restoration more quickly. In some cases, restoration efforts can begin even before a defendant has been formally adjudicated IST. The cost savings can be quite high. While data are still emerging, the daily cost of restoration in a hospital is estimated to be at least 3 times as much as restoration in jail (Ash et al., 2020; Danzer et al., 2019). Given the long waitlists and need for additional restoration services, conducting all restoration in a hospital would also involve the expense of constructing new hospital beds.

However, the jail-based approach has been criticized along a number of lines (Felthous & Bloom, 2018; Kapoor, 2020; Roberson & Vitacco, 2022). The first general critique is that competency restoration is a mental health problem that is simply better done and more therapeutic in a noncorrectional environment and that the defendant's right to speedy restoration implies the defendant should receive the most efficacious treatment (*Trueblood v. Washington*, 2016). Defendants who are referred to JBCR and are not restored or diverted are then typically referred for hospital-based restoration, and arguably the JBCR delayed their restoration. This is particularly relevant for those patients in jurisdictions where they cannot be involuntarily medicated in jail but can receive such medication in a hospital. A second line of critique is that for those incompetent defendants who do not need treatment of inpatient intensity, other programs, such as improved outpatient restoration or residential treatment, could be developed as a continuum of services outside of the correctional system and would allow for treatment of defendants based on their treatment and risk management needs (Kapoor, 2020). Better outcome data of JBCR programs should help inform the debate over how to weigh the cost savings against these other factors.

Summary

JBCR programs were developed in response to demand for restoration services exceeding available hospital beds in many states. While not all programs have reported data, the available data show that a majority of those who receive jail-based restoration were restored in a reasonable time (less than 90 days) at a cost of less than one-third that of hospital-based restoration. The success of programs in reducing costs and shortening waitlists for hospitalization has led to a rapid increase in the number of JBCR programs over the past decade. Programs vary greatly in their procedures, with the most salient difference being between those that provide restoration in the jail's general population and those that have created specialized units in jails. Other variables include selection criteria, the ability to administer involuntary medication, program staffing, and different jurisdictional laws and regulations. Because the wide variety of jail interventions makes the correlation between procedures and outcomes unknown, there is currently no consensus on ideal practices. Despite positive outcomes and cost savings, jail-based restoration remains controversial. Further research is needed to assess best practices for restoration in a jail-based setting.

REFERENCES

Ash, P., Roberts, V. C., Egan, G. J., Coffman, K. L., Schwenke, T. J., & Bailey, K. (2020). A jail-based competency restoration unit as a component of a continuum of restoration services. *Journal of the American Academy of Psychiatry and the Law*, *48*(1), 43–51.

Beltrani, A., & Zapf, P. A. (2020). Competence to stand trial and criminalization: An overview of the research. *CNS Spectrums*, *25*(2), 161–172.

Bloom, J. D., & Kirkorsky, S. E. (2019). Treatment refusal in Arizona's jail-based competency to stand trial restoration programs. *Journal of the American Academy of Psychiatry and the Law Online*, *47*(2), 233–239.

Bloom, J. D., & Kirkorsky, S. E. (2021). The Ninth Circuit Court of Appeals and jail-based competency evaluation and restoration. *Journal of the American Academy of Psychiatry and the Law*, *49*(3), 415–421.

California Penal Code § 2603 (2022).

Danzer, G. S., Wheeler, E. M. A., Alexander, A. A., & Wasser, T. D. (2019). Competency restoration for adult defendants in different treatment environments. *Journal of the American Academy of Psychiatry and the Law*, *47*, 68–81.

Dusky v. United States, 362 U.S. 402 (1960).

Felthous, A. R., & Bloom, J. D. (2018). Jail-based competency restoration. *Journal of the American Academy of Psychiatry and the Law*, *46*(3), 364–372.

Gowensmith, W. N., Frost, L. E., Speelman, D. W., & Therson, D. E. (2016). Lookin' for beds in all the wrong places: Outpatient competency restoration as a promising approach to modern challenges. *Psychology, Public Policy, and Law*, *22*(3), 293–305.

Jackson v. Indiana, 406 U.S. 715 (1972).

Jennings, J. L., & Bell, J. D. (2012). The "ROC" model: Psychiatric evaluation, stabilization and restoration of competency in a jail setting. In L. L'Abate (Ed.), *Mental illnesses—Evaluation, treatments and implications* (pp. 75–88). InTech.

Jennings, J. L., & Rice, K. (2022). The future of jail-based competency treatment: Commentary from 30,000 feet. *Archives of Psychiatry*, *1*(1), 1–6.

Jennings, J. L., Rice, K., & Baglio, C. (2021). Jail-based competency treatment comes of age: Multi-site outcomes and challenges to the implementation of an evidence-based forensic continuum. *Behavioral Sciences & the Law*, *39*(1), 83–105.

Kapoor, R. (2020). A continuum of competency restoration services need not include jail. *Journal of the American Academy of Psychiatry and the Law*, *48*(1), 52–55.

Kirkorsky, S. E., Gable, M., & Warburton, K. (2020). An overview of jail-based competency restoration. *CNS Spectrums*, *25*(5), 624–629.

Lewis, D. E., Jr., Ash, P., Roberts, V. C., Schwenke, T. J., Pagán-González, M., & Egan, G. J. (2023). Jail-based competency restoration services in the United States: The need, the controversy, the impact of COVID-19, and implications for future treatment delivery. *Criminal Justice and Behavior*, *50*(2), 216–234.

McCarthy, M. (2014). US jails hold 10 times more mentally ill people than state hospitals, report finds. *BMJ: British Medical Journal*, *348*, g2705.

Rice, K., & Jennings, J. L. (2014). The ROC program: Accelerated restoration of competency in a jail setting. *Journal of Correctional Health Care*, *20*(1), 59–69.

Roberson, A., & Vitacco, M. J. (2022). Jail-based competency restoration: What's out there and what's missing. *Journal of Correctional Health Care*, *28*(4), 230–235.

Sell v. United States, 539 U.S. 166 (2003).

Trueblood v. Washington State Department of Social and Health, 822 F.3d 1037 (2016).

Wall, B. W., Ash, P., Keram, E., Pinals, D. A., & Thompson, C. R. (2018). *AAPL practice resource for the forensic psychiatric evaluation of competence to stand trial.* http://jaapl.org/content/jaapl/46/3_Supplement/S4.full.pdf

Warburton, K., McDermott, B. E., Gale, A., & Stahl, S. M. (2020). A survey of national trends in psychiatric patients found incompetent to stand trial: Reasons for the reinstitutionalization of people with serious mental illness in the United States. *CNS Spectrums*, *25*(2), 245–251.

Washington v. Harper, 494 U.S. 210 (1990).

Wik, A. (2018). *Alternatives to inpatient competency restoration programs: Jail-based competency restoration programs, 2018.* https://www.nri-inc.org/media/1500/jbcr_website-format_oct2018.pdf

Zapf, P. (2013). *Standardizing protocols for treatment to restore competency to stand trial: Interventions and clinically appropriate time periods* (Document No. 13-01-1901). Washington State Institute for Public Policy. https://www.wsipp.wa.gov/ReportFile/1121/Wsipp_Standardizing-Protocolsfor-Treatment-to-Restore-Competency-to-Stand-Trial-Interventions-andClinically-Appropriate-Time-Periods_Full-Report.pdf

72

International perspectives and practice differences

Lindsay D. G. Thomson and Lindsey Gilling

Introduction

In our practice of correctional psychiatry, what unites us is much greater than what divides us. This chapter examines correctional psychiatry in an international context and explores similarities and differences in our practices and the cultural, political, and economic background to these. Whatever our geographical location, we must learn from other jurisdictions and other systems. Rates of imprisonment, the organization of psychiatric services, and the location of the treatment of mentally disordered offenders all vary, and it is easy to fall into the trap of assuming that your system is the "right" one. Even the use of the term "correctional psychiatry," while recognizable, is not routine in many countries, where the term "forensic psychiatry," although wider in meaning, is more commonly used. This type of psychiatry has been defined as

> a specialty of medicine based on detailed knowledge of relevant legal issues, criminal and civil justice systems, mental health systems, and the relationship between mental disorder, antisocial behavior, and offending. Its purpose is the assessment, care, and treatment of mentally disordered offenders and others requiring similar services; risk assessment and management and the prevention of further victimization are core elements of this. (Nedopil et al., 2012, p. 242)

Correctional psychiatry is, to a degree, dependent on the wider health facilities available and the existence of legislation to move individuals from correctional to health care settings and back, where appropriate. Even the term "prison" has different meanings in different countries. In most of the United States, it refers to correctional facilities in which the population has been convicted of major crimes and given a sentence of more than 1 year, whereas jails largely house people held on bail awaiting trial and serving sentences of less than 1 year. In Europe, no such distinction is made. For the purposes of this chapter, the term "prison" is used generically.

International context

Across the world, 16% of the global burden of disease is attributable to mental, neurological, and substance use disorders (Arias et al., 2022). Individuals with major mental disorders suffer stigma and discrimination, and their rates of employment are low (Baldwin & Marcus, 2010). This stigma is compounded for those who have mental disorders and have also been incarcerated. Approximately 10 million people are held in penal institutions across the world. This has increased by nearly 25% since 2000 but with significant geographical variations: Oceania increased by 82%, the Americas increased by 43%, and Europe decreased by 27% (Fair & Walmsley, 2021).

This chapter deals primarily with wealthier nations with developed systems of correctional psychiatry. In taking an international perspective on our systems of correctional psychiatry, it is important to note the differences in their demographic, political, and economic makeup. Such comparisons, while useful, are complex and limited by many legal, social, and operational differences. Table 72.1 summarizes some of these differences.

Mental health

To consider the context in which we practice correctional psychiatry, Table 72.2 sets out data on mental health and demonstrates that there are significant variations by country in spending on mental health, size of the mental health workforce, and number of mental health beds. Not all countries routinely report information on mental health spending and provision. The actual amount spent on forensic mental health is difficult to determine for most jurisdictions. The Schizophrenia Commission (Andrews et al., 2012) reported that secure and high-dependency services accounted for 19% of NHS England's mental health budget in 2010–2011. The commission recommended a realignment of resources away from prisons and institutional care to community options. It argued that community sentences and community mental health treatment are considerably more cost-effective than imprisonment. Further, given the high rates of recidivism in those currently imprisoned on short-term sentences, community-based alternatives to incarceration are potentially more effective in reducing reoffending behaviors.

The last 30 years have seen a major reduction in psychiatric beds in developed nations and moves toward community care (e.g., Furedi et al., 2006). There is some evidence, however, that other forms of institutional care have taken over, such as residential homes, forensic

Table 72.1 An international overview of psychiatric care for prison populations

Country	Population (millions)*	Government type†	Health care system	Wealth: gross domestic product per capita‡ (USD)	Total / governmental health expenditure per capita§ (USD)	Life expectancy at birth¶	Infant mortality rate**	Prison population rate††
Australia	26.46	Federal parliamentary democracy Constitutional monarchy *Six federated states and 10 federal territories*	Universal publicly funded system (Medicare) with a private health system	$63,487	$5,901 / 4,431	83.28	2.96	167
Belgium	11.91	Federal parliamentary democracy Constitutional monarchy *Three highly autonomous regions*	Mandatory health insurance, publicly subsidized Private care available	$53,656	$5,009 / 3,966	82.06	3.15	93
Canada	38.52	Parliamentary democracy Constitutional monarchy *Federal structure, 10 provinces*	Publicly funded health care organized by provinces	$53,247	$5,619 / 4,213	83.99	4.31	104
China	1,413.14	Communist Party–led state *22 provinces, five autonomous regions, four municipalities, and two special administrative regions*	Basic health insurance covers 95% of population	$12,541	$583 / 319	78.23	6.49	119 Sentenced prisoners only
Denmark	5.95	Parliamentary constitutional monarchy *Five regions*	Universal health care system	$71,402	$6,438 / 5,463	81.87	3.00	72
Germany	84.22	Federal parliamentary republic *16 states*	Mandatory health insurance with 86% covered by statutory insurance, higher earners can opt out and choose private insurance	$52,824	$5,930 / 4,652	81.72	3.14	70
Ireland	5.32	Parliamentary republic	Public health care system with subsidized fees depending on income, age, illness, and need for continuous care	$112,248	$6,092 / 4,802	81.87	3.41	75
Italy	61.02	Parliamentary republic *20 regions, five of which have special autonomous status*	Universal health insurance system	$37,146	$3,057 / 2,326	82.79	3.11	91
Japan	123.72	Parliamentary constitutional monarchy	Universal health insurance system	$33,950	$4,388 / 3,697	85.00	1.88	37
Netherlands	17.46	Parliamentary constitutional monarchy	Mandatory insurance through private insurers, with 84% purchasing complementary insurance	$61,770	$5,846 / 4,022	82.36	3.34	60

Table 72.1 Continued

Country	Population (millions)*	Government type†	Health care system	Wealth: gross domestic product per capita‡ (USD)	Total / governmental health expenditure per capita§ (USD)	Life expectancy at birth¶	Infant mortality rate**	Prison population rate††
New Zealand	5.11	Parliamentary democracy Constitutional monarchy	Universal health coverage in a mostly publicly funded, regionally administered delivery system	$48,072	$4,202 / 3,242	82.74	3.39	164
Russia	141.70	Presidential republic	Universal publicly funded health care system covers basic care Many residents have private insurance	$13,006	$774 / 546	72.72	6.33	326
South Africa	58.05	Parliamentary republic *Nine provinces*	A public and private health care system, operating independently	$6,191	$490 / 304	65.60	24.99	248
United Kingdom	68.14	Parliamentary constitutional monarchy *Devolved administrations for N. Ireland, Wales and Scotland*	National Health Service covers all health care	$48,913	$4,927 / 4,123	82.05	3.79	131 England and Wales 78 Northern Ireland 137 Scotland (~130 United Kingdom)
United States	339.67	Constitutional federal republic *50 state governments and one federal district*	Public health care system (extended by Affordable Care Act 2010) and private insurance	$80,412	$11,702 / 6,643	80.75	5.12	629
European Union	450.86	27 member states	All the member states have either publicly sponsored and regulated universal health care or publicly provided universal health care	$41,114	– / –	77.63	3.47	175 Europe

* National population, 2023 data (Central Intelligence Agency, 2023a).
† Government type (Central Intelligence Agency, 2023b).
‡ Wealth gross domestic product per capita, 2023 data (International Monetary Fund, 2023).
§ Per capita total/domestic government health expenditure at average exchange rate USD, 2020 data (World Health Organization, 2023a, 2023b).
¶ Life expectancy at birth in years, 2023 data (Central Intelligence Agency, 2023c).
** Infant mortality rate (deaths/1,000 live births), 2023 data (Central Intelligence Agency, 2023d).
†† Prison population rate per 100,000, 2021 data (Fair & Walmsley, 2021).

hospitals, and, of particular relevance here, prisons (Priebe et al., 2005). For example, according to the Penrose hypothesis (Penrose, 1939), the availability of psychiatric beds is inversely related to the prison population. Recent evidence from England offers further support for this theory (Wild et al., 2022).

Correctional psychiatry

Ethical codes apply to all who work in correctional psychiatry. The United Nations Principles of Medical Ethics states that the medical professional's role in relation to those deprived of their liberty is to assess, protect, and improve their health (United Nations, 1982). In its code of ethics for psychiatrists, the World Psychiatric Association notes two areas relevant to doctors who practice correctional psychiatry. The first is the dual responsibility to the patient and to legal proceedings inherent in assessing detainees on behalf of a third party, for example, for fitness to stand trial. At the time of assessment, the psychiatrist must disclose this and acknowledge the limits to confidentiality of communicated information. Second, "as physicians who are committed to sustaining and improving people's lives, psychiatrists do not participate in the administration of the death penalty" (World Psychiatric Association, 2020, p. 7). The World Psychiatric Association (2023) and World Medical Association (2018) state that it would be unethical for psychiatrists and physicians, respectively, to participate in capital punishment processes in any way, including in the assessments of competency to be executed. Not all professional organizations agree, however; the American Psychiatric Association and the American Medical Association do not consider participation in the

Table 72.2 International perspective on mental health

Country	Mental health expenditure as proportion of total health budget, %*	Mental health workforce, no. per 100,000 population (psychiatrists / mental health nurses / psychologists)*	Contribution of mental and substance use disorders to global disease burden, %*	Suicide rate, per 100,000 population†	Mental hospital beds/general hospital psychiatric unit beds, per 100,000 population*
Australia	7.6	13.37 / 87.92 / 104.4	13.1	11.25	6.40 / 21.06
Belgium	–	– / – / –	8.9	13.93	118.68 / 36.48
Canada	–	14.39 / 70.28 / 50.24	10.5	10.34	10.98 / 14.85
China	–	2.55 / 5.68 / 0.37	6.8	6.67	35.34 / –
Denmark	–	– / – / –	10.2	7.63	– / –
Germany	13.1	14.22 / 1.20 / 55.08	8.6	8.27	80.98 / 78.89
Ireland	6.0	8.01 / 99.09 / 7.95	12.9	8.9	21.08 / –
Italy	3.6	6.39 / 23.84 / 3.94	8.2	4.33	– / 8.09
Japan	6.2	12.55 / – / 27.81	5.5	12.24	170.35 / 74.92
Netherlands	–	– / – / –	9.6	–	– / –
New Zealand	8.4	8.66 / 71.59 / 9.62	11.1	10.3	– / 18.96
Russia	–	12.73 / – / 3.89	7.6	21.6	87.81 / –
South Africa	5.0	1.59 / 242.62 / 15.36	4.6	23.49	26.74 / 6.99
United Kingdom	–	13.76 / 55.62 / 19.77	10.3	6.88	26.87 / –
United States	–	– / – / –	13.3	14.51	– / –
European Union	–	– / – / –	8.7	--	– / –

* Data reported where available from the Mental Health Atlas 2020.
† Percent of disability-adjusted life years from all causes accounted for by mental disorders and substance use disorders (Global Burden of Disease Network, 2020).

assessment of competency of individuals to be executed unethical (Weinstock et al., 2010).

The World Health Organization Health in Prisons program aims to improve public health by improving health care in prisons and has focused in recent years on generating comparable data on the health of people in prison to bridge the gap between evidence and policy. The latest status report from the World Health Organization Health in Prisons European Database (World Health Organization, 2023c) stated that of the 36 participating nations, responsibility for the delivery of prison health care was shared between the health ministry and justice ministry in 21 countries (58%), assigned to the justice ministry alone in eight (22%), and assigned to the health ministry alone in seven (19%). There is debate around models of governance for prison health care service delivery, chiefly around whether the responsibility and accountability for prison health care should sit with justice or health ministries (McLeod et al., 2020). Those who support health ministries taking on this role state that it is imperative for clinical independence and better facilitates continuity of care between prisons and the community. Some jurisdictions that have transferred responsibility to their ministry of health report that they have seen benefits such as raised clinical standards and greater transparency (Leaman et al., 2017). However, in countries where the responsibility and accountability for health care delivery in prisons have shifted from justice to health, such as Scotland in 2011, the preferred model still requires joint working and a whole-prison approach to health promotion, supported by the prison service. A 2021 national mental health needs analysis of the Scottish prison population found that barriers to effective partnership between justice, health, social work, and third-sector providers, such as charities and volunteer organizations, have led to inadequate and fragmented mental health care (Gilling McIntosh et al., 2023).

Problems that arise in correctional psychiatry

Prisons are designed for containment, public safety, and rehabilitation; they are not designed to provide a therapeutic environment. The rules and environment of a prison can present challenges to a therapist, such as access to patients, provision of medication, sudden transfer of prisoners to another establishment, and poor data collection systems. Services tend to reflect historical arrangements rather than the result of careful design following a systematic assessment of need or a mirroring of those developed in the community. In addition, patients may spend many months in prison acutely psychotic while awaiting transfer to a hospital (Sales et al., 2023).

Often the mental health services in prisons are not truly multidisciplinary, do not reflect the working methods found in community health settings, and are not set up to meet the level of need found in the custodial population. In European countries, the need to develop such services follows from the principle of equivalence of provision of prison mental health services with those established in the community (Levy, 2011). Some argue that we should go beyond this (Exworthy et al., 2011). In the United States, the aim in terms of quality of care is again to provide the same level that should be available in the community (American Psychiatric Association, 2016). Principle 9 of the United Nations Basic Principles for the Treatment of Prisoners states that "Prisoners shall have access to the health services available in the country without discrimination on the grounds of their legal situation." (United Nations, 1990, Principle 9; see Chapter 4).

Suicide is a particular concern in the prison population. A meta-analysis by Fazel, Ramesh, and Hawton (2017) of studies from 24 high-income countries found the risk of suicide in prison to be 3 times greater in male prisoners and 9 times greater in female prisoners than in the community. The authors noted that these rates varied considerably. Countries with lower incarceration rates were found to have higher prison suicide rates, perhaps because prisoners in these countries are more likely to have committed more serious crimes or have higher rates of mental illness, both of which are risk factors for suicide (Fazel, Ramesh, & Hawton, 2017).

The needs of special groups such as women, young offenders, elderly individuals, and those with intellectual disability or comorbid diagnoses present myriad challenges in correctional settings (see Chapters 55, 59, and 60). Co-occurring mental illness and substance misuse is very common in prisoners and increases the risk of suicide, homelessness, violence, recidivism, victimization, and physical ill health. The problem in many jurisdictions is that in prisons, mental illness and substance misuse are treated by different teams; this can lead to inconsistencies and conflict. There needs to be an integrated care model for those with dual diagnosis (see Chapter 48).

Prevalence of psychiatric morbidity in prisoners

The prevalence of mental disorders in prisoners presents a major problem. Studies of mental disorders in prisoners across many countries show increased rates of mental disorders in comparison to those in the community. The range of mental disorders and conditions commonly treated by prison mental health teams has widened in recent years due to an increased focus on diagnosing and supporting individuals with traumatic brain injury and neurodevelopmental disorders including attention-deficit/hyperactivity disorder, autism, and fetal alcohol spectrum disorder. As the prison population is aging in many countries, dementia care is also increasingly required. The results of international meta-analyses and, where the extant research is still too heterogenous for meta-analysis, systematic reviews on the prevalence of these conditions are summarized in Table 72.3.

As well as increased morbidity, increased mortality is a significant issue for offenders, particularly ex-offenders. A meta-analysis of over 1 million offenders (Skinner & Farrington, 2020) found that they were more likely to die prematurely from both natural and unnatural causes than nonoffenders, likely reflecting the effect of their antisocial lifestyle but also the effect of interaction with the correctional system on their mental and physical health.

Models of care in correctional psychiatry

There are three basic models of care for the acutely unwell in correctional psychiatry: prison as the psychiatric hospital, transfer to a psychiatric hospital, and a mixed model. Most countries send those found not guilty by reason of insanity to a psychiatric hospital. Many, however, have no provision for transfer to the psychiatric system for those found to be guilty but whose mental disorder was a major component of the reason for offending (Daigle et al., 2007). Some jurisdictions have no legal mechanisms to transfer acutely unwell psychiatric patients out of prison; instead, psychiatric units exist in the prison to care for these individuals.

In other countries (e.g., the United Kingdom), acutely unwell prisoners are transferred to a hospital. Medication for a mental disorder cannot be given in prison against an individual's wishes. Legislation exists to permit such transfers. There is considerable variation in the length of time it takes to transfer an incarcerated person to a hospital (Sales et al., 2023). In England and Wales, transfer may take many months, whereas in Scotland, the median time from referral to transfer is 17.5 days (L. Thomson, personal communication, February 2, 2024). There are several potential reasons for such a difference, including greater psychiatric bed availability and the cohesion of the forensic service in Scotland, with integration of

Table 72.3 Meta-analyses and systematic reviews of psychiatric morbidity in prison

Mental disorder	Pooled sample	Prevalence (% of people in prison)			Review paper
		Overall	Male	Female	
Meta-analyses					
Psychosis	13,135 adults (~89.5% male)	6.2 (4.0–8.6)	6.6 (3.7–10.2)	5.7 (1.9–11.0)	Baranyi et al. (2019)
	30,625 adults (87.6% males)	3.7 (3.2–4.1)	3.6 (3.1–4.2)	3.9 (2.7–5.0)	Fazel and Seewald (2012)
	27,801 adolescents (87.3% male)	N.R.	2.7 (2.0–3.4)	2.9 (2.4–3.5)	Beaudry et al. (2021)
Depression	13,452 (~89% male)	16.0 (11.7–20.8)	15.9 (11.1–21.4)	19.4 (11.7–28.5)	Baranyi et al. (2019)
	20,049 adults (79.9% male)	11.4 (9.9–12.8)	10.2 (8.8–11.7)	14.1 (10.2–18.1)	Fazel and Seewald (2012)
	18,861 adolescents (84.2% male)	N.R.	10.1 (8.1–12.2)	25.8 (20.3–31.3)	Beaudry et al. (2021)
Alcohol use disorder	18,388 adults (64% male) at reception	24 (21–27)	26 (23–30)	20 (16–24)	Fazel, Yoon, and Hayes (2017)
Substance use disorder	18,388 adults (64% male) at reception	N.R.	30 (22–38)	51 (43–58)	Fazel, Yoon, and Hayes (2017)
Posttraumatic stress disorder	16,136 adolescents (88.4% male)	N.R.	8.6 (6.4–10.7)	18.2 (13.1–23.2)	Beaudry et al. (2021)
Attention-deficit/ hyperactivity disorder	56,221 adult and adolescent offenders (89.2% male)	26.7 (22.7–30.7)	N.R.	N.R.	Baggio et al. (2018)
	28,749 adolescent offenders (86.3% male)	N.R.	17.3 (13.9–20.7)	17.5 (12.1–22.9)	Beaudry et al. (2021)
Fetal alcohol spectrum disorder	171 adult offenders in two studies	14.7 (9.8–20.5)	N.R.	N.R.	Popova et al. (2019)
Personality disorder	Any personality disorder 4,576 adults (33.4% male)	N.R.	65	42	Fazel and Danesh (2002)
	Antisocial personality disorder 13,844 adults (78.0% male)	N.R.	47	21	
	Borderline personality disorder 1,208 adults (100% female)	N.R.	–	25	
Systematic reviews—Research methods in primary studies too heterogenous to conduct meta-analysis					
Dementia	Four studies	0.8–18.8 (included studies range)	N.R.	N.R.	Brooke et al. (2020)
Traumatic brain injury	10 studies	16.5–72.1 (included studies range)	N.R.	N.R.	Hughes et al. (2015)
Intellectual disability	10 studies	0–2.8 (included studies range)	N.R.	N.R.	Fazel et al. (2008)
Autism spectrum disorder	24 studies	0.2–62.8 (included studies range)	N.R.	N.R.	Collins et al. (2023)

Note. N.R. = not reported.

psychiatrists working in local forensic units and local prisons and those working in national prisons with the national high-security hospital.

Other states and countries operate a mixed model, having the ability to transfer patients to a psychiatric hospital and inpatient facilities in the prison setting. For example, the State of Victoria in Australia operates inpatient units in prisons and maintains the ability to transfer an incarcerated person to a secure hospital.

Components of a correctional psychiatry model

Five key elements of effective service provision across the prison care pathway have emerged from the international literature. These are described in the STAIR model, which stands for screening, triage, assessment, intervention, and reintegration (Simpson et al., 2022). This should include, for all people coming into prison, an initial screen from trained mental health staff using validated tools to identify presenting issues that require immediate intervention (e.g., psychosis, suicidality, and substance withdrawal), followed by a subsequent and more detailed second screen. Individuals should be triaged to the appropriate service and level of care following multidisciplinary case discussion of the screening information. Then, a range of culturally competent and evidence-based interventions should be available, tailored to the severity of the individual's needs. Prisoners requiring acute care may be treated according to one of three models of care described above. Finally, planning for community reintegration and specifying the appropriate package of care should begin well in advance of release.

There should also be support for self-help approaches through the chaplaincy service, peer listener programs, and access to tele-mental health programs (e.g., the use of digital platforms, telephones, videoconferencing). The adoption and expansion of tele-mental health programs in many jurisdictions mitigated service delivery disruption during the COVID-19 pandemic and led to much innovation in prison mental health care delivery (Hearty et al., 2023). Videoconferencing technology in particular can be adopted to support remote mental health service delivery and access to specialty services based in the community (see Chapter 21).

Finally, the issue of personality disorder is central to many problem behaviors found in prisons, from failure to take part in therapeutic programs to an excessive drain on health service resources by continual demands for assessment and medication. In these contexts, assessment of individuals for the presence of personality disorder would assist in their subsequent management (see Chapter 37). Mental health professionals need to engage more widely with the therapeutic work of the prison service, including offender-based programs.

Summary

Across the developed world, services for those with mental disorders in prison have been established but are seldom equivalent to those found in the community. There are major differences throughout the world in terms of rates of imprisonment, place of treatment of acutely ill prisoners, and structure of mental health services in prisons. Those requiring hospital care should be transferred out of prison for treatment; independence of health services from correctional services would promote this practice. One challenging issue for correctional psychiatry in some jurisdictions is capital punishment. Ethically, psychiatrists should have no role in executions and should be aware of the ethical stance of the World Psychiatric Association, which differs in some ways from that of the American Psychiatric Association and American Medical Association.

REFERENCES

American Psychiatric Association. (2016). *Psychiatric services in correctional facilities* (3rd ed.).

Andrews, A., Knapp, M., McCrone, P., Parsonage, M., & Trachtenberg, M. (2012). *Effective interventions in schizophrenia the economic case: A report prepared for the Schizophrenia Commission.* Rethink Mental Illness (London School of Economics).

Arias, D., Saxena, S., & Verguet, S. (2022). Quantifying the global burden of mental disorders and their economic value. *EClinicalMedicine, 54*.

Baggio, S., Fructuoso, A., Guimaraes, M., Fois, E., Golay, D., Heller, P., ... Wolff, H. (2018). Prevalence of attention deficit hyperactivity disorder in detention settings: A systematic review and meta-analysis. *Frontiers in Psychiatry, 9*, 331.

Baldwin, M. L., & Marcus, S. C. (2010). Stigma, discrimination, and employment outcomes among persons with mental health disabilities. In I. Z. Schultz & E. S. Rogers (Eds.), *Work accommodation and retention in mental health* (pp. 53–69). Springer.

Baranyi, G., Scholl, C., Fazel, S., Patel, V., Priebe, S., & Mundt, A. P. (2019). Severe mental illness and substance use disorders in prisoners in low-income and middle-income countries: A systematic review and meta-analysis of prevalence studies. *Lancet Global Health, 7*(4), e461–e471.

Beaudry, G., Yu, R., Långström, N., & Fazel, S. (2021). An updated systematic review and meta-regression analysis: Mental disorders among adolescents in juvenile detention and correctional facilities. *Journal of the American Academy of Child & Adolescent Psychiatry, 60*(1), 46–60.

Brooke, J., Diaz-Gil, A., & Jackson, D. (2020). The impact of dementia in the prison setting: A systematic review. *Dementia, 19*(5), 1509–1531.

Central Intelligence Agency. (2023a). *Field listing: Population.* https://www.cia.gov/the-world-factbook/field/population/

Central Intelligence Agency. (2023b). *Field listing: Government type.* https://www.cia.gov/the-world-factbook/field/government-type/

Central Intelligence Agency. (2023c). *Field listing: Life expectancy at birth.* https://www.cia.gov/the-world-factbook/field/life-expectancy-at-birth/

Central Intelligence Agency. (2023d). *Field listing: Infant mortality rate.* https://www.cia.gov/the-world-factbook/field/infant-mortality-rate/

Collins, J., Horton, K., Gale-St. Ives, E., Murphy, G., & Barnoux, M. (2023). A systematic review of autistic people and the criminal justice system: An update of King and Murphy (2014). *Journal of Autism and Developmental Disorders, 53*(8), 3151–3179.

Daigle, M. S., Daniel, A. E., Dear, G. E., Frottier, P., Hayes, L. M., Kerkhof, A., . . . Sarchiapone, M. (2007). Preventing suicide in prisons, part II: International comparisons of suicide prevention services in correctional facilities. *Crisis, 28*(3), 122–130. https://doi.org/10.1027/0227-5910.28.3.122

Exworthy, T., Wilson, S., & Forrester, A. (2011). Beyond equivalence: Prisoners' right to health. *The Psychiatrist, 35*(6), 201–202.

Fair, H., & Walmsley, R. (2021). *World prison population list* (13th ed.). Institute for Crime & Justice Policy Research. https://www.prisonstudies.org/sites/default/files/resources/downloads/world_prison_population_list_13th_edition.pdf

Fazel, S., & Danesh, J. (2002). Serious mental disorder in 23 000 prisoners: A systematic review of 62 surveys. *The Lancet, 359*, 545–550.

Fazel, S., Ramesh, T., & Hawton, K. (2017). Suicide in prisons: An international study of prevalence and contributory factors. *Lancet Psychiatry, 4*(12), 946–952.

Fazel, S., & Seewald, K. (2012). Severe mental illness in 33,588 prisoners worldwide: Systematic review and meta-regression analysis. *British Journal of Psychiatry, 200*, 364–373.

Fazel, S., Xenitidis, K., & Powell, J. (2008). The prevalence of intellectual disabilities among 12 000 prisoners—A systematic review. *International Journal of Law and Psychiatry, 31*(4), 369–373.

Fazel, S., Yoon, I. A., & Hayes, A. J. (2017). Substance use disorders in prisoners: An updated systematic review and meta-regression analysis in recently incarcerated men and women. *Addiction, 112*(10), 1725–1739.

Furedi, J., Mohr, P., Swingler, D., Bitter, I., Gheorghe, M. D., Hotujac, L., ... Sartorius, N. (2006). Psychiatry in selected countries of Central and Eastern Europe: An overview of the current situation. *Acta Psychiatrica Scandinavica, 114*(4), 223–231.

Gilling McIntosh, L., Rees, C., Kelly, C., Howitt, S., & Thomson, L. D. (2023). Understanding the mental health needs of Scotland's prison population: A health needs assessment. *Frontiers in Psychiatry, 14*, 1119228.

Global Burden of Disease Collaborative Network. (2020). *Global Burden of Disease Study 2019 (GBD 2019) results*. Institute for Health Metrics and Evaluation. https://vizhub.healthdata.org/gbd-results/

Hearty, P., Canvin, K., Bellass, S., Hampton, S., Wright, N., & Sheard, L. (2023). Understanding the impact of Covid-19 on the delivery and receipt of prison healthcare: An international scoping review. *Health & Justice, 11*(1), 42.

Hughes, N., Williams, W. H., Chitsabesan, P., Walesby, R. C., Mounce, L. T., & Clasby, B. (2015). The prevalence of traumatic brain injury among young offenders in custody: A systematic review. *Journal of Head Trauma Rehabilitation*, 30(2), 94–105.

International Monetary Fund. (2023). *GDP per capita, current prices*. https://www.imf.org/external/datamapper/NGDPDPC@WEO/OEMDC/ADVEC/WEOWORLD?year=2023

Leaman, J., Richards, A. A., Emslie, L., & O'Moore, E. J. (2017). Improving health in prisons—from evidence to policy to implementation—Experiences from the UK. *International Journal of Prisoner Health, 13*(3–4), 139–167.

Levy, M. (2011). Health services for prisoners. *British Medical Journal, 342*, 351.

McLeod, K. E., Butler, A., Young, J. T., Southalan, L., Borschmann, R., Sturup-Toft, S., . . . Kinner, S. A. (2020). Global prison health care governance and health equity: A critical lack of evidence. *American Journal of Public Health, 110*(3), 303–308.

Nedopil, N., Gunn, J., & Thomson, L. D. G. (2012). Teaching forensic psychiatry in Europe. *Criminal Behaviour and Mental Health, 22*(4), 238–246.

Penrose, L. S. (1939). Mental disease and crime: Outline of a comparative study of European statistics. *British Journal of Medical Psychology, 18*, 1–15.

Popova, S., Lange, S., Shield, K., Burd, L., & Rehm, J. (2019). Prevalence of fetal alcohol spectrum disorder among special subpopulations: A systematic review and meta-analysis. *Addiction, 114*(7), 1150–1172.

Priebe, S., Badesconyi, A., Fioritti, A., Hansson, L., Kilian, R., Torres-Gonzales, F., ... Wiersma, D. (2005). Reinstitutionalisation in mental health care: Comparison of data on service provision from six European countries. *BMJ, 330*(7483), 123–126.

Sales, C. P., Forrester, A., & Tully, J. (2023). Delays in transferring patients from prisons to secure psychiatric hospitals: An international systematic review. *Criminal Behaviour and Mental Health, 33*(5), 371–385.

Simpson, A. I., Gerritsen, C., Maheandiran, M., Adamo, V., Vogel, T., Fulham, L., . . . Jones, R. M. (2022). A systematic review of reviews of correctional mental health services using the STAIR Framework. *Frontiers in Psychiatry, 12*, 747202.

Skinner, G. C., & Farrington, D. P. (2020). A systematic review and meta-analysis of premature mortality in offenders. *Aggression and Violent Behavior, 53*, 101431.

United Nations. (1982). *37/194 Principles of medical ethics. General Assembly—Thirty-seventh session*. https://www.ohchr.org/en/instruments-mechanisms/instruments/principles-medical-ethics-relevant-role-health-personnel#:~:text=Principle%206-,Principle%201,are%20not%20imprisoned%20or%20detained

United Nations. (1990). *Basic principles for the treatment of prisoners. General Assembly Resolution 45/111*. https://www.ohchr.org/en/instruments-mechanisms/instruments/basic-principles-treatment-prisoners

Weinstock, R., Leong, G. B., & Silva, J. A. (2010). Competence to be executed: An ethical analysis post Panetti. *Behavioral Sciences & the Law, 28*(5), 690–706.

Wild, G., Alder, R., Weich, S., McKinnon, I., & Keown, P. (2022). The Penrose hypothesis in the second half of the 20th century: Investigating the relationship between psychiatric bed numbers and the prison population in England between 1960 and 2018–2019. *British Journal of Psychiatry, 220*(5), 295–301.

World Health Organization. (2023a). *Current health expenditure (CHE) per capita in US$: Data by country*. https://apps.who.int/gho/data/view.main.GHEDCHEpcUSSHA2011v

World Health Organization. (2023b). *Domestic general government health expenditure (GGHE-D) per capita in US$: Data by country*. https://apps.who.int/gho/data/node.main.GHEDGGHEDpcUSSHA2011?lang=en

World Health Organization. (2023c). *Status report on prison health in the WHO European Region 2022*. https://www.who.int/europe/publications/i/item/9789289058674

World Medical Association. (2018). *WMA Resolution on prohibition of physician participation in capital punishment*. https://www.wma.net/policies-post/wma-resolution-on-prohibition-of-physician-participation-in-capital-punishment/

World Psychiatric Association. (2020). *Code of ethics for psychiatry*. https://www.wpanet.org/policies#:~:text=It%20is%20a%20universal%20Code,transparency%20and%20accountability%20are%20key

World Psychiatric Association. (2023). *Position statement on mental health and the death penalty*. https://www.wpanet.org/_files/ugd/842ec8_954aafaa000b4ce38c282309ef68b6f9.pdf

SECTION XII

Education, research, and quality improvement

73

Standards and accreditation for jails, prisons, and juvenile facilities

Joseph V. Penn

Introduction

The history of medical and mental health care in America's prisons and jails is replete with examples of gross neglect and indifference. Until the early 1970s, the availability and quality of correctional health care were left to the discretion of correctional officials, with both the courts and society assuming a hands-off policy (Anno, 2001). The result was often woefully inadequate health care. This chapter details the background, evolution, and status of health care standards and provides an overview of accreditation processes for correctional facilities in the United States.

Background

According to a survey of local jails conducted by the American Medical Association (AMA) in 1972, first aid was the only medical care available in two thirds of jails; not even this service was available in about 17% of jails (Steinwald et al., 1973). Only 7% of jails had an infirmary. On-site access to primary care physicians, nurses, other medical and surgical specialists, and other medical personnel was extremely limited. Although most state prisons had some medical facilities, they were typically poorly equipped and staffed primarily by unlicensed physicians and medical assistants (Anno, 2001; U.S. General Accounting Office [GAO], 1978). In some systems, physicians with medical board involvement and resulting disciplinary actions received licensure restrictions that only permitted practice within "institutional" settings such as jails or prisons. In other cases, incarcerated persons (IPs) with no formal medical training dispensed medications, extracted teeth, and even performed minor surgery (McDonald, 1999).

Mental health services in correctional institutions fared no better. With passage of the Mental Retardation Facilities and Community Mental Health Centers Construction Act of 1963, state mental hospitals began releasing thousands of patients with chronic and severe psychiatric disorders into communities that often lacked the resources to provide adequate and accessible alternatives to hospitalization (Lamb & Bachrach, 2001; U.S. GAO, 2000). Unable to access mental health services, large numbers of formerly institutionalized persons with serious mental illness were left homeless, impoverished, and highly symptomatic—a combination of factors that put them at high risk for arrest and criminal prosecution (Lamb & Bachrach, 2001; Stelovich, 1979; Whitmer, 1980). In the wake of deinstitutionalization and new restrictions on civil commitment, the nation's prisons and jails became the de facto psychiatric hospitals (Torrey et al., 2010).

Studies of U.S. prison populations have consistently found elevated rates of serious mental illness relative to the general population (Baillargeon et al., 2010). Very few correctional institutions have had the resources to provide adequate care for this large influx of IPs with potentially impairing and debilitating mental disorders.

Over the past 5 decades, remarkable improvements in correctional health care have occurred thanks, in large part, to increased awareness and the involvement of several health care organizations, along with the federal courts. Due to the increased concern regarding potential risks and deficiencies in health care for the imprisoned, several organizations, including the AMA and the American Public Health Association (APHA, 2003), became involved in developing standards and accreditation programs for health care delivery in prisons and jails in the 1970s (Anno, 2001). Regrettably, these early attempts at health care reform lacked enforcement power, additional funding, or health care staffing and other resources, and many correctional administrators appeared to reject them. During this time, several federal courts began a reversal of a long-held "hands-off" doctrine regarding the rights of IPs to medical care. By 1995, 139 state correctional facilities were under court order or consent decree because of inadequate medical care (Stephan, 1997).

Federal litigation has provided much of the impetus for improved correctional health services, funding, staffing, technologies such as electronic health records, electronic prescribing, telemedicine, telepsychiatry, and other needed resources in jails and prisons. In several class action lawsuits that involved allegations of deficient health care that have gone to trial, state governments have expended considerable resources in resisting health care reforms at enormous cost to taxpayers. Faced with the prospect of such costly litigation, correctional officials have increasingly opted for compliance with national health standards and achieving accreditation (Anno, 2001; Rold, 2008).

Correctional health care standards

According to the International Organization for Standardization (n.d.), a standard is a document that provides requirements, specifications, guidelines, or characteristics that can be used consistently to ensure that materials, products, processes, and services are fit for their purpose. In correctional health care, standards serve that same purpose but also "provide a national process to keep the evolution of correctional health care practices following community-based standards" (Wallenstein, 2004, p. 3). Although correctional and correctional health care standards are often established to support accreditation programs, correctional facilities need not pursue accreditation to benefit from following nationally accepted standards. Many jails, prisons, juvenile facilities, and opioid treatment facilities will cite National Commission on Correctional Health Care (NCCHC) or American Correctional Association (ACA) standards in their policies and procedures. Correctional and correctional health care standards are offered by several organizations, including the ACA (2024a), the NCCHC (2024), the Joint Commission (2024), the APHA (2003), and regional medical state organizations such as the Medical Association of Georgia (1977).

Through a pilot effort in the 1970s, the AMA developed standards of health care delivery for jails, prisons, and juvenile facilities, and it launched an accreditation program for jail health systems. Subsequently, a program was launched to transfer the successful aspects of the pilot effort to other jails in additional states. In this project, the AMA assisted state medical societies in providing technical assistance, coordinating states' efforts, and monitoring progress (Anno, 1981). This AMA Jail Project (Anno, 1981) evolved into the inception of the NCCHC, which promulgates specific dedicated correctional health care standards for jails and prisons (NCCHC, 2018a, 2018b), juvenile detention (NCCHC, 2022), and opioid treatment programs (NCCHC, 2016) in correctional facilities. Updated periodically to remain responsive to contemporary concerns and practices, the NCCHC standards take a holistic approach to health care and integrate mental health services throughout each of these standards: Mental Health Services, Mental Health Screening and Evaluation, Suicide Prevention and Intervention, Restraint and Seclusion, Segregated Inmates, and Emergency Psychotropic Medication. To avoid potential ethical role conflicts (e.g., clinician versus forensic evaluator), there is a specific NCCHC standard (contained in all NCCHC standards), "Therapeutic relationship, forensic information, and disciplinary actions," that details the clinical and nonforensic role for correctional medical and mental health care staff.

Since 2008, due to the unique needs of IPs with mental disorders and serious mental illnesses, the NCCHC has published a separate set of standards specifically for mental health services (NCCHC, 2015). These mental health standards parallel those for jail and prison health (and juvenile) services in format, organization, structure, intent, and substance. However, they make more explicit what the standards require for adequate delivery of mental health services in nine areas: Governance and Administration, Safety, Personnel and Training, Health Care Services and Support, Inmate Care and Treatment, Health Promotion, Special Mental Health Needs and Services, Clinical Records, and Medical–Legal Issues.

Examples of NCCHC mental health standards under the governance and administration section are Access to Care, Responsible Mental Health Authority, Clinical Autonomy, Administrative Meetings and Reports, Policies and Procedures, Continuous Quality Improvement Program, Emergency Response Plan, Communication on Patients' Mental Health Needs, Privacy of Care, Procedure in the Event of an Inmate Death, and Grievance Mechanism for Mental Health Complaints. To illustrate the nature of these standards, the second standard, Responsible Mental Health Authority, specifies that the facility have a designated mental health authority responsible for mental health services. This standard is supported by five compliance indicators that outline the mental health authority's scope of responsibility, minimum qualifications, and other requirements. Terms are defined, and a discussion elaborates the standard's intent.

The ACA accreditation standards (ACA, 2024a) address all aspects of facility operations, including health care. Specifically, they encompass services, programs, and operations essential to good correctional management. These include administrative, staff and fiscal controls, staff training and development, physical plant, safety and emergency procedures, sanitation, food service, rules and discipline, and other subjects that represent good correctional practice.

Accreditation

Accreditation, as defined by the NCCHC, is a process of external peer review in which the NCCHC grants public recognition to detention and correctional institutions that meet nationally established and accepted standards for the provision of health services. The accreditation program renders a professional judgment on the quality of health services provided and assists correctional facilities in their continued improvement (NCCHC, 2024). The ACA also accredits facilities. Among the benefits of accreditation cited by the ACA are improved staff training and development, assessment of program strengths and weaknesses, defense against lawsuits, establishment of measurable criteria for upgrading operations, improved staff morale and professionalism, a safer environment for staff and IPs, reduced liability insurance costs, and performance-based benefits (ACA, 2024b).

There are several types of accreditation available to county, state, and federal correctional facilities and systems, regardless of the size, scope, custody level, and function of a specific facility or system. These include accreditation by the ACA, the NCCHC, the Joint Commission, a combination of these organizations, and state agencies. Accreditation is largely a voluntary process, but there appears to be a national trend toward accreditation related to risk management and the contracting, outsourcing, or "privatization" of correctional health care services to universities, local health centers/systems, or for-profit vendors. Achieving and maintaining accreditation are often contractual obligations or expectations.

It is important for custody and health care leadership, other involved public policy makers, and budget staff to be aware that achieving "voluntary" initial accreditation and maintaining accreditation, regardless of the type, take a great deal of planning, preparation, staff time, and resources. Accreditation types differ depending on the facility's health care mission and its patient population. For example, some correctional systems and leaders may seek to obtain accreditation solely from either the ACA or NCCHC. Some may seek to have their infirmary, acute or tertiary medical units, dialysis centers, or psychiatric facility/unit receive Joint Commission accreditation. Some systems may seek NCCHC accreditation for their psychiatric/mental health facilities without seeking NCCHC accreditation for their medical units. Some facilities/systems seek dual accreditation or have all three (ACA, NCCHC, and Joint Commission). The following descriptions of the primary accrediting bodies are summaries of information provided by the organizations.

National Commission on Correctional Health Care

Today, the NCCHC is the only national organization dedicated solely to improving correctional health care through standards, accreditation, certification, education, and technical assistance. The NCCHC board of directors consists of liaisons from 32 national organizations, including the American Academy of Child and Adolescent Psychiatry (AACAP), the American Academy of Psychiatry and the Law (AAPL), the American Psychiatric Association (APA), and other organizations from the fields of medicine, public health, law, and corrections, as well as state and county associations.

The NCCHC's evidence-based standards represent the organization's requirements for health services (e.g., nursing, medical, dental, and mental health) in state and federal prisons, jails, short-term detention, juvenile detention, and other confinement settings. They are intended for use in evaluating the health services in correctional facilities, including those that are part of larger systems.

Mental health care has been integral to the NCCHC standards and accreditation program from the start. As the number of IPs with mental illness soared, some systems opted to manage mental health services separately from medical services. The NCCHC's mental health standards and accreditation program were designed for correctional facilities in which the legal authority for mental health services is separate from their other health services and both parties are not already accredited under the standards for jails or prisons.

Individuals with substance use disorders are overrepresented in the criminal justice system. To help facilitate universal access to medication treatment and reduce overdose deaths, the White House Office of National Drug Control Policy announced the release of Performance Measures for Medication-Assisted Treatment in Correctional Settings (Legislative Analysis and Public Policy Association, 2023), which is placing a spotlight on the issue in corrections. Additionally, in 2023, the White House expanded access to evidence-based treatment, including for individuals who are incarcerated, through the National Drug Control Strategy (White House, 1989). This strategy is to help ensure that formerly incarcerated people receive the supportive care they need to become productive members of their community.

The NCCHC established an accreditation program in 2004 that enables corrections-based opioid treatment programs to obtain legally required certification from the Substance Abuse and Mental Health Services Administration of the U.S. Department of Health and Human Services. The NCCHC, the only Substance Abuse and Mental Health Services Administration–authorized accrediting body that focuses on corrections, has developed standards (NCCHC, 2016) that are based on federal regulations but tailored for this field. Over the past few years, this has been the NCCHC's fastest growing accreditation program.

Accreditation process

Approximately 500 correctional facilities participate in the NCCHC's accreditation program. These facilities are diverse in terms of jurisdiction, management structure, size, and incarcerated population, ranging from a juvenile facility with an average daily population of 10 to a large metropolitan jail complex housing 9,000 IPs. The average size of an accredited prison is more than 1,300 IPs.

A correctional facility seeking accreditation first reviews the standards relevant to the setting to assess current compliance. The next step is to complete an application, followed by a self-survey questionnaire. Once the facility is ready, a survey is scheduled. The survey duration depends on the facility's size and the complexity of health services provided, but it usually lasts 2 or 3 days.

Survey teams consist of qualified, trained physicians, nurses, health administrators, and other credentialed health professionals certified in correctional health care who understand corrections and combine that knowledge with their professional expertise. They conduct a review of health records, policies, and procedures; interview health staff, correctional officers, and IPs; and tour the facility to gather information. Surveyors use the same compliance indicators listed in each NCCHC standard to measure compliance. At the end of the survey, an exit conference is conducted to discuss their preliminary findings. These reviews are collegial and educational, with the survey team offering suggestions for improvement.

An NCCHC accreditation committee then reviews the survey team's report to evaluate compliance with the standards and make an accreditation decision. The facility receives a comprehensive written report that includes recommendations to assist with standards compliance. Once accredited, the facility submits an annual report with updates on key information. Subsequent on-site visits occur about every 3 years.

American Correctional Association

The ACA's mission is to provide "a professional organization for all individuals and groups, both public and private, that share a common goal of improving the justice system" (ACA, 2024b, Mission section). Approximately 80% of all state departments of corrections and youth services are active ACA members.

The ACA's Standards and Accreditation Department serves a dual mission of providing services for the ACA and the Commission on Accreditation for Corrections. The ACA publishes many standards manuals, primarily administration and standards manuals for the safe, effective, and professional operation of correctional agencies, including local detention facilities and county jails, state and federal prisons, juvenile facilities and/or training schools, private halfway houses or group homes, and probation and parole agencies.

Since 1989, the ACA has developed health care standards for corrections. Beginning in 1999, it began providing what it described as state-of-the-art performance-based standards, an initiative that focuses accreditation on outcome measures that are critical to the consequences of programs. In 2001, the ACA began evaluating compliance of health care against these benchmarks. The standards manuals most relevant to correctional health and mental health staff are the *Performance-Based Standards for Correctional Health Care for Adult Correctional Institutions* (ACA, 2002), *Performance-Based Standards and Expected Practices for Adult Correctional Institutions*

(ACA, 2021), and the *Standards for Adult Correctional Institutions*, Part 4: Institutional Services, Section E: Health Care (ACA, 2003). The stated goal is to "provide appropriate and necessary health services and care for offenders (e.g., incarcerated individuals)" (pp. 1–3). One notable goal of the performance-based health care expected practices is for correctional systems to gain experience in collecting data and providing outcome measures. These standards are under continual revision to reflect changing practice, current case law, new knowledge, and agency experience. These changes are published by the ACA (2008) in the *Standards Supplement*.

Accreditation process

The ACA and the Commission on Accreditation for Corrections administer the only national performance-based accreditation program for all components of the correctional/criminal justice system, including adult correctional institutions (prisons), adult local detention facilities (jails), adult community residential services facilities, adult probation and parole field services, juvenile facilities, and correctional training academies. The accreditation program and process offer the opportunity for correctional agencies to evaluate their operations against national standards, remedy deficiencies, and improve the quality of correctional programs and services. ACA accreditation is available to all adult and juvenile agencies for which standards have been published. The requirements of the accreditation process are the same for all types of agencies: state, county, federal, and private. Correctional administrators initiate accreditation activities voluntarily. When an agency chooses to pursue accreditation, ACA staff provide the agency with relevant information and application materials, including a contract, the applicable standards manual, a policy and procedure manual, and an organization summary.

Accreditation and standards promulgated by other medical organizations

The Joint Commission

The Joint Commission (formerly known as the Joint Commission on Accreditation of Healthcare Organizations, or JCAHO) is an independent, not-for-profit organization whose mission is "to continuously improve health care for the public, in collaboration with other stakeholders, by evaluating health care organizations and inspiring them to excel in providing safe and effective care of the highest quality and value" (Joint Commission, 2024, About the Joint Commission section). It is the nation's oldest and largest standards-setting and accrediting body in health care.

The Joint Commission evaluates and accredits more than 20,000 health care organizations and programs in the United States. Joint Commission accreditation and certification is recognized nationwide as a symbol of quality that reflects an organization's commitment to meeting certain performance standards. Accreditation can be earned by many types of health care organizations, including hospitals, doctor's offices, nursing homes, office-based surgery centers, behavioral health treatment facilities, and providers of home care services.

Providers of health care staffing services can also earn Joint Commission certification. To earn and maintain the Joint Commission's Gold Seal of Approval™, an organization must undergo an on-site survey by a Joint Commission survey team at least every 3 years (laboratories must be surveyed every 2 years). For example, the University of Texas Medical Branch Correctional Managed Care has a unique maximum-security state prison medical surgical hospital and specialty clinic (e.g., Hospital Galveston) in Galveston, Texas, that has achieved Joint Commission accreditation for inpatient and ambulatory health care. Several California Department of Corrections and Rehabilitation facilities have achieved various combinations of Joint Commission accreditation for ambulatory health care, behavioral health care, and nursing care centers. Several other California Department of Corrections and Rehabilitation facilities have applied for Joint Commission accreditation.

American Psychiatric Association and other organizations

The APHA (2003) has promulgated standards for medical, mental health, and other correctional health services. The APA has also developed guidelines. First published in 1989, these guidelines are in their third edition (APA, 2016). Particularly challenging areas covered by the APA guidelines and position statements include the use of seclusion and restraint with IPs with mental disorders (Appelbaum, 2007; Champion, 2007; Metzner et al., 2007) and the housing of IPs with mental illness in solitary confinement, administrative segregation, and other types of restrictive housing units (APA, 2023).

Best health care practices in correctional settings: where are we today?

Psychiatrists and other health care staff who are new to the world of corrections must receive an orientation that helps them understand basic correctional systems, culture, environmental, and personal safety and physical plant issues (see Chapter 13). Topics include security policies and procedures, contraband issues, hostage and other emergency situations, boundaries and communication between IPs and staff, and professionalism. Some relevant examples include the NCCHC standards that focus on personnel and training (NCCHC, 2018) and the ACA standards (ACA, 2003).

Current national standards and/or guidelines for correctional health and specialized mental health care programs emphasize the importance of mental health screening and evaluation performed by qualified mental health personnel on all IPs as part of the admission process to a jail, prison, or juvenile facility (see Chapter 15). Metzner and colleagues (1994) reported data from all 50 state departments of corrections regarding prison mental health screening and evaluation models. They found that most states appeared to have adopted some variation of the most recognized guidelines and/or standards (e.g., APA, NCCHC, APHA) for correctional health care systems.

Position statements of National Commission on Correctional Health Care, the American College of Correctional Physicians, and other organizations

In addition to promulgating standards, the NCCHC, the American College of Correctional Physicians (formerly known as the Society of Correctional Physicians), and other organizations such as the APA, AAPL, AMA, and AACAP periodically adopt position statements on topics of importance for the correctional health care field. Position statements are different from correctional health care or correctional standards. Depending on the organization, some are aspirational in nature, while others set a standard of care. Position statements frequently address newly identified challenges facing correctional staff, health care staff, and facilities and are therefore often used by correctional health and custody administrators and medical and mental health care professionals to update their practices, policies, and procedures. They should be of interest to policy makers and the public because they often frame the social, economic, and political aspects of contemporary correctional health care issues.

Education and certification of correctional health professionals

As awareness grows regarding the specialized needs of health care delivery in correctional settings, national certifications are available for correctional health care professionals, including psychiatrists, other physicians, nurses, dental staff, and others. The NCCHC and the ACA have each established certification processes tailored to these professionals.
The Certified Correctional Health Professional Program provided by the NCCHC includes specialty certifications tailored for different correctional health care professional disciplines. These programs require passing an examination crafted by a committee consisting of peers who are authorities in the field of correctional health care. Lastly, there is also an advanced certification, Certified Correctional Health Professional Program–Advanced, for individuals who have demonstrated excellence, commitment, and contributions to the field of correctional health care and their relative discipline or profession. Furthermore, the NCCHC produces a plethora of correctional health resources, including the peer-reviewed *Journal of Correctional Health Care*.

The ACA has a comprehensive certification program for corrections professionals. There are also three certification categories for nurses: certified corrections nurse manager, certified corrections nurse, and health services administrator.

There is heightened awareness of challenges in the timely delivery of correctional health care. Challenges include the risks of litigation, custody and health care staffing—in particular the challenges in psychiatrist recruitment and retention—escort of patients, growing population on psychotropic medications, and serious mental illness. Associated psychosocial challenges include safely housing individuals with serious mental illness, mobility impairments, and neurocognitive disorders, as well as transgender and other vulnerable individuals, in correctional environments. Other examples include special populations such as youth in adult facilities, pregnant women, postpartum women who are nursing, oncology and dialysis patients, patients needing infirmary and skilled nursing levels of care, terminal patients in hospice care, transgender individuals with or without gender dysphoria, and a growing aging population with resulting medical and psychiatric disease burden and comorbidities. As a result, the APA, AAPL, AACAP, and American College of Correctional Physicians are directing continuing medical educational efforts toward correctional mental health themes, evident through dedicated sessions, panels, and conference presentations that target health care staff, administrators, and custody leadership. There are also creative efforts to raise awareness of the many opportunities in correctional health for medical students, psychiatry residents, and other trainees by establishing clerkships and longitudinal clinic experiences and by encouraging trainees to attend regional and national conferences through scholarships and other programs (see Chapter 76). Lastly, loan repayment and loan forgiveness are some additional strategies to recruit new talent into correctional health care.

Summary

Many challenges confront correctional health care staff in serving the needs of IPs. Effective screening, timely referral, and appropriate treatment are critical. Their implementation requires interagency collaboration, multidisciplinary team approaches, individualized treatment decision-making for patients, adherence to established national correctional standards of care, and implementation of continuous quality improvement practices and research on the health needs of this vulnerable patient population. Effective evaluation and treatment meet vital public health objectives, improve access to care and continuity of health services, and facilitate effective transition into the community upon release. Better correctional health care for IPs, as defined in national standards and accreditation programs, serves the intended goal of treatment and rehabilitation and may have an additional benefit of reducing morbidity, mortality, and the ever-present risk of litigation and court involvement.

REFERENCES

American Correctional Association. (2002). *Performance-based standards for correctional health care for adult correctional institutions.*

American Correctional Association. (2003). *Standards for adult correctional institutions* (4th ed.).

American Correctional Association. (2008). *Standards supplement.*

American Correctional Association. (2021). *Performance-based standards and expected practices for adult correctional institutions.*

American Correctional Association. (2024a). *Standards and accreditation: Benefits of accreditation.* https://www.aca.org/standards/benefits.asp.

American Correctional Association. (2024b). *Vision statement.* https://www.aca.org/common/Uploaded%20files/aca_visionstatement.pdf

American Psychiatric Association. (2016). *Psychiatric services in correctional facilities: A task force report of the American Psychiatric Association* (3rd ed.).

American Psychiatric Association. (2023). *Position statement on restrictive housing of incarcerated adults with serious mental illness.* https://www.psychiatry.org/getattachment/de02560f-34fd-420b-b36a-257f1450558a/Position-Restrictive-Housing-of-Adults.pdf

American Public Health Association. (2003). *Standards for health services in correctional institutions* (3rd ed.).

Anno, B. J. (1981). *Jails' progress in implementing AMA (American Medical Association)* standards—*First evaluation report.* U.S. Department of Justice.

Anno, B. J. (2001). *Correctional health care: Guidelines for the management of an adequate delivery system.* National Institute of Corrections.

Appelbaum, K. L. (2007). Commentary: The use of restraint and seclusion in correctional mental health. *Journal of the American Academy of Psychiatry and the Law, 35*, 431–435.

Baillargeon, J., Penn, J. V., Knight, K., Harzke, A. J., Baillargeon, G., & Becker, E. A. (2010). Risk of reincarceration among prisoners with co-occurring severe mental illness and substance use disorders. *Administration and Policy in Mental Health, 37*(4), 367–374.

Champion, M. K. (2007). Commentary: Seclusion and restraint in corrections—A time for change. *Journal of the American Academy of Psychiatry and the Law*, *35*, 426–430.

International Organization for Standardization. (n.d.). *Standards*. http://www.iso.org/iso/home/standards.htm.

Joint Commission. (2024). *About our standards*. https://www.jointcommission.org/standards/about-our-standards/

Lamb, H. R., & Bachrach, L. L. (2001). Some perspectives on deinstitutionalization. *Psychiatric Services*, *52*, 1039–1045.

Legislative Analysis and Public Policy Association. (2023). *Performance measures for medication-assisted treatment in correctional settings a framework for implementation*. https://legislativeanalysis.org/wp-content/uploads/2022/12/Performance-Measures-for-Medication-assisted-Treatment-in-Correctional-Settings.pdf

McDonald, D. C. (1999). Medical care in prisons. *Crime and Justice*, *26*, 427–478.

Medical Association of Georgia. (1977). *MAG—which developed the standards for evaluating health care in jails and prisons in Georgia—surveys eight jails and 33 prisons*. https://members.mag.org/news/newsarticledisplay.aspx?ArticleID=12

Mental Retardation Facilities and Community Mental Health Centers Construction Act of 1963, Pub. L. No. 88–164, 77 Stat. 282 (1963).

Metzner, J. L., Miller, R. D., & Kleinsasser, D. (1994). Mental health screening and evaluation within prisons. *Bulletin of the American Academy of Psychiatry and the Law*, *22*, 451–457.

Metzner, J. L., Tardiff, K., Lion, J., et al. (2007). Resource document on the use of restraint and seclusion in correctional mental health care. *Journal of the American Academy of Psychiatry and the Law*, *35*, 417–425.

National Commission on Correctional Health Care. (2015). *Standards for mental health services in correctional facilities*.

National Commission on Correctional Health Care. (2016). *Standards for opioid treatment programs in correctional facilities*.

National Commission on Correctional Health Care. (2018a). *Standards for health services in jails*.

National Commission on Correctional Health Care. (2018b). *Standards for health services in prisons*.

National Commission on Correctional Health Care. (2022). *Standards for health services in juvenile detention and confinement facilities*.

National Commission on Correctional Health Care. (2024). *Accreditation programs: Health services: Overview*. https://www.ncchc.org/accreditation/

Rold, W. J. (2008). Thirty years after *Estelle v. Gamble*: A legal retrospective. *Journal of Correctional Health Care*, *14*, 11–20.

Steinwald, C., Alevizos, G., & Aherne, P. (1973). *Medical care in U.S. jails: A 1972 AMA survey*. American Medical Association.

Stelovich, S. (1979). From the hospital to the prison: A step forward in deinstitutionalization? *Hospital and Community Psychiatry*, *30*, 618–620.

Stephan, J. J. (1997). *Census of state and federal correctional facilities, 1995*. U.S. Department of Justice, Bureau of Justice Statistics.

Torrey, E. F., Kennard, A. D., Eslinger, D., Lamb, R., & Pavle, J. (2010). *More mentally ill persons are in jails and prisons than hospitals: A survey of the states*. Treatment Advocacy Center.

U.S. General Accounting Office. (1978). *A federal strategy is needed to help improve medical and dental care in prisons and jails: Report to the Congress*. U.S. Government Printing Office.

U.S. General Accounting Office. (2000). *Mental health: Community-based care increases for people with serious mental illness*. U.S. Government Printing Office.

Wallenstein, A. M. (2004, Fall). Understanding history vital for future success. *CorrectCare*, *18*(4), 3.

White House. (1989, September). *The National Drug Control Strategy*. https://www.ojp.gov/pdffiles1/ondcp/119466.pdf

Whitmer, G. E. (1980). From hospitals to jails: The fate of California's deinstitutionalized mentally ill. *American Journal of Orthopsychiatry*, *50*, 65–75.

74

Systems monitoring and quality improvement

Jeffrey L. Metzner

Introduction

Class action litigation that includes a focus on constitutionally inadequate correctional mental health care has been a major and effective force in jail and prison reform during the past 4 decades. Benefits to correctional mental health systems resulting from such litigation have included increased resources needed to implement basic policies and procedures that are necessary for a constitutionally adequate system (Metzner, 2009a, 2009b). Chapter 3 provides a useful summary regarding the legal basis for requiring adequate mental health services in correctional facilities.

Following the passage of the Prison Litigation Reform Act of 1995, the number of newly initiated consent decrees related to class action litigation involving correctional mental health services significantly decreased. This reduction in litigation followed from limiting the discretion of judges in approving such decrees that were previously allowed. Private settlement agreements and/or memoranda of agreement or their equivalents (the "Agreement") have been substituted for the consent decree process. Although the judicial enforcement of these Agreements is weaker as compared to consent decrees, the monitoring process is similar to that previously used with consent decrees (Metzner, 2009b).

This chapter summarizes the monitoring process frequently involved in an Agreement resulting from a class action lawsuit specific to a correctional mental health care system. Emphasis is placed on the importance of developing a quality improvement (QI) process, which should ultimately eliminate the need for an external monitor.

Phases of class action litigation

One conceptualization of class action litigation in correctional facilities described the following three phases: "the liability phase (legally determining whether constitutional deficiencies exist), the remedial phase (developing a remedy to identified constitutional deficiencies), and the implementation phase (implementing the remedial plan)" (Metzner, 2002).

Occasionally, the parties will agree on joint experts for fact-finding purposes during the liability phase, although monitoring a correctional mental health system in its strictest meaning does not occur during this phase. It is more common that the attorneys for plaintiffs and defendants each have their own psychiatric experts during the liability phase. Since passage of the Prison Litigation Reform Act of 1995, such cases are often settled before trial via a negotiated Agreement or similar process. The remedial plan is generally negotiated between the parties, with each side consulting with its own psychiatric experts. Most Agreements include a provision for the appointment of a monitor.

Although the elements of a remedial plan will vary based on factors specific to the litigation, such as the size and type of correctional facility (e.g., jail or prison), the basic structure of the correctional mental health system that needs to be addressed in a remedial plan is well established. *Ruiz v. Estelle* (1980) mandated six minimal essential elements for such services:

- Systematic screening and evaluation;
- Treatment that is more than mere seclusion or close supervision;
- Participation by trained mental health professionals;
- Accurate, complete, and confidential records;
- Safeguards against psychotropic medication prescribed in dangerous amounts, without adequate supervision, or otherwise inappropriately administered; and
- A suicide prevention program.

National standards, guidelines, and/or court decisions (American Psychiatric Association, 2016, 2023; *Coleman v. Wilson*, 1995; National Commission on Correctional Health Care, 2015, 2018) have provided useful guidelines for addressing these elements in addition to enlarging this framework for a constitutionally adequate correctional mental health system. The expanded framework includes additional elements such as discharge planning, out-of-cell structured therapeutic time for incarcerated persons (IPs) with serious mental illnesses housed in restrictive housing units, mental health rounds in restrictive housing settings, and implementation of a QI process (Metzner, 2009a).

The elements of the remedial plan (i.e., the Agreement) will be operationalized via the facility's mental health care policies and procedures. In addition to the standard topics to be covered by these policies and procedures, such as mission and goals, organizational structure, and training of health care and correctional staff members (Metzner, 1997), they should address the following topics, which are often emphasized and described in detail in the Agreement related to the history of the events leading to the litigation (Metzner, 2009b):

- The screening and evaluation processes for identifying IPs with mental illnesses;
- An adequate physical plant for mental health assessment, treatment, and programming purposes (e.g., clean office space that is safe, with sound privacy and climate controls);
- Staffing credentials and allocations (e.g., adequacy of staff allocations in terms of full-time equivalents);
- Adequacy of an IP's access to the mental health services;
- Treatment programs available, which should specify levels of care available and the quality of these services;
- The use of seclusion and restraints, involuntary medications, and involuntary hospitalization;
- Unique correctional mental health care issues such as treatment requirements for IPs with serious mental illness in lockdown housing units, mental health rounds in such units, and mental health staff's input into the correctional disciplinary process;
- Medication management practices (e.g., administration of medication, documentation of medication administration);
- Suicide prevention program;
- The QI process;
- Training of both mental health and custody staff;
- The working relationships between custody and mental health staff;
- The working relationships between medical (including nursing) and mental health staff; and
- Discharge planning services.

Other issues that should be addressed include obtaining informed consent for treatment and the limits of confidentiality during clinical assessments or interventions.

How the Agreement specifically addresses the details of these areas often depends on the factors that led to the litigation. For example, if one of the alleged deficiencies involved inadequate mental health staffing allocations or the use of mental health workers without appropriate credentials (e.g., licensure), the Agreement may specify caseload ratios and the type of licensure or certification needed for mental health clinicians.

One of the earliest roles of the monitor will be to review and provide consultation to the correctional system's mental health director in the context of developing these policies and procedures. This tedious task, which will require multiple drafts, is crucial because implementation of these policies and procedures will be the focus of both monitoring and the initial stages of the QI process. The more difficult policies and procedures to develop include those involving involuntary treatment (particularly the use of restraints; see Chapter 25), treatment requirements for IPs with a serious mental illness in restrictive housing units, and the details of the treatment programs available, with particular reference to the residential treatment programs. These details should include staffing requirements or periodic staffing needs assessments, minimum required hours per week of structured therapeutic programs offered to IPs requiring a residential level of mental health care (e.g., special needs unit, intermediate care unit), and the minimum frequency of clinical contacts for IPs with their psychiatrist and/or mental health clinician.

If the correctional mental health system does not have an adequate computerized information management system, numerous logbooks and spreadsheets will need to be developed for proof-of-practice purposes to facilitate the monitoring of many elements of these policies and procedures. Staff will often initially embrace such paperwork requirements but will soon find it difficult to keep the paperwork current for many reasons; these can be significantly mitigated with a computerized information system. Without this system, successful implementation of an adequate QI system will be extremely difficult. A properly designed electronic health record system will often serve as a virtual data repository, which can aggregate data elements present in the electronic health record for the information management system.

Roles of a monitor

A monitor (or monitors) is usually appointed prior to the implementation phase. Initially, the monitor's role is to operationalize how the remedial plan will be monitored and interpreted when sections of the plan are vague, unclear, and/or repetitive, which invariably occurs despite everyone's best efforts.

The monitor's role in the implementation phase is critical due to the importance of their interpretations regarding provisions of the remedial plan and assessments relevant to compliance. The monitor helps formulate the various outcome measures to be monitored via record reviews, IP and staff interviews, QI studies, and the like. The Agreement generally defines relevant compliance terms such as noncompliance, partial compliance, and substantial compliance. The relationships the monitor establishes with both parties (i.e., the attorneys), in addition to the key mental health and custody administrators, will have a significant impact on the success of the remedial plan's implementation. When the monitoring process is working well, it is common for the monitor to provide helpful consultation to the correctional mental health care system regarding practices that are not required by the remedial plan. However, recommendations resulting from such a consultative process should clearly be labeled as such, in contrast to being requirements related to the remedial plan (Metzner, 2009b). Thoughtful selection of a monitor and clear delineation of their duties will help avoid dissatisfaction with the monitoring process, which often focuses on unclear or changing outcome measures, costs of the monitoring, and/or perceived monitor bias (i.e., more oriented toward the plaintiff or the defense).

Quality improvement

A key function of the monitor is to help the system develop an adequate QI process, with elements of the Agreement being an initial focus. This learning process will be difficult but rewarding for all involved and requires much patience and mentoring. Common pitfalls initially include inadequate samples due to flawed methodology (e.g., using a completely random sample of IPs rather than a random sample of targeted IPs, such as IPs on the mental health caseload) and QI reports that are produced in a nonsystematic format. QI reports should be stand-alone documents (i.e., the writer should not need to be present for a reader to understand the study purpose, results, and analysis). These reports, which do not need to be lengthy, should have subsections that include the rationale for the issue being studied, the methodology used, results, assessment of the results, and planned actions, if any.

Backhouse and Ogunlayi (2020) summarized many well-established approaches to evaluating and making changes to mental health care services, which included research projects, clinical audits, services assessments, innovation, and QI. These authors conceptualized QI to include "a systematic continuous approach that aims to solve problems in health care, improve service provision, and ultimately provide better outcomes for patients" (Backhouse & Ogunlayi, 2020, p. 1). A QI program has been recognized as an essential component of an adequate correctional mental health care system (National Commission on Correctional Health Care, 2015). Hughes (2008) provided a very useful summary of the evolution of the QI process in the health care field, which included using techniques developed by Deming (1986) in the rebuilding of the manufacturing industry in post–World War II Japan.

Many correctional mental health care systems prior to class action litigation had not developed an adequate QI system, which often contributed to the problems in the system that resulted in the litigation. In correctional mental health care, if a process is not reviewed via a QI mechanism, what is believed to occur is frequently very different from what actually occurs. It is frequently a reflection of an inadequate QI system when a psychiatric expert can identify significant systemic issues during a site visit that were not identified by the system itself. Within a correctional mental health care system, a QI process is crucial in the context of implementing an effective medication management system. Problems that may be addressed include the frequent housing transfers of prisoners and the limited windows of opportunity for medication administration due to mandatory counts, lockdowns, and other competing events.

In a correctional health care setting, the mental health care QI process is most effective when it is part of the facility's health care QI committee that oversees the QI processes for medical, dental, nursing, pharmacy, medical records, and mental health services. Each of these services often has a separate QI subcommittee that reports to the overall health care QI committee on a regular basis, which facilitates resolution of interdisciplinary concerns.

The mental health care subcommittee should include both line and administrative mental health care staff, nursing staff, key custody staff (e.g., deputy warden for health care), and other staff who are directly or indirectly involved with the mental health care delivery system. QI activities should include both process and outcome studies. The effectiveness of a health care delivery process can be assessed by a process QI study. For example, does the sick-call process work, as evidenced by timely triage and clinic appointments? An outcome QI study evaluates whether the goal of a health care intervention was achieved (e.g., decreased symptoms of depression following implementation of treatment).

It is very common for a correctional mental health system to have implemented a quality assurance (QA) program, which is an important component of a QI system but is not an adequate QI system by itself. QA audits are frequently designed to determine the presence or absence of necessary data, such as completion of all the elements of an initial mental health evaluation form. A QI process would not only examine the completion rate of the various elements but also identify barriers to completion of the form, make recommendations relevant to overcoming these barriers, and improve the clinical relevance of the form. A QA audit is typically performed by a designated QA staff person, in contrast to QI studies, which typically involve line staff directly involved with the area being assessed.

A QI indicator is a quantitative measure that gives information about the performance, effectiveness, safety, and/or quality of a health care service (Quentin et al., 2019). Establishing key indicators, especially when they can be measured via software programs, facilitates the development and implementation of an adequate QI system. Key indicators are process, outcome, or structure indicators that are considered essential to assessing high-priority aspects of the health care system. Many of the key indicators will be based on relevant policies and procedures (e.g., timelines for completion of responses to mental health referrals, adequacy of treatment plans, timely access to care). Development of business rules (i.e., specific instructions or constraints on day-to-day actions should be measured) relevant to a specific indicator will require an understanding of the relevant policy and procedure and will be facilitated by reviewing/constructing a workflow chart that is consistent with the applicable policy. The business rules for a specific key indicator need to measure accurately the requirements of the relevant policy and procedures within a reasonable margin of error. The business rule should be written in a manner that ensures the average clinician and/or administrator understands it as quickly, easily, and completely as possible (i.e., using plain language). Among the issues that need to be addressed by a business rule are the population it applies to, triggers (the event that triggers the initiation of the business rule), exceptions, suspending events, relevant time frames, and limitations (D. Potter, personal communication, July 2023).

A data validation process requires detailed specifications on how exactly an indicator and its business rules are intended to work (i.e., do they result in the indicator measuring the relevant requirements as generally defined by the pertinent policy and procedure?). In other words, is the key indicator designed correctly? For systems with a current QI system, an exploratory data analysis can be used to better understand the current data (e.g., discovering patterns, understanding the structure of the data sets, testing clinicians' and administrators' assumptions about how the program operates), which may result in design adjustments to the business rules or creation of a new indicator. The indicator is then programmed according to the business rules. A data verification process, which involves various software tests, determines whether the measurements for the key indicators have been coded correctly. In other words, these tests assist in verifying that the indicator and business rules function as intended.

A data scientist can be very helpful in developing and implementing business rules, as well as the data validity and verification processes. The QI data system needs to be transparent, which means that all updates to the underlying data systems can be tracked and are reviewable. Any significant changes that impact on key indicator measures will need to be revalidated and reverified in the context of such changes.

The monitoring process

Because mental health policies and procedures will contain general provisions, the monitor will need to decide which outcome measures to use to determine whether the facility is in compliance. For example, the policy and procedure relevant to an IP's request for mental health services (i.e., sick call) will generally require the request to be triaged by mental health staff to determine the required response time (e.g., emergent, urgent, or routine). The monitor will need to make clear the time frames required for responses to such referrals. Emergent (response as soon as possible, generally within 4 hours) and urgent (response within 24 hours) referral time frames are usually not controversial, in contrast to the time frame for routine referrals (generally 5 to 10 business days). To establish appropriate outcome measures for time frames, the monitor should obtain feedback from both parties, review national standards of correctional mental health care such as the American Psychiatric Association work group guidelines (American Psychiatric Association, 2016) and National Commission on Correctional Health Care (2015) standards, and consider other systems' practices in addition to the specific system being monitored.

The Agreement invariably addresses the minimum frequency of on-site monitoring, which is usually every 4 to 6 months. The duration of a site visit will depend on the size and mission of the facility and the number of IPs on the mental health caseload. Obtaining pre-site information relevant to the Agreement in a timely manner (e.g., within 1 to 2 weeks) will enable the monitor to significantly reduce the number of on-site days required.

Pre-site information

Pre-site information should include data relevant to monitoring compliance with the Agreement that does not require the monitor to be on-site to review. This will allow the monitor to use the limited and valuable on-site time to interview IPs and staff, observe processes such as the reception center intake assessments, and attend treatment planning team meetings and similar processes. Pre-site information includes staffing allocations and vacancies, new or revised policies and procedures, recent IP population counts, mental health caseload statistics, and pertinent QI studies. Metzner (2009b) has provided a detailed list of recommended pre-site information to obtain.

Probably the most important pre-site information to obtain is a status update (i.e., a written summary that describes the steps taken toward compliance since the last site assessment) on all elements of the Agreement that are still being monitored (i.e., have not met the Agreement criteria for no longer being monitored) with proof of practices. Depending on the nature of the proof of practice (e.g., bulky logbooks), it may only be available during the site visit. Reviewing the pre-site information will raise many questions for the monitor to assess during the site visit and will help provide a focus for the on-site evaluation.

Review of QI reports prior to the site visit should provide information needed in determining compliance with key elements of the Agreement. The timeliness of receiving the pre-site information and the quality and relevance of the content are frequently predictive of the state of compliance with the Agreement. Problems with either the timeliness or content may reflect management issues. The absence of sound QI reports generally predicts significant compliance issues with the Agreement.

The on-site assessment

Site assessments often cause significant anxiety for the mental health and correctional staff, in addition to requiring many hours of preparation. Sensitivity to their anxiety and acknowledgment of their pre-site preparation work will help to establish a collaborative working relationship with the staff.

A joint opening meeting with correctional and mental health leadership provides an opportunity to receive an overview regarding significant changes in the mental health care system since the initiation of the Agreement or since the last site assessment. It is generally helpful during this meeting to review with key custody and clinical staff the issues that were identified when reviewing the pre-site information that involves both groups. This meeting is also useful for scheduling various activities during the site visit, such as interviews with staff and IPs.

Following the opening meeting, it is useful to meet with key mental health staff to review in detail the status updates provided in the pre-site information packet. This review will often guide the monitor to request additional information or help structure questions to be asked of staff and IPs. Proof of practice is essential in determining the accuracy of the status updates provided by the correctional mental health staff. It is common to learn that the staff's perceptions and descriptions of what is occurring are very different from what is actually happening. Such a discrepancy does not usually reflect dishonesty but is related to not having reviewed the issue via adequate management audits or QI processes.

In addition to the pre-site data packet and information obtained from key custody and health care staff, other essential sources of information include the following:

- Interviews with line mental health staff, which includes clerical support staff;
- Interviews with mental health caseload IPs;
- Review of health care and custody records of mental health caseload IPs;
- Interviews with other health care workers whose job responsibilities involve the mental health system, such as nurses, pharmacists, and medical records staff; and
- Interviews with correctional administrators, supervisors, and line correctional officers.

In general, the interviews with IPs and line mental health staff are most efficiently and effectively done in a group setting. It has been the author's experience that obtaining accurate information from both IPs and staff is often challenging. When many IPs provide similar responses to clear and specific questions, it is more likely that their answers are credible; however, the answers still need to be verified via a variety of different ways, such as health care record review and asking similar questions to staff. Line staff responses may be characterized by significant omissions or inaccuracies due to different staff agendas or lack of knowledge. The monitor is more likely to obtain relevant and accurate information via group interviews if they provide a clear explanation regarding the purpose of the interview process and can structure and place limits on the interviewees' responses when necessary.

In general, correctional staff should not be present during group interviews with IPs, and the same usually applies with the mental health staff because the IPs' responses may be limited in the presence of either type of staff. For somewhat similar reasons, it is often not helpful to have supervisors present during group interviews with either custody or mental health staff. Depending on the Agreement and other variables, attorneys from both sides may be present during some of these interviews.

The monitor should directly observe clinical activities relevant to the Agreement. For example, attending mental health treatment team meetings, custody meetings that involve mental health staff (e.g., certain classification review meetings or disciplinary hearings), and group therapy sessions will provide information that often would not otherwise be available to the monitor. It is often helpful to ask the participants questions at the end of the monitor's brief observation to clarify issues that are being monitored.

It is also important for the monitor to visit a representative sample of IPs' housing units, any special needs units or other health care settings, the booking/intake area, and restrictive housing units to answer the following questions:

- Are there environmental and physical plant issues that affect mental health care (e.g., is there adequate office/programming space to ensure sound privacy and safety during clinical assessment/treatment contacts)?
- Is there a mental health staff presence in these units?
- Is there a good working relationship between custody and health care staff and between mental health and medical staff?

The monitor should also observe the mental health rounding process in restrictive housing units for similar reasons, in addition to performing a brief case-finding assessment (i.e., are there IPs with mental illnesses in restrictive housing who had not previously been identified, or are there clinical contraindications for certain IPs in these housing units due to the nature of their mental illnesses?).

At the beginning of the monitoring process, very few of the Agreement provisions will be in compliance. The monitor can provide useful consultation to the director of mental health regarding prioritizing efforts to comply with the Agreement provisions, which often are closely related to staffing allocation and physical plant issues (both of which are often budget driven), risk of harm to IPs or staff if lack of compliance persists, organizational structure of the mental health services, and essential infrastructure issues such as presence or absence of a computerized information management system.

Exit interviews

An exit interview is generally appreciated by the facility leadership because it helps clarify needed steps toward compliance and prepares them for the contents of the monitoring report. There should be few surprises in the exit interview because, throughout the site assessment, the monitor should be providing feedback to staff concerning pertinent findings, especially when the findings have significant ramifications for the mental health care of IPs. Even when the findings are negative, it is important to recognize positive aspects of the program to decrease the risk of the staff becoming demoralized and less motivated to improve the system. Disclaimers should be given during the exit interview about the preliminary nature of the findings, which will be more comprehensive and finalized in the report they will receive.

The monitoring report

The monitoring report should be produced on a timely basis and should address each element of the Agreement. The degree of compliance, which is generally defined in the Agreement, should be stated for each provision. For each provision or group of related provisions, it is often helpful to organize the report with the following subsections:

- Sources of information;
- Findings;
- Assessment of findings; and
- Recommendations.

Production of a timely report will facilitate a more effective response by the facility because the report should serve as a blueprint for achieving compliance.

Summary

Correctional mental health systems have significantly benefited from class action litigation focused on the mental health care system, which often brings increased resources and much-needed external monitoring of policies and procedures. Such monitoring should include facilitating the system's development and implementation of a QI system that will ultimately replace the role of an external monitor and, ideally, will maintain and improve the correctional mental health care system.

REFERENCES

American Psychiatric Association. (2016). *Psychiatric services in correctional facilities* (3rd ed.).

American Psychiatric Association. (2023). *Position statement on restrictive housing of incarcerated adults with serious mental illness.* https://www.psychiatry.org/getattachment/de02560f-34fd-420b-b36a-257f1450558a/Position-Restrictive-Housing-of-Adults.pdf

Backhouse, A., & Ogunlayi, F. (2020). Quality improvement into practice. *BMJ (Clinical Research Ed.)*, *368*, m865.

Coleman v. Wilson, 912 F. Supp. 1282 (E.D. Cal. 1995).

Deming, W. E. (1986). *Out of crisis.* Massachusetts Institute of Technology Center for Advanced Engineering Study.

Hughes, R. G. (2008). Tools and strategies for quality improvement and patient safety. In R. G. Hughes (Ed.), *Patient safety and quality: An evidence-based handbook for nurses* (Publication No. 08-0043; pp. 3:1–3:39). Agency for Healthcare Research and Quality.

Metzner, J. L. (1997). An introduction to correctional psychiatry: Part I. *Journal of the American Academy of Psychiatry and the Law*, *25*, 375–381.

Metzner, J. L. (2002). Class action litigation in correctional psychiatry. *Journal of the American Academy of Psychiatry and the Law*, *30*, 19–29.

Metzner, J. L. (2009a). Monitoring a correctional mental health care system: The role of the mental health expert. *Behavioral Science Law*, *27*, 727–741.

Metzner, J. L. (2009b). Monitoring a correctional mental health system. In C. L. Scott (Ed.), *Handbook of correctional mental health* (2nd ed., pp. 377–394). American Psychiatric Publishing.

National Commission on Correctional Health Care. (2015). *Standards for mental health services in correctional facilities.*

National Commission on Correctional Health Care. (2018). *Standards for health services in prisons.*

Prison Litigation Reform Act of 1995, H.R. 3019, 104th Congress. (Also referenced as Pub. L. No. 104–134, §§ 801–810, 110 Stat.

1321–1366 [1996] [codified as amended in scattered sections of 11, 18, 28, and 42 U.S.C.])

Quentin, W., Partanen, V. M., Brownwood, I., & Klazinga, N. (2019). Measuring healthcare quality. In R. Busse, N. Klazinga, D. Panteli, et al. (Eds.), *Improving healthcare quality in Europe: Characteristics, effectiveness and implementation of different strategies.* Health Policy Series, No. 53. https://www.ncbi.nlm.nih.gov/books/NBK549260/

Ruiz v. Estelle, 503 F. Supp. 1265 (S.D. Texas 1980).

75

Leadership, training, and educational opportunities

Raymond F. Patterson and Marcus R. Patterson

Introduction

Services and programs for the screening, assessment, and treatment of incarcerated persons (IPs) with mental illness in correctional facilities in the United States have changed dramatically since the 1960s. These noteworthy changes can be attributed, in part, to several major legal decisions, including *Estelle v. Gamble* (1976), *Bowring v. Godwin* (1977), and *Ruiz v. Estelle* (1980), which addressed issues regarding the constitutional standard for adequate health and mental health services in correctional facilities (see Chapter 3). Many improvements in the development and administration of mental health services and treatment programs within our jails and prisons have derived from these decisions.

Despite these changes, the absence or limited presence of mental health care providers continues to impact the availability and quality of mental health care services in jails and prisons. Historically, the limited mental health services that were available were often provided by nonpsychiatric physicians, nurses, and/or "counselors" with minimal education, experience, or training in the assessment, diagnosis, or treatment of mental illness or mental conditions. In addition, it was not uncommon for medication management and administration to vary greatly, including administration of medication by custody staff. These staffing and qualification deficiencies continue to plague federal, state, and local correctional facilities and systems. The development of mental health programs was also hindered by the "prison culture" in which IPs who did not adhere to the strict rules of behavior and comportment required of them were considered somehow defective or bad, but not ill or sick. This typically included IPs who exhibited unusual or bizarre behaviors (i.e., disruptive, oppositional, dangerous, or other noncompliant behaviors) that may have been indications of mental illness, IPs who were gender nonconforming, and IPs who engaged in self-harming behaviors, including self-mutilation, serious injurious behaviors, and suicide attempts.

In addition, the passage of the Community Mental Health Centers Construction Act, Mental Retardation Facilities and Construction Act (1963) began with expectations that patients would be released from state psychiatric hospitals into community-based care and treatment that would be available and less expensive to state and municipal governments. Beyond cost savings, this plan would remedy unwarranted or unnecessary "warehousing" of people with mental illness in state facilities, where they had remained for years. Gradually, the release of thousands of patients from state or other mental hospitals, the increasingly strict and/or restrictive criteria for admission to and maintenance in mental hospitals, and limited access to community-based treatment facilities contributed to significant increases in the number of persons with mental illness in jails and prisons (see Chapter 2). In addition, the "War on Drugs" policies, beginning in 1982, contributed to increases in arrests and incarceration of individuals with substance use disorders, including those who also struggled with mental illness. This chapter focuses on the role of psychiatrists in the development and management of mental health services and programs in jails and prisons and, more specifically, on the leadership roles and related training and education opportunities available to psychiatrists who want to work in these facilities.

Leadership

The authors' experiences include providing direct mental health services in jails and prisons and assessing and monitoring mental health programs provided in many correctional systems. From that experience, it is clear that the introduction of mental health professionals into these systems has frequently been met with distrust and cynicism by custody staff. This cynicism appears to come from the combined significant increase in the number of IPs with diagnosable mental illnesses and conditions, along with a history of inadequately trained mental health professionals.

A very informative article by Greifinger (2013), which focuses on cynicism by prison officials and health care professionals, notes that cynicism creates a needless hurdle to access to care and an increased risk of litigation. The authors' experiences are consistent with the view that, in some instances, correctional staff and prison health care providers regard IP complaints about their health care with disbelief or as an attempt to "hustle" the provider for some other desired outcome or secondary gain. This may result in a failure to assess an IP's health care complaints or concerns adequately and is also an endorsement of the frequently encountered correctional culture that presumes IPs are always "gaming" the system. In this case, the presumption is that IPs are attempting to use health care providers to satisfy their needs and wants that are unrelated to health. These perceptions may cause harm through failure to follow established policies and clinical guidelines, including delays in emergency or urgent assessments, delay of an IP's access to an appropriate level of care and treatment, and lapses in continuity and coordination of care. Such cynicism has resulted in foreseeable and/or preventable deaths from suicide (Patterson & Hughes, 2008). It is not accidental that in the federal prison system, sick-call requests are referred to as "cop-outs" by both staff and IPs. Strong clinical leadership by psychiatrists can facilitate positive changes in this unhelpful and often harmful culture.

Psychiatric consultation and monitoring of correctional facilities from a systems perspective is often obtained or court ordered to improve the mental health care delivery system and in response to class action litigation (see Chapter 74). Greifinger (2013) notes that correctional facilities that have demonstrated poor performance often have no stated mission or have a mission statement that is not understood by leadership and staff. Many lack enlightened leadership and/or accountability for health care services, among other deficiencies. Greifinger (2013) opines that among the first solutions to enact is developing or recruiting leadership. Enlightened and aware correctional administrators at the systems and facility levels, as well supervisors and officers on the unit/tier levels, recognize the need for active participation in IP management by their mental health treatment providers. The treatment providers are not considered "guests in the house of corrections" but rather essential correctional health care staff providing treatment and assisting in the management of IPs, particularly those with mental illnesses and others who may exhibit maladaptive behaviors. Such a system contributes to institutional stability, safety, and security and reduces the risks of harm to individual IPs and custody, clinical, and other staff.

Several authors have provided introductions to and descriptions of correctional psychiatry relative to the growing populations and health care needs of persons incarcerated in prisons and jails within the United States (Kapoor et al., 2018; Metzner, 1997a, 1997b, 1998; Metzner et al., 1998; Metzner & Dvoskin, 2006; Morris & West, 2020). Metzner (1997a, 1997b, 1998) described the essential components of adequate correctional mental health systems and the administrative structures of correctional mental health services. He emphasized the need for proper balance between security and treatment and the need for the director of mental health services or their designee to have direct access to the facility's chief administrator regarding all administrative decisions that affect mental health care. These are particularly important components of mental health service delivery in any correctional setting.

The role of psychiatrists as leaders in this process can take a number of avenues. An essential avenue would be for the psychiatrists in leadership to provide direct input to the chief administrator, in addition to providing administrative and direct services. The psychiatrist should also participate in the education, training, and supervision of qualified mental health professionals, as well as collaborative consultations and liaisons with other service providers, custody staff, other administrators, support staff, and the department of mental health as needed.

The involvement of psychiatrists in leadership roles at the facility and central administrative levels presents important opportunities to define, develop, and support the treatment team concept. A psychiatrist in a leadership role may facilitate direct care service delivery and adherence to policies and procedures regarding transfers to higher or lower levels of care based on an individual IP's level of functioning. The level of mental health functioning and the level of mental health care required are determined by the clinical staff. The custody classification is a security determination and may include secure housing units, administrative or punitive segregation, protective custody, and other levels of custody, including maximum-, medium-, and minimum-security levels and "camp" designations. Clinical leadership is needed to educate and work with custody staff in establishing adequate access to all levels of mental health care for IPs as clinically indicated, regardless of their custody classification. Ongoing education and training for both custody and mental health staff are necessary in the context of these principles.

The correctional psychiatrist in a leadership position should demonstrate competence when providing services at multiple levels within the mental health services delivery system. First, the psychiatrist can be the leader for treatment teams that provide direct services to IPs, from intake screening, assessment, and treatment through release and parole. Second would be leadership at the program level, in which the psychiatrist may hold a position as the chief of mental health services, chief of psychiatry, or other titles reflective of the responsibility for supervision and direction of multiple treatment teams within a facility. The third level of leadership would be at the systems level, in which the psychiatrist may be the director of mental health services for multiple facilities within a system. They would therefore have responsibilities not for direct service but for development of policies and procedures, training, implementation of practice guidelines, development of quality management systems including performance indicators, and information managements systems for the measurement of data collection regarding morbidity and mortality, suicide prevention, medication management, treatment services, and peer review. Lastly, the highest level of leadership would be the chief administrative officer, warden, administrator, jailer, or departmental secretary, which, in rare instances, may be a mental health professional, including a psychiatrist or a psychologist, and would be responsible for the health care delivered within the system and for the total operations of the system or correctional facility.

Other opportunities for psychiatric leadership include the quality management of correctional mental health care delivery, which identifies opportunities to improve care and methods to sustain practices that support high quality of care. An adequate quality improvement system integrates mental health assessment and treatment and provides performance measures to evaluate the effectiveness of the treatment and overall management of IPs with mental illness.

Leadership challenges

The criminal justice system provides a full range of administrative and clinical opportunities for psychiatrists. The "front end" of arrest and pretrial determinations has been a long-standing component of forensic practice. The role of expert or opinion witnesses is to provide assistance to the finder of fact (i.e., the judge and/or jury) in pretrial proceedings related to competence, criminal responsibility, diversion, and probation (see Chapter 66). During incarceration, assessment of mental health needs, access to care, provision of treatment, and quality improvement partially constitute the jail and prison components of mental health services. The aftercare aspect of mental health services in correctional psychiatry involves individuals released on probation or parole who need mental health treatment. It further includes individuals who, after serving a sentence in an institutional or community correctional setting, may be civilly committed for treatment as mentally disordered offenders or as sexually violent predators. These aftercare services may be delivered in secure institutional settings. This is particularly the case for IPs committed as sexual psychopaths under sexual psychopathy laws or statutes and for those civilly committed as "mentally disordered offenders" found to be gravely disabled or a continuing threat of harm to themselves or others. Individuals diverted by mental health courts, placed on probation, or placed on parole require community-based services. All these areas provide opportunities for psychiatric leadership, which is often missing. Historically, the lack of psychiatrists working in the criminal justice system on a full-time basis often narrowed their role to medication management, with little opportunity to advance to clinical or administrative leadership positions. Lack of familiarity and discomfort with the correctional environment have also been barriers for psychiatrists who might otherwise assume leadership roles.

The authors' experiences in both traditional (or "free world") and correctional mental health systems have been enlightening with regard to the similarities and the differences of service provision in these two environments. In the traditional community mental health service delivery system, the model might typically be based on treatment or recovery teams composed of practitioners from the disciplines of psychiatry, psychology, social work, and nursing; rehabilitation therapists; counselors; and direct-care service providers (e.g., case managers, milieu staff). Often, the de facto correctional mental health model consists of "physician and other." The physician may or may not be a psychiatrist and the "other" may be any individual defined by local custom, state regulation, or law as the "qualified mental health professional," which can vary remarkably by jurisdiction. Unfortunately, psychiatrists were often only marginally involved in the design, development, and implementation of mental health care delivery systems during the years that the need for such services increased exponentially. As a result, the organizational structure frequently excluded psychiatrists from both clinical and administrative leadership positions and decisions.

The leadership role for psychiatrists working in correctional environments is distinctly different from typical psychiatric venues where the psychiatrist and other mental health professionals are in control and determine what services and practice models will be used. In a correctional environment, the dynamics are different in that the entity in control is not the psychiatrist or other mental health professionals but rather the correctional structure/administration. Within correctional systems, the psychiatric and mental health leadership must understand the nuances and barriers present within "correctional culture" (see Chapter 14). With effective psychiatric leadership, mental health care delivery and its coordination with correctional management of IPs are more likely to be improved.

Educational opportunities

Traditionally, medical school curricula and psychiatric residency programs did not provide experiences and formal training for students and residents in correctional psychiatry other than through electives in later years of training. Fortunately, this lack of training has been significantly remedied since the American Board of Medical Specialties, along with the American Psychiatric Association (APA), recognized forensic psychiatry as a subspecialty in 1992, which eventually resulted in a proliferation of forensic fellowship programs. The target population for these programs is psychiatrists who are treating both traditional forensic patients (e.g., pretrial detainees and "not guilty by reason of insanity" patients) and IPs in correctional facilities. In 2013, there were approximately 42 forensic psychiatry fellowship programs in the United States approved by the Accreditation Council for Graduate Medical Education (ACGME; American Academy of Psychiatry and the Law [AAPL], 2013). By 2019, there were 48 accredited forensic psychiatry fellowship programs (Frierson, 2020), and many required clinical rotations in jails or prisons. In 2024, the ACGME changed its requirements for all forensic fellowships to include a clinical experience in jails, prisons, or lockups (ACGME, 2024), further highlighting the importance of training in this area.

Psychiatrists who are board certified in forensic psychiatry by the American Board of Psychiatry and Neurology are required to participate in continuing education as part of the Maintenance of Certification program to qualify for recertification. The APA, AAPL, and the National Commission on Correctional Health Care (NCCHC) also provide annual conferences with trainings and presentations dedicated to correctional mental health and psychiatry. In addition, the AAPL has established the AAPL Institute for Education and Research to further provide educational opportunities for psychiatrists. Notably, most psychiatric practice has evolved away from long-term hospitalization and long-term outpatient psychiatric treatment toward a community-based model of practice. Unfortunately, while this community-based model has not been realized as intended in the "free world," it has the potential for implementation in correctional systems. Correctional systems have long-term residents who are accessible and often willing to engage in treatment. If the system has adequate human resources, physical plant resources, access to care, and training, the community mental health system model could be realized.

The provision of long-term treatment for psychiatric conditions is more likely to occur in a correctional environment. Disorders encountered in correctional settings often include major mental illnesses such as schizophrenia, bipolar disorder, major depressive disorder, and other mental health conditions, including posttraumatic stress disorder and personality disorders (see Chapter 31). Such exposure and experience can enhance the practitioner's competence in these areas. The opportunities to assist individuals who may have co-occurring disorders, including substance use disorders and medical conditions (including dementias), are extensive. The opportunities for psychiatrists to provide direct services, lead treatment teams, and collaborate with mental health professionals in other disciplines to provide comprehensive assessments and therapeutic interventions are beneficial to IPs and to the psychiatrist's educational and professional development.

Training opportunities

For the psychiatrist practicing in correctional settings, the majority of training takes place inside correctional facilities. Departments of corrections and jail facilities all offer orientation and training for their custody officers and for employees and contractors such as psychiatrists. Corrections-specific training includes such topics as conditions of confinement, hostage negotiations and requirements, contraband, IP counts, restrictive housing, sound confidentiality, and special situations such as lockdowns. In most correctional training that is geared toward custody officers, there is limited training regarding mental health issues. Training typically includes screening of IPs entering the facility, mechanisms to access mental health staff, escort duties for IPs to mental health services, suicide watches and observation by custody officers, medication administration and observation by custody officers, contraband, and emergency procedures for first responders, including cardiopulmonary resuscitation and first aid. For mental health professionals, including psychiatrists, the "custody" training provided by correctional institutions and systems focuses on correctional and custody practices rather than on mental health issues and management, which are presented in very limited formats. Other mental health professionals who have been working at the particular facility usually conduct the clinical, on-the-job training provided to psychiatrists and other mental health professionals.

One major resource that describes the role of the psychiatrist in providing services in jails and prisons is the APA's (2016) *Psychiatric Services in Correctional Facilities*. This work highlights the principles governing the delivery of psychiatric services, offers guidelines for psychiatric services, and discusses special applications for the principles and guidelines. The NCCHC (2015) has also published *Standards for Mental Health Services in Correctional Facilities*, and the Joint Commission on Accreditation of Healthcare Organizations' (2014) *Standards for Behavioral Health Care* are relevant to behavioral health care in corrections. The APA (2016) addresses key areas that include access to mental health care and treatment, quality of care, cultural awareness, suicide prevention, mental health treatment, ethical issues, services in court and other settings, jail diversion, alternatives to incarceration, and research. In addition, there is significant information on education and training that emphasizes the need for professional development for mental health clinicians working in a jail or prison. It references those programs in the facility, as well as continuing medical education activities.

Comprehensive education and training within a correctional facility or system requires substantial cross-training of custody staff by clinical staff and of clinical staff by custody staff. Cross-training should include orientation by custody staff regarding the jail/prison custody culture. Such training supports effective collaboration and includes requirements such as those for mental health screening and evaluation of IPs segregated from the general population (for protective custody, disciplinary sanctions, or administratively for individual or institutional safety). Psychiatrists need to become knowledgeable regarding restrictive housing units due to potential mental health concerns related to the prison environment. Considerable work has been done regarding the conditions of confinement, particularly in restrictive housing environments, and their impact on the mental health functioning of IPs in those settings (Metzner et al., 1998; Patterson & Hughes, 2008). For IPs placed in restrictive housing settings, cell-front rounds no less than once per week by a qualified mental health professional (and more frequently as necessary) should be conducted as an adjunct to determine the need for out-of-cell assessment of the mental health functioning of these IPs, the adequacy of their mental health treatment and management, and their adjustment to restrictive housing conditions.

In addition to in-house training, educational and networking opportunities for correctional psychiatrists are available via the NCCHC, which holds several meetings each year. While it is generally accepted that compliance with the published NCCHC accreditation standards does not guarantee adequate mental health services or compliance with APA guidelines, efforts to achieve accreditation indicate attempts to improve quality of care (APA, 2016; see Chapter 73). Other relevant organizations for similar purposes include the AAPL, the American Correctional Association, and the American College of Correctional Physicians.

Cultural factors and considerations

There have been major efforts in the education and training of mental health professionals to become more aware of and to incorporate consideration of cultural factors in the diagnosis and treatment of mental illness and disorders. Many cultural factors, including but not limited to race, ethnicity, gender identity, sexual orientation, religion, education, socioeconomic status, and life experiences, are all considerations for clinicians to develop comprehensive assessments and treatment. Providing clinical services, training, and leadership in correctional environments should include consideration of these factors and the unique "culture of corrections" (see Chapter 22). Terms such as "prison politics" (interactions between IPs), lockdowns, "the hole" (restrictive housing units), "shot callers" (gang leaders), and "blood in blood out" (gang membership) are often used. The practices of counts, standing at attention when "rank" or "white shirts" (higher ranking/administrative custody staff) are present, wall postings of "no warning shots," and agreement by staff that there be "no hostage trades" for IPs are realities in many systems. Special housing for IPs at risk of harm from other IPs because of their offense (e.g., sexual assault of a child or high-notoriety crime) or status (gang dropout, shot caller, or mental illness) and outside yard activities requiring separation of IPs exist in many systems. While one purpose of incarceration may be "as" punishment for crimes committed, in some systems, the culture supports incarceration "for" punishment while incarcerated.

The psychiatrist must consider that IPs' requests for medical or mental health services may not be for primary gain (i.e., assessment and treatment) but rather for reasons frequently described as secondary gain (i.e., manipulation or malingering). It is extremely important to identify, acknowledge, and incorporate this possibility in assessment and treatment (see Chapter 20). The "two Ms" of manipulation and malingering in a correctional environment may include attempts to avoid or defer responsibility, obtain monetary rewards, or influence a familial, social, or criminal justice outcome. The secondary gain may also be based on threats to an IP's body integrity or social standing (particularly within a gang system), to effect a change in housing, to gain transfer to a mental health treatment environment, and/or to avoid interactions with other IPs or correctional officers. Knowledge of these terms and how to address these issues is usually part of the "on-the-job training" for mental health professionals in correctional environments and needs to be appreciated by clinicians so they can become effective leaders.

Summary

The increase in IPs who require mental health services has created numerous challenges for jail and prison administrators and staff, as well as for professionals caring for individuals in mental health diversion or postrelease programs. The need for dedicated and qualified leadership for mental health services and the importance of providing appropriate education and training in correctional mental health practices is clear. These needs offer remarkable opportunities for psychiatrists to become effective leaders in correctional settings that have historically lacked the benefit of a competent, adequately resourced mental health staff. Fortunately, psychiatrists and other health care professionals can be educated and trained to provide the necessary leadership for these extraordinarily complex systems of care and confinement.

REFERENCES

Accreditation Council for Graduate Medical Education. (2024). *ACGME program requirements for graduate medical education in forensic psychiatry*. https://www.acgme.org/globalassets/pfassets/programrequirements/2024-prs/406_forensic-psychiatry_2024.pdf

American Academy of Psychiatry and the Law. (2013). *Forensic psychiatry fellowships*. http://aapl.org/fellow.php

American Psychiatric Association. (2016). *Psychiatric services in correctional facilities* (3rd ed.).

Bowring v. Godwin, 551 F.2d 44 (1977).

Community Mental Health Centers Construction Act, Mental Retardation Facilities and Construction Act, Pub. L. 88-164, 77 Stat. 282 (1963).

Estelle v. Gamble, 429 U.S. 97 (1976).

Frierson, R. L. (2020). Examining the past and advocating for the future of forensic psychiatry training. *Journal of the American Academy of Psychiatry and the Law*, *48*(1), 16–25.

Greifinger, R. B. (2013). The acid bath of cynicism. *Correctional Law Reporter*, *25*, 3.

Joint Commission on the Accreditation of Healthcare Organizations. (2014). *Standards for behavioral health care*.

Kapoor, R., Dike, C. C., & Norko, M. A. (2018). Psychiatric treatment in forensic hospital and correctional settings. *Psychiatric Annals*, *48*(2), 102–108.

Metzner, J. L. (1997a). An introduction to correctional psychiatry: Part I. *Journal of the American Academy of Psychiatry and the Law*, *25*, 275–281.

Metzner, J. L. (1997b). An introduction to correctional psychiatry: Part II. *Journal of the American Academy of Psychiatry and the Law*, *25*(4), 571–579.

Metzner, J. L. (1998). An introduction to correctional psychiatry: Part III. *Journal of the American Academy of Psychiatry and the Law*, *26*(1), 108–115.

Metzner, J. L., Cohen, F., Grossman, L. S., & Wettstein, R. M. (1998). Treatment in jails and prisons. In R. M. Wettstein (Ed.), *Treatment of offenders with mental disorders* (pp. 217–264). Guilford Press.

Metzner, J. L., & Dvoskin, J. (2006). An overview of correctional psychiatry. *Psychiatric Clinics of North America*, *29*, 761–772.

Morris, N. P., & West, S. G. (2020). Misconceptions about working in correctional psychiatry. *Journal of the American Academy of Psychiatry and the Law*, *48*(2), 251–258.

National Commission on Correctional Health Care. (2015). *Standards for mental health services in correctional facilities*.

Patterson, R. F., & Hughes, K. C. (2008). Review of completed suicides in the California Department of Corrections and Rehabilitation. *Psychiatric Services*, *59*, 676–682.

Ruiz v. Estelle, 503 F. Supp. 1265 (S.D. Tex. 1980).

76

Role of clinical trainees

Charles L. Scott[1]

Introduction

Correctional settings are important and worthy training sites for medical students, general psychiatry residents, child and adolescent psychiatry residents, and forensic psychiatry fellows. Logically, educating future clinicians on how best to treat individuals with mental illness should occur in settings that most commonly treat them. In the United States, there are more than 3 times as many persons with serious mental illness in jails and prisons as in hospitals, making America's jails and prisons the new and largest mental hospitals (Torrey et al., 2010). Correctional institutions now represent the largest providers of mental health care in the United States (Cerny-Suelzer et al., 2019). As a result, more providers trained to work in correctional settings are desperately needed.

Despite an increased need for correctional psychiatrists, most general psychiatry residency programs do not provide training in a correctional site. In an online survey of U.S. general psychiatry residency program training directors, less than one third of responding programs reported that a correctional training site was mandatory for trainees (Fuehrlein et al., 2014). With the significant shift of individuals with mental illness to correctional settings, psychiatric training programs should consider the benefits that such sites can provide for both residents and staff.

Resident benefits of training in a correctional environment

Training in a correctional setting provides medical students, general psychiatry residents, and forensic psychiatry fellows a range of training experiences. First, patients seen in correctional settings typically demonstrate a broad array of psychopathology, which gives trainees the opportunity to hone their diagnostic acumen. Epidemiologic studies indicate that 15% to 24% of U.S. incarcerated persons (IPs) have a severe mental illness (Baillargeon et al., 2009).

In their national survey of IPs, Bronson and colleagues (2017) found that 63% of persons incarcerated in jail and nearly 60% of persons incarcerated in prison met criteria for a substance use disorder (SUD). Lynch and colleagues (2014) conducted a multisite study to examine the prevalence of serious mental illness, posttraumatic stress disorder, and SUD in women in jail. The authors found that 53% had met criteria for posttraumatic stress disorder during their lifetime, with nearly 40% having a serious mental illness and a co-occurring SUD. Mental disorders, personality disorders, and SUD can present phenotypically similarly, with multiple mood, anxiety, and psychotic symptoms, which requires trainees to strengthen their skills in developing and modifying a differential diagnosis.

The constraints of working in a correctional setting can enhance trainees' basic time management and organizational skills. Depending on the specific treatment environment (e.g., general population follow-ups, crisis unit care, parole/probation clinics), a trainee may have to balance the parameters of an evaluation with the needs of the correctional setting and staff. IPs frequently have other obligations, such as meeting with their legal counsel, visiting with family members, and attending court hearings. Similarly, correctional staff's primary obligation is to maintain the safety of the facility. Because of these and other concerns, psychiatric care may not be of primary importance to correctional staff or IPs. Trainees must learn to navigate the environment and use their time wisely in evaluation, treatment, and documentation. Furthermore, the logistical difficulties of traveling through a facility, which can take significant time, demand that the trainee be organized and prepared for the day's workload. A correctional setting, therefore, can serve to bolster trainees' basic skills in time management, documentation, and organization.

Similarly, correctional training sites can teach trainees how to work in a collaborative, team-based model of care. Unique to jails and prisons is the presence of correctional staff that supervise IPs' activities. Psychiatric trainees may gain crucial information important to IP assessment by developing rapport with these staff members, who can report their concerns about the IPs they monitor. Because of this close supervision, correctional staff can provide insights into an IP's hygienic activity, speech, attitude, psychomotor activity, and mood and the presence of odd behaviors that become problematic. These tips can serve as "red flags" for trainees to follow up on, similar to nursing and mental health staff concerns in inpatient psychiatric units in the community.

1. The author acknowledges the contributions of Brian Holoyda, MD, MPH, who was a coauthor of this chapter in the first edition of the textbook.

Learning the principles of psychopharmacology is an essential component of psychiatric training for medical students and residents (Accreditation Council for Graduate Medical Education [ACGME], 2022a). Correctional settings provide trainees with an opportunity to learn basic psychopharmacology, including the use of antidepressants, mood stabilizers, antipsychotics, anxiolytics, antiadrenergic agents, and anticholinergic agents. Correctional settings often have modified drug formularies (see Chapter 27). Psychiatric trainees may be unaware that medications commonly prescribed in the community, including bupropion (Burns, 2009), quetiapine (Tamburello, 2012), and trihexyphenidyl, are frequent substances of abuse in incarcerated populations. Furthermore, some patients may malinger illness to obtain medications, including sedating or activating medications. Lastly, correctional formularies are less likely to include typical substances of abuse, such as stimulants, benzodiazepines, or opioids (Burns, 2009), requiring a trainee to learn creativity and flexibility in prescribing practices to an extent unparalleled in community settings.

Correctional settings also provide opportunities to learn other therapeutic modalities that may benefit patients. The potential to learn about SUD treatments abounds, ranging from detoxification of newly incarcerated individuals to motivational interviewing for drug diversion court participants to pharmacologic and psychotherapeutic interventions for individuals with a history of SUD in parole/probation or general population clinics. There are opportunities to learn and use dialectical behavior therapy and other psychotherapeutic techniques to address borderline personality disorder and self-harm behaviors, which are common in correctional populations (Chaiken et al., 2005; see Chapters 42 and 43). Though the typical inpatient or outpatient correctional treatment setting does not provide time or resources for the most dynamic forms of psychotherapy such as psychoanalysis, the need for supportive psychotherapy is strong. Unfortunately, many systems do not have staffing levels that allow psychiatrists to conduct psychotherapy routinely (beyond those psychotherapeutic interventions provided during appointments to evaluate medication need or treatment response).

As one might expect, there are opportunities to learn about forensic psychiatry within correctional settings. For example, malingering is a common problem among incarcerated individuals (see Chapter 20). Walters (2006) identified seven incentives to malinger in a correctional setting: compensation, avoidance, separation, relocation, entitlement, attention, and amusement. Research (McDermott & Sokolov, 2009) on malingering at a county jail found that 66% of 161 subjects clinically suspected of malingering were confirmed to be malingering using the Structured Interview of Reported Symptoms, with no psychiatric diagnosis (including antisocial personality disorder) predictive of malingering or nonmalingering. This finding indicates the utility of objective assessments to evaluate and potentially confirm suspected malingering. Training in a correctional setting, therefore, provides the trainee an important opportunity to learn the use of both clinical interviewing skills and structured assessment tools to assess suspected malingering.

Given the levels of mental health care available in many correctional systems, psychiatric trainees can practice developing appropriate discharge plans and coordinating follow-up care for their patients, whether it be within the correctional facility, in a parole clinic, or in the community. In fact, correctional settings, with their classification levels and unique housing options, may offer more options than are available in community settings. Following acute hospitalization, the treatment team can work with correctional staff to determine whether an individual will be able to function in the general population, with a cellmate, or under other circumstances and make recommendations based on the patient's mental status. Many correctional settings provide close monitoring and restriction of behaviors for suicidal or self-harming IPs. A correctional setting provides trainees with opportunities for learning the skill of coordinating care for their patients.

Table 76.1 summarizes potential benefits for trainees assigned to a correctional site.

Benefits for correctional staff from academic affiliations

Correctional staff receive many benefits from affiliations with teaching institutions. First, sites that teach medical students and residents create learning environments that help maintain current standards of treatment because supervising staff are expected to impart up-to-date knowledge to trainees. Second, trainees can assist with treatment for IPs, including pharmacotherapy (as appropriate to training level), individual assessment, and group therapy. The additional manpower helps unburden a heavy workload for the correctional staff, and trainees can help deliver high-quality and timely mental health care. Third, academic affiliations give correctional staff a chance to have university appointments and to participate in research and publications. Fourth, correctional staff can help groom and recruit future colleagues through positive learning experiences for trainees.

Matching the requirements of training to correctional rotations

Accreditation organizations set guidelines for required training experiences and competencies that trainees must complete. For graduate medical education, including general adult psychiatry residency and forensic psychiatry fellowship programs, the ACGME (2022a) promulgates these guidelines. There are no specific guidelines for required psychiatric training experiences provided by the ACGME's medical school counterpart, the Liaison Committee on Medical Education. The Liaison Committee on Medical Education provides broad medical education accreditation standards and allows individual medical schools to determine their own graduate competencies and clinical rotations. The Association of Directors of Medical Student Education in Psychiatry (ADMSEP), however, has developed a list of recommended learning objectives in psychiatry

Table 76.1 Potential benefits for trainees assigned to a correctional site

- Improve diagnostic abilities through exposure to a broad array of psychopathology
- Develop efficient time management and organizational skills
- Learn to work in collaborative team-based model of care
- Appreciate role of custody in evaluating incarcerated persons
- Understand potential abuse of prescribed substances
- Enhance ability to utilize clinical skills and structured assessment tools to evaluate malingering

for medical students to meet over the course of their training program (ADMSEP, 2007).

The ADMSEP has outlined learning objectives for medical students, broadly categorized into Clinical Skills; Psychopathology and Psychiatric Disorders; Disease Prevention, Therapeutics, and Management; and Professionalism, Ethics, and the Law (ADMSEP, 2007). Correctional settings offer medical students the opportunity to meet most of these objectives. Leamon and colleagues (2001) found that medical students rotating on an inpatient psychiatric unit in a county jail had the same quality of teaching, level of clinical responsibility, patient variety, and level of clinical observation that they and their colleagues had on other psychiatric services. In addition, the students performed no differently than their peers at other sites on all components of their clerkship grade, including National Board of Medical Examiners exam score, clinical skills grade, and oral examination grade. These findings suggest that jail psychiatric settings can be suitable training sites for medical students.

For correctional settings to serve as appropriate training sites for psychiatric residents, they must meet the requirements set forth by the ACGME. The ACGME identifies six core clinical competencies that must be integrated into a program's curriculum: Patient Care, Medical Knowledge, Practice-Based Learning and Improvement, Interpersonal and Communication Skills, Professionalism, and Systems-Based Practice. Each clinical competency lists requirements that residents must meet during their training. Correctional environments are varied and include inpatient psychiatric units, general population medication clinics, parole or probation clinics, emergency psychiatric evaluations, and consultations with other medical specialties. Many of the ACGME core competency requirements can be met in a correctional site. In fact, depending on the breadth and depth of services available in a system, a residency program could elect to fulfill most of its educational and didactic requirements within the correctional setting.

The ACGME core requirements for child and adolescent psychiatry training are also easily applied to juvenile correctional facilities, including detention facilities and community treatment programs. In addition, the ACGME core program requirements mandate that child and adolescent psychiatrists have "experience in legal issues relevant to child and adolescent psychiatry, which may include forensic consultation, court testimony and/or interaction with a juvenile justice system" (ACGME, 2022b, p. 24).

The ACGME Program Requirements for Graduate Medical Education in Forensic Psychiatry, unlike the general psychiatry and child and adolescent psychiatry requirements, explicitly mandate training related to individuals involved with the criminal justice system (ACGME, 2024). For example, the introduction to these program requirements notes that forensic psychiatry focuses on interrelationships between psychiatry and the law including "the specialized psychiatric treatment by those who have been incarcerated in jails, prisons, or special forensic psychiatric hospitals" (ACGME, 2024, p. 4). Correctional curriculum and training experiences, in addition to criminal and civil forensic evaluations, are heavily emphasized throughout the forensic core requirements, and in 2024, the ACGME added a requirement that trainees' 6-month longitudinal patient care experience include "experiences in jails, prisons, or lock-ups" (ACGME, 2024, p. 24). ACGME forensic program requirements specific to IPs include the following: competence in the evaluation and treatment of IPs, knowledge of the structure and function of correctional systems, knowledge of the structure and function of juvenile systems, knowledge of the theory and practice of sentencing the convicted offender, knowledge of the rights of incarcerated individuals, knowledge of the role of forensic psychiatrists in advocating for reform in forensic systems, evaluating and managing acutely and chronically ill patients in correctional systems, and treating persons involved in the criminal justice system (ACGME, 2024).

In addition to these specific requirements, the forensic program guidelines require that fellows develop skills and habits to analyze practice systematically using quality improvement methods and implement changes with the goal of practice improvement. Jails and prisons provide opportunities for forensic fellows to participate in quality improvement activities. Typical measures of quality improvement include IPs' access to care, appropriateness of suicide risk evaluations, timely delivery of medication, and appropriate medication monitoring.

Factors that increase the positive experience of all trainees' experience in a correctional environment are highlighted in Table 76.2.

Addressing trainees' concerns

Despite the apparent benefits that correctional settings afford psychiatric trainees, medical students and residents may have concerns about such a training experience. One study (Fuehrlein et al., 2012) examined general psychiatry residents' attitudes about correctional psychiatry in a residency program that used a county jail as one of its mandatory training sites. Attitudes were evaluated on a scale with 0 representing "most negative attitude" and 100 representing "most positive attitude." Overall, residents had a neutral attitude toward correctional psychiatry (mean score of 54 out of 100). The residents recognized the need for more psychiatrists to work in jails (mean score of 84 out of 100), but they expressed little likelihood of working in a jail after completing residency (mean score of 22 out of 100). The authors found statistically significant differences in residents' attitudes in the following areas: the professional rewards of working at a jail versus inpatient setting (mean score of 32 versus 60 out of 100), how often patients exaggerate symptoms in a jail versus an inpatient setting (mean score of 65 versus 45 out of 100), the likelihood of negative feelings toward a patient in a jail versus inpatient setting (mean score of 42 versus 28 out of 100), and worries about assault in a jail versus an inpatient setting (mean score

Table 76.2 Factors to maximize positive experience of trainees at correctional site

- Assign supervisors trained in forensic psychiatry with correctional experience
- Provide on-site supervision with weekly meetings with assigned supervisor
- Provide basic training on correctional issues *prior* to site placement. Specific training may include:
- Assessment of suicide risk
- Potential abuse of prescribed medications
- Evaluation of malingering
- Steps to maintain personal safety
- Guidelines to work with custodial staff
- Limits of confidentiality
- Importance of maintaining personal boundaries
- Organize on-site didactic lectures
- Assign teaching responsibilities for general residents and/or medical school students
- Include fellow in quality improvement process

of 52 versus 43 out of 100). Of note, there were no significant differences between the responses of residents who had completed the jail rotation and residents who had not.

These findings raise serious concerns about psychiatric trainees' perspectives on correctional psychiatry. These issues need to be addressed if there is going to be a psychiatric workforce to face the clinical needs of correctional facilities in the future. Foremost among these issues is trainees' perception of their safety. Trainees need to be safe in their work environment; otherwise, they will not enjoy the experience or wish to work in a correctional setting in the future. Although jails can feel safer than general inpatient facilities, given the presence of correctional officers, panic buttons, and restricted movement of IPs (via handcuffs or ankle cuffs), many trainees are nevertheless anxious about this working environment. Because of potential fear of their patients' and their own personal safety, trainees' concerns should be addressed prior to arrival at the training site to lessen fear and increase comfort in the setting.

Another common concern is trainees' enjoyment of the correctional psychiatry experience. Residents and medical students may find it difficult or emotionally draining to treat individuals who have been charged with crimes (Fuehrlein et al., 2012) or those perceived as having a "secondary gain picture" (Bender et al., 1985). These problems are inherent in the correctional milieu, but didactic instruction on the deinstitutionalization movement and resultant influx of persons with mental illness into correctional settings will help assuage trainees' discomfort and negative attitudes toward the incarcerated population. Similarly, lectures on commonly encountered clinical problems in this population (i.e., malingering, antisocial personality disorder, etc.) could increase trainee comfort and serve as points of clinical growth instead of irritating obstacles to patient care.

Morris and West (2020) identified common misconceptions that both residents and trained psychiatrists may have regarding working in correctional psychiatry. These misconceptions include a belief that IPs are less deserving of mental health treatment, that working in a correctional setting signals support for mass incarceration, that correctional psychiatrists are at a greater risk of personal harm compared to psychiatrists who work in noncorrectional settings, that correctional psychiatrists may receive less respect compared to other psychiatric specialties, that the ability to teach in a correctional setting is limited, and that there are few research opportunities when working in a correctional environment. Each of these misconceptions can be easily corrected through direct exposure to correctional experiences as part of training, through a series of educational didactics addressing these beliefs, and through increasing academic affiliation with correctional sites, where teaching and research are key components to an academic appointment.

Logistics of creating academic affiliations with correctional sites

Although a correctional site may be located near a university setting, academic affiliations can be challenging to coordinate. The first logical step when pursuing a potential academic affiliation with a correctional site is determining if the basic components are present or could be developed at the site that meet the necessary criteria by the governing accrediting body. Important factors to consider when determining the appropriateness of the site include distance from teaching institution, expected duty hours, availability of supervisors, willingness by the site to provide coverage for the trainee when off-site, on-call requirements (if any), presence of a quality improvement process, current working relationship between custody and mental health, supervisory responsibilities of forensic fellows for nonphysician mental health providers, availability of emergency psychiatric care, accreditation (or lack thereof) by national organizations, suicide trends, locations to interview IPs, office space, administrative support, current formulary, medical-record-keeping process, and the laboratory monitoring system. The training director should also review current policies and procedures to determine if there is a structure in place to address IPs' mental health needs appropriately and conduct a thorough site visit to evaluate working and safety conditions.

Summary

Increasing numbers of individuals with mental illness receive their treatment in a correctional environment. Correctional settings can provide appropriate and meaningful training opportunities for medical school students, psychiatry residents, and forensic and child and adolescent fellows. Despite the need for psychiatrists trained in correctional psychiatry, such training is not currently available in the majority of residency programs. Future educators interested in developing academic teaching affiliations should anticipate concerns by trainees and be prepared to address those concerns. The opportunities for matching current psychiatric training requirements with correctional settings abound. Providing care to individuals with mental illness where they live increasingly means providing care to those individuals while they are incarcerated in jails and prisons.

REFERENCES

Accreditation Council of Graduate Medical Education. (2022a). *ACGME program requirements for graduate medical education in psychiatry*. https://www.acgme.org/globalassets/pfassets/programrequirements/400_psychiatry_2022_tcc.pdf

Accreditation Council of Graduate Medical Education. (2022b). *ACGME program requirements for graduate medical education in child and adolescent psychiatry*. https://www.acgme.org/globalassets/pfassets/programrequirements/405_childadolescentpsychiatry_2022_tcc.pdf

Accreditation Council for Graduate Medical Education. (2024). *ACGME program requirements for graduate medical education in forensic psychiatry*. https://www.acgme.org/globalassets/pfassets/programrequirements/2024-prs/406_forensic-psychiatry_2024.pdf

Association of Directors of Medical Student Education in Psychiatry. (2007). *Clinical learning objectives guide for psychiatry education of medical students.*

Baillargeon, J., Binswanger, I. A., Penn, J. V., Williams, B. A., & Murray, O. J. (2009). Psychiatric disorders and repeat incarcerations: The revolving prison door. *American Journal of Psychiatry*, *166*, 103–109.

Bender, S. L., Hays, D. S., Klug, R., Matsuzaka, H., & Singleton, P. A. (1985). The teaching of psychiatry in the correctional setting: A new dimension in the medical school curriculum. *Psychiatric Journal of the University of Ottawa, 10*, 139–145.

Bronson, J., Stroop, J., Zimmer, S., & Berzofsky, M. (2017). *Drug use, dependence, and abuse among state prisoners and jail inmates, 2007–2009* (NCJ 250546). Bureau of Justice Statistics. https://bjs.ojp.gov/content/pub/pdf/dudaspji0709.pdf

Burns, K. A. (2009). Commentary: Top ten reasons to limit prescription of controlled substances in prisons. *Journal of the American Academy of Psychiatry and Law, 37*, 50–52.

Cerny-Suelzer, C. A., Ferranti, J., Wasser, T., et al. (2019). Practice resource for forensic training in general psychiatry residency programs. *Journal of the American Academy of Psychiatry and the Law, 47*, S1–S14.

Chaiken, S. B., Thompson, C. R., & Shoemaker, W. (2005). Mental health interventions in correctional settings. In C. Scott & J. Gerbasi (Eds.), *Handbook of correctional mental health* (pp. 122–27). American Psychiatric Publishing.

Fuehrlein, B. S., Jha, M. K., Brenner, A. M., & North, C. S. (2012). Can we address the shortage of psychiatrists in the correctional setting with exposure during residency training? *Community Mental Health, 48*, 756–760.

Fuehrlein, B. S., Jha, M. K., Brenner, A. M., & North, C. S. (2014). Availability and attitudes toward correctional psychiatry training: Results of a national survey of training directors. *Journal of Behavioral Health Services & Research, 41*, 244–250.

Leamon, M. H., Fields, L., Cox, P. D., Scott, C., & Mirassou, M. (2001). Medical students in jail: The psychiatric clerkship in an outpatient correctional setting. *Academic Psychiatry, 25*, 167–172.

Lynch, S. M., DeHart, D. D, Beklnap, J. E., Green, B. L., Dass-Brailsford, P., Johnson, K. A., & Whalley, E. (2014). A multisite study of the prevalence of serious mental illness, PTSD, and substance use disorder of women in jail. *Psychiatric Services, 65*, 670–674.

McDermott, B. E., & Sokolov, G. (2009). Malingering in a correctional setting the use of the Structured Interview of Reported Symptoms in a jail sample. *Behavioral Sciences and the Law, 27*, 753–765.

Morris, N. P., & West, S. G. (2020). Misconceptions about working in correctional psychiatry. *Journal of the American Academy of Psychiatry and the Law, 48*, 251–258.

Tamburello, A. C., Lieberman, J. A., Baum, R. M., & Reeves, R. (2012). Successful removal of quetiapine from a correctional formulary. *Journal of the American Academy of Psychiatry and the Law, 40*, 502–508.

Torrey, E. F., Kennard, A. D., Eslinger, D., et al. (2010, May). *More mentally ill persons are in jails and prisons than in hospitals: A survey of the states.* http://www.treatmentadvocacycenter.org/storage/documents/final_jails_v_hospitals_study.pdf

Walters, G. D. (2006). Coping with malingering and exaggeration of psychiatric symptomatology in offender populations. *American Journal of Forensic Psychology, 24*, 21–40.

77

Correctional mental health research

Nancy Wolff

Introduction

Mental illness, ranging from acute anxiety to schizophrenia, is overrepresented in prisons and jails (Fovet et al., 2023; Prins, 2014). Unlike their free-world counterparts, incarcerated persons (IPs) have a constitutional right to mental health treatment (Metzner, 2002). Yet, despite the need for and right to mental health treatment, remarkably little reliable and valid evidence is available on the nature and severity of mental illness in IPs, the effects of incarceration on symptomatology, the availability and quality of psychoactive medications, cognitive and psychosocial treatment for specific disorders, and how context alters the effectiveness of the treatment that is available. Evidence is absent because corrections-based research is constrained by regulation, financing, and inexperience.

This chapter reviews the history of research involving IPs and the evolution of federal regulations to protect IPs as human subjects. How regulation has affected correctional mental health research (CMHR) is discussed, after first defining what is meant by research and why research is needed to inform policy and practice decisions. This is followed by recommendations for building the CMHR evidence base. The intent is to help researchers within the current regulatory environment and in collaboration with stakeholders to develop, design, and implement research studies and disseminate evidence to advance science and the quality of care available to IPs with mental illnesses.

Value, nature, and requirements of scientific inquiry

Every year, billions of dollars are spent on research (National Institutes of Health [NIH], 2023). The purpose of scientific inquiry is to generate knowledge that will advance our understanding of biological, behavioral, organizational, and social phenomena. Valid and reliable evidence is the hallmark of informed medical decision-making. Without such evidence, medical, clinical, and operational decisions are guided by custom, habit, and idiosyncratic preferences. Decisions made without the benefit of science are likely to misallocate resources toward practices and policies that produce smaller improvements in individual and population well-being.

Empirical evidence is derived from two primary sources: program evaluation and research. Both sources of evidence use scientific designs and qualitative and quantitative methodologies. They differ in their focus and generalizability. Program evaluation investigates the merit of a particular program from the perspective of key stakeholders with the intent to provide information unique to the organization, implementation, or performance of that program as it exists within a dynamic social context. By contrast, research advances scientific inquiry by pursuing theory-driven questions and answering them using controlled designs that produce more generalizable knowledge.

CMHR is a field of scientific inquiry that centers on the etiology, epidemiology, prevention, diagnosis, and treatment of mental disorders in people who reside in a facility under the control of the criminal justice system (e.g., a prison, jail, or juvenile detention center). Table 77.1 summarizes types of CMHR, using posttraumatic stress disorder (PTSD) as an illustration. CMHR is person oriented and seeks to improve the performance of the mental health system in ways that yield better mental health and other ancillary outcomes. It also requires human experimentation. Studying people biologically, diagnostically, behaviorally, cognitively, or socially runs the risk of harming them in known and unknown ways. For this reason, participants in research must understand the risks associated with human experiments and, once fully informed, must be able to choose freely to participate (i.e., without coercion). What makes CMHR controversial is the involvement of IPs in research as human subjects (Gostin et al., 2007).

Evolution of incarcerated persons as a vulnerable population

Whether IPs can make an informed and voluntary choice to participate in research is sharply debated (Christopher et al., 2011; Lazzarini & Attice, 2000). The coercive nature of correctional environments could chill volitional action by IPs. These environments are known for being controlling, manipulative, and disempowering. Cumulatively, they mold individuals into the archetype of "prisoner," making them pliable and acquiescent to those with power. Further, because kindness is scarce and treatment services are a commodity in correctional settings, IPs may be overly responsive to research opportunities that offer relief from deprivation. That is, they may disregard or discount the long-term medical risks associated with human experimentation and inflate near-term, especially humanitarian,

Table 77.1 Examples of correctional mental health research questions related to post-traumatic stress disorder (PTSD)

Etiology of PTSD
What are the risk and preventive factors for PTSD among incarcerated persons (IPs)? How do the conditions of confinement affect the onset and manifestation of PTSD symptoms among IPs?
Epidemiology of Trauma and PTSD
What proportion of IPs have trauma histories? What is the prevalence, type, frequency, and severity of childhood trauma histories among IPs? What is the prevalence of physical, sexual, and emotional trauma during incarceration? How do these rates vary by age, setting, sex, gender identity, sexual orientation, race, ethnicity, and mental disorder? What is the prevalence of PTSD among IPs and how do these rates vary by co-occurring mental disorder and the prison regime?
Prevention of Trauma and PTSD
What stressful conditions within correctional environments trigger or elevate PTSD symptoms? How can these environmental conditions be changed to reduce exposure to trauma during incarceration?
Measurement of Trauma and Diagnosis of PTSD
Are the standard measures of trauma exposure and the instruments used to measure PTSD symptoms and diagnose PTSD in the community reliable and valid for correctional populations?
Treatment of PTSD
Are PTSD interventions effective in community-based populations and settings also effective in correctional settings with IPs? Are group-based PTSD interventions feasible in a correctional setting? Are trauma-processing interventions feasible in correctional settings? Do medications enhance the effectiveness of therapy-based interventions? Is it feasible to provide a safe environment to treat PTSD in correctional settings? Can an effective therapeutic alliance be established between therapists and clients in correctional settings?
Service Delivery and Organization
Is it feasible to provide trauma-informed care to IPs? Can the culture and climate of correctional settings be changed to reflect a trauma-informed approach? How can the correctional system efficiently and effectively screen for PTSD and optimally treat trauma-related symptoms?

benefits (Chwang, 2010). In these ways, IPs are vulnerable to being inadvertently manipulated into research (Sherrer, 1999).

Since the early 1940s, research involving IPs has vacillated between two extremes: fully unrestrained to highly constrained. In recent years, it has become highly constrained, in part because of the extreme abuses of IPs in research prior to the 1980s (Beecher, 1966; Hornblum, 1997). It was customary to use IPs as human subjects during World War II, when there was a growing need to conduct clinical trials on infectious diseases and related vaccines (Hornblum, 1997; Lazzarini & Attice, 2000). By "volunteering" for these medical risks, IPs raised their social status among the public while also advertising their willingness to be the subject of human experimentation (Cislo & Trestman, 2013).

The federal government's permissive use of IPs in clinical studies during World War II, further sanctioned by a report published by the *Journal of the American Medical Association* (Ivy, 1949), signaled a legitimate opportunity in the postwar era for human experimentation by the pharmaceutical industry. IPs were an ideal population for conducting drug trials because they were captives with few advocates, they could be easily recruited at a low cost, they were available in large numbers, and their movements and behavior were highly controlled. In the absence of ethical regulations on research, prisons became the clinical trial center for the pharmaceutical industry (Lazzarini & Attice, 2000; Mitford, 1973). Indeed, by the end of the 1960s, 42 U.S. prisons supplied IPs for clinical trials that tested 85% of new drugs (Kalmbach & Lyons, 2003).

Specific to CMHR, corrections-based medical staff, often in collaboration with federally funded academic researchers, operated institutes or centers for behavioral change (Mitford, 1973). These residential settings were used to coerce IPs into participating in "individualized treatment" designed to "rehabilitate" them. Rehabilitation involved "breaking the person" using punishments that often included social isolation, beatings, electric or insulin shock, hydrotherapy, and other abusive means of inducing privation or severe pain. Behavioral experiments included using IPs to test psychosurgery, psychoactive drugs, surgical and chemical castration, brainwashing techniques, and other putative therapeutic practices that incorporated harsh punitive or disciplinary methods. Many of these behavioral experiments were later deemed cruel and unusual punishment by the courts (Mitford, 1973).

During the 1960s, IPs were recharacterized as a vulnerable population that was susceptible to ethical violations through their involvement in research. Henry Beecher, in an article published in the *New England Journal of Medicine*, highlighted 22 studies that exemplified "unethical or questionably ethical" conduct in research involving IPs. Beecher noted, quoting Pope Pius XII, that "science is not the highest value of which all other orders of values ... should be subordinated" (Beecher, 1966, p. 367). With evidence of exploitation mounting, the 1938 Food, Drug, and Cosmetic Act was amended in 1962 to empower the federal government to regulate drug research. Subsequent amendments to this act established the requirement that clinical investigators obtain informed consent as a condition of participation in research (1963) and articulated the requirements for informed consent (1966).

The National Research Act of 1974 (Pub. L. 93-348) established the National Commission on the Protection of Human Subjects of Biomedical and Behavioral Research, which was responsible for investigating the ethical principles of biomedical and behavioral research involving human subjects. Concurrent with the passage of the National Research Act of 1974, the U.S. Department of Health, Education, and Welfare published a set of regulations, codified as Title 45 of the Code of Federal Regulations (CFR) 46 (summarized in Table 77.2), guiding the use of human subjects in research. Special regulatory provisions protecting IPs as human subjects fell under 45 CFR 46 Subpart C (see Table 77.2; Protection of Human Subjects, 2009). Between 1974 and 1978, the U.S. Department of Health and Human Services (DHHS), the successor to the U.S. Department of Health, Education, and Welfare, revised the 45 CFR 46 regulations in accordance with recommendations advanced by the National Commission in its Belmont Report (National Commission for the Protection of Human Subjects of Biomedical and Behavioral Research, 1979). The DHHS regulations, which became law in 1981, applied only to research funded by the DHHS. By 1991, the NIH, along with 14 other federal agencies, adopted the Federal Policy for the Protection of Human Subjects (45 C.F.R. 46), referred to as the Common Rule.

Table 77.2 Summary of regulations to protect incarcerated persons (IPs) as human subjects

Code of Federal Regulations Title 45, Subpart A (pertains to all adult human subjects)
- Establishes the requirement that research involving human subjects shall be reviewed and approved by an institutional review board (IRB)
- Establishes criteria for IRB approval
- Establishes requirements for informed consent

Code of Federal Regulations Title 45, Subpart C (pertains only to IPs)
- Establishes the requirement that the IRB must include an IP or a representative of IPs
- Limits research to four categories that involve no more than minimal risk
- Study of the causes, effects, and processes of incarceration itself
- Study specifically of institutional structures or IPs
- Study of conditions specifically affecting prisoners as a class
- Study of practices with the intent and reasonable probability of improving the health or well-being of the subject
- Extends the IRB review to include whether and to what extent:
- Benefits of participation are disproportionate to risks
- Risks are comparable to those acceptable to nonincarcerated volunteers
- Subject selection is fair and independent of correctional influence
- Information is presented in an accessible manner
- Subjects understand that participation will have no impact on parole decisions

According to Subpart C, IPs (i.e., "prisoners") are defined as people confined in a penal institution, not those under probation or parole supervision (45 C.F.R. § 46.303), and require additional protections because incarceration "could affect their ability to make a truly voluntary and uncoerced decision whether or not to participate as subjects in research" (45 C.F.R. § 46.302). The approval decisions of local institutional review boards (IRBs) regarding research on IPs funded by some federal agencies (e.g., DHHS, NIH) must be certified as fully compliant with the Common Rule by the sponsoring agency's office that oversees protections of human subjects. For example, the U.S. Office of Human Research Protections must certify research on IPs funded by the NIH. In addition, it is recommended that investigators conducting research on IPs funded by the NIH obtain a certificate of confidentiality—a tool that allows researchers to protect subject data from forced disclosure.

Consequences of the Common Rule

Federal regulation had a swift and progressive impact on research involving IPs. By 1980, only 15% of all drug testing involved incarcerated participants, down from 85% in the 1960s (Kalmbach & Lyons, 2003). Similarly, the number of departments of corrections permitting any medical experiments declined from 46 in 1969 to 12 in 1975 (Hornblum, 1997; Kalmbach & Lyons, 2003). By the late 1990s, a review of institutions in the United States engaged in clinical research found that only 15% involved IPs in their research studies (Christopher et al., 2011). This decline continued into the 21st century. The Institute of Medicine (Gostin et al., 2007) conducted a systematic review of the involvement of IPs in research. According to this report, from 1999 to 2005, the vast majority (94%) of published studies involving IPs were deemed minimal risk and limited to administrative record review (21%), program evaluation (26%), and nontherapeutic social and behavioral inquiry (41%). Articles involving IPs in biomedical studies or medical clinical trials were scarce (6%). This finding is consistent with the fact that only a small number of states allowed therapeutic biomedical research (15 of 48 states), and even fewer allowed nontherapeutic social or behavioral studies involving greater than minimal risk (five of 48; Gostin et al., 2007).

The federal policy designed to protect IPs from exploitation also, collaterally, reduced the amount and type of CMHR. No longer were IPs involved in biomedical or medical studies funded by the federal government. Instead, corrections-based research addressed low-risk behavioral and epidemiological issues funded, in large measure, by small grants from academic institutions, prison systems, private foundations, and state funds (Gostin et al., 2007). These studies provided descriptive information about the need for services and the distribution of disorders but little about how to improve service delivery or the well-being of IPs.

This trend in research funding, however, began to soften in the early 21st century with the passage of the 2003 Prison Rape Elimination Act and the 2007 Second Chance Act, which targeted federal funding to study corrections-based sexual victimization and effective reentry initiatives, respectively. These reforms reinvigorated federal funding in support of scientific investigations into ways to improve the behavioral health and recidivism outcomes of IPs through evidence-based interventions. Because of these funding opportunities, the corrections research base expanded in the areas of substance use disorder treatment (Moore et al., 2019), suicide prevention (Stijelja & Mishara, 2022), trauma-focused treatment (Grady et al., 2023), and reentry initiatives (Berghuis, 2018).

Still, relative to health services research trajectories, federal regulations to protect IPs compressed and shifted scientific inquiry into a shrinking box of lower impact corrections-based research. IPs are now protected from exploitation *and* exploration in ways that sustain the distribution of disease, disorder, and dysfunction in correctional settings. More is known about the distribution of disease there, but little evidence is available to inform choices about how to best treat and manage health and behavioral health problems among those who are incarcerated.

Another consequence of doing less CMHR concerns the development and maintenance of the expertise needed to conduct research in correctional settings (Appelbaum, 2008; Cislo & Trestman, 2013; Wolff & Gerardi, 2007). Correctional environments are unique, both individually and collectively. Gaining access to them requires professional connections. Functioning within them requires an understanding of how they are organized; what motivates organizational and staff behavior; how IPs are engaged, moved, counted, and routinized; and why security is not convenient (see Chapter 13). Once inside, researchers need to know how to engage correctional staff in helpful and respectful ways and keep their own staff safe and productive, while minimizing the burden on correctional staff and respecting the culture of the environment. It also requires specialized training, security clearances, and movement protocols for research materials (e.g., computers, tape recorders). Most importantly, researchers must build an identity that is separate from but respected by correctional staff and known by potential research subjects. Being an "outsider" inside a correctional setting is often met with suspicion by people working and living there; this can impede engagement and the implementation of research (Wolff, 2022). The professional capital and expert knowledge needed to conduct research involving IPs efficiently diminishes with misuse or underuse.

Resetting the balance

Prisoner rights groups, as well as IPs, are advocating for greater inclusion in meaningful prison- and non-prison-based research; they are choosing justice over protection (Gostin et al., 2007). Further, they argue that as an extension of their constitutional right to health care, IPs have a right to participate in research testing treatments that are potentially beneficial to them (Christopher et al., 2011; Thomas, 2010). In a survey of researchers and research ethics committee members in the United Kingdom, the majority of respondents agreed that "prisoners should be treated equally to other members of the population in terms of recruitment into non-prison-specific-research" (Charles et al., 2016, p. 250). A small survey of IPs conducted by Christopher and colleagues (2016) found that less than 20% of participants endorsed statements suggesting that research was exploitive, with the majority endorsing statements that participation in research increased access to treatment and that more opportunities for participation should be offered to IPs. Christopher and colleagues (2011) argued for more influential and inclusionary prison-based research, noting the complexity of their health and mental health problems.

Neither the process of IRB review nor the funding constraints at the federal level prevent high-quality, influential CMHR. Rather, they limit how research is done and what is done. For example, the National Institute of Mental Health funded a large-scale prison-based study that tested the reliability of computer- versus clinician-administered screening for PTSD symptoms and addiction disorders and a randomized, controlled trial of two 12-week manualized PTSD–addiction interventions. This study received local IRB approval in 7 weeks, approval from the Office for Human Research Protections 5 months later, and approval for a certificate of confidentiality within 1 month of the application's submission. This grant was awarded on September 2, 2011, and all IRB requirements were satisfied by October 22, 2011. Subject recruitment began within 6 months of the award date, and 24 laptop computers, 12 research staff, and supportive research materials entered the facility 2 weeks later. Nearly 700 subjects were recruited, 240 were randomly assigned to treatment, and data collection was completed within 28 months of the award date (Wolff, Huening, et al., 2015; Wolff, McHugo, et al., 2015).

The success of this project and others like it requires collaboration, determination, and patience. The following recommendations provide guidance on how to work within Subpart C and the uniqueness of correctional settings to conduct robust, influential, and minimal-risk CMHR:

Publicly connected scholarship: Research is improved when researchers and experience experts (e.g., IPs, corrections staff, administrators) work together to produce new knowledge (Epperson et al., 2023; Wolff, 2022). Build research collaborations and communication networks that include IPs to establish trust between those doing the research and those being researched, as well as to sensitize researchers to issues that affirm or negate voluntary participation (Boghassian et al., 2012). By broadening membership and flattening power hierarchies within the research team, it is possible to foster research practices that empower meaningful participation among IPs while also improving the utility of the research findings (Wolff, 2022). Epperson and colleagues (2023) provide several logic models for building publicly engaged research opportunities in different criminal justice settings.

Research design and orientation: Meet with local departments of corrections and jails to identify their interest in hosting or collaborating in research, the types of research that are permissible, and the research topics that are most appealing. Discuss issues regarding access to data, facilities, and residents, as well as the process by which publications resulting from research are reviewed.

Funding sources: Review funding opportunities for CMHR available through the National Institute of Corrections and Office of Justice Programs, as well as the National Institute for Mental Health and Substance Abuse and Mental Health Services Administration. A good source of funding information is the Office of Justice Programs website, which posts its available funding opportunities (see https://www.ojp.gov/funding/explore/current-funding-opportunities). For each possible funder, contact the project officer to discuss any limitations (e.g., study design, recruitment strategies) associated with funding CMHR.

Human subject review: The goal here is to minimize the effort required to gain IRB approval for research involving IPs. This involves educating yourself and, in some cases, the local IRB on Subpart C. Useful steps include carefully reviewing the regulations for IPs as human subjects, meeting with your IRB administrator to discuss these regulations, requesting samples of approved informed consent forms for IPs, helping your IRB identify a representative of IPs, networking with local researchers who have conducted IRB-approved research involving IPs, and requesting that your IRB conduct a workshop on Subpart C.

Engagement and collaboration: Establishing a presence in the correctional setting where the research will be situated is paramount. The principal investigator (PI), not the research coordinator, needs to be known by the correctional executive and line staff, as well as the people incarcerated at the facility. The PI is the face of the research study; they are the "quarterbacks" (Jutte et al., 2015) who catalyze and sustain the community engagement effort and keep it productive and focused. The more the PI is known, respected, and trusted, the more the organizational leadership, correctional staff, and IPs will accommodate the research study (Wolff, 2022). As outsiders, researchers are reflexively distrusted by correctional staff and IPs alike. Trust is earned by showing respect for the environment, the staff, the IPs, and the culture. IPs look for signs that the researchers are authentic in their concern, independent of the correctional system, and committed to the conditions set forth in the informed consent form. Learning the names of subjects and correctional staff, talking with them in respectful and "normal" ways, and consistently abiding by the rules of the facility and protocols of the research will, over time, foster trust.

Communication: Executive and liaison correctional staff must be kept informed of progress and difficulties. Surprises are unpopular in correctional settings. It is important to update supervisory staff often and succinctly about progress. As a rule, detailed letters should be written periodically to the executive who approved the research. These letters should identify, by name, the people on-site who are fostering the study and how.

Reciprocity: Giving back in meaningful ways to the facility and the people living and working there is central to building productive, enduring collaborations. This might include providing training, workshops, and lectures on topics of interest; facilitating reading clubs; or sponsoring intramural activities. Staying involved with the people living and working there establishes a connection that signals an intent to work together, not just acquire data.

Summary

The current regulatory environment biases correctional scientific inquiry toward research that carries minimal risk. Researchers have not maximized the possibilities for intervention and services research allowable under Subpart C, and the infrastructure for productive research–corrections collaborations has not been well established. The challenge for researchers is to see what is possible and to build the collaborations necessary to design and implement rigorous CMHR that will build the evidence base, improve practice and policy, and benefit IPs. With more debate and empirical exploration, the regulatory environment may change to invite more medical or biomedical research. However, until then, the opportunity for CMHR is vast, limited more by imagination and approach than by federal regulations and funding.

REFERENCES

Appelbaum, K. L. (2008). Correctional mental health research: Opportunities and barriers. *Journal of Correctional Health* Care, *14*, 269–277.

Beecher, H. K. (1966). Ethics and clinical research. *New England Journal of Medicine*, *274*, 367–372.

Berghuis, M. (2018). Reentry programs for adult male offender recidivism and reintegration: A systematic review and meta-analysis. *International Journal of Offender Therapy and Comparative Criminology*, *62*(14), 4655–4676.

Boghassian, P., Glavin, M., O'Connor, T., Boyer, J., & Conway, D. (2012). Prisons, community partnerships, and academia: Sustainable programs and community needs. *Federal Probation*, *76*(1), 30–34.

Charles, A., Rid, A., Davies, H., & Draper, H. (2016). Prisoners as research participants: Current practice and attitudes in the UK. *Journal of Medical Ethics*, *42*, 246–252.

Christopher, P. P., Candilis, P. J., Rich, J. D., & Lidz, C. W. (2011). An empirical ethics agenda for psychiatric research involving prisoners. *AJOB Primary Research*, *2*, 18–25.

Christopher, P. P., Stein, M. D., Johnson, J. E., Rich, J. D., Friedmann, P. D., Clarke, J., & Lidz, C. W. (2016). Exploitation of prisoners in clinical research: Perceptions of study participants. *IRB Ethics and Human Subjects*, *38*(1), 7–12.

Chwang, E. (2010). Against risk-benefit review of prisoner research. *Bioethics*, *24*, 14–22.

Cislo, A. M., & Trestman, R. (2013). Challenges and solutions for conducting research in correctional settings: The U.S. experience. *International Journal of Law and Psychiatry*, *36*, 304–310.

Epperson, M. W., Guz, S., & Sarantakos, S. P. (2023). Fostering community-engaged research on criminal legal innovations with logic models. *Social Work*, *68*(4), 307–319.

Fovet, T., Mundt, A. P., & Fazel, S. (2023). Psychiatry in prisons and corrections. In D. Lecic-Tosevski, D. M. Ndetei, C. H. Ng, et al. (Eds.), *Tasman's psychiatry*. Springer.

Gostin, L. O., Vanchieri, C., Pope, A., & Institute of Medicine Committee on Ethical Considerations for Revisions to DHHS Regulations for Protection of Prisoners Involved in Research (Eds.). (2007). *Ethical considerations for research involving prisoners*. National Academies Press.

Grady, M. D., Tripodi, S., Herod, L., & Rudzinski, M. (2023). Behavioral health interventions for incarcerated adults with histories of trauma: A scoping review. *Research on Social Work Practice*, *34*(4).

Hornblum, A. M. (1997). They were cheap and available: Prisoners as research subjects in twentieth-century America. *British Medical Journal*, *315*, 1437–1440.

Ivy, A. C. (1949). Nazi war crimes of a medical nature: Some conclusions. *Journal of the American Medical Association*, *139*, 131–135.

Jutte, D. P., Miller, J. L., & Erickson, D. J. (2015). Neighborhood adversity, child health, and the role for community development. *Pediatrics*, *135*(Suppl. 2), S48–S57.

Kalmbach, K. D., & Lyons, P. M. (2003). Ethical and legal standards for research in prisons. *Behavioral Sciences and the Law*, *21*, 671–686.

Lazzarini, A., & Altice, F. L. (2000). A review of the legal and ethical issues for the conduct of HIV-related research in prisons. *AIDS & Public Policy Journal*, *15*, 105–135.

Metzner, J. L. (2002). Class action litigation in correctional psychiatry. *Journal of the American Academy of Psychiatry and the Law*, *30*, 19–29.

Mitford, J. (1973). *Kind and usual punishment: The prison business*. Vintage.

Moore, K. E., Roberts, W., Reid, H. H., Smith, K. M. Z., Oberleitner, L. M. S., & McKee, S. A. (2019). Effectiveness of medication assisted treatment for opioid use in prison and jail settings: A meta-analysis and systematic review. *Journal of Substance Abuse Treatment*, *99*, 32–43.

National Commission for the Protection of Human Subjects of Biomedical and Behavioral Research. (1979). *The Belmont report: Ethical principles and guidelines for the protection of human subjects of research*. https://www.hhs.gov/ohrp/regulations-and-policy/belmont-report/read-the-belmont-report/index.html

National Institutes of Health. (2023). *Budget*. https://www.nih.gov/about-nih/what-we-do/budget

National Research Act, 342 Pub. L. 93-348 (1974).

Prins, S. J. (2014). Prevalence of mental illnesses in US State prisons: A systematic review. *Psychiatric Services*, *65*(7), 862–72.

Prison Rape Elimination Act, 42 U.S.C. §§ 15602-15609 (2003).

Protection of Human Subjects, 45 C.F.R. § 46.101 (2009).

Second Chance Act, H.R. 1593 (2007).

Sherrer, H. (1999). The mental torture of American prisoners: Cheaper than lab rats, Part II. *Prison Legal News*, *10*(4), 1–3.

Stijelja, S., & Mishara, B. L. (2022). Preventing suicidal and self-injurious behavior in correctional facilities: A systematic review and meta-analysis. *eClinicalMedicine*, *51*, 101560.

Thomas, D. L. (2010). Prisoner research—Looking back or looking forward. *Bioethics*, *24*(1), 23–26.

Wolff, N. (2022). *The shadow of childhood harm behind the prison wall*. Oxford University Press.

Wolff, N., & Gerardi, D. (2007). Building evidence on best practice through corrections-academic partnerships: Getting to successful practice. *Crime and Justice International*, *23*, 13–22.

Wolff, N., Huening, J., Shi, J., Frueh, B. C., Hoover, D. R., & McHugo, G. (2015). Implementation and effectiveness of integrated trauma and addiction treatment for incarcerated men. *Journal of Anxiety Disorder*, *30*, 66–80.

Wolff, N., McHugo, G., Shi, J., Huening, J., & Frueh, B. C. (2015). Screening for PTSD among incarcerated men: A comparative analysis of computer-administered and interviewer-administered modalities. *Criminal Justice and Behavior*, *42*(2), 219–236.

78

The future of correctional psychiatry: Evolving and recommended standards

Jeffrey L. Metzner, Reena Kapoor, Anthony C. Tamburello, and James L. Knoll IV[1]

Introduction

In recent decades, mental health services in jails and prisons have seen many advances in the knowledge base and practice standards. The "Future of Correctional Psychiatry" chapter in the first edition of this textbook expected further progress in these areas, as well as clearer guidance regarding ethical standards for psychiatrists practicing in correctional settings. In this chapter, we discuss developments in these areas since the first edition and briefly summarize promising new models for correctional settings. As part of our review, we describe what we believe the future may hold for our subspecialty.

Where things stand

The broad range of topics covered in this textbook attest to the growing complexity of the field of correctional psychiatry. As reflected in some of the chapters, correctional psychiatry has areas that lack consensus or a well-established evidence base. These deficiencies take on greater significance because of the high prevalence of psychiatric disorders among incarcerated persons (IPs); many individuals with the most serious mental illnesses reside in jails and prisons. The psychiatric profession, via the American Psychiatric Association (APA), has increasingly attempted to address the needs of these IPs by establishing treatment guidelines and advocacy efforts (APA, 2016). Examples include position statements addressing the use of restrictive housing units (RHUs) for IPs with serious mental illness and guidelines regarding the use of restraints for clinical reasons (APA, 2023; Metzner et al., 2007). Despite these steady efforts at standardization and professionalization of correctional psychiatry, much work remains to be done.

Relatively little research has been done in correctional psychiatry compared to other areas of psychiatric practice (Cislo & Trestman, 2013; see Chapter 77). Some of that research has relied on community-based tools and methods that do not necessarily adapt well to jail- and prison-based studies. For example, much of the basic epidemiologic data on the prevalence of mental illnesses among IPs has used screening instruments developed for use with community populations. Symptoms and behaviors suggestive of pathology in the community (e.g., hypervigilance, anxiety, aggression, and loss of interests or libido) can represent normal and adaptive findings among individuals in jails and prisons. These and other limitations have led many correctional mental health researchers to conclude that we need to greatly expand the empirical foundation of the field (Appelbaum, 2008). A significant impediment to increasing research in correctional facilities is existing federal regulations, which were appropriately developed in response to significant violations of informed consent principles for vulnerable research subjects (Gostin et al., 2007) but now sometimes pose a barrier to full participation of IPs in research studies.

In addition to the need for targeted research, untapped prospects for innovation in assessment and intervention abound in correctional psychiatry. For example, different models of behavioral intervention programs exist, but we lack robust findings that allow us to differentiate which programs work best for specific populations of IPs or in specific settings. Such knowledge is crucial for improving the treatment and management of IPs diagnosed with personality disorders who frequently engage in self-injurious or disruptive behaviors (e.g., throwing body waste at staff, openly masturbating) and take up a disproportionate share of mental health and custody resources. In another example, even as a consensus has emerged about specific standards for RHUs (e.g., number of hours per week for out-of-cell structured and unstructured activities for IPs with mental illness), the standards often lack an evidence-based foundation. The recommended programming levels for IPs with a serious mental illness in RHU settings have arisen largely from a cascade of imitative

1. The authors acknowledge the contributions of Kenneth L. Appelbaum and Robert L. Trestman, who were coauthors of the first edition of this chapter.

court decisions without research data to support their specificity, although they are based on pragmatic considerations.

The challenge of impediments to critical research in correctional facilities must be met for progress to occur. Fortunately, the increasing sophistication of quality improvement systems that have been implemented in some correctional health care systems has provided a mechanism for evaluating and improving processes and outcomes. As correctional systems mature in their identity and sense of professionalism, their ability and desire to utilize quality improvement programs to enhance health care provision will also grow.

The future of correctional psychiatric practice and standards

At the most basic level, correctional psychiatrists must grapple with several questions. First, should ethics standards differ in correctional settings compared to other practice venues? The APA's (2016) practice guideline on psychiatric services in correctional facilities discusses ethics, especially in the context of dual agency, though provides limited guidance. Second, should clinical standards differ in correctional settings compared to other practice venues? If disparate standards are warranted, how will we establish those standards? The APA and the National Commission on Correctional Health Care (NCCHC) have taken the lead in establishing correctional mental health standards (APA, 2016; NCCHC, 2015, 2018), which specifically address mental health care. Third, how will our profession support correctional practitioners who find themselves under pressure to act in ways inconsistent with clinical and ethical standards? Correctional psychiatrists have gained a larger role in both the APA and the American Academy of Psychiatry and the Law due to their increasing numbers and the growth of forensic fellowship programs utilizing jails and prisons as training sites. These professional affiliations have all facilitated increased support for psychiatrists practicing in correctional settings while also shining a light on the work being done there.

Before considering whether psychiatric practice in correctional settings should have unique clinical and ethics standards, we should first determine whether differences already exist. In what ways, if any, does our work in jails and prisons vary from what we do in other settings, or at least come under pressure to diverge from community-based customs? Several examples come to mind.

Confidentiality is an essential condition for psychiatric care. It is akin to creating a sterile field in surgery. It may yield under emergency circumstances but remains a prerequisite at all other times. Frequent exceptions to privacy, however, occur in some correctional settings, especially RHUs or other lockdown units. Routine cell-front clinical encounters breach confidentiality in a way that would never be tolerated outside of correctional facilities.

Pharmacological practices in correctional settings also tend to stray from community standards. Significant, and understandable, concerns arise about prescription of controlled and even some noncontrolled substances to IPs (Burns, 2009; Tamburello et al., 2017). Many of those concerns, however, have parallels to risks associated with controlled substances for patients in the community. Nevertheless, correctional formularies often include de facto exclusions that rarely have counterparts in community medication access. This is not always a bad thing, especially in the context of an opioid epidemic that has ravaged the United States in the past decade and has been attributed, in part, to prescription opioids (Pieters, 2023). It does, however, raise questions about why incarcerated people, as a group, should have access to a narrower range of pharmacologic options than individuals in the community.

IPs sometimes need clinical seclusion or restraints (Metzner et al., 2007). Jails, prisons, and community outpatient settings often lack the staffing and therapeutic environments to provide seclusion or restraint in a way consistent with prevailing standards. In the community, outpatients who need such emergency interventions typically are admitted for hospital care; however, the same does not always occur for IPs who may have clinical restraints applied in minimally therapeutic environments with less capacity to respond to medical complications, fewer procedural protections, and less oversight (Appelbaum, 2007). Furthermore, many jails and prisons rarely use therapeutic restraints at all, instead employing security tools and protocols (e.g., capsaicin spray, metal handcuffs, waist chains) to manage behaviors like self-injury.

Correctional psychiatrists may come under pressure to endorse denials of services for individual IPs or specific disorders in general (e.g., personality disorders, gender dysphoria). Such pressure can place psychiatrists in conflict with prevailing clinical standards in psychiatry and medicine that explicitly support access to care (American Medical Association, 2022; APA, 2018; NCCHC, 2020).

In relation to ethics standards and practices, correctional psychiatrists are asked to do things that have no parallel in community settings. Along with other mental health staff, they may be asked to evaluate IPs prior to or while being housed in an RHU for psychiatric contraindications to such placement. A growing international consensus, however, has called for the abolition of or significant restrictions on the use of solitary confinement, sometimes describing the use of isolation for periods exceeding several weeks as akin to torture (Metzner & Fellner, 2010; NCCHC, 2016). In many instances, placement in an RHU has an explicitly punitive purpose. Assessing the capacity of individuals to tolerate punishment under conditions of intentionally unpleasant and stressful deprivations, and subsequently providing clinical clearances to place them under such conditions, let alone participation in torture, has no equivalent in community practice.

Similar concerns arise with hunger strikes, which frequently occur in jails and prisons (see Chapter 69). Hunger strikes are vexing for correctional officers and administrators, who may pressure health care staff to participate in forcibly ending a protest via medical means. Participation in forcibly feeding a competent IP has long been considered unethical by the World Medical Organization (2017), though the motives and mental states of hunger strikers and the psychological sequelae of hunger strikes are complicated. Wei and Brendel (2010) conclude that psychiatrists have a critical role to play in managing hunger strikes, especially when the IP requires current mental health treatment.

Should clinical and ethics standards differ in correctional settings?

As discussed above, jails and prisons are unique environments. IPs differ from patients in the community in that IPs have been charged with crimes or adjudicated guilty of those crimes, and the institutional mission is focused on containment and public safety. Do such differences warrant clinical and ethics standards for psychiatric practice that diverge from community standards? If the institutional mission was exclusive, or even just paramount, that might sway the answer. Medical and psychiatric care for IPs, however, plays as integral a role in correctional policy and procedure. The U.S. Supreme Court has recognized a constitutional mandate for clinical services (*Bowring v. Godwin*, 1977; *Estelle v. Gamble*, 1976). The right to psychiatric care is fundamental, not ancillary. This suggests that justifications, if any, for divergent standards of care must be compelling.

Convenience or resource constraints provide a poor basis for disparity. Transferring IPs from RHU cells to private interview rooms, for example, requires available space and takes time and staff. Other needs compete for those resources, but confidentiality is a core component of psychiatric care, and failure to provide it falls below acceptable professional, if not constitutional, standards. Comparable considerations have relevance to an analysis of clinical procedures for seclusion, restraint, and other practices.

Public safety and security considerations may also have relevance to clinical services such as the availability of medications for psychiatric disorders, including substance use disorders. Potential compromises to safety and security must be balanced with the clinical consequences of a more narrow, cautious treatment approach. Resource limitations are also a poor justification for substandard care. Reasonable adaptations other than clinical restrictions (e.g., adequate budgeting, providing settings where transgender IPs can safely receive treatment, ensuring sufficient numbers of custody staff on duty to transfer IPs to confidential rooms for clinical encounters) require full implementation before reconsidering the balance between clinical and security needs.

Where and how to draw an ethical line poses especially thorny challenges. Correctional systems in the United States do not always follow the most progressive management practices. Individual psychiatrists may balk at working in settings where they perceive progress to be limited or that their autonomy to practice is diminished. It would be an extreme and counterproductive reaction, however, for the profession to withdraw from serving an underserved population. One can do good work even in faulty settings. If psychiatrists, however, are required to play a role in punitive or psychologically harmful correctional practices, a thoughtful review becomes necessary. Whether these practices ultimately advance security or other penological interests is a question for custody officials to grapple with. However, even if punishment serves legitimate correctional purposes, participation by psychiatrists may not be appropriate. Does it make a difference that RHU evaluations screen some fragile IPs out of that placement when others are screened in? Does it matter that some IPs tolerate prolonged RHU placement without showing signs of significant distress or lasting psychological harm? If ongoing monitoring of IPs in RHUs can identify and remove those who begin to show significant distress, does this lessen ethics concerns about providing mental health clearances for placement in these units?

If disparate standards are warranted, how will we establish them?

An infrastructure already exists for consideration of correctional psychiatry guidelines and practice standards, but extant resources have their limitations. The APA's (2016) practice guideline provides useful general principles and assumes compliance with the NCCHC's (2015) Standards for Mental Health Services in Correctional Facilities. Neither, however, addresses in adequate detail the type of challenging questions identified above. For example, NCCHC Standard MH-A-09 states that "clinical encounters are conducted in private" (NCCHC, 2015, p. 23) but considers this only an "important," not an "essential," standard. Essential standards generally represent "the critical components of a mental health care system" in the context of NCCHC facility accreditation (NCCHC, 2015, p. 148). Thus, the lack of privacy for clinical encounters would not necessarily impede accreditation.

The APA (2016, p. 5) report states, "The fundamental policy goal for correctional mental health care is to provide the same level of mental health services to each patient in the criminal justice process that *should be available* in the community." It further states that "a full range of psychotropic medications [should be available] with a capacity to administer them, including involuntarily in an emergency where state law allows" (APA, 2016, p. 35). The NCCHC (2015) has more general essential requirements that IPs "have access to care to meet their serious mental health needs" (MH-A-01, p. 3) and that "custody staff supports the implementation of clinical decisions" (MH-A-03, p. 7). Taken collectively, these standards could be read as providing support for IP access to controlled substances, treatment for gender dysphoria, and other interventions that correctional psychiatrists deem clinically indicated. Unfortunately, this does not always happen in actual practice.

Currently, guidelines sometimes conflict with each other, reflecting the lack of consensus—or at least the evolution of thinking—around certain aspects of correctional mental health care. For example, both the APA (2016) report and the NCCHC (2015, see standard MH-E-07) continue to require mental health assessments for clearance purposes prior to placing IPs in an RHU setting. Yet, an NCCHC (2016, p. 4) position statement specific to solitary confinement states, "Health staff must not be involved in determining whether adults or juveniles are physically or psychologically able to be placed in isolation." These two ideas appear incongruous, and it remains to be seen whether the NCCHC's guidelines and standards will eventually follow its position statement.

Organizations such as the APA and NCCHC that have a vested interest in correctional mental health standards need to clarify, refine, and expand their positions in a way that offers explicit, consistent guidance and support to practitioners and correctional programs. Fortunately, both organizations have systems in place to update their guidelines and standards periodically.

How will our profession support correctional practitioners who act in ways consistent with clinical and ethical standards?

Many correctional psychiatrists work in settings where they have no on-site peer support, especially in jails and smaller prisons. They might find allies among medical colleagues and mental health professionals from other disciplines, but they often provide the sole voice on clinical and ethics standards for their own practice. Pressure from custody staff and other clinicians to bend, if not break, those standards may sometimes become intense. This underscores the need for explicit professional guidelines that directly address the situations that correctional psychiatrists often face, such as the use of restraint and seclusion (Metzner et al., 2007). Guidelines provide practitioners with defensible, sound, nonidiosyncratic bases for their positions if challenged.

Professional organizations can play a more proactive role. Many of our patients who are most in need of treatment have become incarcerated, and we need to have a strong voice on their behalf. This might entail outreach and advocacy efforts by professional societies, such as supporting psychiatrists in jails and prisons in their efforts to explain professional standards to correctional administrators. It may also include more formal review and commentary on policies and practices in local and national settings, holding facilities accountable with standards that best serve the health care needs of IPs. Professional organizations also play an important role in creating a community of correctional psychiatrists nationally and internationally, combating the physical and emotional isolation that often accompanies work in correctional settings (see Chapter 65).

Reimagining incarceration

During the past 5 years, correctional officials have paid increasing attention to the so-called "Norway model" of incarceration. This model, in contrast to most correctional systems in the United States, is characterized by a progressive partnership between the line custody staff and correctional administrators, extensive training requirements to be certified as a correctional officer, and a 1:1.1 custody staff–to–IP ratio. The Norway model uses the principle of normalcy, which means that the more normal the experience of incarceration is, the more likely it will be rehabilitative (One Voice United, 2023). Aspects of this model are being introduced in departments of correction within the states of Oregon, North Dakota, Washington, and California (University of California, San Francisco, 2023). Barriers to implementation will include institutional culture, union objections, staffing shortages, and larger numbers of IPs in a typical U.S. prison as compared to Norway. However, it is very encouraging that such changes are in the process of development and implementation.

Technological advances are frequently not available, or belatedly made available, to IPs related to security and budgetary concerns. In recent years, many correctional systems have provided tablet computers to IPs, which has facilitated access to limited emails, phone calls with families, educational opportunities, leisure activities, and electronic requests for services, including health care. The tablets have been well received by the IPs and frequently have resulted in an improved milieu related to increased connectedness and decreased idleness and boredom.

The use of tele-mental health has greatly expanded related to the COVID-19 pandemic and subsequent exacerbation of mental health staff vacancies. Increasing access to mental health services for IPs via the use of tele-mental health is certainly a positive factor. However, it has led to many correctional mental health clinicians having minimal to no experience working in a correctional environment, which means they will have less influence on changing the nature of the correctional environment. Psychiatrists are more effective in this regard when they establish relationships with front-line correctional officers and administrators, which gives them credibility and makes it more likely that their concerns are included in policy development and implementation. A hybrid model that includes a significant percentage of time with the clinician working on-site will hopefully emerge.

The use of artificial intelligence in correctional psychiatry will be inevitable, although it will require collaboration among many different disciplines such as mental health clinicians, ethicists, engineers, information technology professionals, and others to develop and implement (Ray et al., 2022). Machine learning has been a technique increasingly used in research on large data sets to assist in diagnosis and to make predictions, such as stratifying risk for suicide (Dwyer et al., 2018; Gradus et al., 2020). The applications for machine learning with correctional electronic medical record databases are potentially limitless, though excitement should be tempered by the need to develop an evidence base to support acting on insights (Fazel & O'Reilly, 2020).

Psychiatry's potential role in the future of incarceration

Having considered the continued evolution of clinical and ethical standards of psychiatric practice with IPs, we turn to another important question: Might psychiatrists also have something to offer in terms of reforming the nature of incarceration itself? Thoughtful but mostly abortive attempts to do this have been made in the not-so-distant past (Menninger, 1970; Gilligan & Lee, 2005). Continued high incarceration rates, burgeoning costs, and concerns about racial inequities have created fertile ground for a new wave of reforms.

Even in the absence of psychiatric input, alternative-to-incarceration programs will continue to expand. Management of many nonviolent criminals or those with only substance-related crimes may shift to community settings. Psychiatrists can play a central role in designing and implementing interventions for these populations, though caution must be exercised when promoting such programs as the answer to the problem of mass incarceration. Over the past decade, criminal justice systems have begun to appreciate what many correctional psychiatrists have long understood: that criminal behavior is often multifactorial, even for individuals with serious mental illness. Although some people are arrested and incarcerated for behaviors directly resulting from a mental illness (e.g., hearing voices directing them to engage in violence), many others commit criminal offenses in the same context of poverty, limited education, poor job prospects, antisocial peers, and communities with high rates of violence that plague those without mental illness (see Chapter 6). Thus, merely diverting individuals with mental illness into traditional treatment pathways (i.e., therapy and medication) is likely insufficient to ease the burden of mental illness in correctional settings; attention to the social determinants of mental health and criminal justice involvement is also needed (Wasser, 2023). Without this shift in thinking and devotion of resources, correctional populations will continue to include large numbers of people needing intensive mental health treatment.

Even if diversion to community programs for less violent criminal offenses is successful, this will not necessarily lead to a decreased need for mental health services in jails and prisons. As individuals with nonviolent offenses are diverted, a greater percentage of people who become incarcerated may have aggressive behaviors. As currently occurs, some of these IPs will have underlying mental disorders that contribute to their challenging behaviors. Thus, the proportion of jail and prison IPs who need psychiatric services will increase, enhancing the central role that psychiatrists and other mental health professionals already have in these facilities.

Along with treating high rates of mental illness among IPs, psychiatrists may have contributions to make toward mitigating violent tendencies more broadly. This might entail development and expansion of behavioral programs that help people learn skills to manage emotions and avoid violence when discharged back to the community. On a more fundamental level, psychiatric insights could help correctional administrators modify some punitive and security-based policies and practices that do not reduce the risk of future inappropriate behaviors and may even exacerbate that risk (e.g., excessive use of RHUs; Metzner & Fellner, 2010).

Finally, criminal justice and mental health systems are increasingly recognizing that a period of incarceration is just one part of an individual's life, and their recovery from mental illness must include smooth transitions between correctional and community-based care. In countries that have or adopt a one-payer system of health care or those that have multiple but well-integrated systems, inclusion of seamless insurance coverage for IPs would allow for greater coordination and continuity of care across community and criminal justice settings. A well-functioning national electronic medical record system must also be implemented to ensure efficient, safe treatment. We envision a time in the near future when IPs will have routine access to electronic intranet systems for health care purposes (e.g., for submission of sick-call requests or for psychoeducational materials). In some systems, that time has already come via tablet computers. Developments such as these will expand opportunities for psychiatrists to provide services to criminal justice populations that rival the best available community services.

Summary

The questions and dilemmas that we have presented do not all lend themselves to easy consensus. They do, however, require attention and resolution. Custodial and clinical practices in correctional settings continue to evolve and change. Psychiatrists should stake out a place in the forefront of the ongoing debate, as both leaders and teachers (Knoll, 2011; Metzner, 2011). By being proactive instead of reactive, on both individual and professional organization levels, we will have a greater chance of influencing the outcomes and fulfilling our responsibilities to the IPs we serve. No one can predict with certainty what the future holds. We feel safe, however, in predicting that incremental and perhaps revolutionary changes will occur in correctional psychiatry. We hope that this textbook paints a picture of where things stand and projects a vision of where we need to go.

REFERENCES

American Medical Association. (2022). *Removing financial barriers to care for transgender patients, H-185.950*. https://policysearch.ama-assn.org/policyfinder/detail/Removing%20Financial%20Barriers%20to%20Care%20for%20Transgender%20Patients%20H-185.950?uri=%2FAMADoc%2FHOD.xml-0-1128.xml

American Psychiatric Association. (2016). *Psychiatric services in correctional facilities* (3rd ed.).

American Psychiatric Association. (2018). *Position statement on access to care for transgender and gender diverse individuals*. https://www.psychiatry.org/getattachment/d3ef4763-8a0e-4da3-ab01-efe932ca9478/Position-2018-Access-to-Care-for-Transgender-and-Gender-Diverse-Individuals.pdf

American Psychiatric Association. (2023). *Position statement on restrictive housing of incarcerated adults with serious mental illness*. https://www.psychiatry.org/getattachment/de02560f-34fd-420b-b36a-257f1450558a/Position-Restrictive-Housing-of-Adults.pdf

Appelbaum, K. L. (2007). Commentary: The use of restraint and seclusion in correctional mental health. *Journal of the American Academy of Psychiatry & the Law, 35*(4), 431–435.

Appelbaum, K. L. (2008). Correctional mental health research: Opportunities and barriers. *Journal of Correctional Health Care, 14*(4), 269–277.

Bowring v. Godwin, 551 F.2d 44 (1977).

Burns, K. A. (2009). The top ten reasons to limit prescription of controlled substances in prisons. *Journal of the American Academy of Psychiatry & the Law, 37*(1), 50–52.

Cislo, A. M., & Trestman, R. (2013). Challenges and solutions for conducting research in correctional settings: The U.S. experience. *International Journal of Law and Psychiatry, 36*(3–4), 304–310.

Dwyer, D. B., Falkai, P., & Koutsouleris, N. (2018). Machine learning approaches for clinical psychology and psychiatry. *Annual Review of Clinical Psychology, 14*, 91–118.

Estelle v. Gamble, 429 U.S. 97 (1976).

Fazel, S., & O'Reilly, L. (2020). Machine learning for suicide research—Can it improve risk factor identification? *JAMA Psychiatry, 77*(1), 13–14.

Gilligan, J., & Lee, B. (2005). The Resolve to Stop the Violence Project: Reducing violence in the community through a jail-based initiative. *Journal of Public Health (Oxford, England), 27*(2), 143–148.

Gostin, L. O., Vanchieri, C., & Pope, A. (Eds). (2007). *Institute of Medicine (US) Committee on Ethical Considerations for Revisions to DHHS Regulations for Protection of Prisoners Involved in Research*. National Academies Press.

Gradus, J. L., Rosellini, A. J., Horváth-Puhó, E., et al. (2020). Prediction of sex-specific suicide risk using machine learning and single-payer health care registry data from Denmark. *JAMA Psychiatry, 77*(1), 25–34.

Knoll, J. (2011). The correctional psychiatrist: Healer–teacher–leader. *Correctional Mental Health Report, 13*(3), 47–48.

Menninger, K. (1970). The crime of punishment. *International Journal of Law and Psychiatry, 9*, 541–551.

Metzner, J. (2011). The role of psychiatrist in the correctional mental healthcare systems. *Correctional Mental Health Report, 13*(3), 38–39.

Metzner, J. L., & Fellner, J. (2010). Solitary confinement and mental illness in U.S. prisons: A challenge for medical ethics. *Journal of the American Academy of Psychiatry and the Law, 38*(1), 104–108.

Metzner, J. L., Tardiff, K., Lion, J., et al. (2007). Resource document on the use of restraint and seclusion in correctional mental health care. *Journal of the American Academy of Psychiatry & the Law, 35*(4), 417–425.

National Commission on Correctional Health Care. (2015). *Standards for mental health services in correctional facilities*.

National Commission on Correctional Health Care. (2016). *Position statement: Solitary confinement (isolation)*. https://www.ncchc.org/wp-content/uploads/Solitary-Confinement-Isolation.pdf

National Commission on Correctional Health Care. (2018). *Standards for health services in prisons*.

National Commission on Correctional Health Care. (2020). *Position statement: Transgender and gender diverse health care in correctional settings*. https://www.ncchc.org/position-statements/transgender-and-gender-diverse-health-care-in-correctional-settings-2020/

One Voice United. (2023). *Reimagining incarceration: American corrections professionals explore the "Norway model."* Corrections One. https://www.corrections1.com/re-entry-and-recidivism/articles/reimagining-incarceration-american-corrections-professionals-explore-the-norway-model-Zdfhuro1mFaQFG5l/

Pieters, T. (2023). The imperative of regulation: The co-creation of a medical and non-medical US opioid crisis. *Psychoactives*, *2*(4), 317–336.

Ray, A., Bhardwaj, A., Malik, Y. K., Singh, S., & Gupta, R. (2022). Artificial intelligence and psychiatry: An overview. *Asian Journal of Psychiatry*, *70*, 103021.

Tamburello, A. C., Kathpal, A., & Reeves, R. (2017). Characteristics of inmates who misuse prescription medication. *Journal of Correctional Health Care: Official Journal of the National Commission on Correctional Health Care*, *23*(4), 449–458.

University of California, San Francisco. (2023). *How Norway is helping to restore humanity inside US prisons.* https://phys.org/news/2023-08-norway-humanity-prisons.html.

Wasser, T. D. (2023). A saturation point for criminal legal diversion. *Psychiatric Services*, *74*(1), 1.

Wei, M., & Brendel, R. W. (2010). Psychiatry and hunger strikes. *Harvard Human Rights Journal*, *23*, 75–109.

World Medical Association. (2017). *Declaration on hunger strikers (Declaration of Malta).* Amended October 2017. https://www.wma.net/policies-post/wma-declaration-of-malta-on-hunger-strikers/

Appendix
Resources

Anthony C. Tamburello and Jeffrey L. Metzner[1]

This appendix covers a selected range of references and resources available to support correctional health care, including accrediting bodies, professional organizations, relevant journals, practice guidelines, and practice resources.

Accrediting organizations

Organization	Website	Resources
American Correctional Association (ACA)	http://www.aca.org	Standards and accreditation Professional development Conferences Certification Publications and resources Correctional health care
The Joint Commission (TJC)	http://www.jointcommission.org	Accreditation Educational programs Certification Publications and resources Technical assistance
National Commission on Correctional Health Care (NCCHC)	http://www.ncchc.org	Accreditation Educational programs Certification Publications and resources Standards and position statements Technical assistance

Selected professional bodies and governmental agencies

Organization	Website	Resources
American Civil Liberties Union	http://www.aclu.org/	Publications and resources
American Civil Liberties Union National Prison Project	http://www.aclu.org/documents/aclu-national-prison-project	Publications and resources Court cases
Bureau of Justice Statistics	http://www.bjs.gov	Educational programs Publications and resources
Centers for Disease Control and Prevention	http://www.cdc.gov	Educational programs Publications and resources Technical assistance
Correctional Leaders Association	http://www.correctionalleaders.com/cla-headquarters	Resources
Correctional Peace Officers Foundation	http://www.cpof.org	Publications and resources
Justice Center of the Counsel of State Governments	http://csgjusticecenter.org	Publications and resources
Federal Bureau of Prisons	http://www.bop.gov	Publications and resources
Criminal Justice Testing and Evaluation Consortium	http://www.nlectc.org	Equipment standards Publications
Liman Center (Yale)	http://seeingsolitary.limancenter.yale.edu/research/	Publications on restricted housing
National Archive of Criminal Justice Data	http://www.icpsr.umich.edu/icpsrweb/NACJD	Data on crime and justice
National Association of State Mental Health Program Directors	http://nasmhpd.org	Publications and training
National Center for Missing and Exploited Children	http://www.missingkids.com/home	Focus on child protection issues
National Center for State Courts	http://www.ncsc.org	Courses and resources
National Center for Victims of Crime	http://www.victimsofcrime.org	Publications and resources
National Correctional Industries Association	http://www.nationalcia.org	Publications, training, and resources
National Criminal Justice Association	http://ncja.org	Publications and resources
National Domestic Violence Hotline	http://thehotline.org	Publications and resources

[1] The authors acknowledge the contributions used from the original version of this appendix by Stacey K. Rich and Robert L. Trestman.

Organization	Website	Resources
National Institute of Corrections	http://www.nicic.gov	Educational programs Publications and resources Technical assistance
National Institute of Justice (NIJ)	http://www.nij.gov	Research and evaluation Publications
Pew Research Center	http://www.pewresearch.org	Publications and resources
Prison Legal News	http://www.prisonlegalnews.org	Publications and case law
Prison Policy Initiative	http://www.prisonpolicy.org	Publications and resources
Prison Reform Trust	http://www.prisonreformtrust.org.uk	Publications and resources
Substance Abuse and Mental Health Services Administration GAINS Center	http://www.samhsa.gov/gains-center	Training and resources
Treatment Advocacy Center	http://www.treatmentadvocacycenter.org	Publications and resources
U.S. Department of Justice, Civil Rights Division, Special Litigation Section	https://www.justice.gov/crt/special-litigation-section	Publications, resources, cases, and findings letters
Vera Institute for Justice	http://www.vera.org	Publications

Professional organizations

Organization	Website	Resources
Academic Consortium on Criminal Justice Health	http://www.accjh.org	Educational programs Publications and resources
Academy of Correctional Health Professionals	http://www.correctionalhealth.org	Educational programs Publications and resources
American Academy of Child and Adolescent Psychiatry	http://www.aacap.org/web/aacap	Educational programs Publications and resources Board certification
American Academy of Psychiatry and the Law	http://www.aapl.org	Educational programs Publications and resources Landmark cases
American Bar Association	http://www.americanbar.org/aba.html	Educational programs Publications and resources
American College of Correctional Physicians	http://accpmed.org	Educational programs Resources
American Jail Association	http://www.americanjail.org	Educational programs Publications and resources
American Probation and Parole Association	http://www.appa-net.org/eweb	Publications and resources
American Psychiatric Association	http://www.psych.org	Educational programs Publications and resources Position papers Board certification
American Psychology-Law Society	http://www.ap-ls.org	Educational programs Publications and resources Position papers
Corrections Technology Association	http://www.correctionstech.org	Publications and resources
International Association for Correctional and Forensic Psychology	http://myiacfp.org	Publications and resources
International Association of Forensic Mental Health Services	http://www.iafmhs.org	Publications and resources
International Association of Forensic Psychotherapy	http://www.forensicpsychotherapy.org	Educational programs Publications and resources
International Association of Law and Mental Health	http://ialmh.org	Educational programs
International Corrections and Prisons Association	http://icpa.org	Publications and resources
Office for Victims of Crime	http://www.ojp.usdoj.gov/ovc	Publications and resources
Victim Law	http://www.victimlaw.org	Publications and resources

Selected relevant journals

Journal	Website
American Journal of Bioethics	http://www.bioethics.net
American Journal of Public Health	http://ajph.aphapublications.org
Behavioral Sciences and the Law	http://onlinelibrary.wiley.com/journal/10990798
Corrections Today Magazine	http://www.aca.org/publications
Criminal Justice and Behavior	http://journals.sagepub.com/home/cjb
European Journal of Psychotherapy & Counseling	http://www.tandfonline.com/toc/rejp20/current
International Journal of Forensic Psychotherapy	http://pep-web.org/browse/IJFP/volumes
International Journal of Law and Psychiatry	http://www.sciencedirect.com/journal/international-journal-of-law-and-psychiatry

Journal	Website
International Journal of Offender Therapy and Comparative Criminology	http://ijo.sagepub.com
Journal of Clinical Psychiatry	http://www.psychiatrist.com
Journal of Correctional Health Care	http://home.liebertpub.com/publications/journal-of-correctional-health-care/664/overview
Journal of Medical Systems	http://link.springer.com/journal/10916
Journal of Offender Rehabilitation	http://www.tandfonline.com/journals/wjor20
Journal of Psychiatric Research	http://www.journalofpsychiatricresearch.com
Journal of the American Academy of Psychiatry and the Law	http://www.jaapl.org
Law and Human Behavior	http://www.apa.org/pubs/journals/lhb
Prison Journal	http://tpj.sagepub.com
Psychiatric Services	http://ps.psychiatryonline.org/journal/ps
Violence and Gender	http://home.liebertpub.com/publications/violence-and-gender/620/overview

Guidelines and practice resources

Resource	Website
American Correctional Association, Performance-Based Health Care Standards	https://www.aca.org/ACA_Member/ACA/ACA_Member/Standards_and_Accreditation/StandardsInfo_Home.aspx
American Psychiatric Association, Psychiatric Services in Correctional Facilities (Third Edition)	https://www.appi.org/psychiatric_services_in_correctional_facilities_third_edition
American Academy of Psychiatry and the Law Practice Resource for Prescribing in Corrections	http://jaapl.org/content/50/4_Supplement/S1
American Society of Addiction Medicine, Treatment in Correctional Settings Toolkit	http://www.asam.org/advocacy/advocacy-in-action/toolkits/treatment-in-correctional-settings
Federal Clinical Guidelines	http://www.ncchc.org/federal-clinical-guidelines
National Commission on Correctional Health Care, Standards	http://www.ncchc.org/standards
National Commission on Correctional Health Care, Jail Guidelines for the Medical Treatment of Substance Use Disorders	https://www.ncchc.org/wp-content/uploads/2025-MAT-Guidelines-for-Substance-Use-Disorders-3-6-25.pdf
World Professional Organization for Transgender Health, Standards of Care Version 8	http://www.wpath.org/soc8

Index

For the benefit of digital users, indexed terms that span two pages (e.g., 52–53) may, on occasion, appear on only one of those pages

Tables, figures, and boxes are indicated by an italic *t*, *f*, and *b* following the page number